D1391329

TARGETING PROTEIN KINASES FOR CANCER THERAPY

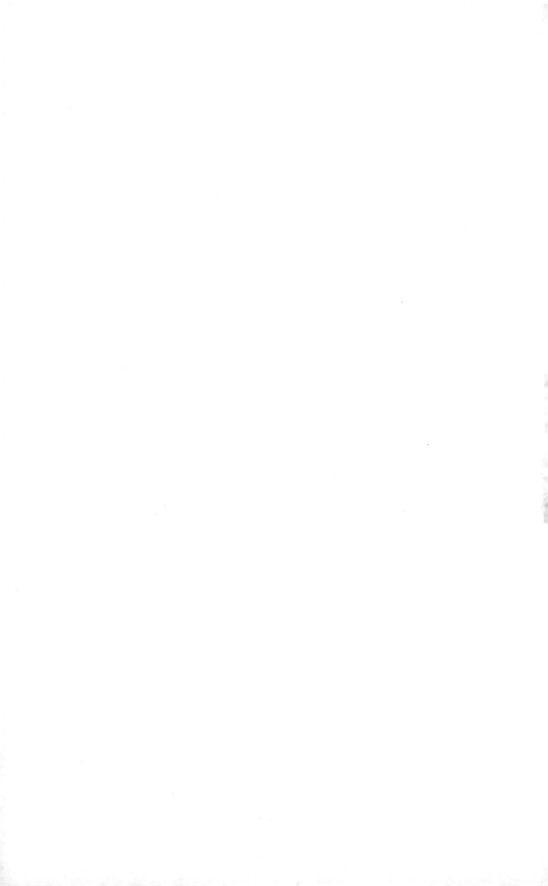

TARGETING PROTEIN KINASES FOR CANCER THERAPY

David J. Matthews

Mary E. Gerritsen

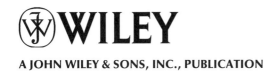

A JOHN WILEY & SONS, INC., PUBLICATION

Published by John Wiley & Sons, Inc., Hoboken, New Jersey
Published simultaneously in Canada.

For general information on our other products and services or for technical support, please contact our Customer Care Department within the United States at (800) 762-2974, outside the United States at (317) 572-3993 or fax (317) 572-4002.

Wiley also publishes its books in a variety of electronic formats. Some Content that appears in print may not be available in electronic formats. For more information about Wiley products, visit our web site at www.wiley.com.

Library of Congress Cataloging-in-Publication Data:
Matthews, David J. (David John), 1965–
    Targeting protein kinases for cancer therapy / David J. Matthews, Mary E. Gerritsen.
      p. ; cm.
    Includes bibliographical references and index.
    ISBN 978-0-470-22965-1 (cloth)
    1. Protein kinases–Inhibitors–Therapeutic use. 2. Antineoplastic agents. 3. Protein kinases. I. Gerritsen, Mary E. II. Title.
    [DNLM: 1. Neoplasms–drug therapy. 2. Protein Kinase Inhibitors–therapeutic use. 3. Drug Discovery. 4. Drug Resistance, Neoplasm. 5. Protein Kinases–physiology. 6. Protein-Tyrosine Kinases–antagonists & inhibitors. QZ 267 M438t 2009]
    RC271.P76M38 2009
    615′.798–dc22

                                                                                    2009020804

Printed in the United States of America

10 9 8 7 6 5 4 3 2 1

CONTENTS

11 CURRENT CHALLENGES AND FUTURE DIRECTIONS

These Appendices referred to in the text can be found on Wiley ftp site at the following address:

ftp://ftp.wiley.com/public/sci_tech_med/protein_kinase

PREFACE

Protein kinases are among the most critical and widely studied cellular signaling molecules and regulate essentially all processes central to the growth, development, and homeostasis of eukaryotic cells. In the 1980s, protein kinases were first shown to have an important role in oncogenesis and tumor progression, and since then they have received increasing attention as targets for anticancer drugs. Several kinase inhibitors are now approved for the treatment of cancer, and many more are advancing through clinical trials. In *Targeting Protein Kinases for Cancer Therapy*, we provide an integrated view of kinase cancer targets and the drugs that inhibit them, with a focus on small molecule inhibitors. We have sought to cover the field broadly, and although some targets, pathways, and drugs are covered in depth, some have of necessity only been covered briefly. We have included many references to both review articles and primary literature, but apologize to colleagues whose work could not be cited due to limitations of space.

Throughout this book, proteins are denoted by their most widely accepted abbreviation in capital letters (see List of Abbreviations) and often additional names by which the protein is known are also provided. The human genes (using the abbreviations of the Human Genome Nomenclature Committee (www.genenames.org)) are denoted by italic capital letters. Genes from lower organisms are denoted by italic lowercase letters. Viral proteins or genes are denoted by the prefix v-. Protein kinase structures (discussed mainly in Chapters 2 and 7) are referenced by their protein data bank (PDB) accession code and can be accessed at www.rcsb.org.

In Chapter 1, we review the human kinome—the superfamily of over 500 protein kinases, many of which have been implicated in tumorigenesis and the proliferation and survival of cancer cells. We also consider various approaches for the discovery and validation of kinase cancer targets, and some of the therapeutic modalities that have been employed apart from small molecule inhibitors of kinase domains. Here we meet a recurring theme: many kinases appear to be dual agents with regard to cancer, in that depending on the cellular context in which they operate, they can either promote or inhibit tumor formation and progression. Chapter 2 introduces the structural features of protein kinases. We discuss various modes of receptor:ligand interaction used by receptor tyrosine kinases, then turn our attention to the catalytic properties and various regulatory mechanisms of the kinase catalytic domain itself. Chapter 3 presents a review of some prominent receptor tyrosine kinases, which to date have received the most attention as cancer targets. In Chapter 4, we move inside the cell membrane and focus on the non-receptor tyrosine kinases. Chapters 5 and 6 introduce various intracellular kinase signaling pathways that are dysregulated in tumor cells and that have received significant attention for the development of anticancer drugs. These include a complex, interconnected signaling network downstream of cell surface receptors, as well as circuits that control transit through the cell cycle, cell division, and DNA repair. In Chapter 7, we revisit kinase structure but with a focus on the design of small molecule inhibitors. Various binding modes have been discovered and are discussed along with their implications for achieving potency and selectivity. Chapters 8–10 discuss many of the kinase inhibitors that have entered clinical trials for treatment of cancer, with an emphasis on those molecules that have progressed to late stage clinical trials and, in a few cases, to market. We have categorized these drugs by their primary cognate targets: tumor cell tyrosine kinase inhibitors in Chapter 8, angiogenesis ("angiokinase") inhibitors in Chapter 9, and intracellular pathway inhibitors in Chapter 10. However, since many of the inhibitors discussed have multiple targets, there are many overlaps between these categories, as indicated by the extensive cross-referencing between these chapters. In Chapter 11, we conclude by considering some of the challenges facing the field of oncology kinase inhibitor discovery. Although there have been some notable successes, drug resistance has emerged as a substantial impediment to achieving profound and durable responses in patients. We consider some of the strategies to address this, in particular, the use of combination therapy regimens that may simultaneously target multiple pathways and mechanisms. Such approaches rely on a thorough understanding of the underlying biology, and we focus on two prominent areas that are driving this knowledge forward: systems biology and translational medicine.

DAVID J. MATTHEWS
MARY E. GERRITSEN

So. San Francisco, California
November 2009

ACKNOWLEDGMENTS

Many of our colleagues have provided indispensable assistance in the preparation of this work. We thank Glenn Hammonds and Joanne Adamkewicz for help with bioinformatics and preparation of figures (in particular, the dendrograms in Chapter 1, the kinase domain diagrams throughout the book, and the appendices), and Thomas Stout for the molecular graphics figures on the front cover and in Chapters 2, 5 and 7; thanks also to Dr. Marat Valiev for supplying Figure 2.5B. Michael Ollmann wrote much of the target validation discussion (Chapter 1); Robert Blake provided helpful suggestions regarding target validation and also contributed to the section on SRC kinase (Chapter 4). Kwang-Ai Won and Timothy Heuer provided much of the cyclin-dependent kinase review (Chapter 6); Ross Francis, Peiwen Yu, Vanessa Lemahieu, Sophia Kuo, Michael Ollmann, Scott Detmer, Timothy Heuer, and Garth McGrath assisted in preparation of the appendices. We thank Paul Foster, Stuart Johnston, and Scott Robertson, whose work formed the basis for the discussions of PI-3 kinase, RAF/MEK kinases, and CDC7, respectively. We also thank Dana Aftab for helpful discussions regarding translational medicine, and Peter Lamb and Michael Morrissey for their encouragement and support. Many others have provided expert review of various chapters (although we take sole responsibility for any errors herein), including Robert Blake, Richard Cutler, Scott Detmer, Art Hanel, Timothy Heuer, Douglas Laird, Sophia Kuo, Vanessa Lemahieu, Nicole Miller, John Nuss, Michael Ollmann, Obdulio Piloto, Thomas Stout, Valentina Vysotskaia, Ron Weitzman, Kwang-Ai Won, and Peiwen Yu.

The views expressed in this book are those of the authors and do not represent the views of Exelixis, Inc.

D. J. M.
M. E. G.

CHAPTER *1*

KINASES AND CANCER

1.1 A BRIEF HISTORY OF PROTEIN PHOSPHORYLATION

The importance of phosphorus in cellular metabolism has been appreciated for over 100 years, since inorganic phosphate was shown to be a prerequisite for fermentation by yeast (1). Over the ensuing decades high energy phosphate esters, in particular, adenosine triphosphate (ATP), were recognized as central sources of cellular free energy. ATP is present in cells at a concentration of 1 to 5 mM (2, 3), and its hydrolysis to adenosine diphosphate (ADP) and inorganic phosphate is central to almost all cellular processes and pathways.

By the early 1950s, it was clear that proteins could incorporate phosphorus into their structures. Moreover, it appeared that the phosphorus in the "phospho-protein fraction" was labile and was rapidly turned over in living cells (4, 5). The site of protein phosphorylation was initially shown to be serine residues (6), and in 1954 George Burnett and Eugene Kennedy described an enzyme extract from rat liver mitochondria that catalyzed the phosphorylation of a protein substrate (casein) by ATP (7). Around this time, Edmond Fischer and Edwin Krebs were studying the biochemistry of glycogen phosphorylase from skeletal muscle, an enzyme that releases glucose from intracellular glycogen stores and plays a critical role in the cellular energy supply. Glycogen phosphorylase was known to exist in two forms: the inactive glycogen phosphorylase *b* and the active glycogen phosphorylase *a*. Fischer and Krebs showed that the conversion of glycogen phosphorylase *b* to *a* was catalyzed by an enzyme that they called phosphorylase kinase, which transferred the γ-phosphate of ATP to the protein (8, 9) (Figure 1.1). This was the first demonstration that protein kinases play a key role in regulating biochemical signaling pathways, and in 1992 Krebs and Fischer were awarded the Nobel Prize in physiology/medicine "for their discoveries concerning reversible protein phosphorylation as a biological regulatory mechanism" (10, 11).

Phosphorylase kinase was subsequently found to be phosphorylated and activated by another kinase, cAMP-dependent protein kinase (PKA) (12). This was the first demonstration of a protein kinase cascade, which has since been found to be a

Targeting Protein Kinases for Cancer Therapy, by David J. Matthews and Mary E. Gerritsen
Copyright © 2010 John Wiley & Sons, Inc.

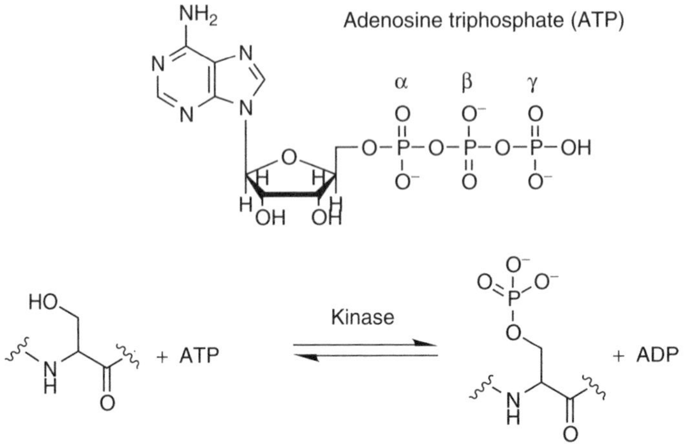

Figure 1.1   The protein kinase phosphotransfer reaction. Protein kinases catalyze the transfer of the adenosine triphosphate (ATP) γ-phosphate to the hydroxyl group of an amino acid within the peptide/protein substrate, yielding a phosphopeptide and adenosine diphosphate (ADP). The figure shows a serine residue as the phosphate acceptor.

widespread mechanism for controlling the diversity and specificity of intracellular kinase signaling pathways. PKA represents a landmark in kinase research in several other ways. It was the first kinase for which a consensus substrate sequence was identified (R-R-X-S-X, where X represents any amino acid (13–16)), and the first kinase for which the complete amino acid sequence was determined (17). Furthermore, in 1991 Susan Taylor and colleagues determined the structure of PKA using X-ray crystallography, providing the first insight into the molecular architecture of protein kinases and the structural basis for their activity (18).

In the early 1980s, the repertoire of protein kinase functions was expanded with the discovery that some kinases phosphorylate tyrosine residues instead of serines. It had previously been shown that the oncogenic Rous sarcoma virus encoded a gene with homology to protein kinases, and that the product of this gene, designated pp60[SRC], was responsible for the oncogenicity of the virus (19–21). Tony Hunter and colleagues showed that pp60[SRC] is a tyrosine kinase, and that its kinase activity is critical for cellular transformation by the virus (22, 23). In the same year, Stanley Cohen and colleagues showed that epidermal growth factor receptor (EGFR) is also a tyrosine kinase (24). Many tyrosine kinases of both the receptor and non receptor variety have subsequently been identified, and in addition to performing critical cellular signaling functions in normal cells they have emerged as a particularly important group of kinases in multiple aspects of tumor biology. Although most kinases can broadly be classified as either serine/threonine or tyrosine kinases, there are several instances of kinases that can accept either serine/threonine or tyrosine as a substrate. Notable examples include the mitogen activated protein kinase kinases (MAPKKs, or MAP2Ks), which phosphorylate their substrates on both threonine and tyrosine residues of a T-X-Y motif. Protein kinases are highly conserved among mammalian species and have significant homology with related proteins from other metazoans, yeast, plants, and all of the major eukaryotic kingdoms. (Lower eukaryotes also express protein histidine kinases, which autophosphorylate on histidine residues and transfer the phosphate group to an aspartate residue in a receiver protein (25). These are related to prokaryotic proteins with similar function but are not part of the protein kinase superfamily, and we will not consider them further.)

Eukaryotic protein kinase domains are comprised of 250–300 amino acids residues and have characteristic regions of conserved sequence that have been used to both characterize functionally important regions and to determine phylogenetic relationships between the various kinases (26, 27). Initial sequence analysis of kinases from various eukaryotes revealed the presence of 12 conserved subdomains (typically referred to by roman numerals I–XI; subdomain VI is further divided into VIA and VIB). X-ray crystal structures subsequently revealed that kinase domains are comprised of two major lobes, with the ATP binding site and catalytic machinery lying at the interface of the two lobes (Figure 2.3). Subdomains I–V constitute the N-terminal lobe of the kinase and subdomains V–XI the C-terminal lobe. Of particular note, subdomain I contains a conserved glycine-rich region that forms part of the nucleotide binding site. Subdomains II and III contain a highly conserved lysine and glutamate residue, respectively, which together form a salt bridge that interacts with ATP. The formation and disruption of this salt bridge forms an important part of the regulatory mechanism for many kinases. Subdomain VIB contains an invariant aspartate residue that acts as the catalytic base and a conserved asparagine that helps to orient the catalytic aspartate. Subdomain VII contains a characteristic "DFG" sequence, which marks the start of the so-called activation segment, another important feature in regulation of kinase activity. The aspartate of the DFG motif is another important catalytic residue that coordinates a divalent cation in the active site. Further details of protein kinase structure and catalytic mechanism are presented in Chapter 2.

In summary, investigations over the past 50 years have shown protein phosphorylation to be a universal switching mechanism that regulates the activity of almost all cellular processes. It should also be noted that the inverse reaction—dephosphorylation of proteins by protein phosphatases—is also a crucial aspect of this regulatory switching. We mention several important phosphatases during our discussions of protein kinases, although a thorough description of these enzymes is beyond the scope of this book.

1.2   KINASES AND CANCER

Cancer is a group of diseases characterized by aberrations in cellular growth, proliferation, and survival pathways, resulting in uncontrolled expansion of cancer cells and tumor formation. Collectively, these diseases represent one of the most pressing health challenges of the 21st century. The American Cancer Society estimated that, in 2008, over 1,437,000 cases of cancer were diagnosed in the United States alone and that over 565,000 people died from their disease (28). The National Institutes of Health estimate that the cumulative cost of cancer, including direct medical costs and loss of productivity, amounted to $219.2 billion in 2007. The 5-year survival rate for all patients diagnosed between 1996 and 2003 is 66%, although this includes patients who still have active disease or who have relapsed but are still alive. Survival rates vary widely between different kinds of cancer and the stage of the disease at diagnosis, with later stage diagnosis and metastatic disease invariably corresponding to poorer survival. For example, in women with breast cancer who are diagnosed when the tumor is confined to the immediate tissue of origin, the 5-year survival rate is 98%: however, if diagnosis is not made until distal metastases are present, 5-year survival drops to only 27% (28). The prognosis for pancreatic cancer is particularly dismal, with 5-year survival of only 20% for patients with local disease and 1.7% for metastatic disease. The prevalence of tumor sites varies between the sexes: in men, the most common forms of cancer are prostate, lung, colorectal, bladder, and non Hodgkin's lymphoma (NHL), whereas in women they are breast, lung, colorectal, uterine, and NHL. However, the major causes of death are lung, prostate, colorectal, pancreatic, and liver cancer (men), and lung, breast, colorectal, pancreatic, and ovarian (women). It is notable that different populations throughout the world have markedly different incidences of certain tumor types, indicating that hereditary, cultural, and environmental factors play a significant role in disease risk. About 10,700 pediatric tumors were diagnosed in the United States in 2008, with almost 1500 deaths estimated to occur in children aged 0–14, the most common disease and cause of death being leukemia. Nevertheless, cancer is primarily a disease of old age, as the cumulative probability of acquiring multiple tumorigenic mutations at some site within the body (discussed later) increases with increasing years. The incidence rates for all cancers in the United States (adjusted for age, i.e., normalized to account for the different population size for each group) range from 145 per 100,000 in the 20–49 age group to 2465 per 100,000 in the over 75 age group (SEER17 survey, year 2000; seer.cancer.gov).

Cancer arises most commonly in epithelial tissues, which give rise to carcinomas (broadly subdivided into adenocarcinoma, which originate in secretory cells, and squamous cell carcinoma, derived from the layer(s) of cells coating basement membranes). Other cancers of nonepithelial origin include sarcomas (arising from mesenchymal cells), hematological malignancies (leukemia, myeloma, and lymphoma), neurally derived tumors (such as glioma and glioblastoma), and melanoma (cancer of melanocytes, or pigmented skin cells). The initial (primary) tumor can present significant health problems and morbidity: however, the lethality of cancer is most frequently associated with invasion and metastasis, whereby malignant cells can migrate from their initial site of development and colonize both local and distal sites within the body.

Why do we get cancer? It may be more appropriate to ask why we don't get cancer, for it is one of the most amazing aspects of life that a metazoan organism as large and complex as a human can develop and remain viable for many decades. The adult human body contains an estimated 10^{13}–10^{14} cells, each of which has responded to environmental and endogenous signals to occupy its specific developmental niche within the organism. Moreover, each cell division entails the faithful replication of its entire complement of DNA (over 6 billion base pairs per diploid cell), and the accurate segregation of the chromosomes between the two daughter cells. A complex molecular network of proofreading and regulatory checkpoint machinery ensures that the overwhelming majority of cell divisions occur in an orderly manner. However, in some cases errors arise, leading to loss of control of critical cellular pathways. Occasionally, a single mutation or translocation may be the primary driver of disease, the most prominent example being constitutive activation of ABL kinase via the "Philadelphia" chromosome translocation in chronic myelogenous leukemia (CML) (29). In most cases, though, tumorigenesis seems to be a multistage process, with the accumulation of multiple genetic lesions leading to increasingly dysregulated cell growth (30). The accumulation of genetic and epigenetic changes affecting key cellular homeostasis mechanisms is a hallmark of malignancy. In many cases, the cell's genomic surveillance and regulatory apparatus can be compromised, leading to increased rates of mutation, widespread chromosomal instability, and aneuploidy (the acquisition of an abnormal number of chromosomes) (31). This genetic and epigenetic plasticity presents one of the principal challenges to targeted therapy, in that it can facilitate the intracellular "rewiring" of signaling pathways, both during tumor development and in response to treatment.

Given the central role of protein kinases in mediating diverse intracellular signaling pathways, it is not surprising that aberrant kinase activity is a common feature of tumors and that kinase inhibitors have attracted significant attention as targets for cancer drugs. Some of these dysregulated kinases are bona fide oncogenes—drivers of tumor growth. In addition to the case of ABL in CML mentioned above, other prominent examples include the ERBB2 receptor in breast cancer, the KIT receptor in gastrointestinal stromal tumors, and the intracellular RAF kinase in melanoma and thyroid cancer. In other cases, dysregulated kinase activity may play more of an indirect role. Many kinases in pathways downstream of activated oncogenes are only rarely found to be mutated or overexpressed in tumors, but are critical regulators of oncogenic signaling: examples include AKT, mTOR, and MEK. Other kinase-related pathways may be required to maintain the rapid growth and proliferation of tumor cells, often in the presence of extensive DNA damage (cyclin-dependent kinases, mitotic kinases, and cell cycle checkpoint kinases). Finally, some kinases play a more indirect role such as the VEGFR2 receptor, which is present on vascular endothelial cells and promotes tumor angiogenesis, increasing tumor oxygenation, nutrient supply, and growth. In a landmark review (32), Hanahan and Weinberg outlined the key characteristics of cancer cells, most of which can be promoted or exacerbated by dysregulation of kinase signaling (Figure 1.2). These features include the following.

- **Growth factor independence and unregulated proliferation.** The receptor tyrosine kinases (RTKs) are the primary cellular effectors of mitogenic growth factors, initiating complex and interconnected intracellular signaling cascades that promote cell growth, proliferation, and survival. Many of the nonreceptor tyrosine kinases (NRTKs) are tightly coupled to other extracellular receptors (e.g., cytokine receptors and cellular adhesion proteins) and may also be thought of as effectors of extracellular signals. Aberrant activation of

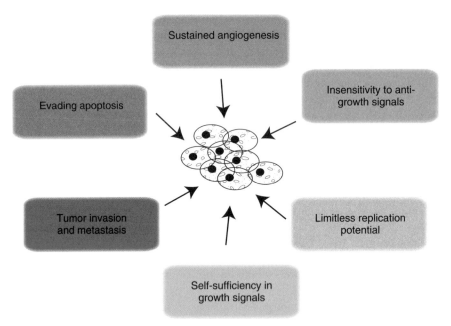

Figure 1.2 The hallmarks of cancer. (Adapted from (32). Copyright © 2000 with permission from Elsevier.).

these receptors (and/or kinases in downstream pathways, such as the PI3K and RAS/MAPK signaling cascades) decouples their activity from control by extracellular ligands and has been linked to tumor initiation, progression, and resistance to therapeutic intervention.

- **Resistance to cell death signals.** Many RTKs and intracellular kinases are important regulators of prosurvival signaling and are frequently activated in tumors, conferring resistance to apoptosis. The intracellular kinases signal through various mechanisms including the Forkhead and NFκB transcription factors, caspases, and BCL2 family proteins. Conversely, members of the TGFβ receptor family of membrane-bound serine/threonine kinases play an important role in transduction of antiproliferative and proapoptotic signals and activate tumor suppressor mechanisms that are frequently lost in some tumor types.

- **Insensitivity to antigrowth signals; unabated cell cycle progression.** Control of cell growth and division is orchestrated by a complex and precisely choreographed network of kinases, which mediate the mechanics of gene transcription and translation as well as the progression through different phases of the cell cycle and, ultimately, cell division. Cell cycle progression is largely directed by the cyclin-dependent kinases (CDKs) and their regulatory partners, the cyclins: a subset of the CDKs also plays a key role in transcriptional control. Dysregulation of these kinases is a common feature of tumor cells. Additional kinases, including the Aurora family and polo-like kinase 1 (PLK1), are involved in mitosis and are often dysregulated in tumors in order to promote cell division in the face of aneuploidy and other genomic aberrations. The cell cycle checkpoint kinases respond to genotoxic stress and initiate DNA repair programs or, in the event of catastrophic damage, trigger cell death. These cell cycle checkpoints are key guardians of the genome, but if tumor cells escape their surveillance they may contribute to productive cell division under conditions of endogenous or chemotherapy-induced genotoxic stress.

- **Sustained angiogenesis.** One of the key requirements of tumor growth is access to the vasculature and its supply of oxygen and nutrients. Several RTKs (notably the receptors for the growth factors VEGF, PDGF, FGF, and HGF) are important mediators of vascular recruitment, development, and support and have received significant attention as targets for anticancer drugs. Furthermore, intracellular protein kinase pathways (notably those involving AKT and mTOR) serve to integrate growth factor and nutrient signaling and respond to hypoxia and other sources of environmental stress by promoting tumor neovascularization.

- **Unlimited replicative potential.** Normal cells have a limit to the number of growth and division cycles that they can undergo, after which they either enter senescence or undergo apoptosis. Tumors frequently circumvent this limit via multiple mechanisms. Expression of telomerase in tumor cells can help to protect against the chromosomal damage produced by critically short telomeres. The antiapoptotic, promitotic, and cell cycle checkpoint mechanisms discussed earlier may support continued replication in the presence of widespread chromosomal aberrations. Furthermore, the persistent activation of CDKs, discussed previously, overcomes the cell cycle arrest that accompanies replicative senescence.

- **Tumor invasion and metastasis.** As indicated earlier, the most lethal aspect of advanced tumors is their ability to invade adjacent tissues and migrate to distal sites within the body, where they can implant and undergo metastatic growth. The acquisition of an invasive phenotype by tumors is intimately linked to the phenomenon of epithelial–mesenchymal transition (EMT), a form of transcriptional reprogramming whereby epithelial cells acquire characteristics of mesenchymal cells. This transition has been linked to signaling through growth factor receptors such as EGFR and IGF1R, expression of which is often lost during EMT. When cells migrate to a new environment, they may undergo reversion to an epithelial phenotype and reinitiate tumor formation. Several other characteristics are essential to the invasive, metastatic phenotype and are controlled by protein kinases. The MET receptor plays a particularly important role, promoting cell migration and working in concert with VEGF/VEGF receptor signaling to promote tumor invasion to better oxygenated tissue. In order for cells to effectively migrate they must also become anchorage independent, and several kinases are important mediators of anchorage-dependent growth signaling.

An additional feature of tumor cells that has received increasing attention in recent years is their altered bioenergetic pathways. It has been appreciated for over 80 years that tumors exhibit altered glycolytic metabolism compared to normal cells (33). Even in the presence of abundant oxygen, some tumors preferentially generate ATP via glycolysis rather than oxidative phosphorylation. Although this process (termed aerobic glycolysis) is less efficient than oxidative phosphorylation, it may provide the tumor cells with a competitive advantage when hypoxic conditions arise, as they often do during tumor growth. Furthermore, switching to aerobic glycolysis causes acidification of the extracellular milieu, which may further select for growth of tumor cells at the expense of the surrounding tissue (34). Oncogenic activation of the PI3K pathway (in particular, AKT) promotes glucose uptake and utilization and may be a driver of the aerobic glycolysis phenotype (35). As well as providing further rationale for targeting the PI3K/AKT/mTOR axis, this "glycolytic switch" in tumor cells suggests that additional small molecule kinases that control glycolysis (such as various isoforms of hexokinase and phosphofructokinase) may be novel targets for cancer treatment. Tumor cells also exhibit additional changes in metabolic fluxes, including increased fatty acid synthesis and glutamine metabolism (36).

In the remainder of this chapter, we take a tour of the kinase family tree and identify some of the kinases that have been implicated in promoting tumorigenesis and tumor growth, survival, and metastasis. Although some kinases have a clear tumor-promoting or tumor suppressor role, we encounter several examples of kinases that appear to have both of these properties. The question of which property will be manifest in a given tumor is clearly of great importance to target validation and drug discovery and may depend critically on the genetic background of the tumor, its microenvironment, and the stage of tumor development.

1.3 A TOUR OF THE HUMAN PROTEIN KINASE SUPERFAMILY

An analysis of the human kinome by Manning and colleagues in 2002 remains the canonical point of reference for the identification and classification of human protein kinases (37). In this study, data mining of various human gene sequence repositories revealed 518 putative protein kinases, collectively comprising about 1.7% of all human genes (Table 1.1). In addition, 106 kinase pseudogenes were identified. Of the 518 protein kinase genes, 478 can be classified into 9 groups, designated TK, TKL, STE, CK1, AGC, CAMK, CMGC, RGC, and Other (with this last group consisting of a diverse collection of kinases that do not fall into one of the former groups). Within most groups, a number of families have been identified, with some families further divided into subfamilies. The remaining 40 kinases that do not fall into the above groups are substantially divergent in sequence from the main kinase superfamily and form the atypical kinase group.

One somewhat surprising finding from this catalog of human kinase sequences was the fact that about 10% of all sequences contained amino acid substitutions in one of three residues known to be critical to catalytic function:

TABLE 1.1   Classification of the Human Kinome

Group	Total kinase domains	Families	Family members
		ABL	2
		ACK	2
		ALK	2
		AXL	3
		CCK4	1
		CSK	2
		DDR	2
		EGFR	4
		EPH	14
		FAK	2
		FER	2
		FGFR	4
		INSR	3
		JAK	8^a
TK	94	LMR	3
		MET	2
		MUSK	1
		PDGFR	5
		RET	1
		ROR	2
		RYK	1
		SEV	1
		SRC	11
		SYK	2
		TEC	5
		TIE	2
		TRK	3
		VEGFR	3
		TK-unique	1
		IRAK	4
		LISK	4
		LRRK	2
TKL	43	MLK	10
		RAF	5
		RIPK	5
		STKR	12
		TKL-unique	1

(continued)

TABLE 1.1   Classification of the Human Kinome (*Continued*)

Group	Total kinase domains	Families	Family members
STE	48	STE7	7
		STE11	8
		STE20	30
		STE-unique	3^b
CK1	12	CK1	7
		TTBK	2
		VRK	3
AGC	59	AKT	3
		DMPK	7
		GRK	7
		MAST	5
		NDR	4
		PKA	5
		PKB	1
		PKC	9
		PKG	2
		PKN	3
		RSK	9
		RSKL	2
		SGK	3
		YANK	3
CAMK	82	CAMK1	5
		CAMK2	4
		CAMKL	20
		CASK	1
		DAPK	5
		DCAMKL	3
		MAPKAPK	5
		MLCK	5
		PHK	2
		PIM	3
		PKD	3
		PSK	2
		RAD53	1
		RSK	6^c
		TRBL	3
		TRIO	6^d
		TSSK	5
		CAMK-unique	3
		CDK	20
		CDKL	5
		CLK	4

TABLE 1.1 (*Continued*)

Group	Total kinase domains	Families	Family members
CMGC	61	DYRK	10
		GSK	2
		MAPK	14
		RCK	3
		SRPK	3
RGC	5	RGC	5
Other	83	AUR	3
		BUB	2
		Bud32	1
		CAMKK	2
		CDC7	1
		CK2	2
		Haspin	1
		IKK	4
		IRE	2
		MOS	1
		NAK	4
		NEK	11
		NKF1	3
		NKF2	1
		NKF3	2
		NKF4	2
		NKF5	2
		NRBP	2
		PEK	4
		PLK	4
		SCY1	3
		Slob	1
		TBCK	1
		TLK	2
		TOPK	1
		TTK	1
		ULK	5
		VPS15	1
		WEE	3
		WNK	4
		Other—unique	7

[a] Includes four active kinase domains and four inactive, regulatory domains.
[b] Includes one second kinase domain.
[c] Includes the second kinase domains of RSK1,2,3,4 and MSK1,2.
[d] Includes two second kinase domains.

K30, D125, and D143 (PKA numbering). Some of these so-called pseudokinase domains (not to be confused with the pseudogenes mentioned above) may be truly inactive but nevertheless serve a regulatory role (38). Perhaps the most notable example in the field of cancer-associated kinases is ERBB3 (Chapter 3), a member of the EGFR/ERBB family that lacks intrinsic catalytic activity but forms heterodimers with other ERBB family members and is an important mediator of ERBB signaling. The STRADα/STRADβ kinases (also called STLK5 and STLK6) are also catalytically inactive but are required to form an active complex with LKB1, an important regulator of cellular energy levels (39). In other cases there have been reports of kinase activity despite the lack of canonical catalytic residues. Members of the WNK kinase family lack a critical conserved lysine residue that is important in establishing the architecture of the protein kinase active site: however, the X-ray crystal structure of WNK1 shows that another lysine residue can take its place, and it has been demonstrated to have kinase activity (40, 41). The attribution of enzymatic activity remains controversial for several pseudokinases, including KSR (kinase suppressor of RAS) and ILK (integrin-linked kinase).

Over half (260) of the kinases identified by Manning et al. (37) contain little or no sequence apart from the kinase domain. The remaining kinases vary widely in size and contain over 80 known protein domains. The largest kinase by far is the muscle protein Titin, which is the largest known protein and contains 26,926 amino acids. The most common sequence motifs include extracellular receptor domains such as immunoglobulin (Ig) domains (present in 30 genes), fibronectin type III domains (28 genes), and ephrin receptor binding domains (14 genes). Common domains in intracellular signaling proteins include SH2 (25 genes), SH3 (27 genes), pleckstrin homology (23 genes), diacylglycerol binding (23 genes), and calmodulin binding (23 genes). A few kinase proteins possess two kinase domains. For example, members of the p90RSK family (RSK1, RSK2, RSK3, and RSK4) have two functional kinase domains: an AGC kinase at the N terminus and a CAMK kinase at the C terminus. The Janus kinase family members (JAK1, JAK2, JAK3, and TYK2) each possess a functional kinase and a catalytically inactive pseudokinase domain, which is thought to play a regulatory role.

Over half of the kinase genes identified can be mapped to genetic loci that are associated with disease, and 164 kinases are associated with amplicons that are frequently found in tumors, further underscoring the importance of the protein kinase family in cellular signaling and the relevance of their dysregulation to tumor biology. Next, we introduce some of the most important kinases that have been implicated in cancer and also review some additional interesting kinases that, for reasons of space, are not discussed in later chapters.

1.3.1 Tyrosine Kinase Group

Tyrosine kinases (TKs) are one of the most widely studied and important kinase families with respect to cancer biology. In humans, there are around 90 distinct tyrosine kinases, which can broadly be divided into 58 receptor tyrosine kinases (RTKs) and 32 nonreceptor tyrosine kinases (NRTKs).

Receptor Tyrosine Kinases   On the basis of sequence homology and the structure of their extracellular domains, RTKs have been classified into approximately 20 families (Table 1.2; Figures 1.3 and 1.4) (42). Collectively, members of the RTK family perform the critical function of transducing signals from extracellular ligands to intracellular signaling pathways (Figure 1.5). Depending on the tissues/cells and ligands/receptors involved, these signals may modulate such diverse processes as mitogenesis, metabolism, migration, and angiogenesis. Examples of these extracellular signals include epidermal growth factor (EGF), insulin, fibroblast growth factor (FGF), vascular endothelial growth factor (VEGF), and nerve growth factor (NGF). Engagement of extracellular ligands results in receptor aggregation and/or conformational change, and phosphorylation of multiple tyrosine residues in the kinase domain and C-terminal regions of the receptor's intracellular domain. The C-terminal phosphotyrosine residues couple the receptors to multiple downstream signaling events, including protein kinase pathways, various phospholipid signaling mechanisms, and nuclear transcription factors. Dysregulation of RTKs (and, consequently, of their associated phenotypic effects) is a common feature of tumor biology, and Chapter 3 is devoted to a detailed description of some of the more prominent RTKs that have been implicated in cancer.

Class I RTKs (Epidermal Growth Factor Receptor Family)   The EGFR/ERBB family of RTKs was the first to be implicated in cancer, when EGFR was found to be closely related to the viral oncogene *v-ERBB* (48). Subsequent investigation of EGFR and the other members of the Class I RTK family have revealed a rich and diverse signaling network: at least ten receptor ligands interact with four cell surface receptors (which can form various heterodimers and homodimers), resulting in activation of multiple downstream signaling pathways that can promote mitogenesis, differentiation, migration, and survival. Dysregulation of ERBB signaling is a prominent feature of many tumor types and can be caused by multiple mechanisms, including mutational activation of the receptor and receptor/ligand overexpression. ERBB receptors were among the first to be targeted with both small molecule and antibody-based therapeutics, and several anti-ERBB therapeutics have been approved in recent years following demonstration of clinical benefit in several tumor types. Structural studies on the EGFR kinase domain and extracellular domains are presented in Chapter 2, and the biology of ERBB receptors is discussed in detail in Chapter 3. Chapter 7 includes a description of the structural basis for small molecule ERBB kinase inhibitors, and the inhibitors currently undergoing clinical evaluation are discussed in Chapter 8.

Class II RTKs (Insulin Receptor Family)   The insulin receptor (IR) and IGF1 receptor (IGF1R) differ from most other RTKs in that they exist as preformed dimers on the cell surface in the absence of ligand. Nevertheless, they are somewhat structurally related to Class I (EGFR) receptors and, like the Class I receptors, can also form both homodimeric and heterodimeric complexes. Insulin receptor is a key mediator of glucose uptake and mobilization, whereas IGF1 receptor is more prominently involved in growth hormone signaling and development. Both of these mechanisms can be dysregulated in tumor cells; IGF1 signaling has widely been

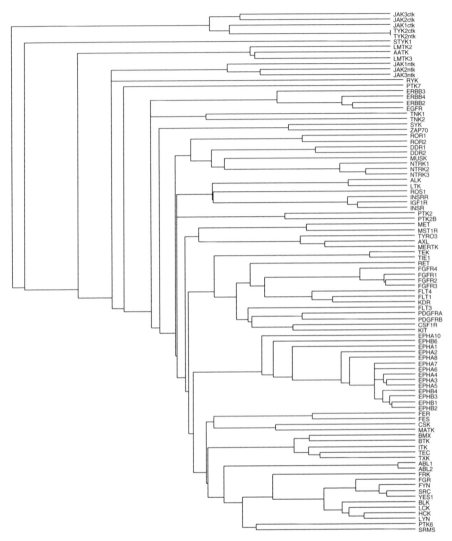

Figure 1.3 The TK kinase group. Similarity of kinase sequences within the TK group. Kinase domain sequences and groups were those described (37) as updated at KinBase (www.kinase.com). These sequences were checked versus Entrez Gene Refseq (43) and gene symbols were updated accordingly. Only 14 kinase sequences remain without HGNC symbol assignments (44). All sequences within each group were aligned using muscle v3.6 (www.drive5.com/muscle (45, 46)) with default settings; newick trees were produced using the -tree2 option of muscle. Trees were visualized in ATV/Forester 4.0.5 (47) and printed to PDF files without editing. Final editing was performed in Adobe Illustrator.

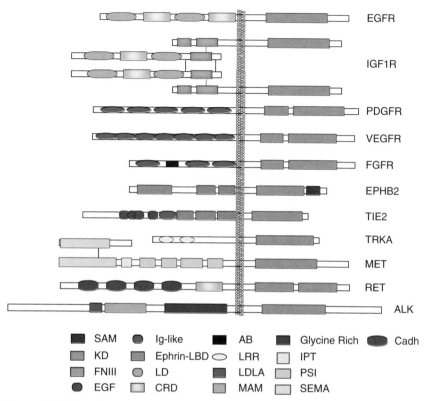

Figure 1.4 Domain structures for selected RTKs. There is substantial diversity in the structure of the extracellular domains: however, all RTKs have an intracellular kinase domain and C-terminal "tail." In some cases, such as PDGF and FGF receptors, there is an insert of ~70 amino acids in the kinase domain.

associated with tumor development, survival, and drug resistance, and high levels of glucose uptake and utilization have been recognized as a hallmark of cancer cells for many years. Further details of Class II RTKs and inhibitors thereof can be found in Chapters 3 and 8, respectively.

Class III RTKs (PDGF Receptor Family) Together with Class V RTKs, the Class III family is characterized by a "split" kinase domain, with an insertion of approximately 70 amino acids in the C-terminal half of the domain. The platelet-derived growth factor (PDGF) receptors are mediators of diverse biological effects in mesenchymal cells, including proliferation, migration, matrix synthesis, and cytokine production. As discussed in Chapter 3, PDGF receptors are found in multiple tumor types, including glioblastoma and gastrointestinal stromal tumors (GIST); furthermore, PDGFR signaling plays an important role in recruitment and assembly of pericytes in tumor vasculature. Disruption of both vascular endothelial growth factor receptor (VEGFR) signaling in endothelial cells and PDGFR signaling in pericytes has been shown to be more effective than blocking either

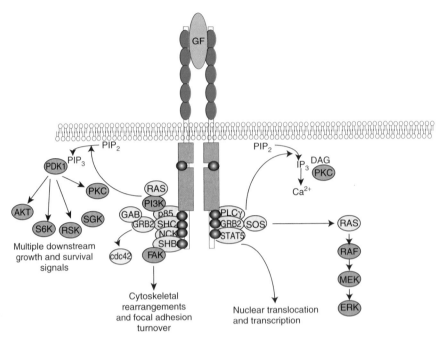

Figure 1.5 Signal transduction by RTKs. Binding of growth factor ligands (GF) to the receptor promotes receptor aggregation (typically dimerization), kinase activation, and phosphorylation of tyrosine residues (glowing grey circles) in the intracellular domain of the kinase. When phosphorylated, these tyrosine residues recruit specific receptor substrates (yellow proteins) by virtue of their SH2 domains, which bind to specific phosphotyrosine containing peptide sequences of the C-terminal domain of the RTK. The receptor substrates either undergo phosphorylation or engage additional downstream components via protein:protein interactions. Many of these activate other intracellular kinases (blue proteins), which in turn modulate various cellular processes including cellular growth, proliferation, survival, differentiation, motility, and invasion.

receptor alone, and many of the antiangiogenic agents in development ("angiokinase inhibitors"; Chapter 9) exhibit dual inhibition of PDGF and VEGF receptors. Another important member of Class III includes the stem cell factor receptor KIT, which is expressed in many tumors including small cell lung carcinoma, melanoma, acute myelogenous leukemia, and over 90% of GIST. Another family member, FLT3, is involved in hematopoiesis and is often mutationally activated in acute myeloid and lymphocytic leukemias. Mutations are usually either an internal tandem duplication in the juxtamembrane region or a point mutation in the kinase domain. PDGFR, KIT, and FLT3 are discussed further in Chapter 3.

Class IV RTKs (FGF Receptor Family) The fibroblast growth factors (FGFs) are a large family of peptide growth factors that promote cellular proliferation, differentiation, survival, and migration and play key roles in embryonic development and tissue repair. There are four FGF receptor tyrosine kinases (FGFR1–4), which

TABLE 1.2   **Classification of Receptor Tyrosine Kinases**[a]

Class	Family name	Members
I	EGFR/ERBB receptor	EGFR (ERBB1, HER1), ERBB2 (HER2), ERBB3 (HER3), ERBB4 (HER4)
II	Insulin receptor	IR (INSR), IGF1R, IRR
III	PDGF receptor	FLT3, FMS, KIT, PDGFRα, PDGFRβ
IV	FGF receptor	FGFR1, FGFR2, FGFR3, FGFR4
V	VEGF receptor	VEGFR1 (FLT1), VEGFR2 (KDR), VEGFR3 (FLT4)
VI	HGF receptor	MET, RON
VII	TRK receptor	TRKA (NTRK1), TRKB (NTRK2) TRKC (NTRK3)
VIII	EPH receptor	EPHA1, EPHA2, EPHA3, EPHA4, EPHA5, EPHA6, EPHA7, EPHA8, EPHA10, EPHB1, EPHB2, EPHB3, EPHB4, EPHB6
IX	AXL receptor	AXL, MER, TYRO3
X	LTK (leukocyte tyrosine kinase) receptor	ALK, LTK
XI	TIE (angiopoietin) receptor	TIE1, TIE2
XII	ROR receptor	ROR1, ROR2
XIII	DDR receptor	DDR1, DDR2
XIV	RET receptor	RET
XV	KLG/CCK receptor	CCK4
XVI	RYK receptor	RYK
XVII	MuSK	MUSK

[a]Only a subset of families within the TK group are shown, although these include most of the receptors that have been implicated in cancer.

exist as multiple isoforms due to differential splicing. These receptors are frequently amplified or overexpressed in tumors. Germline mutations of FGFR2 are found in craniosynostosis syndromes and some of these mutations have also been identified in solid tumors; a translocation involving the *FGFR3* gene is also found in about 15% of multiple myeloma cases. In addition, FGFR can promote angiogenesis and may be able to support tumor vascular development in the absence of VEGFR signaling, suggesting that FGFR inhibitors may also have value as antiangiogenic agents. FGF receptors are discussed further in Chapter 3.

Class V RTKs (VEGF Receptor Family)   VEGF (vascular endothelial growth factor) receptors are the most important mediators of endothelial cell proliferation, survival, migration, and morphogenesis. Of the three VEGF receptors, VEGFR2 (also known as KDR) plays the most prominent role in angiogenesis; VEGFR3 (FLT4) is primarily involved in lymphatic development.

Tumor neovascularization—the "angiogenic switch"—is a key factor in allowing the expansion of solid tumors. Under conditions of low pH, hypoxia, poor nutrient availability, and inflammatory stimuli, both cancer cells and tumor stromal cells produce VEGF and other proangiogenic factors, promoting the recruitment of new blood capillaries that can further support tumor growth. The concept of tumor angiogenesis was first proposed in the 1970s (49), and over the past decade many antivascular agents have been evaluated as anticancer therapies in the clinic. These efforts have met with some success, and both antibody and small molecule drugs targeting angiogenesis have been approved in several oncology indications. The biology of the VEGF family of growth factors and its receptors is discussed in Chapter 3, and clinical studies involving "angiokinase" inhibitors are reviewed in Chapter 9.

Class VI RTKs (HGF Receptor Family) Hepatocyte growth factor receptor, or MET, has received significant attention as a cancer target in recent years, prompting the development of several small molecule and antibody therapeutics that are in various stages of clinical evaluation. Overexpression of MET has widely been documented in many human tumor types, amplification is found in gastric and colorectal tumors, and activating MET mutations have been identified in hereditary and sporadic papillary renal cell carcinoma. MET activation has widely been associated with poor prognosis, reflecting its multiple roles in tumor pathology. In addition to promoting tumor cell growth and survival, MET is strongly implicated in tumor invasion and metastasis and also promotes angiogenesis in endothelial cells. Furthermore, MET and VEGF receptor signaling may act synergistically to promote tumor invasion and vascularization: in response to hypoxia, HIF transcription factors promote the expression of VEGF and MET, thereby both promoting tumor angiogenesis and facilitating the migration of tumor cells to better oxygenated regions. A closely related MET homolog, RON, is the receptor for macrophage stimulating protein (MSP) and may also promote invasive growth in tumor cells. MET and RON are discussed in Chapter 3, and small molecule MET inhibitors are described in Chapter 8.

Class VII RTKs (TRK Receptors) The Class VII RTKs are known as tropomyosin-related kinases (TRKs), since the founder member of the family, TRKA, was originally found as a fusion protein with a nonmuscle tropomyosin in colon carcinoma (50). TRKA was subsequently shown to be a receptor for nerve growth factor (NGF) (51), and all three TRK family members (TRKA/NTRK1, TRKB/NTRK2, and TRKC/NTRK3) are now known to be receptors for neurotrophins—pleiotropic growth factors that promote outgrowth and survival of neural cells and thereby regulate development and maturation of the central and peripheral nervous systems. The extracellular domain of each receptor comprises a cysteine-rich domain followed by a leucine-rich domain and another cysteine-rich domain, then two IgG-like domains; the intracellular region contains the kinase domain and a C-terminal tail. Each receptor has several isoforms that exhibit variations to this structure. Neuronal TRKA has a short insertion in the extracellular domain near the membrane, and both TRKB and TRKC have isoforms that lack the intracellular kinase domain.

The full-length TRK proteins have been found and implicated in growth and survival of a number of tumor types. In neuroblastoma, TRKA expression may actually be a good prognostic marker, since it can lead to growth arrest and differentiation: however, an oncogenic form of the receptor has also been identified in this tumor type (52). Autocrine NGF/TRKA signaling has also been reported in prostate and breast cancer, where it is implicated in tumor survival and proliferation (53, 54). TRKB is also often overexpressed in neuroblastoma (55), as well as tissues of nonneuronal origin including pancreatic carcinoma, prostate carcinoma, and multiple myeloma (56). TRKA and TRKC (but not TRKB) have also been found as fusion proteins in various tumors. In addition to the original tropomyosin (TPM3) fusion found in colon cancer, TRKA is found as a fusion to the *TPR* and *TFG* gene products in papillary thyroid tumors, both of which lead to constitutive dimerization and activation of the oncoproteins (57). TRKC is found as a fusion protein with the *ETV6* gene in several tumor types including congenital fibrosarcoma, congenital mesoblastic nephroma, secretory breast carcinoma, and acute myelogenous leukemia (58).

Class VIII RTKs (EPH Receptors)   EPH receptors (named for erythropoietin-producing hepatocellular carcinoma, where EPHA1 was first identified (59)) are the largest subfamily of receptor tyrosine kinases, comprising 14 human genes: EPHA1–8, EPHA10, EPHB1–4, and EPHB6. The A-class EPH receptors are attached to the cell membrane via a glycosylphosphatidylinositol (GPI) anchor, whereas the B-class receptors each contain a transmembrane domain. The ligands of EPH receptors are the ephrins, also a class of plasma membrane-bound proteins. There is evidence that ephrin:EPH receptor activation is bidirectional, so that EPH receptors can act as ligands for ephrins as well as vice versa: ephrin:EPH receptor signaling is defined as "forward" and EPH receptor ephrin as "reverse." Ephrin:EPH receptors contribute to diverse cellular processes such as cell boundary formation, cell migration, and tissue morphogenesis. They are also important regulators of vascular development, working in concert with the VEGF and angiopoietin receptors. EPH receptors and their ligands regulate positional guidance of the developing vascular system and are required for arteriovenous differentiation (60). In this context, arterial expression of ephrin B2 and venous EPHB4 appear to be the most important isoforms (61–63). Given this range of activities, dysregulated EPH receptor function has been implicated in tumorigenesis, tumor angiogenesis, and metastasis (64). Although all EPH receptor members have been found in tumors, EPHA2 appears to be frequently dysregulated and, in some cases, correlated with tumor stage (65–67). However, there are conflicting data on the molecular mechanisms of EPH receptor signaling in cancer: both tumorigenic and tumor suppressor roles have been described, often involving the same receptor (68). Some of these contradictions undoubtedly stem from the inherent complexity of the system: the bidirectionality of ephrin EPH receptor signaling and the potential involvement of tumor, endothelial, and/or stromal cells.

Other RTKs Implicated in Cancer   The anaplastic lymphoma kinase (ALK) gene is commonly translocated in anaplastic large cell lymphoma, resulting in expression of a constitutively active fusion protein with nucleophosmin (NPM-ALK). However, its cognate ligand has not conclusively been identified and it remains an orphan receptor. Wild-type ALK is overexpressed and has been implicated in the growth of several solid tumor types, and another ALK fusion protein, EML4-ALK, has been reported in a small fraction of non small cell lung carcinomas. RET (rearranged in transfection) is a Class XIV RTK that has gained prominence as a cancer target, particularly in thyroid cancer. Activating RET translocations are a common feature of papillary thyroid tumors, and activating point mutations in RET are found in the inherited form of medullary thyroid carcinoma. Further discussion of RET and ALK can be found in Chapter 3.

TIE1 and TIE2 (tyrosine kinase with Ig and EGF homology domains) comprise the Class XI family of receptor tyrosine kinases (69). No cognate ligand has been identified for TIE1: however, it is important for vascular development since mice lacking TIE1 die in utero or perinatally due to edema and hemorrhage (70). TIE2 is activated by angiopoietins, a small family of secreted proteins that coordinate with other endothelial regulators to orchestrate angiogenesis and vascular remodeling. The angiopoietin ANG1 is responsible for activation of TIE2: however, it appears to induce migration and angiogenic sprouting rather than proliferation (71). The ANG2 ligand antagonizes the effects of ANG1 and is expressed at sites of vascular remodeling (72). Although initially identified as vascular remodeling factors, both TIE1 and TIE2 are also found in other cell types and may contribute directly to tumor cell growth (73).

Nonreceptor Tyrosine Kinases   The nonreceptor tyrosine kinases are cytoplasmic proteins that do not directly interact with extracellular ligands: nevertheless, they are tightly coupled to signaling cascades downstream of a diverse range of RTKs, G-protein coupled receptors, and cytokine receptors. The SRC family comprises that largest subset of NRTKs with 11 members (Table 1.3; Figure 1.3). Members of the SRC, ABL, and TEC families have a common core domain structure, with an N-terminal SH3 domain followed by an SH2 domain, then the kinase domain. Other important NRTK families with members implicated in cancer include JAK kinases (which have a regulatory pseudokinase domain in addition to the functional kinase) and FAK, in which the kinase domain is flanked by N-terminal integrin-binding and C-terminal focal adhesion-targeting domains.

SRC Family Kinases   As noted previously, SRC was the first tyrosine kinase to be identified and also the first human proto-oncogene. Despite this, adoption of SRC as a cancer drug target has been relatively slow, perhaps due to the complexity of its biology and the lack of mutational activation in most tumors (although SRC enzyme activity is frequently increased in tumors relative to normal cells (74)). SRC has a multitude of both upstream effectors and downstream cellular substrates including various docking and adaptor proteins, other tyrosine kinases, GPCRs, and various proteins involved in focal adhesion and cellular junction signaling. Correspondingly, SRC mediates many cellular effects that are implicated

TABLE 1.3   Nonreceptor Tyrosine Kinase Families

Family	Members
SRC	BLK, BRK, FGR, FRK, FYN, HCK, LCK, LYN, SRC, SRM, YES
TEC	BMX, BTK, ITK, TEC, TXK
ABL	ABL, ARG
CSK	CSK, CTK
JAK	JAK1, JAK2, JAK3, TYK2
SYK	SYK, ZAP70

in tumor growth, including morphological transformation, mobility and invasion, growth factor independence, and proliferation. These various effects may be modulated to varying extents at different times in the evolution of tumor, for example, uncontrolled proliferation at early stages and invasion and metastasis later (75). Of particular relevance is the collaboration of SRC with FAK (see later discussion) in mediating anoikis, loss of density inhibition, and migration. The structure and regulation of SRC has been elucidated by X-ray crystallography and complementary functional studies and is discussed in Chapter 2. The many facets of SRC biology are explored in more detail in Chapter 4, and SRC inhibitors are described in Chapter 8.

Breast tumor kinase (BRK) is a SRC-like nonreceptor tyrosine kinase that has attracted attention as a potential factor in breast cancer and several other tumor types. The protein was first identified in metastatic breast tumor tissue and is overexpressed in approximately two-thirds of breast tumors (76, 77). BRK promotes signaling through the ERBB receptor family (78) and is amplified in concert with ERBB2, another major factor in breast tumor progression and survival (79). It may also promote migration and invasion, via interaction with the focal adhesion protein paxillin and activation of RHO GTPases (80, 81).

ABL Kinase   ABL kinase (in the form of the BCR-ABL fusion protein) holds a special place in the field of kinase inhibitor research: it is the primary target of imatinib (Gleevec), a small molecule kinase inhibitor that has revolutionized the treatment of chronic myelogenous leukemia (CML) and spurred much of the current interest in kinase inhibitors as anticancer drugs. ABL is a widely expressed and tightly controlled kinase that regulates cytoskeletal function, progression through the cell cycle, myogenic differentiation, and cell death. CML is almost invariably associated with a translocation fusion of the *BCR* (breakpoint cluster region) gene to the *ABL* gene, producing in a fusion protein with constitutive kinase activity. This results in aberrant expansion of CML cells, due to enhanced cell proliferation, disrupted cell adhesion, and resistance to apoptosis. Clinical evaluation of the ABL inhibitor imatinib in CML showed that it was both well tolerated and produced dramatically better responses than the previous standard of care. ARG, a closely related member of the ABL family, has also been found as a fusion protein in several leukemia samples. ABL and ARG are discussed in detail in Chapter 4;

imatinib is covered in Chapter 8, and the structural basis for imatinib inhibition is discussed in Chapter 7.

FAK Family Kinases Focal adhesion kinase (FAK) and the homologous proline-rich tyrosine kinase 2 (PYK2) are centrally involved in linking integrin signaling to intracellular protein kinase signaling pathways. The heterodimeric integrins are cell surface receptors for various extracellular matrix proteins such as fibronectin, collagen, and laminin and are important mediators of cellular adhesion and anchorage-dependent growth. FAK is associated with integrin receptor clusters at points of cellular adhesion, and its activity is stimulated by engagement of integrins with the extracellular matrix. Both FAK and PYK2 have tyrosine phosphorylation sites that mediate interactions with the adaptor protein p130^{Cas}, and together with SRC kinase this complex connects to various intracellular pathways including the RAS/MAPK cascade, PI3K, and RHO family GTPases. The ensuing phenotypic effects include cell adhesion, spreading, motility, proliferation, and survival. Consequently, in addition to their role in development, FAK and PYK2 have been associated with increased invasion and metastasis in tumors, and inhibiting this pathway has been proposed as a strategy for blocking invasive growth and tumor metastasis. These kinases are discussed in more detail in Chapter 4.

JAK Family Kinases Collectively, JAK kinases are activated by many cytokines and other growth factors (e.g., interferons, interleukins, growth hormone (GH), and erythropoietin (EPO)). JAK1, JAK2, and TYK2 are ubiquitously expressed, whereas JAK3 is restricted to hematopoietic cells. The JAK kinases are associated with the C-terminal regions of the receptors, and receptor activation leads to their transphosphorylation and activation. The active JAK kinases subsequently phosphorylate additional proteins, including the cytokine receptors and STAT (signal transducer and activator of transcription) proteins. STAT proteins are the major downstream effectors of JAK signaling, and phoshorylation results in their dimerization, nuclear translocation, and regulation of gene expression. There is much crosstalk between the various receptors, JAKs and STATs (Figure 1.6). In general, interferon α/β signaling is associated with JAK1, TYK2, and STAT1/STAT2, whereas interferon γ signals through JAK1/JAK2 and STAT1; interleukins mostly engage JAK1 and/or JAK3 in concert with STAT3, STAT5, or STAT6. Together, these interferon and interleukin signals mediate host defense, allergic response, and inflammation. JAK2 is the primary mediator of GH, EPO, and other growth factor signals and couples downstream to STAT3 and STAT5. In cancer, JAK2 activation has been found in many different solid tumors; however, it has received particular attention following the discovery of a highly prevalent activating mutation (V617F) in various myeloproliferative disorders. JAK2 is discussed in more detail in Chapter 4, and JAK2 inhibitors are reviewed in Chapter 8.

1.3.2 TKL (Tyrosine Kinase-like) Group

As suggested by the group name, the TKL kinases have homology to the TK family although they are predominantly serine/threonine kinases (Figure 1.7). Among

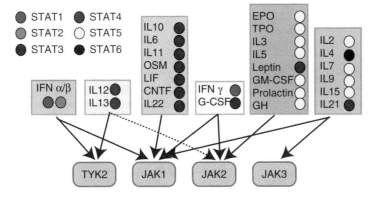

Figure 1.6 JAK/STAT signaling.

the most prominent members of this group are the RAF family kinases, including ARAF, BRAF, and CRAF. These kinases are important components of the RAS/MAPK signaling pathway, acting as key conduits from the RAS GTPase to the downstream MEK kinases. RAS and BRAF kinase are frequently dysregulated in tumors, and the role of RAF kinases in cancer biology is discussed further in Chapter 5. Also within this family are the kinase-suppressor-of-RAS (KSR) proteins, KSR1 and KSR2. These proteins appear to have a role in RAF signaling, although it is not clear that they have intrinsic kinase activity themselves.

Integrin-linked kinase (ILK) is another member of the TKL family that is implicated in cancer biology, although as in the case of KSR the evidence for intrinsic activity is controversial. ILK lacks two aspartate residues that participate in the catalytic function of most kinases, and it therefore seems likely that it is a pseudokinase (38): nevertheless, it has also been reported to have catalytic function (82). Regardless of its enzymatic activity, there are extensive data implicating ILK protein:protein interactions in the interactions between integrin receptors and the actin cytoskeleton, with consequent functions in cellular adhesion, migration, and morphology (83).

TGFβ Receptors   The TKL group is also home to the transforming growth factor β (TGFβ) receptors, TGFβR1 and TGFβR2. TGFβ signaling has an enigmatic role in cancer biology and has been characterized as both a tumor suppressor mechanism and a potential target for therapeutic intervention (84). TGFβR1 and TGFβR2 form a single heterodimeric receptor for TGFβ, which exists as three isoforms. Binding of dimeric TGFβ ligands to TGFβR2 leads to recruitment of TGFβR1 and transphosphorylation of the GS (glycine–serine) sequence in the TGFβR1 juxtamembrane region by TGFβR2. The receptor also phosphorylates SMAD2/3 proteins, which translocate to the nucleus, form a complex with SMAD4, and initiate a potent antiproliferative transcriptional program. Specific effects include upregulation of cyclin-dependent kinase (CDK) inhibitors and subsequent G1 arrest, suppression of c-MYC, and induction of apoptosis. Consequently, the TGFβ pathway has a tumor suppressor function, and loss of TGFβ receptor function (by mutation or

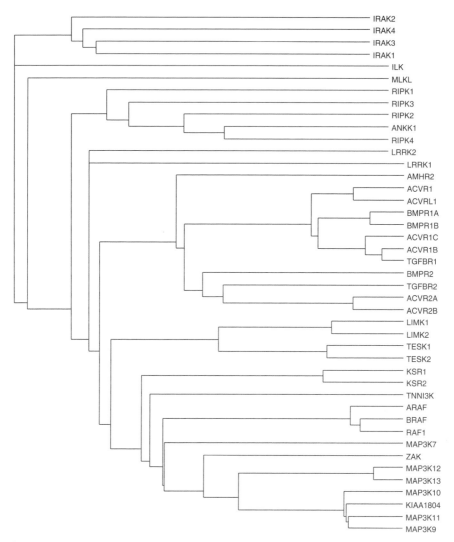

Figure 1.7 The TKL kinase group. The figure was produced as described in Figure 1.3 legend.

deletion of the receptor itself or of the downstream SMAD proteins) is a feature of several tumor types, including colon, gastric, and pancreatic carcinomas. As well as directly suppressing tumor cell growth, TGFβ can block expression of mitogens in stromal cells and suppress inflammatory responses.

In contrast to its antiproliferative, tumor suppressor function, TGFβ signaling can also promote tumor invasion and metastasis. TGFβ can stimulate EMT in tumor cells, via increased expression of the SLUG, SNAIL, and TWIST transcription factors (85). This fundamental change in the biochemical program of tumor cells leads to increased invasiveness, motility, and anoikis (anchorage-independent growth). When such tumor cells implant in distal sites of metastasis (such as bone), TGFβ signaling may promote a positive feedback loop of increased cytokine and TGFβ production between tumor and host cells, resulting in further invasive growth (86). Furthermore, the immunosuppressive effects of TGFβ signaling may also lead to escape from immune surveillance in some tumor cells. Downstream signaling through the TGFβ receptor also involves another TKL group kinase, TGFβ-associated kinase (TAK1). TAK1 mediates signaling of TGFβ receptor to the JNK and p38 MAPK pathways and also couples TGFβ signaling to the NFκB signaling pathway (87, 88).

Finally, it should be noted that the TGFβ family and its associated receptors are part of a larger cytokine/receptor family. This family includes the bone morphogenetic proteins (BMPs) and their TKL family receptors, BMPR1A, BMPR1B, and BMPR2. These factors are important for bone growth and repair and, although not as broadly studied as TGFβ in the field of oncology, may also have a role in tumor metastasis (89).

1.3.3 STE Group

The STE kinases are human homologs of the yeast STE20, STE11, and STE7 kinases and derive their name from the fact that deletion of the ancestral gene in yeast leads to sterility (Figure 1.8). Many members of this group are important for activation of mitogen activated protein kinase (MAPK) signaling; although the MAPKs themselves are found in the CMGC group (see Section 1.3.7), the MAPK kinases (MAP2Ks) and MAP2K kinases (MAP3Ks) are STE kinases. In multicellular organisms, there are four characterized MAPK pathway modules: extracellular signal regulated kinase (ERK), c-JUN NH_2-terminal kinase (JNK), p38, and ERK5 (90). Each pathway responds to different extracellular signals, which stimulate an intracellular pathway activator. This activator initiates a phospho-relay system composed of three sequentially activated kinases: MAP3K, MAP2K, and finally the MAPK for which the pathway is named. Selectivity of MAPK activation is mediated by docking interactions between MAPKs and MAP2Ks, as well as the sequence surrounding the TXY dual phosphorylation motif. The various MAP3K and MAP2K enzymes and pathways are shown in Figure 1.9, and their cellular activities are further discussed along with their associated MAPKs in Section 1.3.7.

The PAK (p21-activated kinase) family comprises six proteins, subdivided into PAKA (PAK1, PAK2, PAK3) and PAKB (PAK4, PAK5, PAK6). They respond to various extracellular stimuli (via RTKs and G-protein coupled receptors) and are primarily associated with regulating cytoskeleton dynamics and cellular morphology. PAK1 is an effector of the small molecule GTPases RAC1 and CDC42 and stimulates cellular motility and invasion. Downstream of PAK1, cellular responses are evoked via the MAPK, JNK, and IKK pathways, as well as by direct transcriptional regulation in concert with steroid hormone receptors (91). Of the PAK family, PAK1 is the most prominently associated with cancer. Increased PAK1 expression and activity has been documented in multiple tumor types including breast cancer, where the level of overexpression correlates with tumor invasiveness and has

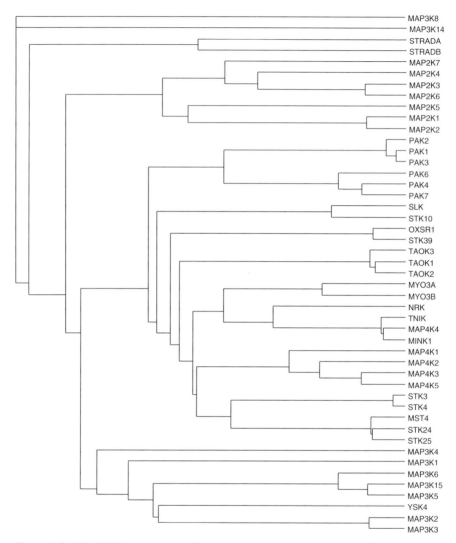

Figure 1.8 The STE kinase group. The figure was produced as described in Figure 1.3 legend.

also been associated with resistance to tamoxifen (92, 93). Other tumor types with amplified or overexpressed PAK1 include ovarian, colon, bladder, brain, and T-cell lymphoma (91). In addition, PAK1 is implicated in the NF2 form of inherited neurofibromatosis. PAK1 phosphorylates and inactivates Merlin (the product of the *NF2* tumor suppressor gene), which is an inhibitor of PAK1; loss of Merlin in NF2 thus leads to aberrant activation of PAK1 (94). As well as promoting tumor invasion by phosphorylating cytoskeletal proteins, PAK1 (and other PAK family members) can inactivate BCL2 and NFκB-dependent apoptotic pathways, although PAK2 has also been reported to have proapoptotic activity. Additional functions

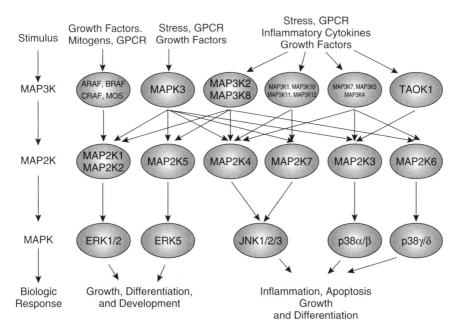

Figure 1.9 MAPK signaling pathways.

of PAKs include regulation of epithelial–mesenchymal transition (downstream of TGFβ) and regulation of microtubule assembly in mitosis.

1.3.4 CSNK1 Group

CSNK1 (casein kinase 1, also known as CK1) is one of the smaller protein kinase groups, with 12 members divided between 3 families (Figure 1.10). The largest of these families, also called CSNK1, has 7 members: CSNK1A1, CSNK1A1L, CSNK1D, CSNK1E, CSNK1G1, CSNK1G2, and CSNK1G3. These kinases are widely and constitutively expressed and are regulated by a series of autophosphorylation sites in the C-terminal domain of the protein. CNSK1 kinases preferentially phosphorylate serine/threonine substrates that have been "primed" by another phosphorylation event on the N-terminal side of their target phosphorylation residue, or which have a cluster of acidic residues (Asp or Glu) in this region. A wide range of functionally diverse CSNK1 substrates has been identified, including cytoskeletal proteins, receptors, and transcription factors (95). One particularly intriguing CSNK1 function is regulation of the circadian rhythm, first identified in the *Drosophila* CSNK1 homolog *doubletime* (96, 97). This may have implications in tumor biology: a lentiviral kinome-wide RNAi screen recently identified the CSNK1E gene (*CSNK1E*) as a regulator of cancer cell growth, and growth inhibition by a small molecule CSNK1E inhibitor could be rescued by inhibiting expression of the circadian clock protein PER2 (98). CSNK1 isoforms (in particular, CSNK1A1, CSNK1D, and CSNK1E) have also been associated with other

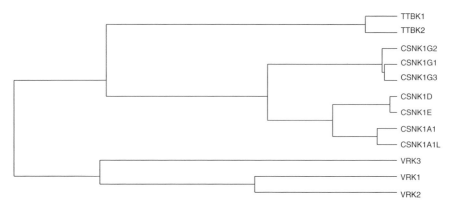

Figure 1.10 The CK1 kinase group. The figure was produced as described in Figure 1.3 legend.

aspects of tumor cell biology, although like many of the kinases discussed here it has been ascribed both tumorigenic and tumor suppressor functions. These include phosphorylation of p53 and its regulator MDM2 (99–102), resistance to apoptosis (103, 104), and regulation of WNT/β-catenin and Hedgehog signaling (105).

1.3.5 AGC Group

The AGC group is named for three of its constituent families: PK<u>A</u> (*PRKA*), PK<u>G</u> (*PRKG*), and PK<u>C</u> (*PRKC*) (Figure 1.11). PDK1 (3-phosphoinositide-dependent protein kinase 1, *PDPK1*) has a central role in this group: it is a proximal effector of PI-3 kinase signaling and is implicated in the activation of many other group members including PKC, AKT, SGK, p90RSK, and p70S6K. The PKB subfamily, also known as AKT, is comprised of AKT1, AKT2, and AKT3 and constitutes a key signaling node downstream of PI-3 kinase and PDK1. AKT proteins phosphorylate a wide range of substrates, promoting diverse phenotypic sequelae including cellular proliferation, survival, and glucose uptake/glycogen mobilization (106). AKT signaling is broadly implicated in cancer cell biology and, in addition to promoting tumorigenesis, tumor growth, and survival, is thought to mediate resistance to both targeted and genotoxic therapies. The closely related serum and glucocorticoid activated kinases (SGK1, SGK2, and SGK3) have somewhat overlapping functions with AKT, particularly with respect to cell survival. The ribosomal S6 kinases are also important regulators of cellular growth and survival, falling into two subfamilies: the p70S6 kinases (S6K1 and S6K2) and the RSK family (RSK1(*RPS6KA1*), RSK2 (*RPS6KA2*), RSK3(*RPS6KA3*), and RSK4 (*RPS6KA6*)). S6K1 (*RPS6KB1*) and S6K2 (*RPS6KB2*) are activated downstream of both PDK1 and the atypical kinase mTOR and promote biogenesis via multiple mechanisms including activation of the ribosomal protein translation complex and enhancing translation of spliced mRNAs. RSKs have a C-terminal CAMK domain in addition to the N-terminal AGC kinase: these domains are substrates for the

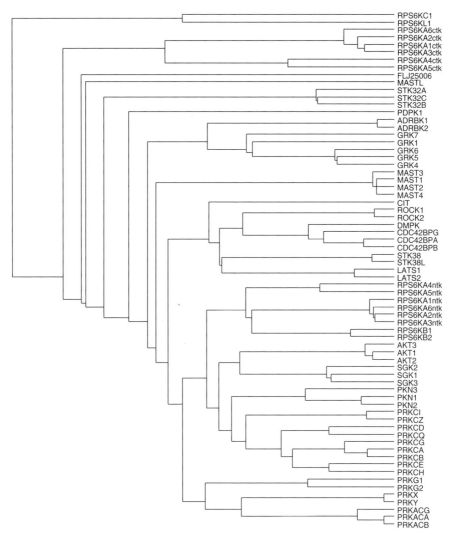

Figure 1.11 The AGC kinase group. The figure was produced as described in Figure 1.3 legend.

mitogen-activated protein kinase (MAPK) ERK and the AGC group "master regulator" kinase PDK1, respectively. Therefore RSKs serve as a node of convergence between the PI3K and RAS/MAPK signaling pathways. The mitogen and stress activated kinases (MSK1(*RPS6KA5*) and MSK2 (*RPS6KA4*)) are another example of signaling proteins with two kinase domains; they are downstream effectors of the ERK and p38 MAPKs (see Section 1.3.7). Protein kinase C is an additional important AGC family, containing 10 proteins with diverse mechanisms of activation and complex roles in the proliferation and survival of both normal and transformed cells. These important intracellular signaling proteins are all discussed in more detail in Chapter 5.

The "A" of the AGC group is PKA, which regulates a plethora of effects in a tissue-specific manner. It is principally an effector of G-protein coupled receptors. The specific phenotypic effects elicited by PKA signaling include stimulation of glycogenolysis and gluconeogenesis in hepatocytes and muscle cells, and dopamine signaling in the brain.

PRKs (PRK1 (*PNK1*) and PRK2 (*PKN2*)) are AGC family kinases that have been implicated in signaling downstream of the GTPase RHO. In particular, PRKs have been shown to stimulate androgen receptor (AR) activity even in the presence of specific AR antagonists and may therefore play a role in development of prostate cancer (107).

The GRKs are important for regulation of G-protein coupled receptor (GPCR) signaling. Following ligand stimulation of GPCRs, GRKs phosphorylate the receptors, leading to recruitment of arrestins, blockade of G-protein coupled responses, and in some cases initiation of alternative downstream signaling events.

1.3.6 CAMK Group

This group, named for the Ca^{2+}/calmodulin-dependent protein kinase, contains a diverse array of kinases with varied structure and function (Figure 1.12). As the name suggests, several members of this group are effectors of intracellular calcium signaling. In the latent state, kinase activity is restrained by an autoinhibitory domain; binding of the Ca^{2+}:calmodulin complex relieves this autoinhibition and stimulates kinase activity (108, 109). The CAMKII isoform was identified over 30 years ago (110) and has since been studied extensively. There are four human CAMKII genes (*CAMK2A, CAMK2B, CAMK2D, CAMK2G*), each encoding a protein of 50–60 kDa, which can assemble into homomeric and heteromeric multimers; in addition to Ca^{2+}:calmodulin binding, these complexes can be regulated further by autophosphorylation (108, 111). CAMKII is ubiquitously expressed but is particularly abundant in neuronal tissue, where it is implicated in synaptic plasticity and memory (112). Many other physiological processes are regulated by intracellular calcium and calcium-dependent kinases, including muscle contraction (myosin light chain kinase, MLCK (113)), lymphocyte activation (CAMKIV (*CAMPK4*) (114)), and calcium channel function (CAMKII (115)). The CAMK family contains the second (C-terminal) kinase domains of the RSKs and MSKs, as mentioned earlier. The RSKs are sometimes referred to as isoforms of MAPKAPK1 (MAPK-activated protein kinase 1) and should not be confused with the p38-activated kinase MAPKAPK2 (MK2), which contains a single CAMK domain.

The DNA damage/cell cycle checkpoint kinases CHK1 (*CHEK1*) and CHK2 (*CHEK2*) are also found in the CAMK group; more recently, MAPKAPK2 (MK2) has also been implicated in DNA damage repair, although with a somewhat distinct mode of activation compared to CHK1 and CHK2. Collectively, the cell cycle checkpoint kinases are activated in response to DNA damage and phosphorylate members of the CDC25 phosphatase family, leading to their degradation (CDC25A) or cytoplasmic sequestration (CDC25B/C). This in turn causes accumulation of hyperphosphorylated, inactive cyclin-dependent kinases, inducing cell cycle arrest and enabling DNA repair mechanisms to be invoked. The role of these kinases in

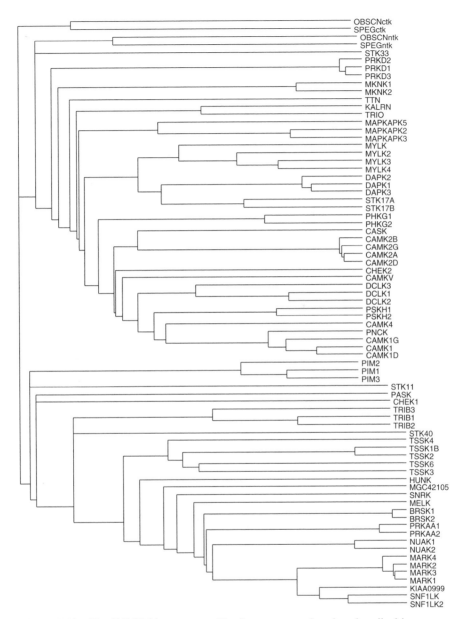

Figure 1.12 The CAMK kinase group. The figure was produced as described in Figure 1.3 legend.

DNA repair and resistance to chemotherapy is reviewed in more detail in Chapter 6. The CAMK group also includes AMP-dependent kinase (AMPK (*PRKAA*)) and its upstream regulator LKB1 (*STK11*). AMPK plays an important role in signaling the energetic status of the cell: when ATP levels are low and the AMP:ATP ratio is high, AMPK is activated and conveys an inhibitory signal to mTOR, which serves as an integrator of mitogenic and nutrient signaling in cells (Chapter 5). The activity of AMPK is also dependent on LKB1, the product of a tumor suppressor gene that is deleted or inactivated in a significant fraction of non small cell lung carcinomas (116). In fact, LKB1 can phosphorylate and activate almost all of the CAMKs that are most closely related to AMPK (117). These include the MARKs (MARK1, 2, 3, and 4), which are microtubule-associated proteins that control cell polarity and may contribute to pathologies such as cancer and Alzheimer disease (118, 119).

Protein kinase D (PKD, *PRKD*) was initially considered to be a member of the protein kinase C (PKC) family—it is also known as PKCµ—but its kinase domain sequence places it in the CAMK group (120). However, its overall structure has many similarities with the PKC proteins (Chapter 5): there are two N-terminal cysteine-rich regions implicated in diacylglycerol binding, a pleckstrin homology domain, and a C-terminal kinase domain (121). Also, many studies have demonstrated that PKD is an effector of PKC signaling: it is activated in response to tumorigenic phorbol esters and is directly phosphorylated by novel PKC isoforms (122). There are three PKD isozymes: PKD1(*PRKD1*), PKD2 (*PRKD21*), and PKD3(*PRKD3*). PKDs mediate multiple cellular signaling pathways including stimulation of the RAS/MAPK pathway, inhibition of the JNK stress-activated kinase pathway, and various functions relating to cell motility and adhesion (121). PKD has been implicated in proliferation and invasion of several tumor cell types, including pancreatic carcinoma (123), small cell lung carcinoma (124), chronic myelogenous leukemia (125), and lymphoma (126). It is also involved in VEGF-mediated endothelial cell proliferation and migration (127, 128). A selective, non ATP-competitive small molecule inhibitor of PKD was recently reported (129).

The PIM kinases (PIM1, PIM2, and PIM3) have been implicated in a number of solid and hematological tumors and are reviewed in Chapter 5.

1.3.7 CMGC Group

The CMGC family is named for its primary constituent groups: cyclin-dependent kinases (CDKs), mitogen-activated protein kinases (MAPKs), glycogen synthase kinases (GSKs), and CDK-like kinases (CLKs) (Figure 1.13).

CDKs CDKs (cyclin-dependent kinases) can be divided into two broad groups: those that mediate cell cycle progression (e.g., CDK1 (*CDC2*), CDK2, CDK4, CDK6) and those that regulate transcription (e.g., CDK7, CDK9). The CDKs are regulated by their partner proteins, the cyclins: while CDK expression remains relatively constant, cyclin levels vary throughout the cell cycle and restrict activity of their partner CDKs to specific intervals. Hence tumor cells are often characterized by aberrant expression of cyclins rather than of the cell cycle CDKs themselves. During interphase, cell cycle progression is mediated by CDK4, CDK6, CDK2, and CDK3, whereas entry into mitosis is dependent on CDK1. Remarkably, however, it appears that only CDK1 is absolutely essential for completion of the cell cycle (130). CDK7, CDK8, and CDK9 are all involved in promoting mRNA

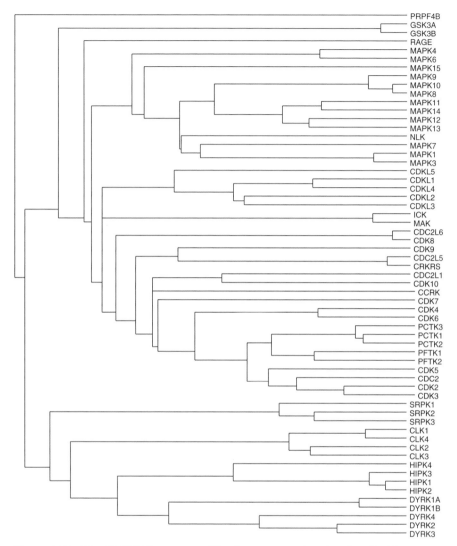

Figure 1.13 The CMGC kinase group. The figure was produced as described in Figure 1.3 legend.

transcription by RNA polymerase II, which directs expression of multiple proteins that are essential for proliferation and survival; other CDK proteins modulate diverse processes including RNA splicing (CDK11 (*CDC2L1*), CDK12 (*CRKRS*)) and neuronal function (CDK5, CDK10). Further details on CDKs can be found in Chapter 6. In addition to the CDKs, several other important kinases are found in the CMGC group, most notably the mitogen-activated protein kinases.

Mitogen-Activated Protein Kinases (MAPKs)   The MAPKs are the downstream effectors of an ancient signaling mechanism that is highly conserved from yeast to humans. Collectively, these kinases control diverse intracellular signaling pathways in response to changing cellular conditions. Such factors include nutrient levels, growth factors, cytokines, and environmental stress such as osmotic potential and genotoxic insult. There are four canonical MAPK pathways: ERK, JNK, p38, and ERK5 (Figure 1.9). In the ERK pathway, the RAS GTPase stimulates activity of the TKL group RAF kinases, which activate the STE group kinases MEK1 and MEK2, which finally activate ERK1 (*MAPK3*) and ERK2 (*MAPK1*). Activated ERK phosphorylates a number of additional cytoplasmic signaling kinases, such as RSK and MSK, and also translocates to the nucleus where it regulates gene expression through the activation of several key transcription factors (131, 132). The ERK/MAPK pathway and its role in cancer are reviewed in detail in Chapter 5.

The p38 MAPK family kinases are mediators of inflammation and the immune response and are activated by multiple stress signals (133). Together with the JNKs (see later discussion), p38 family members are also referred to as stress-activated protein kinases (SAPKs). There are four isoforms: p38α (*MAPK14*), β (*MAPK11*), γ (MAPK12), and δ (*MAPK13*) of which α is the best characterized. All p38 isoforms are widely expressed, although p38α is most prominent in skeletal muscle and p38δ is particularly found in testis, small intestine, kidney, and pancreas (134). The immediate upstream regulators of p38 are the MAPK kinases (MAP2Ks) MKK3 and MKK6, which are highly selective for p38 compared to the JNK family kinases; MKK4 activates both p38 and JNK. p38 exerts negative effects on cell proliferation, and most of the data indicate that it is a tumor suppressor. Inactivation of p38 supports cellular transformation, and increased p38 expression suppresses tumorigenesis (135, 136). In particular, oncogenic activation of the RAS pathway promotes proliferation via the ERK/MAPK pathway but also triggers senescence in premalignant cells, mediated by MKK3, MKK6, p38, and their downstream effectors p16^{INK4A} and p53 (136–139). It was recently proposed that p38 signaling in response to oncogene activation is triggered by generation of reactive oxygen species (140). p38 is also a mediator of the DNA damage response, via phosphorylation of MAPKAPK2 (Chapter 6). Like may kinases, however, p38 has a dark side, and in tumors that have managed to subvert the reactive oxygen species stress response, p38 may have a protumorigenic role by promoting angiogenesis and tissue invasion (133).

The c-JUN N-terminal kinases (JNKs) initiate a diverse range of transcriptional activities in response to ultraviolet radiation, inflammatory cytokines, and other mechanisms of cellular stress (141, 142). As indicated by the name, JNKs phosphorylate c-JUN, a component of the AP-1 transcription factor complex. There are three JNKs—JNK1 (*MAPK8*), JNK2 (*MAPK9*), and JNK3 (*MAPK10*)—each of which can exist as differentially spliced isoforms. There is evidence that the different splice forms may respond to different upstream activators, phosphorylate different substrates, and thereby enhance the diversity of JNK signaling (143). JNK1 and JNK2 are widely expressed, whereas JNK3 expression is restricted to the brain, heart, and testes. JNK kinases are the downstream effectors of a signaling cascade comprising the MAP2Ks MKK4 and MKK7, and at least 14 MAP3Ks. These MAP2K and MAP3K pathways have significant overlap with each other and in some cases also communicate with p38 MAPK signaling. MAP3K signaling may be initiated by diverse factors including the RAC1 and CDC42 GTPases (144, 145) and other kinases (MAP3Ks, or MAP4Ks), including the PAKs (146, 147). In addition to these levels of selectivity, further specification of signaling is provided by various scaffolding proteins including the JIP (JNK interacting protein) family and POSH (plenty of SH3 domains). In general, JNK signaling is associated with promoting apoptosis and has been particularly implicated in excitotoxic neuronal cell death and ischemic injury in multiple tissues. Consequently, JNK inhibition has been proposed as a strategy for treating neurodegenerative diseases and ischemia/reperfusion injury. The role for JNK signaling in cancer is complex. On one hand, the proapoptotic role of JNK signaling suggests that its inhibition would be counterproductive as an antitumor strategy (148): indeed, the upstream JNK activator MKK4 has been identified as a putative tumor suppressor that is inactivated in different tumor types, including breast, pancreatic, ovarian, and prostate cancer (149). However, MKK4 and JNK may also promote tumor cell growth in some cellular context, and several cancer cell lines express high levels of JNK (150). As in the case of p38, context is critical, and in order to target these kinases therapeutically it will be important to understand which tumor types and stages of tumor development use JNK as a tumor progression factor rather than a tumor suppressor.

GSK3α/β Glycogen synthase kinase 3 (GSK3) is a multifunctional kinase existing as two isoforms (GSK3α and GSK3β) encoded by distinct genes (*GSK3A* and *GSK3B*). It is found in all eukaryotes and, as suggested by its name, was first identified as a regulator of glycogen synthesis (151). GSK3 (in particular, GSK3β) has since been implicated in many additional cellular processes involved in proliferation, differentiation, and survival and has been pursued as a therapeutic target in diabetes, neurological disorders, and inflammation. The regulation of GSK3 differs from many kinases in that phosphorylation (at S9) results in inhibition of enzyme activity; as described in Chapter 2, this mechanism of regulation is intimately related to the substrate specificity of GSK3, which preferentially phosphorylates serine residues that have a "priming" phosphoserine located 4 residues C-terminal to the target serine. As well as inhibiting glycogen synthesis, GSK3 is a key regulator of the WNT/β-catenin pathway. In the basal state, a fraction of cellular GSK3 is present in the adenomatous polyposis coli (APC) complex, where it phosphorylates β-catenin, targeting it for destruction. Activation of the WNT pathway leads to dephosphorylation and nuclear translocation of β-catenin, where it promotes morphogenetic signaling: however, aberrant WNT signaling has been associated with tumor formation. Furthermore, GSK3 phosphorylates the cell cycle regulators cyclin D1 and MYC, also initiating their destruction. Accordingly, effectors of growth factor signaling pathways, including AKT, RSK, and p70S6K, can phosphorylate GSK3 on S9 and downregulate its activity. Hence, in many contexts, GSK3 suppresses growth, promotes apoptosis, and is a negative regulator of tumorigenesis, so it might be regarded as a target to avoid in anticancer drugs. As with many signaling proteins involved in cancer, however, GSK may be a double-edged sword and in some instances GSK3β has been associated with promoting tumor development. Elevated levels of GSK3β have been detected in ovarian tumors, and inhibition of GSK3β has been shown to suppress ovarian tumor cell growth in vitro and in vivo (152); similar results have been demonstrated in colon and pancreatic cancer (153, 154). The conflicting roles of GSK3 in tumor biology have recently been reviewed (155).

1.3.8 RGC Group

The smallest group of human protein kinases is the RGC (receptor guanylate cyclase) group, consisting of a single family with five members (Figure 1.14). The members of this group are all pseudokinases and include the atrial natriuretic peptide (ANP) receptors (*NPR1, NPR2*). The kinase domain provides an ANP- and ATP-dependent regulatory function for the neighboring guanylate cyclase domain (156).

1.3.9 Others

Several important kinases do not have sufficiently close sequence similarity to assign them to one of the previously described groups (Figure 1.15). These include several important families such as the PLK and Aurora kinases, which are important regulators of mitosis and are discussed in Chapter 6. Some additional "other" kinases that have been associated with cancer biology are listed next.

CK2 CK2 (*CSNK2*) is a ubiquitous and highly conserved protein kinase that was originally named casein kinase II. However, it is notable for its very broad specificity: over 300 CK2 substrates have been identified both in vitro and/or in cells (157). Although these substrates primarily contain a serine or threonine residue at the phosphorylation site, tyrosine residues can also be phosphorylated (158). In addition, CK2 is a rare example of a kinase that can use GTP as a phosphate donor in addition to ATP; the structural basis for this dual specificity has been elucidated by X-ray crystallography (159). CK2 exists as a tetramer comprised of two catalytic domains (α) and two regulatory subunits (β). There are two catalytic domain isoforms CK2α (*CSNK2A1*) and CK2α′ (*CSNK2A2*); intact CK2 tetramers may contain two CK2α, two CK2α′, or one of each. The C-terminal regions of CK2α and CK2α′ are quite distinct and may confer functional specialization on

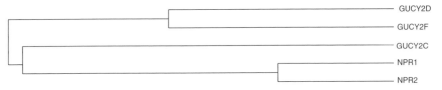

GUCY2D
GUCY2F
GUCY2C
NPR1
NPR2

Figure 1.14 The RGC kinase group. The figure was produced as described in Figure 1.3 legend.

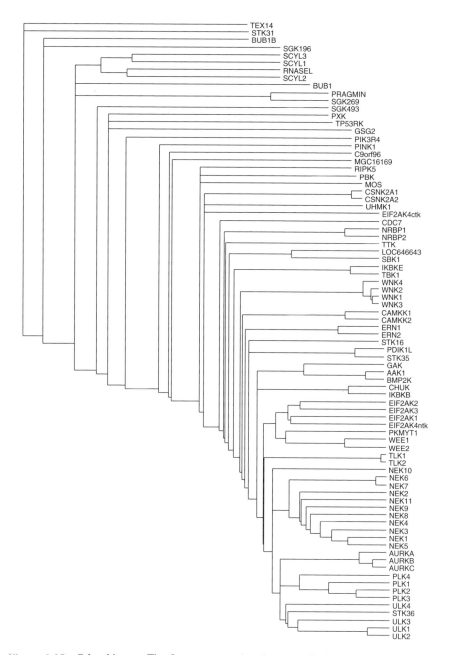

Figure 1.15 Other kinases. The figure was produced as described in Figure 1.3 legend.

the individual isoforms: for example, CK2α (but not CK2α′) is phosphorylated in mitotic cells and interacts with the peptidyl-prolyl isomerase PIN1 (160). Elucidation of the role of CK2 in cancer is complicated by the fact that it phosphorylates so many substrates. The list includes cell cycle proteins, apoptotic regulators, and stress signaling pathways and is further extended by the observation that CK2 phosphorylates the molecular chaperone CDC37, promoting its stabilization of a wide range of protein kinases (161). CK2 may also play a role in the complex relationship between inflammation and cancer and was identified as a regulator of IKKε (see later discussion) in inflammatory breast cancer (162). Downregulation of CK2 by antisense was shown to promote apoptosis in cancer cells both in vit-roand in vivo (163). Although no small molecule CK2 inhibitors have advanced into the clinic, structural studies have illuminated the binding modes of several natural product CK2 inhibitors (164), and more recently a series of highly potent small molecules was also identified (165).

CDC7 CDC7 is an evolutionarily conserved serine–threonine kinase with homology to CK2 and to the CMGC group of cyclin-dependent kinases (CDKs). CDC7 phosphorylates and activates components of the DNA replication complexes, playing a critical role in the initiation of DNA synthesis and in cell cycle checkpoint control. As in the case of the CDKs, the monomeric CDC7 enzyme is inactive and it requires association with a regulatory subunit (ASK) for catalytic activity. Activated CDC7 phosphorylates and activates MCM2, a component of the hexameric MCM complex, which is a replicative helicase required for DNA replication (166, 167) (Figure 1.16). CDC7 function is absolutely required for DNA replication to proceed, and its activity is often upregulated in cancer cells, either by overexpression of either CDC7 kinase itself or the regulatory ASK subunit (167, 168). Inhibition of CDC7 leads to a block in replication and a halt to cell cycle progression, and in many tumor cell lines inhibition of CDC7 function leads to apoptosis (169). CDC7 inhibition may also be useful in combination with chemotherapy agents. Inhibition of CDC7 by siRNA in HeLa cells and A2780 ovarian carcinoma cells in conjunction with treatment with hydroxyurea or etoposide leads to increased cell death, suggesting that CDC7 activity is required for protecting cells from apoptosis during replication stress (170). CDC7 also plays a role in cell cycle checkpoint responses and, as discussed further in Chapter 6, seems to be required for the activation of CHK1 in response to DNA damage (171).

IκB Kinase (IKK) The IκB kinases (IKKα (*CHUK*) and IKKβ (*IKBKB*)) are important regulators of inflammatory signaling and are downstream effectors of the Toll-like receptors and other mediators of the innate immune response. Chronic inflammation has long been associated with cancer, and as many as 20% of cancer deaths have been attributed to inflammatory responses to underlying infectious diseases (172). The NFκ B family of transcription factors has been proposed as a key mediator of this link between inflammation and cancer (173). Dimeric NFκB proteins promote the expression of inflammatory cytokines and also orchestrate an antiapoptotic, growth-promoting program, which not only supports the expansion of tumor cells but may protect them against chemotherapy and other anticancer treatments. The activity of NFκB is restrained by the IκB proteins, which bind to NFκB dimers and inhibit their translocation to the nucleus. The IKK complex consists of two catalytic domains (IKKα and IKKβ) and a regulatory IKKγ subunit (Figure 1.17). IKK phosphorylates the IκB proteins, which targets them for

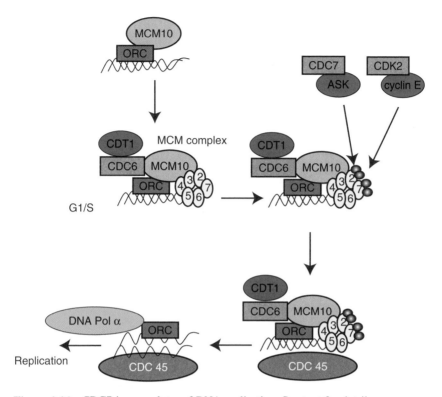

Figure 1.16   CDC7 is a regulator of DNA replication. See text for details.

ubiquitination and degradation: this unmasks the nuclear localization site in NFκB and enables it to translocate to the nucleus and regulate gene transcription. Both IKKα and IKKβ are involved in NFκB activation, although their relative importance depends on the nature of the external stimulus and the specific IκB/NFκB substrate.

Following the identification of IKK, two additional IKK-related proteins have been discovered, both of which can also play a role in NFκB regulation (reviewed in (174)). TBK1 (TANK binding kinase 1) was shown to act upstream of NFκB in response to PKCε and is both constitutively and ubiquitously expressed; in contrast, IKKε (*IKBKE*) is restricted to pancreas and lymphoid tissues and is induced as part of the inflammatory response. The IKK-related kinases have also been placed downstream of RAS, in particular, as effectors of RALGEF (TBK1) and PI3K (IKKε), and may therefore have a tumorigenic function independent of their role in inflammation. TBK1 is overexpressed in tumor cell lines and under hypoxic conditions and promotes expression of proangiogenic factors as well as inflammatory cytokines (175). Its disruption using RNA interference promotes apoptosis in tumor cells but not in normal epithelial cells, further supporting its role in tumor growth and survival (176). IKKε was recently linked to breast cancer, where it emerged

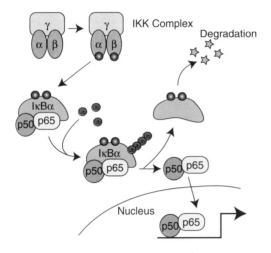

Figure 1.17 The IKK signaling pathway. See text for details.

as an important effector of AKT signaling; furthermore, the locus encompassing *IKBKE* was found to be amplified in 16% of breast cancer cell lines (177).

NEK The NEKs are orthologs of the fungal kinase NIMA (never-in-mitosis-A), identified as a regulator of mitosis in *Aspergillus nidulans* (178–180). There are 11 human NEK family members, each comprising a conserved N-terminal kinase domain and highly variable C-terminal region. Only a few of the NEKs have been extensively characterized (181). NEK2 is perhaps the most widely studied and, together with NEK6, NEK7, and NEK9, appears to be a regulator of mitosis like the ancestral fungal protein. NEK2 is expressed in S and G2 phases where it localizes to the centrosome and promotes centrosome separation during mitosis (182). There are several splice forms of NEK2, which may have distinct roles in mitosis. The most prominent splice variant, NEK2A, is degraded soon after mitotic entry, but NEK2B is present in late mitosis and may help to regulate mitotic exit (183). NEK2 is abnormally expressed in a variety of tumors, including lymphoma, breast, cervical, and prostate cancer, and given its physiological role in mitotic regulation it may contribute to the chromosomal abnormalities that are characteristic of many tumor cells (184). NEK9 (also called NERCC1) is expressed throughout the cell cycle. It has an extended C-terminal region that includes an RCC1 (GTPase exchange factor) homology domain and has been shown to interact with the RAN GTPase: however, it is not clear that the RCC1 domain actually modulates GTPase activity (185). Its substrates include NEK6 and NEK7, and together these kinases function to regulate mitotic spindle assembly (186). Like NEK9, NEK7 is expressed throughout the cell cycle: however, NEK6 appears to be upregulated during mitosis. NEK1 also localizes to centrosomes but, in contrast to the aforementioned NEKs, depletion of NEK1 prevents activation of the checkpoint kinases CHK1 and CHK2 in response to genotoxic insults. Hence NEK1 may be an important regulator of the cell cycle checkpoint/DNA damage response (187).

1.3.10 Atypical Protein Kinases

The atypical kinases (Figure 1.18) are somewhat divergent in sequence from the canonical protein kinase family but have nevertheless been shown in many cases to have protein kinase activity. Of these, the most important subgroup with regard to cancer biology is the PIKK (phosphatidylinositol-3′ kinase-related kinase) family. Members of this family are large proteins containing a phosphatidylinositol-3′ kinase (PI3K) domain, an N-terminal FAT domain, and a C-terminal FATC domain. The mTOR (mammalian target of rapamycin, *FRAP1*) kinase is perhaps the most prominent member and is extensively reviewed in Chapter 5. This protein is conserved in all eukaryotes, including yeast, and acts as a central cellular integrator of mitogenic signaling, cellular energy, and nutritional status. Two distinct mTOR complexes have been identified (mTORC1 and mTORC2), each of which has a distinct mode of regulation, spectrum of substrates, and role in mediating cellular proliferation and survival. The macrolide rapamycin, from which mTOR derives its name, specifically inhibits the mTORC1 complex, and a derivative of rapamycin has been approved for treatment of metastatic renal cell carcinoma with poor prognostic factors. Other important members of the atypical kinase family are DNAPK (DNA-activated protein kinase, *PRKDC*), ATM (ataxia telangiectasia-mutated), and ATR (ataxia telangiectasia and RAD3 related), all of which are involved in sensing DNA damage and activating cellular DNA damage checkpoints. These kinases are discussed further in Chapter 6.

1.3.11 Nonprotein Kinases

Although our focus is on protein kinases, the activities of several lipid kinases are intimately related to protein kinase signaling pathways. Most notable are the kinases that modulate phosphoinositides, particularly the Class I phosphatidylinositol-3 kinase (PI3K) family (188). These lipid kinases provide a crucial connection between extracellular signals (conveyed through RTKs or G-protein coupled receptors) and intracellular protein kinase signal transduction cascades. Phosphatidylinositol (4,5) bisphosphate (PIP_2) has long been known to be an important signaling molecule and is hydrolyzed to the second messengers diacylglycerol and inositol (1,4,5) trisphosphate, the latter of which promotes release of intracellular calcium. In the late 1980s, Lew Cantley and co-workers showed that stimulation of smooth muscle cells with PDGF led to increases in cellular levels of phosphatidylinositol (3,4,5) trisphosphate (PIP_3), implicating this molecule in mitogenic signaling (189). The catalytic subunit of PI3Kα (p110α) was subsequently cloned and characterized (190) and, together with the other members of the Class I PI3K family, has since been intensively studied. There are four Class I kinases (PI3Kα, PI3Kβ, PI3Kγ, and PI3Kδ) and a corresponding family of regulatory/adaptor proteins, which couple PI3K enzymes to upstream activators such as RTKs (Figure 1.19). The primary role of Class I PI3Ks in mitogenic signaling is to catalyze the conversion of PIP_2 to PIP_3 (Figure 1.19), leading to engagement of multiple effector proteins at the cell membrane via their PIP_3 binding pleckstrin homology (PH) domains. Conversely, several

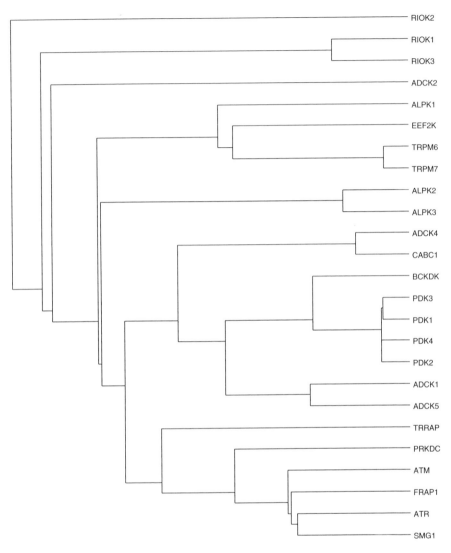

Figure 1.18 Atypical kinases. The figure was produced as described in Figure 1.3 legend.

phospholipid phosphatases have been shown to oppose the action of PI3K and dephosphorylate PIP$_3$. Activating p110α mutations have been found in many different tumors, highlighting the importance of this signaling pathway in cancer biology. Furthermore, the PTEN phosphatase, which specifically removes the 3′ phosphate from PIP$_3$, is inactivated in many tumors and provides a second proximal mechanism for dysregulation of PIP$_3$ signaling. Further details of the structure and function of the Class I PI3K proteins and their role in cancer are found in Chapter 5.

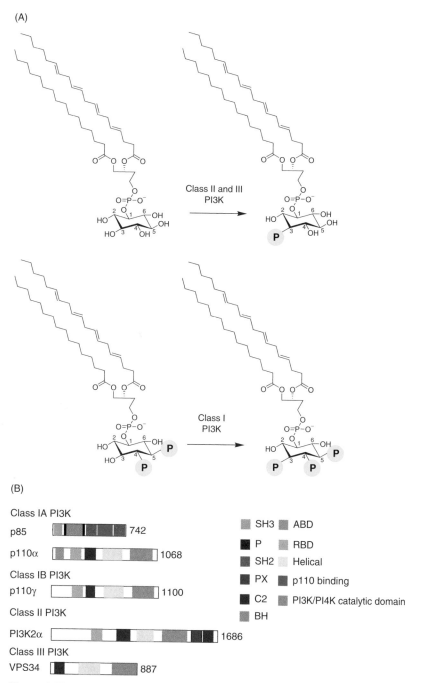

Figure 1.19 Structure and activity of phosphatidylinositol 3-kinases (PI3Ks). (A) PI3Ks catalyze the transfer of phosphate (yellow circle) to the 3-position of the substrate phosphoilipid. (B) Domain structures of different PI3K enzymes. ABD, adaptor binding domain; RBD, RAS binding domain; P, proline-rich domain; PX, PHOX homology domain; BH, breakpoint cluster region-homology domain.

The Class II PI3Ks (PI3K-C2α, PI3K-C2β, and PI3K-C2γ) are less well characterized than Class I (Figure 1.19). They are functional monomers as opposed to the Class I heterodimers and are distinguished by a C2 domain similar to that found in PKC enzymes, which is responsible for Ca^{2+} and/or phospholipid binding. Class II PI3Ks have been placed downstream of growth factor and cytokine signaling (191–193) and are implicated in membrane trafficking, cell migration, muscle contraction, and survival (194–198). The precise phospholipids modified by Class II enzymes have remained somewhat obscure, although PI3K-C2α was shown to specifically phosphorylate PI at the 3-position (Figure 1.19), producing PI(3)P. This study also implicated the small GTPase TC10 in activation of PI3K-C2α in response to insulin (199). Recently, PI3K-C2α has been implicated in protecting tumor cells from apoptosis, suggesting that inhibiting this isoform may have direct effects on tumor cell survival and sensitize them to proapoptotic therapeutic agents (200).

PI3K Class III contains a single member, known as VPS34 (vacuolar protein sorting 34; Figure 1.19). VPS34 regulates endosomal trafficking via local production of its product, phosphatidylinositol-3-phosphate (PI3P) from unphosphorylated phosphatidylinositol (201, 202). The principal functions associated with VPS34 with respect to tumor cell survival are nutrient signaling and initiation of autophagy. VPS34 is implicated in nutrient signaling: it promotes cellular growth in response to mitogenic factors and is thought to play a role in the nutrient sensing mechanisms that feed in to the mTOR kinase (203–205). Autophagy is a process of cellular self-digestion, whereby cells can sequester portions of their cytoplasm and subcellular organelles in large vesicles (autophagosomes). These vesicles fuse with lysosomes and proceed to digest the enclosed components, leading to release of amino acids, fatty acids, and other cellular nutrients. When driven to completion, autophagy can be a route to cell death: however, autophagy appears to be a tumor suppressor mechanism that protects cells from damage under conditions of metabolic stress (206–208). This tumor suppression may paradoxically be subverted in established tumors: cancer cells frequently find themselves in hostile environments (including low pH, low oxygen and nutrient supply, and assault by genotoxic drugs), and autophagy may represent a mechanism for the cells to survive until more favorable conditions allow them to emerge from this "hibernating" state and resume neoplastic growth. Hence VPS34 inhibitors may have utility in promoting tumor cell death, particularly in combination with other agents that disrupt the tumor nutrient supply or promote genotoxic and other forms of cellular stress.

Several other lipid kinases are also emerging as potentially important regulators of cancer cell growth and survival, in particular, the various kinases that regulate production of bioactive sphingolipids. Sphingolipids such as sphingosine, ceramide, and their phosphorylated derivatives are components of cellular membranes and, like phosphoinositides, are also important mediators of diverse cellular functions including cell growth, death, senescence, adhesion, and migration (209). Ceramide can be cleaved by ceramidase to produce sphingosine, and both ceramidase and sphingosine can be phosphorylated by ceramide kinase and one of two sphingosine kinases, respectively (Figure 1.20). Ceramide-1-phosphate and sphingosine-1-phosphate (S1P) are mitogenic and proinflammatory and promote cell survival; conversely, ceramide and sphingosine promote cell cycle arrest

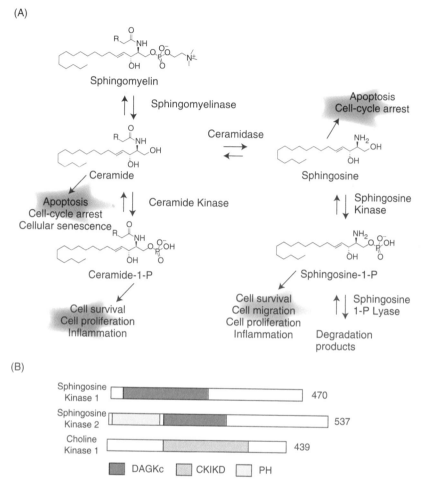

Figure 1.20 Lipid kinases. (A) The sphingosine–ceramide "rheostat": interconversion of (phospho)sphingolipids promotes various cellular responses including cell survival, proliferation, cell cycle arrest, and apoptosis. (B) Domain structures of sphingosine kinase 1, sphingosine kinase 2, and choline kinase. DAGKc, diacylglycerol kinase domain; CK1KD, choline kinase 1 catalytic domain; PH, pleckstrin homology domain.

and apoptosis (210). Furthermore, secreted S1P is the ligand for a family of five G-protein coupled receptors (S1PR$_{1-5}$). In particular, S1PR$_1$ signaling regulates lymphocyte trafficking and collaborates with the PI3K pathway in vascular endothelial cells to promote adherens junction assembly and increase vascular integrity (211, 212). Inhibitors of sphingosine or ceramide kinases may therefore have utility in promoting apoptosis in tumor cells and also as vascular disrupting agents. Several small molecule sphingosine kinase inhibitors have been reported to have antitumor activity (213).

Choline kinase (CHOK, also known as CHK) is another lipid kinase that has attracted attention as a cancer target. CHOK is encoded by two separate genes

(*CHKA* and *CHKB*) and expressed as three isoforms: CHOKα1, CHOKα2, and CHOKβ. Phosphorylation of choline produces phosphocholine, which is essential for biosynthesis of phosphatidylcholine (PC). CHOK is overexpressed and activated in several different tumor types including lung, breast, colon, and prostate (214), and generation of phosphocholine has been associated with oncogenic transformation and tumor cell growth (215–217). A series of compounds with CHOK inhibitory activity have been reported, and some of these molecules have shown activity in cancer cells and xenograft models (218–220).

1.4 STRATEGIC CONSIDERATIONS FOR SELECTING KINASES AS DRUG TARGETS

Selective killing of tumor cells requires the identification of drug targets critical to pathways that drive or support cancer progression. A conceptual framework for identifying and selecting drug targets that meet this requirement suggests four general tracks to consider when evaluating a potential target (221):

1. *Oncogene addiction*, in which mutational activation of a gene drives tumor development and dependency on that gene for tumor cell survival (222). For example, the efficacy of inhibitors of mutated receptor tyrosine kinases such as EGFR and ABL may be attributable to oncogene addiction (discussed in Chapter 8).

2. *Lineage addiction*, in which a gene required for development of a tissue is later required for survival of a tumor cell derived from that tissue (223). While regulators of transcription like the androgen receptor or MITF appear to act in this manner, few kinases have been proposed to act by this mechanism.

3. *Synthetic lethality*, in which inhibition or activation of two genes together has a deleterious effect not seen with either gene alteration alone (224). Drugs that achieve synthetic lethality in combination with loss of a tumor suppressor, for example, could provide an excellent therapeutic window, as has been shown for PARP inhibitors and BRCA deficiency in some models (225–227).

4. *Host factors*, which exploit tumor dependency on surrounding normal tissues for growth/survival signals and processes like angiogenesis. The development of kinase-directed antiangiogenic therapies has received particular attention in recent years and is discussed in Chapter 9.

All of these tracks apply to kinase-based drug discovery and each calls for a different approach to target identification and validation. For example, blocking angiogenesis as a host factor supporting tumorigenesis has been the goal of many efforts, and a suite of assays has been developed to quantify angiogenic phenotypes (228). In addition, large-scale screening efforts and algorithms for detecting synergy have been developed to identify rare targets and compounds with relevant synthetic lethal interactions (229, 230).

Most often, evidence for oncogene addiction has provided the therapeutic rationale for kinase-based drug discovery efforts (231). Technological advances and coordinated efforts to define gene copy number alterations, gene expression differences, point mutations, and epigenetic changes in tumors have implicated many kinases as likely drivers of tumorigenesis in discrete patient populations. For example, recurring activating mutations in BRAF in melanoma guided the development and clinical application of BRAF inhibitors, and evidence for gene amplification and overexpression of ERBB2/HER2 in breast cancer supported successful drug discovery efforts. Recent collaborative efforts seek to fully define the range of genetic alterations in tumors, including large-scale efforts like the Cancer Genome Anatomy Project. These efforts have already identified kinases with previously unknown roles in specific cancers (232–234), but they have also highlighted the difficulty of distinguishing "driver" mutations from the large number of "passenger" mutations inherent in unstable cancer genomes (235–237). Furthermore, even recurring mutations that drive cancer may not prove to be relevant drug targets, if they are only required at an early stage of tumorigenesis. This highlights the fact that, as with other approaches for target selection, the therapeutic rationale provided by tumor genomics requires preclinical validation in model systems in order to prioritize drug discovery efforts.

Model systems such as yeast (*Saccharomyces cerevisiae* and *Schizosaccharomyces pombe*), fruit flies (*Drosophila melanogaster*), zebrafish (*Danio rerio*), and nematodes (*Caenorhabditis elegans*) have proved useful for both target identification and validation, oftentimes providing the initial links for a novel gene to cancer relevant pathways and processes. These systems offer powerful tools for exploring conserved pathways and rapidly uncovering gene functions but are clearly limited in their ability to fully model the biology of human tumors. To extend results to more relevant mammalian systems, transgenic mice overexpressing a protein or "knockout" mice lacking gene function have been employed to identify and validate drug targets. For target validation using mouse models, it remains challenging to manipulate gene function at the time and in the tissues needed to model a human tumor. However, recent advances in conditional knockout techniques and viral delivery methods have sparked development of genetically engineered mouse models that more faithfully recapitulate human cancers (238), offering uniquely powerful tools for target identification and validation. For certain targets, however, the mouse ortholog of the human gene may not exist, and additionally, if there is a known ortholog in the mouse, it may have different functions.

Most commonly, studies in cultured mammalian cell lines are the tool of choice for target validation, due to the breadth of phenotypes that can be examined and the availability of a wide range of human tumor cell lines. Traditionally, overexpression and transformation assays have been powerful tools for uncovering novel oncogenes and tumor suppressors, particularly when activating or dominant negative mutations can be employed to model gain or loss of function. These approaches have been expanded upon in more recent studies through use of cell lines with genetically defined backgrounds and kinome-wide expression libraries, as in the efforts by Boehm et al. (177) to identify potentially oncogenic kinases.

The discovery of RNA interference (RNAi) as a tool for gene knockdown ushered in a new era of target validation by providing a straightforward method for inhibiting gene function in human cells. Introduction into cells of small double-stranded RNA known as short interfering RNA (siRNA) or overexpression of short hairpin constructs (shRNA) results in knockdown of genes with sequence matching the small double-stranded RNA, albeit with well-established off-target effects that can complicate analyses (239). One advantage of siRNA is that it can mimic the partial knockdown of gene function often seen with small molecule inhibitors of a target, with the caveat that RNAi acts at the level of mRNA and protein and does not fully mimic the enzymatic inhibition provided by a drug. Kinome-wide siRNA and shRNA libraries are now broadly used for kinase target identification and validation, including efforts to identify essential genes (240) and screens to identify targets appropriate for combination therapies with existing chemotherapeutics (229).

Given that neither RNAi nor knockouts in model organisms can fully model the enzymatic inhibition provided by a drug, it is beneficial to use tool compounds developed in the drug discovery process to assist in target validation. Profiling the effect of compounds on tumor cell lines, particularly when combined with an understanding of the gene alterations in specific cell lines, has been used effectively to demonstrate that the enzymatic activity of a particular kinase is required for tumor cell survival (241, 242). Furthermore, tool compounds allow critical in vivo studies using genetically engineered mouse models or xenografts in immuno-compromised mice. Incorporating tool compounds to prove that target modulation has the expected effects can validate the therapeutic rationale for a target while assisting in identification of desirable chemical scaffolds, an approach described by Collins and Workman (243) as the "pharmacologic audit trail."

Using these approaches, the role of protein kinases in promoting and maintaining tumor growth has been well established in many cases, indicating that many of these proteins may be appropriate targets for development of targeted therapeutics. However, even the most compelling target validation data only addresses one aspect of the tractability of a given target. Various additional aspects governing target value and tractability may be divided into intrinsic and extrinsic factors, either or both of which may have positive or negative effects on our evaluation. We define intrinsic factors as properties of the protein itself that we cannot change, such as subcellular localization, physical properties, and enzymological characteristics. As a trivial example, the availability of an extracellular domain on the cell surface determines whether a kinase might be an appropriate target for a therapeutic antibody. Extrinsic factors are additional features of the selected target that do not depend on the protein directly but may influence the efficacy of a therapeutic agent developed against it: as an example, the presence of redundant signaling mechanisms may enable the effects of target inhibition to be circumvented. Several intrinsic and extrinsic factors are considered next in more detail.

Intrinsic Properties   Most of the kinase inhibitors in clinical and preclinical development are competitive with ATP. The value of K_M^{ATP} for different kinases (where K_M^{ATP} represents the Michaelis constant, an approximate estimate of the ATP binding affinity) varies over a wide range, from <1 μM to ~ 1000 μM

TABLE 1.4 K_M^{ATP} Values[a] for Selected Protein Kinases

Kinase	K_M^{ATP} (μM)	Reference
c-ABL	12	244
Aurora-A	50	245
CDK2/cyclin A	31	246
CDK4/cyclin D1	25	246
CHK1	120	246
EGFR	5	247
ERBB2	13	247
IGF1R (0P, 1P, 2P, 3P) [b]	720, 527, 148, 107	248
IKKβ	0.1	249
MEK1	5.6	250
MTOR	1000	251
CRAF	11.6	252
VEGFR2 (0P, 5P)[b]	600, 150	253

[a] Note that these numbers may not be directly comparable to each other and may differ from other literature values due to differences in substrates and methodologies. However, they indicate the wide range of ATP binding interactions between different kinases

[b] Different phosphorylation states

(Table 1.4; a more comprehensive list can be found in the supplementary material for reference 254). However, cellular ATP levels are approximately 1–5 mM (2, 3). Under these conditions, a small molecule kinase inhibitor with the same inhibition constant (K_I) for two kinases will cause greater inhibition of the kinase with the higher K_M^{ATP} value, since ATP binding is weaker for this enzyme. So, for ATP-competitive inhibitors, targets with higher K_M^{ATP} might be expected to be more tractable in terms of achieving potent cellular activity. Alternatively, if a high value target is identified with a very low K_M^{ATP}, it might be worthwhile to consider screening for non ATP-competitive compounds. By a judicious choice of enzyme and ATP concentrations, it is often possible to favor discovery of ATP-competitive or noncompetitive compounds, either in primary screening or in medium–high throughput lead validation assays. (In practice, more complex modes of inhibition often occur, including uncompetitive inhibition—where the inhibitor only binds to the enzyme:substrate complex—and mixed inhibition.) The relationship between IC_{50} and K_I at different substrate (ATP) concentrations is given by the following equations, where [S] is the substrate concentration and K_M is the Michaelis constant for the substrate (255):

$$\text{Competitive}: \quad IC_{50} = K_I(1 + [S]/K_M) \qquad (1.1)$$

$$\text{Noncompetitive}: \quad IC_{50} = K_I \qquad (1.2)$$

Hence screening or follow-up testing at high concentrations of ATP (relative to the K_M for ATP) will preferentially identify noncompetitive inhibitors, whereas using low ATP concentrations will favor ATP-competitive molecules. As an illustration of this, Wei et al. (256) performed a series of high-throughput mode-of-inhibition assays using hits from a kinase-directed high-throughput screening campaign. Kinase inhibitors were found to be broadly segregated into two populations: ATP-noncompetitive (where $IC_{50}^{low\ substrate} \approx IC_{50}^{high\ substrate}$) and ATP-competitive (where $IC_{50}^{low\ substrate} < IC_{50}^{high\ substrate}$).

Physical properties of the target protein (or the isolated kinase domain of the target protein) have a substantial impact on its tractability as a molecular target. In particular, good solubility and stability properties are important in the development of robust screening and follow-up assays and are even more relevant in pursuing crystallographic and other biophysical analyses (257). There are now numerous examples of protein kinase domain expression in bacterial and eukaryotic expression systems, although the speed and ease with which this can be accomplished may be a limitation in some cases.

Extrinsic Properties   One of the key requirements for successful drug lead optimization is demonstration of cellular activity for lead compounds and subsequent translation of this cellular activity into pharmacodynamic target modulation in vivo. In order to accomplish this, it is necessary to establish a mechanistic cellular assay that is specific for the target in question. Ideally, the chosen cellular substrate should be phosphorylated by the target protein alone, so that potential interference by off-target activity can be excluded. The choice of cellular substrate is obvious in some cases (as in the case of MEK kinase, for which the primary cellular substrate is ERK; Chapter 5) but can be more complex, since cellular signaling networks are often multiple, redundant mechanisms. For example, the proapoptotic BCL2 family member BAD is phosphorylated at two main sites, S112 and S136. At least two kinases (p90RSK and mitochondrial-anchored PKA) are known to phosphorylate the S112 site, and two additional kinases (AKT and p70S6K) can phosphorylate S136; moreover, there is evidence that PIM kinases can phosphorylate both sites (258). In such cases, analysis of several independent substrates is preferable in order to confirm specific cellular inhibition of the target kinases.

Is it sufficient to target the protein of interest alone, or will it be necessary to simultaneously target other kinases/pathways in order to obtain therapeutic benefit? There are several examples of single kinases that represent the predominant underlying driver of disease; however, most tumors have multiple dysregulated pathways and moreover can "rewire" their cellular signaling if a single pathway is blocked. Although this does not preclude a given kinase from being chosen as a target, it will be important to consider whether additional kinases need to be targeted in parallel (either with a single multitargeted inhibitor or by combining two or more agents), in order for an effective therapeutic regimen to be developed.

Having amassed sufficient data to nominate a target, there are additional questions of drug lead validation, which depend on the available molecule(s) emerging from high-throughput screening or other methods of lead discovery (e.g., fragment-based drug design (259)). Can we actually discover inhibitors with the appropriate profile? In other words, is the chemical scaffold sufficiently malleable that a desirable kinase specificity profile can be achieved? In addition, there are many additional challenges that are common to most contemporary drug discovery programs: for example, do the inhibitors get into the cell? Are they bioavailable, do they have appropriate pharmacokinetic properties, and can any metabolic and toxicological liabilities be overcome? It is worth noting that the process of drug lead validation may have substantial overlap with target validation. Compounds emerging from lead discovery/screening campaigns may have substantial utility in validating the cognate target. Early on in the course of a drug lead optimization project involving a novel target, correlations between cellular mechanistic activity (e.g., inhibition of kinase substrate phosphorylation) and phenotypic activity (e.g., inhibition of proliferation or apoptosis) may provide valuable confirmation that small molecule inhibitors (in particular, the small molecule series chosen for optimization) are able to phenocopy the effects seen in target validation studies with, for example, RNAi experiments.

1.5   COMPARISON OF KINASE INHIBITOR THERAPEUTIC STRATEGIES

1.5.1   Small Molecule Versus Antibody-Directed Therapies

The two main modalities currently employed to inhibit kinase activity are small organic molecules and antibodies. Small molecules (typically with molecular weight <1000 Da) are almost always produced by organic synthesis, although some examples of natural products exist (e.g., the mTOR inhibitor rapamycin, described in Chapter 9). Small molecule inhibitors range from the highly specific (with a single target) to highly promiscuous ("multitargeted"), and the relative merits of inhibiting one versus many kinases are discussed further in Chapter 7. To date, all therapeutic antibodies are monoclonal and recognize a single epitope on a single target. Since these proteins are not cell permeable, their utility with regard to kinases is restricted to cell surface receptors or the ligands thereof. Some of the more prominent examples are the anti-HER2 (ERBB2) antibody trastuzumab (Herceptin®), the anti-EGFR antibody cetuximab (Erbitux®), and the anti-VEGF antibody bevacizumab (Avastin®). A comparison of various attributes of small molecule inhibitors and antibodies is presented in Table 1.5 and is further discussed in (260).

1.5.2   Alternative Strategies for Kinase Inhibition

Our focus in this book is primarily on small molecule inhibitors of protein kinase domains, discussed in Chapters 7–10. However, several alternative approaches may be used for inhibiting kinase function in cells, some of which being evaluated clinically and others that are useful research tools for dissecting the roles of various kinases in both normal and pathogenic cellular function.

Targeting Domains Other than the Kinase Domain   Many protein kinases contain functional modules apart from the kinase domain that are critical for normal cellular function. In some cases, small molecule drugs may be developed to inhibit the function of these domains, thereby blocking cellular kinase activity without

TABLE 1.5 Comparison of Antibody and Small Molecule Kinase Inhibitors

	Kinase inhibitors	Antibodies
Mechanism		
Site of action	Kinase domain	Ligand binding domain
Number of targets/specificity	Selective or multitargeted	Selective
Kinases amenable to approach	All	Cell surface receptors only
Molecular mechanism	Inhibits catalytic activity	Inhibits ligand binding and/or receptor activation
May promote antibody-dependent cell-mediated cytotoxicity	No	Yes
Can conjugate to radioligand or toxin	No	Yes
Effect of kinase domain mutations	May sensitize or impart resistance	No direct effect; may be indirect effects?
Effect of ligand binding domain mutations	None	May inhibit binding
Pharmacokinetics		
Mode of delivery	Oral/parenteral	Parenteral
Half-life	Usually short (hours)	Long (days/weeks)
Enterohepatic recirculation	Yes	No
Tumor penetration	High	Low
Cross blood–brain barrier?	Yes or no	No
Drug–drug interaction potential	High	Low
Interpatient variability in exposure	High	Low
Cost of manufacture and dosing	Low	High

directly interfering with the kinase active site. Two notable examples are the discovery of AKT (protein kinase B) inhibitors that are dependent on the pleckstrin homology (PH) domain of this kinase, and inhibitors of SH2 domains.

PH Domain Antagonists The AKT kinases (AKT1, AKT2, and AKT3) fulfill a central role in signaling downstream of PI3K and modulate myriad functions including cellular growth, survival, and glycolytic metabolism (Chapter 5). The major functional regions of the AKT protein are an N-terminal PH domain and a C-terminal kinase domain. The PH domain is important for recruitment to the plasma membrane via interaction with phosphoinositides, and phosphorylation sites within and adjacent to the kinase domain provide an additional layer of regulation. A number of small molecules have been reported to inhibit AKT function in a PH domain-dependent manner (261, 262). A bisphenyl quinoxaline lead compound derived from high-throughput screening, subsequently referred to as

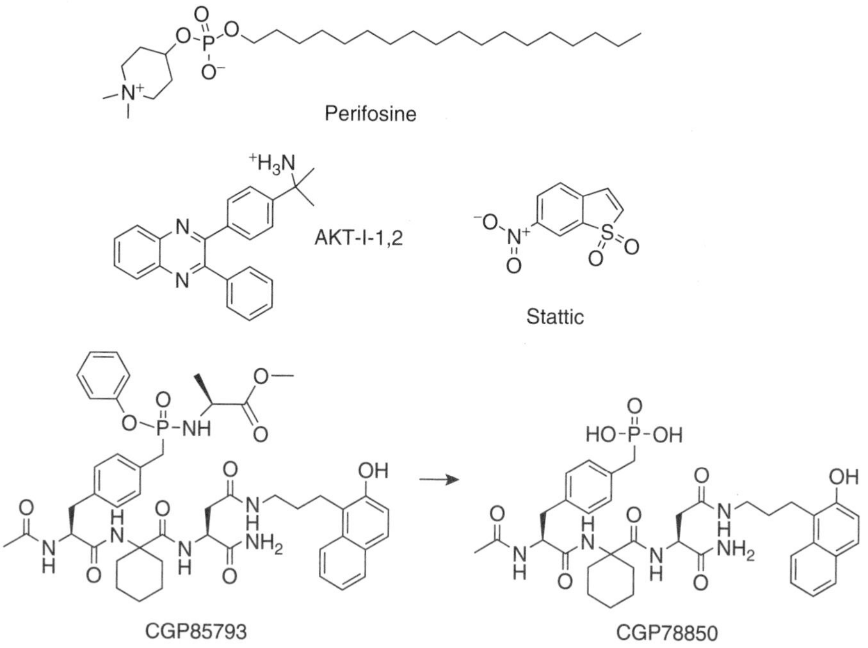

Figure 1.21 Selected small molecule kinase inhibitors that bind to regions other than the kinase catalytic domain.

Akt-I-1,2 (Figure 1.21), was found to specifically inhibit AKT1 (IC_{50} = 2.7 μM), with weaker activity toward AKT2 and no activity toward AKT3 or related AGC family kinases. Enzymological characterization showed that inhibition was not competitive with either ATP or substrate, and an AKT1 protein lacking the PH domain was insensitive to Akt-I-1,2 but retained sensitivity to the ATP-competitive inhibitor staurosporine. Moreover, antibodies to the PH domain and the "hinge" region between the PH and kinase domains also blocked inhibitor activity (262). In cellular assays, treatment with Akt-I-1,2 inhibited AKT phosphorylation and modulated downstream pathways. Optimization of these initial lead compounds resulted in potent dual inhibitors of AKT1 and AKT2, with one example molecule having in vitro IC_{50} values of 3.5 nM and 42 nM for AKT1 and AKT2, respectively, and antitumor activity in an A2780 xenograft model (263). Related AKT inhibitors were also shown to sensitize tumor cells to apoptotic stimuli such as chemotherapy (camptothecin, doxorubicin), γ-radiation, and biological agents including the anti-ERBB2 antibody trastuzumab and the tumor necrosis factor apoptosis-inducing ligand TRAIL (264). The high specificity of this class of inhibitors makes them particularly useful tools for probing the role of AKT in tumor cell biology: for example, breast cancers with PI3K mutation or HER2 amplification were recently shown to be highly dependent on AKT signaling and susceptible to treatment with Akt-I-1,2 in xenograft models (265). No clinical development has been reported for these inhibitors, although recent medicinal chemistry has produced analogs with improved pharmacokinetics and other pharmaceutical properties (266–269).

Perifosine (Figure 1.21) is an alkylphospholipid that has also been described as an AKT inhibitor, although its effects on cellular signaling are likely to involve a broader range of mechanisms such as induction of the DR4 and DR5 "death" receptors (270). Treatment of cells with perifosine results in dose-dependent inhibition of AKT phosphorylation, correlating with loss of AKT membrane localization. A myristoylated form of AKT (which does not depend on the PH domain for membrane localization) was found to be resistant to the effects of perifosine, suggesting that the synthetic phospholipid abrogates the interaction of the AKT PH domain with the plasma membrane (271). Preclinical data show that perifosine has antitumor activity in multiple cell lines, including multiple myeloma, non small cell lung cancer, and prostate carcinoma (272–274). Perifosine was originally developed by AEterna Zentaris and licensed to Access Oncology/Keryx Biopharmaceuticals for development in the United States, Canada, and Mexico. Multiple Phase I studies have been conducted and Phase II trials are currently ongoing in several indications, both as single agent therapy and in combination with other chemotherapy agents.

SH2 Domain Antagonists SH2 (SRC homology region 2) domains are ubiquitous and important signaling modules of ~100 amino acids that bind to specific peptide sequences with phosphorylated tyrosine residues. Specificity is determined by the sequence immediately C-terminal to the phosphotyrosine. SH2 domains couple receptor tyrosine kinases to various intracellular signaling pathways and are also found as components of a number of kinases (notably SRC, from which they derive their name), where they regulate enzyme activation, subcellular localization, and coupling to other signaling components. Targeting specific phosphopeptide:SH2 interactions has been proposed as a strategy for inhibiting oncogenic signaling and may, for example, allow specific downregulation of one signaling cascade downstream of RTKs without significantly impacting others (275). Although a number of peptidic and nonpeptidic small molecule SH2 inhibitors have been reported, none have yet progressed to clinical testing. This may reflect the difficulty in producing specific, high affinity inhibitors that mimic the negatively charged phosphotyrosine moiety: such molecules typically have poor physicochemical and pharmacological properties. Nevertheless, the identification of SH2 domain inhibitors has potential utility in dissecting the effects of specifically downregulating SH2-mediated signaling, and several such molecules have been shown to have cellular activity. As an example, we consider some inhibitors of the GRB2 and STAT3 SH2 domains.

GRB2 is an adaptor molecule comprising two SH3 domains that flank a single SH2 domain. GRB2 is particularly important for relaying mitogenic signals from RTKs to the RAS/RAF/MEK/ERK signaling cascade. The consensus sequence for binding to the GRB2 SH2 domain is pY-X-N-X, with an asparagine residue at the pY+2 position being a key determinant of specificity (276). Discovery of small molecules that compete with phosphopeptide binding has largely been based on a peptidomimetic, structure-based design strategy, and many crystallographic and NMR structures are available for both apo and ligand bound forms of GRB2 (277, 278). Optimization of a pY-I-N tripeptide sequence by modification of the N terminus and isoleucine yielded several inhibitors with nanomolar binding affinities (279, 280). Further analogs were derived with cellular activity: in particular, CGP78850 and a prodrug version of this compound that masks the phosphate charge (CGP85793; Figure 1.21) blocked HGF and EGF receptor-mediated effects on signal transduction, cytoskeletal rearrangement, cell motility, and anchorage-independent growth (281–283).

A small molecule inhibitor of the STAT3 SH2 domain, named Stattic (Figure 1.21), has also been reported (284). STAT3 is an important mediator of cytokine/JAK kinase signaling (Chapter 4) and is implicated in tumor growth and survival. Stattic is a nonpeptidic small molecule identified by screening a chemical library for competitive binding to STAT3 using a fluorescently labeled phosphopeptide. Binding was found to be temperature dependent (with an IC_{50} of 5 μM at 37°C but weaker affinity at lower temperatures) and time dependent, pointing to an irreversible mode of inhibition. Selective inhibition of STAT3 phosphorylation and induction of apoptosis was demonstrated in cells; although this activity is unlikely to be sufficiently potent for pharmacological development, it may be a useful tool for dissecting STAT3 SH2-dependent signaling.

Indirect Kinase Inhibitors: Receptor Ligand Modulators   An alternative approach for inhibition of receptor tyrosine kinase function is to block the activity of the receptor ligands rather than the receptors themselves. This is a clinically validated strategy: the anti-VEGF antibody bevacizumab (Avastin®) has been shown to modulate VEGF receptor function in numerous preclinical studies and was the first FDA approved therapy designed to inhibit angiogenesis. Proof of principle was initially provided by a monoclonal antibody that specifically binds to VEGFA, which was subsequently developed into a clinical formulation (285). Bevacizumab is approved by the FDA for the first and second line treatment of patients with metastatic colorectal cancer in combination with intravenous 5-FU, for first line treatment of patients with unresectable, locally advanced, recurrent or metastatic nonsquamous, non small cell lung cancer in combination with carboplatin and paclitaxel, and for treatment of metastatic HER2-negative breast cancer in combination with paclitaxel. A second example of targeting ligand rather than receptor function is inhibition of sheddases—proteases that catalyze the release of ligands from cells and trigger RTK signaling. The ADAM family of sheddases (particularly ADAM10 and ADAM17) plays a key role in the release of ERBB receptor ligands from cells, discussed further in Chapter 3. These processed ligands may then act in an autocrine or paracrine fashion to activate ERBB receptors on tumor cells. Several ADAM protease inhibitors have been described, including INCB3619 and INCB7839, two small molecule inhibitors of ADAM10, ADAM17, and several other metalloproteinases (286). These molecules were found to inhibit the shedding of the EGFR ligand amphiregulin in breast cancer cells and augmented the growth inhibitory properties of the EGFR/ERBB2 inhibitor lapatinib both in vitro and in vivo. However, this activity may not be dependent exclusively on inhibition of amphiregulin secretion, since ADAM metalloproteinases are also implicated in shedding of the ERBB2 extracellular domain, resulting in a constitutively activated receptor.

Indirect Kinase Inhibitors: HSP90 Inhibitors   HSP90 is a key component of a molecular chaperone complex that promotes the conformational maturation and stabilization of diverse cellular proteins (287). Chaperones are particularly important in maintaining correct protein folding under conditions of stress, including hypoxia, acidosis, and nutrient deprivation. These conditions are frequently present in tumors, so it is perhaps not surprising that HSP90 and other chaperones are often overexpressed in cancer cells (288). Moreover, HSP90 extracted from tumor cells appears to exist in a hyperactivated state with elevated ATPase activity, which is highly sensitive to HSP90 inhibition compared to the largely latent form found in normal cells (289). The chaperone substrates, or "client" proteins of HSP90, include many of the kinases discussed in Chapters 3–6 that are implicated in tumor initiation, survival, and invasion. (An updated list of HSP90 clients, including proteins other than kinases, is maintained at http://www.picard.ch/downloads/downloads.htm.) Furthermore, mutant oncogenic proteins may be particularly dependent on the molecular chaperone machinery for correct folding and stabilization. For example, although wild-type BRAF kinase is an HSP90 client, the BRAF V600E activating mutant is critically dependent on HSP90 for stability and function and shows increased sensitivity to the HSP90 inhibitor 17-AAG (290, 291). Therefore HSP90 acts as a biochemical buffer in tumor cells, maintaining homeostasis in the face of environmental stress, genomic derangement, and aberrant activation of intracellular signaling. Inhibition of HSP90 may therefore act as a multitargeted kinase inhibitor, with the added benefit of being somewhat specific for the overexpressed, hyperactivated form of HSP90 in tumor cells. There has been much recent interest in the development of HSP90 inhibitors as cancer therapeutics, and therapeutic validation of HSP90 as an anticancer drug target has been provided by ATP-competitive inhibitors of HSP90 (292–296). The geldanamycin derivative 17-AAG (17-allylamino-17-desmethoxy-geldanamycin) was the first molecule to undergo clinical testing, and several different formulations have been developed in an attempt to overcome the poor physicochemical properties of this molecule. Modest activity has been reported as a single agent in melanoma; more robust activity was found in combination with the proteasome inhibitor bortezomib in multiple myeloma, where 9/19 patients with relapsed or refractory multiple myeloma achieved a minor, partial, or complete response to therapy (297). Encouraging activity was also reported in a Phase II study of HER2-positive breast cancer patients who had progressed on trastuzumab therapy. Twenty-five patients were treated with both tanespimycin (a formulation of 17-AAG developed by Kosan Biosciences, now part of Bristol Myers Squibb) and trastuzumab. One partial response, four minor responses, and four cases of disease stabilization were achieved (298). Another more soluble derivative of geldanamycin, IPI-504 (retaspimycin; Infinity Pharmaceuticals), has shown some encouraging activity in treatment of kinase inhibitor-resistant gastrointestinal stromal tumors, with 78% of patients achieving disease stabilization (299). Several second generation non-ansamycin inhibitors are also being evaluated in the clinic.

Antisense and Related Approaches to Kinase Inhibition Several other approaches to kinase inhibition have been pursued in both the laboratory and the clinic, most notably antisense inhibitors. Antisense oligonucleotides (ASOs) are short (~20 base pairs) nucleic acid molecules that are complementary to the RNA of a target gene and inhibit its expression. Multiple mechanisms of inhibition have been proposed, including direct blockade of DNA transcription, direct blockade of RNA translation, inhibition of RNA splicing and maturation, interference with ribosome activity, and targeting RNA for degradation by RNAse H (300). In theory, antisense drugs are able to target any cellular protein whose RNA includes a region that is accessible for complexation with an ASO and offers the requisite specificity relative to homologous genes. However, a number of practical challenges have limited the development of antisense therapies, in particular, the generation of nucleic acid-derived polymers that are sufficiently stable, tolerable, and bioavailable to be used as drugs.

Several kinases have been targeted in clinical studies using antisense technology, including CRAF and PKCα. The potential utility of CRAF antisense for treating tumors was demonstrated as early as 1989 (301), but such molecules have only been evaluated in humans relatively recently. CGP-69846A (ISIS 5132; Isis Pharmaceuticals) is an ASO targeting the 5′ untranslated region of the CRAF gene. In preclinical studies, CGP-69846A demonstrated antitumor activity following daily intravenous administration to mice bearing xenograft tumors, both as a single agent and in combination with various chemotherapy treatments (302, 303). In a Phase I clinical study employing a 2-hour infusion three times weekly, the drug was rapidly cleared with a half-life of ~60 minutes, although some suppression of CRAF expression was noted in peripheral blood cells (304). Continuous dosing was also evaluated and was well tolerated with some signs of clinical activity, but no target suppression or activity was seen following a weekly 24-hour infusion regimen (305, 306). Several Phase II studies were initiated in prostate, lung, colorectal, and ovarian cancers, but the lack of clear response in these studies precluded further development (307–310). LERafAON (Neopharm Inc.) is a liposome-encapsulated preparation of CRAF antisense that is suitable for intravenous administration (311). In preclinical studies, multiple daily injections of this formulation were relatively well tolerated in mice, rabbits, and monkeys. CRAF expression was inhibited in xenograft tumors and surrogate tissues, and antitumor activity was demonstrated in combination with radiation and multiple chemotherapy drugs (311–313). However, clinical testing produced infusion-related hypersensitivity reactions across all dose groups, suggesting that the liposomal carrier may be poorly tolerated in humans and that reformulation was necessary (314, 315).

Another ASO from Isis Pharmaceuticals was directed at the 5′ untranslated region of the gene encoding PKCα. ISIS 3521 (aprinocarsen; LY-900003) demonstrated preclinical activity as a single agent and in combination with chemotherapy in mouse xenograft models (316, 317). Phase I studies were conducted using a 2-hour infusion three times weekly, or a continuous 21-day infusion. As with the CRAF antisense inhibitor, these studies demonstrated a short half-life; however, significant activity was seen in patients with non Hodgkin's lymphoma and ovarian cancer (318, 319). The activity in ovarian cancer was recapitulated in a Phase II study (320), and additional trials were undertaken in various other tumor types and in combination with chemotherapy. However, no recent development activity has been reported for this drug.

Two additional related approaches are worth mentioning. The advent of RNA silencing technology (siRNA) has provided a powerful tool for inhibiting gene expression in model systems and may serve as a platform for a new generation of expression-modulating drugs. This relatively new technology is now in clinical testing, with the most advanced compound, Bevasarinib (an siRNA targeting *VEGFA* in development by Acuity Pharmaceuticals), in Phase III trials for age-related macular degeneration. Early stage compounds are in evaluation for a variety of indications including various cancers.

An alternative to the antisense/siRNA approach is to discover small molecules that interfere with post-transcriptional processing of a given target gene. PTC299 (PTC Therapeutics) is an orally bioavailable small molecule that is reported to selectively inhibit tumor VEGF production. A Phase I study in healthy volunteers demonstrated that the drug could safely be administered at plasma exposures associated with preclinical activity (321).

REFERENCES

1. Harden A, Young W. The alcoholic ferment of yeast-juice. Proc R Soc Lond Ser B 1905;77:405–420.
2. Gribble FM, Loussouarn G, Tucker SJ, Zhao C, Nichols CG, Ashcroft FM. A novel method for measurement of submembrane ATP concentration. J Biol Chem 2000;275(39):30046–30049.
3. Traut TW. Physiological concentrations of purines and pyrimidines. Mol Cell Biochem 1994;140(1):1–22.
4. Davidson JN, Frazer SC, Hutchison WC. Phosphorus compounds in the cell. I. Protein-bound phosphorus fractions studied with the aid of radioactive phosphorus. Biochem J 1951;49(3):311–321.
5. Johnson RM, Albert S. Incorporation of P32 into the phosphoprotein fraction of mammalian tissue. J Biol Chem 1953;200(1):335–344.
6. Kennedy EP, Smith SW. The isolation of radioactive phosphoserine from phosphoprotein of the Ehrlich ascites tumor. J Biol Chem 1954;207(1):153–163.
7. Burnett G, Kennedy EP. The enzymatic phosphorylation of proteins. J Biol Chem 1954;211(2):969–980.
8. Fischer EH, Graves DJ, Crittenden ER, Krebs EG. Structure of the site phosphorylated in the phosphorylase *b* to *a* reaction. J Biol Chem 1959;234(7):1698–1704.
9. Fischer EH, Krebs EG. Conversion of phosphorylase *b* to phosphorylase *a* in muscle extracts. J Biol Chem 1955;216(1):121–132.
10. Fischer EH. Protein Phosphorylation and Cellular Regulation, II. Ringertz N, editor. Singapore: World Scientific Publishing Co.; 1997.
11. Krebs EG. Protein Phosphorylation and Cellular Regulation, I. Ringertz N, editor. Singapore: World Scientific Publishing Co.; 1997.
12. Walsh DA, Perkins JP, Krebs EG. An adenosine 3′,5′-monophosphate-dependant protein kinase from rabbit skeletal muscle. J Biol Chem 1968;243(13):3763–3765.
13. Daile P, Carnegie PR, Young JD. Synthetic substrate for cyclic AMP-dependent protein kinase. Nature 1975;257(5525):416–418.
14. Kemp BE, Bylund DB, Huang TS, Krebs EG. Substrate specificity of the cyclic AMP-dependent protein kinase. Proc Natl Acad Sci U S A 1975;72(9):3448–3452.

15. Kemp BE, Graves DJ, Benjamini E, Krebs EG. Role of multiple basic residues in determining the substrate specificity of cyclic AMP-dependent protein kinase. J Biol Chem 1977;252(14):4888–4894.

16. Zetterqvist O, Ragnarsson U, Humble E, Berglund L, Engstrom L. The minimum substrate of cyclic AMP-stimulated protein kinase, as studied by synthetic peptides representing the phosphorylatable site of pyruvate kinase (type L) of rat liver. Biochem Biophys Res Commun 1976;70(3):696–703.

17. Shoji S, Parmelee DC, Wade RD, Kumar S, Ericsson LH, Walsh KA, Neurath H, Long GL, Demaille JG, Fischer EH, Titani K. Complete amino acid sequence of the catalytic subunit of bovine cardiac muscle cyclic AMP-dependent protein kinase. Proc Natl Acad Sci U S A 1981;78(2):848–851.

18. Knighton DR, Zheng JH, Ten Eyck LF, Xuong NH, Taylor SS, Sowadski JM. Structure of a peptide inhibitor bound to the catalytic subunit of cyclic adenosine monophosphate-dependent protein kinase. Science 1991;253(5018):414–420.

19. Brugge JS, Erikson RL. Identification of a transformation-specific antigen induced by an avian sarcoma virus. Nature 1977;269(5626):346–348.

20. Collett MS, Erikson RL. Protein kinase activity associated with the avian sarcoma virus src gene product. Proc Natl Acad Sci U S A 1978;75(4):2021–2024.

21. Levinson AD, Oppermann H, Levintow L, Varmus HE, Bishop JM. Evidence that the transforming gene of avian sarcoma virus encodes a protein kinase associated with a phosphoprotein. Cell 1978;15(2):561–572.

22. Hunter T, Sefton BM. Transforming gene product of Rous sarcoma virus phosphorylates tyrosine. Proc Natl Acad Sci U S A 1980;77(3):1311–1315.

23. Sefton BM, Hunter T, Beemon K, Eckhart W. Evidence that the phosphorylation of tyrosine is essential for cellular transformation by Rous sarcoma virus. Cell 1980;20(3):807–816.

24. Ushiro H, Cohen S. Identification of phosphotyrosine as a product of epidermal growth factor-activated protein kinase in A-431 cell membranes. J Biol Chem 1980;255(18):8363–8365.

25. Thomason P, Kay R. Eukaryotic signal transduction via histidine–aspartate phosphorelay. J Cell Sci 2000;113(Pt 18):3141–3150.

26. Hanks SK, Hunter T. Protein kinases 6. The eukaryotic protein kinase superfamily: kinase (catalytic) domain structure and classification. FASEB J 1995;9(8):576–596.

27. Hanks SK, Quinn AM, Hunter T. The protein kinase family: conserved features and deduced phylogeny of the catalytic domains. Science 1988;241(4861):42–52.

28. Cancer Facts and Figures 2008. Altanta: American Cancer Society; 2008.

29. Rowley JD. Letter: A new consistent chromosomal abnormality in chronic myelogenous leukaemia identified by quinacrine fluorescence and Giemsa staining. Nature 1973;243(5405):290–293.

30. Knudson AG. Two genetic hits (more or less) to cancer. Nat Rev Cancer 2001;1(2):157–162.

31. Loeb LA. Mutator phenotype may be required for multistage carcinogenesis. Cancer Res 1991;51(12):3075–3079.

32. Hanahan D, Weinberg RA. The hallmarks of cancer. Cell 2000;100(1):57–70.

33. Warburg O. On the origin of cancer cells. Science 1956;123(3191):309–314.

34. Gatenby RA, Gillies RJ. Why do cancers have high aerobic glycolysis? Nat Rev Cancer 2004;4(11):891–899.

35. Elstrom RL, Bauer DE, Buzzai M, Karnauskas R, Harris MH, Plas DR, Zhuang H, Cinalli RM, Alavi A, Rudin CM, Thompson CB. Akt stimulates aerobic glycolysis in cancer cells. Cancer Res 2004;64(11):3892–3899.

36. DeBerardinis RJ, Lum JJ, Hatzivassiliou G, Thompson CB. The biology of cancer: metabolic reprogramming fuels cell growth and proliferation. Cell Metab 2008;7(1):11–20.

37. Manning G, Whyte DB, Martinez R, Hunter T, Sudarsanam S. The protein kinase complement of the human genome. Science 2002;298(5600):1912–1934.

38. Boudeau J, Miranda-Saavedra D, Barton GJ, Alessi DR. Emerging roles of pseudokinases. Trends Cell Biol 2006;16(9):443–452.

39. Baas AF, Boudeau J, Sapkota GP, Smit L, Medema R, Morrice NA, Alessi DR, Clevers HC. Activation of the tumour suppressor kinase LKB1 by the STE20-like pseudokinase STRAD. EMBO J 2003;22(12):3062–3072.

40. Lenertz LY, Lee BH, Min X, Xu BE, Wedin K, Earnest S, Goldsmith EJ, Cobb MH. Properties of WNK1 and implications for other family members. J Biol Chem 2005;280(29):26653–26658.

41. Min X, Lee BH, Cobb MH, Goldsmith EJ. Crystal structure of the kinase domain of WNK1, a kinase that causes a hereditary form of hypertension. Structure 2004;12(7):1303–1311.

42. Robinson DR, Wu YM, Lin SF. The protein tyrosine kinase family of the human genome. Oncogene 2000;19(49):5548–5557.

43. Maglott D, Ostell J, Pruitt KD, Tatusova T. Entrez Gene: gene-centered information at NCBI. Nucleic Acids Res 2005;33(Database issue): D54–58.

44. Bruford EA, Lush MJ, Wright MW, Sneddon TP, Povey S, Birney E. The HGNC Database in 2008: a resource for the human genome. Nucleic Acids Res 2008;36(Database issue): D445–448.

45. Edgar RC. MUSCLE: a multiple sequence alignment method with reduced time and space complexity. BMC Bioinformatics 2004;5: 113.

46. Edgar RC. MUSCLE: multiple sequence alignment with high accuracy and high throughput. Nucleic Acids Res 2004;32(5):1792–1797.

47. Zmasek CM, Eddy SR. ATV: display and manipulation of annotated phylogenetic trees. Bioinformatics 2001;17(4):383–384.

48. Downward J, Yarden Y, Mayes E, Scrace G, Totty N, Stockwell P, Ullrich A, Schlessinger J, Waterfield MD. Close similarity of epidermal growth factor receptor and v-erb-B oncogene protein sequences. Nature 1984;307(5951):521–527.

49. Folkman J. Tumor angiogenesis: therapeutic implications. N Engl J Med 1971;285(21): 1182–1186.

50. Martin-Zanca D, Hughes SH, Barbacid M. A human oncogene formed by the fusion of truncated tropomyosin and protein tyrosine kinase sequences. Nature 1986;319(6056):743–748.

51. Klein R, Jing SQ, Nanduri V, O'Rourke E, Barbacid M. The trk proto-oncogene encodes a receptor for nerve growth factor. Cell 1991;65(1):189–197.

52. Tacconelli A, Farina AR, Cappabianca L, Desantis G, Tessitore A, Vetuschi A, Sferra R, Rucci N, Argenti B, Screpanti I, Gulino A, Mackay AR. TrkA alternative splicing: a regulated tumor-promoting switch in human neuroblastoma. Cancer Cell 2004;6(4):347–360.

53. Djakiew D, Delsite R, Pflug B, Wrathall J, Lynch JH, Onoda M. Regulation of growth by a nerve growth factor-like protein which modulates paracrine interactions between a neoplastic epithelial cell line and stromal cells of the human prostate. Cancer Res 1991;51(12):3304–3310.

54. Dolle L, Adriaenssens E, El Yazidi-Belkoura I, Le Bourhis X, Nurcombe V, Hondermarck H. Nerve growth factor receptors and signaling in breast cancer. Curr Cancer Drug Targets 2004;4(6):463–470.

55. Nakagawara A, Azar CG, Scavarda NJ, Brodeur GM. Expression and function of TRK-B and BDNF in human neuroblastomas. Mol Cell Biol 1994;14(1):759–767.

56. Geiger TR, Peeper DS. The neurotrophic receptor TrkB in anoikis resistance and metastasis: a perspective. Cancer Res 2005;65(16):7033–7036.

57. Pierotti MA, Greco A. Oncogenic rearrangements of the NTRK1/NGF receptor. Cancer Lett 2006;232(1):90–98.

58. Lannon CL, Sorensen PH. ETV6-NTRK3: a chimeric protein tyrosine kinase with transformation activity in multiple cell lineages. Semin Cancer Biol 2005;15(3):215–223.

59. Hirai H, Maru Y, Hagiwara K, Nishida J, Takaku F. A novel putative tyrosine kinase receptor encoded by the eph gene. Science 1987;238(4834):1717–1720.

60. Heroult M, Schaffner F, Augustin HG. Eph receptor and ephrin ligand-mediated interactions during angiogenesis and tumor progression. Exp Cell Res 2006;312(5):642–650.

61. Wang HU, Chen ZF, Anderson DJ. Molecular distinction and angiogenic interaction between embryonic arteries and veins revealed by ephrin-B2 and its receptor Eph-B4. Cell 1998;93(5):741–753.

62. Adams RH, Wilkinson GA, Weiss C, Diella F, Gale NW, Deutsch U, Risau W, Klein R. Roles of ephrinB ligands and EphB receptors in cardiovascular development: demarcation of arterial/venous domains, vascular morphogenesis, and sprouting angiogenesis. Genes Dev 1999;13(3):295–306.

63. Gerety SS, Wang HU, Chen ZF, Anderson DJ. Symmetrical mutant phenotypes of the receptor EphB4 and its specific transmembrane ligand ephrin-B2 in cardiovascular development. Mol Cell 1999;4(3):403–414.

64. Surawska H, Ma PC, Salgia R. The role of ephrins and Eph receptors in cancer. Cytokine Growth Factor Rev 2004;15(6):419–433.
65. Walker-Daniels J, Hess AR, Hendrix MJ, Kinch MS. Differential regulation of EphA2 in normal and malignant cells. Am J Pathol 2003;162(4):1037–1042.
66. Zelinski DP, Zantek ND, Stewart JC, Irizarry AR, Kinch MS. EphA2 overexpression causes tumorigenesis of mammary epithelial cells. Cancer Res 2001;61(5):2301–2306.
67. Ogawa K, Pasqualini R, Lindberg RA, Kain R, Freeman AL, Pasquale EB. The ephrin-A1 ligand and its receptor, EphA2, are expressed during tumor neovascularization. Oncogene 2000;19(52):6043–6052.
68. Noren NK, Pasquale EB. Paradoxes of the EphB4 receptor in cancer. Cancer Res 2007;67(9):3994–3997.
69. Sato T, Qin Y, Kozak C, Audus K. Tie-1 and Tie-2 define another class of putative receptor tyrosine kinase genes expressed in early embryonic vascular system. Proc Natl Acad Sci U S A 1993;90:9355–9358.
70. Sato TN, Tozawa Y, Deutsch U, Wolburg-Buchholz K, Fujiwara Y, Gendron-Maguire M, Gridley T, Wolburg H, Risau W, Qin Y. Distinct roles of the receptor tyrosine kinases Tie-1 and Tie-2 in blood vessel formation. Nature 1995;376(6535):70–74.
71. Davis S, Aldrich TH, Jones PF, Acheson A, Compton DL, Jain V, Ryan TE, Bruno J, Radziejewski C, Maisonpierre PC, Yancopoulos GD. Isolation of angiopoietin-1, a ligand for the TIE2 receptor, by secretion-trap expression cloning. Cell 1996;87(7):1161–1169.
72. Maisonpierre PC, Suri C, Jones PF, Bartunkova S, Wiegand SJ, Radziejewski C, Compton D, McClain J, Aldrich TH, Papadopoulos N, Daly TJ, Davis S, Sato TN, Yancopoulos GD. Angiopoietin-2, a natural antagonist for Tie2 that disrupts in vivo angiogenesis. Science 1997;277(5322):55–60.
73. Makinde T, Agrawal DK. Intra and extravascular transmembrane signalling of angiopoietin-1-Tie2 receptor in health and disease. J Cell Mol Med 2008;12(3):810–828.
74. Bolen JB, Veillette A, Schwartz AM, DeSeau V, Rosen N. Activation of pp60c-src protein kinase activity in human colon carcinoma. Proc Natl Acad Sci U S A 1987;84(8):2251–2255.
75. Frame MC. Src in cancer: deregulation and consequences for cell behaviour. Biochim Biophys Acta 2002;1602(2):114–130.
76. Barker KT, Jackson LE, Crompton MR. BRK tyrosine kinase expression in a high proportion of human breast carcinomas. Oncogene 1997;15(7):799–805.
77. Mitchell PJ, Barker KT, Martindale JE, Kamalati T, Lowe PN, Page MJ, Gusterson BA, Crompton MR. Cloning and characterisation of cDNAs encoding a novel non-receptor tyrosine kinase, brk, expressed in human breast tumours. Oncogene 1994;9(8):2383–2390.
78. Kamalati T, Jolin HE, Mitchell PJ, Barker KT, Jackson LE, Dean CJ, Page MJ, Gusterson BA, Crompton MR. Brk, a breast tumor-derived non-receptor protein-tyrosine kinase, sensitizes mammary epithelial cells to epidermal growth factor. J Biol Chem 1996;271(48):30956–30963.
79. Xiang B, Chatti K, Qiu H, Lakshmi B, Krasnitz A, Hicks J, Yu M, Miller WT, Muthuswamy SK. Brk is coamplified with ErbB2 to promote proliferation in breast cancer. Proc Natl Acad Sci U S A 2008;105(34):12463–12468.
80. Chen HY, Shen CH, Tsai YT, Lin FC, Huang YP, Chen RH. Brk activates rac1 and promotes cell migration and invasion by phosphorylating paxillin. Mol Cell Biol 2004;24(24):10558–10572.
81. Shen CH, Chen HY, Lin MS, Li FY, Chang CC, Kuo ML, Settleman J, Chen RH. Breast tumor kinase phosphorylates p190RhoGAP to regulate rho and ras and promote breast carcinoma growth, migration, and invasion. Cancer Res 2008;68(19):7779–7787.
82. Hannigan G, Troussard AA, Dedhar S. Integrin-linked kinase: a cancer therapeutic target unique among its ILK. Nat Rev Cancer 2005;5(1):51–63.
83. Legate KR, Montanez E, Kudlacek O, Fassler R. ILK, PINCH and parvin: the tIPP of integrin signalling. Nat Rev Mol Cell Biol 2006;7(1):20–31.
84. Massague J. TGFbeta in Cancer. Cell 2008;134(2):215–230.
85. Thuault S, Valcourt U, Petersen M, Manfioletti G, Heldin CH, Moustakas A. Transforming growth factor-beta employs HMGA2 to elicit epithelial–mesenchymal transition. J Cell Biol 2006;174(2):175–183.

86. Kingsley LA, Fournier PG, Chirgwin JM, Guise TA. Molecular biology of bone metastasis. Mol Cancer Ther 2007;6(10):2609–2617.

87. Karin M, Greten FR. NF-kappaB: linking inflammation and immunity to cancer development and progression. Nat Rev Immunol 2005;5(10):749–759.

88. Yamaguchi K, Shirakabe K, Shibuya H, Irie K, Oishi I, Ueno N, Taniguchi T, Nishida E, Matsumoto K. Identification of a member of the MAPKKK family as a potential mediator of TGF-beta signal transduction. Science 1995;270(5244):2008–2011.

89. Bailey JM, Singh PK, Hollingsworth MA. Cancer metastasis facilitated by developmental pathways: Sonic hedgehog, Notch, and bone morphogenic proteins. J Cell Biochem 2007;102(4):829–839.

90. Johnson GL, Lapadat R. Mitogen-activated protein kinase pathways mediated by ERK, JNK, and p38 protein kinases. Science 2002;298(5600):1911–1912.

91. Kumar R, Gururaj AE, Barnes CJ. p21-activated kinases in cancer. Nat Rev Cancer 2006;6(6):459–471.

92. Balasenthil S, Sahin AA, Barnes CJ, Wang RA, Pestell RG, Vadlamudi RK, Kumar R. p21-activated kinase-1 signaling mediates cyclin D1 expression in mammary epithelial and cancer cells. J Biol Chem 2004;279(2):1422–1428.

93. Holm C, Rayala S, Jirstrom K, Stal O, Kumar R, Landberg G. Association between Pak1 expression and subcellular localization and tamoxifen resistance in breast cancer patients. J Natl Cancer Inst 2006;98(10):671–680.

94. Kissil JL, Wilker EW, Johnson KC, Eckman MS, Yaffe MB, Jacks T. Merlin, the product of the Nf2 tumor suppressor gene, is an inhibitor of the p21-activated kinase, Pak1. Mol Cell 2003;12(4):841–849.

95. Knippschild U, Gocht A, Wolff S, Huber N, Lohler J, Stoter M. The casein kinase 1 family: participation in multiple cellular processes in eukaryotes. Cell Signal 2005;17(6):675–689.

96. Kloss B, Price JL, Saez L, Blau J, Rothenfluh A, Wesley CS, Young MW. The *Drosophila* clock gene double-time encodes a protein closely related to human casein kinase I epsilon. Cell 1998;94(1):97–107.

97. Price JL, Blau J, Rothenfluh A, Abodeely M, Kloss B, Young MW. Double-time is a novel *Drosophila* clock gene that regulates PERIOD protein accumulation. Cell 1998;94(1):83–95.

98. Yang WS, Stockwell BR. Inhibition of casein kinase 1-epsilon induces cancer-cell-selective, PERIOD2-dependent growth arrest. Genome Biol 2008;9(6): R92.

99. Sakaguchi K, Saito S, Higashimoto Y, Roy S, Anderson CW, Appella E. Damage-mediated phosphorylation of human p53 threonine 18 through a cascade mediated by a casein 1-like kinase. Effect on Mdm2 binding. J Biol Chem 2000;275(13):9278–9283.

100. Dumaz N, Milne DM, Meek DW. Protein kinase CK1 is a p53-threonine 18 kinase which requires prior phosphorylation of serine 15. FEBS Lett 1999;463(3):312–316.

101. Alsheich-Bartok O, Haupt S, Alkalay-Snir I, Saito S, Appella E, Haupt Y. PML enhances the regulation of p53 by CK1 in response to DNA damage. Oncogene 2008;27(26):3653–3661.

102. Winter M, Milne D, Dias S, Kulikov R, Knippschild U, Blattner C, Meek D. Protein kinase CK1delta phosphorylates key sites in the acidic domain of murine double-minute clone 2 protein (MDM2) that regulate p53 turnover. Biochemistry 2004;43(51):16356–16364.

103. Izeradjene K, Douglas L, Delaney A, Houghton JA. Influence of casein kinase II in tumor necrosis factor-related apoptosis-inducing ligand-induced apoptosis in human rhabdomyosarcoma cells. Clin Cancer Res 2004;10(19):6650–6660.

104. Desagher S, Osen-Sand A, Montessuit S, Magnenat E, Vilbois F, Hochmann A, Journot L, Antonsson B, Martinou JC. Phosphorylation of bid by casein kinases I and II regulates its cleavage by caspase 8. Mol Cell 2001;8(3):601–611.

105. Price MA. CKI, there's more than one: casein kinase I family members in Wnt and Hedgehog signaling. Genes Dev 2006;20(4):399–410.

106. Mitsiades CS, Mitsiades N, Koutsilieris M. The Akt pathway: molecular targets for anti-cancer drug development. Curr Cancer Drug Targets 2004;4(3):235–256.

107. Metzger E, Muller JM, Ferrari S, Buettner R, Schule R. A novel inducible transactivation domain in the androgen receptor: implications for PRK in prostate cancer. EMBO J 2003;22(2):270–280.

108. Hudmon A, Schulman H. Structure-function of the multifunctional Ca^2+/calmodulin-dependent protein kinase II. Biochem J 2002;364(Pt 3):593–611.

109. Soderling TR. The Ca-calmodulin-dependent protein kinase cascade. Trends Biochem Sci 1999;24(6):232–236.

110. Schulman H, Greengard P. Stimulation of brain membrane protein phosphorylation by calcium and an endogenous heat-stable protein. Nature 1978;271(5644):478–479.

111. Griffith LC. Regulation of calcium/calmodulin-dependent protein kinase II activation by intramolecular and intermolecular interactions. J Neurosci 2004;24(39):8394–8398.

112. Griffith LC. Calcium/calmodulin-dependent protein kinase II: an unforgettable kinase. J Neurosci 2004;24(39):8391–8393.

113. Kohama K, Ye LH, Hayakawa K, Okagaki T. Myosin light chain kinase: an actin-binding protein that regulates an ATP-dependent interaction with myosin. Trends Pharmacol Sci 1996;17(8):284–287.

114. Racioppi L, Means AR. Calcium/calmodulin-dependent kinase IV in immune and inflammatory responses: novel routes for an ancient traveller. Trends Immunol 2008;29(12):600–607.

115. Anderson ME. Calmodulin kinase and L-type calcium channels; a recipe for arrhythmias? Trends Cardiovasc Med 2004;14(4):152–161.

116. Makowski L, Hayes DN. Role of LKB1 in lung cancer development. Br J Cancer 2008;99(5):683–688.

117. Lizcano JM, Goransson O, Toth R, Deak M, Morrice NA, Boudeau J, Hawley SA, Udd L, Makela TP, Hardie DG, Alessi DR. LKB1 is a master kinase that activates 13 kinases of the AMPK subfamily, including MARK/PAR-1. EMBO J 2004;23(4):833–843.

118. Espinosa L, Navarro E. Human serine/threonine protein kinase EMK1: genomic structure and cDNA cloning of isoforms produced by alternative splicing. Cytogenet Cell Genet 1998;81(3–4):278–282.

119. Trinczek B, Brajenovic M, Ebneth A, Drewes G. MARK4 is a novel microtubule-associated proteins/microtubule affinity-regulating kinase that binds to the cellular microtubule network and to centrosomes. J Biol Chem 2004;279(7):5915–5923.

120. Valverde AM, Sinnett-Smith J, Van Lint J, Rozengurt E. Molecular cloning and characterization of protein kinase D: a target for diacylglycerol and phorbol esters with a distinctive catalytic domain. Proc Natl Acad Sci U S A 1994;91(18):8572–8576.

121. Rozengurt E, Rey O, Waldron RT. Protein kinase D signaling. J Biol Chem 2005;280(14):13205–13208.

122. Waldron RT, Rozengurt E. Protein kinase C phosphorylates protein kinase D activation loop Ser744 and Ser748 and releases autoinhibition by the pleckstrin homology domain. J Biol Chem 2003;278(1):154–163.

123. Guha S, Lunn JA, Santiskulvong C, Rozengurt E. Neurotensin stimulates protein kinase C-dependent mitogenic signaling in human pancreatic carcinoma cell line PANC-1. Cancer Res 2003;63(10):2379–2387.

124. Paolucci L, Rozengurt E. Protein kinase D in small cell lung cancer cells: rapid activation through protein kinase C. Cancer Res 1999;59(3):572–577.

125. Mihailovic T, Marx M, Auer A, Van Lint J, Schmid M, Weber C, Seufferlein T. Protein kinase D2 mediates activation of nuclear factor kappaB by Bcr-Abl in Bcr-Abl+ human myeloid leukemia cells. Cancer Res 2004;64(24):8939–8944.

126. Kovalevska LM, Yurchenko OV, Shlapatska LM, Berdova GG, Mikhalap SV, Van Lint J, Sidorenko SP. Immunohistochemical studies of protein kinase D (PKD) 2 expression in malignant human lymphomas. Exp Oncol 2006;28(3):225–230.

127. Wong C, Jin ZG. Protein kinase C-dependent protein kinase D activation modulates ERK signal pathway and endothelial cell proliferation by vascular endothelial growth factor. J Biol Chem 2005;280(39):33262–33269.

128. Qin L, Zeng H, Zhao D. Requirement of protein kinase D tyrosine phosphorylation for VEGF-A165-induced angiogenesis through its interaction and regulation of phospholipase C gamma phosphorylation. J Biol Chem 2006;281(43):32550–32558.

129. Sharlow ER, Giridhar KV, Lavalle CR, Chen J, Leimgruber S, Barrett R, Bravo-Altamirano K, Wipf P, Lazo JS, Wang QJ. Potent and selective disruption of protein kinase D functionality by a Benzoxoloazepinolone. J Biol Chem 2008;283(48):33516–33526.

130. Santamaria D, Barriere C, Cerqueira A, Hunt S, Tardy C, Newton K, Caceres JF, Dubus P, Malumbres M, Barbacid M. Cdk1 is sufficient to drive the mammalian cell cycle. Nature 2007;448(7155):811–815.

131. Downward J. Targeting RAS signalling pathways in cancer therapy. Nat Rev Cancer 2003;3(1):11–22.

132. Yoon S, Seger R. The extracellular signal-regulated kinase: multiple substrates regulate diverse cellular functions. Growth Factors 2006;24(1):21–44.

133. Cuenda A, Rousseau S. p38 MAP-kinases pathway regulation, function and role in human diseases. Biochim Biophys Acta 2007;1773(8):1358–1375.

134. Goedert M, Cuenda A, Craxton M, Jakes R, Cohen P. Activation of the novel stress-activated protein kinase SAPK4 by cytokines and cellular stresses is mediated by SKK3 (MKK6); comparison of its substrate specificity with that of other SAP kinases. EMBO J 1997;16(12):3563–3571.

135. Timofeev O, Lee TY, Bulavin DV. A subtle change in p38 MAPK activity is sufficient to suppress in vivo tumorigenesis. Cell Cycle 2005;4(1):118–120.

136. Bulavin DV, Phillips C, Nannenga B, Timofeev O, Donehower LA, Anderson CW, Appella E, Fornace AJ Jr. Inactivation of the Wip1 phosphatase inhibits mammary tumorigenesis through p38 MAPK-mediated activation of the p16(Ink4a)–p19(Arf) pathway. Nat Genet 2004;36(4):343–350.

137. Iwasa H, Han J, Ishikawa F. Mitogen-activated protein kinase p38 defines the common senescence-signalling pathway. Genes Cells 2003;8(2):131–144.

138. Wang W, Chen JX, Liao R, Deng Q, Zhou JJ, Huang S, Sun P. Sequential activation of the MEK-extracellular signal-regulated kinase and MKK3/6-p38 mitogen-activated protein kinase pathways mediates oncogenic ras-induced premature senescence. Mol Cell Biol 2002;22(10):3389–3403.

139. Sun P, Yoshizuka N, New L, Moser BA, Li Y, Liao R, Xie C, Chen J, Deng Q, Yamout M, Dong MQ, Frangou CG, Yates JR 3rd, Wright PE, Han J. PRAK is essential for ras-induced senescence and tumor suppression. Cell 2007;128(2):295–308.

140. Dolado I, Swat A, Ajenjo N, De Vita G, Cuadrado A, Nebreda AR. p38 alpha MAP kinase as a sensor of reactive oxygen species in tumorigenesis. Cancer Cell 2007;11(2):191–205.

141. Weston CR, Davis RJ. The JNK signal transduction pathway. Curr Opin Cell Biol 2007;19(2):142–149.

142. Johnson GL, Nakamura K. The c-jun kinase/stress-activated pathway: regulation, function and role in human disease. Biochim Biophys Acta 2007;1773(8):1341–1348.

143. Gupta S, Barrett T, Whitmarsh AJ, Cavanagh J, Sluss HK, Derijard B, Davis RJ. Selective interaction of JNK protein kinase isoforms with transcription factors. EMBO J 1996;15(11):2760–2770.

144. Coso OA, Chiariello M, Yu JC, Teramoto H, Crespo P, Xu N, Miki T, Gutkind JS. The small GTP-binding proteins Rac1 and Cdc42 regulate the activity of the JNK/SAPK signaling pathway. Cell 1995;81(7):1137–1146.

145. Minden A, Lin A, Claret FX, Abo A, Karin M. Selective activation of the JNK signaling cascade and c-Jun transcriptional activity by the small GTPases Rac and Cdc42Hs. Cell 1995;81(7):1147–1157.

146. Brown JL, Stowers L, Baer M, Trejo J, Coughlin S, Chant J. Human Ste20 homologue hPAK1 links GTPases to the JNK MAP kinase pathway. Curr Biol 1996;6(5):598–605.

147. Zhang S, Han J, Sells MA, Chernoff J, Knaus UG, Ulevitch RJ, Bokoch GM. Rho family GTPases regulate p38 mitogen-activated protein kinase through the downstream mediator Pak1. J Biol Chem 1995;270(41):23934–23936.

148. Dhanasekaran DN, Reddy EP. JNK signaling in apoptosis. Oncogene 2008;27(48):6245–6251.

149. Whitmarsh AJ, Davis RJ. Role of mitogen-activated protein kinase kinase 4 in cancer. Oncogene 2007;26(22):3172–3184.

150. Kennedy NJ, Davis RJ. Role of JNK in tumor development. Cell Cycle 2003;2(3):199–201.

151. Frame S, Cohen P. GSK3 takes centre stage more than 20 years after its discovery. Biochem J 2001;359(Pt 1):1–16.

152. Cao Q, Lu X, Feng YJ. Glycogen synthase kinase-3 beta positively regulates the proliferation of human ovarian cancer cells. Cell Res 2006;16(7):671–677.

153. Shakoori A, Ougolkov A, Yu ZW, Zhang B, Modarressi MH, Billadeau DD, Mai M, Takahashi Y, Minamoto T. Deregulated GSK3 beta activity in colorectal cancer: its association with tumor cell survival and proliferation. Biochem Biophys Res Commun 2005;334(4):1365–1373.

154. Ougolkov AV, Fernandez-Zapico ME, Bilim VN, Smyrk TC, Chari ST, Billadeau DD. Aberrant nuclear accumulation of glycogen synthase kinase-3 beta in human pancreatic cancer: association with kinase activity and tumor dedifferentiation. Clin Cancer Res 2006;12(17):5074–5081.

155. Luo J. Glycogen synthase kinase 3 beta (GSK3 beta) in tumorigenesis and cancer chemotherapy. Cancer Lett 2008;273(2):194–200.

156. Chinkers M, Garbers DL. The protein kinase domain of the ANP receptor is required for signaling. Science 1989;245(4924):1392–1394.

157. Meggio F, Pinna LA. One-thousand-and-one substrates of protein kinase CK2? FASEB J 2003;17(3):349–368.

158. Vilk G, Weber JE, Turowec JP, Duncan JS, Wu C, Derksen DR, Zien P, Sarno S, Donella-Deana A, Lajoie G, Pinna LA, Li SS, Litchfield DW. Protein kinase CK2 catalyzes tyrosine phosphorylation in mammalian cells. Cell Signal 2008;20(11):1942–1951.

159. Niefind K, Putter M, Guerra B, Issinger OG, Schomburg D. GTP plus water mimic ATP in the active site of protein kinase CK2. Nat Struct Biol 1999;6(12):1100–1103.

160. Messenger MM, Saulnier RB, Gilchrist AD, Diamond P, Gorbsky GJ, Litchfield DW. Interactions between protein kinase CK2 and Pin1. Evidence for phosphorylation-dependent interactions. J Biol Chem 2002;277(25):23054–23064.

161. Miyata Y, Nishida E. CK2 controls multiple protein kinases by phosphorylating a kinase-targeting molecular chaperone, Cdc37. Mol Cell Biol 2004;24(9):4065–4074.

162. Eddy SF, Guo S, Demicco EG, Romieu-Mourez R, Landesman-Bollag E, Seldin DC, Sonenshein GE. Inducible I kappa B kinase/I kappa B kinase epsilon expression is induced by CK2 and promotes aberrant nuclear factor-kappa B activation in breast cancer cells. Cancer Res 2005;65(24):11375–11383.

163. Ahmad KA, Wang G, Slaton J, Unger G, Ahmed K. Targeting CK2 for cancer therapy. Anticancer Drugs 2005;16(10):1037–1043.

164. Sarno S, Moro S, Meggio F, Zagotto G, Dal Ben D, Ghisellini P, Battistutta R, Zanotti G, Pinna LA. Toward the rational design of protein kinase casein kinase-2 inhibitors. Pharmacol Ther 2002;93(2–3):159–168.

165. Nie Z, Perretta C, Erickson P, Margosiak S, Almassy R, Lu J, Averill A, Yager KM, Chu S. Structure-based design, synthesis, and study of pyrazolo[1,5-a][1,3,5]triazine derivatives as potent inhibitors of protein kinase CK2. Bioorg Med Chem Lett 2007;17(15):4191–4195.

166. Jares P, Donaldson A, Blow JJ. The Cdc7/Dbf4 protein kinase: target of the S phase checkpoint? EMBO Rep 2000;1(4):319–322.

167. Nambiar S, Mirmohammadsadegh A, Hassan M, Mota R, Marini A, Alaoui A, Tannapfel A, Hegemann JH, Hengge UR. Identification and functional characterization of ASK/Dbf4, a novel cell survival gene in cutaneous melanoma with prognostic relevance. Carcinogenesis 2007;28(12):2501–2510.

168. Hess GF, Drong RF, Weiland KL, Slightom JL, Sclafani RA, Hollingsworth RE. A human homolog of the yeast CDC7 gene is overexpressed in some tumors and transformed cell lines. Gene 1998;211(1):133–140.

169. Montagnoli A, Tenca P, Sola F, Carpani D, Brotherton D, Albanese C, Santocanale C. Cdc7 inhibition reveals a p53-dependent replication checkpoint that is defective in cancer cells. Cancer Res 2004;64(19):7110–7116.

170. Tenca P, Brotherton D, Montagnoli A, Rainoldi S, Albanese C, Santocanale C. Cdc7 is an active kinase in human cancer cells undergoing replication stress. J Biol Chem 2007;282(1):208–215.

171. Kim JM, Kakusho N, Yamada M, Kanoh Y, Takemoto N, Masai H. Cdc7 kinase mediates Claspin phosphorylation in DNA replication checkpoint. Oncogene 2007;27(24):3475–3482.

172. Kuper H, Adami HO, Trichopoulos D. Infections as a major preventable cause of human cancer. J Intern Med 2000;248(3):171–183.

173. Karin M, Cao Y, Greten FR, Li ZW. NF-kappaB in cancer: from innocent bystander to major culprit. Nat Rev Cancer 2002;2(4):301–310.

174. Clement JF, Meloche S, Servant MJ. The IKK-related kinases: from innate immunity to oncogenesis. Cell Res 2008;18(9):889–899.

175. Korherr C, Gille H, Schafer R, Koenig-Hoffmann K, Dixelius J, Egland KA, Pastan I, Brinkmann U. Identification of proangiogenic genes and pathways by high-throughput functional genomics: TBK1 and the IRF3 pathway. Proc Natl Acad Sci U S A 2006;103(11):4240–4245.

176. Chien Y, Kim S, Bumeister R, Loo YM, Kwon SW, Johnson CL, Balakireva MG, Romeo Y, Kopelovich L, Gale M Jr, Yeaman C, Camonis JH, Zhao Y, White MA. RalB GTPase-mediated activation of the I kappa B family kinase TBK1 couples innate immune signaling to tumor cell survival. Cell 2006;127(1):157–170.

177. Boehm JS, Zhao JJ, Yao J, Kim SY, Firestein R, Dunn IF, Sjostrom SK, Garraway LA, Weremowicz S, Richardson AL, Greulich H, Stewart CJ, Mulvey LA, Shen RR, Ambrogio L, Hirozane-Kishikawa T, Hill DE, Vidal M, Meyerson M, Grenier JK, Hinkle G, Root DE, Roberts TM, Lander ES, Polyak K, Hahn WC. Integrative genomic approaches identify IKBKE as a breast cancer oncogene. Cell 2007;129(6):1065–1079.

178. Oakley BR, Morris NR. A mutation in *Aspergillus nidulans* that blocks the transition from interphase to prophase. J Cell Biol 1983;96(4):1155–1158.

179. Osmani SA, May GS, Morris NR. Regulation of the mRNA levels of nimA, a gene required for the G2-M transition in *Aspergillus nidulans*. J Cell Biol 1987;104(6):1495–1504.

180. Osmani SA, Pu RT, Morris NR. Mitotic induction and maintenance by overexpression of a G2-specific gene that encodes a potential protein kinase. Cell 1988;53(2):237–244.

181. O'Regan L, Blot J, Fry AM. Mitotic regulation by NIMA-related kinases. Cell Div 2007;2: 25.

182. Fry AM, Meraldi P, Nigg EA. A centrosomal function for the human Nek2 protein kinase, a member of the NIMA family of cell cycle regulators. EMBO J 1998;17(2):470–481.

183. Fletcher L, Cerniglia GJ, Yen TJ, Muschel RJ. Live cell imaging reveals distinct roles in cell cycle regulation for Nek2A and Nek2B. Biochim Biophys Acta 2005;1744(2):89–92.

184. Hayward DG, Fry AM. Nek2 kinase in chromosome instability and cancer. Cancer Lett 2006;237(2):155–166.

185. Roig J, Mikhailov A, Belham C, Avruch J. Nercc1, a mammalian NIMA-family kinase, binds the Ran GTPase and regulates mitotic progression. Genes Dev 2002;16(13):1640–1658.

186. Belham C, Roig J, Caldwell JA, Aoyama Y, Kemp BE, Comb M, Avruch J. A mitotic cascade of NIMA family kinases. Nercc1/Nek9 activates the Nek6 and Nek7 kinases. J Biol Chem 2003;278(37):34897–34909.

187. Chen Y, Chen PL, Chen CF, Jiang X, Riley DJ. Never-in-mitosis related kinase 1 functions in DNA damage response and checkpoint control. Cell Cycle 2008;7(20):3194–3201.

188. Engelman JA, Luo J, Cantley LC. The evolution of phosphatidylinositol 3-kinases as regulators of growth and metabolism. Nat Rev Genet 2006;7(8):606–619.

189. Auger KR, Serunian LA, Soltoff SP, Libby P, Cantley LC. PDGF-dependent tyrosine phosphorylation stimulates production of novel polyphosphoinositides in intact cells. Cell 1989;57(1):167–175.

190. Hiles ID, Otsu M, Volinia S, Fry MJ, Gout I, Dhand R, Panayotou G, Ruiz-Larrea F, Thompson A, Totty NF, et al. Phosphatidylinositol 3-kinase: structure and expression of the 110kD catalytic subunit. Cell 1992;70(3):419–429.

191. Arcaro A, Zvelebil MJ, Wallasch C, Ullrich A, Waterfield MD, Domin J. Class II phosphoinositide 3-kinases are downstream targets of activated polypeptide growth factor receptors. Mol Cell Biol 2000;20(11):3817–3830.

192. Brown RA, Domin J, Arcaro A, Waterfield MD, Shepherd PR. Insulin activates the alpha isoform of class II phosphoinositide 3-kinase. J Biol Chem 1999;274(21):14529–14532.

193. Ktori C, Shepherd PR, O'Rourke L. TNF-alpha and leptin activate the alpha-isoform of class II phosphoinositide 3-kinase. Biochem Biophys Res Commun 2003;306(1):139–143.

194. Arcaro A, Khanzada UK, Vanhaesebroeck B, Tetley TD, Waterfield MD, Seckl MJ. Two distinct phosphoinositide 3-kinases mediate polypeptide growth factor-stimulated PKB activation. EMBO J 2002;21(19):5097–5108.

195. Domin J, Gaidarov I, Smith ME, Keen JH, Waterfield MD. The class II phosphoinositide 3-kinase PI3K-C2 alpha is concentrated in the trans-Golgi network and present in clathrin-coated vesicles. J Biol Chem 2000;275(16):11943–11950.

196. Zhao Y, Gaidarov I, Keen JH. Phosphoinositide 3-kinase C2 alpha links clathrin to microtubule-dependent movement. J Biol Chem 2007;282(2):1249–1256.

197. Yoshioka K, Sugimoto N, Takuwa N, Takuwa Y. Essential role for class II phosphoinositide 3-kinase alpha-isoform in Ca^2+-induced, Rho- and Rho kinase-dependent regulation of myosin phosphatase and contraction in isolated vascular smooth muscle cells. Mol Pharmacol 2007;71(3):912–920.

198. Wang Y, Yoshioka K, Azam MA, Takuwa N, Sakurada S, Kayaba Y, Sugimoto N, Inoki I, Kimura T, Kuwaki T, Takuwa Y. Class II phosphoinositide 3-kinase alpha-isoform regulates Rho, myosin phosphatase and contraction in vascular smooth muscle. Biochem J 2006;394(Pt 3):581–592.

199. Falasca M, Hughes WE, Dominguez V, Sala G, Fostira F, Fang MQ, Cazzolli R, Shepherd PR, James DE, Maffucci T. The role of phosphoinositide 3-kinase C2 alpha in insulin signaling. J Biol Chem 2007;282(38):28226–28236.

200. Elis W, Triantafellow E, Wolters NM, Sian KR, Caponigro G, Borawski J, Gaither LA, Murphy LO, Finan PM, Mackeigan JP. Down-regulation of class II phosphoinositide 3-kinase alpha expression below a critical threshold induces apoptotic cell death. Mol Cancer Res 2008;6(4):614–623.

201. Siddhanta U, McIlroy J, Shah A, Zhang Y, Backer JM. Distinct roles for the p110 alpha and hVPS34 phosphatidylinositol 3′-kinases in vesicular trafficking, regulation of the actin cytoskeleton, and mitogenesis. J Cell Biol 1998;143(6):1647–1659.

202. Johnson EE, Overmeyer JH, Gunning WT, Maltese WA. Gene silencing reveals a specific function of hVps34 phosphatidylinositol 3-kinase in late versus early endosomes. J Cell Sci 2006;119 (Pt 7):1219–1232.

203. Nobukuni T, Joaquin M, Roccio M, Dann SG, Kim SY, Gulati P, Byfield MP, Backer JM, Natt F, Bos JL, Zwartkruis FJ, Thomas G. Amino acids mediate mTOR/raptor signaling through activation of class 3 phosphatidylinositol 3OH-kinase. Proc Natl Acad Sci U S A 2005;102(40):14238–14243.

204. Byfield MP, Murray JT, Backer JM. hVps34 is a nutrient-regulated lipid kinase required for activation of p70S6 kinase. J Biol Chem 2005;280(38):33076–33082.

205. Gulati P, Gaspers LD, Dann SG, Joaquin M, Nobukuni T, Natt F, Kozma SC, Thomas AP, Thomas G. Amino acids activate mTOR complex 1 via Ca^2+/CaM signaling to hVps34. Cell Metab 2008;7(5):456–465.

206. Levine B, Kroemer G. Autophagy in the pathogenesis of disease. Cell 2008;132(1):27–42.

207. Hippert MM, O'Toole PS, Thorburn A. Autophagy in cancer: good, bad, or both? Cancer Res 2006;66(19):9349–9351.

208. Jin S, White E. Tumor suppression by autophagy through the management of metabolic stress. Autophagy 2008;4(5):563–566.

209. Hannun YA, Obeid LM. Principles of bioactive lipid signalling: lessons from sphingolipids. Nat Rev Mol Cell Biol 2008;9(2):139–150.

210. Wymann MP, Schneiter R. Lipid signalling in disease. Nat Rev Mol Cell Biol 2008;9(2):162–176.

211. Komarova YA, Mehta D, Malik AB. Dual regulation of endothelial junctional permeability. Sci STKE 2007;2007(412): re8.

212. Rosen H, Sanna MG, Cahalan SM, Gonzalez-Cabrera PJ. Tipping the gatekeeper: S1P regulation of endothelial barrier function. Trends Immunol 2007;28(3):102–107.

213. French KJ, Upson JJ, Keller SN, Zhuang Y, Yun JK, Smith CD. Antitumor activity of sphingosine kinase inhibitors. J Pharmacol Exp Ther 2006;318(2):596–603.

214. Ramirez de Molina A, Rodriguez-Gonzalez A, Gutierrez R, Martinez-Pineiro L, Sanchez J, Bonilla F, Rosell R, Lacal J. Overexpression of choline kinase is a frequent feature in human tumor-derived cell lines and in lung, prostate, and colorectal human cancers. Biochem Biophys Res Commun 2002;296(3):580–583.

215. Ramirez de Molina A, Gallego-Ortega D, Sarmentero J, Banez-Coronel M, Martin-Cantalejo Y, Lacal JC. Choline kinase is a novel oncogene that potentiates RhoA-induced carcinogenesis. Cancer Res 2005;65(13):5647–5653.

216. Jimenez B, del Peso L, Montaner S, Esteve P, Lacal JC. Generation of phosphorylcholine as an essential event in the activation of Raf-1 and MAP-kinases in growth factors-induced mitogenic stimulation. J Cell Biochem 1995;57(1):141–149.

217. Cuadrado A, Carnero A, Dolfi F, Jimenez B, Lacal JC. Phosphorylcholine: a novel second messenger essential for mitogenic activity of growth factors. Oncogene 1993;8(11):2959–2968.

218. Al-Saffar NM, Troy H, Ramirez de Molina A, Jackson LE, Madhu B, Griffiths JR, Leach MO, Workman P, Lacal JC, Judson IR, Chung YL. Noninvasive magnetic resonance spectroscopic pharmacodynamic markers of the choline kinase inhibitor MN58b in human carcinoma models. Cancer Res 2006;66(1):427–434.

219. Hernandez-Alcoceba R, Saniger L, Campos J, Nunez MC, Khaless F, Gallo MA, Espinosa A, Lacal JC. Choline kinase inhibitors as a novel approach for antiproliferative drug design. Oncogene 1997;15(19):2289–2301.

220. Rodriguez-Gonzalez A, Ramirez de Molina A, Fernandez F, Ramos MA, del Carmen Nunez M, Campos J, Lacal JC. Inhibition of choline kinase as a specific cytotoxic strategy in oncogene-transformed cells. Oncogene 2003;22(55):8803–8812.

221. Benson JD, Chen YN, Cornell-Kennon SA, Dorsch M, Kim S, Leszczyniecka M, Sellers WR, Lengauer C. Validating cancer drug targets. Nature 2006;441(7092):451–456.

222. Weinstein IB. Cancer. Addiction to oncogenes—the Achilles heal of cancer. Science 2002;297(5578):63–64.

223. Garraway LA, Sellers WR. Lineage dependency and lineage-survival oncogenes in human cancer. Nat Rev Cancer 2006;6(8):593–602.

224. Kaelin WG Jr. The concept of synthetic lethality in the context of anticancer therapy. Nat Rev Cancer 2005;5(9):689–698.

225. Bryant HE, Schultz N, Thomas HD, Parker KM, Flower D, Lopez E, Kyle S, Meuth M, Curtin NJ, Helleday T. Specific killing of BRCA2-deficient tumours with inhibitors of poly(ADP-ribose) polymerase. Nature 2005;434(7035):913–917.

226. Evers B, Drost R, Schut E, de Bruin M, van der Burg E, Derksen PW, Holstege H, Liu X, van Drunen E, Beverloo HB, Smith GC, Martin NM, Lau A, O'Connor MJ, Jonkers J. Selective inhibition of BRCA2-deficient mammary tumor cell growth by AZD2281 and cisplatin. Clin Cancer Res 2008;14(12):3916–3925.

227. Rottenberg S, Jaspers JE, Kersbergen A, van der Burg E, Nygren AO, Zander SA, Derksen PW, de Bruin M, Zevenhoven J, Lau A, Boulter R, Cranston A, O'Connor MJ, Martin NM, Borst P, Jonkers J. High sensitivity of BRCA1-deficient mammary tumors to the PARP inhibitor AZD2281 alone and in combination with platinum drugs. Proc Natl Acad Sci U S A 2008;105(44):17079–17084.

228. Orgaz JL, Martinez-Poveda B, Fernandez-Garcia NI, Jimenez B. Following up tumour angiogenesis: from the basic laboratory to the clinic. Clin Transl Oncol 2008;10(8):468–477.

229. Turner NC, Lord CJ, Iorns E, Brough R, Swift S, Elliott R, Rayter S, Tutt AN, Ashworth A. A synthetic lethal siRNA screen identifying genes mediating sensitivity to a PARP inhibitor. EMBO J 2008;27(9):1368–1377.

230. Chou TC. Preclinical versus clinical drug combination studies. Leuk Lymphoma 2008;49(11):2059–2080.

231. Sharma SV, Settleman J. Oncogene addiction: setting the stage for molecularly targeted cancer therapy. Genes Dev 2007;21(24):3214–3231.

232. Parsons DW, Jones S, Zhang X, Lin JC, Leary RJ, Angenendt P, Mankoo P, Carter H, Siu IM, Gallia GL, Olivi A, McLendon R, Rasheed BA, Keir S, Nikolskaya T, Nikolsky Y, Busam DA, Tekleab H, Diaz LA Jr, Hartigan J, Smith DR, Strausberg RL, Marie SK, Shinjo SM, Yan H, Riggins GJ, Bigner DD, Karchin R, Papadopoulos N, Parmigiani G, Vogelstein B, Velculescu VE, Kinzler KW. An integrated genomic analysis of human glioblastoma multiforme. Science 2008;321(5897):1807–1812.

233. Jones S, Zhang X, Parsons DW, Lin JC, Leary RJ, Angenendt P, Mankoo P, Carter H, Kamiyama H, Jimeno A, Hong SM, Fu B, Lin MT, Calhoun ES, Kamiyama M, Walter K, Nikolskaya T, Nikolsky Y, Hartigan J, Smith DR, Hidalgo M, Leach SD, Klein AP, Jaffee EM, Goggins M, Maitra A, Iacobuzio-Donahue C, Eshleman JR, Kern SE, Hruban RH, Karchin R, Papadopoulos N, Parmigiani G, Vogelstein B, Velculescu VE, Kinzler KW. Core signaling pathways in human pancreatic cancers revealed by global genomic analyses. Science 2008;321(5897):1801–1806.

234. Ding L, Getz G, Wheeler DA, Mardis ER, McLellan MD, Cibulskis K, Sougnez C, Greulich H, Muzny DM, Morgan MB, Fulton L, Fulton RS, Zhang Q, Wendl MC, Lawrence MS, Larson DE,

Chen K, Dooling DJ, Sabo A, Hawes AC, Shen H, Jhangiani SN, Lewis LR, Hall O, Zhu Y, Mathew T, Ren Y, Yao J, Scherer SE, Clerc K, Metcalf GA, Ng B, Milosavljevic A, Gonzalez-Garay ML, Osborne JR, Meyer R, Shi X, Tang Y, Koboldt DC, Lin L, Abbott R, Miner TL, Pohl C, Fewell G, Haipek C, Schmidt H, Dunford-Shore BH, Kraja A, Crosby SD, Sawyer CS, Vickery T, Sander S, Robinson J, Winckler W, Baldwin J, Chirieac LR, Dutt A, Fennell T, Hanna M, Johnson BE, Onofrio RC, Thomas RK, Tonon G, Weir BA, Zhao X, Ziaugra L, Zody MC, Giordano T, Orringer MB, Roth JA, Spitz MR, Wistuba II, Ozenberger B, Good PJ, Chang AC, Beer DG, Watson MA, Ladanyi M, Broderick S, Yoshizawa A, Travis WD, Pao W, Province MA, Weinstock GM, Varmus HE, Gabriel SB, Lander ES, Gibbs RA, Meyerson M, Wilson RK. Somatic mutations affect key pathways in lung adenocarcinoma. Nature 2008;455(7216):1069–1075.

235. Rubin AF, Green P. Comment on "The consensus coding sequences of human breast and colorectal cancers." Science 2007;317(5844): 1500.

236. Getz G, Hofling H, Mesirov JP, Golub TR, Meyerson M, Tibshirani R, Lander ES. Comment on "The consensus coding sequences of human breast and colorectal cancers." Science 2007;317(5844): 1500.

237. Forrest WF, Cavet G. Comment on "The consensus coding sequences of human breast and colorectal cancers." Science 2007;317(5844): 1500; author reply 1500.

238. Singh M, Johnson L. Using genetically engineered mouse models of cancer to aid drug development: an industry perspective. Clin Cancer Res 2006;12(18):5312–5328.

239. Jackson AL, Burchard J, Schelter J, Chau BN, Cleary M, Lim L, Linsley PS. Widespread siRNA "off-target" transcript silencing mediated by seed region sequence complementarity. RNA 2006;12(7):1179–1187.

240. Luo B, Cheung HW, Subramanian A, Sharifnia T, Okamoto M, Yang X, Hinkle G, Boehm JS, Beroukhim R, Weir BA, Mermel C, Barbie DA, Awad T, Zhou X, Nguyen T, Piqani B, Li C, Golub TR, Meyerson M, Hacohen N, Hahn WC, Lander ES, Sabatini DM, Root DE. Highly parallel identification of essential genes in cancer cells. Proc Natl Acad Sci U S A 2008;105(51):20380–20385.

241. McDermott U, Iafrate AJ, Gray NS, Shioda T, Classon M, Maheswaran S, Zhou W, Choi HG, Smith SL, Dowell L, Ulkus LE, Kuhlmann G, Greninger P, Christensen JG, Haber DA, Settleman J. Genomic alterations of anaplastic lymphoma kinase may sensitize tumors to anaplastic lymphoma kinase inhibitors. Cancer Res 2008;68(9):3389–3395.

242. McDermott U, Sharma SV, Dowell L, Greninger P, Montagut C, Lamb J, Archibald H, Raudales R, Tam A, Lee D, Rothenberg SM, Supko JG, Sordella R, Ulkus LE, Iafrate AJ, Maheswaran S, Njauw CN, Tsao H, Drew L, Hanke JH, Ma XJ, Erlander MG, Gray NS, Haber DA, Settleman J. Identification of genotype-correlated sensitivity to selective kinase inhibitors by using high-throughput tumor cell line profiling. Proc Natl Acad Sci U S A 2007;104(50):19936–19941.

243. Collins I, Workman P. New approaches to molecular cancer therapeutics. Nat Chem Biol 2006;2(12):689–700.

244. Liu Y, Witucki LA, Shah K, Bishop AC, Shokat KM. Src-Abl tyrosine kinase chimeras: replacement of the adenine binding pocket of c-Abl with v-Src to swap nucleotide and inhibitor specificities. Biochemistry 2000;39(47):14400–14408.

245. Cheetham GM, Knegtel RM, Coll JT, Renwick SB, Swenson L, Weber P, Lippke JA, Austen DA. Crystal structure of aurora-2, an oncogenic serine/threonine kinase. J Biol Chem 2002;277(45):42419–42422.

246. Zhao B, Bower MJ, McDevitt PJ, Zhao H, Davis ST, Johanson KO, Green SM, Concha NO, Zhou BB. Structural basis for Chk1 inhibition by UCN-01. J Biol Chem 2002;277(48):46609–46615.

247. Brignola PS, Lackey K, Kadwell SH, Hoffman C, Horne E, Carter HL, Stuart JD, Blackburn K, Moyer MB, Alligood KJ, Knight WB, Wood ER. Comparison of the biochemical and kinetic properties of the type 1 receptor tyrosine kinase intracellular domains. Demonstration of differential sensitivity to kinase inhibitors. J Biol Chem 2002;277(2):1576–1585.

248. Favelyukis S, Till JH, Hubbard SR, Miller WT. Structure and autoregulation of the insulin-like growth factor 1 receptor kinase. Nat Struct Biol 2001;8(12):1058–1063.

249. Sadler TM, Achilleos M, Ragunathan S, Pitkin A, LaRocque J, Morin J, Annable R, Greenberger LM, Frost P, Zhang Y. Development and comparison of two nonradioactive kinase assays for I kappa B kinase. Anal Biochem 2004;326(1):106–113.

250. Horiuchi KY, Scherle PA, Trzaskos JM, Copeland RA. Competitive inhibition of MAP kinase activation by a peptide representing the alpha C helix of ERK. Biochemistry 1998;37(25):8879–8885.

251. Dennis PB, Jaeschke A, Saitoh M, Fowler B, Kozma SC, Thomas G. Mammalian TOR: a homeostatic ATP sensor. Science 2001;294(5544):1102–1105.

252. Force T, Bonventre JV, Heidecker G, Rapp U, Avruch J, Kyriakis JM. Enzymatic characteristics of the c-Raf-1 protein kinase. Proc Natl Acad Sci U S A 1994;91(4):1270–1274.

253. Parast CV, Mroczkowski B, Pinko C, Misialek S, Khambatta G, Appelt K. Characterization and kinetic mechanism of catalytic domain of human vascular endothelial growth factor receptor-2 tyrosine kinase (VEGFR2 TK), a key enzyme in angiogenesis. Biochemistry 1998;37(47):16788–16801.

254. Knight ZA, Shokat KM. Features of selective kinase inhibitors. Chem Biol 2005;12(6):621–637.

255. Cheng Y, Prusoff WH. Relationship between the inhibition constant (K_1) and the concentration of inhibitor which causes 50 per cent inhibition (I_{50}) of an enzymatic reaction. Biochem Pharmacol 1973;22(23):3099–3108.

256. Wei M, Wynn R, Hollis G, Liao B, Margulis A, Reid BG, Klabe R, Liu PC, Becker-Pasha M, Rupar M, Burn TC, McCall DE, Li Y. High-throughput determination of mode of inhibition in lead identification and optimization. J Biomol Screen 2007;12(2):220–228.

257. Stout TJ, Foster PG, Matthews DJ. High-throughput structural biology in drug discovery: protein kinases. Curr Pharm Des 2004;10(10):1069–1082.

258. Macdonald A, Campbell DG, Toth R, McLauchlan H, Hastie CJ, Arthur JS. Pim kinases phosphorylate multiple sites on Bad and promote 14–3-3 binding and dissociation from Bcl-XL. BMC Cell Biol 2006;7:1.

259. Rees DC, Congreve M, Murray CW, Carr R. Fragment-based lead discovery. Nat Rev Drug Discov 2004;3(8):660–672.

260. Imai K, Takaoka A. Comparing antibody and small-molecule therapies for cancer. Nat Rev Cancer 2006;6(9):714–727.

261. Lindsley CW, Zhao Z, Leister WH, Robinson RG, Barnett SF, Defeo-Jones D, Jones RE, Hartman GD, Huff JR, Huber HE, Duggan ME. Allosteric Akt (PKB) inhibitors: discovery and SAR of isozyme selective inhibitors. Bioorg Med Chem Lett 2005;15(3):761–764.

262. Barnett SF, Defeo-Jones D, Fu S, Hancock PJ, Haskell KM, Jones RE, Kahana JA, Kral AM, Leander K, Lee LL, Malinowski J, McAvoy EM, Nahas DD, Robinson RG, Huber HE. Identification and characterization of pleckstrin-homology-domain-dependent and isoenzyme-specific Akt inhibitors. Biochem J 2005;385(Pt 2):399–408.

263. Bilodeau MT, Balitza AE, Hoffman JM, Manley PJ, Barnett SF, Defeo-Jones D, Haskell K, Jones RE, Leander K, Robinson RG, Smith AM, Huber HE, Hartman GD. Allosteric inhibitors of Akt1 and Akt2: a naphthyridinone with efficacy in an A2780 tumor xenograft model. Bioorg Med Chem Lett 2008;18(11):3178–3182.

264. DeFeo-Jones D, Barnett SF, Fu S, Hancock PJ, Haskell KM, Leander KR, McAvoy E, Robinson RG, Duggan ME, Lindsley CW, Zhao Z, Huber HE, Jones RE. Tumor cell sensitization to apoptotic stimuli by selective inhibition of specific Akt/PKB family members. Mol Cancer Ther 2005;4(2):271–279.

265. She QB, Chandarlapaty S, Ye Q, Lobo J, Haskell KM, Leander KR, DeFeo-Jones D, Huber HE, Rosen N. Breast tumor cells with PI3K mutation or HER2 amplification are selectively addicted to Akt signaling. PLoS ONE 2008;3(8): e3065.

266. Hartnett JC, Barnett SF, Bilodeau MT, Defeo-Jones D, Hartman GD, Huber HE, Jones RE, Kral AM, Robinson RG, Wu Z. Optimization of 2,3,5-trisubstituted pyridine derivatives as potent allosteric Akt1 and Akt2 inhibitors. Bioorg Med Chem Lett 2008;18(6):2194–2197.

267. Siu T, Li Y, Nagasawa J, Liang J, Tehrani L, Chua P, Jones RE, Defeo-Jones D, Barnett SF, Robinson RG. The design and synthesis of potent and cell-active allosteric dual Akt 1 and 2 inhibitors devoid of hERG activity. Bioorg Med Chem Lett 2008;18(14):4191–4194.

268. Siu T, Liang J, Arruda J, Li Y, Jones RE, Defeo-Jones D, Barnett SF, Robinson RG. Discovery of potent and cell-active allosteric dual Akt 1 and 2 inhibitors. Bioorg Med Chem Lett 2008;18(14):4186–4190.

269. Zhao Z, Robinson RG, Barnett SF, Defeo-Jones D, Jones RE, Hartman GD, Huber HE, Duggan ME, Lindsley CW. Development of potent, allosteric dual Akt1 and Akt2 inhibitors with improved physical properties and cell activity. Bioorg Med Chem Lett 2008;18(1):49–53.

270. David E, Sinha R, Chen J, Sun SY, Kaufman JL, Lonial S. Perifosine synergistically enhances TRAIL-induced myeloma cell apoptosis via up-regulation of death receptors. Clin Cancer Res 2008;14(16):5090–5098.

271. Kondapaka SB, Singh SS, Dasmahapatra GP, Sausville EA, Roy KK. Perifosine, a novel alkylphospholipid, inhibits protein kinase B activation. Mol Cancer Ther 2003;2(11):1093–1103.

272. Elrod HA, Lin YD, Yue P, Wang X, Lonial S, Khuri FR, Sun SY. The alkylphospholipid perifosine induces apoptosis of human lung cancer cells requiring inhibition of Akt and activation of the extrinsic apoptotic pathway. Mol Cancer Ther 2007;6(7):2029–2038.

273. Floryk D, Thompson TC. Perifosine induces differentiation and cell death in prostate cancer cells. Cancer Lett 2008;266(2):216–226.

274. Hideshima T, Catley L, Yasui H, Ishitsuka K, Raje N, Mitsiades C, Podar K, Munshi NC, Chauhan D, Richardson PG, Anderson KC. Perifosine, an oral bioactive novel alkylphospholipid, inhibits Akt and induces in vitroand in vivo cytotoxicity in human multiple myeloma cells. Blood 2006;107(10):4053–4062.

275. Garcia-Echeverria C. Inhibitors of signaling interfaces: targeting Src homology 2 domains in drug discovery. In: Fabbro D, McCormick F, editors. Protein Tyrosine Kinases: From Inhibitors to Useful Drugs, Cancer Drug Discovery and Development. Totowa, NJ: Humana Press Inc.; 2006. pp.31–52.

276. Songyang Z, Shoelson SE, McGlade J, Olivier P, Pawson T, Bustelo XR, Barbacid M, Sabe H, Hanafusa H, Yi T, et al. Specific motifs recognized by the SH2 domains of Csk, 3BP2, fps/fes, GRB-2, HCP, SHC, Syk, and Vav. Mol Cell Biol 1994;14(4):2777–2785.

277. Rahuel J, Gay B, Erdmann D, Strauss A, Garcia-Echeverria C, Furet P, Caravatti G, Fretz H, Schoepfer J, Grutter MG. Structural basis for specificity of Grb2-SH2 revealed by a novel ligand binding mode. Nat Struct Biol 1996;3(7):586–589.

278. Thornton KH, Mueller WT, McConnell P, Zhu G, Saltiel AR, Thanabal V. Nuclear magnetic resonance solution structure of the growth factor receptor-bound protein 2 Src homology 2 domain. Biochemistry 1996;35(36):11852–11864.

279. Furet P, Gay B, Garcia-Echeverria C, Rahuel J, Fretz H, Schoepfer J, Caravatti G. Discovery of 3-aminobenzyloxycarbonyl as an N-terminal group conferring high affinity to the minimal phosphopeptide sequence recognized by the Grb2-SH2 domain. J Med Chem 1997;40(22):3551–3556.

280. Garcia-Echeverria C, Furet P, Gay B, Fretz H, Rahuel J, Schoepfer J, Caravatti G. Potent antagonists of the SH2 domain of Grb2: optimization of the X+1 position of 3-amino-Z-Tyr(PO3H2)-X+1-Asn-NH2. J Med Chem 1998;41(11):1741–1744.

281. Furet P, Gay B, Caravatti G, Garcia-Echeverria C, Rahuel J, Schoepfer J, Fretz H. Structure-based design and synthesis of high affinity tripeptide ligands of the Grb2-SH2 domain. J Med Chem 1998;41(18):3442–3449.

282. Gay B, Suarez S, Weber C, Rahuel J, Fabbro D, Furet P, Caravatti G, Schoepfer J. Effect of potent and selective inhibitors of the Grb2 SH2 domain on cell motility. J Biol Chem 1999;274(33):23311–23315.

283. Gay B, Suarez S, Caravatti G, Furet P, Meyer T, Schoepfer J. Selective GRB2 SH2 inhibitors as anti-Ras therapy. Int J Cancer 1999;83(2):235–241.

284. Schust J, Sperl B, Hollis A, Mayer TU, Berg T. Stattic: a small-molecule inhibitor of STAT3 activation and dimerization. Chem Biol 2006;13(11):1235–1242.

285. Kim KJ, Li B, Winer J, Armanini M, Gillett N, Phillips HS, Ferrara N. Inhibition of vascular endothelial growth factor-induced angiogenesis suppresses tumour growth in vivo. Nature 1993;362(6423):841–844.

286. Witters L, Scherle P, Friedman S, Fridman J, Caulder E, Newton R, Lipton A. Synergistic inhibition with a dual epidermal growth factor receptor/HER-2/neu tyrosine kinase inhibitor and a disintegrin and metalloprotease inhibitor. Cancer Res 2008;68(17):7083–7089.

287. Wegele H, Muller L, Buchner J. Hsp70 and Hsp90—a relay team for protein folding. Rev Physiol Biochem Pharmacol 2004;151:1–44.

288. Sreedhar AS, Kalmar E, Csermely P, Shen YF. Hsp90 isoforms: functions, expression and clinical importance. FEBS Lett 2004;562(1–3):11–15.

289. Kamal A, Thao L, Sensintaffar J, Zhang L, Boehm MF, Fritz LC, Burrows FJ. A high-affinity conformation of Hsp90 confers tumour selectivity on Hsp90 inhibitors. Nature 2003;425(6956):407–410.

290. da Rocha Dias S, Friedlos F, Light Y, Springer C, Workman P, Marais R. Activated B-RAF is an Hsp90 client protein that is targeted by the anticancer drug 17-allylamino-17-demethoxygeldanamycin. Cancer Res 2005;65(23):10686–10691.

291. Grbovic OM, Basso AD, Sawai A, Ye Q, Friedlander P, Solit D, Rosen N. V600E B-Raf requires the Hsp90 chaperone for stability and is degraded in response to Hsp90 inhibitors. Proc Natl Acad Sci U S A 2006;103(1):57–62.

292. Bagatell R, Whitesell L. Altered Hsp90 function in cancer: a unique therapeutic opportunity. Mol Cancer Ther 2004;3(8):1021–1030.

293. Isaacs JS, Xu W, Neckers L. Heat shock protein 90 as a molecular target for cancer therapeutics. Cancer Cell 2003;3(3):213–217.

294. Powers MV, Workman P. Targeting of multiple signalling pathways by heat shock protein 90 molecular chaperone inhibitors. Endocr Relat Cancer 2006;13 Suppl 1: S125–135.

295. Sharp SY, Prodromou C, Boxall K, Powers MV, Holmes JL, Box G, Matthews TP, Cheung KM, Kalusa A, James K, Hayes A, Hardcastle A, Dymock B, Brough PA, Barril X, Cansfield JE, Wright L, Surgenor A, Foloppe N, Hubbard RE, Aherne W, Pearl L, Jones K, McDonald E, Raynaud F, Eccles S, Drysdale M, Workman P. Inhibition of the heat shock protein 90 molecular chaperone in vitroand in vivo by novel, synthetic, potent resorcinylic pyrazole/isoxazole amide analogues. Mol Cancer Ther 2007;6(4):1198–1211.

296. Solit DB, Rosen N. Hsp90: a novel target for cancer therapy. Curr Top Med Chem 2006;6(11):1205–1214.

297. Richardson PG, Chanan-Khan A, Lonial S, Krishman A, Carroll M, Cropp GF, Kersey K, Abitar M, Johnson RG, Hannah AL, Anderson KC. Tanespimycin (T) + bortezomib (BZ) in multiple myeloma (MM): confirmation of the recommended dose using a novel formulation. ASH Annual Meeting Abstracts 2007;110(11):Abstr 1165.

298. Modi S, Sugarman S, Stopeck A, Linden H, Ma W, Kersey K, Johnson RG, Rosen N, Hannah AL, Hudis CA. Phase II trial of the Hsp90 inhibitor tanespimycin (Tan) + trastuzumab (T) in patients (pts) with HER2-positive metastatic breast cancer (MBC). J Clin Oncol 2008;26 (May 20 suppl):Abstr 1027.

299. Wagner AJ, Morgan JA, Chugh R, Rosen LS, George S, Gordon MS, Devine CM, Van den Abbeele AD, Grayzel D, Demetri GD. Inhibition of heat shock protein 90 (Hsp90) with the novel agent IPI-504 in metastatic GIST following failure of tyrosine kinase inhibitors (TKIs) or other sarcomas: clinical results from phase I trial. J Clin Oncol 2008;26(May 20 suppl):Abstr 10503.

300. Gleave ME, Monia BP. Antisense therapy for cancer. Nat Rev Cancer 2005;5(6):468–479.

301. Kasid U, Pfeifer A, Brennan T, Beckett M, Weichselbaum RR, Dritschilo A, Mark GE. Effect of antisense c-raf-1 on tumorigenicity and radiation sensitivity of a human squamous carcinoma. Science 1989;243(4896):1354–1356.

302. Geiger T, Muller M, Monia BP, Fabbro D. Antitumor activity of a C-raf antisense oligonucleotide in combination with standard chemotherapeutic agents against various human tumors transplanted subcutaneously into nude mice. Clin Cancer Res 1997;3(7):1179–1185.

303. Monia BP, Sasmor H, Johnston JF, Freier SM, Lesnik EA, Muller M, Geiger T, Altmann KH, Moser H, Fabbro D. Sequence-specific antitumor activity of a phosphorothioate oligodeoxyribonu-cleotide targeted to human C-raf kinase supports an antisense mechanism of action in vivo. Proc Natl Acad Sci U S A 1996;93(26):15481–15484.

304. Stevenson JP, Yao KS, Gallagher M, Friedland D, Mitchell EP, Cassella A, Monia B, Kwoh TJ, Yu R, Holmlund J, Dorr FA, O'Dwyer PJ. Phase I clinical/pharmacokinetic and pharmaco-dynamic trial of the c-raf-1 antisense oligonucleotide ISIS 5132 (CGP 69846A). J Clin Oncol 1999;17(7):2227–2236.

305. Cunningham CC, Holmlund JT, Schiller JH, Geary RS, Kwoh TJ, Dorr A, Nemunaitis J. A phase I trial of c-Raf kinase antisense oligonucleotide ISIS 5132 administered as a continuous intravenous infusion in patients with advanced cancer. Clin Cancer Res 2000;6(5):1626–1631.

306. Rudin CM, Holmlund J, Fleming GF, Mani S, Stadler WM, Schumm P, Monia BP, Johnston JF, Geary R, Yu RZ, Kwoh TJ, Dorr FA, Ratain MJ. Phase I trial of ISIS 5132, an antisense oligonucleotide inhibitor of c-raf-1, administered by 24-hour weekly infusion to patients with advanced cancer. Clin Cancer Res 2001;7(5):1214–1220.

307. Oza AM, Elit L, Swenerton K, Faught W, Ghatage P, Carey M, McIntosh L, Dorr A, Holmlund JT, Eisenhauer E. Phase II study of CGP 69846A (ISIS 5132) in recurrent epithelial ovarian cancer: an NCIC clinical trials group study (NCIC IND.116). Gynecol Oncol 2003;89(1):129–133.

308. Cripps MC, Figueredo AT, Oza AM, Taylor MJ, Fields AL, Holmlund JT, McIntosh LW, Geary RS, Eisenhauer EA. Phase II randomized study of ISIS 3521 and ISIS 5132 in patients with locally advanced or metastatic colorectal cancer: a National Cancer Institute of Canada clinical trials group study. Clin Cancer Res 2002;8(7):2188–2192.

309. Coudert B, Anthoney A, Fiedler W, Droz JP, Dieras V, Borner M, Smyth JF, Morant R, de Vries MJ, Roelvink M, Fumoleau P. Phase II trial with ISIS 5132 in patients with small-cell (SCLC) and non-small cell (NSCLC) lung cancer. A European Organization for Research and Treatment of Cancer (EORTC) Early Clinical Studies Group report. Eur J Cancer 2001;37(17):2194–2198.

310. Tolcher AW, Reyno L, Venner PM, Ernst SD, Moore M, Geary RS, Chi K, Hall S, Walsh W, Dorr A, Eisenhauer E. A randomized phase II and pharmacokinetic study of the antisense oligonucleotides ISIS 3521 and ISIS 5132 in patients with hormone-refractory prostate cancer. Clin Cancer Res 2002;8(8):2530–2535.

311. Gokhale PC, Zhang C, Newsome JT, Pei J, Ahmad I, Rahman A, Dritschilo A, Kasid UN. Pharmacokinetics, toxicity, and efficacy of ends-modified raf antisense oligodeoxyribonucleotide encapsulated in a novel cationic liposome. Clin Cancer Res 2002;8(11):3611–3621.

312. Mewani RR, Tang W, Rahman A, Dritschilo A, Ahmad I, Kasid UN, Gokhale PC. Enhanced therapeutic effects of doxorubicin and paclitaxel in combination with liposome-entrapped ends-modified raf antisense oligonucleotide against human prostate, lung and breast tumor models. Int J Oncol 2004;24(5):1181–1188.

313. Pei J, Zhang C, Gokhale PC, Rahman A, Dritschilo A, Ahmad I, Kasid UN. Combination with liposome-entrapped, ends-modified raf antisense oligonucleotide (LErafAON) improves the anti-tumor efficacies of cisplatin, epirubicin, mitoxantrone, docetaxel and gemcitabine. Anticancer Drugs 2004;15(3):243–253.

314. Rudin CM, Marshall JL, Huang CH, Kindler HL, Zhang C, Kumar D, Gokhale PC, Steinberg J, Wanaski S, Kasid UN, Ratain MJ. Delivery of a liposomal c-raf-1 antisense oligonucleotide by weekly bolus dosing in patients with advanced solid tumors: a phase I study. Clin Cancer Res 2004;10(21):7244–7251.

315. Dritschilo A, Huang CH, Rudin CM, Marshall J, Collins B, Dul JL, Zhang C, Kumar D, Gokhale PC, Ahmad A, Ahmad I, Sherman JW, Kasid UN. Phase I study of liposome-encapsulated c-raf antisense oligodeoxyribonucleotide infusion in combination with radiation therapy in patients with advanced malignancies. Clin Cancer Res 2006;12(4):1251–1259.

316. Geiger T, Muller M, Dean NM, Fabbro D. Antitumor activity of a PKC-alpha antisense oligonucleotide in combination with standard chemotherapeutic agents against various human tumors transplanted into nude mice. Anticancer Drug Des 1998;13(1):35–45.

317. Dean N, McKay R, Miraglia L, Howard R, Cooper S, Giddings J, Nicklin P, Meister L, Ziel R, Geiger T, Muller M, Fabbro D. Inhibition of growth of human tumor cell lines in nude mice by an antisense of oligonucleotide inhibitor of protein kinase C-alpha expression. Cancer Res 1996;56(15):3499–3507.

318. Yuen AR, Halsey J, Fisher GA, Holmlund JT, Geary RS, Kwoh TJ, Dorr A, Sikic BI. Phase I study of an antisense oligonucleotide to protein kinase C-alpha (ISIS 3521/CGP 64128A) in patients with cancer. Clin Cancer Res 1999;5(11):3357–3363.

319. Nemunaitis J, Holmlund JT, Kraynak M, Richards D, Bruce J, Ognoskie N, Kwoh TJ, Geary R, Dorr A, Von Hoff D, Eckhardt SG. Phase I evaluation of ISIS 3521, an antisense oligodeoxynucleotide to protein kinase C-alpha, in patients with advanced cancer. J Clin Oncol 1999;17(11):3586–3595.

320. Advani R, Peethambaram P, Lum BL, Fisher GA, Hartmann L, Long HJ, Halsey J, Holmlund JT, Dorr A, Sikic BI. A phase II trial of aprinocarsen, an antisense oligonucleotide inhibitor of protein

kinase C alpha, administered as a 21-day infusion to patients with advanced ovarian carcinoma. Cancer 2004;100(2):321–326.

321. Hirawat S, Elfring GL, Northcutt VJ, Paquette-Lamontagne N, Davis T, Weetall M, Babiak J, Miller LL. Phase 1 studies assessing the safety, PK, and VEGF-modulating effects of PTC299, a novel VEGF expression inhibitor. J Clin Oncol (Meeting Abstracts) 2007;25(18 suppl):Abstr 3562.

CHAPTER 2

PROTEIN KINASE STRUCTURE, FUNCTION, AND REGULATION

Understanding the molecular basis for activation, regulation, and inhibition of protein kinases is of paramount importance, not only in dissecting the role of various kinases in cancer but also for the design of kinase inhibitors. Over the past 15–20 years a vast body of structural data has been generated, mainly from X-ray crystallography, with additional contributions from NMR spectroscopy and other biophysical techniques. These studies have proved tremendously useful, even though, in most cases, they are of necessity based on somewhat artificial systems: the protein expression constructs used may not correspond to the complete, intact native protein, crystallization may occur only under distinctly nonphysiological conditions, and crystal packing interactions may suggest adventitious interactions that are not relevant in the native cellular environment. Nevertheless, in many cases site-directed mutagenesis studies and biochemical analyses have provided complementary support for structure-based hypotheses, and collectively these data have helped to illuminate many of the diverse structural and mechanistic features of protein kinases.

We begin this chapter by considering the interaction of native protein ligands with the extracellular receptor domains of receptor tyrosine kinases. Structural studies with many of these receptors, ligands, and receptor:ligand complexes have revealed a diverse range of binding mechanisms, which have obvious implications for the development of biotherapeutic agents targeting the kinase extracellular domains. The remainder of the chapter is focused on the structure, catalytic function, and diverse regulatory mechanisms of protein kinase domains. The critical role played by kinases in signal transduction requires that their activity must be exquisitely controlled, and we explore some of the more important mechanisms employed by protein kinases to upregulate and downregulate their activity, with particular reference to kinases that are implicated in the initiation and progression of cancer. Understanding protein kinase catalytic machinery and regulatory mechanisms has been, and continues to be, important for the design of small molecule kinase inhibitors. This theme is further developed in Chapter 7, where we consider some of the binding modes employed by such inhibitors.

2.1   LIGAND BINDING TO RECEPTOR TYROSINE KINASES

Receptor tyrosine kinases (RTKs) are one of the most important and widely studied kinase families and perform the critical function of transducing signals from extracellular ligands to diverse intracellular signaling pathways (1). The domain structures of selected RTKs are shown in Figure 1.4. Each receptor comprises an extracellular ligand binding domain, a single transmembrane region, and an intracellular kinase domain. The extracellular domains are highly diverse in both sequence and structure and employ a diverse range of structural motifs to bind an equally diverse range of ligands. In most instances, ligand binding leads to receptor aggregation (frequently dimerization, although higher order aggregates are also known to occur). The exact molecular mechanism whereby ligand binding translates into activation of intracellular domains remains somewhat obscure, although in a few cases structural studies have supported some promising hypotheses. In some cases, a simple increase in local receptor density may be sufficient to promote phosphorylation and activation of intracellular domains, although some studies indicate that, at least for some RTKs, the precise disposition of one receptor relative to another is of paramount importance in the activation process. Ligand binding may also promote a substantial change in receptor structure, which may be necessary for signal transduction. Indeed, in the case of insulin and insulin-like growth factor signaling the receptors appear to exist as covalently crosslinked, preformed dimers on the cell surface, such that ligand binding does not promote receptor aggregation and activation occurs via another mechanism.

2.1.1   EGF:EGF Receptor Interactions

The epidermal growth factor receptors, comprising the eponymous EGF receptor (EGFR/HER1/ERBB1) and related family members HER2/ERBB2, HER3/ERBB3, and HER4/ERBB4, are strongly implicated in the pathogenesis of multiple tumor types (Chapter 3). There also exists a wealth of structural data on the extracellular domains of these receptors, illuminating the mechanism of their ligand-mediated activation. X-ray crystal structures are available for the extracellular domains of EGFR, ERBB2, ERBB3, and ERBB4 in various states of activation and with various ligands. Further structural studies of these receptors in complex with therapeutic antibodies have shown how these molecules achieve their therapeutic effects and provided additional insight into receptor function (2).

The EGF receptor extracellular region comprises four distinct, heavily glycosylated domains, arranged as a tandem repeat of L (large, or leucine-rich repeat) and CR (cysteine-rich) domains (2, 3). Receptor dimerization appears to be critical for activation, although higher order complexes may also be involved (4). Ligands (e.g., EGF or TGFα) bind the receptor in a 2:2 stoichiometry, with the two L domains in each receptor chain comprising a discontinuous ligand binding site. As depicted in Figure 2.1A, the ligands do not participate in receptor dimerization, which is largely mediated by one of the CR domains (CR1) from each receptor. The CR1 domains possess a hairpin loop known as the "dimerization arm," each of which

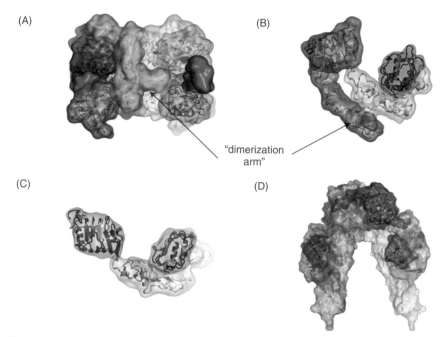

Figure 2.1   EGFR and IGFR structures. (A) Complex between EGF and the EGFR extracellular domain. Two EGF molecules interact with two receptors. Receptor L domains are shown in dark blue (receptor 1) and dark green (receptor 2), and the CR1 domains are shown in cyan (receptor 1) and yellow (receptor 2). Most of the CR2 domain is not present in the crystallized protein. The two EGF ligands (red) bind on opposite sides of the dimeric complex, and the receptor:receptor interaction is mediated by the "dimerization arms" of the receptors. (PDB accession code 1IVO.) (B) Inactive conformation of EGF receptor extracellular domain. The L domains are in blue and the CR1 domain is cyan; CR2 is shown in orange. The dimerization arm of CR1 interacts with the CR2 domain, blocking receptor activation. (PDB accession code 1NQL.) (C) The first three domains of the IGF1 receptor are shown in similar orientation to the EGFR inactive conformation (compare with panel B). Coloring of the L1, CR1, and L2 domains is as for EGFR in panel B. (PDB accession code 1IGR.) (D) Structure of the insulin receptor ectodomain dimer. The two monomers in the crystal structure both contain L1, CR1, and L2 domains as well as three FNIII domains. In one monomer, the L and CR domains are colored as in panel C, with the FNIII domains in green; in the other monomer, the L, CR, and FNIII domains are red, orange, and yellow, respectively. Insulin is thought to bind at the interface between the L1 domain from one monomer and the FNIII domains of the other monomer. (PDB accession code 2DTG.)

interacts with the CR1 domain in its dimeric partner. These dimerization arms serve a dual purpose, since in the inactive, monomeric form of the receptor they interact with the CR2 domain and stabilize the inactive conformation (Figure 2.1B). This inactive conformation has been observed for EGFR (5), ERBB3 (6), and ERBB4 (7). Although the inactive form predominates in the ensemble of inactive receptors, sampling of alternative conformations (including the active state) is likely to occur. However, EGFR mutants wherein the CR1-CR2 domain interaction is disrupted are not constitutively active, and ligand engagement appears to be necessary to stabilize the active conformation and promote intracellular signaling (2, 8). Although there are no structures of the complexes between the ERBB3/ERBB4 receptors and their ligands, mutagenesis and proteolytic fragmentation studies suggest that the binding of cognate ligands (neuregulins) to these receptors is somewhat different from the EGF:EGFR complex, with more prominent contacts involving the receptor L1 domain (9, 10).

HER2/ERBB2 differs from the other three EGF receptors in that it has no cognate ligand: hence ERBB2 signaling is dependent on formation of heterodimeric complexes with other EGFR family members. Structural studies have shown that this is because the CR2 domain cannot sequester the CR1 dimerization arm, and the two L domains interact with each other directly, occluding the ligand binding site that is found in EGFR (Figure 2.1A,B). The CR1 domains of ERBB2 show little propensity to dimerize, possibly due to repulsion between the ERBB2 CR1 domains. Thus the receptor constitutively adopts a more active-like conformation that is primed for dimerization, providing an explanation for why ERBB2 is such a potent activator of EGFR family signaling and a preferred binding partner for other family members (11–13).

X-ray crystal structures have been solved for several antibody:ERBB receptor complexes. These structures include therapeutic antibodies that have been evaluated for oncology indications in the clinic and have revealed quite distinct mechanisms of action for each antibody. The anti-EGFR antibody cetuximab (Erbitux®) binds to the L2 domain of EGF receptor and directly competes for ligand binding (14). In contrast, the anti-ERBB2 antibody pertuzumab (Omnitarg®) interacts with the CR1 domain and sterically blocks receptor dimerization (12). In the case of trastuzumab (Herceptin®), the antibody epitope is located in the CR2 domain and does not appear to have a direct role in either blocking ligand binding or preventing receptor dimerization (11). In this case, mechanisms such as receptor endocytosis or antibody-mediated cytotoxicity are likely to make substantial contributions to efficacy.

2.1.2 Insulin:Insulin Receptor and IGF1:IGF1R

In contrast to other RTKs discussed in this chapter, where ligand engagement results in receptor aggregation, insulin and insulin-like growth factor 1 (IGF1) receptors exist on the cell surface as preformed dimers. The insulin/IGF1 receptor extracellular domains bear some resemblance to those of the EGF family receptors, although the mechanism of receptor activation appears to be quite distinct (15, 16). Like EGFR, the insulin/IGF1 receptor extracellular domain comprises two L domains,

L1 and L2, separated by a cysteine-rich (CR) domain; however, the second CR domain found in the EGF receptors is replaced by the first of the three fibronectin type III (FnIII) domains in insulin/IGF1 receptor. The second FnIII domain encompasses a proteolytic site, cleavage of which produces the α ectodomain (N-terminal fragment) and the membrane-spanning β chain (C-terminal fragment) (Figure 1.4). Disulfide bridges are found within the FnIII domains, connecting the α and β chains and also linking the α chains together, thus producing preassembled dimers on the cell surface (17). The structure of the IGF1R ectodomain provided some initial clues as to how IGF1 may interact with the receptor (18). In the crystal structure, the L1-CR-L2 domains adopt a "question mark" conformation, somewhat reminiscent of the first three domains in the inactive EGFR structure (Figure 2.1C). The L1 and CR domains have an extensive interface and are likely to form a rigid structure: however, CR and L2 are connected by a more flexible linker region, which may serve to encapsulate the ligand. Mutagenesis and domain swapping studies subsequently identified the L1 and CR regions as being important mediators of ligand binding (19–22). More recently, the structure of the L1-CR-L2 domains of the insulin receptor have provided further insight into how insulin/IGF specificity may be determined, with the conformation of F39 in the L1 domain of the insulin receptor and a loop within the CR domain playing important roles (23). Finally, the crystal structure of the entire dimeric insulin receptor ectodomain has been solved, revealing that the L1-CR-L2 ensemble of each monomer folds back on the fibronectin domains of the adjacent monomer to form a double inverted "V" shape (Figure 2.1D) (24). Although some ambiguities remain to be resolved, this structure is consistent with several features of insulin binding and a model of the insulin:IR ectodomain interaction has been proposed, providing a potential molecular explanation for the negative cooperativity observed for binding of insulin to its receptor (24).

2.1.3   FGF:FGF Receptor (Heparin/Heparan Sulfate) Interactions

Several structures of fibroblast growth factors (FGFs) in complex with their receptors (FGFRs) have revealed the molecular mechanism of receptor binding and also illuminated the role of heparin/heparan sulfate proteoglycans in regulating FGF/FGFR signaling. The FGFR extracellular region is comprised of three Ig-like domains (Figure 1.4), of which domains 2 and 3 are most important for ligand binding and on which structural studies have focused. The structures of FGF1:FGFR2 (25), FGF1:FGFR1 (26), and FGF2:FGFR2 (26) all show that FGF binds at the junction of immunoglobulin (Ig) domains 2 and 3, involving residues from both domains and the interdomain linker (Figure 2.2A). Structures of FGF:FGFR in complex with heparin (27, 28) led to two alternative (and possibly coexisting) models for assembly of the signaling complex (29). However, more recent data appears to support the "two-end" model, wherein two 1:1 FGF:FGFR complexes form a back-to-back symmetrical complex with the FGF moieties facing outwards from the receptor:receptor interface (30, 31). The proteoglycan moieties in the structure occupy a basic groove formed by the surfaces of both FGF and domain D2 of the receptor, acting cooperatively with the growth factor and receptor to assemble the active signaling complex and providing an additional level of specificity and functional control (32). Binding of both FGF and heparin-derived oligosaccharides may also be negatively regulated by the presence of N-glycosylation on the receptor (33).

2.1.4 VEGF:VEGF Receptor Interactions

Vascular endothelial growth factor (VEGF) and its various cell surface receptors are key modulators of tumor angiogenesis (Chapter 3). The anti-VEGF antibody bevacizumab (Avastin®) has been instrumental in demonstrating the potential benefit of antiangiogenic therapy for cancer treatment, and a multitude of small molecule VEGF receptor kinase inhibitors have also been developed (discussed in Chapter 9). The VEGF ligand adopts an antiparallel homodimeric structure, with each monomer comprised largely of β strands and stabilized by a disulfide knot motif (34, 35). In addition to the intramolecular disulfide knot, two symmetrically disposed intermolecular disulfide bridges link the monomers together. Mutagenesis studies demonstrated that the key residues in VEGF for binding to VEGFR2 are located at either end of the dimeric ligand, suggesting that the ligand promotes symmetric or pseudosymmetric dimerization of the receptor. The extracellular domain of each of the three VEGF receptors (VEGFR1, VEGFR2, and VEGFR3) is comprised of seven immunoglobulin-like (Ig) domains. The structure of VEGF in complex with one of the Ig domains from VEGFR1 supports this hypothesis (36). In this structure, each end of the dimeric VEGF ligand interacts with VEGFR1 Ig domain 2 (Figure 2.2C). (Domain 2 was shown to contain the major determinants for VEGF binding, although domain 3 is also likely to be involved.) Based on homology and mutagenesis data, binding of VEGF to VEGFR2 is proposed to be similar. The structure of placental growth factor (PlGF) bound to VEGFR1 has also been determined and is globally similar to the VEGF:VEGFR1 structure (37); however, mutagenesis studies suggest that, in contrast to VEGF, glycosylation may be important in mediating PlGF binding (38). Also, the platelet-derived growth factors (PDGFs) are structurally similar to VEGF and the PDGF receptor extracellular regions contain five Ig domains, suggesting that a similar dimerization pattern may occur in this case.

2.1.5 Angiopoietin2:TIE2 Receptor Interactions

The TIE2 receptor and its ligands, the angiopoietins (ANGs), are important in both developmental and tumor-associated angiogenesis. TIE2 comprises three epidermal growth factor (EGF) domains, three immunoglobulin (Ig) domains, and three fibronectin type III domains (Figure 1.4), of which the Ig and EGF domains have been implicated in ligand binding (39, 40). The angiopoietins each contain an N-terminal domain implicated in ligand clustering, a coiled coil domain, and a C-terminal fibrinogen-like region that binds the TIE2 receptor (41, 42). The crystal structure of the TIE2 extracellular domain (excluding the FnIII domains) shows that the two N-terminal Ig domains and the EGF domains pack together into a roughly conical shape, which in turn packs against the third Ig domain (43). The

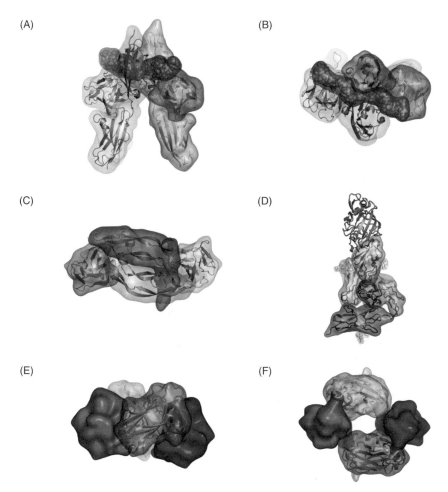

Figure 2.2   Receptor tyrosine kinase ligand interactions. (A) Interaction of FGF2 with
FGFR1; side view (with the cell membrane toward the bottom of the figure). FGF2
(orange) binds at the junction of two Ig domains in each of the receptor chains (teal and
green). Two heparan sulfate molecules are shown in red CPK rendering. (PDB accession
code 1FQ9.) (B) View from the top of the FGF2:FGFR1 complex (i.e., looking toward the
cell surface) shows the cooperative assembly of two receptor Ig domains, two FGF2
ligands, and two proteoglycan moieties. Coloring is as for panel A. (C) The VEGF dimer
is depicted in red and orange: the VEGFR1 receptor Ig domains are in blue and green. The
top view is shown, that is, looking from above the complex toward the cell surface. (PDB
accession code 1FLT.) (D) ANG2:TIE2 complex. The receptor binding domain of ANG2
is shown in red: the three EGF-like domains of TIE2 are green and the TIE2 Ig domain is
shown in blue. ANG2 binding is mediated largely via the second EGF domain. Several
N-linked carbohydrates are also visible in the structure, shown in ball-and-stick rendering.
(PDB accession code 2GY7.) (E) Ephrin B2:EPHB2 receptor complex. The ephrin ligands
(red) and EPH receptors (teal and green) form a tetrameric assembly. The side view is
shown, with the C-terminal tails of the receptors pointing down (i.e., toward the cell
membrane). (PDB accession code 1KGY.) (F) Top view of the ephrin B2:EPHB2 receptor
complex, showing the pseudosymmetric arrangement of the ligands and receptors.
Coloring is as for panel E.

fibrinogen-like region of ANG2 binds to the second Ig domain of TIE2 with 1:1 stoichiometry, and receptor aggregation is achieved via the tetrameric or higher order multimeric state of the ANG2 ligands (41, 42, 44) (Figure 2.2D).

2.1.6 Ephrin:EPH Receptor Interactions

EPH receptors (EPHRs) comprise the largest subfamily of tyrosine kinase receptors and, together with their cognate ligands (ephrins), play an important role in cell boundary formation, cell movement, and tissue morphogenesis (45). Ephrin:EPHR complexes are unique among the examples in this section, in that both receptor and ligand are membrane-tethered proteins. Furthermore, there is evidence that ephrin/EPH receptor signaling is bidirectional, so that EPH receptors can act as ligands for ephrins as well as vice versa. Biophysical studies have suggested that receptor aggregation is a multistep process, involving initial formation of ephrin:EPH complexes and subsequent aggregation into tetrameric complexes. The X-ray crystal structure of the EPHB2 receptor and ephrin B2 extracellular domains (46) shows that the tetramers form a ring-like structure, with the C termini of the ephrins on one side of the ring and the C termini of the EPHRs on the other. This arrangement is physiologically plausible, in that the ephrins and EPHRs may interact while being anchored in neighboring cells (Figure 2.2E,F). The ephrin extracellular domains adopt a "Greek key" β-barrel fold, whereas the EPHR globular domain has a "jelly roll" β-sandwich structure, reminiscent of several carbohydrate binding proteins. In addition to the globular domain, the EPHR extracellular region comprises a cysteine-rich linker and two fibronectin type III domains. Hence there is likely to be a sizeable spacer region between the ephrin:EPHR interface and the EPHR cell membrane. The crystal structure of EPHB4, a family member that may have particular relevance to cancer biology, has also been solved in complex with ephrin B2 (47).

2.1.7 The Role of Transmembrane Domains

Compared to studies with extracellular receptor domains and intracellular kinase domains, the transmembrane domains of receptor tyrosine kinases have received scant attention. However, these integral receptor components may play a significant role in both normal and pathological signaling (48). The *Neu* oncogene (encoding the rat homolog of ERBB2) provided some of the first evidence for the potential role of transmembrane domains in oncogenic receptor activation. Mutations of V664 in the transmembrane region of *Neu* were found to promote constitutive receptor aggregation and activation (49, 50), and similar polymorphisms of the human ERBB2 (I654V and V655I) may be associated with increased and decreased risk of breast cancer, respectively (51, 52). Additionally, there is evidence that EGF receptors may exist as preformed dimers on the cell surface, and that the relative orientation of the transmembrane domains plays a key role in activation (53). Indeed, computational modeling of ERBB2 transmembrane dimers suggests that two stable conformations are possible (54), and that transition between these arrangements is feasible (55). As a further example, multiple mutations in the transmembrane region of FGFR3 have been associated with bladder cancer (56).

2.2 PROTEIN KINASE DOMAIN STRUCTURE AND FUNCTION

The first kinase domain structure to be determined by X-ray crystallography (in 1991) was that of a serine/threonine kinase, protein kinase A (PKA) (57), and in 1994 the first receptor tyrosine kinase structure (human insulin receptor kinase, IR) was reported (58). Since then, over 800 kinase structures have been deposited in the protein data bank (PDB), representing various activation states, structural forms, and complexes with at least 140 distinct kinase domains. These structures include representatives from all of the major protein kinase families, providing insight into their many similarities and differences. (In addition, there are undoubtedly thousands of additional structures of drug-like molecules in complex with various kinases in the proprietary archives of various drug discovery companies.) Our initial overview of kinase structure focuses on IR; the major structural and functional features described are broadly conserved in other serine/threonine and tyrosine kinases.

Protein kinase domains are comprised of two subdomains or lobes (Figure 2.3). The N-terminal subdomain is dominated by a series of β strands (often folded into an orthogonal barrel-like structure), with at least one absolutely conserved α helix. The C-terminal lobe varies in size, sequence, and topology but is larger than the N-terminal domain and predominantly α-helical. (In PKA and several other members of the AGC kinase family, a C-terminal tail traces around the outside of the kinase domain and interacts with a hydrophobic region

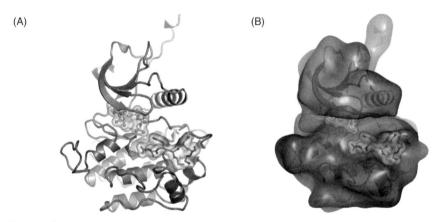

(A)   (B)

Figure 2.3 Global features of insulin receptor kinase domain structure. (A) The N-terminal lobe (olive) contains mostly β-strand structures, with one prominent α helix. The C-terminal lobe (teal) is predominantly α-helical and connects to the N-terminal lobe via a linker, or hinge region. ATP (shown in ball-and-stick rendering) binds at the junction between the two lobes, and the substrate peptide (red) is located on a "platform" formed by components of the C-terminal domain. (PDB accession code 1IR3.) (B) Surface representation of the insulin receptor kinase domain, showing ATP buried in the cleft between the two lobes and the substrate peptide binding site in the C-terminal domain. The color scheme is as in panel A.

in the N-terminal domain.) A short polypeptide chain (commonly referred to as the linker, or hinge region) connects the two domains. This linker region is a key element of the ATP nucleotide binding site, which lies in a cleft formed at the junction of the N- and C-terminal lobes. (This cleft is somewhat deeper in tyrosine kinases compared to serine/threonine kinases, consistent with accommodation of the longer tyrosine side chain.) The adenosine moiety of ATP generally forms two hydrogen bonds with main chain atoms in the linker region, and the nucleotide also interacts with a glycine-rich, phosphate binding loop (sometimes called the P-loop) that borders the N-terminal β-strand region (Figure 2.4B,C, and D). Immediately N-terminal to the linker sequence is an amino acid residue commonly referred to as the "gatekeeper" residue. This amino acid (methionine in IR) varies between kinases but is usually somewhat bulky (never glycine or alanine). The gatekeeper residue is an important determinant of the size of the ATP binding site and is particularly relevant to the binding and specificity of small molecule kinase inhibitors (described in Chapter 7). The side chain of the residue following the gatekeeper is directed away from the ATP binding site but may play an important role in regulating the activation of several kinases, including FGF, VEGF, and PDGF receptors (Figure 2.4E). This residue (Glu in many receptor tyrosine kinases) forms a conserved hydrogen bond network with several neighboring residues that has been proposed to stabilize the unphosphorylated state, serving as a "molecular brake" and restraining the structural plasticity necessary for activation, thereby reducing inappropriate kinase activity (59).

Due to its critical role in binding and orienting ATP, it is not surprising that the backbone conformation in the linker region is virtually identical in almost all known kinases. Notable exceptions are the PIM kinases, in which a two residue insertion and a unique proline residue introduce a prominent kink in the linker region. The structure of PIM1 in complex with an ATP analog shows that the ATP binding site is substantially enlarged, and the ATP adenosine interaction with the linker region is missing one of the hydrogen bonds that is present in other structures (60–62). The PIM kinases appear to compensate for the lost H-bond through an enhanced K_M for ATP, driven largely by electrophilic residues surrounding the phosphate binding site. Although almost all kinases employ ATP as the source of phosphate groups, it is worth noting that a few kinases, for example, CK2 (formerly known as casein kinase), can also use GTP. The structures of CK2 with ATP and GTP reveals that a water molecule may participate in hydrogen bonding between the GTP carbonyl moiety and a carbonyl of the enzyme backbone, in place of the exocyclic amine of ATP, which binds to the same backbone residue (63). The physiological relevance of this mechanism, however, is not clear.

The conserved α helix in the N-terminal domain, termed the C helix, is an important regulator of activation. (The name "C helix" derives from the fact that PKA, the first protein kinase structure to be solved, has two additional helices (A and B) located N-terminal to the C helix: however, most kinases lack these additional helices.) Firstly, the C helix contributes a glutamate residue, the side chain of which forms an ion pair interaction with a lysine residue in a neighboring β strand (in IR, these residues are E1047 and K1030, respectively). This ion pair interaction is critical for maintaining the proper conformation and function of the kinase

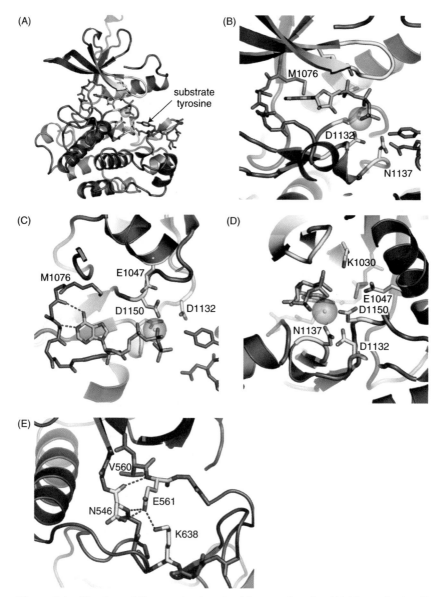

Figure 2.4 Structure of the receptor tyrosine kinase active site. (A) The entire insulin receptor kinase domain in complex with an ATP analog, Mg^{2+} ion and peptide substrate; (B) the active site is expanded. (C) A $90°$ rotation about the horizontal axis relative to (B); (D) a $90°$ rotation about the vertical axis relative to (B). The substrate peptide is in red, with the phospho-acceptor tyrosine pointing toward the catalytic site. Key catalytic Asp and Asn residues and the Glu-Lys ion pair are in yellow, and the Mg^{2+} ion is represented by a transparent sphere; the main chain of the "linker region" is shown in stick representation. (PDB accession code 1IR3.) (E) Three residues on the "back side" of the ATP binding pocket may act as a molecular brake to restrain kinase activation. In FGFR1, the gatekeeper residue is V560 (shown in orange). E561 forms a hydrogen bond network with N546 and K638, which is hypothesized to impair activation. Note that in the PDB file the numbering differs by one, for example, the gatekeeper residue is V561. (PDB accession code 1FGK.)

active site and also plays a role in stabilizing and orienting the phosphate groups of ATP (Figure 2.4). Several important kinase regulatory mechanisms, discussed later, involve the formation or disruption of this interaction by displacement of the C helix.

The C-terminal lobe of the kinase domain is responsible for substrate binding, and many structures of different kinases are now available with a peptide bound in the substrate binding groove. The C-terminal domain also contributes some of the key residues involved in catalysis. In particular, substrate phosphorylation is critically dependent on an aspartate residue (D1132 in IR), which interacts with the target —OH. The catalytic aspartate is stabilized and oriented by a neighboring residue (IR N1137) which, together with a second aspartate residue (IR D1150), chelates a divalent cation associated with ATP. The second aspartate residue (IR D1150) marks the start of the kinase activation segment, a regulatory sequence of 20–35 residues starting with the consensus sequence DFG. . . and ending with . . .APE. As the name suggests, the conformation of this region plays a critical role in regulating the activation state of many kinases. Kinase activation often involves phosphorylation of one or more residues in a loop within this region, promoting a structural rearrangement in the activation segment (Section 2.4.1). The active conformation moves key residues into the optimal configuration for catalysis, removes steric hinderance from the ATP and/or substrate binding sites, and, together with additional residues from the C-terminal domain, helps to form a "platform" for substrate binding and orientation. Notably, the overall conformation of the activation segment is quite similar in all active structures that have been determined, although the unactivated conformations vary widely (64). The activation loop is also a key determinant of binding for many small molecule inhibitors: while many inhibitors target the activated form of the kinase, several bind preferentially (and in some cases exclusively) to the inactive form, thereby preventing activation. In cases where the inhibitor exclusively targets the inactive form of the kinase, a relatively high degree of specificity for the kinase may be achieved since the inactive conformations are less well conserved than the active, catalytically competent conformations. However, mutations that increase the propensity of the activation loop to adopt the active conformation may confer resistance to such inhibitors. In fact, such mutations have been discovered both in the laboratory and in the clinic: this issue is revisited in later chapters.

Several receptor tyrosine kinases, collectively referred to as split kinase domain kinases, have an inserted sequence of approximately 70 additional residues (the kinase insert domain, or KID) between two of the helices in the C-terminal domain. These kinases include the VEGF and PDGF receptors, as well as KIT and CSF1R. The inserted sequence does not appear to be critical for catalytic activity but may contribute to receptor turnover and interactions with partner proteins (65–68). The structures of the VEGFR2, KIT, and CSF1R kinase domains have been determined (69–71), although in each case the KID was excised from the protein in order to facilitate crystallization. However, the TIE2 structure (see Figure 2.9) has been solved with an intact kinase insert domain (72).

The many kinase crystal structures solved to date, including multiple conformational and activation states of the same enzyme, have revealed a high degree of flexibility in the kinase domain. This structural plasticity is important for regulation of catalytic activity and is likely shared to some degree by all members of the protein kinase superfamily (73). In particular, the transition from inactive to active kinase results in a profound rearrangement of the activation segment, helix C and, in some cases, the relative orientation of the N- and C-terminal lobes (described earlier and in Section 2.4). The structural mobility is likely to be important not only for a switch-like transformation from the inactive to active state, but for the catalytic process itself.

2.3   CATALYTIC ACTIVITY OF PROTEIN KINASES

Protein kinases catalyze the transfer of the γ-phosphate of ATP to the hydroxyl acceptor group on either a tyrosine, serine, or threonine residue in the substrate protein (Figure 2.5). Many of the fundamental insights into protein kinase chemistry and enzymology were initially derived from studies on cAMP-dependent protein kinase (PKA), and much of our discussion (particularly with reference to the chemistry of protein phosphorylation and the role of different active site residues in catalysis) focuses on this enzyme. Due to the considerable conservation of both structure and key amino acid residues in the active site, the general mechanistic principles are likely to be conserved across the superfamily. In contrast, kinetic analyses have shown that the relative substrate binding affinities and catalytic efficiencies may differ considerably between kinases: for example, the Michaelis constant for ATP (K_M^{ATP}) varies over at least three orders of magnitude, from ~1 nM to ~1000 nM (74). Such variability is also reflected in the high diversity of substrate specificity between different kinases, consistent with the broad range of cellular substrates and functions that they modify.

2.3.1   Steady State Kinetics

There are numerous examples of kinetic characterization of protein kinases: readers are referred to the online supplement of reference 74, which contains a helpful list of references to studies with almost 100 protein kinases. In general, the precise reaction scheme (in terms of order of binding and release of substrates and products) may vary between different members of the kinase superfamily. Initial studies with PKA demonstrated a random bi-bi mode of substrate binding; that is, either ATP or peptide/protein may bind first, and both remain bound during the conversion to ADP and phosphorylated peptide (75–77). However, due to the high intracellular concentration of ATP (1–5 mM, substantially greater than most active kinase K_M values) and relatively low intracellular abundance of substrates, mass action dictates that many if not most reactions are likely to involve ATP binding first, followed by engagement of the peptide/protein substrate and subsequent catalysis. Product release appears to be ordered in the case of PKA, with the phosphopeptide dissociating first followed by ADP (78). In general, however, the relative binding order and contribution of each step in the reaction to the overall rate may vary from kinase to kinase. Several studies with various kinases other

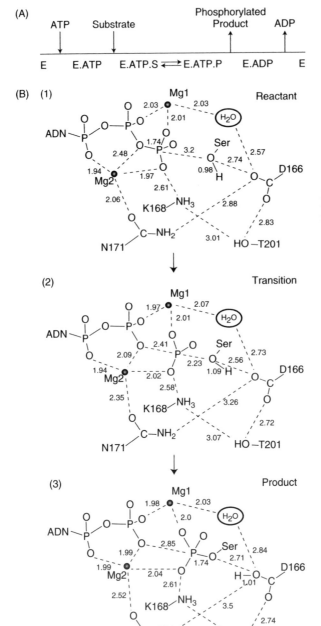

Figure 2.5 The protein kinase phosphoryltransfer reaction. (A) General scheme for the protein kinase catalytic reaction. E, enzyme; S, peptide substrate; P, phosphorylated product. The reaction scheme indicates that ATP binds before substrate, and product is released before ADP: although this has been shown to be true for many kinases, some reactions may involve a different order of binding and release. (B) Structures of (1) reactant, (2) transition state, and (3) product as determined from quantum mechanical/molecular mechanics simulation. Numbers indicate optimized bond lengths for the respective structures. ADN; adenosine. Reproduced with permission from (88). Copyright © 2007 American Chemical Society.

than PKA have also suggested an ordered bi-bi mechanism, with either ATP or peptide binding first. Also, for some enzymes there is strong evidence to suggest that product release is rate limiting, whereas in other cases phosphoryl transfer and product release appear to have more similar rate constants (79). A general reaction scheme is shown in Figure 2.5A.

Most kinases phosphorylate either serine/threonine residues or tyrosine residues, although several "dual specificity" kinases have also been identified. In the case of Ser/Thr kinases, there appears to be an overall preference for serine over threonine in the cellular environment (80). The primary substrate recognition sites typically extend to three or four residues on the N-terminal and/or C-terminal side of the Ser/Thr/Tyr phospho-acceptor residue, and investigations of both known substrates and peptide libraries have helped to define the consensus sequences for many important kinases (Table 2.1). For reasons of experimental tractability, most enzymological characterization of protein kinases has been performed using model peptide substrates, which can readily be quantitated in both substrate and product form. However, most phosphorylation reactions in the cellular environment involve extended protein substrates, which may also interact with the kinase in regions that are distal from the catalytic center. Such interactions may help to direct the kinase toward specific cellular substrates, serve to increase the local substrate concentration at the active site, or enable allosteric control of kinase activation. The structural features contributing to protein kinase substrate specificity have been comprehensively reviewed in (96).

2.3.2   Chemistry of Protein Kinase Catalysis

The reaction path for protein kinase-mediated catalysis has been studied using a variety of experimental and theoretical techniques, and some general properties of the mechanism can be inferred. For an extensive discussion of protein kinase chemistry (with specific emphasis on the mechanism of PKA), the reader is referred to reference 79, which provides an excellent overview.

The role of the catalytic aspartate residue has been the subject of particularly close scrutiny, with the initial analysis of PKA providing many key insights. Structural studies of PKA in complex with ADP and a substrate peptide showed clear evidence for hydrogen bond formation between the catalytic D166 carboxylate and the substrate serine hydroxyl Oγ, suggesting a role for D166 as a catalytic base (97); a similar interaction was observed in the crystal structure of PKA in complex with a transition state analog (98). In contrast, various mechanistic studies indicated that the D166 side chain is not sufficiently basic to accept the hydroxyl proton, leading to the idea that the D166 side chain plays more of a structural role, orienting the substrate —OH toward the ATP γ-phosphate (99, 100). Quantum mechanical calculations and molecular dynamics simulations have provided additional insight into the mechanism and offered a potential explanation for these differences (101–103). Furthermore, results from the most recent and most comprehensive simulation are in good concordance with empirical data (103). In these models, the D166 carboxylate is proposed to act as a proton acceptor late in the reaction process, after the ATP γ-phosphate:serine Oγ bond is substantially formed

TABLE 2.1 Substrate Specificity for Selected Protein Kinases[a]

Kinase	Motif	Reference
Abl	EAI**Y***AAPF	81
	EEI**Y***EEPY	81
	EXI**Y***XXPX	81
	EEI**Y***YYVH	81
	ERI**Y***ARTK	81
	[IVL]**Y***XX[PF]	82
	AEV[ILVF]**Y***AA[PF]F	83
CAMKII	RXX[**ST***]	82
	RXX[**ST***]V	82
CDK2–cyclin A	[**ST***]PX[RK]	82
CK1	**S***(P)XX[**ST***]	82
CK2	[**ST***]XXE	82
CSK	EE[DE]I**Y***FFFF	84
Dual specificity MAPK	**T***X**Y***	85
EGFR	[EDRA][ED][ED]EDI]**Y***[FVIE][EF][LIFV]V	86
	X[ED]**Y***X	82
	Y*IPP	87
ERK	PX[**ST***]P	82
	XX[**ST***]P	88
FGFR	A[EA]EE**Y***FV]F[LFMIV]F	86
GSK3	**S***XXX**S***(P)	82
IR	**Y***MXM	89
	EE[END]**Y***[MF][MF][MFIE][MF]	86
JAK2	**Y***XX[LIV]	90
JNK	**T***P**Y***	91
LCK	EX[IVLF]**Y***[GA]V[LVFI][FLVI]	86
PDGFR	[LN][RI]T**Y***	92
	[ED][ED][ED][ED]**Y***[VEI]F[IVF]	86
PKA	RX[**ST***]R[RK]X[**ST***]	82
SRC	D[EC][EDG][IVL]**Y***[GE]E [FI]F	86
SRC family kinase	TX**Y***XXVI	93
v-SRC	[ED][ED][EDG][IVL]**Y***[GED]E[FILV]	86
SRC family kinase "ITAM motif"	[ED]XXXXXXX[ED]XX**Y***XXLXXXX	94
SRC family kinase "ITIM motif"	[IVLS]X**Y***XX[LI]	95
SRC family kinase "ITSM motif"	TX**Y***XX[VI]	(93, 95)

[a]Bold letters with the asterisk refer to the phosphorylated amino acid; letters in square brackets indicate either/or. Abbreviations: A, alanine; R, arginine; N, asparagine; D, aspartic acid; C, cysteine; E, glutamine; G, glycine; H, histidine; I, isoleucine; L, leucine; K, lysine; M, methionine; F, phenylalanine; P, proline; S, serine; T, threonine; W, tryptophan; Y, tyrosine; V, valine; X, any amino acid.

(Figure 2.5B). Furthermore, the protonated D166 carboxylate may act to promote product release at the end of the reaction cycle by transferring the proton to the phosphate on the newly phosphorylated substrate peptide. These molecular simulation data, together with empirical evidence, also indicated that the catalytic mechanism exhibits more of a dissociative than associative character, meaning that the hydroxyl group of the substrate and the transferred phosphate do not make substantial bonds with each other before the leaving group (ADP) is released. There is also experimental evidence for a dissociative transition state in kinases other than PKA, including linear free energy relationships for phosphorylation of a series of fluorotyrosine peptides by the nonreceptor tyrosine kinase C-terminal SRC kinase (CSK) (104), structural and kinetic studies with the insulin receptor kinase (IR) and a tetrafluorotyrosine substrate (105), and structural and kinetic studies with CDK2/cyclin A and a nitrate transition state analog (106).

Several other residues in the kinase active site play critical roles in supporting catalysis, most of which are highly conserved across all kinases. In PKA, these residues include K72 (from the canonical Glu-Lys ion pair), which interacts with the α- and β-phosphates of ATP; K168, which is hydrogen bonded to the ATP γ-phosphate; and N171, which, together with a conserved water molecule, appears to help orient the catalytic D166. A high affinity divalent cation (usually Mg^{2+}) is also intimately involved in the catalytic process. This Mg^{2+} ion is most likely associated with ATP prior to binding of ATP at the active site, and in PKA it is coordinated by the side chain of D184 and the ATP β- and γ-phosphates (Figure 2.5B). This Mg^{2+} ion may be involved in maintaining the correct conformation of ATP and stabilizing charge transfer during the catalytic process. A second, lower affinity divalent cation is also observed in some high-resolution crystal structures and has also been inferred from metal ion titration studies. In PKA, this ligand is coordinated by the ATP α- and γ-phosphates and the D184/N171 side chains, and it appears to affect both k_{cat} (decreased in the presence of high Mg^{2+}) and K_M^{ATP} (increased in the presence of high Mg^{2+}). Recent calculations indicate that this second Mg^{2+} may act as a Lewis acid and attack the oxygen linkage between the β- and γ-phosphates (103), but the effect of metal ion binding at this site is not consistent between kinases. For example, Mg^{2+} titration studies with CSK, SRC, and FGFR have shown increased V_{max} and increased $K_M^{peptide}$ in the presence of high Mg^{2+} (107), and both FGFR and IR have decreased K_M^{ATP} in the presence of increasing Mg^{2+} (107, 108). Notably, the ATP conformation and its interaction with the second magnesium ion may be different in these other kinases: in the structure of FGFR2 the Mg^{2+}: ATP interaction is via the α- and β-phosphates rather than the β- and γ-phosphates (59).

2.4 PROTEIN KINASE REGULATION

Structural analyses of protein kinase domains in various states of phosphorylation and activation have indicated that the active conformations share many common features, including the conformation of the activation loop, formation of the conserved Glu-Lys ion pair interaction (and the associated positioning of the C helix), and the degree of openness of the catalytic cleft. However, there are many diverse means of downregulating and/or blocking kinase activity, and many kinases use various combinations of these mechanisms to regulate their function. Clearly, cell surface receptor kinases have a fundamental control mechanism involving ligand binding, as reviewed above: here, however, we concern ourselves with interactions proximal to and within the kinase domain itself. Several excellent reviews have surveyed the structural basis of protein kinase regulation, and the reader is referred to these for additional examples, references, and insight (64, 73, 109–111).

Perhaps the most common mechanism is phosphorylation of the activation segment, which is required for activation of many (but not all) kinases (Section 2.4.1). A diverse range of additional regulatory mechanisms has emerged from structural and mutagenesis studies. These include phosphorylation of regions outside (but adjacent to) the canonical kinase domain, steric and dynamic influence of distal domains within the same polypeptide chain, and interactions of the kinase domain with other polypeptide chains. In many cases, the regulatory peptides, domains, or proteins combine multiple functions into the same structural motif. For example, the regulatory domain may repress catalytic function in one conformational or phosphorylation state: in the alternate state, the kinase is activated and the regulatory domain also provides an additional function (such as providing a partner protein docking site or displaying a nuclear localization signal). Later, we consider several mechanisms associated with kinases that have N-terminal regulatory regions (FLT3, TGFβI, EPH receptors, and GSK3β) or C-terminal regulatory regions (MAPKAPK2 and TIE2). In many kinases, additional structural domains within the same polypeptide chain are found to regulate enzymatic activity. The multiple domains of SRC family kinases employ several interdependent mechanisms to govern kinase activity, and the recent structure of focal adhesion kinase (FAK) demonstrates how autoinhibition is achieved via its N-terminal domain. Finally, we consider the role of protein:protein interactions in modulating the activation state of protein kinase domains. Some of these mechanisms promote kinase activity, as in the case of the interaction of cyclins with cyclin-dependent kinase (CDK) domains and the asymmetric interactions that have been proposed to regulate EGF receptor activation. It should be noted that the various mechanisms listed here are by no means mutually exclusive: most kinases are subject to multiple regulatory mechanisms.

2.4.1 Regulation Via Activation Segment Phosphorylation

The phosphorylation and conformation of the activation segment region is centrally important to regulating the activity of many serine/theronine and tyrosine kinases (64). Almost all tyrosine kinases have between one and three tyrosine residues in their activation loops, and the combination of X-ray crystal structures and elegant biochemical and biophysical experiments have shed light on how some of these kinases regulate their activity by trans-autophosphorylation. As an illustrative example of activation segment phosphorylation, we revisit the structure of insulin receptor (IR); similar results have also been described for the insulin-like growth factor receptor (IGF1R) kinase (112–115).

The activation segment starts with a highly conserved "DFG" sequence, the "D" (aspartate) playing a key role in chelating a Mg^{2+} ion and orienting the ATP phosphates for catalysis. Many kinase structure conformations are described in terms of the orientation of the DFG peptide, particularly with respect to drug binding modes (Chapter 7). "DFG-in" or "Phe-in" refers to the active state, with the Asp residue positioned for catalysis and the Phe buried in a hydrophobic pocket below the C helix (Figure 2.6A). In the inactive ("DFG-out" or "Phe-out") structure of IR, the aspartate side chain of the DFG sequence at the start of the activation loop points away from the ATP adenosine binding site, and the adjacent phenylalanine can no longer be accommodated in the hydrophobic pocket between the C helix and the C-terminal lobe. Instead, the phenylalanine side chain rotates into the ATP binding pocket and the resulting displacement forces the C helix away from the active site, separating E1047 from its ion pair partner, K1030 (Figure 2.6B). (Other inactive kinase structures have shown the DFG peptide to be entirely inverted, with the phenylalanine side chain wholly exposed to solvent.) Next in the activation segment is a short peptide sequence, which forms a β strand in active kinases and couples the activation loop to the N-terminal side of the catalytic loop. This is followed by a loop region of variable sequence and length (the activation loop or

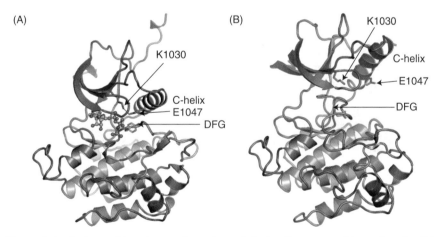

Figure 2.6 Active and inactive conformations of the insulin receptor kinase domain. (A) Active structure (PDB accession code 1IR3.) (B) Inactive structure (PDB accession code 1IRK.) The structures are shown in a similar orientation, aligned by residues in the C-terminal domain; the activation segments are in orange and ATP is shown in ball-and-stick representation in the active structure. Major structural transitions between the active and inactive conformations include repositioning of the activation segment (orange), including the "DFG" sequence to expose the active site cleft, rotation of the C helix toward the ATP/substrate binding site, and a coordinated "clamping" of the ATP binding site by the N-terminal domain.

T-loop), which is the most labile part of the activation region and, in kinases regulated by activation loop phosphorylation, contains the phosphate acceptor residues. Although the activation loops in active kinases follow broadly similar trajectories, the diverse lengths and sequences of these regions likely contribute to the distinct modes of activation and substrate specificities of each kinase.

In the unphosphorylated, unactivated structure of IR the activation segment fills the space normally occupied by the ATP phosphate groups in active kinase structures and also occludes the substrate binding region, thus inactivating the kinase (58). The kinase domain has three tyrosine residues in the activation loop, which are autophosphorylated in an ordered manner, with Y1162 followed by Y1158 followed by Y1163 (116) (Figure 2.7B). Phosphorylation results in destabilization of the autoinhibitory conformation and a dramatic rearrangement of the

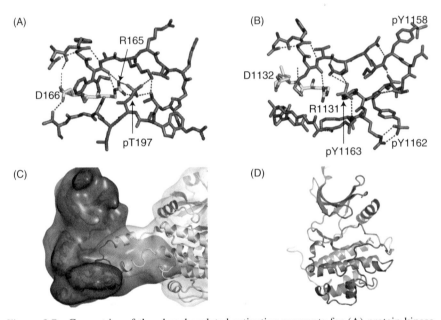

Figure 2.7 Geometries of the phosphorylated activation segments for (A) protein kinase A (PKA), (B) insulin receptor (IR), (C) CHK2, and (D) CHK1. Relative to the kinase domain orientation in Figure 2.4, this view is looking down on the activation segment from above. The RD dipeptide segment is shown in yellow and is situated below the activation segment. (A, B) The primary phosphorylation site (phosphothreonine in PKA, phosphotyrosine in IR) occupies a similar spatial region in each structure, although the hydrogen bond interactions vary. (PDB accession codes 1ATP and 1IR3.) (C) Structure of the CHK2 activation segment. Two CHK2 kinase domains are shown in teal and yellow. The extended activation loops from each domain form a pseudosymmetrical interaction with a neighboring molecule (highlighted in red). The conformation of the activation segment from the neighboring molecule mimics the intramolecular conformation of the activation segment in other active Ser/Thr kinases such as CHK1. (D) CHK1 is shown for comparison (in blue, with part of the activation segment highlighted in red). (PDB accession codes 2CN5 and 1IA8.)

activation segment, opening up the active site and enabling ATP and substrate binding. As discussed earlier, the DFG aspartate is repositioned such that it can interact with the ATP phosphates and the DFG phenylalanine side chain rotates through approximately $90°$, with concomitant repositioning of the C helix and formation of the canonical Glu-Lys ion pair. Interactions between activation loop residues and other elements of the kinase subsequently stabilize the active conformation. In particular, phospho-Y1162 (pY1162) interacts with R1164 and pY1163 interacts with R1155 within the activation loop; the activation segment is also anchored to elements in and around the catalytic loop in the C-terminal lobe (112). Of particular note, pY1163 also packs adjacent to R1131, which is the residue preceding the catalytic aspartate, D1132. This interaction between the activation loop phospho-acceptor site and a conserved basic pocket is a common feature of kinases that are regulated by activation loop phosphorylation. All kinases that are regulated by activation loop phosphorylation have an arginine before the catalytic aspartate and are termed "RD kinases" (111); however, not all RD kinases are subject to activation loop phospho-regulation. This relationship holds for both serine/threonine and tyrosine kinases, although the geometries of the phosphorylated activation loops are distinct (Figure 2.7). The activation segment terminates with the consensus sequence . . . APE in a region historically called the P+1 loop, due to its role in binding the P+1 residue (i.e., the residue following the phospho-acceptor) in the PKA substrate. Although not conserved in sequence, the region C-terminal to the . . . APE sequence also moves in concert with the activation loop during the active/inactive structural rearrangement. Overall, conversion from the unphosphorylated to the triple phosphorylated form of IR results in decreases in K_M for ATP, decreased K_M with respect to the substrate peptide interaction and increased reaction rate (116).

Not all kinases are activated by phosphorylation of the activation segment, perhaps the most notable example being EGF receptor. An alternative activation mechanism for EGFR involving an asymmetric interaction of two kinase domains is discussed in Section 2.4.4. The structure of ACK1 has also been determined with and without activation loop phosphorylation and adopts essentially identical, active-like conformations in either case (117). CSK has no activation loop tyrosines and activation is mediated by the SH2 domain and related sequences within the protein, although in a manner different from that of SRC kinase discussed later (118, 119).

The crystal structure of the DNA damage mediator kinase CHK2 (discussed further in Chapter 6) reveals an additional regulatory mechanism involving the activation loop (120). The CHK2 protein consists of a SCD (serine–glutamine/threonine–glutamine cluster domain) at the N terminus, followed by an FHA (Forkhead-associated) domain and a C-terminal kinase domain. Using a truncated CHK2 construct comprising just the kinase domain, the CHK2 activation loop was found to be unphosphorylated but nevertheless adopted an extended, active-like conformation containing two short helical segments. This extended loop forms a symmetrical dimer interaction with another CHK2 molecule, such that the tip of the trans activation loop adopts a similar orientation and conformation to that of the cis activation loop in kinases such as PKA (57) and CHK1 (121) (Figure 2.7).

The dimeric molecule is competent to bind ATP: in fact, an ADP molecule is bound in the crystal structure (120). CHK2 activation is initiated by T68 phosphorylation in the N-terminal domain, which was previously shown to mediate CHK2 dimerization (122, 123): this then enables trans-autophosphorylation in the activation loop, which is proposed to stabilize the active form by binding to the "RD" binding pocket (120).

2.4.2 Regulation by N-Terminal Sequences and Domains

The crystal structures of FLT3, CSF1R, and KIT have been instrumental in demonstrating the role of a small juxtamembrane (JM) domain in regulating the activity of these kinases. In the autoinhibited FLT3 structure (124), a 30-amino acid region between the kinase domain and the cell membrane makes extensive interactions with both the N-terminal and C-terminal lobes of the kinase, with the hydroxyl groups of two tyrosine residues (Y589 and Y591) appearing to anchor the JM domain to the C-terminal lobe (Figure 2.8). These interactions lock the C helix and the activation loop in an inactive conformation, with the key regulatory tyrosine residue of the activation loop pointing toward the active site in a position normally occupied by a substrate tyrosine. However, due to the inaccessibility of the catalytic machinery (notably the catalytic D829) and steric hindrance to ATP binding, phosphorylation cannot occur. More recently, the structure of the closely related CSF1R kinase has been solved: the autoinhibitory mechanism appears to be essentially identical, despite the fact that CSF1R has only one of the tyrosine "anchor" residues (70). The anchor residues are known phosphorylation sites for this family of kinases, suggesting that phosphorylation of the JM domain may relieve its inhibitory effects. Such a mechanism is supported by the structure of KIT, which was solved in both an inactive form similar to that of FLT3 (125) and an activated form where the tyrosine "anchor" residues are phosphorylated (71). In the active KIT structure, most of the JM domain is disordered and not in contact with the kinase domain: however, one of the JM phosphotyrosines binds in trans to the active site of an adjacent kinase molecule in the crystal lattice. Although the activation loop is not phosphorylated, it adopts an open conformation that is amenable to ATP and substrate peptide binding, while the C helix is rotated to form the conserved Glu-Lys ion pair that coordinates the ATP α- and β-phosphates. Furthermore, although a structure for PDGF receptor has not yet been reported, mutagenesis of the PDGFRβ JM domain has highlighted amino acids that are functionally implicated in regulation of kinase activity (126), and these are in good agreement with the structures of FLT3, KIT, and CSF1R.

EPH receptor signaling is initiated by engagement of ephrin ligands as described previously but is also subject to direct regulation of kinase activity. EPHR activity is controlled in part by phosphorylation of the activation loop, but also by phosphorylation of residues in the juxtamembrane (JM) domain. This domain is immediately N-terminal to the kinase domain, although it is structurally quite dissimilar from that of FLT3, KIT, and CSF1R. Mutagenesis and crystallographic studies with the EPHB2 receptor indicate that the juxtamembrane domain (immediately N-terminal to the kinase domain) binds to the N-terminal

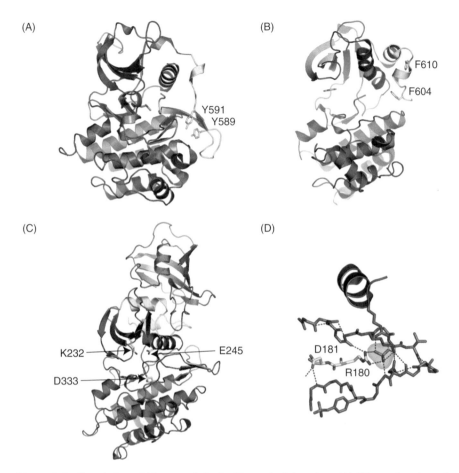

Figure 2.8 Regulation of kinase activity by N-terminal domains. (A) Kinase domain and juxtamembrane region of FLT3. The activation segment (orange) occludes the ATP binding site, and the inactive form is stabilized by interactions with the juxtamembrane region (yellow), specifically involving two tyrosine residues. (PDB accession code 1RJB.) (B) The juxtamembrane region of EPHA2 (yellow) also impairs activation. Although the conformation is very different from that of FLT3, two tyrosine residues (mutated to phenylalanine in the structure) also play an important regulatory role. The activation segment (orange) is mostly disordered, and the ATP binding site is not occluded: the adenosine ring is visible in the structure. (PDB accession code 1JPA.) (C) In the case of TGFβ1 receptor, the N-terminal GS domain (yellow) forms a binding site for the immunophilin FKBP12 (orange), which distorts the structure (in particular, the C helix) and blocks activation. (PDB accession code 1B6C.) (D) The GSK3β activation loop, RD dipeptide, and an arginine residue from the C helix form an anion binding pocket, in place of the canonical phospho-Ser/Thr/Tyr site (compare with Figures 2.8A and 2.8B). In the crystal structure, a sulfonate is located at this site (highlighted in red); in the full-length protein, it is likely occupied by the phosphorylated S9 residue. (PDB accession code 1GNG.)

lobe of the adjacent kinase domain, making extensive contact with the EPHB2 C helix and forcing the kinase domain to adopt an unproductive conformation (Figure 2.8) (127, 128). However, this interaction does not occlude the ATP binding site: in fact, the double mutant protein binds ATP with similar affinity to the native protein. Phosphorylation of two tyrosine residues in the JM domain disrupts the JM:kinase interaction and enables catalytic function to occur.

TGFβR1 is a receptor serine/threonine kinase that is also subject to regulation by an N-terminal juxtamembrane domain. This juxtamembrane domain, termed the GS (glycine–serine) region, is comprised of two α helices connected by a hairpin loop. In complex with the immunophilin FKBP12, the unphosphorylated GS region interacts with the N-terminal lobe of TGFβR1 kinase. This forces the N-lobe into an unproductive conformation, displacing the C helix, constricting the ATP binding site and displacing the E245-K232 ion pair from the catalytic D333 (129) (Figure 2.8). Phosphorylation of the GS region prevents FKBP12 from binding and also creates a binding site for the FHA domain of the TGFβ receptor substrate SMAD2 (130).

Glycogen synthase kinase-3β (GSK3β) is a key regulator of several important biochemical processes including WNT signaling, insulin signaling, cell adhesion, and cell cycle progression (131). In contrast to the juxtamembrane regulatory regions described earlier, phosphorylation of the N-terminal region of GSK3β (S9) leads to inhibition rather than activation of kinase activity (132). S9 phosphorylation can be mediated by several kinases including AKT, p70S6K, and p90RSK, and the crystal structure of GSK3β suggests a molecular explanation for the resulting inhibition (133, 134). In two independent structural studies, GSK3β was crystallized in the absence of activation loop phosphorylation: however, the resulting structures showed that the activation loop nevertheless adopts an active conformation. Several residues within and adjacent to the activation loop form an anion binding site (the "RD" sequence binding pocket described earlier), which, in the protein crystals, is occupied by a phosphate ion (134) or the sulfonate moiety of a HEPES buffer molecule (133) (Figure 2.8D). The N terminus of the protein is disordered in both structures: however, based on biochemical (133) and mutagenesis experiments (135), it is likely that phosphorylation of S9 enables it to engage this binding site and prevent substrate binding, with P5 occupying the catalytic phospho-acceptor site. Thus S9 may play a role that is analogous to the primary phospho-Ser/Thr/Tyr residue in kinases that are regulated by activation loop phosphorylation (see earlier discussion). Moreover, the anion binding site explains the preference of GSK3β for "preprimed" substrates, that is, substrates that already have a phosphorylated residue as part of their recognition sequence. This phosphorylated residue is at the P+4 position (where P represents the target residue for GSK3β phosphorylation) and is accommodated by the anion binding site.

2.4.3   C-Terminal Regulatory Regions

C-Terminal Inhibitory Domains   TIE2 and MAPKAPK2 represent two examples of kinases that are autoinhibited by protein segments immediately C-terminal to the kinase domain. In both cases, the C-terminal tail not only inhibits the enzyme but also occludes binding sites for effector proteins, thus combining two inhibitory functions in one regulatory region. TIE2 is the receptor for the angiogenic factor ANG1, an important regulator of vascular remodeling (Chapter 1). The crystal structure of the inactive TIE2 tyrosine kinase domain reveals that a ~15-residue C-terminal tail folds along the surface of the kinase domain C-lobe and interferes with the substrate binding site (72) (Figure 2.9A). In

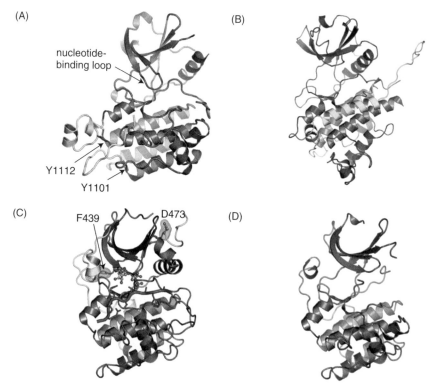

Figure 2.9 Regulation of kinase activity by C-terminal domains. (A) Crystal structure of TIE2 kinase domain. The kinase insert domain and C-terminal peptide are shown in yellow; Tyr1101 and Tyr1112 are in red. The C-terminal peptide packs against the substrate binding region and kinase insert domain, partially burying the two tyrosine residues. Also of note, the nucleotide binding loop dips into a region normally occupied by the ATP α- and β-phosphates. (PDB accession code 1FVR.) (B) In the crystal structure of MAPKAPK2, the C-terminal peptide (yellow) adopts a helical conformation, occluding the substrate binding site. (PDB accession code 1KWP.) (C) Active structure of AKT, with substrate peptide in red and ATP bound at the active site. The C-terminal tail of AKT (yellow) extends up past the ATP binding site and around the N-terminal lobe, although the central portion of the tail is disordered and not visible. The phosphorylated S473 (mutated to Asp in the structure, shown in orange) engages the PIF pocket in the N-terminal lobe and stabilizes the active conformation. (PDB accession codes 1O6K.) (D) In the inactive structure of AKT, S473 is unphosphorylated and does not interact with the N-terminal lobe. The C helix is disordered, and the ATP binding site is obscured. (PDB accession code 1MRV.)

addition, this C-terminal tail contains tyrosine residues (Y1101 and Y1112), which, when phosphorylated, become binding sites for SH2 domains and other downstream effector proteins. These sites are buried in the inactive structure and presumably only become accessible for phosphorylation when receptor activation occurs. Several additional modulatory mechanisms are apparent in the inactive TIE2 kinase domain structure. Although the activation loop appears to be in an active-like conformation, the DFG region may occlude the ATP binding site; furthermore, the nucleotide binding loop also occupies the region normally bound by the α- and β-phosphates of ATP. In addition, the C helix is positioned such that the residues comprising the canonical Glu-Lys ion pair are too far apart to form an ATP binding pocket.

MAPKAPK2 is an important mediator of cellular stress response and inflammation and is a substrate of p38 MAP kinase. Recently, MAPKAPK2 was also shown to play a role in cell cycle checkpoint regulation (136) (Chapter 6). Like TIE2, MAPKAPK2 also contains a C-terminal regulatory region; however, in contrast to the extended conformation of the TIE2 C-terminal tail, the MAPKAPK2 C terminus adopts a helical structure that packs against the substrate binding site (137) (Figure 2.9). This C-terminal helix also contains nuclear localization and nuclear export sequences. In the inactive state, the substrate binding site and nuclear export sequences are occluded while the nuclear localization sequence is exposed. Phosphorylation of the C-terminal helix by p38 leads to increased substrate binding and catalytic rate, as well as unmasking the nuclear export sequence (138). Hence the MAPKAPK2 regulatory region may serve a dual purpose, modulating both kinase activity and cellular localization. Several other kinases possess helical C-terminal autoinhibitory segments, including calcium/calmodulin-dependent kinase I (139), and the serine kinase domain from the giant muscle filament protein Titin (140). In both of these cases, the C-terminal tail extends across both the N- and C-terminal lobes of the kinase domain, forming multiple interactions with both the protein substrate and ATP binding regions.

C-Terminal Activation Domains: AGC Kinases   Several AGC family kinases play a critical role in cellular growth, survival, and proliferation and are frequently dysregulated in cancer. In particular, PDK1 and AKT kinases, discussed in Chapter 5, are important effectors of Class I phosphatidylinositol 3-kinase (PI3K) signaling. PDK and AKT are both comprised of a pleckstrin homology (PH) domain and a kinase domain, although the order is reversed: PDK1 has an N-terminal kinase domain and a C-terminal PH domain, while the kinase is at the C terminus of AKT. Both PDK1 and AKT are regulated by interaction of their PH domains with phosphoinositides, in particular, phosphatidylinositol(3,4,5)trisphosphate (PIP$_3$). Most AGC kinases contain a C-terminal hydrophobic motif with a conserved Ser/Thr residue, and phosphorylation of this residue is necessary for optimal kinase activity (141). In active AGC kinases (e.g., AKT), the phosphorylated C-terminal tail loops around the kinase and engages a hydrophobic/phosphopeptide binding pocket in the N-lobe of the kinase, termed the PIF (PDK1-interacting fragment) pocket. Engagement of the phosphorylated C-terminal peptide with the PIF pocket stabilizes the C-helix conformation and the active state, with the ATP binding site exposed and key active site residues positioned for catalysis (142) (Figure 2.9C). In the structure of the inactive form of AKT, the PIF pocket is disordered and unavailable to bind the C-terminal tail; correspondingly, the C helix is disordered and the ATP binding pocket obscured (143, 144) (Figure 2.9D).

PDK1 also has a PIF pocket in its N-terminal lobe: however, it lacks the corresponding C-terminal hydrophobic region/phosphorylation site. The lack of this motif in PDK1 seems to be intimately related to its role as a key activator of many AGC kinases (145, 146). The results of many X-ray crystallographic, site-directed mutagenesis, and other biochemical studies indicate that PDK1 substrates such as AKT are activated by a two-step process (Figure 2.10). First, the conserved Ser/Thr in the C-terminal hydrophobic motif is phosphorylated, either constitutively or in response to signaling by a kinase other than PDK1. (In the case of AKT, this kinase has been shown to be the mTOR:Rictor complex (147), although DNAPK

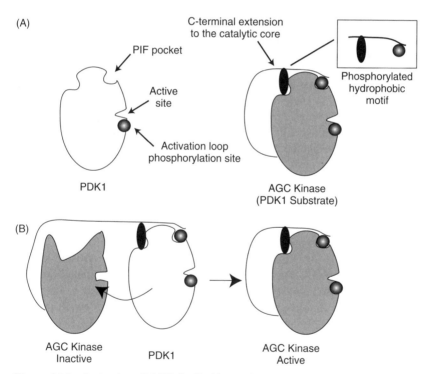

Figure 2.10 Activation of AGC family kinases by PDK1. Phosphorylated residues are denoted by gray spheres. (A) PDK1 and its substrates in the AGC kinase group contain a hydrophobic/phosphopeptide binding region (the PIF pocket), but PDK1 lacks the corresponding regulatory hydrophobic motif region found in the C-terminal region of other AGC kinases. (B) Phosphorylation of the AGC kinase C-terminal region creates a binding site for PDK1, which subsequently phosphorylates the activation loop of the substrate AGC kinase. The C-terminal region of the fully activated AGC kinase then binds to its own PIF pocket, displacing PDK1. Adapted with permission from (130). Copyright © 2001 The Biochemical Society.

and/or PKCβII may also play a role in some cellular contexts.) This leads to engagement of active PDK1, via interaction of the substrate C-terminal tail with the binding pocket in the N-terminal domain of PDK1. Following PDK1-mediated phosphorylation of the activation loop, it is likely that the C-terminal region of the substrate disengages from PDK1 and binds to its own hydrophobic/phosphopeptide binding pocket. An additional phosphorylation site in the C-terminal region of AGC kinases is less well characterized than either the activation segment or the hydrophobic motif site. This site is constitutively phosphorylated in AKT, p70S6K, and PRK2 kinases and inducibly phosphorylated in RSK2 and MSK1. Mutagenesis and molecular modeling studies suggest that this site docks to a basic region in the N-terminal lobe of AGC kinases and facilitates their activation via engagement of the hydrophobic motif site (148).

How is the activity of PDK1 regulated? It has long been established that PDK1 localizes to the cell membrane via binding of its pleckstrin homology (PH) domain to 3-phosphoinositides—in particular, phosphatidylinositol(3,4,5)tris-phosphate, the product of PI3K (149, 150). This membrane localization is likely to be the key factor in promoting activation of AKT, since AKT also localizes in plasma membranes via its own PH domain. However, the intrinsic kinase activity of PDK1 appears to be constitutive, in that neither growth factor stimulation nor binding to phosphoinositides affects catalytic activity. Instead, it is likely that PDK1 activation is mediated by autophosphorylation *in trans* (151). PDK1 also regulates the activity of multiple substrates that reside in the cytosolic compartment. Crystallographic studies with the PDK1 PH domain have suggested that binding to D6-phosphorylated phosphoinositides may explain how PDK1 can promote activation of substrate kinases away from the cell membrane (152) and may also play a direct role in nuclear signaling (153, 154).

2.4.4   Regulation by Other Domains and Partner Proteins

SRC Family Kinases   The SRC family members are nonreceptor tyrosine kinases that signal downstream of cell surface proteins, including other tyrosine kinases and cytokine receptors. Extensive crystallographic studies with isolated domains and holoenzymes of SRC and related tyrosine kinases have provided a rich source of data to explain the multiple mechanisms by which these multidomain proteins are regulated (155–158). In addition to SRC and ABL (which are discussed later), additional SRC family members with available X-ray structures include HCK (159, 160), LCK (161), and FYN (162).

The SRC protein structure comprises an N-terminal region followed by an SH3 domain, an SH2 domain, the catalytic kinase domain and an important C-terminal tail region. These domains all collaborate to provide multiple layers of functional regulation. The structures of nearly full-length chicken and human SRC (163–165) provided a clear picture of how the various domains of SRC interact with each other and regulate activity (Figure 2.11; in this figure and the following discussion, residue numbers correspond to the chicken SRC sequence, which was the first SRC structure solved). First, one level of regulation is provided by activation segment autophosphorylation on Y416. In the inactive SRC structure

(A)

L255

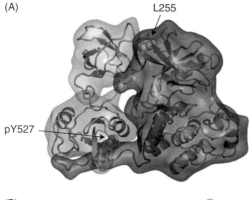

pY527

(B)

L255

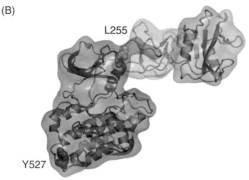

Y527

Figure 2.11   Structure of SRC kinase. (A) In the autoinhibited structure, the domains are locked in a rigid, compact conformation. The SH3 domain is in yellow, the SH2 domain is in orange, and the kinase domain is in teal blue. Two key residues that contribute to autoinhibition are shown in CPK representation: L255 (yellow) and (phospho)Y527 (red). (B) In the activated structure (shown partially rotated relative to panel A), the SH2-SH3 domain assembly adopts an extended conformation (L255 is colored cyan in this image). The unphosphorylated Y527 packs into a pocket in the C-terminal lobe of the kinase domain, which may also represent a docking site for the N-terminal myristate moiety. (PDB accession codes 1FMK and 1Y57.)

Y416 is on a short helical region within the activation loop, and the side chain is buried within a hydrophobic pocket in the N-terminal lobe of the kinase. Second, the SH3 domain packs against the linker between the SH2 and kinase domains. This linker region—and, in particular, L255—makes an important contribution to the inhibitory mechanism (166) and results in displacement of the C helix out of the active site, preventing formation of the Glu-Lys ion pair interaction. Third, the SH2 domain is anchored to the C-terminal kinase domain via a tyrosine residue in the C-terminal tail (Y527). Phosphorylation of Y527 by CSK is known to repress catalytic activity (167, 168), and the structure shows that this residue is sequestered by the SH2 domain's phosphopeptide binding site. Collectively, the SH2 and SH3 domains form a "clamp" (156), which rigidifies the kinase domain, inhibiting activity and preventing activation loop phosphorylation. Finally, the N-terminal domain of SRC contains a myristylation site that is important for membrane localization and biological activity (169). Structural studies with an unphosphorylated form of SRC (in complex with an analog of the ABL kinase inhibitor imatinib) have led to a possible explanation for how the myristate moiety contributes to activation (170). In the unphosphorylated SRC structure, the SH3 domain still binds to the SH2-kinase linker region but the linker, including the critical L255 residue, is disengaged from the back side of the N-terminal kinase lobe. The SH3-SH2 assembly adopts an extended conformation and no longer restrains the kinase domain

(Figure 2.11). Although the kinase activation loop is unphosphorylated, it adopts an active-like configuration. Of particular note, the unphosphorylated C-terminal tail binds to a hydrophobic pocket in the C-lobe of the kinase domain. In full-length SRC, this pocket may be a binding site for the N-terminal myristate (which is missing in the N-terminally truncated protein used for crystallization). Indeed, NMR experiments showed that myristate does not interact with unphosphorylated SRC but binds to the same protein after phosphorylation of Y527, consistent with this hypothesis (170). Furthermore, such a mechanism has also been found in an isoform of the SRC family kinase ABL (171, 172), which lacks the C-terminal phosphorylation site of SRC. The availability of multiple layers of regulation may enable kinases such as SRC to engage different downstream pathways depending on the mode of activation. For example, there is evidence for the SRC family member HCK that activation via engagement of the SH3 domain may not necessarily disrupt the SH2:C-terminal tail interaction, perhaps favoring activation of non-SH2-related pathways (173). Conversely, activation by dephosphorylation of the C-terminal tail may loosen the SH3-SH2 "clamp" but not fully expose the SH3 domain (174).

FAK Focal adhesion kinase (FAK; Chapter 4) is a nonreceptor tyrosine kinase that regulates adhesion and growth factor-mediated cellular signaling and may play an important role in tumor progression (175). From N terminus to C terminus, FAK is comprised of a ∼350-residue FERM domain, a 40-residue linker region, a kinase domain, a proline-rich domain, and a C-terminal focal adhesion targeting (FAT) domain. FAK is regulated by either intramolecular or intermolecular autophosphorylation of Y397 in the linker region (176, 177). The phosphorylated Y397 site recruits binding of SH2 domain-containing proteins including SRC kinase, which subsequently phosphorylates activation loop tyrosine residues in FAK (178). The isolated human FAK kinase domain structure was determined for the unphosphorylated form in complex with ATP and is notable for a short-range disulfide bond between C456 and C459 (179). The structure of a large fragment of avian FAK, encompassing the FERM domain, linker region, and kinase domain, shows how the FERM domain interacts with and regulates kinase domain activity, both directly and in concert with SRC kinase (180). In the autoinhibited structure, the FERM domain packs against the C-terminal lobe of the kinase domain, preventing phosphorylation of the activation loop and blocking access of substrates to the active site. Y397 is located in a β-strand region of the linker that forms a β sheet with the N-terminal end of the FERM domain. Displacement of the FERM domain, perhaps by associated signaling proteins such as growth factor receptors or integrins, is thought to disengage the linker region. This enables autophosphorylation of Y397, engagement of the SRC SH2 domain (and SH3 domain, which binds to a proline-rich segment of the linker region), and activation of the kinase via activation loop phosphorylation.

CDK2:cyclin A Cyclin-dependent kinases (CDKs) and their regulatory cyclin binding partners are critical for orchestrating cellular transit through the cell cycle (Chapter 6). The CDK2:cyclin A complex is critical for regulating transit through S phase, and multiple structures of CDK2 in different activation states have revealed some of the mechanisms underlying the stringent regulation of its activity. The CDK2 protein comprises the kinase domain with short N- and C-terminal extensions, and the structure of unphosphorylated, isolated CDK2 shows that it adopts an inactive conformation (181). In particular, the activation segment forms a short helix followed by a loop that occludes the active site, and the C helix is twisted out (relative to the canonical position observed in active kinases) such that the Glu-Lys ion pair (E51-K33) is not formed (Figure 2.12A). The N terminus of the C helix and adjacent regions also show significant disorder and mobility in the structure. The structure of a ~260 amino acid fragment of cyclin A has been solved alone (182) and in complex with CDK2 (183). This fragment contains two structurally homologous five-helix bundles and is highly similar in both the isolated and CDK2-bound states. In contrast, CDK2 undergoes substantial structural changes on cyclin binding. Cyclin A packs against the C

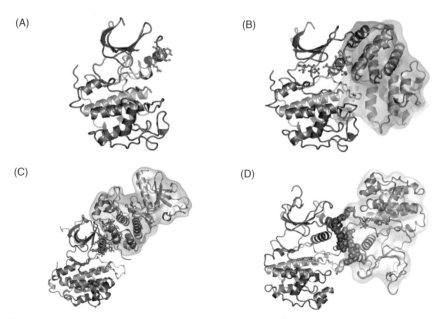

Figure 2.12   Regulation of CDK2, EGFR, and ERK2 by protein:protein interactions. (A) Inactive structure of CDK2, with activation segment in yellow and PSTAIRE sequence in orange ball-and-stick representation (PDB accession code 1HCL.) (B) Active CDK2:cyclin A complex with ATP. The PSTAIRE sequence interacts with cyclin A (blue), rotating the C helix and forming a competent active site (PDB accession code 1FIN.) (C) Structure of the active EGFR kinase domain (teal). The activation segment is in yellow and the C helix is in orange. The neighboring, "cyclin-like" EGFR molecule is in blue and its activating helix is in red (PDB accession code 2GS2.) (D) Structure of active ERK2. The activation segment is shown in yellow for one monomer. Residues from the activation segment and a C-terminal extension in ERK2 (shown as red and orange spheres) interact to form a symmetrical dimer (PDB accession code 2ERK.)

helix and binds to a PSTAIRE sequence, which is a conserved motif in the CDK family. The C helix is repositioned closer to the β-sheet region and E51 is now within ion pairing distance of K33, thus forming this key component of the ATP binding site. At the same time, the short helix in the activation segment is unwound and this region adopts a conformation similar to that of other active kinases (Figure 2.12). In this conformation, T160 in the activation segment is amenable to phosphorylation by the CDK7:cyclin H:MAT1 complex, although the ability of CDK2 to autophosphorylate has also recently been demonstrated (184). Phosphorylation at T160 leads to further rearrangement of the activation segment, optimizing the "platform" for substrate binding and priming the active site for catalysis (185, 186). There is also emerging evidence that, in addition to its role in activation, cyclin binding may also modulate CDK substrate specificity (187). Since the initial determination of the CDK2:cyclin A structure, several additional CDK and/or cyclin structures have been solved, further enriching our structural understanding of cell cycle regulation. Among these are cyclin H (188, 189), cyclin B (190), cyclin K (191), CDK2:cyclin E (192), CDK2:cyclin B (187), CDK6:cyclin D (in complex with p18^{INK4c}) (193), CDK6:viral cyclin (194), and the inactive form of the CDK activating kinase, CDK7 (195). Cyclin-dependent kinases have also attracted significant interest as cancer drug targets: consequently, there are also many structures of small molecule inhibitors in complex with various CDK proteins.

EGF Receptor   Crystallographic and biochemical data have suggested a potential role for asymmetric dimers of the EGFR kinase domain in receptor activation. EGF receptor is unusual among receptor tyrosine kinases in that activation loop phosphorylation is not required for activity (196), and the initial crystal structure of the unphosphorylated EGFR kinase domain confirmed that it adopts an active-like conformation (197). However, the EGFR activation loop is not locked in this state and can also adopt an inactive conformation, as demonstrated crystallographically by the complex of the kinase domain with the inhibitor lapatinib (198). A mechanism whereby an asymmetric dimer of kinase domains might promote activation was initially proposed based on sequence comparisons and homology modeling, prior to the EGFR kinase structure being available (199). Such an asymmetric dimer was subsequently noticed in the crystals of the active structure, providing empirical evidence for a mechanism whereby one kinase domain might promote and/or stabilize the active conformation of another (200). This asymmetric dimer is reminiscent of the interactions found in the CDK2:cyclin A complex, in that the primary interaction involves an α-helical ("cyclin-like") region from the C-terminal domain of one kinase interacting with the C helix of the activated kinase, promoting formation of the conserved Glu-Lys ion pair and a more closed, active configuration (Figure 2.12C). Mutagenesis studies involving the putative contact residues confirmed that this was likely to be a relevant physiological mechanism rather than a factitious crystal packing interaction. Moreover, the structure of an EGFR mutant with a compromised "cyclin-like" region (V924R) adopts an inactive conformation, with the C helix rotated outward and the Glu738-Lys721 ion pair interaction disrupted. This model elegantly explains how the ERBB3 kinase domain can act as a potent activator of signaling in complex with other EGFR family members, although it cannot be activated itself due to sequence differences in its own C-helix interface and substitution of highly conserved residues in the catalytic domain, including the substitution of asparagine for the catalytic aspartate (D834).

ERK2   Investigation of the mitogen-activated protein (MAP) kinase ERK2 has revealed a somewhat distinct role for modulation of kinase activity by dimerization (201). ERK2 has a similar topology to other protein kinases, but contains a 50-residue insertion in the C-terminal domain and an extended C-terminal tail, which culminates in a helix that packs against the C helix in the N-terminal domain (202). In the crystal structure of active ERK2, a portion of this extended C-terminal tail and the tip of the phosphorylated activation loop form a symmetrical dimerization interface (Figure 2.12). The phosphorylated protein forms high affinity dimers ($K_D = 7.5$ nM), in contrast to unphosphorylated protein ($K_D = 20$ µM). Moreover, dimerization appears to have important biological consequences: it appears to be a prerequisite for nuclear translocation, and the twofold symmetry offers a plausible mechanism for efficient phosphorylation of dimeric leucine zipper transcription factors such as c-FOS:c-JUN (203).

REFERENCES

1. Schlessinger J. Cell signaling by receptor tyrosine kinases. Cell 2000;103(2):211–225.
2. Burgess AW, Cho HS, Eigenbrot C, Ferguson KM, Garrett TP, Leahy DJ, Lemmon MA, Sliwkowski MX, Ward CW, Yokoyama S. An open-and-shut case? Recent insights into the activation of EGF/ErbB receptors. Mol Cell 2003;12(3):541–552.
3. Jorissen RN, Walker F, Pouliot N, Garrett TP, Ward CW, Burgess AW. Epidermal growth factor receptor: mechanisms of activation and signalling. Exp Cell Res 2003;284(1):31–53.
4. Clayton AH, Walker F, Orchard SG, Henderson C, Fuchs D, Rothacker J, Nice EC, Burgess AW. Ligand-induced dimer–tetramer transition during the activation of the cell surface epidermal growth factor receptor-A multidimensional microscopy analysis. J Biol Chem 2005;280(34):30392–30399.
5. Ferguson KM, Berger MB, Mendrola JM, Cho HS, Leahy DJ, Lemmon MA. EGF activates its receptor by removing interactions that autoinhibit ectodomain dimerization. Mol Cell 2003;11(2):507–517.
6. Cho HS, Leahy DJ. Structure of the extracellular region of HER3 reveals an interdomain tether. Science 2002;297(5585):1330–1333.
7. Bouyain S, Longo PA, Li S, Ferguson KM, Leahy DJ. The extracellular region of ErbB4 adopts a tethered conformation in the absence of ligand. Proc Natl Acad Sci USA 2005;102(42): 15024–15029.
8. Ferguson KM. Active and inactive conformations of the epidermal growth factor receptor. Biochem Soc Trans 2004;32(Pt 5):742–745.
9. Kim JH, Saito K, Yokoyama S. Chimeric receptor analyses of the interactions of the ectodomains of ErbB-1 with epidermal growth factor and of those of ErbB-4 with neuregulin. Eur J Biochem 2002;269(9):2323–2329.
10. Singer E, Landgraf R, Horan T, Slamon D, Eisenberg D. Identification of a heregulin binding site in HER3 extracellular domain. J Biol Chem 2001;276(47):44266–44274.
11. Cho HS, Mason K, Ramyar KX, Stanley AM, Gabelli SB, Denney DW Jr, Leahy DJ. Structure of the extracellular region of HER2 alone and in complex with the Herceptin Fab. Nature 2003;421(6924):756–760.

12. Franklin MC, Carey KD, Vajdos FF, Leahy DJ, de Vos AM, Sliwkowski MX. Insights into ErbB signaling from the structure of the ErbB2–pertuzumab complex. Cancer Cell 2004;5(4):317–328.

13. Garrett TP, McKern NM, Lou M, Elleman TC, Adams TE, Lovrecz GO, Kofler M, Jorissen RN, Nice EC, Burgess AW, Ward CW. The crystal structure of a truncated ErbB2 ectodomain reveals an active conformation, poised to interact with other ErbB receptors. Mol Cell 2003;11(2):495–505.

14. Li S, Schmitz KR, Jeffrey PD, Wiltzius JJ, Kussie P, Ferguson KM. Structural basis for inhibition of the epidermal growth factor receptor by cetuximab. Cancer Cell 2005;7(4):301–311.

15. De Meyts P, Whittaker J. Structural biology of insulin and IGF1 receptors: implications for drug design. Nat Rev Drug Discov 2002;1(10):769–783.

16. Ward CW, Lawrence MC, Streltsov VA, Adams TE, McKern NM. The insulin and EGF receptor structures: new insights into ligand-induced receptor activation. Trends Biochem Sci 2007;32(3):129–137.

17. Sparrow LG, McKern NM, Gorman JJ, Strike PM, Robinson CP, Bentley JD, Ward CW. The disulfide bonds in the C-terminal domains of the human insulin receptor ectodomain. J Biol Chem 1997;272(47):29460–29467.

18. Garrett TP, McKern NM, Lou M, Frenkel MJ, Bentley JD, Lovrecz GO, Elleman TC, Cosgrove LJ, Ward CW. Crystal structure of the first three domains of the type-1 insulin-like growth factor receptor. Nature 1998;394(6691):395–399.

19. Kristensen C, Wiberg FC, Andersen AS. Specificity of insulin and insulin-like growth factor I receptors investigated using chimeric mini-receptors. Role of C-terminal of receptor alpha subunit. J Biol Chem 1999;274(52):37351–37356.

20. Sorensen H, Whittaker L, Hinrichsen J, Groth A, Whittaker J. Mapping of the insulin-like growth factor II binding site of the Type I insulin-like growth factor receptor by alanine scanning mutagenesis. FEBS Lett 2004;565(1–3):19–22.

21. Whittaker J, Groth AV, Mynarcik DC, Pluzek L, Gadsboll VL, Whittaker LJ. Alanine scanning mutagenesis of a type 1 insulin-like growth factor receptor ligand binding site. J Biol Chem 2001;276(47):43980–43986.

22. Whittaker J, Sorensen H, Gadsboll VL, Hinrichsen J. Comparison of the functional insulin binding epitopes of the A and B isoforms of the insulin receptor. J Biol Chem 2002;277(49):47380–47384.

23. Lou M, Garrett TP, McKern NM, Hoyne PA, Epa VC, Bentley JD, Lovrecz GO, Cosgrove LJ, Frenkel MJ, Ward CW. The first three domains of the insulin receptor differ structurally from the insulin-like growth factor 1 receptor in the regions governing ligand specificity. Proc Natl Acad Sci USA 2006;103(33):12429–12434.

24. McKern NM, Lawrence MC, Streltsov VA, Lou MZ, Adams TE, Lovrecz GO, Elleman TC, Richards KM, Bentley JD, Pilling PA, Hoyne PA, Cartledge KA, Pham TM, Lewis JL, Sankovich SE, Stoichevska V, Da Silva E, Robinson CP, Frenkel MJ, Sparrow LG, Fernley RT, Epa VC, Ward CW. Structure of the insulin receptor ectodomain reveals a folded-over conformation. Nature 2006;443(7108):218–221.

25. Stauber DJ, DiGabriele AD, Hendrickson WA. Structural interactions of fibroblast growth factor receptor with its ligands. Proc Natl Acad Sci USA 2000;97(1):49–54.

26. Plotnikov AN, Hubbard SR, Schlessinger J, Mohammadi M. Crystal structures of two FGF–FGFR complexes reveal the determinants of ligand-receptor specificity. Cell 2000;101(4):413–424.

27. Pellegrini L, Burke DF, von Delft F, Mulloy B, Blundell TL. Crystal structure of fibroblast growth factor receptor ectodomain bound to ligand and heparin. Nature 2000;407(6807):1029–1034.

28. Schlessinger J, Plotnikov AN, Ibrahimi OA, Eliseenkova AV, Yeh BK, Yayon A, Linhardt RJ, Mohammadi M. Crystal structure of a ternary FGF–FGFR–heparin complex reveals a dual role for heparin in FGFR binding and dimerization. Mol Cell 2000;6(3):743–750.

29. Harmer NJ, Ilag LL, Mulloy B, Pellegrini L, Robinson CV, Blundell TL. Towards a resolution of the stoichiometry of the fibroblast growth factor (FGF)–FGF receptor–heparin complex. J Mol Biol 2004;339(4):821–834.

30. Mohammadi M, Olsen SK, Goetz R. A protein canyon in the FGF–FGF receptor dimer selects from an a la carte menu of heparan sulfate motifs. Curr Opin Struct Biol 2005;15(5):506–516.

31. Mohammadi M, Olsen SK, Ibrahimi OA. Structural basis for fibroblast growth factor receptor activation. Cytokine Growth Factor Rev 2005;16(2):107–137.

32. Wu ZL, Zhang L, Yabe T, Kuberan B, Beeler DL, Love A, Rosenberg RD. The involvement of heparan sulfate (HS) in FGF1/HS/FGFR1 signaling complex. J Biol Chem 2003;278(19): 17121–17129.

33. Duchesne L, Tissot B, Rudd TR, Dell A, Fernig DG. N-glycosylation of fibroblast growth factor receptor 1 regulates ligand and heparan sulfate co-receptor binding. J Biol Chem 2006;281(37):27178–27189.

34. Muller YA, Li B, Christinger HW, Wells JA, Cunningham BC, de Vos AM. Vascular endothelial growth factor: crystal structure and functional mapping of the kinase domain receptor binding site. Proc Natl Acad Sci USA 1997;94(14):7192–7197.

35. Starovasnik MA, Christinger HW, Wiesmann C, Champe MA, de Vos AM, Skelton NJ. Solution structure of the VEGF-binding domain of Flt-1: comparison of its free and bound states. J Mol Biol 1999;293(3):531–544.

36. Wiesmann C, Fuh G, Christinger HW, Eigenbrot C, Wells JA, de Vos AM. Crystal structure at 1.7 Å resolution of VEGF in complex with domain 2 of the Flt-1 receptor. Cell 1997;91(5):695–704.

37. Christinger HW, Fuh G, de Vos AM, Wiesmann C. The crystal structure of placental growth factor in complex with domain 2 of vascular endothelial growth factor receptor-1. J Biol Chem 2004;279(11):10382–10388.

38. Errico M, Riccioni T, Iyer S, Pisano C, Acharya KR, Persico MG, De Falco S. Identification of placenta growth factor determinants for binding and activation of Flt-1 receptor. J Biol Chem 2004;279(42):43929–43939.

39. Barton WA, Tzvetkova D, Nikolov DB. Structure of the angiopoietin-2 receptor binding domain and identification of surfaces involved in Tie2 recognition. Structure 2005;13(5):825–832.

40. Fiedler U, Krissl T, Koidl S, Weiss C, Koblizek T, Deutsch U, Martiny-Baron G, Marme D, Augustin HG. Angiopoietin-1 and angiopoietin-2 share the same binding domains in the Tie-2 receptor involving the first Ig-like loop and the epidermal growth factor-like repeats. J Biol Chem 2003;278(3):1721–1727.

41. Davis S, Papadopoulos N, Aldrich TH, Maisonpierre PC, Huang T, Kovac L, Xu A, Leidich R, Radziejewska E, Rafique A, Goldberg J, Jain V, Bailey K, Karow M, Fandl J, Samuelsson SJ, Ioffe E, Rudge JS, Daly TJ, Radziejewski C, Yancopoulos GD. Angiopoietins have distinct modular domains essential for receptor binding, dimerization and superclustering. Nat Struct Biol 2003;10(1):38–44.

42. Procopio WN, Pelavin PI, Lee WM, Yeilding NM. Angiopoietin-1 and -2 coiled coil domains mediate distinct homo-oligomerization patterns, but fibrinogen-like domains mediate ligand activity. J Biol Chem 1999;274(42):30196–30201.

43. Barton WA, Tzvetkova-Robev D, Miranda EP, Kolev MV, Rajashankar KR, Himanen JP, Nikolov DB. Crystal structures of the Tie2 receptor ectodomain and the angiopoietin-2–Tie2 complex. Nat Struct Mol Biol 2006;13(6):524–532.

44. Kim KT, Choi HH, Steinmetz MO, Maco B, Kammerer RA, Ahn SY, Kim HZ, Lee GM, Koh GY. Oligomerization and multimerization are critical for angiopoietin-1 to bind and phosphorylate Tie2. J Biol Chem 2005;280(20):20126–20131.

45. Pasquale EB. Eph receptor signalling casts a wide net on cell behaviour. Nat Rev Mol Cell Biol 2005;6(6):462–475.

46. Himanen JP, Rajashankar KR, Lackmann M, Cowan CA, Henkemeyer M, Nikolov DB. Crystal structure of an Eph receptor–ephrin complex. Nature 2001;414(6866):933–938.

47. Chrencik JE, Brooun A, Kraus ML, Recht MI, Kolatkar AR, Han GW, Seifert JM, Widmer H, Auer M, Kuhn P. Structural and biophysical characterization of the EphB4*ephrinB2 protein–protein interaction and receptor specificity. J Biol Chem 2006;281(38):28185–28192.

48. Li E, Hristova K. Role of receptor tyrosine kinase transmembrane domains in cell signaling and human pathologies. Biochemistry 2006;45(20):6241–6251.

49. Bargmann CI, Hung MC, Weinberg RA. Multiple independent activations of the neu oncogene by a point mutation altering the transmembrane domain of p185. Cell 1986;45(5):649–657.

50. Weiner DB, Liu J, Cohen JA, Williams WV, Greene MI. A point mutation in the neu oncogene mimics ligand induction of receptor aggregation. Nature 1989;339(6221):230–231.

51. Frank B, Hemminki K, Wirtenberger M, Bermejo JL, Bugert P, Klaes R, Schmutzler RK, Wappenschmidt B, Bartram CR, Burwinkel B. The rare ERBB2 variant Ile654Val is associated with an increased familial breast cancer risk. Carcinogenesis 2005;26(3):643–647.

52. Xie D, Shu XO, Deng Z, Wen WQ, Creek KE, Dai Q, Gao YT, Jin F, Zheng W. Population-based, case–control study of HER2 genetic polymorphism and breast cancer risk. J Natl Cancer Inst 2000;92(5):412–417.

53. Moriki T, Maruyama H, Maruyama IN. Activation of preformed EGF receptor dimers by ligand-induced rotation of the transmembrane domain. J Mol Biol 2001;311(5):1011–1026.

54. Fleishman SJ, Schlessinger J, Ben-Tal N. A putative molecular-activation switch in the transmembrane domain of erbB2. Proc Natl Acad Sci USA 2002;99(25):15937–15940.

55. Enosh A, Fleishman SJ, Ben-Tal N, Halperin D. Prediction and simulation of motion in pairs of transmembrane alpha-helices. Bioinformatics 2007;23(2): e212–218.

56. van Rhijn BW, van Tilborg AA, Lurkin I, Bonaventure J, de Vries A, Thiery JP, van der Kwast TH, Zwarthoff EC, Radvanyi F. Novel fibroblast growth factor receptor 3 (FGFR3) mutations in bladder cancer previously identified in non-lethal skeletal disorders. Eur J Hum Genet 2002;10(12):819–824.

57. Knighton DR, Zheng JH, Ten Eyck LF, Xuong NH, Taylor SS, Sowadski JM. Structure of a peptide inhibitor bound to the catalytic subunit of cyclic adenosine monophosphate-dependent protein kinase. Science 1991;253(5018):414–420.

58. Hubbard SR, Wei L, Ellis L, Hendrickson WA. Crystal structure of the tyrosine kinase domain of the human insulin receptor. Nature 1994;372(6508):746–754.

59. Chen H, Ma J, Li W, Eliseenkova AV, Xu C, Neubert TA, Miller WT, Mohammadi M. A molecular brake in the kinase hinge region regulates the activity of receptor tyrosine kinases. Mol Cell 2007;27(5):717–730.

60. Kumar A, Mandiyan V, Suzuki Y, Zhang C, Rice J, Tsai J, Artis DR, Ibrahim P, Bremer R. Crystal structures of proto-oncogene kinase Pim1: a target of aberrant somatic hypermutations in diffuse large cell lymphoma. J Mol Biol 2005;348(1):183–193.

61. Jacobs MD, Black J, Futer O, Swenson L, Hare B, Fleming M, Saxena K. Pim-1 ligand-bound structures reveal the mechanism of serine/threonine kinase inhibition by LY294002. J Biol Chem 2005;280(14):13728–13734.

62. Qian KC, Wang L, Hickey ER, Studts J, Barringer K, Peng C, Kronkaitis A, Li J, White A, Mische S, Farmer B. Structural basis of constitutive activity and a unique nucleotide binding mode of human Pim-1 kinase. J Biol Chem 2005;280(7):6130–6137.

63. Niefind K, Putter M, Guerra B, Issinger OG, Schomburg D. GTP plus water mimic ATP in the active site of protein kinase CK2. Nat Struct Biol 1999;6(12):1100–1103.

64. Nolen B, Taylor S, Ghosh G. Regulation of protein kinases; controlling activity through activation segment conformation. Mol Cell 2004;15(5):661–675.

65. Carlberg K, Tapley P, Haystead C, Rohrschneider L. The role of kinase activity and the kinase insert region in ligand-induced internalization and degradation of the c-fms protein. EMBO J 1991;10(4):877–883.

66. Heidaran MA, Pierce JH, Lombardi D, Ruggiero M, Gutkind JS, Matsui T, Aaronson SA. Deletion or substitution within the alpha platelet-derived growth factor receptor kinase insert domain: effects on functional coupling with intracellular signaling pathways. Mol Cell Biol 1991;11(1):134–142.

67. Lev S, Givol D, Yarden Y. Interkinase domain of kit contains the binding site for phosphatidylinositol 3′ kinase. Proc Natl Acad Sci USA 1992;89(2):678–682.

68. Kazlauskas A, Cooper JA. Autophosphorylation of the PDGF receptor in the kinase insert region regulates interactions with cell proteins. Cell 1989;58(6):1121–1133.

69. McTigue MA, Wickersham JA, Pinko C, Showalter RE, Parast CV, Tempczyk-Russell A, Gehring MR, Mroczkowski B, Kan CC, Villafranca JE, Appelt K. Crystal structure of the kinase domain of human vascular endothelial growth factor receptor 2: a key enzyme in angiogenesis. Structure 1999;7(3):319–330.

70. Walter M, Lucet IS, Patel O, Broughton SE, Bamert R, Williams NK, Fantino E, Wilks AF, Rossjohn J. The 2.7 Å crystal structure of the autoinhibited human c-Fms kinase domain. J Mol Biol 2007;367(3):839–847.

71. Mol CD, Lim KB, Sridhar V, Zou H, Chien EY, Sang BC, Nowakowski J, Kassel DB, Cronin CN, McRee DE. Structure of a c-kit product complex reveals the basis for kinase transactivation. J Biol Chem 2003;278(34):31461–31464.

72. Shewchuk LM, Hassell AM, Ellis B, Holmes WD, Davis R, Horne EL, Kadwell SH, McKee DD, Moore JT. Structure of the Tie2 RTK domain: self-inhibition by the nucleotide binding loop, activation loop, and C-terminal tail. Structure 2000;8(11):1105–1113.

73. Huse M, Kuriyan J. The conformational plasticity of protein kinases. Cell 2002;109(3):275–282.

74. Knight ZA, Shokat KM. Features of selective kinase inhibitors. Chem Biol 2005;12(6):621–637.

75. Adams JA, Taylor SS. Energetic limits of phosphotransfer in the catalytic subunit of cAMP-dependent protein kinase as measured by viscosity experiments. Biochemistry 1992;31(36):8516–8522.

76. Kong CT, Cook PF. Isotope partitioning in the adenosine 3′,5′-monophosphate dependent protein kinase reaction indicates a steady-state random kinetic mechanism. Biochemistry 1988;27(13):4795–4799.

77. Cook PF, Neville ME Jr, Vrana KE, Hartl FT, Roskoski R Jr. Adenosine cyclic 3′,5′-monophosphate dependent protein kinase: kinetic mechanism for the bovine skeletal muscle catalytic subunit. Biochemistry 1982;21(23):5794–5799.

78. Shaffer J, Adams JA. Detection of conformational changes along the kinetic pathway of protein kinase A using a catalytic trapping technique. Biochemistry 1999;38(37):12072–12079.

79. Adams JA. Kinetic and catalytic mechanisms of protein kinases. Chem Rev 2001;101(8):2271–2290.

80. Olsen JV, Blagoev B, Gnad F, Macek B, Kumar C, Mortensen P, Mann M. Global, in vivo, and site-specific phosphorylation dynamics in signaling networks. Cell 2006;127(3):635–648.

81. Wu JJ, Afar DE, Phan H, Witte ON, Lam KS. Recognition of multiple substrate motifs by the c-ABL protein tyrosine kinase. Comb Chem High Throughput Screen 2002;5(1):83–91.

82. Pearson R, Kemp B. Protein kinase phosphorylation site sequences and consensus specificity motifs: tabulations. In: Hunter TaS, editor. Methods in Enzymology, Volume 200. San Diego: Academic Press; 1991. pp. 62–81.

83. Songyang Z, Carraway KL 3rd, Eck MJ, Harrison SC, Feldman RA, Mohammadi M, Schlessinger J, Hubbard SR, Smith DP, Eng C, et al. Catalytic specificity of protein-tyrosine kinases is critical for selective signalling. Nature 1995;373(6514):536–539.

84. Sondhi D, Xu W, Songyang Z, Eck MJ, Cole PA. Peptide and protein phosphorylation by protein tyrosine kinase Csk: insights into specificity and mechanism. Biochemistry 1998;37(1):165–172.

85. Tonks NK, Neel BG. Combinatorial control of the specificity of protein tyrosine phosphatases. Curr Opin Cell Biol 2001;13(2):182–195.

86. Songyang Z, Margolis B, Chaudhuri M, Shoelson SE, Cantley LC. The phosphotyrosine interaction domain of SHC recognizes tyrosine-phosphorylated NPXY motif. J Biol Chem 1995;270(25):14863–14866.

87. Seta K, Sadoshima J. Phosphorylation of tyrosine 319 of the angiotensin II type 1 receptor mediates angiotensin II-induced trans-activation of the epidermal growth factor receptor. J Biol Chem 2003;278(11):9019–9026.

88. Davis RJ. The mitogen-activated protein kinase signal transduction pathway. J Biol Chem 1993;268(20):14553–14556.

89. Garcia P, Shoelson SE, George ST, Hinds DA, Goldberg AR, Miller WT. Phosphorylation of synthetic peptides containing Tyr-Met-X-Met motifs by nonreceptor tyrosine kinases in vitro. J Biol Chem 1993;268(33):25146–25151.

90. Argetsinger LS, Kouadio JL, Steen H, Stensballe A, Jensen ON, Carter-Su C. Autophosphorylation of JAK2 on tyrosines 221 and 570 regulates its activity. Mol Cell Biol 2004;24(11):4955–4967.

91. Tournier C, Dong C, Turner TK, Jones SN, Flavell RA, Davis RJ. MKK7 is an essential component of the JNK signal transduction pathway activated by proinflammatory cytokines. Genes Dev 2001;15(11):1419–1426.

92. Chan PM, Keller PR, Connors RW, Leopold WR, Miller WT. Amino-terminal sequence determinants for substrate recognition by platelet-derived growth factor receptor tyrosine kinase. FEBS Lett 1996;394(2):121–125.

93. Mikhalap SV, Shlapatska LM, Yurchenko OV, Yurchenko MY, Berdova GG, Nichols KE, Clark EA, Sidorenko SP. The adaptor protein SH2D1A regulates signaling through CD150 (SLAM) in B cells. Blood 2004;104(13):4063–4070.

94. Flaswinkel H, Barner M, Reth M. The tyrosine activation motif as a target of protein tyrosine kinases and SH2 domains. Semin Immunol 1995;7(1):21–27.

95. Sidorenko SP, Clark EA. The dual-function CD150 receptor subfamily: the viral attraction. Nat Immunol 2003;4(1):19–24.

96. Ubersax JA, Ferrell JE Jr. Mechanisms of specificity in protein phosphorylation. Nat Rev Mol Cell Biol 2007;8(7):530–541.

97. Madhusudan, Trafny EA, Xuong NH, Adams JA, Ten Eyck LF, Taylor SS, Sowadski JM. cAMP-dependent protein kinase: crystallographic insights into substrate recognition and phosphotransfer. Protein Sci 1994;3(2):176–187.

98. Madhusudan, Akamine P, Xuong NH, Taylor SS. Crystal structure of a transition state mimic of the catalytic subunit of cAMP-dependent protein kinase. Nat Struct Biol 2002;9(4):273–277.

99. Adams JA, Taylor SS. Phosphorylation of peptide substrates for the catalytic subunit of cAMP-dependent protein kinase. J Biol Chem 1993;268(11):7747–7752.

100. Zhou J, Adams JA. Is there a catalytic base in the active site of cAMP-dependent protein kinase? Biochemistry 1997;36(10):2977–2984.

101. Diaz N, Field MJ. Insights into the phosphoryl-transfer mechanism of cAMP-dependent protein kinase from quantum chemical calculations and molecular dynamics simulations. J Am Chem Soc 2004;126(2):529–542.

102. Valiev M, Kawai R, Adams JA, Weare JH. The role of the putative catalytic base in the phosphoryl transfer reaction in a protein kinase: first-principles calculations. J Am Chem Soc 2003;125(33):9926–9927.

103. Valiev M, Yang J, Adams JA, Taylor SS, Weare JH. Phosphorylation reaction in cAPK protein kinase-free energy quantum mechanical/molecular mechanics simulations. J Phys Chem B 2007;111(47):13455–13464.

104. Kim K, Cole PA. Measurement of a Brønsted nucleophile coefficient and insights into the transition state for a protein tyrosine kinase. J Am Chem Soc 1997;119: 11096–11097.

105. Ablooglu AJ, Till JH, Kim K, Parang K, Cole PA, Hubbard SR, Kohanski RA. Probing the catalytic mechanism of the insulin receptor kinase with a tetrafluorotyrosine-containing peptide substrate. J Biol Chem 2000;275(39):30394–30398.

106. Cook A, Lowe ED, Chrysina ED, Skamnaki VT, Oikonomakos NG, Johnson LN. Structural studies on phospho-CDK2/cyclin A bound to nitrate, a transition state analogue: implications for the protein kinase mechanism. Biochemistry 2002;41(23):7301–7311.

107. Sun G, Budde RJ. Requirement for an additional divalent metal cation to activate protein tyrosine kinases. Biochemistry 1997;36(8):2139–2146.

108. Vicario PP, Saperstein R, Bennun A. Role of divalent metals in the kinetic mechanism of insulin receptor tyrosine kinase. Arch Biochem Biophys 1988;261(2):336–345.

109. Hubbard SR. Juxtamembrane autoinhibition in receptor tyrosine kinases. Nat Rev Mol Cell Biol 2004;5(6):464–471.

110. Hubbard SR, Till JH. Protein tyrosine kinase structure and function. Annu Rev Biochem 2000;69: 373–398.

111. Johnson LN, Noble ME, Owen DJ. Active and inactive protein kinases: structural basis for regulation. Cell 1996;85(2):149–158.

112. Favelyukis S, Till JH, Hubbard SR, Miller WT. Structure and autoregulation of the insulin-like growth factor 1 receptor kinase. Nat Struct Biol 2001;8(12):1058–1063.

113. Pautsch A, Zoephel A, Ahorn H, Spevak W, Hauptmann R, Nar H. Crystal structure of bis-phosphorylated IGF-1 receptor kinase: insight into domain movements upon kinase activation. Structure 2001;9(10):955–965.

114. Munshi S, Hall DL, Kornienko M, Darke PL, Kuo LC. Structure of apo, unactivated insulin-like growth factor-1 receptor kinase at 1.5 Å resolution. Acta Crystallogr D Biol Crystallogr 2003;59(Pt 10):1725–1730.

115. Munshi S, Kornienko M, Hall DL, Reid JC, Waxman L, Stirdivant SM, Darke PL, Kuo LC. Crystal structure of the Apo, unactivated insulin-like growth factor-1 receptor kinase. Implication for inhibitor specificity. J Biol Chem 2002;277(41):38797–38802.

116. Wei L, Hubbard SR, Hendrickson WA, Ellis L. Expression, characterization, and crystallization of the catalytic core of the human insulin receptor protein-tyrosine kinase domain. J Biol Chem 1995;270(14):8122–8130.

117. Lougheed JC, Chen RH, Mak P, Stout TJ. Crystal structures of the phosphorylated and unphosphorylated kinase domains of the Cdc42-associated tyrosine kinase ACK1. J Biol Chem 2004;279(42):44039–44045.

118. Lamers MB, Antson AA, Hubbard RE, Scott RK, Williams DH. Structure of the protein tyrosine kinase domain of C-terminal Src kinase (CSK) in complex with staurosporine. J Mol Biol 1999;285(2):713–725.

119. Ogawa A, Takayama Y, Sakai H, Chong KT, Takeuchi S, Nakagawa A, Nada S, Okada M, Tsukihara T. Structure of the carboxyl-terminal Src kinase, Csk. J Biol Chem 2002;277(17):14351–14354.

120. Oliver AW, Paul A, Boxall KJ, Barrie SE, Aherne GW, Garrett MD, Mittnacht S, Pearl LH. Trans-activation of the DNA-damage signalling protein kinase Chk2 by T-loop exchange. EMBO J 2006;25(13):3179–3190.

121. Chen P, Luo C, Deng Y, Ryan K, Register J, Margosiak S, Tempczyk-Russell A, Nguyen B, Myers P, Lundgren K, Kan CC, O'Connor PM. The 1.7 Å crystal structure of human cell cycle checkpoint kinase Chk1: implications for Chk1 regulation. Cell 2000;100(6):681–692.

122. Ahn J, Prives C. Checkpoint kinase 2 (Chk2) monomers or dimers phosphorylate Cdc25C after DNA damage regardless of threonine 68 phosphorylation. J Biol Chem 2002;277(50):48418–48426.

123. Xu X, Tsvetkov LM, Stern DF. Chk2 activation and phosphorylation-dependent oligomerization. Mol Cell Biol 2002;22(12):4419–4432.

124. Griffith J, Black J, Faerman C, Swenson L, Wynn M, Lu F, Lippke J, Saxena K. The structural basis for autoinhibition of FLT3 by the juxtamembrane domain. Mol Cell 2004;13(2):169–178.

125. Mol CD, Fabbro D, Hosfield DJ. Structural insights into the conformational selectivity of STI-571 and related kinase inhibitors. Curr Opin Drug Discov Dev 2004;7(5):639–648.

126. Irusta PM, Luo Y, Bakht O, Lai CC, Smith SO, DiMaio D. Definition of an inhibitory juxtamembrane WW-like domain in the platelet-derived growth factor beta receptor. J Biol Chem 2002;277(41):38627–38634.

127. Wybenga-Groot LE, Baskin B, Ong SH, Tong J, Pawson T, Sicheri F. Structural basis for autoinhibition of the Ephb2 receptor tyrosine kinase by the unphosphorylated juxtamembrane region. Cell 2001;106(6):745–757.

128. Binns KL, Taylor PP, Sicheri F, Pawson T, Holland SJ. Phosphorylation of tyrosine residues in the kinase domain and juxtamembrane region regulates the biological and catalytic activities of Eph receptors. Mol Cell Biol 2000;20(13):4791–4805.

129. Huse M, Chen YG, Massague J, Kuriyan J. Crystal structure of the cytoplasmic domain of the type I TGF beta receptor in complex with FKBP12. Cell 1999;96(3):425–436.

130. Huse M, Muir TW, Xu L, Chen YG, Kuriyan J, Massague J. The TGF beta receptor activation process: an inhibitor- to substrate-binding switch. Mol Cell 2001;8(3):671–682.

131. Frame S, Cohen P. GSK3 takes centre stage more than 20 years after its discovery. Biochem J 2001;359(Pt 1):1–16.

132. Cross DA, Alessi DR, Cohen P, Andjelkovich M, Hemmings BA. Inhibition of glycogen synthase kinase-3 by insulin mediated by protein kinase B. Nature 1995;378(6559):785–789.

133. Dajani R, Fraser E, Roe SM, Young N, Good V, Dale TC, Pearl LH. Crystal structure of glycogen synthase kinase 3 beta: structural basis for phosphate-primed substrate specificity and autoinhibition. Cell 2001;105(6):721–732.

134. ter Haar E, Coll JT, Austen DA, Hsiao HM, Swenson L, Jain J. Structure of GSK3 beta reveals a primed phosphorylation mechanism. Nat Struct Biol 2001;8(7):593–596.

135. Frame S, Cohen P, Biondi RM. A common phosphate binding site explains the unique substrate specificity of GSK3 and its inactivation by phosphorylation. Mol Cell 2001;7(6):1321–1327.

136. Manke IA, Nguyen A, Lim D, Stewart MQ, Elia AE, Yaffe MB. MAPKAP kinase-2 is a cell cycle checkpoint kinase that regulates the G2/M transition and S phase progression in response to UV irradiation. Mol Cell 2005;17(1):37–48.

137. Meng W, Swenson LL, Fitzgibbon MJ, Hayakawa K, Ter Haar E, Behrens AE, Fulghum JR, Lippke JA. Structure of mitogen-activated protein kinase-activated protein (MAPKAP) kinase 2 suggests a bifunctional switch that couples kinase activation with nuclear export. J Biol Chem 2002;277(40):37401–37405.

138. Underwood KW, Parris KD, Federico E, Mosyak L, Czerwinski RM, Shane T, Taylor M, Svenson K, Liu Y, Hsiao CL, Wolfrom S, Maguire M, Malakian K, Telliez JB, Lin LL, Kriz RW, Seehra J, Somers WS, Stahl ML. Catalytically active MAP KAP kinase 2 structures in complex with staurosporine and ADP reveal differences with the autoinhibited enzyme. Structure 2003;11(6):627–636.

139. Goldberg J, Nairn AC, Kuriyan J. Structural basis for the autoinhibition of calcium/calmodulin-dependent protein kinase I. Cell 1996;84(6):875–887.

140. Mayans O, van der Ven PF, Wilm M, Mues A, Young P, Furst DO, Wilmanns M, Gautel M. Structural basis for activation of the titin kinase domain during myofibrillogenesis. Nature 1998;395(6705):863–869.

141. Gold MG, Barford D, Komander D. Lining the pockets of kinases and phosphatases. Curr Opin Struct Biol 2006;16(6):693–701.

142. Yang J, Cron P, Good VM, Thompson V, Hemmings BA, Barford D. Crystal structure of an activated Akt/protein kinase B ternary complex with GSK3-peptide and AMP-PNP. Nat Struct Biol 2002;9(12):940–944.

143. Balendran A, Casamayor A, Deak M, Paterson A, Gaffney P, Currie R, Downes CP, Alessi DR. PDK1 acquires PDK2 activity in the presence of a synthetic peptide derived from the carboxyl terminus of PRK2. Curr Biol 1999;9(8):393–404.

144. Huang X, Begley M, Morgenstern KA, Gu Y, Rose P, Zhao H, Zhu X. Crystal structure of an inactive Akt2 kinase domain. Structure 2003;11(1):21–30.

145. Biondi RM, Nebreda AR. Signalling specificity of Ser/Thr protein kinases through docking-site-mediated interactions. Biochem J 2003;372(Pt 1):1–13.

146. Mora A, Komander D, van Aalten DM, Alessi DR. PDK1, the master regulator of AGC kinase signal transduction. Semin Cell Dev Biol 2004;15(2):161–170.

147. Sarbassov DD, Guertin DA, Ali SM, Sabatini DM. Phosphorylation and regulation of Akt/PKB by the rictor-mTOR complex. Science 2005;307(5712):1098–1101.

148. Hauge C, Antal TL, Hirschberg D, Doehn U, Thorup K, Idrissova L, Hansen K, Jensen ON, Jorgensen TJ, Biondi RM, Frodin M. Mechanism for activation of the growth factor-activated AGC kinases by turn motif phosphorylation. EMBO J 2007;26(9):2251–2261.

149. Alessi DR, James SR, Downes CP, Holmes AB, Gaffney PR, Reese CB, Cohen P. Characterization of a 3-phosphoinositide-dependent protein kinase which phosphorylates and activates protein kinase B alpha. Curr Biol 1997;7(4):261–269.

150. Stokoe D, Stephens LR, Copeland T, Gaffney PR, Reese CB, Painter GF, Holmes AB, McCormick F, Hawkins PT. Dual role of phosphatidylinositol-3,4,5-trisphosphate in the activation of protein kinase B. Science 1997;277(5325):567–570.

151. Wick MJ, Ramos FJ, Chen H, Quon MJ, Dong LQ, Liu F. Mouse 3-phosphoinositide-dependent protein kinase-1 undergoes dimerization and trans-phosphorylation in the activation loop. J Biol Chem 2003;278(44):42913–42919.

152. Komander D, Fairservice A, Deak M, Kular GS, Prescott AR, Peter Downes C, Safrany ST, Alessi DR, van Aalten DM. Structural insights into the regulation of PDK1 by phosphoinositides and inositol phosphates. EMBO J 2004;23(20):3918–3928.

153. Lian Z, Di Cristofano A. Class reunion: PTEN joins the nuclear crew. Oncogene 2005;24(50):7394–7400.

154. Kikani CK, Dong LQ, Liu F. "New" clear functions of PDK1: beyond a master kinase in the cytosol? J Cell Biochem 2005;96(6):1157–1162.

155. Boggon TJ, Eck MJ. Structure and regulation of Src family kinases. Oncogene 2004;23(48):7918–7927.

156. Harrison SC. Variation on an Src-like theme. Cell 2003;112(6):737–740.

157. Sicheri F, Kuriyan J. Structures of Src-family tyrosine kinases. Curr Opin Struct Biol 1997;7(6):777–785.

158. Hubbard SR. Src autoinhibition: let us count the ways. Nat Struct Biol 1999;6(8):711–714.

159. Moarefi I, LaFevre-Bernt M, Sicheri F, Huse M, Lee CH, Kuriyan J, Miller WT. Activation of the Src-family tyrosine kinase Hck by SH3 domain displacement. Nature 1997;385(6617):650–653.

160. Sicheri F, Moarefi I, Kuriyan J. Crystal structure of the Src family tyrosine kinase Hck. Nature 1997;385(6617):602–609.

161. Zhu X, Kim JL, Newcomb JR, Rose PE, Stover DR, Toledo LM, Zhao H, Morgenstern KA. Structural analysis of the lymphocyte-specific kinase Lck in complex with non-selective and Src family selective kinase inhibitors. Structure 1999;7(6):651–661.

162. Kinoshita T, Matsubara M, Ishiguro H, Okita K, Tada T. Structure of human Fyn kinase domain complexed with staurosporine. Biochem Biophys Res Commun 2006;346(3):840–844.

163. Xu W, Doshi A, Lei M, Eck MJ, Harrison SC. Crystal structures of c-Src reveal features of its autoinhibitory mechanism. Mol Cell 1999;3(5):629–638.

164. Xu W, Harrison SC, Eck MJ. Three-dimensional structure of the tyrosine kinase c-Src. Nature 1997;385(6617):595–602.

165. Williams JC, Weijland A, Gonfloni S, Thompson A, Courtneidge SA, Superti-Furga G, Wierenga RK. The 2.35 Å crystal structure of the inactivated form of chicken Src: a dynamic molecule with multiple regulatory interactions. J Mol Biol 1997;274(5):757–775.

166. Gonfloni S, Frischknecht F, Way M, Superti-Furga G. Leucine 255 of Src couples intramolecular interactions to inhibition of catalysis. Nat Struct Biol 1999;6(8):760–764.

167. Nada S, Okada M, MacAuley A, Cooper JA, Nakagawa H. Cloning of a complementary DNA for a protein-tyrosine kinase that specifically phosphorylates a negative regulatory site of p60c-src. Nature 1991;351(6321):69–72.

168. Okada M, Nakagawa H. A protein tyrosine kinase involved in regulation of pp60c-src function. J Biol Chem 1989;264(35):20886–20893.

169. Resh MD. Myristylation and palmitylation of Src family members: the facts of the matter. Cell 1994;76(3):411–413.

170. Cowan-Jacob SW, Fendrich G, Manley PW, Jahnke W, Fabbro D, Liebetanz J, Meyer T. The crystal structure of a c-Src complex in an active conformation suggests possible steps in c-Src activation. Structure 2005;13(6):861–871.

171. Hantschel O, Nagar B, Guettler S, Kretzschmar J, Dorey K, Kuriyan J, Superti-Furga G. A myristoyl/phosphotyrosine switch regulates c-Abl. Cell 2003;112(6):845–857.

172. Nagar B, Hantschel O, Young MA, Scheffzek K, Veach D, Bornmann W, Clarkson B, Superti-Furga G, Kuriyan J. Structural basis for the autoinhibition of c-Abl tyrosine kinase. Cell 2003;112(6):859–871.

173. Lerner EC, Smithgall TE. SH3-dependent stimulation of Src-family kinase autophosphorylation without tail release from the SH2 domain in vivo. Nat Struct Biol 2002;9(5):365–369.

174. Young MA, Gonfloni S, Superti-Furga G, Roux B, Kuriyan J. Dynamic coupling between the SH2 and SH3 domains of c-Src and Hck underlies their inactivation by C-terminal tyrosine phosphorylation. Cell 2001;105(1):115–126.

175. McLean GW, Carragher NO, Avizienyte E, Evans J, Brunton VG, Frame MC. The role of focal-adhesion kinase in cancer—a new therapeutic opportunity. Nat Rev Cancer 2005;5(7): 505–515.

176. Schaller MD, Hildebrand JD, Shannon JD, Fox JW, Vines RR, Parsons JT. Autophosphorylation of the focal adhesion kinase, pp125FAK, directs SH2-dependent binding of pp60src. Mol Cell Biol 1994;14(3):1680–1688.

177. Toutant M, Costa A, Studler JM, Kadare G, Carnaud M, Girault JA. Alternative splicing controls the mechanisms of FAK autophosphorylation. Mol Cell Biol 2002;22(22):7731–7743.

178. Calalb MB, Polte TR, Hanks SK. Tyrosine phosphorylation of focal adhesion kinase at sites in the catalytic domain regulates kinase activity: a role for Src family kinases. Mol Cell Biol 1995;15(2):954–963.

179. Nowakowski J, Cronin CN, McRee DE, Knuth MW, Nelson CG, Pavletich NP, Rogers J, Sang BC, Scheibe DN, Swanson RV, Thompson DA. Structures of the cancer-related Aurora-A, FAK, and EphA2 protein kinases from nanovolume crystallography. Structure 2002;10(12):1659–1667.

180. Lietha D, Cai X, Ceccarelli DF, Li Y, Schaller MD, Eck MJ. Structural basis for the autoinhibition of focal adhesion kinase. Cell 2007;129(6):1177–1187.

181. De Bondt HL, Rosenblatt J, Jancarik J, Jones HD, Morgan DO, Kim SH. Crystal structure of cyclin-dependent kinase 2. Nature 1993;363(6430):595–602.

182. Brown NR, Noble ME, Endicott JA, Garman EF, Wakatsuki S, Mitchell E, Rasmussen B, Hunt T, Johnson LN. The crystal structure of cyclin A. Structure 1995;3(11):1235–1247.

183. Jeffrey PD, Russo AA, Polyak K, Gibbs E, Hurwitz J, Massague J, Pavletich NP. Mechanism of CDK activation revealed by the structure of a cyclin A–CDK2 complex. Nature 1995;376(6538):313–320.

184. Abbas T, Jha S, Sherman NE, Dutta A. Autocatalytic phosphorylation of CDK2 at the activating Thr160. Cell Cycle 2007;6(7):843–852.

185. Russo AA, Jeffrey PD, Pavletich NP. Structural basis of cyclin-dependent kinase activation by phosphorylation. Nat Struct Biol 1996;3(8):696–700.

186. Brown NR, Noble ME, Lawrie AM, Morris MC, Tunnah P, Divita G, Johnson LN, Endicott JA. Effects of phosphorylation of threonine 160 on cyclin-dependent kinase 2 structure and activity. J Biol Chem 1999;274(13):8746–8756.

187. Brown NR, Lowe ED, Petri E, Skamnaki V, Antrobus R, Johnson LN. Cyclin B and cyclin A confer different substrate recognition properties on CDK2. Cell Cycle 2007;6(11):1350–1359.

188. Kim KK, Chamberlin HM, Morgan DO, Kim SH. Three-dimensional structure of human cyclin H, a positive regulator of the CDK-activating kinase. Nat Struct Biol 1996;3(10):849–855.

189. Andersen G, Busso D, Poterszman A, Hwang JR, Wurtz JM, Ripp R, Thierry JC, Egly JM, Moras D. The structure of cyclin H: common mode of kinase activation and specific features. EMBO J 1997;16(5):958–967.

190. Petri ET, Errico A, Escobedo L, Hunt T, Basavappa R. The crystal structure of human cyclin B. Cell Cycle 2007;6(11):1342–1349.

191. Baek K, Brown RS, Birrane G, Ladias JA. Crystal structure of human cyclin K, a positive regulator of cyclin-dependent kinase 9. J Mol Biol 2007;366(2):563–573.

192. Honda R, Lowe ED, Dubinina E, Skamnaki V, Cook A, Brown NR, Johnson LN. The structure of cyclin E1/CDK2: implications for CDK2 activation and CDK2-independent roles. EMBO J 2005;24(3):452–463.

193. Jeffrey PD, Tong L, Pavletich NP. Structural basis of inhibition of CDK–cyclin complexes by INK4 inhibitors. Genes Dev 2000;14(24):3115–3125.

194. Schulze-Gahmen U, Kim SH. Structural basis for CDK6 activation by a virus-encoded cyclin. Nat Struct Biol 2002;9(3):177–181.

195. Lolli G, Lowe ED, Brown NR, Johnson LN. The crystal structure of human CDK7 and its protein recognition properties. Structure 2004;12(11):2067–2079.

196. Gotoh N, Tojo A, Hino M, Yazaki Y, Shibuya M. A highly conserved tyrosine residue at codon 845 within the kinase domain is not required for the transforming activity of human epidermal growth factor receptor. Biochem Biophys Res Commun 1992;186(2):768–774.

197. Stamos J, Sliwkowski MX, Eigenbrot C. Structure of the epidermal growth factor receptor kinase domain alone and in complex with a 4-anilinoquinazoline inhibitor. J Biol Chem 2002;277(48):46265–46272.

198. Wood ER, Truesdale AT, McDonald OB, Yuan D, Hassell A, Dickerson SH, Ellis B, Pennisi C, Horne E, Lackey K, Alligood KJ, Rusnak DW, Gilmer TM, Shewchuk L. A unique structure for epidermal growth factor receptor bound to GW572016 (lapatinib): relationships among protein conformation, inhibitor off-rate, and receptor activity in tumor cells. Cancer Res 2004;64(18):6652–6659.

199. Groenen LC, Walker F, Burgess AW, Treutlein HR. A model for the activation of the epidermal growth factor receptor kinase involvement of an asymmetric dimer? Biochemistry 1997;36(13):3826–3836.

200. Zhang X, Gureasko J, Shen K, Cole PA, Kuriyan J. An allosteric mechanism for activation of the kinase domain of epidermal growth factor receptor. Cell 2006;125(6):1137–1149.

201. Cobb MH, Goldsmith EJ. Dimerization in MAP-kinase signaling. Trends Biochem Sci 2000;25(1):7–9.

202. Zhang F, Strand A, Robbins D, Cobb MH, Goldsmith EJ. Atomic structure of the MAP kinase ERK2 at 2.3 Å resolution. Nature 1994;367(6465):704–711.

203. Khokhlatchev AV, Canagarajah B, Wilsbacher J, Robinson M, Atkinson M, Goldsmith E, Cobb MH. Phosphorylation of the MAP kinase ERK2 promotes its homodimerization and nuclear translocation. Cell 1998;93(4):605–615.

CHAPTER *3*

RECEPTOR TYROSINE KINASES

RECEPTOR TYROSINE kinases (RTKs) are one of the most important and widely studied subgroups of protein kinases and have particular relevance to cancer. These receptors are key sensors of the extracellular environment, transducing signals from a vast array of ligands to diverse intracellular signaling networks. Broadly, each RTK contains an N-terminal extracellular (growth factor binding) segment, a transmembrane segment, and a C-terminal intracellular segment containing the kinase domain and a series of tyrosine phosphorylation sites. Binding of growth factor typically promotes receptor aggregation (most commonly dimerization) and kinase activation, with subsequent *trans*-phosphorylation of tyrosine residues in the intracellular domain. These phosphorylation sites include regulatory sequences within and adjacent to the kinase domain, which modulate receptor activation and kinase activity (see Chapter 2). In addition, autophosphorylation occurs on a series of phosphotyrosine residues in the C-terminal tails of the receptors, coupling them to various intracellular signaling pathways. The receptor substrates either undergo phosphorylation or engage additional downstream components via protein:protein interactions. The protein:protein interactions are often mediated by SH2 (SRC homology 2) domains, which bind to specific phosphotyrosine-containing peptide sequences in the receptors. In some cases, additional intracellular kinases can also phosphorylate and regulate the biological function of the receptors. Signal transduction can be downregulated by several mechanisms, including dephosphorylation by protein tyrosine phosphatases and receptor internalization, lysosomal translocation, and degradation.

The biological processes mediated by RTKs include cellular growth, proliferation, survival, differentiation, motility, and invasion and are manifest in all cell types, including epithelial, endothelial, mesenchymal, and hematopoietic lineages. Given the critical role of RTKs in directing cellular fates, it is not surprising that the dysregulation of one or more of these receptors has been implicated in the initiation and progression of almost all kinds of cancer (1). The

Targeting Protein Kinases for Cancer Therapy, by David J. Matthews and Mary E. Gerritsen
Copyright © 2010 John Wiley & Sons, Inc.

epidermal growth factor receptor (EGFR) was the first RTK to be implicated in oncogenesis in the 1980s, with the discovery that it had been co-opted in mutant form by the avian erythroblastosis virus, resulting in the *v-ERBB* oncogene (2); this was soon followed by the identification of the related *ERBB2/HER2* (*neu*) oncogene (3–5). Since then, many RTKs (including those of the EGFR/ERBB family) have been found to be overexpressed, amplified, mutated, and/or translocated in human tumors. These factors, together with autocrine growth factor production, are important in promoting the autonomous growth and proliferation, evasion of apoptosis, and invasive phenotype that are characteristic of tumor cells (6). RTKs are also critical in promoting tumor angiogenesis, the inhibition of which was proposed as an anticancer strategy over 30 years ago (7). Accordingly, RTKs were among the first kinases to be targeted for therapeutic intervention: several RTK antagonists (both antibodies and small molecules) are currently approved for treatment of cancer and a dizzying array of new RTK inhibitors are now under evaluation in the clinic (Chapters 8 and 9). In this chapter we discuss some of the RTKs that have been shown to play a role in tumor formation and progression, as well as various receptors that help to maintain tumor viability by promoting tumor angiogenesis.

3.1 EGF/ERBB RECEPTORS

The epidermal growth factor receptor (EGFR, ERBB1, HER1) and related paralogs ERBB2 (HER2), ERBB3 (HER3), and ERBB4 (HER4) collectively comprise the Type I subfamily of receptor tyrosine kinases. The ERBB pathway is an ancient metazoan signaling mechanism: orthologs of EGF receptor are found in *Caenorhabditis elegans* (let-23 (8)) and *Drosophila melanogaster* (DER/torpedo (9, 10)). In mammals, the four ERBB receptors play an important role in development and are active in epithelial, mesenchymal, and neuronal cells. ERBB receptors promote cellular proliferation, migration, survival, and differentiation, and the dysregulation of one or more ERBB receptors is a common feature in tumor cells. As such, the development of anti-ERBB therapies—both antibodies and small molecules—has received substantial attention in recent years. Here we discuss these four receptors collectively, since both homodimers and heterodimers of ERBB family members play an important role in normal cellular homeostasis and in tumor development and progression.

As noted earlier, EGFR was the first tyrosine kinase receptor to be linked to cancer (reviewed in (11)). The EGFR gene is located on chromosome 7p12 and comprises 28 exons distributed over approximately 200 kb of genomic DNA (12). The receptor is a 170-kDa glycoprotein comprising an extracellular ligand binding domain (arranged as a tandem repeat of L (large, or leucine-rich repeat) and CR (cysteine-rich) domains), a transmembrane region, an intracellular kinase domain, and a C-terminal tail that contains multiple phosphorylation sites involved in downstream signaling. (X-ray crystal structures of the EGFR ectodomains and kinase domain are discussed further in Chapter 2.) The overall domain structure of EGFR is shared by ERBB2, ERBB3, and ERBB4. The genes encoding each of the receptors are found on different chromosomes: *ERBB2* is located at 17q12 (13), ERBB3 is on chromosome 12 (12q13) (14), and *ERBB4* is on chromosome 2 (2q33–34) (15). Notably, ERBB4 exists as several different splice forms with varying sequences adjacent to the membrane in the extracellular domain (16, 17); these variants have distinct expression patterns and signaling mechanisms.

ERBB receptor signaling is triggered by a family of at least ten growth factor ligands, with varying receptor specificities (18). Each ligand contains a small (60 amino acid) domain with three disulfide bonds and homology to epidermal growth factor (EGF). Broadly, the ligands can be segregated into three groups (Figure 3.1). Members of the first group, including EGF, transforming growth factor-α (TGFα), and amphiregulin, bind only to EGFR; the second group (betacellulin, heparin binding EGF (HB-EGF), and epiregulin) are dual specificity ligands, recognizing both EGFR and ERBB4. The third group, the neuregulins (also known as heregulins), is a large family of growth factors arising from alternate splicing of four genes. Neuregulins either bind to both ERBB3 and ERBB4 (NRG1 and NRG2) or

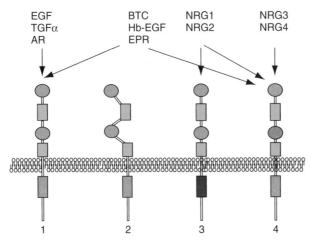

Figure 3.1 Common domain structures and features of the ERBB family of receptors. The ERBB receptors share common domain features, including an extracellular region with tandem repeats of leucine-rich repeats (green ovals) and cysteine-rich repeats (tan rectangles) in the extracellular domain, a single transmembrane spanning region, a short juxtamembrane region, followed by a kinase region (blue rectangle) and a cytoplasmic tail of varying length with multiple tyrosine phosphorylation sites. ERBB receptors are activated by a family of ligands, with varying specificities for each receptor. There are no cognate ligands for ERBB2: however, it adopts a conformation that enables it to form heterodimers with other ERBB receptors. The kinase domain of ERBB3 is inactive, although this receptor forms potent heterodimeric signaling complexes with other ERBB family members.

are specific for ERBB4 (NRG3 and NRG4); an additional ERBB4 ligand called tomoregulin has also been reported.

Notably, no ligands bind ERBB2 (HER2), so it is perhaps not a bona fide receptor in the most literal sense. As discussed in Chapter 2, the structure of the ERBB2 extracellular domain is incompatible with ligand binding but adopts a "preactivated" conformation, making it an ideal partner for homodimerization with other family members. ERBB3 is also unique among the EGFR family in that it has no intrinsic kinase activity. However, ERBB3 can act as a potent activator of other family members, and in fact the ERBB2/ERBB3 heterodimer appears to be the most potent signaling complex of all the possible homo/heterodimers (19). An additional mechanism of ERBB2 activation involves metalloproteinase-mediated cleavage of the receptor extracellular domain (ECD), leaving a constitutively active membrane-tethered fragment (20–22). High levels of ERBB2 ECD in the serum of cancer patients correlates with poor prognosis (22, 23), and may also confer resistance to anti-ERBB2 therapeutic antibodies by competition with cell surface receptors (24).

Receptor tyrosine kinase ligand engagement is typically envisaged as binding of a soluble growth factor to a membrane-bound receptor: however, the ERBB ligands are synthesized as membrane-associated proteins (18). In fact, the tethered ligand and transmembrane receptor may promote direct ("juxtacrine") cell–cell signaling in some circumstances (25): for example, pro-TGFα on the surface of murine bone marrow stromal cells was shown to interact with EGFR expressed on adjacent hematopoietic progenitor cells (26). Both autocrine and paracrine ERBB activation pathways employ a common mechanism of ligand activation termed ectodomain shedding (27). (To avoid confusion, it should be noted that ectodomain shedding is also sometimes used to describe the proteolytic cleavage of the ERBB2 *receptor* extracellular domains, described previously.) Ectodomain shedding in EGF family proteins involves activation of a metalloproteinase belonging to the ADAM (a disintegrin and metalloproteinase) family, which in turn cleaves the extracellular portions of the membrane-bound ERBB ligand. The liberated extracellular ligand can then bind to its cognate ERBB receptor, promoting autocrine or paracrine receptor activation and signaling (Figure 3.2). The fact that this mechanism can operate in an autocrine fashion may be particularly important in promoting the autonomous growth of tumor cells. Studies in mouse embryonic fibroblasts lacking various ADAM metalloproteinases have implicated ADAM17 (TACE) in the shedding of HB-EGF, TGFα, and amphiregulin, and ADAM10 in the processing of EGF and betacellulin (28), although the proteinase specificity may vary in different cellular contexts.

In addition to ERBB family homo- and heterodimerization, several other cellular proteins and pathways have been implicated in ERBB transactivation. Various G-protein coupled receptors (GPCRs) appear to mediate this process by triggering the ADAM-mediated ectodomain shedding of ERBB ligands (29). For example, estrogen receptor (ER) signaling appears to transactivate EGFR via the GPR30 receptor and release of pro HB-EGF (30), although GPR30 can also attenuate EGFR-mediated MAPK (ERK1/2) activity by stimulation of adenylyl cyclase and cAMP-dependent signaling (31). Another ER/GPCR/EGFR transactivation pathway

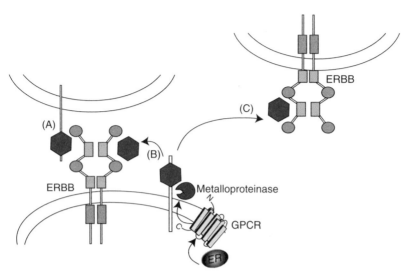

Figure 3.2 Juxtacrine, autocrine, and paracrine activation of ERBB receptors. (A) EGF family ligands (purple hexagon) are synthesized as membrane-associated proteins and may directly activate receptors on neighboring cells (juxtacrine signaling). (B) Autocrine signaling entails release of ligands from the cell surface and subsequent engagement with receptors on the surface of the same cell. (C) In paracrine signaling, EGF ligands are released from one cell and activate receptors on the surface of nearby cells. In both autocrine and paracrine signaling, ligands are released from the cell surface by the activity of ADAM metalloproteinases, which is often mediated by G-protein coupled receptor signaling.

was shown to involve release of sphingosine-1 phosphate (S1P), activation of the S1P receptor EDG-3, and subsequent metalloproteinase-mediated ectodomain shedding (32). Notably, the selective estrogen receptor modulator tamoxifen, used in treatment of hormone receptor positive breast cancer, can also promote EGFR transactivation and may thus blunt the antiproliferative effects of tamoxifen in tumor cells (33). Conversely, ERBB4 has been implicated in transactivation of ER, and ERBB4 expression is regulated by ER: thus a potent positive feedback loop between estrogen and ERBB signaling may contribute to growth of ER and ERBB4-positive breast tumors (34). The WNT receptor (Frizzled) has also been implicated in EGFR transactivation in mammary cells (35). EGFR and ERBB2 can also interact with the gp130 chain of IL6 receptor, and IL6 may promote ERBB receptor phosphorylation in some tumor types (36, 37). More recently, the β4−integrin receptor was shown to interact with ERBB2, promoting tumorigenesis and invasive growth in a mouse mammary carcinoma model (38). Additional transactivation mechanisms involve phosphorylation of ERBB receptors by intracellular kinases other than ERBB family members. In particular, SRC is both an upstream mediator and a downstream effector of EGFR and was shown to phosphorylate EGFR in both the catalytic domain and C-terminal tail, increasing receptor function (39, 40). EGFR and ERBB2 can also be phosphorylated by JAK2, which is activated by the growth hormone family of cytokine receptors (41–43). PKC phosphorylates EGFR in the juxtamembrane region and may thereby negatively regulate downstream signaling (44). Furthermore, phosphorylation by ABL kinase has been shown to inhibit CBL-mediated receptor endocytosis (45).

Engagement of ligands with ERBB extracellular domains promotes receptor dimerization and *trans*-phosphorylation of cytoplasmic tyrosine residues, which couples receptor activation to intracellular signaling networks. The combination of tissue-specific receptor expression, multiple activating ligands and transactivation mechanisms, various hetero- and homodimeric receptor complexes, and coupling to diverse intracellular signaling cascades results in a rich, multilayered, and flexible signaling network (46). Signaling is highly time dependent, and some tyrosine residues can be phosphorylated and dephosphorylated within minutes. Historically, the association of specific phosphotyrosines with downstream signaling pathways has been deduced using immunoprecipitation/Western blot analysis of specific proteins following growth factor stimulation. More recently, proteomic approaches (including mass spectrometry and protein microarrays) have allowed a much broader survey of the ERBB "interactome," revealing some global properties of ERBB signaling that were not apparent from earlier, more focused studies.

A schematic overview of phosphorylation sites and their associated intracellular signaling effects is shown in Figure 3.3. Each ERBB family member couples to a distinct but overlapping set of downstream adaptor and effector proteins, leading to activation of many intracellular signaling networks including the RAS/MAPK and PI3K pathways (Chapter 5). EGFR has multiple autophosphorylation sites in its C-terminal tail, some of which are quite promiscuous and others that are highly selective in their binding partners. Collectively, these sites couple to multiple signal transduction adaptor proteins containing PTB (phosphotyrosine binding) or SH2 (SRC homology region 2) domains. These adaptor proteins include SHC (SRC homology 2-containing) and GRB2 (growth factor receptor-bound), which both couple to RAS/MAPK signaling (and, via RAS, to PI3K signaling). As well as directly interacting with EGFR, GRB2 can also signal downstream by interracting with EGFR-bound SHC. The GAB1 adaptor protein can also couple EGFR to the PI3K pathway, though it appears that this may not be the predominant mechanism in tumor cells, which rely substantially on ERBB3 (47). In addition to autophosphorylation, EGFR is also phosphorylated by SRC (39); conversely, EGFR downstream signals can promote SRC and PAK1 kinase activation and actin cytoskeleton signaling (48). EGFR can also directly activate PLCγ (phospholipase C, which promotes phospholipid cleavage, Ca^{2+} release, and PKC activation) and the STAT1/STAT5 (signal transduction and transcription) factors. EGFR phosphotyrosines also mediate inhibitory interactions, and EGFR undergoes efficient endocytosis and lysosomal degradation following ligand binding and dimerization. The GRB2 adaptor protein and the CBL ubiquitin ligases play important roles in the complex process of receptor internalization and trafficking (reviewed in (49)), and an additional phospho-EGFR binding protein, EPS15, is proposed to mediate internalization via clathrin-coated pits (50). Notably, the fate of internalized EGFR can depend on the ligand to which it is bound: TGFα becomes dissociated from EGFR in the endosomal compartment and the receptors are recycled to the cell

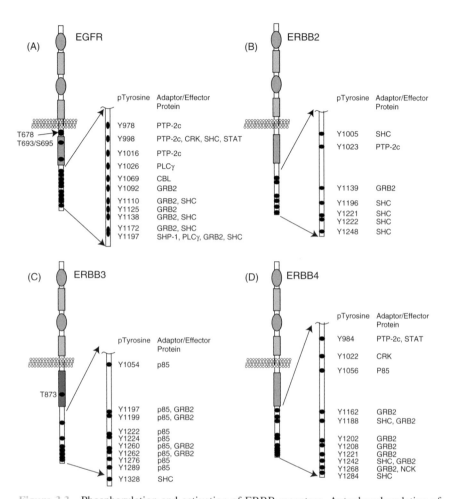

Figure 3.3 Phosphorylation and activation of ERBB receptors. Autophosphorylation of ERBB receptor C-terminal tyrosines recruits many different proteins, signaling to diverse downstream effectors. (A) In the case of EGFR, PTP-2c binds to Y978, Y998, and Y1016; SHC to Y998, Y1110, Y1138, Y1172 and Y1197; CRK to Y998; STAT to Y998; PLCγ to Y1026 and Y1197; SHP-1 to Y1197; and GRB2 to Y1102, Y1110, Y1125, Y1138, Y1172, and Y1197. EGFR is also phosphorylated by SRC kinase (Y845 and Y1101), PKC (T654), and ERK/p38 MAP kinase (T669). (B) ERBB2 has no cognate ligand but is phosphorylated following heterodimerization with other ERBB family members. In this case phosphorylation of Y1005, Y1196, Y1221, Y1222, and Y1248 recruits SHC; phosphorylation of Y1023 rercruits PTP-2c; and phosphorylation of Y1139 recruits GRB2. (C) When ERBB3 is activated by ligand binding, phosphorylation of Y1054, Y1197, Y1199, Y1222, Y1224, Y1260, Y1262, Y1276, and Y1289 results in the binding of the p85 subunit of PI3K. Phosphorylation of Y1197, Y1199, Y1260, and Y1262 recruits GRB2, and phosphorylated Y1328 recruits SHC. (D) Activation of ERBB4 results in the phosphorylation of a number of tyrosines in the C terminus, which recruit a variety of binding partners. Phosphorylated Y984 recruits STAT and PTP-2c, phosphorylated Y1022 recruits CRK, and phosphorylated Y1056 recruits the p85 subunit of PI3K. GRB2 binds to phosphorylated Y1162, Y1188, Y1202, Y1208, Y1221, Y1242, and Y1268; SHC binds to phosphorylated Y1188, Y1242, and Y1284. NCK binds to phosphorylated Y1268. Note that, for EGFR and ERBB3, alternative numbering schemes (starting after the signal peptide) are sometimes used, resulting in amino acid numbers that are 24 (EGFR) or 19 (ERBB3) less than those indicated here.

surface, whereas EGF-bound receptors are transported to lysosomes and degraded (51, 52). EGFR is also regulated by Ser/Thr kinases. PKC phosphorylates a threonine residue in the juxtamembrane region that promotes kinase deactivation (53), and a neighboring site is a substrate for ERK/p38 MAP kinases (54).

Like EGFR, ERBB2 also couples to the RAS pathway via SHC and GRB2 and can also signal to PLCγ but does not directly activate PI3K in tumor cells. Additional adaptor proteins linked to ERBB2 signaling include DOK-R and CRKII. ERBB2 is internalized and downregulated less efficiently than EGFR, and so EGFR:ERBB2 heterodimers may confer elevated levels of signaling compared to EGFR homodimers (55). A genome-wide survey of the interactions of PTB/SH2-containing proteins with ERBB phosphotyrosines suggests that, in general, ERBB2 phosphotyrosines are more promiscuous than those of other ERBB family members. Furthermore, this study indicated that as receptor concentration is increased (and the threshold for binding to a given phosphotyrosine thereby lowered), EGFR and ERBB2 can recruit more and more binding partners, whereas the ERBB3 interactome shows relatively little change (56). This increased diversity (in addition to increased amplitude and duration of signaling) may explain the frequent overexpression in tumor cells of EGFR and ERBB2, but not ERBB3. However, only a small fraction of these potential interactions may actually be manifest in a given cellular context, and a recent survey of ERBB phosphopeptide-interacting proteins in HeLa cells by mass spectrometry identified only a relatively small set of proteins as ERBB2 binders (57).

ERBB3 has particular importance in signaling through the PI3K pathway, as it has at least six phosphotyrosine sites that are recognized by the PI3K p85 regulatory subunit (Chapter 5). In addition, ERBB3 can associate with GRB2/GRB7 and SHC adaptor proteins, thereby also coupling this receptor to the RAS/MAPK pathway. Three of the GRB2/GRB7 sites are adjacent to PI3K p85 binding sites in a YEY motif, where the first tyrosine binds p85 and the second GRB2. Hence there may be competition between the downstream signaling pathways; GRB2 binding is weaker when both sites are phosphorylated, but it is not clear if this is physiologically relevant (57). ERBB3 is emerging as a critical component of oncogenic EGFR signaling in non small cell lung cancer (NSCLC), since sensitivity of NSCLC cells to EGFR inhibitors is correlated with coupling of PI3K to ERBB3 (58). It is not clear whether direct EGFR:ERBB3 complexes are involved, or if there is an indirect signaling mechanism involving formation of an initial EGFR:ERBB2 complex, followed by a "handoff" of ERBB2 to form a secondary heterodimer with ERBB3 (59). Although ERBB2 and ERBB3 are both intrinsically disabled due to lack of ligand binding and kinase activity, respectively, the ERBB2:ERBB3 heterodimer is a particularly potent signaling complex (60). Complexation of ERBB3 with ERBB2 appears to increase ligand promiscuity and binding affinity such that, in addition to neuregulins, EGF and betacellulin can also bind to and activate the receptor. The dimeric receptor is a strong activator of multiple growth and survival signals, including those mediated by the RAS/MAPK and PI3K pathways. ERBB3 may also help tumor cells evade the effects of EGFR and ERBB2 inhibition, due to an AKT-mediated feedback mechanism that upregulates ERBB3 and decreases receptor dephosphorylation following chronic treatment with small molecule EGFR/ERBB2 inhibitors (61).

ERBB4 has until recently been less widely studied than the other ERBB receptors, although it is known to bind to SHC and PI3K p85 and was more recently shown to interact with STAT1 (62). Although it has 19 potential tyrosine phosphorylation sites (compared to 12, 8, and 11 for EGFR, ERBB2, and ERBB3, respectively), ERBB4 appears to couple to a relatively small subset of downstream signaling proteins (average of 2.2 per site, compared to 9.8 (EGFR), 18.4 (ERBB2), and 11.4 (ERBB3)) (56, 62). This relative paucity of downstream signaling may explain why ERBB4 is associated with protective, antitumor effects and favorable prognosis in several types of cancer, including bladder and breast tumors: heterodimerization with ERBB4 may serve to buffer the oncogenic effects of signaling through other ERBB receptors.

In addition to the canonical phosphotyrosine-mediated modes of signaling, ERBB receptors may also directly signal to the nucleus (63, 64). EGFR has been reported to translocate to the nucleus and activate transcription factors in a ligand-dependent manner (65). Alternatively, ligand binding or PKC activation can induce one of the splice forms of ERBB4 to undergo metalloproteinase-mediated processing, resulting in translocation of the cytoplasmic fragment to nuclei and mitochondria (66, 67). This fragment is catalytically active and regulates gene expression via STAT5A (67). Remarkably, the ERBB4 cytoplasmic fragment appears to contain a BCL2 homology (BH3) domain near the C-terminal end of the kinase domain, revealing a functional connection to proapoptotic BCL2 family members such as BID, BIM, NOXA, and PUMA (68). The BH3 homology domain interacts with BCL2 and promotes apoptotic cell death via BAK-mediated mitochondrial permeabilization.

ERBB receptors are critical to developmental morphogenesis and regulate cell proliferation and migration as well as differentiation. In particular, EGF family growth factor signaling is a key driver of epithelial–mesenchymal transitions, which not only play a key role in embryonic development but are a major factor in metastasis of tumor cells (69, 70). The role of specific ERBB receptors in mammalian development has been illuminated by studies with transgenic knockout mice. Defects in any of the *erbb* receptors are embryonic or perinatally lethal in mice, underscoring the crucial role that they play in development. Mice lacking *egfr* die either during gestation or soon after birth due to respiratory problems and defects in the gastrointestinal tract, skin, and hair (71, 72), with additional defects in the CNS and other organs. ERBB2 is important in adult mammary gland development, foreshadowing its role in breast cancer initiation and progression (73). Furthermore, *erbb2* knockout mice die in utero due to heart abnormalities, indicating a role for this receptor in cardiac development (74); these embryos also show impaired neural development. *erbb3* knockout mice also die in utero due to cardiac and neural dysfunction (75). A similar phenotype is found with *ERBB4* knockout mice (76), and both ERBB2 and ERBB4 are expressed in the myocardium: hence, since ERBB2 has no cognate ligands, ERBB2:ERBB4 heterodimers may be involved. ERBB4 signaling is implicated in neural development and is also important in promoting differentiation and lactation in breast tissue, particularly in late pregnancy and at parturition (77). As discussed earlier, ERBB4 undergoes metalloproteinase-mediated cleavage resulting in nuclear and mitochondrial accumulation of the cytoplasmic fragment (66, 67). The nuclear form of ERBB4 is important in regulating astrogenesis in the developing brain (78) and induces differentiation in mammary epithelial cells (79, 80).

3.1.1 ERBB Receptors and Cancer

Multiple mechanisms have been implicated in the dysregulation of ERBB receptor function in tumors. In general, aberrant activation of EGFR appears to occur largely through mutation, whereas gene amplification and overexpression is the main driver of ERBB2-mediated malignancy. However, overexpression and mutation are frequently found to occur together in many tumors.

EGFR EGFR is often overexpressed in many tumor types including breast, colon, lung, head and neck, and bladder cancers and glioblastoma multiforme (GBM). Amplification occurs frequently in GBM but is also found to a lesser extent in other tumors such as non small cell lung carcinoma (NSCLC) (81). Expression of EGFR in head and neck cancer has been clearly correlated with poor response to therapy and overall survival, and similar trends have been observed in ovarian, cervical, bladder, and esophageal cancers (82). However, the prognostic significance of EGFR expression has been less clear in other disease settings (including breast, lung, and colorectal cancers), with some studies indicating a correlation between EGFR expression and poor prognosis and others showing no significant relationship. Some of this variability may be due to different techniques for measuring EGFR expression (such as radioligand binding and immunohistochemistry). There is probably also an underlying biological reason, stemming from the fact that EGFR signaling is tightly coupled to that of other ERBB family members, as well as the status of receptor ligands such as TGFα, other RTKs, and downstream intracellular signaling pathways. Further complications arise from the observation that expression of EGFR in primary tumors does not necessarily correlate with expression at metastatic sites in the same patient (83).

Mutations in EGFR have been described in many tumor types, but are perhaps most prevalent and best characterized in GBM (84) and NSCLC (85). Various EGFR exon deletions and tandem duplications are found in GBM, the most common of which is the EGFRvIII variant. EGFRvIII comprises over 50% of mutations found in GBM and has an in-frame deletion of exons 2–7, resulting in loss of most of the extracellular domain and ligand-independent activation. Moreover, this variant is frequently expressed at high levels, and EGFRvIII overexpression in the presence of EGFR amplification is associated with particularly poor survival (86). EGFRvIII has also been infrequently reported in breast, ovarian, and lung tumors (87). Two further deletion variants, EGFRvII (lacking exons 14 and 15) and EGFRvV (truncated in the intracellular domain), are each found in ~15% of GBM samples (88). Both of these variants retain ligand dependency but likely confer a selective growth advantage over the wild-type receptor (84).

In contrast to the large genomic rearrangements found in GBM, EGFR variants in NSCLC are typically point mutations or small in-frame insertions/deletions (89). These mutations were first uncovered in clinical studies with the small molecule EGFR inhibitors gefitinib and erlotinib (90–92). Although response rates to these inhibitors in NSCLC were relatively low (around 10%), a very high proportion of responders were found to harbor mutant forms of EGFR in their tumors. Further analysis indicated that mutations were particularly prevalent in nonsmokers, in women, in East Asians, and in adenocarcinomas with bronchioloalveolar histology. The most common mutations associated with drug sensitivity are small deletions within exon 19 (e.g., ΔE746-A750) and point mutations in the activation loop (exon 21, in particular, L858R and, to a lesser extent, L861Q). These mutations are generally thought to enhance kinase activity, though not necessarily to the level of ligand independence (90–92). Additional drug-sensitizing mutations are found in the nucleotide binding loop (exon 18, particularly G719). A single mutation in exon 20, T790M, has been associated with acquired resistance to EGFR inhibitors (93, 94). This mutation confers resistance to gefitinib and erlotinib, although it also promotes receptor activity and may potentiate the effects of other mutations (95). T790M was also shown to be a rare germline allele associated with susceptibility to lung cancer (96, 97) and has been detected in tumor samples prior to drug exposure, suggesting that drug treatment imposes selective pressure for growth of cells harboring this mutation. Tumor-derived mutations in EGFR are summarized in Appendix I.

ERBB2   Amplification and overexpression of ERBB2 is an important event in tumorigenesis, particularly in breast cancer, but also in ovarian and gastric tumors (98, 99). ERBB2 gene amplification and/or overexpression is strongly linked to poor outcome in breast tumors with lymph node metastasis. Gene amplification appears to be an early event in tumorigenesis and is maintained through progression to invasive and metastatic disease: as such, ERBB2-positive tumors constitute a clinically defined subset of breast cancer that display sensitivity not just to anti-ERBB therapies but to certain cytotoxic therapies as well (100). ERBB2 amplification and overexpression has also been demonstrated in other tumor types, including bladder, lung, prostate, esophageal, and endometrial tumors. Coexpression of EGFR and ERBB2 has also been linked to poor prognosis in breast and lung tumors (101–103). However, in contrast to EGFR, ERBB2 mutations have only rarely been noted in various tumors such as non small cell lung, gastric, and breast carcinomas (104, 105). In particular, several small insertions were observed in NSCLC tumors in a region adjacent to the homologous exon 19 substitutions in EGFR (e.g., insertion of YVMA at residue 776) (106, 107). This insertion was shown to increase kinase activity and constitutively transactivate EGFR, promoting resistance to the EGFR inhibitors gefitinib and erlotinib (108). A summary of tumor-derived ERBB2 mutations is shown in Appendix II.

ERBB3   ERBB3 is frequently overexpressed in parallel with EGFR and/or ERBB2 in breast cancer (109). This has important significance for neoplastic transformation and tumor progression because, as discussed previously, ERBB3 is a potent signaling partner for other ERBB family members, coupling strongly to the PI3K signaling pathway. Consistent with this, ERBB3 expression is associated with histological grade and/or poor prognosis in multiple tumor types, including breast, bladder, and pancreatic cancers. The role of mutations in ERBB3 is poorly understood. ERBB3 mutations are reported to be rare in lung, breast, and colon carcinomas (110) and, given the lack of intrinsic ERBB3 catalytic activity, mutational activation of this receptor is unlikely. However, ERBB3 plays an important role in mediating signaling from mutationally activated EGFR, in particular, activation of the PI3K pathway (58).

ERBB4 In contrast to its carcinogenic cousins, there is evidence that ERBB4 may help promote tumor cell death rather than survival. However, this function is not universal and there are also reports correlating ERBB4 expression with poor prognosis and advanced tumor grade, particularly in combination with other ERBB family members. ERBB4 signaling has been associated with antiproliferative effects and improved differentiation in breast cancer cells (111). The antiproliferative activity is dependent on metalloproteinase-mediated release of the C-terminal intracellular domain (112). As discussed previously, ERBB4 intracellular fragment can stimulate STAT5A-mediated gene expression, a key regulator of mammary epithelial differentiation (80). This domain can function at mitochondria as a proapoptotic BH3-only protein, inducing cell death and suppressing tumor formation. Consequently, in contrast to ERBB2, ERBB4 expression is reported to be inversely correlated with tumor grade, recurrence, and survival in breast cancer (113–115), although some reports suggest that this might not be a general phenomenon (116). ERBB4 somatic mutations have been reported to occur with low frequency (1–3%) in gastric, colorectal, NSCLC, and breast tumors from Korean patients (117). These include residues in the activation loop and C helix, regions where mutations in EGFR have been shown to affect activity. However, the role (if any) of these mutations in ERBB4 remains unclear.

3.2 INSULIN/IGF RECEPTORS

The insulin receptor (IR) tyrosine kinase is one of the primary regulators of cellular metabolism. Insulin is secreted from pancreatic β cells in response to high blood glucose, promoting cellular glucose uptake and a broad range of anabolic processes. Insulin signaling is predominantly active in terminally differentiated cells, in particular, liver, muscle, and fat tissue. Cells from these tissues integrate signals from the insulin receptor with other mitogenic pathways, enabling cellular growth, proliferation, and survival. The insulin-like growth factors IGF1 and IGF2, together with the IGF1 receptor (IGF1R), also play a key role in regulating cell growth and survival. In contrast to insulin signaling, IGF1R signaling predominates in proliferating cells. IGF1 is a primary effector of human growth hormone (hGH) and its growth stimulatory effects are particularly critical during embryogenesis and postnatal development. Given their critical role in signaling cellular growth and proliferation, it is perhaps not surprising that overexpression and activation of IR and/or IGF1R is a common feature of tumor cell lines and primary human tumors. Generally, IGF1R signaling is more strongly implicated in cancer than IR, and our focus therefore is primarily on the IGF/IGF1R axis. However, as discussed later, IR may also have an important role in tumor biology, both as a homodimeric receptor and in heterodimeric complex with IGF1R.

The insulin and IGF1 receptors have strong structural and functional homology, generating an integrated cellular response to extracellular nutrient and growth signals. Three homologous ligands (insulin, IGF1, and IGF2) participate in various interactions with three homologous receptors: two insulin receptor splice forms (IR_A and IR_B) and IGF1R. An additional homologous receptor, the insulin-related receptor (IRR), has also been identified (118, 119). IRR is expressed in kidney, stomach, and brain but does not bind to insulin, IGF1, or IGF2; nevertheless, some reports have suggested a role for IRR in mediating IGF1R signaling (120, 121). The insulin/IGF signaling network is further diversified by the formation of receptor heterodimers and the interaction of IGF2 with a structurally distinct receptor (IGF2R, also known as the mannose 6-phosphate receptor). Downregulation of IR/IGF1R signaling is achieved via several mechanisms, including receptor dephosphorylation by protein tyrosine phosphatases (such as PTP1B) and binding of various proteins such as the suppressor of cytokine signaling proteins SOCS1 and SOCS3 (122). Ligand-stimulated internalization of both IR and IGF1R also occurs (123), although in the case of IGF1R this has been associated with sustained activation rather than inhibition of downstream signaling pathways (124). IGF signaling is subject to additional regulation by at least six IGF binding proteins, which bind to circulating IGF1 with varying affinities and may also elicit cellular responses independent of IGF1R (125). IGFBP3 appears to play the most prominent role and importantly binds to IGF1 with higher affinity than the IGF1R—hence imposing strict regulation of the availability of this potent growth factor.

The insulin receptor is located on chromosome 19p13.3-p13.2, and spans over 120 kb, comprising 11 exons each for the α and β chains (126, 127). Insulin receptor exists in two distinct splice forms, differing by the absence (IR_A) or presence (IR_B) of exon 11, which encodes a 12 amino acid sequence at the C terminus of the α subunit (128, 129). These isoforms differ in their expression patterns: IR_A is the major isoform in most fetal cells, adult hematopoietic cells, and tumors, whereas IR_B is predominant in liver and somewhat higher in myocytes and adipocytes (128, 130, 131). The IGF1R gene maps to 15q25-q26, spans ~100 kb, and contains 21 exons (lacking the alternatively spliced exon 11 of insulin receptor) (132, 133). Both IR and IGF1R are heterotetrameric receptors, comprising dimers of disulfide-linked α and β chains that are derived from a single polypeptide precursor (Chapter 2). Each α chain has a molecular weight of ~130 kDa, whereas the β chains are ~90 kDa. The dimers are assembled in the endoplasmic reticulum prior to cleavage into α and β subunits by prohormone convertases such as furin (134, 135).

Signaling through IR and IGF1R is initiated by binding of insulin, IGF1, or IGF2 to the receptor extracellular domain. Insulin is a small disulfide-linked protein (molecular weight ~6 kDa) and has ~50% amino acid identity with IGF1 and IGF2; IGF1 and IGF2 are ~70% identical to each other. Each ligand binds to each type of receptor (and to hybrid receptors) with varying affinities, although the mode

of binding is complex and may involve multiple binding sites and negative cooperativity (136–138). Insulin has very high affinity ($IC_{50} < 1$ nM) for both the IR_A and
IR_B isoforms but does not appreciably interact with IGF1R ($IC_{50} > 1000$ nM). Conversely, IGF1 and IGF2 bind tightly to IGF1R ($IC_{50} < 1$ nM) but have 10–100-fold
weaker affinity for insulin receptor, with somewhat higher affinity for the IR_A form
compared to IR_B. Nevertheless, IGF2 can signal effectively via IR_A even in cell
backgrounds that are null for IGF1R (139). Conflicting data have been generated
using hybrid receptors (comprising one chain each from IR and IGF1R). IGFR-IR_B
hybrids have been reported to have significantly lower affinity for all ligands compared to IGFR-IR_A (140): however, more recent data suggests that hybrid receptors
bind tightly to IGF1 and IGF2 irrespective of the IR isoform involved, but have
intermediate potency ($IC_{50} \sim 70$ nM) for insulin (141, 142).

Binding of ligand to IR or IGF1R promotes autophosphorylation of the kinase
domain (see Chapter 2) and subsequent activation of diverse intracellular pathways. IR and IGF1R can phosphorylate several intracellular substrates including
SHC (143, 144), GAB1 (145), focal adhesion kinase (146), and JAK1/JAK2 (147).
However, the primary substrates and intracellular transducers of insulin/IGF signaling are the IRS (insulin receptor substrate) proteins (148). There are at least six IRS
proteins (IRS1–6), although IRS-1 and IRS-2 appear to be the predominant effectors of IR/IGF1R and are the most widely characterized. IRS proteins contain an
N-terminal pleckstrin homology (PH) domain and protein tyrosine binding (PTB)
domain, responsible for membrane localization and receptor binding, respectively.
The C-terminal region of IRS proteins is of variable length and contains multiple
tyrosine phosphorylation sites that engage SH2 domains of downstream adaptor
proteins, including SHP2 (149), GRB2 (150, 151), and the p85 subunit of PI3K
(152). IRS proteins also undergo serine phosphorylation by multiple proteins, in
both the protein tyrosine binding domain and C-terminal region (Figure 3.4). In particular, phosphorylation by kinases downstream of IR/IGF1R (e.g., p70S6K) blunts
IRS signaling, creating a negative feedback loop (153). Like many other RTKs,
the primary intracellular effectors of IR and IGF1R are the PI3K and RAS/MAPK
pathways (Chapter 5). Intriguingly, the two IR splice forms may signal via different
downstream effectors: in pancreatic β cells, IR_A was found to activate PI3K Class
I signaling, whereas IR_B was linked to PI3K Class II (154). Additional targets of
IGF1R include integrin signaling (155) and expression of extracellular proteinases
(156), which contribute to cell motility and, in the context of tumor cells, may
promote invasion and metastasis.

Insulin is secreted by pancreatic β cells and acts as a signal of nutritional
abundance, particularly for muscle, fat, and liver cells that are centrally involved
in the storage, mobilization, and utilization of glucose. The activation of AKT
downstream of insulin receptor in these tissues promotes the uptake of glucose
(via translocation of the GLUT4 glucose transporter) and glycogen synthesis (via
inhibitory phosphorylation of glycogen synthase kinase 3 (GSK3) and subsequent
activation of glycogen synthase). In addition, AKT can also mediate hexokinase activity, phosphofructokinase activity, and glycolysis (157). Diminished
insulin receptor signaling in humans is associated with various pathological
conditions depending on the extent of the defect, including varying degrees

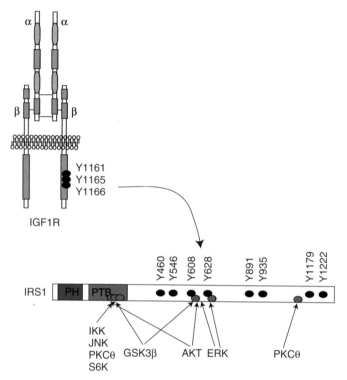

Figure 3.4   Structure and activation of IGF1R. The IGF1R comprises a preformed heterotetramer, with dimers of disulfide-linked α and β chains that are derived from a single polypeptide. Signaling through IGF1 (and insulin) receptors is largely mediated by insulin receptor substrate (IRS) proteins. Following ligand binding, autophosphorylation of IGF1R in the kinase domain activates the kinase, and subsequent tyrosine phosphorylation in the C-terminal domain of IRS proteins creates binding sites for downstream effectors. For IRS1 these include PI3K (Y608, Y628, Y891, and Y935), GRB2 (Y891), and SHP2 (Y1179 and Y1222). IRS proteins are also phosphorylated on serine residues by various kinases including AKT, IKK, JNK, PKC, p70S6K, ERK, and GSK3β. These phosphorylation events disrupt interactions between IGF1R and IRS, attenuating downstream signaling.

of insulin resistance, Rabson–Mendenhall syndrome, and Donohue syndrome (leprechaunism).

IGF1 and IGF2 are primarily produced in the liver, although they are also synthesized and secreted by other normal and malignant tissues (158). The factors regulating their production are complex, but growth hormone plays a dominant role in regulation of hepatic IGF1 production. Mice with specific ablation of IGF1 in the liver show relatively normal growth, suggesting that local autocrine/paracrine signaling may be able to compensate for the lack of hepatic IGF1 production (159). IGF signaling is important in both embryonic and postnatal signaling, and mice lacking IGF1R die at birth with severe developmental defects (160). Rare mutations in human IGF1R have been reported, leading to diminished IGF signaling and retarded intrauterine and postnatal growth (161, 162). In contrast, increased IGF1R copy number has been found to lead to dysmorphic features and increased rate of linear growth (162).

3.2.1 Insulin/IGF Receptors and Cancer

IGF1R is required for transformation of fibroblasts by classical oncogenes such as SV40 large T antigen, SRC, EGFR, PDGFR, and RAS (reviewed in (163)); moreover, overexpression of IGF1R alone is sufficient to transform fibroblasts, and overexpression of a constitutively activated IGF1R transgene in mice leads to rapid tumor development (164). IR and IGF1R are frequently overexpressed and activated in tumors, including multiple myeloma, melanoma, lung, breast, prostate, colon, ovarian, endometrial, bladder, and pancreatic cancers (131, 165–172). IGF1R expression may also be influenced by p53 status. Mutant p53 has a stimulatory effect on the IGF1R promoter activity, whereas wild-type p53 suppresses promoter activity (173). Apart from receptor overexpression, several other mechanisms can also lead to dysregulation of IGF signaling in cancer (reviewed in (174)). Epidemiological studies show a positive association between high IGF1 levels and/or low levels of IGFBP3 with tumor development (175), and individuals with acromegaly (who produce excess growth hormone and thus have high levels of IGF1) have an increased risk of cancer (176). Activating mutations of IGF1R or IR in tumor cells have not been reported. However, loss of heterozygosity and/or mutation of IGF2R have been found in breast, colon, lung, and hepatocellular carcinomas with high frequencies (30–70%) (177–180). Loss of IGF2 imprinting is also a common feature of tumor cells, resulting in activation of the normally silent maternal allele and increased expression of IGF2 (181). Furthermore, obesity has been consistently associated with increased cancer risk, and dysregulation of IGF and insulin pathways in obese individuals may play a role in this predisposition (182). Consistent with this, dietary restriction leads to a reduction in IGF1 levels and slows tumor progression in rodents (183), although the validity of a similar strategy in humans is not clear (184). It is also noteworthy that hyperinsulinemic syndromes have been associated with an increased risk of developing colon cancer (185). As noted earlier, insulin and IR play a pivotal role in stimulating cellular glucose uptake and utilization. Cancer cells have been known for many years to exhibit very high rates of glucose utilization (186), and enhanced glucose uptake resulting from IR activity may represent an important survival mechanism for some tumors. Inhibition of IGF1R activity using various modalities (siRNA, receptor decoys, monoclonal antibodies, and small molecule kinase inhibitors) has been shown to inhibit growth of many tumor cells both in vitro and in vivo, thus further validating this pathway as a target for cancer therapeutics. (166, 170, 187–190). Furthermore, signaling through IGF1R has been implicated in resistance to a wide range of cancer therapies (reviewed in (191)), including radiation (192, 193), diverse chemotherapy agents (194, 195), and targeted therapies such as EGFR inhibitors (196, 197). Hence inhibition of

IGF1R signaling may be an attractive strategy both as a single agent and in combination with current standards of clinical care.

Due to the high expression of IGF1 and the role of IGF1R signaling from embryogenesis through puberty, it is perhaps not surprising that several pediatric tumors have appropriated this pathway to maintain their proliferation and survival. These include Ewing's sarcoma, Wilms' tumor, and neuroblastoma. Ewing's sarcoma is a bone or soft tissue sarcoma occurring predominantly in children and teenagers, resulting predominantly from a t(11;22) translocation that fuses the 5' end of the EWS (RNA binding protein) gene to the 3' end of the gene encoding the ETS family transcription factor FLI1 (198). The EWS-FLI1 fusion leads to aberrant transcriptional activation, including upregulation of IGF1 and repression of IGFBP3 and IGFBP5 expression (199). Consistent with this, EWS-FLI1 tumors secrete IGF1 and rely on autocrine IGF1 signaling for proliferation and survival (200). Several preclinical studies with small molecule IGF1R antagonists have supported this hypothesis (201–203), and there are some early clinical data with an anti-IGF1R antibody suggesting that IGF1R inhibition may have utility in Ewing's sarcoma (204). Wilms' tumor is another form of pediatric malignancy in which IGF1R signaling has been implicated, also involving a t(11;22) translocation. In this form of renal cancer, the 5' end of EWS is fused to the 3' end of WT1, a tumor suppressor gene that normally represses IGF1R expression but is converted to an IGF1R activator in the mutant form (205–207). Furthermore, loss of IGF2 imprinting is a frequent feature of these tumors, creating a potent autocrine signaling loop (208, 209). An EWS-WT1 fusion protein is also implicated in desmoplastic small round cell tumors (205, 210). IGF1R signaling has also been shown to contribute to tumorigenicity of rhabdomyosarcoma (211–213) and neuroblastoma (214–216).

IGF1R signaling also appears to act in a concerted manner with other growth factor receptors involved in cancer, including receptor tyrosine kinases and hormone receptors. Crosstalk with EGFR may occur via direct physical interaction between the receptors (217, 218) and/or regulation of autocrine/paracrine ligand production (219). IGF1R function is required for cellular transformation by EGFR (220, 221), and preclinical studies suggest that targeting both the EGF and IGF axis may be necessary for potent antitumor activity (196, 222). However, the EGF/IGF relationship is complex and clinical translation of this concept may not be so simple. For example, a study of non small cell lung cancer patients found that expression of IGF1R had no effect on response to the EGFR inhibitor gefitinib and was actually associated with longer median survival (223). IGF1R and MET were shown to cooperate to promote mitogenesis in a rat model of hepatocellular carcinoma (224) and have also been implicated in migration and invasion of pancreatic carcinoma cells (225). Steroid hormones can also modulate and be modulated by IGF1R signaling, with particular implications for estrogen signaling in breast cancer and androgen signaling in prostate cancer (226–232). IGF1R activation results in phosphorylation and activation of both the androgen and estrogen receptors and sensitizes them to their cognate ligands (233, 234): conversely, androgens and estrogens upregulate both IGF1R and IGFs (231, 235).

3.3 ANAPLASTIC LYMPHOMA KINASE

Anaplastic lymphoma kinase (ALK), a gene located on 2p23, encodes a protein of 1620 amino acids with a molecular weight of 177 kDa. The mature glycoprotein is about 220 kDa, due to glycosylation. ALK is composed of an extracellular domain, a transmembrane domain, and an intracellular domain containing the tyrosine kinase catalytic site and 18 tyrosine residues forming potential sites of phosphorylation. The ligand for ALK is still controversial. As discussed later, there are several reports that pleiotrophin and the related protein midkine may be ligands for ALK (236–239), but ALK is still considered an orphan tyrosine kinase receptor, with some homology to the neurotrophin receptors and MET. Receptor crosslinking with an antibody directed against the extracellular domain results in the recruitment and phosphorylation of the adaptor proteins SHC and FRS2 (fibroblast receptor substrate-2). SHC is recruited to the consensus phosphotyrosine site NPTpY1507 and FRS2 is thought to be recruited to a novel nonorthodox phosphotyrosine site within ALK (240). The most detailed study of ALK expression was carried out using in situ hybridizations for the detection of ALK mRNA and protein in the mouse at different developmental stages. This study demonstrated the absence of transcripts at all developmental stages in nearly all nonneural tissue, and restricted expression in neural structures of the central and peripheral nervous system, initiating at day 12. ALK was expressed in the eye, nasal epithelium, olfactory nerve, tongue, and skin, as well as tissue surrounding the esophagus, stomach, and midgut, but not the hindgut. Expression was also noted in the testis and ovary. After a peak in expression during neonatal development, receptor expression declines markedly (241).

ALK has been proposed to be the physiological receptor for pleiotrophin (PTN), a 136 amino acid cytokine with diverse functions. Initially this appeared surprising as earlier studies had demonstrated the receptor protein tyrosine phosphatase PTPβ/ζ to be a functional receptor for PTN. Insights from model organisms did not clarify the situation: in *Drosophila*, *Jelly Belly* (*Jeb*) was identified as a ligand for ALK (242, 243), and *Jeb* has no homology with PTN and does not activate human ALK (244). Conversely, there is no homolog of *Jeb* in the human genome databases. Additionally, neither the *Drosophila* homologs of PTN (*Miple1*) or midkine (*Miple 2*) showed any spatial or temporal correlation with the *Drosophila* ALK (*DAlk*) during development (cf. (238)). Mooog-Lutz et al. (245) published conflicting evidence using anti-ALK monoclonal antibodies which activated ALK; under the experimental conditions of these authors, no activation of ALK by PTN was observed. A recent report by Perez-Pinera et al. (238) provided some new insights into this controversy. In cells not stimulated by PTN, PTPβ/ζ dephosphorylates ALK at the site of autophosphorylation. In contrast, when stimulated by PTN, PTPβ/ζ is inactivated and the sites of ALK phosphorylation are not dephosphorylated, allowing for a rapid increase in ALK phosphorylation. Thus this appears to be the first demonstration of a cytokine-dependent inactivation of a transmembrane tyrosine phosphatase, resulting in the activation of transmembrane receptor tyrosine kinase.

3.3.1 ALK and Cancer

ALK first came to light as a possible oncogene when the t(2;5)(p23;q25) translocation was described by several groups as a frequent translocation observed in anaplastic large cell lymphoma (ALCL), a form of high grade, T-cell non Hodgkin's lymphoma, which accounts for about 40% of NHL diagnoses in pediatric patients (246–248). In 1994, the product of this translocation was identified as ALK fused to nucleophosmin (NPM1) (249). The resulting fusion protein, NPM-ALK, consists of the N-terminal portion of NPM fused to the catalytic domain of ALK (Figure 3.5). The N-terminal region of NPM contributes

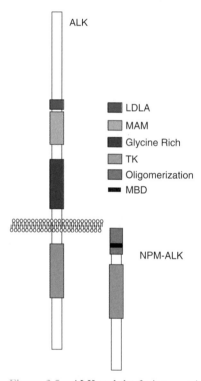

Figure 3.5   ALK and the fusion protein NPM-ALK. ALK is a single transmembrane spanning RTK, with a large extracellular domain, a hydrophobic transmembrane domain, and a tyrosine kinase domain. There are 16 consensus sites for N-linked glycosylation sites in the extracellular domain. Computer-assisted domain analysis reveals an LDL receptor A domain (aa 423–471; a cysteine-rich repeat similar to that found in the low-density lipoprotein (LDL) receptor), a MAM domain (aa 480–636; meprin/A5-protein/PTPμ; a homophilic binding site for PTPμ), and a glycine-rich region (aa 738–940). A putative EGF-Ca domain is also predicted at aa 990–1021. The NPM-ALK fusion protein results from the 2;5 translocation creating a fusion gene consisting of the 3′ half of ALK derived from chromosome 2 fused to the 5′ portion of NPM from chromosome 5. The resulting protein contains the oligomerization domain of NPM, fused to the intracellular domain of ALK, containing the tyrosine kinase and tyrosine phosphorylation sites. The resulting 80-kDa protein is hypophosphorylated and associated with oncogene activity. MBD; methylated DNA binding domain.

the promoter and oligomerization domain of NPM, and the fusion results in deletion of the extracellular and transmembrane domains of the normal ALK protein. Consequently, the NPM-ALK fusion protein is constitutively activated due to autophosphorylation and is also aberrantly expressed (in terms of both cell type and cellular compartment). Normally, ALK is only expressed in the nervous system, and thus immunohistochemical detection of the catalytic domain of ALK became a way of detecting aberrant expression of this fusion protein in ALCL. It was soon realized though that immunohistochemical staining for ALK did not always correlate with expression of NPM-ALK by reverse transcriptase–polymerase chain reaction. Subsequently, a number of additional translocations in which ALK is fused to other partners have been described and are summarized in Table 3.1. In most of the cases identified to date, the 5′end partner fused to the ALK tyrosine kinase supplies domains that promote dimerization, favoring holo- and heterocomplexes, promoting ALK transphosphorylation and autoactivation. The different chimeras, however, localize to different cellular compartments and thus may promote different biological activities. Between 70% and 80% of ALK-positive ALCL express the NPM-ALK fusion protein. The TPM3-ALK fusion is the next most common, accounting for about 12–18% of ALK$^+$ALCL. ALK fusion proteins have also been identified in inflammatory myofibroblastic tumors (IMTs) and in diffuse large B cell lymphoma (DLBCL). About 50% of IMTs display clonal rearrangements in which the ALK is fused to either TPM3 or TPM4. Several other ALK fusion proteins have also been identified in IMT, including RANBP2-ALK, SEC31L1-ALK, and CARS-ALK (see Table 3.1). Dysregulated expression of ALK also occurs in B-cell NHL, although ALK$^+$ DLBCL is quite rare (∼1%). Most reported cases of ALK$^+$ DLBCL are characterized by t(2;17)(p23;q23) involving the clathrin gene (254, 255).

Constitutive activation of ALK as a consequence of gene amplification has also been reported in several cell lines derived from neuroblastomas (266), although ALK amplification was only detected in 1/85 neuroblastoma samples (267). Recently, a number of publications by multiple laboratories have reported that germline mutations in ALK are responsible for the majority of hereditary neuroblastomas. Additionally, activating mutations may also be somatically acquired. These mutations result in constitutive phosphorylation, and targeted knockdown of ALK with siRNA inhibits proliferation in cell lines harboring mutant or amplified ALK, as well as also inhibiting proliferation in cell lines overexpressing wild-type ALK (268–272). Tumor-associated mutations in ALK are summarized in Appendix III.

Wild-type ALK has been implicated in the pathogenesis of a number of nonhematological cancers including rhabdomyosarcomas (273), neuroblastoma and neuroectodermal tumors (274), glioblastomas (239), and melanomas (275). Recently, Perez-Pinera et al. (276) reported that ALK was strongly expressed in different histological subtypes of human breast cancer. Protein was both nuclear and cytoplasmic, and with the "dotted" pattern characteristic of ALK fusion proteins in ALCL. Earlier studies have shown that PTN is expressed in breast cancers and in cell lines derived from breast cancers (277), and moreover, a dominant negative PTN was shown to reverse the malignant phenotype of human

TABLE 3.1   ALK Fusion Proteins

Chromosomal translocation	Partner protein	Fusion protein	Type of tumor	Reference
t(2;5)(p23;q35)	Nucleophosmin (NPM)	NPM-ALK	ALK$^+$ ALCL, ALK$^+$ DLBCL	246–248
t(1;2)(125;p23)	Tropomyosin-3 (TPM3)	TPM3-ALK	ALK$^+$ ALCL and IMT	258
t(2;3)(p23;q21)	TRK-fused gene (TFG)	TFG-ALK	ALK$^+$ ALCL	251, 252
inv(2)(p23;q35)	5-Aminoimidazole-4-carboxamide ribonucleotide formyltrans-ferase/IMP cyclohydrolase (ATIC)	ATIC-ALK	ALK$^+$ ALCL and IMT	253
t(2;17)(p23;q23)	Clathrin heavy chain-like 1 (CLTC1)	CLTC1-ALK	ALK$^+$ ALCL, IMT, and ALK$^+$ DLBCL	254, 255
t(2;X)(p23;q11–12)	Moesin (MSN)	MSN-ALK	ALK$^+$ ALCL	256, 257
t(2;19)(p23;p13)	Tropomyosin-4 (TPM4)	TPM4-ALK	ALK$^+$ ALCL, IMT	258, 259
t(2;17)(p23;q25)	ALK lymphoma oligomerization partner on chromosome 17 (ALO-17)	ALO-17-ALK	ALK$^+$ ALCL	260
t(2;2)(p23;q13) or inv(2)(p23;q11–13)	RAN binding protein 2 (RANPBP2)	RANBP2-ALK	IMT	261
t(2;22)(p23;q11.2)	Nonmuscle myosin heavy chain (MYH9)	MYH9-ALK	ALK$^+$ ALCL	262
t(2;11;2)(p23;p15;q31)	Cysteinyl-tRNA synthetase (CARS)	CARS-ALK	IMT	263
t(2;4)(p23;q21)	SEC31 homolog A (SEC31L1)	SEC31L1-ALK	IMT	264
Inv(2)(p21;p23)	Echinoderm microtubule associated protein-like 4 (EML4)	AML4-ALK	NSCLC	265

Source: Adapted from reference 250.

breast cancer cells in vivo (278), suggesting the constitutive PTN signaling might contribute to the pathogenesis of breast cancer.

Soda et al. (265) recently identified a novel fusion protein, EML4-ALK, in non small cell lung cancer (NSCLC). The predicted fusion protein has the N-terminal half of EML4 encompassing the basic region, the HELP domain, and a portion of the WD-repeat region fused to the intracellular juxtamembrane region of ALK. Both EML4 and ALK map to the short arm of chromosome 2 (2p21 and 2p23, respectively) but are oriented in opposing directions. At present it remains undetermined as to whether the fusion protein results from a simple inversion (2)(p21p23) or if more complex translocations involving 2p are responsible. Transfection of NIH 3T3 cells with EML4-ALK, but not wild-type ALK, or EML4-ALK(K589M) (kinase dead) constructs was shown to transform the 3T3 cells, demonstrating that EML4-ALK has transforming activity that is dependent on its catalytic activity. Moreover, the EML4-ALK fusion protein exhibits a cytoplasmic distribution, in contrast to the membrane-restricted distribution of the wild-type ALK. A limited sampling of EML4-ALK frequency indicated that the fusion occurred in 9.1% (3/33 NSCLC patients), and that the expression of the fusion gene did not overlap with NSCLC patients harboring EGFR mutations, suggesting that EML4-ALK positive cancer may be a novel subclass of NSCLC. Wild-type ALK mRNA was detectable in 24% of the specimens examined. These authors screened for the fusion gene in 261 other cancer specimens, including acute myeloid leukemia, non Hodgkin's leukemia, gastric carcinoma, and colorectal carcinoma, but were unable to identify the fusion gene in any of these other cancers. A second independent study using fluorescence in situ hybridization to detect fusions examined over 600 NSCLC specimens and found EML4-ALK fusions occur in less than 3% of NSCLC samples and that EML4 and/or ALK amplifications also occur (279).

As discussed earlier, fusions of ALK have been demonstrated to have oncogenic potential, with the aberrant tyrosine kinase activity sufficient to enhance cell proliferation, survival, cytoskeletal rearrangements, and alterations in cell shape. This transforming activity is mediated by interactions with intracellular signaling cascades; the best characterized being the RAS/ERK pathway, the JAK/STAT pathway, and the PI3K/AKT pathway (recently reviewed in (250)).

3.4   VEGF RECEPTORS (VEGFR1, VEGFR2, VEGFR3)

The concept that tumor growth depends on angiogenesis, the formation of new blood vessels, was first proposed by Judah Folkman in 1971 (7) and is now widely accepted. The concomitant growth of new blood vessels (or a means to effectively co-opt existing capillary networks) allows tumors to expand beyond a size regulated by diffusional distances, to invade local tissues, and to metastasize to distant sites. Vascular endothelial growth factor (VEGF) now has a well-established role in this process. An essential growth and survival factor for endothelial cells, VEGF promotes endothelial survival, proliferation, migration, and morphogenesis into tube-like structures. Tumor-derived VEGF is thought to play a critical role in the recruitment and formation of a vasculature that will support tumor growth.

Additionally, constitutive autocrine production of VEGF by normal endothelial cells seems to be required for some essential endothelial functions. Traditionally, VEGF was thought to be an endothelial restricted mitogen, but in recent years it has become clear that other cells, including platelets, megakaryocytes, smooth muscle cells, hematopoietic progenitor cells, and certain tumor cells also express VEGF receptors and exhibit various associated biological responses. VEGF plays multiple roles in the process of tumor angiogenesis, promoting the proliferation, migration, and invasion of endothelial cells, organization of the endothelial cells into functional tubular structures, recruiting circulating endothelial cells and progenitor cells to sites of neovascularization, and also inducing vascular permeability. The hyperpermeability characteristic of tumor vasculature allows the leakage of plasma proteins including fibrinogen and other clotting proteins, which further transforms the stroma into a proangiogenic environment.

There are five human VEGF family members (existing as different splice forms and/or proteolytic fragments) and three VEGF receptors. The VEGF ligands are VEGF A, B, C, D and placental growth factor (PlGF); the receptors are VEGFR1 (FLT1), VEGFR2 (KDR), and VEGFR3 (FLT4). Each of the VEGFs has a characteristic receptor binding pattern. VEGFA, VEGFB, and PlGF bind to VEGFR1; VEGFA binds to VEGFR2, and VEGFC and VEGFD bind to VEGFR3 (Figure 3.6, reviewed in (280)). Proteolytic processing of VEGFC and VEGFD results in forms that do bind to VEGFR2, albeit with lower affinity than to VEGFR3. A class of coreceptors, the neuropilins, are transmembrane glycoproteins with short cytoplasmic domains and also interact with some of the members of the VEGF family.

VEGFA stimulates endothelial proliferation, migration, and increased vascular permeability and promotes cell survival, primarily through the activation of VEGFR2. The critical importance of VEGFA was initially realized when deletion of even one allele of VEGFA resulted in embryonic lethality due to defective vascular development (281). The human *VEGFA* gene has been mapped to chromosome 6p21.3 (282). The coding region is approximately 14 kb and contains eight exons. VEGFA undergoes alternative splicing resulting in a number of different isoforms, which are named by their amino acid number (human): $VEGFA_{206}$, $VEGFA_{189}$, $VEGFA_{183}$, $VEGFA_{165}$, $VEGFA_{145}$, and $VEGFA_{121}$. The isoforms vary in their patterns of expression and their binding properties for heparan sulfate proteoglycans (HSPGs) and the coreceptors, neuropilin 1 and 2. For example, $VEGFA_{121}$ binds neither HSPGs nor the neuropilins, whereas $VEGFA_{145}$ and $VEGFA_{165}$ do (reviewed in (280)). Differences in the interactions with neuropilins and HSPG contribute to the differences in the biological activity of the different isoforms (283–289). Alternative splicing also plays an important role in the regulation of the bioavailability of VEGFA. The shortest form, $VEGFA_{121}$, which does not bind to HSPGs, is freely diffusible. In contrast, $VEGFA_{189}$ is almost completely sequestered in the extracellular matrix (ECM) through its HSPG interactions. Enzymes such as heparinase or plasmin can release $VEGFA_{189}$ from the ECM. An alternative splice variant, $VEGFA_{165b}$, has reently been identified; this variant acts as an inhibitor of VEGF signaling in vitro and in vivo (290, 291). The VEGFAs are secreted as covalently linked homodimers, stabilized by intra- and interchain disulfide bonds.

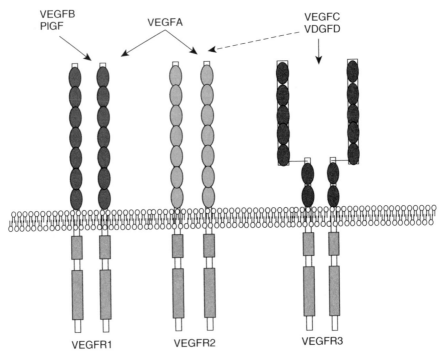

Figure 3.6 Binding of the VEGF family members to the VEGF receptor family members. VEGFA binds to VEGFR1 and VEGFR2 homodimers as well as VEGFR1/VEGFR2 heterodimers. VEGFB and PlGF bind only to VEGFR1 homodimers, and VEGFC and VEGFD bind to both VEGFR2 and VEGFR3 homo- and heterodimers, although binding to VEGFR2 homodimers requires proteolytic processing of VEGFC and VEGFD.

In humans, VEGFA$_{165}$ is the predominant form, occurring as a 46-kDa homodimer with two 23-kDa subunits. VEGFA is produced by many different cell types, including most tumor cells and cells in the tumor stroma. Expression of VEGF is strongly upregulated by hypoxia, due to the presence of a hypoxia-regulated element in the 5′ UTR.

VEGFB, which shares about 43% amino acid sequence identity with VEGFA$_{165}$, is also alternatively spliced (VEGFB$_{167}$ and VEGFB$_{186}$), resulting in a frame shift and two nonhomologous C termini. The predominant isoform seems to be VEGFB$_{167}$ (292, 293). Unlike other VEGF family members, VEGFB does not contain any N-linked carbohydrates. VEGFB$_{167}$ is not glycosylated, while the longer form, VEGFB$_{186}$, is O-glycosylated. The function of VEGFB remains poorly characterized, and at present there are few links to cancer. Deletion of VEGFB results in a mild cardiac phenotype (294).

Both VEGFC and VEGFD have less homology to VEGFA than VEGFB but are potent mitogens for vascular endothelial cells in vitro and can stimulate angiogenesis in vivo. Mice with homozygous deletion of VEGFC die prenatally as a consequence of a lack of lymphatic vessels resulting in fluid accumulation in tissues

(295). In contrast, the deletion of VEGFD does not have a severe phenotype. Mice that are *vegfd*$^{-/-}$ develop normally, although there is a slight reduction of lymphatics adjacent to lung bronchioles (296). VEGFC and VEGFD bind VEGFR2 and VEGFR3 as well as neuropilins (297, 298). VEGFR3 becomes highly restricted to lymphatic endothelial cells during embryogenesis (299, 300). VEGFC and VEGFD specifically stimulate the proliferation of lymphatic endothelial cells, an activity not possessed by VEGFA (301, 302). VEGFC is synthesized as a precursor protein, which undergoes proteolytic processing. The C-terminal domain is cleaved upon secretion but remains associated with the N-terminal domain by disulfide bonds, thus giving rise to a disulfide linked tetramer composed of 29-kDa and 31-kDa polypeptides. Upon processing of the N-terminal propeptide, a smaller "mature" form is released, which consists of two 21-kDa polypeptide chains. These polypeptide chains correspond to the VEGF homology domain. Additional proteolytic processing generates two additional fragments with apparent Mr of 15 and 43 kDa. The full-length and "mature" form of VEGFC binds to VEGFR3 with high affinity. In contrast, high affinity interactions with VEGFR2 require proteolytic processing (303, 304).

Although PlGF was originally identified from extracts of the placenta, it is quite widely expressed and secreted by many cell types. PlGF also undergoes alternative splicing, and to date, four different isoforms have been described which differ in size and in their binding properties: PlGF1 (PlGF$_{131}$), PlGF2 (PlGF$_{153}$), PlGF3 (PlGF$_{203}$), and PlGF4 (PlGF$_{224}$). PlGF2 and PlGF4 both contain an insertion of 21 amino acids at the carboxy terminus, which confers the ability to bind polyanionic substances such as HSPG and also the coreceptors neuropilin 1 and 2 (305, 306). PlGF appears to play a role in pathological angiogenesis. Indeed, loss of PlGF impairs angiogenesis in ischemic retina, limb, and heart, in wounded skin, and in cancer, without affecting physiological angiogenesis (281).

The VEGFRs are members of the RTK superfamily, most closely related to PDGFRs, FGFRs, FLT3, and KIT. These glycosylated, Type I integral membrane proteins have seven immunoglobulin-like domains forming the extracellular portion and a split tyrosine kinase domain forming the interior portion. The Ig domain 2 constitutes the ligand binding site on the receptor, although Ig domain 3 also plays a role in ligand binding specificity (Chapter 2). Alternative splicing and/or proteolytic processing of VEGFRs also gives rise to secreted forms of VEGFR1 and VEGFR2.

VEGFR1 (also known as FLT1) has a fairly restricted expression, currently known to include hematopoietic stem cells, monocytes, macrophages, trophoblasts, osteoclasts, Muller cells, Leydig cells of the testis, certain tumor cells, and vascular endothelial cells. VEGFR1 has been mapped to chromosome 13q12 (307) and encodes a full-length receptor of 1338 aa. Deletion of VEGFR1 results in embryonic lethality, characterized by increased endothelial precursors and vascular disorganization (308). However, in a gene targeting study in which the entire cytoplasmic region of VEGFR1 was deleted, the knockin truncated VEGFR1 mice developed normally (309). VEGFR1 has been described as a "kinase-impaired" RTK (310) and may only signal in the context of receptor heterodimers. Although VEGFR1 has the highest affinity of the VEGF receptors for VEGFA, in endothelial cells, at least, it appears to function as a decoy receptor (311, 312). However, PlGF, which specifically binds VEGFR1, can promote heterodimerization of VEGFR1 with VEGFR2, leading to transactivation of VEGFR2 and promotion of angiogenesis (305).

VEGFR2 (also known as KDR) was originally thought to be an endothelial-specific receptor that mediates most if not all of the known activities of VEGFA on this cell type (recently reviewed in (313)). Biologic activities linked to VEGFR2 activation include stimulation of endothelial proliferation, migration, morphogenesis, survival, vascular permeability, and vasodilatation. The human *VEGFR2* gene is located on chromosome 4q11-q12 and encodes a full-length receptor of 1356 aa. *vegfr2*$^{-/-}$ mice are embryonic lethal, due to defective development of blood islands, endothelial cells, and hematopoietic cells (314). VEGFR2 is expressed predominantly by endothelial cells, although in recent years expression by neuronal cells, megakaryocytes, and hematopoietic stem cells has been reported. There are also reports of VEGFR2 expression in a few tumor types, including hematopoietic malignancies (315) and melanoma (316, 317). The affinity of VEGFA for VEGFR2 is approximately tenfold lower than that of VEGFR1. However, upon ligand binding to VEGFR2, receptor dimerization is induced, resulting in autophosphorylation. Mapping studies have shown that tyrosines Y801, Y951, Y996, Y1054, Y1059, Y1175, and Y1214 are phosphorylated (Figure 3.7, reviewed in (280)). Phosphorylation of Y1054 and Y1059, in the activation loop of the kinase domain, is critical for the catalytic activity of the receptor. Phosphorylation of Y1175 creates a binding site for a number of signaling proteins, including PLCγ (318), and the adaptor proteins SHB (319) and SCK (320). Phosphorylation of Y1214 creates a binding site for the adaptor protein NCK (321). Y951 is a binding site for the signaling adaptor VRAP (322, 323), which appears to be important in VEGF-induced endothelial migration and tumor angiogenesis (322). VRAP is thought to

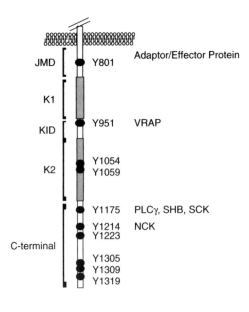

Figure 3.7 Schematic of the cytoplasmic domain of VEGFR2, illustrating the juxtamembrane domain (JMD), the split kinase domains (K1 and K2), the kinase insert domain (KID), and the C-terminal tail. Phosphotyrosine sites are indicated by the black circles. Binding of the ligand (e.g., VEGFA) to VEGFR2 results in receptor dimerization and tyrosine phosphorylation. The phosphorylated receptors recruit interacting proteins, inducing the activation of signaling pathways.

regulate SRC activation and vascular permeability induced by VEGF (324). Additionally, phosphorylation of Y1223, Y1305, Y1309, and Y1319 has been reported, although the function of these residues is unclear at present. The carboxy terminus of VEGFR2 also contains putative serine phosphorylation sites, which may play a role in receptor downregulation. In contrast to many of the other RTKs, VEGFR2 promotes phosphorylation of CBL (325), but activation, ubiquitination, and downregulation of VEGFR2 are not influenced by CBL activity. Downregulation of VEGFR results from a distinct mechanism involving PKC phosphorylation and requires a region of 39 amino acids within the carboxyl-terminal domain, immediately C-terminal to the kinase domain (326).

Structurally, VEGFR3 (also known as FLT4) is somewhat different from the other VEGF RTKs in that the fifth Ig homology domain of the extracellular region is proteolytically cleaved and the resulting polypeptides linked by two disulfide bonds. VEGFR3 is found almost exclusively in lymphatic endothelial cells in the adult (although reports of expression in other tissues such as corneal epithelium are starting to emerge). During development, VEGFR3 expression is first detected at day 8.5 (mouse) in the angioblasts of the head mesenchyme, the cardinal vein, and the allontois. As the mouse develops, however, VEGFR3 expression gradually becomes more restricted, at first to the venous endothelium and subsequently to the lymphatic vessels. The *VEGFR3* gene has been mapped to chromosome 5q33-q35, and the full-length form of the protein is 1298 aa. The coding sequence of the gene has 31 exons and corresponds to the genomic organization of *VEGFR2*. VEGFR3 appears to be unique among the VEGF RTKs in that it is the only receptor for which germline missense mutations have been identified and associated with disease (familial early onset lymphedema) (327–329). Mice deficient in VEGFR3 die at E9.5 of cardiovascular failure, due to an impairment in the remodeling and maturation of large vessels (330).

VEGFR3 has a number of tyrosines that become phosphorylated upon ligand binding. Phosphorylation of Y1063 and Y1068 is thought to regulate the kinase activity (280) (Figure 3.8). Phosphorylation of Y1337 results in association of the SHC:GRB2 complex (331). The roles of the other phosphotyrosines (Y1240, Y1231, Y1265, Y1337, and Y1363) are not known at the present time. Processed VEGFC will induce VEGFR3 to form homodimers or heterodimers with VEGFR2 (332). The heterodimeric complexes are thought to occur in lymphatic endothelial cells and also in some specialized vascular endothelial cells (e.g., fenestrated endothelial cells), which are known to express both receptor types. In the heterodimeric complex, VEGFR3 is not phosphorylated at Y1337 (the SHC binding site) and Y1363, suggesting different downstream signaling pathways may be activated (332). Activation of VEGFR3 has been shown to activate ERK1/2 in a PKC-dependent manner and also to activate the PI3K/AKT pathway (302). The coreceptor neuropilin 2 is an important modulator of VEGFR3 signaling as evidenced by the phenotype of the *neuropilin 2* $^{-/-}$ mice, which are embryonic lethal due to a failure to form lymphatic vessels and capillaries (333).

Overexpression of VEGFR3 ligands in tumor xenograft models induces intratumoral and peritumoral lymphangiogenesis and increases metastasis to peripheral lymph nodes (298, 301, 334–336). Soluble VEGFR3, which inhibits the signaling

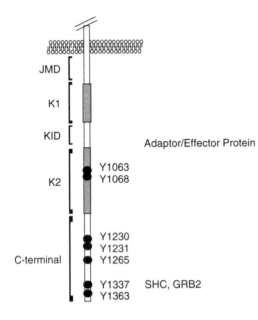

Figure 3.8 Schematic diagram of the cytoplasmic domain of VEGFR3, illustrating the juxtamembrane domain (JMD), the split kinase domains (K1 and K2), the kinase insert domain (KID), and the C-terminal tail. Phosphotyrosine sites are indicated by the black circles. Binding of the ligand (VEGFC or VEGFD) results in receptor dimerization and tyrosine phosphorylation, and the phosphorylated receptors in turn recruit interacting proteins, activating several signal transduction pathways.

of both VEGFC and VEGFD, inhibits both lymphangiogenesis and metastasis (334, 337–339). VEGFR3 may also contribute to tumor angiogenesis; anti-VEGFR3 inhibits the growth of several human tumor xenografts in immunocompromised mice and also reduces the vascular density of the tumors (340).

3.5 PDGF RECEPTORS

Platelet-derived growth factor (PDGF) family members are involved in the control of proliferation, survival, and motility of various mesenchymal cell types. Overexpression or constitutive activation of PDGF signaling has been linked to various diseases involving excessive cell proliferation, including atherosclerosis, various fibroses, and cancer. In addition, PDGF signaling is important for maintenance of the perivascular structure that surrounds and supports tumor blood vessels, leading to interest in PDGF receptors as targets for antiangiogenic cancer therapy.

PDGF is a disulfide linked dimer of which there are now five known isoforms—homodimers of A, B, C, and D polypeptide chains and a heterodimer (PDGFAB). All of the polypeptide chains are synthesized as inactive precursors. The A and B chains are cleaved during secretion from the producing cell and thus are present as active forms in the extracellular milieu (reviewed in (341)). In contrast, the C and D chains are secreted as inactive forms containing N-terminal CUB domains, which must be activated by proteases (tissue plasminogen activator and urokinase plasminogen activator) in order to bind the receptor (342).

Activation of the PDGF receptors follows ligand binding-induced dimerization, which allows autophosphorylation in *trans* between the receptor subunits.

Phosphorylation of multiple tyrosine residues in both the activation loop of the kinase and other regions of the cytoplasmic tail is involved in the regulation of catalytic activity and downstream signaling pathways. The PDGFAA, PDGFAB, and PDGFCC isoforms all bind to and activate the PDGFRα receptor homodimers. The PDGFBB and PDGFDD isoforms bind the PDGFRβ homodimer, and PDGFDD, PDGFBB, and PDGFAB bind to and activate the PDGFRα-PDGFRβ heterodimer (Figure 3.9). All of the receptor homo- and heterodimers stimulate cell proliferation, whereas only PDGFRββ and PDGFRαβ mediate smooth muscle cell and fibroblast chemotaxis.

At least ten different SH2 domain-containing molecules have been shown to bind to different phosphorylation sites of PDGFRα (Figure 3.10) and PDGFRβ (Figure 3.11), including PI3K, PLCγ, SRC, SHP2, GAP, GRB2, SHC, NCK, GRB7, CRK, and STATs. The p85 subunit of PI3K interacts with phosphoryated Y731 and Y742 of PDGFRα, and phosphorylated Y740 and Y751 of PDGFRβ. SRC interacts with phosphorylated Y572 of PDGFRα, and Y579 of PDGFRβ. PLCγ binds to phosphorylated Y988 and Y1018 of PDGFRα, and Y1009 and Y1021 of PDGFRβ. STAT5 has been shown to interact with phosphorylated Y579, Y581, and Y775 of PDGFRβ. SHP2 binds to phosphorylated Y720 and Y754 of PDGFRα and Y763 and Y1009 of PDGFRβ. When activated, the phosphorylated

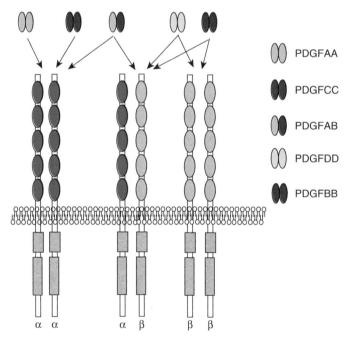

Figure 3.9 Binding of the PDGF receptor family members to their receptors. There are five known forms of PDGF dimers: PDGFAA (binds only to PDGFRα homodimers), PDGFAB (binds to PDGFRα homodimers and PDGFRα/PDGFRβ heterodimers), PDGFBB (binds only to PDGFRβ homodimers), PDGFCC (binds to PDGFα heterodimers), and PDGFDD (binds to PDGFRβ, PDGFRα/PDGFRβ heterodimers).

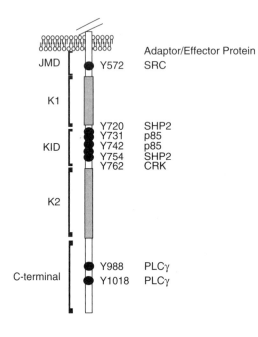

Figure 3.10 Schematic diagram of the cytoplasmic domain of PDGFRα, illustrating the juxtamembrane domain (JMD), the split kinase domains (K1 and K2), the kinase insert domain (KID), and the C-terminal tail. Phosphotyrosine sites are indicated by the black circles. Binding of the ligand (PDGFAA, PDGFAB, or PDGFBB) results in receptor dimerization and tyrosine phosphorylation, and the phosphorylated receptors in turn recruit interacting proteins, activating several signal transduction pathways.

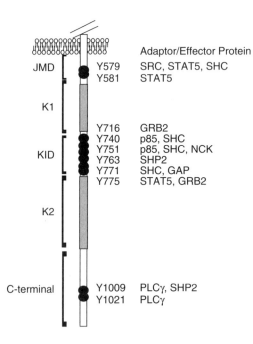

Figure 3.11 Schematic diagram of the cytoplasmic domain of PDGFRβ, illustrating the juxtamembrane domain (JMD), the split kinase domains (K1 and K2), the kinase insert domain (KID), and the C-terminal tail. Phosphotyrosine sites are indicated by the black circles. Binding of the ligand (PDGFBB or PDGFDD) results in receptor dimerization and tyrosine phosphorylation, and the phosphorylated receptors in turn recruit interacting proteins, activating several signal transduction pathways.

Y762 of PDGFRα binds to CRK. SHC binds to phosphorylated Y579, Y740, Y751, and Y771; GRB2 to Y716 and Y775; NCK to Y751; and GAP to Y771 of PDGFRβ (reviewed in (343)).

The best characterized downstream signaling pathways activated by PDGF are the RAS/MAPK pathway (which modulates cell proliferation, migration, and differentiation) and the PI3K/AKT pathway (which promotes cell survival). CBL also binds to PDGFRα via its N-terminal PTB domain, and is believed to regulate PDGFRα signaling. Studies from many groups have now established that CBL, a cytoplastmic, 120-kDa polypeptide, becomes rapidly phosphorylated on tyrosine residues following ligand stimulation. Its mechanism of association with the PDGFRα receptor is via the GRB2 adaptor protein, which binds to the proline-rich region of CBL via SH3 domains and to the PDGFRα by its SH2 domain. At least one mechanism of CBL-negative regulation of the PDGFRα is that CBL promotes ubiquitination and degradation of the PDGFRα (344). For more detailed reviews of PDGFR signaling the reader is referred to a review (343).

3.5.1   PDGFRs and Cancer

Gastrointestinal Stromal Tumors   Gastrointestinal stromal tumors (GISTs) are mesenchymal neoplasms that arise in the wall of the gut (stomach 60%, small intestine 25%, rectum 5%, esophagus 2%, and a variety of other locations including appendix, gallbladder, pancreas, mesenter, omentum, and retroperitoneum (345)) and generally have a spindle cell, epithelioid, and rarely pleomorphic morphology. They are typically characterized by the expression of the oncogene *KIT* (CD117) and the majority (up to 92%) have gain of function *KIT* mutations (346–353). However, there is a small subset of GISTs without *KIT* mutations, and some with low to no KIT expression. This subset can be divided into two groups: those with gain of function mutations in *PDGFRA*, which appear to be mutually exclusive of the *KIT* gain of function mutation; and those without identified kinase mutations (354). The gain of function mutations in PDGFRα occur in the activation loop (exon 18) and in the juxtamembrane region (exon 12). Familial GIST is a rare autosomal dominant genetic disorder, which has been associated with germline mutations in *KIT*; however, a kindred of GIST patients with a *PDGFRA* germline mutation (D846Y) was recently identified (355). Tumor-associated mutations in PDGFRα are summarized in Appendix IV.

PDGFRα, Hypereosinophilic Syndrome, and Chronic Eosinophilic Leukemia   Hypereosinophilic syndrome (HES) was originally coined to describe patients with prolonged eosinophilia of unknown cause (356) and was extended to require exclusion of reactive causes of eosinophilia, malignancies in which eosinophilia is reactive or part of the neoplastic clone, and T-cell disorders associated with abnormalities of immunophenotype and cytokine production (357). Chronic eosinophilia is distinguished from HES by the presence of increased peripheral blood or marrow blasts, or the demonstration of a clonal cytogenetic abnormality in the myeloid lineage (357). However, recently, a fusion protein, FIPIL1-PDGFRα, has been identified in patients diagnosed with both forms of the disease, questioning the somewhat arbitrary division of the two diagnoses. This fusion gene is created by the del (4)(q12q12), an 800-bp deletion on chromosome 4q12. Such a deletion is not detectable using standard cytogenetic banding techniques, providing an explanation as to why most HES patients with this fusion have an apparently normal karyotype. The deletion disrupts both the *FIP1L1* and *PDGFRA* genes, fusing the 5′ region of *FIP1L1* to the 3′ end of *PDGFRA*. The breakpoints vary from patient to patient, but the fusions are in frame. Disruption in *FIP1L1* occurs over a region of 40 kb, whereas the breakpoint in *PDGFRA* is found over a much smaller region involving exon 12 (juxtamembrane region). Interruption of the juxtamembrane region is strictly required to activate the kinase activity of FIP1L1–PDGFRα (358). FIP1L1 itself is a 520 amino acid protein of unknown function; however, it has a region (the Fip1 motif) with homology to FIP1, a yeast protein with synthetic lethal function involved in polyadenylation. The product of the fusion, FIP1L1-PDGFRα, is a constitutively active tyrosine kinase capable of transforming hematopoietic cells in vitro and in vivo; interestingly, the FIP1L1-PDGFRα fusion protein is predicted to be cytoplasmic and it does not activate the mitogen-activated protein kinase pathway, in contrast to PDGFRα (for a recent review see (359)). Additional *PDGFRA* fusion genes have recently been reported (Table 3.2), two in chronic eosinophilic leukemia, *STRN-PDGFRA* (t(2;4)(p24;q12)) (362) and *ETV6-PDGFRA* (t(4;12)(q2?3;p1?2) (362), and a third in HES, *KIF5B-PDGFRA* (365). All three fusion proteins appear to confer constitutive activity, and patients diagnosed thus far with these fusion proteins have been imatinib sensitive. *RHE-PDGFRA* was identified as a genetic rearrangement in the eosinophilic cell line EOL-1 that occured as a consequence of the expression of a fusion

TABLE 3.2   PDGFA Fusion Proteins

Chromosomal translocation	Fusion gene	Clinical syndrome	Reference
t(4;22)(q12;q11.2)	BCR-PDGFRA	Atypical chronic myeloid leukemia BCR-ABL negative	360, 361
t(4;12)(q2?3;p1?2)	ETV6-PDGFRA	Chronic eosinophilic leukemia	362
Del(4)(q12q12)	FIP1L1-PDGFRA	Idiopathic hypereosinophilic syndrome; chronic eosinophilic leukeumia	363
t(2;4)(p24;q12)	STRN-PDGFRA	Chronic eosinophilic leukemia	362
Del(4)(q11q12)	RHE-PDGFRA	Idiopathic hypereosinophilic syndrome	364

protein encoded by a gene of unknown function (NM_30917; rearranged in hypereosinophilia, RHE) and a C-terminal region derived from PDGFRα. The fusion gene was also detected in blood cells of two patients with hypereosinophilic syndrome. The fusion is produced by deletion of a region of chromosome 4, linking RHE to exon 12 of PDGFRA on chromosome 4q12. The resulting fusion kinase is constitutively active and confers IL3-independent growth in BaF3 cells. This fusion kinase is inhibited by imatinib, vatalanib, and THRX-165724 (364).

PDGFRα and Glioblastoma   Malignant gliomas are among the most highly aggressive and invasive human cancers; following diagnosis, the median survival time is just 9–12 months, a statistic that has remained unchanged despite multiple clinical trials. A common defect in brain tumors at all stages is the establishment of an activated PDGF autocrine loop (366). Both PDGFA and PDGFRα are overexpressed by glial tumor cells and all grades of astrocytomas have increased levels of PDGFRA; glioblastoma is the highest. A small subset (8–16%) may have PDGFRα amplification (367). The novel PDGFR ligands, PDGFC and PDGFD, are also expressed in glioma cells and primary glioblastoma tissues, but very low or absent in normal adult and fetal brain (368).

PDGFRα and Malignant Peripheral Nerve Sheath Tumors   Malignant peripheral nerve sheath tumors (MPNSTs) are an aggressive tumor type associated with a poor prognosis. MPNSTs are most common in the deep soft tissue, usually in close proximity of a nerve trunk. The most common sites include the sciatic nerve, brachial plexus, and sacral plexus. The majority of them are associated with neurofibromatosis type 1, a hereditary tumor syndrome. These patients have germline mutations in *NF1* (neurofibromatosis type 1, neurofibromin). Neurofibromin is a negative regulator of RAS and, as such, acts as a tumor suppressor. Mutations in the *NF1* gene lead to the production of a nonfunctional version of neurofibromin that cannot regulate cell growth and division. Until recently, other than *NF1* mutations, little was known about genetic aberrations in neurofibromas. Holtkamp et al. (369) reported higher than normal expression of PDGFRα in MPNSTs than in benign nerve sheath tumors and, in a later study, found gene amplification of *PDGFRA* in 6 out of 31 patients and, additionally, two somatic *PDGFRA* mutations (both in the extracellular domain) (370). These observations led to the suggestion that imatinib (and other drugs that inhibit PDGFRα) might offer new treatment options for MPNST patients.

PDGFRβ Fusion Proteins   Eosinophilia is a common feature of several myeloproliferative disorders (MPDs), including chronic myelogenous leukemia (CML) and the 8p11 myeloproliferative syndrome. However, eosinophilias associated with translocations involving chromosome band 5q31–33 have been observed, and cloning of these translations revealed consistent targeting of the *PDGFRB* gene. To date, at least 15 fusion partners of *PDGFRB* have been identified (Table 3.3). In most of the chromosomal aberrations, the breakpoint in the *PDGFRB* gene is located in the intron immediately 3′ to the exon encoding the transmembrane

TABLE 3.3 PDGFRB Fusion Proteins

Chromosomal translocation	Fusion gene	Clinical syndrome	Reference
t(5;15)(q33;q22)	53BP-1-PDGFRB	Chronic myeloid leukemia-like disorder associated with eosinophilia	371
t(5; 14)(q33; q32)	CEV14-PDGFRB	Acute myeloid leukemia with eosinophilia	372
t(17;22)(q22;q13.1)	COL1A1-PDGFB	Dermatofibrosarcoma protuberans	373
t(5;12)(q31–33;q24)	GIT2-PDGFRB	BCR-ABL negative chronic myeloproliferative disorder	374
Complex rearrangement involving chromosomes 1, 5, and 11	GPIAP1-PDGFRB	BCR-ABL negative chronic myeloproliferative disorder	374
t(5;10)(q33;q22)	H4-PDGFRB	ACML	375
t(5;7)(q33;q11.2)	HIP1-PDGFRB	CML	376
t(5;17)(q33;p11.2)	HMOGT1-PDGFRB	JMML	377
t(5;14)(q33;q32)	KIAA1509-PDGFRB	CML	378
t(1;5)(q23;q33)	Myomegalin-PDGFRB	Myeloproliferative disorder associated with eosinophilia	379
t(5;14)(q33;q24)	NIN-PDGFRB	Chronic myeloproliferative disorder with eosinophlia	380
t(4;5;5)(q23;q31;q33)	PRKG2-PDGFRB	BCR-ABL negative chronic myeloproliferative disorder	374
t(5;17)(q33;p13)	Rabaptin-5-PDGFRB	CML	381
t(5;12)(q33;p13)	TEL-PDGFRB	CML	382

region of PDGFRβ. These fusion proteins are believed to provide homodimerization domains, promoting dimerization and constitutive activation of PDGFRβ.

The ETV6-PDGFRβ fusion protein results from a t(5;12)(q31–33;p13) translocation and, while rare, is the most frequent of the known PDGFRβ fusion genes. It was also the first to be identified (382). *ETV6-PDGFRB* is most frequently seen in patients with chronic myelomonocytic leukemia, atypical chronic myeloid leukemia, or chronic eosinophilic leukemia. Interestingly, most of the patients present with peripheral blood or bone marrow eosinophilia. Notably, the t(5;12)(q31–33;p13) confirmation of *ETV6-PDGFRB* is important for clinical management with imatinib since many of the patients with this disease have no involvement of PDGFRβ. ETV6, also known as TEL, is a member of ETS family of transcription factors. It is characterized by a HLH domain (exons 3 and 4) and an ETS domain. The *ETV6-PDGFRB* fusion gene is formed by the translocation of the region encoding the amino terminus of ETV6 to the transmembrane and cytoplasmic domains of PDGFRβ. The HLH domain of ETV6 homodimerizes, and the fusion protein leads to the constitutive activation of the PDGFRβ receptor tyrosine kinase and stimulation of subsequent signaling pathways important in cell proliferation (382). In mice, ETV6-PDGFRβ is sufficient to produce a chronic myeloproliferative disorder (383, 384). Several distinct ETV6-PDGFRβ fusion proteins have been described, and additional gene translocations/PDGFRβ fusion proteins have been associated with various myeloproliferative disorders (Table 3.2).

PDGFRβ and Dermatofibrosarcoma Protuberans   Dermatofibrosarcoma protuberans (DFSB) is a relatively uncommon cutaneous malignancy that arises from the dermis. While metastases are rare, this is a local and highly aggressive tumor. Molecular studies have shown that more than 90% of these tumors are associated with a translocation (t(17;22)) affecting the *PDGFB* gene. These fusion genes display a consistent structure where N-terminal parts of *COL1A1* of variable length are fused to the N-terminal prosequence of *PDGFB*. These fusion proteins are processed to functional PDGFBB. These rearrangements lead to constitutive activation of PDGFR signaling as a consequence of deregulated ligand expression. Recently, imatinib has been reported to induce complete or partial remissions in most patients treated for advanced DFSP (385).

PDGFRβ and Pericytes   PDGF signaling plays a prominent role in supporting tumor vasculature. Although PDGFRβ is expressed on some endothelial cells, the major role of vascular PDGFR signaling is thought to involve recruitment of pericytes, which are important for stabilization and integrity of blood vessels. This "scaffolding" composed of pericytes and basement membranes may enable regrowth of vessels following antiangiogenic therapy, so targeting PDGFR signaling in addition to VEGFR signaling may be expected to provide added benefit. Indeed, preclinical studies have highlighted the benefits of this combination. In an angiogenic model of pancreatic islet cell carcinogenesis, blockade of both VEGFR signaling in endothelial cells and PDGFR signaling in pericytes was shown to be more effective than either therapy alone, both in preventing tumor formation and in regressing established tumors (386).

3.6   FGF RECEPTORS

The human fibroblast growth factor (FGF) family contains 22 related peptide growth factors (FGF1 to FGF23; the human equivalent of the mouse FGF15 has not been identified(387)), although four of them (FGF11–14) are probably not canonical FGFs. FGFs influence the proliferation and differentiation of many different cell types. Increased FGF signaling is associated with several skeletal disorders, including dwarfism and craniosynostosis syndromes. In adult organisms, FGFs have been implicated in both physiological (e.g., in response to exercise, wound healing) and pathological (e.g., tumors, retinopathies) angiogenesis. The majority of the FGFs (FGF3–8, 10,15, 17–19, and 21–23) have N-terminal signal peptides and are readily secreted. In addition, despite the lack of obvious signal sequences, FGFs 9, 16, and 20 are also secreted. FGF9 has a noncleaved amino-terminal hydrophobic sequence that is required for secretion. A third set of FGFs (FGF11–14) lack signal sequences and are believed to remain inside the cell.

FGF1 and FGF2 were originally designated acidic and basic FGF, respectively, based on their isoelectric points. FGF1 binds with high affinity to all of the known receptor isoforms (388), a property that distinguishes it from the other FGF family members. Although FGF1 and FGF2 lack a signal peptide at their 5' ends and are found in the cytosol, both growth factors seem to be released from cells through a nonclassical secretory pathway (389, 390) as they are found on the surface of cells as well as deposited in the extracellular matrix. FGF1 and FGF2 are also present in the cell nucleus. A putative nuclear localization signal has been identified at the 5' end of the FGF1 protein (391). Higher molecular weight isoforms of FGF2, derived from alternative translation initiation sites in the 5' region of the *FGF2* gene, also localize to the nucleus (389, 392). However, the precise role of these nuclear forms of FGF1 and FGF2 remains unclear.

FGF2 regulates many cellular functions including cell proliferation, differentiation, survival, adhesion, migration, motility, and apoptosis. In vivo, FGF2 is involved in processes such as limb formation, wound healing, tumorigenesis, angiogenesis, vasculogenesis, and blood vessel remodeling. With respect to the vascular cells, FGF2 is a potent mitogen and chemotactic factor for endothelial and smooth muscle cells and stimulates pericyte proliferation. FGF2 also stimulates plasminogen activator production and matrix metalloproteinase (MMP) expression, which play an important role in vessel destabilization and breakdown of the extracellular matrix (see later discussion). However, despite this broad spectrum of activity, $fgf2^{-/-}$ mice are viable with only mild cardiovascular, skeletal, and neuronal abnormalities (393–395). Similarly, neither $fgf1^{-/-}$ nor $fgf1/fgf2^{-/-}$ (double knockout) mice exhibit vascular abnormalities. However, wound healing is delayed in $fgf2^{-/-}$ and $fgf1/fgf2^{-/-}$ mice (396).

The diverse effects of the FGFs are mediated by a family of receptor tyrosine kinases. Structurally, the FGF receptors (FGFR1–4) are characterized by an extracellular ligand binding region consisting of three immunoglobulin-like (Ig) domains (D1 to D3), a single transmembrane helix, and a split cytoplasmic tyrosine kinase domain (Figure 3.12). These related, but distinct FGFRs consist of multiple isoforms that are generated by alternative mRNA splicing. Multiple FGFs can activate each receptor, and moreover, most of the FGFs activate more than one receptor. The exception is FGF7, which is known only to activate the FGFR2 IIIB isoform. FGFR dimers may be both homodimers and heterodimers. Recently, a fifth FGFR family member was described, FGFR5. Unlike the canonical FGFRs, FGFR5 lacks a cytoplasmic tyrosine kinase domain (397). FGFR5β binds FGF2, although with lower affinity than FGF2 binds to its cognate receptor FGFR2 (398).

One splicing event results in the skipping of the exons encoding D1, resulting in a shorter form of the receptor containing only two Ig-like domains. The binding specificity for the different FGF family members resides in the D2 and D3 Ig domains as well as a short linker between D2 and D3 (Chapter 2). The shorter form of the receptor may have a higher affinity for some FGFs than the long form. Another splicing site specifies the sequence of the carboxy-terminal half of D3, resulting in either the 3b (IIIb) or 3c (IIIc) isoform of the FGFR. FGFR splicing

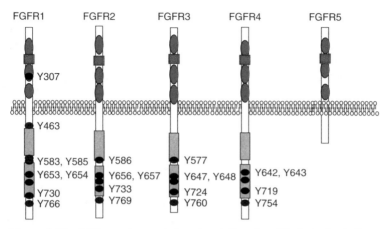

Figure 3.12 FGF receptors and phosphorylation sites. Black circles indicate positions of tyrosine residues. The D1, D2, and D3 domains are indicated by the red ovals and the acid box domain by the black rectangle.

appears to be tissue specific, with exon IIIb found in epithelial cells while IIIc is associated with mesenchymal-derived cells. For example, the keratinocyte growth factor receptor (KGFR), also known as FGFR2IIIb, is predominantly localized in epithelial cells and is activated by KGF (FGFR7) that is primarily synthesized by mesenchymal cells.

Although receptor dimerization is necessary for activity, FGF signaling also requires heparin or heparan sulfate proteoglycans (HSPGs). HSPGs have long been thought to play a role as a coreceptors for heparin binding growth factors such as FGFs. Interaction with HSPG or heparin stabilizes FGFs to thermal denaturation and proteolysis and moreover restricts the diffusion distance from the site of FGF production. The cell surface heparan sulfates are carried on membrane-bound core proteins (e.g., syndecans and glypicans). Recent studies now suggest that some of the core proteins, and not just the heparan sulfate chains, may also play important roles in signal transduction. Syndecan-4, for example, can bind and activate protein kinase Cα (PKCα) following FGF2-induced oligomerization (399). The full activity of FGF requires not only receptor interactions but also internalization of the ligand. The internalization of FGF2 in endothelial cells has been shown to occur via a syndecan-4-dependent activation of a RAS and CDC42-dependent macropinocytotic pathway (400).

With respect to FGFR signaling, FGFR1 is the best characterized of the FGF receptors. The *FGFR1* gene (also known as *FLT2* and *FLG*) has been mapped to chromosome 8p11.2-p11.1. The full-length gene encodes a protein of 822 amino acids and results in a 100–135-kDa glycoprotein from a 90–115-kDa protein core. There are seven tyrosine residues in the cytoplasmic tail of FGFR1. Y653 and Y654 have been shown to be important for the catalytic activity and are essential for signaling (401). Y766 binds the SH2 domain of PLCγ and is required for FGFR activation (402). However, the other potential tyrosine phosphorylation sites on FGFR1 can be mutated to phenylalanine residues without inhibiting MAPK or mitogenic signaling in rat fibroblasts, although this may be cell type dependent. For example, CRK, an SH2/SH3 containing protein, binds through its SH2 domain to Y463 of the activated FGFR which when mutated to a phenylalanine, abrogates FGF-induced proliferation and ERK2 and JNK activation in endothelial cells (403).

It is now thought that FGFs mediate signal transduction by at least two independent pathways: the traditional tyrosine kinase SH2 pathway linking to PLCγ and CRK (discussed earlier) and a second pathway through an interaction in the JM region. Both the wild-type and mutant FGFR1 lacking all noncatalytic tyrosine residues phosphorylate a 90-kDa protein, known as SNT1/FRS2. When activated, SNT1/FRS2 recruits the adaptor protein GRB2, which in turn recruits SOS, leading to activation of the RAS/MAPK pathway. Activated FRS2 also binds the protein tyrosine phosphates SHP2, and further SHP2 is associated with the docking protein GAB1 leading to recruitment and activation of the PI3K pathway. FRS2 may also link FGFR activation to atypical protein kinase C isotypes (reviewed in (404)).

3.6.1 FGFRs and Cancer

Numerous studies now support a role for altered FGF/FGFR signaling in tumorigenesis, ranging from the overexpression of FGF and FGFR family members to activating mutations, translocations, and amplifications of FGFRs. Additionally, alterations in FGFR isoforms, changes in coreceptors, and downregulation of negative regulators such as the Sprouty proteins have been reported. FGFR1, 3, and 4 are frequently overexpressed in prostate cancer cell lines and tumors (405) and breast and ovarian tumors. Increased expression of FGF2 and FGF7 has also been found in a high proportion of prostate cancers and has been correlated with tumor stage, shorter postoperative survival, and the presence of lymph node metastases. Thus FGFs/FGFRs have been proposed to form an autocrine or paracine loop. FGFR1 is amplified in 8–10% of breast cancers (406–413) and is overexpressed and occasionally amplified in oral and esophageal squamous carcinomas (414, 415), prostate cancer (405), and some bladder carcinomas (416). Amplifications have also been observed in ovarian tumors (413, 417, 418). FGFR1 is overexpressed in primary rhabdomyosarcomas (419) and occasionally amplified in nonsmall cell lung carcinomas (420) and primary cutaneous CD30[+] anaplastic large cell lymphoma (C-ALCL) (421). Potentially activating FGFR1 mutants have been reported in glioblastoma, lung, colon, and gastric carcinomas and other malignancies (422) (see Appendix V). A translocation at the 8p11 locus leading to a constitutively active FGFR1 fused to one of 8 fusion partners causes 8p11 myeloproliferative syndrome, an atypical stem cell myeloproliferative disorder typically characterized by eosinophilia and often an associated T- or B-cell lymphoma (423). Loss of function mutations in this *FGFR1* have been associated with dominant Kallmann syndrome 2, whereas gain of function mutations have been associated with Pfeiffer syndrome, Jackson–Weiss syndrome, and some other syndromes related to skeletal defects.

Fibroblast growth factor receptor 2 (FGFR2, KGFR) and FGF7 have been implicated in cancer growth as well as in tissue development and repair. In pancreatic ductal adenocarcinoma, FGFR2 and FGF7 expression/immunoreactivity correlated with venous invasion, VEGFA expression, and poor prognosis (424). FGF10, which also signals through FGFR2IIIb, is also expressed in stromal cells surrounding pancreatic tumors and in in vitro studies was shown to induce expression of MMPs and pancreatic tumor cell migration and invasion (425). The chromosomal location of FGFR2 has been mapped to 10q25.3-q26. C-terminally truncated FGFR2 splicing variants that were constitutively phosphorylated and spontaneously dimerized have been identified in a number of cancer cell lines, including those from gastric cancer (426) and breast cancer (427). Additionally, there may be a suppressor role for normal FGFR2. Epigenetic silencing of FGFR2 through DNA methylation has been noted in gastric cancer (428) and pituitary adenomas (429). A tumor suppressor role for the FGFR2IIIb (KGFR) isoform has been proposed in the skin (173), bladder, and other tumors (430). Several genome-wide association studies have linked FGFR2 alleles with breast cancer (427, 431–438).

However, the vast majority of the literature regarding activating missense mutations in FGFR2 concerns the role of this receptor in a variety of craniosynostosis syndromes. Most mutations have been found in either exon IIIa or IIIc or in the intronic sequence preceding exon IIIc. For example, germline gain of function mutations in FGFR2 (usually S252W or P253R) result in Apert syndrome (a relatively uncommon craniofacial anomaly, occurring with a frequency of 1/160,000 live births). The clinical features include early fusion of skull bones, mainly coronal, sometimes lambdoid, midface regression, and webbed digits (syndactyly; both fingers and toes). Such mutations may predispose these patients to ovarian and other tumors (439): indeed, several mutations found in craniosynostosis syndromes (including S267P and W290C) have also been identified in various solid tumors (Appendix VI). Other craniosynostosis syndromes associated with FGFR2 mutations include Crouzon, Pfeiffer, Antley–Bixler, Beare–Stevenson cutis gyrata, and Jackson–Weiss syndromes. Somatic missense mutations, of which several are also detected in the aforementioned congenital skeletal disorders, as well as FGFR2 gene amplification have been identified in endometrial, lung, breast, gastric, and ovarian cancers (see Appendix VI). In addition, isoform switching from FGFR2B to 2C is linked to malignant progression of prostate and bladder cancer. Endometrial carcinomas were recently reported to have frequent activating mutations in FGFR2 that parallel those associated with craniosynostosis and skeletal dysplasia syndromes (440).

FGFR3, similar to other members of the FGFR family, is activated by oligomerization induced by ligand binding resulting in trans-autophosphorylation at tyrosine residues in the cytoplasmic domain. *FGFR3* is located at chromosome 4p16.3 and is thought to play an important role in the pathogenesis and disease progression of a number of hematopoietic malignancies. Most notably, a t(4;14) translocation involving *FGFR3* has been identified in up to 15% of multiple myeloma patients (441). FGFR3 is also involved in a form of peripheral T-cell lymphoma that progresses into acute myeloid leukemia. These patients have a t(4;12)(p16;p13) translocation that generates the TEL-FGFR3 fusion protein with constitutive tyrosine kinase activity. A few patients with multiple myeloma have also been found to have activating mutations in addition to the t(4:12) translocation (442). A lethal, hereditary syndrome (thanatophoric dysplasia type II) occurs with germline expression of the *FGFR3* gene containing an activating mutation (K650E) (443). In addition, in common with other FGF receptors, mutational activation of FGFR3 is involved in several craniosynostosis syndromes including Muenke syndrome, coronal craniosynostosis, Crouzon's dermoskeletal syndrome, hypochondroplasia, SADDAN (severe achondroplasia with developmental delay and acanthosis nigricans), and thanatophoric dysplasia type I. Several of these FGFR3 activating mutations have also been identified in human cancers including multiple myeloma, colorectal cancer, oral squamous cell carcinoma, bladder carcinoma (40–60%), and cervical cancer (442); see Appendix VII. Differential splicing is also associated with malignant transformation. For example, a soluble splice variant FGFR3IIIs is frequently expressed in tumors but rarely in normal cells (444).

The genomic organization of *FGFR4* differs slightly from the other members of the FGFR family. The gene for FGFR4 encompasses 18 exons, and although alternative splicing has been observed, there is no evidence that the C-terminal half of the IgIII domain varies between three alternate forms, in contrast to FGFR1–3. The chromosomal location of FGFR4 is 5q35.1-qter. FGFR4 preferentially binds FGF1 and FGF8. FGFR4 is overexpressed in breast, ovarian, and prostate tumors, suggesting possible roles in tumorigenesis in these tissues (445–447). One report suggests that up to 10% of breast tumors may show two- to fourfold amplification of FGFR4, with amplification occuring more frequently in estrogen- and progesterone receptor-positive tumors and in tumors with high lymph node involvement (448). The FGFR4 allele R388 is associated with both an increased incidence and clinical aggressiveness of prostate cancer (446, 449) and has been associated with a poor prognosis for node-positive breast cancer (450, 451), high-grade soft-tissue sarcoma (452), lung adenocarcinoma (453), colon carcinoma, and head and neck squamous cell carcinoma (454). However, there are conflicting reports in breast, lung, and colorectal cancers (455–457). The polymorphism is apparently not relevant for node-negative breast (450), bladder (458), or glioma (459) cancer prognosis. This allele has been suggested to be a marker for melanoma progression (460). FGFR4 with the R388 polymorphism has been shown to have increased receptor stability and sustained receptor activation, suggesting that this polymorphism may contribute to the oncogenic state (461). FGFR4 may also have a role in human thyroid cancer (462) and hepatocellular carcinoma progression (463, 464). Somatic mutations in the kinase domain have recently been identified in lung adenocarcinoma (325, 465), suggesting the possibility that FGFR4 mutations might have a role in a subset of lung adenocarcinomas. (Tumor-associated FGFR4 mutations are summarized in Appendix VIII.)

3.7   KIT

KIT, also known as CD117, is a 145-kDa transmembrane tyrosine kinase. It is the cellular counterpart of the transforming gene of the Hardy–Zuckerman feline sarcoma virus c-KIT (466). KIT is constitutively expressed in certain normal tissues including hematopoietic stem cells, mast cells, basal cells of the skin, melanocytes, epithelial cells of the breast, germ cells, interstitial cells of Cajal, and certain regions of the central nervous system. In contrast, KIT expression is very low or not detectable in normal squamous epithelium or the glandular epithelium of the endocervix, prostate, stomach, intestine, and pancreas. However, many tumors express KIT, including GISTs, mast cell tumors, seminomas, melanomas, endometrial carcinomas, ovarian carcinomas, chromophobe renal cell carcinomas, small cell carcinomas of the lung, and occasionally AML and ductal breast carcinomas.

KIT is a member of the tyrosine kinase subclass III family that includes PDGFRα, PDGFRβ, CSF1R, and FLT3. The characteristic features of Type III receptors include the presence of five immunoglobulin (Ig)-like domains in the extracellular domain, and a 70–100 residue cytoplasmic domain containing a characteristic kinase insert domain. The *KIT* gene is located on human chromosome 4 (4cen-q21) and is encoded by 21 exons; it encodes at least three different mRNAs with three corresponding protein variants. Two of the protein variants are derived from alternate splicing a 5.5-kb mRNA and are distinguished by an in-frame insertion of four amino acid residues (GNNK) in the extracellular region at the exon/intron junction of exon 9. The shorter form has an increased basal level of autophosphorylation (467, 468). The third form of *KIT* is an alternate 3.2-kb mRNA derived from alternative promoter usage; this isoform is only expressed in postmeiotic germ cells of the testis (469). This form is called tr-*KIT* and encodes a form with a truncated cytoplasmic region (469).

The ligand for KIT has several names including mast cell growth factor, steel factor, and stem cell factor (SCF, the most widely accepted name). SCF is a noncovalent homodimer occuring in two major isoforms, both of which present as both membrane bound and soluble forms. The first membrane isoform is a 45-kDa, 248 amino acid glycoprotein that is cleaved by proteases to generate a 31-kDa, 163 aa soluble protein. In this isoform, the cleavage site (VVAS; aa 163–166) is encoded by exon 6. The second SCF isoform occurs as the result of alternate splicing around exon 6. This isoform is a 32-kDa, 220 aa glycoprotein that lacks exon 6 and is primarily membrane bound, although it can be shed by proteases to yield a soluble form. Activation of KIT by SCF is highly species specific, even though the murine SCF shows 83% homology to the human SCF (470). Binding of SCF to KIT leads to rapid receptor dimerization and autophosphorylation (activation) of the tyrosine kinase moiety. Mutations in the murine locus for the ligand (SCF) and its receptor (KIT) have revealed pleiotrophic functions for this pathway; the mutations lead to defects in melanogenesis, gametogenesis, and hematopoiesis.

SCF binding to KIT results in receptor dimerization or oligomerization, activation of the tyrosine kinase activity, and rapid, transient tyrosine phosphorylation of several cellular proteins, including KIT. Activated KIT becomes autophosphorylated on a number of tyrosine residues, mostly located outside the kinase domain; these sites serve as docking sites for various signal transduction molecules including the p85 subunit of PI3K, PLCγ, and SHP2. Phosphorylated Y568 and Y570 bind to CBL, SHC, and SHP1 and SHP2 (Figure 3.13). CBL, once phosphorylated, recruites E3 ligase, mediating the ubiquitination and degradation of KIT. SHP1 and SHP2 also play a role in the negative modulation of KIT. Phosphorylated Y703 recruits GRB2, Y721, the p85 subunit of PI3K; Y730 binds to PLCγ, Y900 interacts with CRK, and Y936 binds GRB2 and PLCγ. These and other interactions

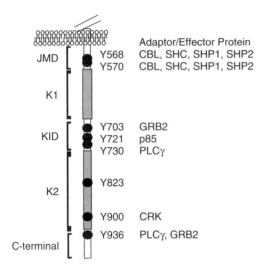

Adaptor/Effector Protein

| JMD | Y568 | CBL, SHC, SHP1, SHP2 |
| | Y570 | CBL, SHC, SHP1, SHP2 |

K1

KID	Y703	GRB2
	Y721	p85
	Y730	PLCγ

| K2 | Y823 | |

| | Y900 | CRK |
| C-terminal | Y936 | PLCγ, GRB2 |

Figure 3.13 Schematic diagram of the cytoplasmic domain of KIT, illustrating the juxtamembrane domain (JMD), the split kinase domains (K1 and K2), the kinase insert domain (KID), and the C-terminal tail. Phosphotyrosine sites are indicated by the black circles. Binding of the ligand (SCF) results in receptor dimerization and tyrosine phosphorylation, and the phosphorylated receptors in turn recruit interacting proteins, activating several signal transduction pathways.

lead to the activation of the SRC kinase family, PI3K, JAK/STAT, RAS/MAPK, and PLCγ pathways. (For a recent review, see (471).)

Interaction of SCF and KIT is critical for mast cell development, survival, homeostasis, and function. Transgenic mice in which KIT or SCF is abrogated are mast cell deficient. Similarly, in human cell culture the differentiation of mast cells from progenitor cells and continued survival of mast cells is dependent on the presence of SCF (472–474). Additionally, SCF is chemotactic and it has been suggested that another role for SCF is to modulate the location of mast cells to the appropriate site within tissues and organs (475). When KIT is inappropriately activated, accumulation of mast cells in tissues results in mastocytosis (described later).

3.7.1 KIT and Cancer

Gastrointestinal Stromal Tumors (GISTs) GISTs are the most common mesenchymal tumor of the human gastrointestinal tract, accounting for roughly 5000 new cases/year in the United States. Until recently, surgical resection was the only effective treatment for patients (and only those with operable tumors). GISTs are highly resistant to chemotherapeutic agents, including newer approved drugs such as temozolomide. In the majority of cases, surgery was not possible and for patients with operable tumors the 5-year survival rate was 35–65%. Worse was the prognosis for patients with unresectable disease, who had a median survival of only 10–20 months following diagnosis.

GISTs provide an excellent example of a disease in which understanding the molecular pathology led to remarkable advances in therapy. Early microscopic studies of GISTs led investigators to propose that these tumors were neoplasms of smooth muscle origin and thus were often classified as leiomyomas, leiomyosarcomas, or leiomyoblastomas. More powerful microscopes enabled high power studies, and these results were inconsistent with tumors of smooth muscle origin. Studies of various markers revealed that a subset of gastrointestinal stromal tumors stained for neural crest markers (e.g., S-100, neuron-specific enolase, and PGP.5), fostering a longstanding debate over the origin of these mesenchymal tumors of the gut wall. With the increasing use of antibodies to study markers, investigators began to make new observations about the nature of these tumors. A key early observation was the positive staining for CD34 in GISTs (476, 477), which enabled better diagnosis of GIST. However, the curious overlap of both smooth muscle and neural features of GISTs led investigators to speculate that these tumors might be related to a small subset of rather poorly characterized, spindle-shaped cells in the gut wall, the so-called interstitial cells of Cajal (ICC). ICC in the stomach and intestine also frequently express CD34, embryonic smooth muscle myosin heavy chain, and nestin (478–480); curiously, these cells failed to develop in mice deficient in either KIT or SCF, strongly suggesting the critical role of the KIT-SCF axis in the development of these cells (481, 482). The observation that ICC were KIT (CD117) positive, followed by the discovery that KIT is strongly expressed in most GISTs (483–487), provided both a marker for the diagnosis of GISTs and a suggestion of their molecular pathology (although it should be noted that GISTs have a relatively broad morphologic and antigenic spectrum: approximately 95% of GISTs stain positively for KIT; other markers, somewhat more variable include BCL2 (80%), CD34 (70%), muscle-specific actin (50%), smooth muscle actin (20–30%) (355), S-100 (10%), and desmin (5%) (345)).

A critical publication by Hirota and co-workers in 1998 (351) documented that not only did GISTs express KIT, but many of the GISTs also had mutations in the juxtamembrane domain of the *KIT* gene. Of the tumors examined by this group, 5/6 had exon 11 mutations, four in-frame deletions, and a fifth a missense mutation. When expressed in vitro, the mutant KIT isoforms exhibited constitutive activation, and all five KIT mutations transformed Ba/F3 cells in a nude mouse tumorigenesis assay (351). It is now known that the juxtamembrane region of KIT functions to inhibit receptor dimerization in the absence of ligand (SCF) and thus small in-frame deletions, insertions, or point mutations have the potential to disrupt this function and promote constitutive activation. The reported frequency of exon 11 mutations in GISTs was initially somewhat variable (ranging from as low as 20% to as high as 83%), possibly due to technical issues arising from the source of the tumor DNA (fresh frozen versus paraffin imbedded). More recent estimates with better controlled technical analysis suggest the rate may be 65–80% (discussed in (345)). Additional mutations in KIT have also been described in the extracellular domain, the kinase I domain, and the activation loop (summarized in Appendix IX). Familial (germline) mutations have also been identified. One of the first familial mutations to be reported was in the juxtamembrane region of KIT. Kindred of a Japanese family had deletions of one or two consecutive valine residues (codon 559 or 560); affected individuals had hyperpigmentations of the perineal skin and developed multiple benign and malignant GISTs (488). Substitution of V599A has also been described in two regions—one in Italy and another in Japan (489, 490). Affected members in both kindreds had pigmented macules on the skin of the perineum, axilla, hands, and face. In addition, affected patients in both families developed numerous GISTs in the stomach and the small bowel. A germline V599A KIT mutation has been identified, which also manifests in skin pigmentation and multiple GISTs (491). Other identified germline mutations associated with GISTs include W557R (492), K642E (kinase I domain) (493), and D820Y (activation loop). A common feature of patients harboring germline activating mutations of KIT is that they develop multiple GISTs, but generally not until early adulthood, suggesting that mutations in other genes are required for a stromal tumor to become distinguished from a background of hyperplasia of the interstitial cells of Cajal. Karyotype studies have shown that many GISTs demonstrate either monosomy 14 or possible loss of 14q; also loss of the long arm of chromosome 22. Losses on chromosomes 1p, 9p, and 11p, while less common, are more often associated with malignancy (for a more comprehensive review, see (345)). A small percentage of GISTs are KIT negative; some of these harbor PDGFRA mutations whereas other tumors have either low or no KIT expression and do not harbor identified PDGFRA mutations. GISTs that harbor KIT mutations exhibit strong KIT phosphorylation, particularly of the GRB2 and PI3K binding sites (Y703 and Y721), and also exhibit activation of several downstream signaling pathways including RAS/MAPK, PI3K/AKT, mTOR/p70S6K, and STAT1 and STAT3 (although the JNK and STAT5 pathways are not activated). Inhibitor studies have suggested that the activation of the PI3K/mTOR pathway, but not the MAPK pathway appears to be essential for KIT-mediated tumorigenesis.

Mastocytosis   Mastocytosis is a disorder resulting from pathological accumulation and activation of mast cells in tissues such as skin, bone marrow, liver, spleen, and lymph nodes. The clinical spectrum of mastocytosis is variable and may range from a self-limited disease confined to skin in children to progressive and life-threatening variants associated with poor prognosis. The WHO consensus classification for mastocytosis includes three major categories. (1) Cutaneous mastocytosis, a benign disease in which mast cell infiltration is confined to the skin. This form is preferentially seen in young children and exhibits a marked tendency to regress spontaneously. (2) Systemic mastocytosis (SM), more commonly found in adults, includes four major subtypes: (i) indolent SM, the most common form involving mainly skin and bone marrow); (ii) SM with an associated non mast cell clonal hematological disease, (iii) aggressive SM usually presenting without skin lesions, and (iv) mast cell leukemia. (3) The extremely rare localized extracutaneous mast cell neoplasms, either presenting as malignant mast cell sarcoma or as benign extracutaneous mastocytoma. The symptoms observed in mastocytosis are thought to be due to the spontaneous or triggered release of mast cell mediators or the consequences of the clonal expansion of the hematopoietic clone giving rise to mast cells. Mastocytosis is reported in 1000–8000 patients in the United States every year. Activating mutations (see Appendix IX) in KIT have been reported in a variety of patients with mastocytosis. The majority of these mutations map to the kinase domain of KIT. More than 90% of patients with systemic mastocytosis have the D816V KIT mutation (494). Activating mutations are more common in adult than pediatric patients.

Pediatric mastocytosis falls into three categories. The first class of patients has an activating mutation in codon 816 of KIT. The second class of patients that were identified (495) have a novel inactivating mutation at codon 839 of KIT, resulting in substitution of a lysine with glutamic acid. The third class of patients has no known mutations. Mutations found in pediatric mastocytosis are associated with a higher risk of advanced disease. Familial mastocytosis may also occur in the absence of KIT mutations (495).

In addition to mutations in KIT, increased levels of SCF may also be involved in mastocytosis. High levels of SCF are prevalent in the dermis and extracellular spaces between keratinocytes in skin from mastocytosis patients (496). Altered distribution of SCF in the skin also occurs in patients with cutaneous mastocytosis.

The release of mast cell mediators in the tissues and the response to these mediators result in varied clinical manifestations; although this usually chronic disease progresses slowly, it can progress into malignant disease. Mast cell leukemia, one of the rarest forms of leukemia (but very lethal), occurs in a small subset of patients with mastocytosis. Normal mast cell development requires the interaction of SCF and KIT; and as discussed earlier, mice harboring mutations in either ligand or receptor had markedly reduced mast cells in tissues (497). Mast cells are also one of the few hematopoietic cell lineages that retain KIT expression following differentiation from progenitors; these cells also proliferate in response to KIT activation. In the adult, sporadic forms of mastocytosis, activating mutations of KIT, characteristically occur—the most dominant form being the D816V mutation, which is resistant to imatinib (495). There are some additional rare mutations, notably D816Y and D816F, which do retain at least some sensitivity to the KIT kinase inhibitors.

Small Cell Lung Cancer (SCLC)   About 25,000 patients develop SCLC every year in the United States, thus representing a significant minority of the total number of lung cancers (15–25%). In most cases, SCLC presents as an extensive-stage disease (metastasized outside the chest) and has a highly aggressive clinical course. Despite treatment with combination chemotherapy, patients have a median survival of less than 10 months, and less than 1% are alive after 5 years. SCLC is often initially highly responsive to cisplatin-based combination therapy, but most patients present with disease recurrence within a few months after completion of the initial therapy and succumb to the disease shortly thereafter.

In the search for new therapeutic approaches for SCLC, there has been considerable interest in the identification of possible molecular targets. One of these is KIT. KIT overexpression is quite common in SCLC (~70%) (498–500), although there is some controversy whether KIT expression is of prognostic significance (501–503). There is little to no data about the activation state of KIT in SCLC, and to date, no activating mutations in KIT have been identified in SCLC tumors or cell lines. SCF can stimulate migration in SCLC cell lines expressing KIT (500, 504).

Melanoma   The KIT receptor plays an important role in the normal development and function of melanocytes during embryogenesis and postnatal development (505, 506). This is exemplified by the white spotting phenotype of mice and humans with loss of function mutations in either KIT or SCF (507–509). KIT is expressed in normal melanocytes, and by benign nevi and in situ melanoma, but is often downregulated in invasive and metastatic melanomas (510, 511), suggesting the possibility that KIT signaling might be important in the regulation of cell differentation and morphogenesis, and that the loss of its expression might contribute to melanoma progression. However, there have been isolated reports of activating KIT mutations in melanoma patients. Several groups have identified a L576P KIT mutation in acral melanomas (512) and K642E and K642E/N566D double mutations as well as KIT amplifications have also been noted in mucosal, acral, and melanomas on skin with chronic sun damage (513). Other KIT mutations identified in these subtypes of melanoma include Y553N, R634W, V599A, D816H, and A829P. Of these, the K642E, L576P, V599A, Y553N, and N566D mutations occur in the juxtamembrane region and would be predicted (or have already been shown) to promote KIT dimerization in the absence of ligand, resulting in constitutive activation. No mutations in KIT were identified in melanomas on skin without chronic sun-induced damage (513).

Acute Myelogenous Leukemia   A number of studies have suggested a role for KIT in leukemogenesis, with high expression of KIT in AML (60–80%) (514, 515) as well as point mutations in core binding factor AML with inv (16) (33–45%) and AML M2 with t(8;21) (13–47%) (516, 517). A more recent paper, which characterized KIT abnormalities through whole gene resequencing, showed that KIT mutations were closely correlated with t(8;21) leukemia with a mutation rate of 48.1% (518). In total, seven different point mutations (I748T (1), L773S (1), D816Y (4), D816V (3), D816H (2), N822K (10), V825I (1)), three internal tandem duplication type mutations (AFNF repeat, I571+14 (1), Q575+17 (1)), and one amino acid deletion (D419) were characterized. The ITD-type mutations occured in the juxtamembrane region (I571+14 and Q575+17) and in the extracellular domain (AFNF repeat). Only one of the mutations was in the kinase insert sequence (I748T), while the point mutations at L733, D816, N822, and V825 are clustered at the enzymatic pocket of KIT.

Sinonasal Natural Killer/T-Cell Lymphoma   Sinonasal lymphoma is a clinical condition of lethal, midline granuloma, a progressive destructive lesion that affects the midline of the face. It is more common in Asian countries than Western countries and has been shown to be highly associated with Epstein–Barr virus infections. Molecular studies of the disease have been difficult due to the massive necrosis associated with the disease, and the consequent limited availability of viable tumor tissue. A landmark paper by Hongyo et al. (519) describes the analysis of KIT mutations in 23 cases of this disease, 14 from Beijing, China, and 9 cases from Osaka, Japan. Ten of the Chinese cases (71.4%) had mutations at exon 11 or exon 17 of *KIT*; in contrast, only 2 of the Japanese cases had mutations. Seven of the 8 mutations in exon 17 occured at codon 825 (V825A) and three of the four mutations in exon 11 occurred at codon 561 (Q561K (2); Q561Q (1 silent)). These mutations are unique to this disorder and have not been reported in other human studies. However, transfection studies suggested that the V825A mutation was not a gain of function mutation (519). Later studies in Korean and Indonesian populations also identified KIT mutations in cases of natural killer/T-cell lymphoma populations (520, 521).

Testicular Germ Cell Tumors (TGCTs)   TGCTs are the most frequent cancer type in young men. These cancers are divided into two major subgroups, seminoma and nonseminoma. The seminoma type accounts for about 50% of TGCTs, and the typical form has the histological appearance of sheets of large cells with abundant cytoplasm and round, hyperchromatic nuclei with prominent nucleoli. KIT and SCF are known to be essential for germ cell development and spermatogenesis. There have been a few reports of KIT mutations in germ cell tumors; one fairly comprehensive survey of KIT mutations in germ cell tumors was published by Kemmer et al. (522). The activating mutations of KIT in testicular seminoma appear to be localized to exon 17. Fourteen of the seminomas (25.9% of those examined) contained point mutations in exon 17 (D816V, 6 cases; D816H, 3 cases; Y823D, 2 cases; and single examples of Y823G, N822K, and T801L mutations). Two of the mutants were imatanib sensitive (N822K and Y823D), whereas D816V and D816H were resistant to imatinib. Other authors have reported additional mutations including D820V and K818R (523). Biochemical evidence of KIT activation, as assessed by KIT phosphorylation and KIT association with PI3K, was largely confined to those seminomas with a genomic KIT mutation. However, KIT mutations were not observed in nonseminomatous germ cell tumors. While it might seem logical to treat seminomas with a KIT kinase inhibitor, the current medical treatment of seminoma results in a very high cure rate; thus development of KIT inhibitors in this disease setting is likely to have a more restricted utility.

3.8   FLT3

FLT3 (FMS-like tyrosine kinase 3, also known as CD135, FLK2, and STK1) is a Class III receptor tyrosine kinase, structurally related to PDGFR, KIT, and FMS. This receptor class has five immunoglobulin-like extracellular domains, and an intracellular tyrosine kinase domain with a characteristic hydrophobic kinase insert domain splitting the tyrosine kinase domain. Upon immunoprecipitation of human FLT3, two bands are usually seen; a minor band of molecular weight 130,000 (the immature high mannose containing form) and a major band of 155,000–160,000 (representing the mature, N-glycosylated form). FLT3 is expressed on bone marrow CD34 positive cells (which correspond to multipotential, myeloid, and B-lymphoid progenitor cells) and expression is lost as hematopoietic cells differentiate. Human FLT3 is expressed in human pro-B and pre-B cell lines (524–526) but is not expressed in myeloma cell lines (524), erythroid or erythroblastic (524, 526), NK, Hodgkin's lymphoma cell lines, or T-cell lines (524–526). FLT3 is also expressed by many human myeloid and monocytic cell lines (524–526). The gene encoding FLT3 has been mapped to chromosome 13q12 (527), near the VEGFR1 locus.

The ligand for FLT3 is called the "FLT3 ligand" (FL). The primary translation product of the FL gene is a Type I transmembrane protein, and the human protein contains 235 amino acids. The first 26 amino acids constitute a signal peptide (absent from the mature protein), a 156 aa extracellular domain, a 23 aa TM domain, and a 30 aa cytoplasmic tail. At the amino acid level, the human protein is 72% identical to the murine (528) and the cytoplasmic domains of murine and human FL are quite divergent (only 52% identical). Nevertheless, the murine and human FL can each stimulate the proliferation of either murine or human primitive hematopoietic cells. The human FL protein is N-glycosylated and exists as a noncovalently bound homodimer. There are several isoforms of FL, including a soluble form generated by proteolytic cleavage of the extracellular domain, and a second, soluble FL isoform generated by an alternatively spliced sixth exon, which introduces a stop codon near the end of the extracellular domain (this form appears to be quite rare). The binding affinity of FL for FLT3 is 200–500 pM (529). FL is widely expressed in human tissues, in fact, in almost every tissue analyzed (528, 530, 531). The human FL has been mapped to chromosome 19q13.3–13.4 (532).

Clues to the role of FLT3 in normal hematopoiesis have come from murine gene deletion studies of either FLT3 (533) or FL (534). Both mouse genotypes are viable, with normal litter sizes and the expected Mendelian ratio. The mice have normal life spans and no notable hematological diseases. The mice do show reduced numbers of B progenitors, NK cells, and dendritic cells (DCs). FLT3 expression is usually lost upon hematopoietic stem cell differentiation, with the exception of DCs, which display persistent FLT3 expression. In vivo treatment of mice with FL greatly expands the number of myeloid and lymphoid-derived DCs in the bone marrow, spleen, GI tract, skin, and lymph nodes in vivo, and also stimulates DC expansion in vitro. The important role of FL in DC generation is also supported by the observed reduced numbers of DCs in FL-deficient mice (534). FLT3 responses are dependent on the cell type as well as costimulation with other growth factors. For example, FL stimulation without the addition of other growth factors promotes the monocytic differentiation of early hematopoietic progenitor cells (without a marked proliferative response) (535, 536); FL in combination with other growth factors such as IL3, GSF3, CSF1, GM-CSF, EPO, and SCF results in a more vigorous proliferative response and enhanced development of granulocytic–monocytic colony forming units (535–537). FL in combination with IL7 promotes the stromal cell independent growth of pro-B cells and differentiation of pro-B cells to pre-B cells (538), while the combination of IL3, IL6, IL7, and FL increases primitive thymic progenitors (539).

Similar to other Class II RTKs, FLT3 is activated by FL-dependent dimerization and transphosphorylation of tyrosine residues (540), leading to the association and/or phosphorylation of a number of cytoplasmic substrates including the p85 subunit of PI3K, RAS/GTP activating protein, PLCγ, VAV, SHC, GRB2, CBL and CBLB (the CBL related protein), and SHP2 (Figure 3.14). However, SHP2 does not associate directly with FLT3; it binds directly to GRB2 in response to FL stimulation. GRB2 also associates with FLT3 and SHC after FL stimulation, and SHP2 becomes tyrosine phosphorylated and binds to tyrosine phosphorylated SHC. In contrast, SHP1, another tyrosine phosphatase that binds KIT, is not phosphorylated by FLT3, nor does it bind to the FLT3 receptor. Downstream pathways activated by FL-FLT3 include RAS/MAPK, STAT5, and PI3K/AKT. Other proteins reported to be phosphorylated following FL-FLT3 activation include GAB1, GAB2, AKT, FOXO3A, LYN, GAP, p90RSK, BAD, and C/EBPα.

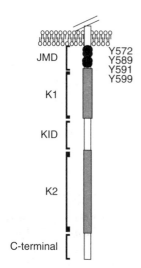

Figure 3.14 Schematic diagram of the cytoplasmic domain of FLT3, illustrating the juxtamembrane domain (JMD), the split kinase domains (K1 and K2), the kinase insert domain (KID), and the C-terminal tail. Phosphotyrosine sites are indicated by the black circles. Binding of the ligand (FL) results in receptor dimerization and tyrosine phosphorylation, and the phosphorylated receptors in turn recruit interacting proteins, activating several signal transduction pathways.

3.8.1 FLT3 and Cancer

Leukemia At the level of both RNA and protein, FLT3 is overexpressed in most B lineage and acute myeloid leukemias, a smaller subset of T-acute lymphocytic leukemia (ALL), and in CML blast crises. Leukemic cells of the B lineage ALL and AML frequently coexpress FL, creating an autocrine or paracine signaling loop contributing to constitutive and chronic activation of FLT3. In addition, FL stimulates the proliferation of many leukemia-derived cell lines.

FLT3 mutations are the most frequent somatic mutations in AML and have been found in over 30% of AML patients. Two major types of mutation are observed. The more common form (23% of AML patients) is the internal tandem duplication (ITD) of 3–400 bp (541–543). These are always in frame and map to the juxtamembrane region. The second form is a point mutation, most frequently involving D835 of the kinase domain (544), although other point mutations have been found. There have been additional insertion/deletion mutations reported that affect the juxtamembrane region. Children with AML have a lower incidence of ITD but a similar rate of kinase domain point mutations as adults; FLT3 ITD mutations also occur in ALL but are much less frequent (<1%), occurring primarily in cases that are termed biphenotypic leukemia (a form of leukemia with characteristics of both myeloid and lymphoid lineages; for a recent review, see (545)). FLT3 activating mutations have been reported to occur more frequently in ALL patients with MLL rearrangements and hyperdiploidy (546). Both the kinase domain and ITD mutations result in constitutive activation of FLT3 in the absence of ligand.

ITD mutations are associated with a poor prognosis for both pediatric and adult patients; for example, in one study, the event-free survival rate was 44% for patients without a FLT3 ITD mutation compared to just 7% for those harboring the mutation (547). The prognosis is even worse for patients who have the ITD mutation and have lost the wild-type copy of FLT3. In contradistinction, the kinase domain point mutant does not seem to portend this grim prognosis (548), perhaps due to some differences in downstream signaling events. Interestingly, there are also reports of AML patients who did not have FLT3 mutations at time of diagnosis, but acquired them at time of relapse (549). FLT3 mutations have also been seen in a small percentage (3–5%) of patients with myelodysplastic sysndrome, and acquisition of FLT3 mutations may be an important component of progression to AML (550). Appendix X summarizes reported tumor-associated mutations in FLT3.

3.9 RET

The RET (rearranged during transfection) proto-oncogene encodes a receptor tyrosine kinase for members of the glial cell line-derived neurotrophic factors (GDNFs). The gene for RET is localized to chromosome 10 (10q11.2). The RET gene contains 21 exons and spans more than 60 kb of genomic DNA, and the mRNA can be alternatively spliced to produce up to ten protein isoforms. The three most common are defined as RET51, RET43, and RET9, referring to 51, 43, and 9 amino acids in the C-terminal tail. RET51 and RET9 are the best characterized (551).

A schematic diagram of the common domain structure is provided in Figure 3.15. The N-terminal extracellular domain contains four cadherin-like repeats and a cysteine-rich region. The extracellular domain contains nine N-glycosylation sites. There is a hydrophobic transmembrane domain, and a cytoplasmic tyrosine kinase domain split by an insertion of 27 amino acids. Within the cytoplasmic tyrosine kinase domain, the RET51 isoform has 18 tyrosines, and the RET9 isoform has 16. Tyr1090 and Tyr1096 are specific to the RET51 isoform.

During embryogenesis, RET is expressed by various neuronal subsets of the central and peripheral nervous system. Additionally, RET is expressed in the

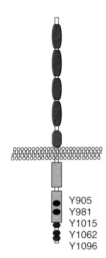

Y905
Y981
Y1015
Y1062
Y1096

Figure 3.15 Schematic diagram of the RET receptor. The four cadherin domains are indicated by dark blue ovals and the cysteine-rich domain by the violet oval. The kinase domain is indicated by the cyan colored rectangles. Sites of tyrosine phosphorylation are depicted as black circles.

Wolffian duct, budding ureter, and later in the tips of the renal collecting tubules. The expression pattern of the receptor reflects the distribution and in most cases RET and GDNF are expressed in adjacent cells or tissues. Both GDNF null mice and RET null mice are born alive but die during the first postnatal day because of renal aplasia or hypodysplasia (552). Both knockouts also lack enteric nervous plexuses in both their small and large bowels (552). The RET protein is also necessary for spermatogenesis (553). Mice deficient in the RET co-receptor (GFRα1, discussed next) have a similar phenotype to that of the RET and GDNF deficient mice (554).

Overexpression of RET in human embryonic fibroblasts and rat olfactory neuroblast cell lines induces apoptosis, a phenotype that can be rescued by treatment with the RET ligand, GDNF. RET-induced apoptosis appears to result from RET-induced caspase cleavage exposing a proapoptotic domain of RET (555). RET signaling may also be essential for Peyer's patch formation since deficiency of GFRα3 results in impairment of Peyer's patch development, suggesting a role for RET/GFRα3/ARTM. The RET ligand ARTM can recruit gut hematopoietic cells to induce the formation of ectopic Peyer's patch-like structures (556).

Binding and activation of RET requires coreceptors (GFRs) α1–4, a family of glycosylphosphatidylinositol anchored proteins with preferentially high affinity for selective ligands. For example, GDNF primarily associates with GFRα1, neurturin with GFRα2, artemin (ARTN) with GFRα3, and persephin with GFRα4 (557). Differential tissue specificity and regulated expression during development suggest that these ligands and coreceptors have distinct roles, despite all activating the RET tyrosine kinase with similar kinetics.

Following ligand-induced activation of the RET receptor, the receptors form homodimers and undergo autophosphorylation of intracellular tyrosines 905, 981, 1015, 1062, and 1096. These phosphotyrosine residues in turn serve as docking sites for downstream signal transduction pathways (318). Y1062 seems to be particularly critical (558, 559), acting as a multifunctional docking site for many adaptor proteins including SHC, SHCC, FRS1, IRS1/2, DPK1, DOK4/5, DOK6, Enigma, and protein kinase C (recently reviewed in (560)). Of note, GRB2 binds directly to Y1096, a residue that is only present in the RET splicing variant RET51 (as reviewed in (560)). Multiple signaling pathways are activated by RET. Upon SHC binding to RET, the recruitment of the GRB2/SOS complex leads to activation of the RAS/MEK/ERK pathway, promoting cell cycle progression (561, 562). Assembly of GRB2 and GAB1/2 with SHC recruits the p85 subunit of phosphatidylinositol 3-kinase, and subsequent activation of the PI3K/AKT pathway, promoting enhanced cell survival, motility, and cell cycle progression (561–564). The JNK pathway can be activated by DOK1 and NCK assembly on phosphorylated Y1062; the p38 MAPK and ERK5 pathways are also activated by RET Y1062 activation (563, 564). Phosphorylation of other tyrosine residues leads to activation of the JAK/STAT and protein kinase C pathways (565, 566).

3.9.1   RET and Thyroid Carcinoma

Approximately 25,000 new cases of thyroid cancer are diagnosed in the United States each year, and the majority of these are papillary thyroid carcinomas (PTCs).

In both sporadic and radiation-induced PTCs, chromosomal translocations lead to the fusion of one of several heterologous genes to the 5′ end of the RET intracellular domain coding sequence, leading to constitutive dimerization, cytoplasmic localization, and activation of RET. For example, activating RET translocations (collectively described as RET/PTC rearrangements) have been found to be prevalent in thyroid tumors of children exposed to radiation following the Chernobyl nuclear reactor accident in 1986 (567–570).

A more uncommon disorder (5–8% of the total thyroid cancers) is medullary thyroid cancer (MTC), which develops from the parafollicular epithelial cells (the calcitonin secreting cells) of the thyroid gland. Approximately 75–80% of the MTC cases are sporadic. However, a small number are inherited as part of a familial cancer syndrome termed multiple endocrine neoplasia type 2 (MEN2). MEN2 is further divided into three distinct clinical forms: MEN2A, MEN2B, and familial MTC (FMTC). Germline mutations in the RET proto-oncogene have been identified as the underlying cause in nearly all MEN2 syndromes (571, 572); indeed, 98% of MEN2 cases and 25–50% of sporadic MTC cases are associated with RET mutations (573). The MEN2A subtype is characterized by MTC and lower incidence of pheochromocytoma and hyperparathyroidism. MEN2B is a more aggressive subtype of the disease and is characterized by earlier clinical manifestation as well as pheochromocytoma and ganglioneuromatosis. In MEN2A patients, the mutations identified affect one of the six cysteine residues in the cysteine-rich extracellular domain of RET, leading to ligand-independent homodimers and constitutive activation of RET (574). In contradistinction, the mutations associated with the RET gene in MEN2B patients affect residues in the tyrosine kinase domain, promoting constitutive activation of the monomeric receptor and altered substrate specificity (575); increased phosphorylation of Y1062 has been described in patients with MEN2B (576, 577). In particular, MEN2B mutations appear to elicit enhanced activation of PI3K, RAS/MEK/ERK, and JNK signaling and also promote signaling via the STAT3 transcription factor. In FMTC patients, mutations in both the cysteine-rich extracellular domain and tyrosine kinase domain have been identified, which leads to low-level activation of RET, and possibly explains the more indolent penetrance phenotype of FMTC (578). Tumor-associated mutations in RET are summarized in Appendix XI.

3.10 MET AND RON

3.10.1 MET

The MET receptor tyrosine kinase was initially identified as a proto-oncogene (579). A fairly large gene, human *MET* is located on 7q21-q31, spanning more than 120 kb in length and consisting of 21 exons separated by 20 introns (580). Like its ligand, hepatocyte growth factor (HGF, also known as scatter factor), MET is a disulfide linked heterodimer. The primary MET transcript produces a 150-kDa polypeptide that is subsequently glycosylated, producing a 170-kDa precursor protein. This precursor is further glycosylated then cleaved at a furin site located between residues 307 and 308. The mature form of MET consists of a 50-kDa extracellular α chain, and a longer, 140-kDa β chain; the two are disulfide linked. The β subunit contains extracellular, transmembrane, and tyrosine kinase domains.

A schematic diagram of the domain structure is provided in Figure 3.16. The N terminus contains a "SEMA" domain (similar to that of the semaphorin axon-guidance proteins) and furin cleavage site; after cleavage, the α subunit and first 212 residues of the β subunit function to bind the ligand HGF. Working toward the C terminus, one finds the PSI domain, IPT repeats (also known as TIG domains), the transmembrane domain, juxtamembrane (JM) domains, and the C-terminal intracellular tyrosine kinase domain. MET has been classified as the prototype member of a RTK family that includes RON and SEA, based on shared

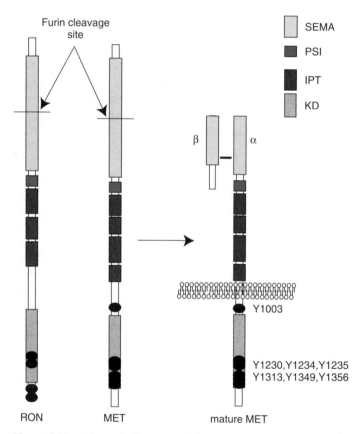

Figure 3.16 Schematic diagrams of the unprocessed forms of the MET and RON receptors and the mature form of the MET receptor. The SEMA domain (a protein domain of approximately 450 amino acids identified in the semaphorins) is depicted as the chartreuse rectangle, the PSI (plexin/semaphorin/integrin) domain is indicated by the deep pink rectangle, the IPT (Ig-like/plexin/transcription factors) domains are in dark blue, and the kinase domain is shown in cyan. Tyrosine phosphorylation sites are shown as black circles.

structural homology. The tyrosine kinase domain of MET also shares homology with molecules of the TYRO3 family (including AXL, TYRO3, and MER) and with IGF1R.

Upon ligand binding, MET undergoes autophosphorylation of specific tyrosine residues in the cytoplasmic region of the molecule. Phosphorylation of Y1230, Y1234, and Y1235 in the activation loop of the tyrosine kinase domain results in activation of the intrinsic kinase activity of MET. The phosphorylation of Y1313 is critical in the recruitment and binding of PI3K, and phosphorylation of Y1349 and Y1356 in the C terminus activates the so-called bidentate, multisubstrate signal transducer docking site ($Y^{1349}VHVX_3Y^{1356}VNV$), which contains docking sites for SH2 domains, PTB domains, and MET binding domains for signal transducers and adaptor proteins.

When phosphorylated, the bidentate docking site of MET binds substrates such as GAB1, GRB2, PI3K, and others. Most of these proteins contain SH2 domains, which often mediate the interactions. Although two substrates are not thought to simultaneously bind to this site in one MET molecule, GAB1 can bind to phosphorylated Y1349 on one molecule and GRB2 to Y1356 on a second. Thus interactions between GAB1 and GRB2 can occur on MET dimers or multimers. Compelling evidence for the critical role of this site in MET signal transduction was provided by chimeric studies, which demonstrated that transfer of the bidentate site to other receptor tyrosine kinases was sufficient to confer typical MET phenotypic responses (581).

GAB1, the most crucial substrate for MET signaling (582, 583), is a scaffolding adaptor protein. The interaction with tyrosine phosphorylated MET is mediated by the "MET binding site" in GAB1. This sequence of 13 amino acids is distinct from the classical SH2 and phosphotyrosine binding domains and is not present in other GAB family members. This binding site allows a direct and robust interaction between GAB1 and MET and results in prolonged GAB1 phosphorylation in response to HGF/SF. In turn, phosphorylated GAB1 binds various signal-relay molecules, including the SH2 domain containing protein tyrosine phosphatase (SHP2), PI3K, PLCγ, and CRK through their SH2 domains. SHP2 has low constitutive tyrosine phosphatase activity as a consequence of allosteric inhibition by its amino terminal SH2 domain. However, when the two phosphorylated residues of GAB1 bind the SH2 domains of SHP2, this inhibition is relieved and SHP then upregulates the ERK/MAPK pathway (for a review, see (584)).

Another key residue in MET signaling/regulation is Y1003, and the surrounding amino acids that comprise an additional docking site. This residue is found in the juxtamembrane region and acts as a negative regulator of MET activity. CBL, an E3 ubiquitin ligase, binds to phosphorylated Y1003. This, in turn, results in the ubiquitination of MET, MET endocytosis, translocation to the endosomal compartment, and, ultimately, MET degradation (585–587). Therefore CBL-mediated degradation provides a means to attenuate or terminate MET signaling.

HGF is a potent mitogen for a variety of tumor cells derived from ovarian, gastric, CNS, lung, pancreatic, colorectal, prostate, and breast cancers. It is also a potent endothelial mitogen and thus plays an important role in the angiogenesis required to support tumor growth. HGF can also act as a survival factor for many tumor cells and also endothelial cells, preventing apoptosis under serum starved or other stress conditions. Epithelial cells, exemplified by the Madin–Darby canine kidney (MDCK) cell line, respond to HGF/SF by "scattering" (hence the early name "scatter factor"). HGF causes cells that normally grow in sheets (such as epithelial and endothelial cells) to separate into single cells that move apart from one another. When dissociated, cells more readily invade collagen matrices, providing an assay often used to quantitate the invasive capacity of cells. Another activity programmed by the HGF–MET signaling axis leads to a coordinated consortium of biological responses resulting in invasive growth, tubulogenesis, and branching morphogenesis.

Many investigators have attempted to delineate the role of individual downstream signaling pathways in specific cellular responses. For example, inhibitors of both PI3K and ERK/MAPK inhibit epithelial scattering (588), implicating these pathways in disassembly of adherens junctions, cell spreading, cell motility, and cytoskeletal rearrangements. MET also activates RAS, RAC1, and p21-activated kinase (PAK) and this pathway plays a role in cytoskeletal rearrangements and cell adhesion (589, 590). GSB1/CRK/RAP1 signaling has also been implicated in the control of cell motility (591, 592). The cell survival activity of HGF is mediated primarily through PI3K/AKT (593, 594), whereas activation of the GAB1/SHP2/ERK/MAPK cascade is thought to regulate cell proliferation, junctional competence, and motility (583, 589, 590, 595–599).

MET/HGF and Cancer   In recent years, dysregulation of the HGF/MET axis has emerged as a common feature of many human cancers. This dysregulation can occur at one or more levels including translocation, amplification, overexpression, and activating mutations. Experimentally, expression of HGF, MET, or mutant MET confers malignant properties on normal cells (e.g., increased motility, invasiveness, tumorigenicity). Moreover, HGF/SF overexpression correlates with poor prognosis in a number of different malignancies (600). Cooperative interactions between MET and VEGF receptor signaling may have specific significance in promoting tumor neoangiogenesis. The expression of both MET and VEGF are regulated by HIF1 in response to hypoxia (601). Hence hypoxic regions within tumors may serve to both recruit new blood vessels and promote tumor cell motility, thus increasing the invasive and metastatic potential of the tumor (602). MET overexpression can also induce VEGF production, and HGF and VEGF act synergistically to promote vascular tube formation and activate multiple intracellular signaling pathways involved in endothelial cell proliferation (603, 604). More recently, loss of TGFβII receptor in mouse stromal cells has been associated with upregulated secretion of HGF (in addition to TGFα and macrophage stimulating factor) (605). This was associated with activation of MET and other RTKs in implanted breast cancer cells leading to increased growth and invasion, which was suppressed by MET inhibition (606). MET has also emerged as a mediator of resistance to RTK inhibitors in lung tumors and was found to be amplified in 22% of tumor samples that had acquired resistance to gefitinib (607). In a separate study, EGFR inhibitor-resistant cells that overexpressed MET were shown to be sensitive to a small molecule MET inhibitor (608).

The oncogenic potential of MET was initially identified by the discovery of the fusion gene, TPR-MET. TPR-MET was originally identified as the product of a chromosomal rearrangement induced by the treatment of a human osteogenic sarcoma line with the carcinogen N-methyl-N'-nitronitrosoguanidine, fusing two genetic loci: a translocated promoter region from chromosome 1q25, encoding a dimerization motif, and MET, from chromosome 7q31. In the resulting protein product of this fusion gene, the extracellular, transmembrane, and juxtamembrane portions of MET are replaced by the N-terminal amino acids of the TPR gene product. The TPR domain is a coiled-coil domain derived from the nucleopore complex. TPR-MET is constitutively dimerized resulting in ligand-independent transphosphorylation and constitutive activation of the MET kinase. Additionally, the lack of the juxtamembrane domain of MET excludes the fusion protein from the CBL ubiquitination/degradation pathway (609). Thus the inability to be targeted to the lysosomal degradative pathway may also contribute to the oncogenic activity of TPR-MET. The TPR-MET translocation may also occur naturally, although at fairly low frequency, in a number of nonhematopoietic malignancies. There are conflicting reports about the frequency of TPR-MET in gastric carcinomas (610–613).

Elevated MET expression is observed in many human tumors. Activation of MET in cancer often occurs through ligand-dependent autocrine or paracrine mechanisms. For example, both osteosarcomas and glioblastoma multiforme express both MET and HGF. Many carcinomas express or overexpress MET, but in this case, the ligand is not expressed by the tumor cells themselves, but by the surrounding stroma, resulting in paracrine activation of MET. In tumors expressing high levels of MET, ligand-independent activation of MET may also occur. MET amplification occurs in 5–10% of gastric cancers (614–616), 4% of esophageal cancers (617), and 4% of lung cancers (420); MET amplification and MET and/or HGF overexpression have been correlated with poor clinical outcome in a variety of cancers (584).

Missense mutations of *MET* have been reported in a variety of cancers, with the majority of the mutations identified in the activation loop tyrosine kinase domain (summarized in Appendix XII). Patients with hereditary papillary renal carcinoma (HPRC) have a predisposition to multiple, bilateral papillary type 1 renal tumors; genetic studies revealed that these patients inherited activating missense mutations in the tyrosine kinase domain of the MET proto-oncogene (618). Activating mutations in the tyrosine kinase domain of MET have also been identified in a subset of tumors from patients with sporadic type 1 papillary renal carcinoma (619, 620). Additionally, HPRC-associated type 1 papillary renal carcinomas are also characterized by trisomy 7 with a nonrandom duplication of the mutant *MET* allele (621).

Activating mutations of MET in the juxtamembrane domain, the semaphorin domain, and insertions and alternative splice forms involving the juxtamembrane and extracellular domains have been identified in small cell lung cancers (622). Additional mutations in the semaphorin domain, the juxtamembrane domain, and alternative splice products of MET have also been identified in non small cell lung cancers (623) (Appendix XII). MET mutations have also been found in gastric cancers (306, 624), ovarian tumors (625), glioma (626), lymph node and pulmonary metastases (627), head and neck squamous cell carcinomas (593, 628), breast tumors (629), childhood hepatocellular carcinomas (619), melanoma (630), and pleural mesotheliomas (631).

3.10.2 RON

Recepteur d'origine Nantais (RON) (also known as macrophage stimulating 1 receptor, MST1R) is a member of the MET receptor family (632). The RON gene contains 20 exons and 19 introns and is located on chromosome 3p21 (632), a region frequently altered in cancer (633). RON is a heterodimeric glycoprotein with disulfide linked α and β chains derived from the proteolytic cleavage of a common precursor of 170 kDa (634). The α chain is completely extracellular, whereas the β chain has regions that are extracellular, transmembrane, and intracellular. The β chain contains the intracellular tyrosine kinase and regulatory elements. The α chain possesses a specialized sema domain, with a conserved pattern of cysteine residues, amino acid sequences, and a potential glycosylation site, and it is this region that contains the ligand binding site. Only RON and MET have sema domains in the extracellular portions of the proteins (635, 636). RON signaling occurs when RON forms either homodimers or heterodimers with other receptors. RON is a specific cell surface receptor for macrophage stimulating protein (MSP), a protein that is structurally related to HGF (634, 637, 638). Binding of MSP to RON stimulates the intrinsic tyrosine kinase activity and phosphorylation of the docking site, leading to binding of multiple SH2 domain-containing signal transducing and adaptor proteins.

MSP, also known as HGF-like protein or scatter factor 2, is an 80-kDa heterodimer, composed of a 53-kDa α chain and a 30-kDa β chain, linked by a disulfide bond. HGF and MSP belong to the plasminogen–prothrombin gene family, characterized by multiple kringle domains that are identified by triple disulfide loop structures in the N-terminal domain (639). Neither MSP nor HGF has proteolytic activity. The major source of MSP is the hepatocyte, and the protein is secreted as in an inactive precursor form, pro-MSP (640). Pro-MSP is proteolytically cleaved at R483-V484 (641), leading to its activation, and a number of enzymes have been shown to do this including coagulation cascade enzymes such as factors XIa, XIIa, and kallikrein. There is also a pro-MSP convertase that has been found in wound fluid exudates and on the surface of macrophages (640).

Both RON and MET trigger complex morphogenic programs of epithelial cells that lead to invasive growth—under physiological conditions contributing to organ development and regeneration and, in cancer cells, contributing to cell invasion and metastasis. The RON receptor is expressed in epithelial and hematopoietic cells. Biological responses attributed to RON include regulation of tissue macrophage motility, epithelial scattering, and matrix invasion. Addition of MSP to macrophages inhibits LPS-induced expression of inflammatory mediates such as inducible nitric oxide and prostaglandins, suggesting an inhibitory role of RON in regulating inflammation (642, 643). In keratinocytes, MSP phosphorylates RON and activates cell adhesion, motility, and antiapoptotic and proliferative responses (644, 645). RON is regulated through CBL ubiquitin ligase, which binds to phosphorylated RON, leading to its endocytosis and subsequent degradation (646).

RON and Cancer   RON signaling has been shown to augment papilloma growth and malignant transformation in vivo, and it has been suggested that the malignant skin tumors in animal models resemble squamous cell carcinomas and malignant fibrous histiocytomas, suggesting a possible role of RON in these cancer types (647).

RON is overexpressed and amplified in various human cancers (648–657). Although activating missense mutations in the tyrosine kinase domain, similar to those that occur in MET, have not been identified in tumor samples to date, introduction of activating mutations such as D1232V and M1254T mutations is sufficient to increase receptor phosphorylation resulting in a tumorigenic phenotype (658, 659)

In addition to the full-length form of RON, biologically active RON variants have been identified in various tumor cells. Currently, three RON mRNA splicing variants have been described. RONΔ165 (also known as ΔRON) has a molecular mass of 165 kDa and has been identified in gastric cancer cell lines (650) and later in normal and malignant colon tissue samples (660). In the gastric carcinoma cell line KATO-III, ΔRON is translated into an uncleaved precursor protein with an uneven number of cysteine residues, and because of this aberrant intermolecular disulfide bridge formation, this form of the protein oligomerizes in the intracellular compartment and is constitutively activated (650). Expression of ΔRON is found in additional gastric and lung tumor cell lines (634, 661). Aberrerant ΔRON expression leads to altered morphology and motility of breast cancer cell lines, an outcome more striking than overexpression of the full sized RON receptor (662). The transformed phenotype of cells expressing ΔRON is associated with a loss of E-cadherin (662). A few other naturally occuring RON variants have been described with oncogenic potential (663). The second RON variant, RONΔ160, was originally cloned from the colon cancer cell lines HT29 and SW837 (664, 665). RONΔ160 has an in-frame deletion of 109 amino acids in the extracellular domain of the β chain; the deletion of the 109 amino acids results in unbalanced numbers of cysteine residues in the extracellular domain, resulting in abnormal dimerization and constitutive activation. The third novel RON variant, RONΔ155, has a deletion of 158 amino acids from the extracellular domain resulting from splicing with deletion of exons 5, 6, and 11. This isoform is also constitutively active, with autophosphorylation of tyrosine residues. This is a nonprocessed single chain protein that is retained in the cytoplasm (666). All of these in-frame deletions lead to constitutive activation and are associated with activation of cell growth in transformation assays and cell motility in invasion assays.

Additional lines of evidence suggest that RON may be a good cancer target. Downregulation of RON in RON-expressing cancer cell lines was shown to have an antiproliferative effect. RON has also been shown to synergize with known oncogenes such as polyoma middle T and RAS (647, 667). Additionally, neutralizing antibodies to RON were shown to have antitumor activity in HT29 (colon), NCI-H292 (lung), and BXPC3 (pancreatic) xenograft models, and to exhibit synergistic activity when combined with an EGFR inhibitor cetuximab in the BXPC3 xenograft model (668).

REFERENCES

1. Blume-Jensen P, Hunter T. Oncogenic kinase signalling. Nature 2001;411(6835):355–365.
2. Lin CR, Chen WS, Kruiger W, Stolarsky LS, Weber W, Evans RM, Verma IM, Gill GN, Rosenfeld MG. Expression cloning of human EGF receptor complementary DNA: gene amplification and three related messenger RNA products in A431 cells. Science 1984;224(4651):843–848.
3. Coussens L, Yang-Feng TL, Liao YC, Chen E, Gray A, McGrath J, Seeburg PH, Libermann TA, Schlessinger J, Francke U, et al. Tyrosine kinase receptor with extensive homology to EGF receptor shares chromosomal location with neu oncogene. Science 1985;230(4730):1132–1139.
4. King CR, Kraus MH, Aaronson SA. Amplification of a novel v-erbB-related gene in a human mammary carcinoma. Science 1985;229(4717):974–976.
5. Schechter AL, Hung MC, Vaidyanathan L, Weinberg RA, Yang-Feng TL, Francke U, Ullrich A, Coussens L. The neu gene: an erbB-homologous gene distinct from and unlinked to the gene encoding the EGF receptor. Science 1985;229(4717):976–978.
6. Hanahan D, Weinberg RA. The hallmarks of cancer. Cell 2000;100(1):57–70.
7. Folkman J. Tumor angiogenesis: therapeutic implications. N Engl J Med 1971;285(21): 1182–1186.
8. Aroian RV, Koga M, Mendel JE, Ohshima Y, Sternberg PW. The let-23 gene necessary for *Caenorhabditis elegans* vulval induction encodes a tyrosine kinase of the EGF receptor subfamily. Nature 1990;348(6303):693–699.
9. Price JV, Clifford RJ, Schupbach T. The maternal ventralizing locus torpedo is allelic to faint little ball, an embryonic lethal, and encodes the *Drosophila* EGF receptor homolog. Cell 1989;56(6):1085–1092.
10. Schejter ED, Shilo BZ. The *Drosophila* EGF receptor homolog (DER) gene is allelic to faint little ball, a locus essential for embryonic development. Cell 1989;56(6):1093–1104.
11. Gschwind A, Fischer OM, Ullrich A. The discovery of receptor tyrosine kinases: targets for cancer therapy. Nat Rev Cancer 2004;4(5):361–370.
12. Reiter JL, Threadgill DW, Eley GD, Strunk KE, Danielsen AJ, Sinclair CS, Pearsall RS, Green PJ, Yee D, Lampland AL, Balasubramaniam S, Crossley TD, Magnuson TR, James CD, Maihle NJ. Comparative genomic sequence analysis and isolation of human and mouse alternative EGFR transcripts encoding truncated receptor isoforms. Genomics 2001;71(1):1–20.
13. Popescu NC, King CR, Kraus MH. Localization of the human erbB-2 gene on normal and rearranged chromosomes 17 to bands q12–21.32. Genomics 1989;4(3):362–366.
14. Kraus MH, Issing W, Miki T, Popescu NC, Aaronson SA. Isolation and characterization of ERBB3, a third member of the ERBB/epidermal growth factor receptor family: evidence for overexpression in a subset of human mammary tumors. Proc Natl Acad Sci U S A 1989;86(23):9193–9197.
15. Zimonjic DB, Alimandi M, Miki T, Popescu NC, Kraus MH. Localization of the human HER4/erbB-4 gene to chromosome 2. Oncogene 1995;10(6):1235–1237.
16. Elenius K, Corfas G, Paul S, Choi CJ, Rio C, Plowman GD, Klagsbrun M. A novel juxtamembrane domain isoform of HER4/ErbB4. Isoform-specific tissue distribution and differential processing in response to phorbol ester. J Biol Chem 1997;272(42):26761–26768.
17. Sundvall M, Peri L, Maatta JA, Tvorogov D, Paatero I, Savisalo M, Silvennoinen O, Yarden Y, Elenius K. Differential nuclear localization and kinase activity of alternative ErbB4 intracellular domains. Oncogene 2007;26(48):6905–6914.
18. Harris RC, Chung E, Coffey RJ. EGF receptor ligands. Exp Cell Res 2003;284(1):2–13.
19. Holbro T, Beerli RR, Maurer F, Koziczak M, Barbas CF 3rd, Hynes NE. The ErbB2/ErbB3 heterodimer functions as an oncogenic unit: ErbB2 requires ErbB3 to drive breast tumor cell proliferation. Proc Natl Acad Sci U S A 2003;100(15):8933–8938.
20. Liu PC, Liu X, Li Y, Covington M, Wynn R, Huber R, Hillman M, Yang G, Ellis D, Marando C, Katiyar K, Bradley J, Abremski K, Stow M, Rupar M, Zhuo J, Li YL, Lin Q, Burns D, Xu M, Zhang C, Qian DQ, He C, Sharief V, Weng L, Agrios C, Shi E, Metcalf B, Newton R, Friedman S, Yao W, Scherle P, Hollis G, Burn TC. Identification of ADAM10 as a major source of HER2 ectodomain sheddase activity in HER2 overexpressing breast cancer cells. Cancer Biol Ther 2006;5(6):657–664.

21. Codony-Servat J, Albanell J, Lopez-Talavera JC, Arribas J, Baselga J. Cleavage of the HER2 ectodomain is a pervanadate-activable process that is inhibited by the tissue inhibitor of metalloproteases-1 in breast cancer cells. Cancer Res 1999;59(6):1196–1201.

22. Pupa SM, Menard S, Morelli D, Pozzi B, De Palo G, Colnaghi MI. The extracellular domain of the c-erbB-2 oncoprotein is released from tumor cells by proteolytic cleavage. Oncogene 1993;8(11):2917–2923.

23. Hudelist G, Kostler WJ, Attems J, Czerwenka K, Muller R, Manavi M, Steger GG, Kubista E, Zielinski CC, Singer CF. Her-2/neu-triggered intracellular tyrosine kinase activation: in vivo relevance of ligand-independent activation mechanisms and impact upon the efficacy of trastuzumab-based treatment. Br J Cancer 2003;89(6):983–991.

24. Brodowicz T, Wiltschke C, Budinsky AC, Krainer M, Steger GG, Zielinski CC. Soluble HER-2/neu neutralizes biologic effects of anti-HER-2/neu antibody on breast cancer cells in vitro. Int J Cancer 1997;73(6):875–879.

25. Singh AB, Harris RC. Autocrine, paracrine and juxtacrine signaling by EGFR ligands. Cell Signal 2005;17(10):1183–1193.

26. Anklesaria P, Teixido J, Laiho M, Pierce JH, Greenberger JS, Massague J. Cell–cell adhesion mediated by binding of membrane-anchored transforming growth factor alpha to epidermal growth factor receptors promotes cell proliferation. Proc Natl Acad Sci U S A 1990;87(9):3289–3293.

27. Sanderson MP, Dempsey PJ, Dunbar AJ. Control of ErbB signaling through metalloprotease mediated ectodomain shedding of EGF-like factors. Growth Factors 2006;24(2):121–136.

28. Sahin U, Weskamp G, Kelly K, Zhou HM, Higashiyama S, Peschon J, Hartmann D, Saftig P, Blobel CP. Distinct roles for ADAM10 and ADAM17 in ectodomain shedding of six EGFR ligands. J Cell Biol 2004;164(5):769–779.

29. Fischer OM, Hart S, Gschwind A, Ullrich A. EGFR signal transactivation in cancer cells. Biochem Soc Trans 2003;31(Pt 6):1203–1208.

30. Filardo EJ, Quinn JA, Bland KI, Frackelton AR Jr. Estrogen-induced activation of Erk-1 and Erk-2 requires the G protein-coupled receptor homolog, GPR30, and occurs via trans-activation of the epidermal growth factor receptor through release of HB-EGF. Mol Endocrinol 2000;14(10):1649–1660.

31. Filardo EJ, Quinn JA, Frackelton AR Jr, Bland KI. Estrogen action via the G protein-coupled receptor, GPR30: stimulation of adenylyl cyclase and cAMP-mediated attenuation of the epidermal growth factor receptor-to-MAPK signaling axis. Mol Endocrinol 2002;16(1):70–84.

32. Sukocheva O, Wadham C, Holmes A, Albanese N, Verrier E, Feng F, Bernal A, Derian CK, Ullrich A, Vadas MA, Xia P. Estrogen transactivates EGFR via the sphingosine 1-phosphate receptor Edg-3: the role of sphingosine kinase-1. J Cell Biol 2006;173(2):301–310.

33. Vivacqua A, Bonofiglio D, Recchia AG, Musti AM, Picard D, Ando S, Maggiolini M. The G protein-coupled receptor GPR30 mediates the proliferative effects induced by 17beta-estradiol and hydroxytamoxifen in endometrial cancer cells. Mol Endocrinol 2006;20(3):631–646.

34. Zhu Y, Sullivan LL, Nair SS, Williams CC, Pandey AK, Marrero L, Vadlamudi RK, Jones FE. Coregulation of estrogen receptor by ERBB4/HER4 establishes a growth-promoting autocrine signal in breast tumor cells. Cancer Res 2006;66(16):7991–7998.

35. Civenni G, Holbro T, Hynes NE. Wnt1 and Wnt5a induce cyclin D1 expression through ErbB1 transactivation in HC11 mammary epithelial cells. EMBO Rep 2003;4(2):166–171.

36. Badache A, Hynes NE. Interleukin 6 inhibits proliferation and, in cooperation with an epidermal growth factor receptor autocrine loop, increases migration of T47D breast cancer cells. Cancer Res 2001;61(1):383–391.

37. Qiu Y, Ravi L, Kung HJ. Requirement of ErbB2 for signalling by interleukin-6 in prostate carcinoma cells. Nature 1998;393(6680):83–85.

38. Guo W, Pylayeva Y, Pepe A, Yoshioka T, Muller WJ, Inghirami G, Giancotti FG. Beta 4 integrin amplifies ErbB2 signaling to promote mammary tumorigenesis. Cell 2006;126(3):489–502.

39. Biscardi JS, Maa MC, Tice DA, Cox ME, Leu TH, Parsons SJ. c-Src-mediated phosphorylation of the epidermal growth factor receptor on Tyr845 and Tyr1101 is associated with modulation of receptor function. J Biol Chem 1999;274(12):8335–8343.

40. Tice DA, Biscardi JS, Nickles AL, Parsons SJ. Mechanism of biological synergy between cellular Src and epidermal growth factor receptor. Proc Natl Acad Sci U S A 1999;96(4):1415–1420.

41. Huang Y, Li X, Jiang J, Frank SJ. Prolactin modulates phosphorylation, signaling and trafficking of epidermal growth factor receptor in human T47D breast cancer cells. Oncogene 2006;25(58):7565–7576.

42. Kim SO, Houtman JC, Jiang J, Ruppert JM, Bertics PJ, Frank SJ. Growth hormone-induced alteration in ErbB-2 phosphorylation status in 3T3-F442A fibroblasts. J Biol Chem 1999;274(50):36015–36024.

43. Yamauchi T, Ueki K, Tobe K, Tamemoto H, Sekine N, Wada M, Honjo M, Takahashi M, Takahashi T, Hirai H, Tushima T, Akanuma Y, Fujita T, Komuro I, Yazaki Y, Kadowaki T. Tyrosine phosphorylation of the EGF receptor by the kinase Jak2 is induced by growth hormone. Nature 1997;390(6655):91–96.

44. Davis RJ. Independent mechanisms account for the regulation by protein kinase C of the epidermal growth factor receptor affinity and tyrosine-protein kinase activity. J Biol Chem 1988;263(19):9462–9469.

45. Tanos B, Pendergast AM. Abl tyrosine kinase regulates endocytosis of the epidermal growth factor receptor. J Biol Chem 2006;281(43):32714–32723.

46. Oda K, Matsuoka Y, Funahashi A, Kitano H. A comprehensive pathway map of epidermal growth factor receptor signaling. Mol Syst Biol 2005;1: 2005 0010.

47. Sithanandam G, Smith GT, Fields JR, Fornwald LW, Anderson LM. Alternate paths from epidermal growth factor receptor to Akt in malignant versus nontransformed lung epithelial cells: ErbB3 versus Gab1. Am J Respir Cell Mol Biol 2005;33(5):490–499.

48. Yang Z, Bagheri-Yarmand R, Wang RA, Adam L, Papadimitrakopoulou VV, Clayman GL, El-Naggar A, Lotan R, Barnes CJ, Hong WK, Kumar R. The epidermal growth factor receptor tyrosine kinase inhibitor ZD1839 (Iressa) suppresses c-Src and Pak1 pathways and invasiveness of human cancer cells. Clin Cancer Res 2004;10(2):658–667.

49. Sorkin A, Goh LK. Endocytosis and intracellular trafficking of ErbBs. Exp Cell Res 2008;314(17):3093–3106.

50. Torrisi MR, Lotti LV, Belleudi F, Gradini R, Salcini AE, Confalonieri S, Pelicci PG, Di Fiore PP. Eps15 is recruited to the plasma membrane upon epidermal growth factor receptor activation and localizes to components of the endocytic pathway during receptor internalization. Mol Biol Cell 1999;10(2):417–434.

51. Ouyang X, Gulliford T, Huang G, Epstein RJ. Transforming growth factor-alpha short-circuits downregulation of the epidermal growth factor receptor. J Cell Physiol 1999;179(1):52–57.

52. French AR, Tadaki DK, Niyogi SK, Lauffenburger DA. Intracellular trafficking of epidermal growth factor family ligands is directly influenced by the pH sensitivity of the receptor/ligand interaction. J Biol Chem 1995;270(9):4334–4340.

53. Thiel KW, Carpenter G. Epidermal growth factor receptor juxtamembrane region regulates allosteric tyrosine kinase activation. Proc Natl Acad Sci U S A 2007;104(49):19238–19243.

54. Northwood IC, Gonzalez FA, Wartmann M, Raden DL, Davis RJ. Isolation and characterization of two growth factor-stimulated protein kinases that phosphorylate the epidermal growth factor receptor at threonine 669. J Biol Chem 1991;266(23):15266–15276.

55. Worthylake R, Opresko LK, Wiley HS. ErbB-2 amplification inhibits down-regulation and induces constitutive activation of both ErbB-2 and epidermal growth factor receptors. J Biol Chem 1999;274(13):8865–8874.

56. Jones RB, Gordus A, Krall JA, MacBeath G. A quantitative protein interaction network for the ErbB receptors using protein microarrays. Nature 2006;439(7073):168–174.

57. Schulze WX, Deng L, Mann M. Phosphotyrosine interactome of the ErbB-receptor kinase family. Mol Syst Biol 2005;1: 2005 0008.

58. Engelman JA, Janne PA, Mermel C, Pearlberg J, Mukohara T, Fleet C, Cichowski K, Johnson BE, Cantley LC. ErbB-3 mediates phosphoinositide 3-kinase activity in gefitinib-sensitive non-small cell lung cancer cell lines. Proc Natl Acad Sci U S A 2005;102(10):3788–3793.

59. Graus-Porta D, Beerli RR, Daly JM, Hynes NE. ErbB-2, the preferred heterodimerization partner of all ErbB receptors, is a mediator of lateral signaling. EMBO J 1997;16(7):1647–1655.

60. Citri A, Skaria KB, Yarden Y. The deaf and the dumb: the biology of ErbB-2 and ErbB-3. Exp Cell Res 2003;284(1):54–65.

61. Sergina NV, Rausch M, Wang D, Blair J, Hann B, Shokat KM, Moasser MM. Escape from HER-family tyrosine kinase inhibitor therapy by the kinase-inactive HER3. Nature 2007; 445(7126):437–441.

62. Kaushansky A, Gordus A, Budnik BA, Lane WS, Rush J, MacBeath G. System-wide investigation of ErbB4 reveals 19 sites of Tyr phosphorylation that are unusually selective in their recruitment properties. Chem Biol 2008;15(8):808–817.

63. Massie C, Mills IG. The developing role of receptors and adaptors. Nat Rev Cancer 2006;6(5):403–409.

64. Carpenter G. Nuclear localization and possible functions of receptor tyrosine kinases. Curr Opin Cell Biol 2003;15(2):143–148.

65. Lin SY, Makino K, Xia W, Matin A, Wen Y, Kwong KY, Bourguignon L, Hung MC. Nuclear localization of EGF receptor and its potential new role as a transcription factor. Nat Cell Biol 2001;3(9):802–808.

66. Ni CY, Murphy MP, Golde TE, Carpenter G. gamma -Secretase cleavage and nuclear localization of ErbB-4 receptor tyrosine kinase. Science 2001;294(5549):2179–2181.

67. Vidal GA, Naresh A, Marrero L, Jones FE. Presenilin-dependent gamma-secretase processing regulates multiple ERBB4/HER4 activities. J Biol Chem 2005;280(20):19777–19783.

68. Naresh A, Long W, Vidal GA, Wimley WC, Marrero L, Sartor CI, Tovey S, Cooke TG, Bartlett JM, Jones FE. The ERBB4/HER4 intracellular domain 4ICD is a BH3-only protein promoting apoptosis of breast cancer cells. Cancer Res 2006;66(12):6412–6420.

69. Thiery JP, Chopin D. Epithelial cell plasticity in development and tumor progression. Cancer Metastasis Rev 1999;18(1):31–42.

70. Wilkins-Port CE, Higgins PJ. Regulation of extracellular matrix remodeling following transforming growth factor-beta1/epidermal growth factor-stimulated epithelial–mesenchymal transition in human premalignant keratinocytes. Cells Tissues Organs 2007;185(1–3):116–122.

71. Sibilia M, Wagner EF. Strain-dependent epithelial defects in mice lacking the EGF receptor. Science 1995;269(5221):234–238.

72. Threadgill DW, Dlugosz AA, Hansen LA, Tennenbaum T, Lichti U, Yee D, LaMantia C, Mourton T, Herrup K, Harris RC, et al. Targeted disruption of mouse EGF receptor: effect of genetic background on mutant phenotype. Science 1995;269(5221):230–234.

73. Stern DF. ErbBs in mammary development. Exp Cell Res 2003;284(1):89–98.

74. Lee KF, Simon H, Chen H, Bates B, Hung MC, Hauser C. Requirement for neuregulin receptor erbB2 in neural and cardiac development. Nature 1995;378(6555):394–398.

75. Erickson SL, O'Shea KS, Ghaboosi N, Loverro L, Frantz G, Bauer M, Lu LH, Moore MW. ErbB3 is required for normal cerebellar and cardiac development: a comparison with ErbB2-and heregulin-deficient mice. Development 1997;124(24):4999–5011.

76. Gassmann M, Casagranda F, Orioli D, Simon H, Lai C, Klein R, Lemke G. Aberrant neural and cardiac development in mice lacking the ErbB4 neuregulin receptor. Nature 1995;378(6555):390–394.

77. Jones FE, Golding JP, Gassmann M. ErbB4 signaling during breast and neural development: novel genetic models reveal unique ErbB4 activities. Cell Cycle 2003;2(6):555–559.

78. Sardi SP, Murtie J, Koirala S, Patten BA, Corfas G. Presenilin-dependent ErbB4 nuclear signaling regulates the timing of astrogenesis in the developing brain. Cell 2006;127(1):185–197.

79. Muraoka-Cook RS, Sandahl M, Husted C, Hunter D, Miraglia L, Feng SM, Elenius K, Earp HS 3rd. The intracellular domain of ErbB4 induces differentiation of mammary epithelial cells. Mol Biol Cell 2006;17(9):4118–4129.

80. Long W, Wagner KU, Lloyd KC, Binart N, Shillingford JM, Hennighausen L, Jones FE. Impaired differentiation and lactational failure of Erbb4-deficient mammary glands identify ERBB4 as an obligate mediator of STAT5. Development 2003;130(21):5257–5268.

81. Hirsch FR, Varella-Garcia M, Bunn PA Jr, Di Maria MV, Veve R, Bremmes RM, Baron AE, Zeng C, Franklin WA. Epidermal growth factor receptor in non-small-cell lung carcinomas: correlation between gene copy number and protein expression and impact on prognosis. J Clin Oncol 2003;21(20):3798–3807.

82. Nicholson RI, Gee JM, Harper ME. EGFR and cancer prognosis. Eur J Cancer 2001;37 (Suppl 4): S9–15.

83. Scartozzi M, Bearzi I, Berardi R, Mandolesi A, Fabris G, Cascinu S. Epidermal growth factor receptor (EGFR) status in primary colorectal tumors does not correlate with EGFR expression in related metastatic sites: implications for treatment with EGFR-targeted monoclonal antibodies. J Clin Oncol 2004;22(23):4772–4778.

84. Frederick L, Wang XY, Eley G, James CD. Diversity and frequency of epidermal growth factor receptor mutations in human glioblastomas. Cancer Res 2000;60(5):1383–1387.

85. Riely GJ, Politi KA, Miller VA, Pao W. Update on epidermal growth factor receptor mutations in non-small cell lung cancer. Clin Cancer Res 2006;12(24):7232–7241.

86. Shinojima N, Tada K, Shiraishi S, Kamiryo T, Kochi M, Nakamura H, Makino K, Saya H, Hirano H, Kuratsu J, Oka K, Ishimaru Y, Ushio Y. Prognostic value of epidermal growth factor receptor in patients with glioblastoma multiforme. Cancer Res 2003;63(20):6962–6970.

87. Pedersen MW, Meltorn M, Damstrup L, Poulsen HS. The type III epidermal growth factor receptor mutation. Biological significance and potential target for anti-cancer therapy. Ann Oncol 2001;12(6):745–760.

88. Nicholas MK, Lukas RV, Jafri NF, Faoro L, Salgia R. Epidermal growth factor receptor-mediated signal transduction in the development and therapy of gliomas. Clin Cancer Res 2006;12(24):7261–7270.

89. Sharma SV, Bell DW, Settleman J, Haber DA. Epidermal growth factor receptor mutations in lung cancer. Nat Rev Cancer 2007;7(3):169–181.

90. Lynch TJ, Bell DW, Sordella R, Gurubhagavatula S, Okimoto RA, Brannigan BW, Harris PL, Haserlat SM, Supko JG, Haluska FG, Louis DN, Christiani DC, Settleman J, Haber DA. Activating mutations in the epidermal growth factor receptor underlying responsiveness of non-small-cell lung cancer to gefitinib. N Engl J Med 2004;350(21):2129–2139.

91. Paez JG, Janne PA, Lee JC, Tracy S, Greulich H, Gabriel S, Herman P, Kaye FJ, Lindeman N, Boggon TJ, Naoki K, Sasaki H, Fujii Y, Eck MJ, Sellers WR, Johnson BE, Meyerson M. EGFR mutations in lung cancer: correlation with clinical response to gefitinib therapy. Science 2004;304(5676):1497–1500.

92. Pao W, Miller V, Zakowski M, Doherty J, Politi K, Sarkaria I, Singh B, Heelan R, Rusch V, Fulton L, Mardis E, Kupfer D, Wilson R, Kris M, Varmus H. EGF receptor gene mutations are common in lung cancers from "never smokers" and are associated with sensitivity of tumors to gefitinib and erlotinib. Proc Natl Acad Sci U S A 2004;101(36):13306–13311.

93. Kobayashi S, Boggon TJ, Dayaram T, Janne PA, Kocher O, Meyerson M, Johnson BE, Eck MJ, Tenen DG, Halmos B. EGFR mutation and resistance of non-small-cell lung cancer to gefitinib. N Engl J Med 2005;352(8):786–792.

94. Pao W, Miller VA, Politi KA, Riely GJ, Somwar R, Zakowski MF, Kris MG, Varmus H. Acquired resistance of lung adenocarcinomas to gefitinib or erlotinib is associated with a second mutation in the EGFR kinase domain. PLoS Med 2005;2(3):e73.

95. Mulloy R, Ferrand A, Kim Y, Sordella R, Bell DW, Haber DA, Anderson KS, Settleman J. Epidermal growth factor receptor mutants from human lung cancers exhibit enhanced catalytic activity and increased sensitivity to gefitinib. Cancer Res 2007;67(5):2325–2330.

96. Vikis H, Sato M, James M, Wang D, Wang Y, Wang M, Jia D, Liu Y, Bailey-Wilson JE, Amos CI, Pinney SM, Petersen GM, De Andrade M, Yang P, Wiest JS, Fain PR, Schwartz AG, Gazdar A, Gaba C, Rothschild H, Mandal D, Kupert E, Seminara D, Viswanathan A, Govindan R, Minna J, Anderson MW, You M. EGFR-T790M is a rare lung cancer susceptibility allele with enhanced kinase activity. Cancer Res 2007;67(10):4665–4670.

97. Bell DW, Gore I, Okimoto RA, Godin-Heymann N, Sordella R, Mulloy R, Sharma SV, Brannigan BW, Mohapatra G, Settleman J, Haber DA. Inherited susceptibility to lung cancer may be associated with the T790M drug resistance mutation in EGFR. Nat Genet 2005;37(12):1315–1316.

98. Shawver LK, Slamon D, Ullrich A. Smart drugs: tyrosine kinase inhibitors in cancer therapy. Cancer Cell 2002;1(2):117–123.

99. Park JB, Rhim JS, Park SC, Kimm SW, Kraus MH. Amplification, overexpression, and rearrangement of the erbB-2 protooncogene in primary human stomach carcinomas. Cancer Res 1989;49(23):6605–6609.

100. Ross JS, Fletcher JA, Linette GP, Stec J, Clark E, Ayers M, Symmans WF, Pusztai L, Bloom KJ. The Her-2/neu gene and protein in breast cancer 2003: biomarker and target of therapy. Oncologist 2003;8(4):307–325.

101. Brabender J, Danenberg KD, Metzger R, Schneider PM, Park J, Salonga D, Holscher AH, Danenberg PV. Epidermal growth factor receptor and HER2-neu mRNA expression in non-small cell lung cancer is correlated with survival. Clin Cancer Res 2001;7(7):1850–1855.

102. DiGiovanna MP, Stern DF, Edgerton SM, Whalen SG, Moore D 2nd, Thor AD. Relationship of epidermal growth factor receptor expression to ErbB-2 signaling activity and prognosis in breast cancer patients. J Clin Oncol 2005;23(6):1152–1160.

103. Wiseman SM, Makretsov N, Nielsen TO, Gilks B, Yorida E, Cheang M, Turbin D, Gelmon K, Huntsman DG. Coexpression of the type 1 growth factor receptor family members HER-1, HER-2, and HER-3 has a synergistic negative prognostic effect on breast carcinoma survival. Cancer 2005;103(9):1770–1777.

104. Lee JW, Soung YH, Seo SH, Kim SY, Park CH, Wang YP, Park K, Nam SW, Park WS, Kim SH, Lee JY, Yoo NJ, Lee SH. Somatic mutations of ERBB2 kinase domain in gastric, colorectal, and breast carcinomas. Clin Cancer Res 2006;12(1):57–61.

105. Stephens P, Hunter C, Bignell G, Edkins S, Davies H, Teague J, Stevens C, O'Meara S, Smith R, Parker A, Barthorpe A, Blow M, Brackenbury L, Butler A, Clarke O, Cole J, Dicks E, Dike A, Drozd A, Edwards K, Forbes S, Foster R, Gray K, Greenman C, Halliday K, Hills K, Kosmidou V, Lugg R, Menzies A, Perry J, Petty R, Raine K, Ratford L, Shepherd R, Small A, Stephens Y, Tofts C, Varian J, West S, Widaa S, Yates A, Brasseur F, Cooper CS, Flanagan AM, Knowles M, Leung SY, Louis DN, Looijenga LH, Malkowicz B, Pierotti MA, Teh B, Chenevix-Trench G, Weber BL, Yuen ST, Harris G, Goldstraw P, Nicholson AG, Futreal PA, Wooster R, Stratton MR. Lung cancer: intragenic ERBB2 kinase mutations in tumours. Nature 2004;431(7008):525–526.

106. Buttitta F, Barassi F, Fresu G, Felicioni L, Chella A, Paolizzi D, Lattanzio G, Salvatore S, Camplese PP, Rosini S, Iarussi T, Mucilli F, Sacco R, Mezzetti A, Marchetti A. Mutational analysis of the HER2 gene in lung tumors from Caucasian patients: mutations are mainly present in adenocarcinomas with bronchioloalveolar features. Int J Cancer 2006;119(11):2586–2591.

107. Shigematsu H, Takahashi T, Nomura M, Majmudar K, Suzuki M, Lee H, Wistuba II, Fong KM, Toyooka S, Shimizu N, Fujisawa T, Minna JD, Gazdar AF. Somatic mutations of the HER2 kinase domain in lung adenocarcinomas. Cancer Res 2005;65(5):1642–1646.

108. Wang SE, Narasanna A, Perez-Torres M, Xiang B, Wu FY, Yang S, Carpenter G, Gazdar AF, Muthuswamy SK, Arteaga CL. HER2 kinase domain mutation results in constitutive phosphorylation and activation of HER2 and EGFR and resistance to EGFR tyrosine kinase inhibitors. Cancer Cell 2006;10(1):25–38.

109. Naidu R, Yadav M, Nair S, Kutty MK. Expression of c-erbB3 protein in primary breast carcinomas. Br J Cancer 1998;78(10):1385–1390.

110. Jeong EG, Soung YH, Lee JW, Lee SH, Nam SW, Lee JY, Yoo NJ, Lee SH. ERBB3 kinase domain mutations are rare in lung, breast and colon carcinomas. Int J Cancer 2006;119(12):2986–2987.

111. Sartor CI, Zhou H, Kozlowska E, Guttridge K, Kawata E, Caskey L, Harrelson J, Hynes N, Ethier S, Calvo B, Earp HS 3rd. Her4 mediates ligand-dependent antiproliferative and differentiation responses in human breast cancer cells. Mol Cell Biol 2001;21(13):4265–4275.

112. Feng SM, Sartor CI, Hunter D, Zhou H, Yang X, Caskey LS, Dy R, Muraoka-Cook RS, Earp HS 3rd. The HER4 cytoplasmic domain, but not its C terminus, inhibits mammary cell proliferation. Mol Endocrinol 2007;21(8):1861–1876.

113. Barnes NL, Khavari S, Boland GP, Cramer A, Knox WF, Bundred NJ. Absence of HER4 expression predicts recurrence of ductal carcinoma in situ of the breast. Clin Cancer Res 2005;11(6):2163–2168.

114. Kew TY, Bell JA, Pinder SE, Denley H, Srinivasan R, Gullick WJ, Nicholson RI, Blamey RW, Ellis IO. c-erbB-4 protein expression in human breast cancer. Br J Cancer 2000;82(6):1163–1170.

115. Suo Z, Risberg B, Kalsson MG, Willman K, Tierens A, Skovlund E, Nesland JM. EGFR family expression in breast carcinomas. c-erbB-2 and c-erbB-4 receptors have different effects on survival. J Pathol 2002;196(1):17–25.

116. Lodge AJ, Anderson JJ, Gullick WJ, Haugk B, Leonard RC, Angus B. Type 1 growth factor receptor expression in node positive breast cancer: adverse prognostic significance of c-erbB-4. J Clin Pathol 2003;56(4):300–304.

117. Soung YH, Lee JW, Kim SY, Wang YP, Jo KH, Moon SW, Park WS, Nam SW, Lee JY, Yoo NJ, Lee SH. Somatic mutations of the ERBB4 kinase domain in human cancers. Int J Cancer 2006;118(6):1426–1429.

118. Hanze J, Berthold A, Klammt J, Gallaher B, Siebler T, Kratzsch J, Elmlinger M, Kiess W. Cloning and sequencing of the complete cDNA encoding the human insulin receptor related receptor. Horm Metab Res 1999;31(2–3):77–79.

119. Shier P, Watt VM. Primary structure of a putative receptor for a ligand of the insulin family. J Biol Chem 1989;264(25):14605–14608.

120. Elmlinger MW, Rauschnabel U, Koscielniak E, Haenze J, Ranke MB, Berthold A, Klammt J, Kiess W. Correlation of type I insulin-like growth factor receptor (IGF-I-R) and insulin receptor-related receptor (IRR) messenger RNA levels in tumor cell lines from pediatric tumors of neuronal origin. Regul Pept 1999;84(1–3):37–42.

121. Weber A, Huesken C, Bergmann E, Kiess W, Christiansen NM, Christiansen H. Coexpression of insulin receptor-related receptor and insulin-like growth factor 1 receptor correlates with enhanced apoptosis and dedifferentiation in human neuroblastomas. Clin Cancer Res 2003;9(15):5683–5692.

122. Ueki K, Kondo T, Kahn CR. Suppressor of cytokine signaling 1 (SOCS-1) and SOCS-3 cause insulin resistance through inhibition of tyrosine phosphorylation of insulin receptor substrate proteins by discrete mechanisms. Mol Cell Biol 2004;24(12):5434–5446.

123. Foti M, Moukil MA, Dudognon P, Carpentier JL. Insulin and IGF-1 receptor trafficking and signalling. Novartis Found Symp 2004;262: 125–141; discussion 141–127, 265–128.

124. Romanelli RJ, LeBeau AP, Fulmer CG, Lazzarino DA, Hochberg A, Wood TL. Insulin-like growth factor type-I receptor internalization and recycling mediate the sustained phosphorylation of Akt. J Biol Chem 2007;282(31):22513–22524.

125. Firth SM, Baxter RC. Cellular actions of the insulin-like growth factor binding proteins. Endocr Rev 2002;23(6):824–854.

126. Seino S, Seino M, Nishi S, Bell GI. Structure of the human insulin receptor gene and characterization of its promoter. Proc Natl Acad Sci U S A 1989;86(1):114–118.

127. Yang-Feng TL, Francke U, Ullrich A. Gene for human insulin receptor: localization to site on chromosome 19 involved in pre-B-cell leukemia. Science 1985;228(4700):728–731.

128. Moller DE, Yokota A, Caro JF, Flier JS. Tissue-specific expression of two alternatively spliced insulin receptor mRNAs in man. Mol Endocrinol 1989;3(8):1263–1269.

129. Nagaoka I, Someya A, Iwabuchi K, Yamashita T. Expression of insulin-like growth factor-IA and factor-IB mRNA in human liver, hepatoma cells, macrophage-like cells and fibroblasts. FEBS Lett 1991;280(1):79–83.

130. Mosthaf L, Grako K, Dull TJ, Coussens L, Ullrich A, McClain DA. Functionally distinct insulin receptors generated by tissue-specific alternative splicing. EMBO J 1990;9(8):2409–2413.

131. Denley A, Wallace JC, Cosgrove LJ, Forbes BE. The insulin receptor isoform exon 11- (IR-A) in cancer and other diseases: a review. Horm Metab Res 2003;35(11–12):778–785.

132. Abbott AM, Bueno R, Pedrini MT, Murray JM, Smith RJ. Insulin-like growth factor I receptor gene structure. J Biol Chem 1992;267(15):10759–10763.

133. Francke U, Yang-Feng TL, Brissenden JE, Ullrich A. Chromosomal mapping of genes involved in growth control. Cold Spring Harb Symp Quant Biol 1986;51 (Pt 2):855–866.

134. Bravo DA, Gleason JB, Sanchez RI, Roth RA, Fuller RS. Accurate and efficient cleavage of the human insulin proreceptor by the human proprotein-processing protease furin. Characterization and kinetic parameters using the purified, secreted soluble protease expressed by a recombinant baculovirus. J Biol Chem 1994;269(41):25830–25837.

135. Robertson BJ, Moehring JM, Moehring TJ. Defective processing of the insulin receptor in an endoprotease-deficient Chinese hamster cell strain is corrected by expression of mouse furin. J Biol Chem 1993;268(32):24274–24277.

136. De Meyts P, Whittaker J. Structural biology of insulin and IGF1 receptors: implications for drug design. Nat Rev Drug Discov 2002;1(10):769–783.

137. Hao C, Whittaker L, Whittaker J. Characterization of a second ligand binding site of the insulin receptor. Biochem Biophys Res Commun 2006;347(1):334–339.

138. Surinya KH, Forbes BE, Occhiodoro F, Booker GW, Francis GL, Siddle K, Wallace JC, Cosgrove LJ. An investigation of the ligand binding properties and negative cooperativity of soluble insulin-like growth factor receptors. J Biol Chem 2007;283(9):5335–5563.

139. Scalia P, Heart E, Comai L, Vigneri R, Sung CK. Regulation of the Akt/glycogen synthase kinase-3 axis by insulin-like growth factor-II via activation of the human insulin receptor isoform-A. J Cell Biochem 2001;82(4):610–618.

140. Pandini G, Frasca F, Mineo R, Sciacca L, Vigneri R, Belfiore A. Insulin/insulin-like growth factor I hybrid receptors have different biological characteristics depending on the insulin receptor isoform involved. J Biol Chem 2002;277(42):39684–39695.

141. Benyoucef S, Surinya KH, Hadaschik D, Siddle K. Characterization of insulin/IGF hybrid receptors: contributions of the insulin receptor L2 and Fn1 domains and the alternatively spliced exon 11 sequence to ligand binding and receptor activation. Biochem J 2007;403(3):603–613.

142. Slaaby R, Schaffer L, Lautrup-Larsen I, Andersen AS, Shaw AC, Mathiasen IS, Brandt J. Hybrid receptors formed by insulin receptor (IR) and insulin-like growth factor I receptor (IGF-IR) have low insulin and high IGF-1 affinity irrespective of the IR splice variant. J Biol Chem 2006;281(36):25869–25874.

143. Kharbanda S, Bharti A, Pei D, Wang J, Pandey P, Ren R, Weichselbaum R, Walsh CT, Kufe D. The stress response to ionizing radiation involves c-Abl-dependent phosphorylation of SHPTP1. Proc Natl Acad Sci U S A 1996;93(14):6898–6901.

144. Gustafson TA, He W, Craparo A, Schaub CD, O'Neill TJ. Phosphotyrosine-dependent interaction of SHC and insulin receptor substrate 1 with the NPEY motif of the insulin receptor via a novel non-SH2 domain. Mol Cell Biol 1995;15(5):2500–2508.

145. Lehr S, Kotzka J, Herkner A, Sikmann A, Meyer HE, Krone W, Muller-Wieland D. Identification of major tyrosine phosphorylation sites in the human insulin receptor substrate Gab-1 by insulin receptor kinase in vitro. Biochemistry 2000;39(35):10898–10907.

146. Baron V, Calleja V, Ferrari P, Alengrin F, Van Obberghen E. p125Fak focal adhesion kinase is a substrate for the insulin and insulin-like growth factor-I tyrosine kinase receptors. J Biol Chem 1998;273(12):7162–7168.

147. Gual P, Baron V, Lequoy V, Van Obberghen E. Interaction of Janus kinases JAK-1 and JAK-2 with the insulin receptor and the insulin-like growth factor-1 receptor. Endocrinology 1998;139(3):884–893.

148. Taniguchi CM, Emanuelli B, Kahn CR. Critical nodes in signalling pathways: insights into insulin action. Nat Rev Mol Cell Biol 2006;7(2):85–96.

149. Myers MG Jr, Mendez R, Shi P, Pierce JH, Rhoads R, White MF. The COOH-terminal tyrosine phosphorylation sites on IRS-1 bind SHP-2 and negatively regulate insulin signaling. J Biol Chem 1998;273(41):26908–26914.

150. Dey BR, Frick K, Lopaczynski W, Nissley SP, Furlanetto RW. Evidence for the direct interaction of the insulin-like growth factor I receptor with IRS-1, Shc, and Grb10. Mol Endocrinol 1996;10(6):631–641.

151. Tartare-Deckert S, Sawka-Verhelle D, Murdaca J, Van Obberghen E. Evidence for a differential interaction of SHC and the insulin receptor substrate-1 (IRS-1) with the insulin-like growth factor-I (IGF-I) receptor in the yeast two-hybrid system. J Biol Chem 1995;270(40):23456–23460.

152. Myers MG Jr, Backer JM, Sun XJ, Shoelson S, Hu P, Schlessinger J, Yoakim M, Schaffhausen B, White MF. IRS-1 activates phosphatidylinositol 3′-kinase by associating with src homology 2 domains of p85. Proc Natl Acad Sci U S A 1992;89(21):10350–10354.

153. Harrington LS, Findlay GM, Gray A, Tolkacheva T, Wigfield S, Rebholz H, Barnett J, Leslie NR, Cheng S, Shepherd PR, Gout I, Downes CP, Lamb RF. The TSC1-2 tumor suppressor controls insulin-PI3K signaling via regulation of IRS proteins. J Cell Biol 2004;166(2):213–223.

154. Leibiger B, Leibiger IB, Moede T, Kemper S, Kulkarni RN, Kahn CR, De Vargas LM, Berggren PO. Selective insulin signaling through A and B insulin receptors regulates transcription of insulin and glucokinase genes in pancreatic beta cells. Mol Cell 2001;7(3):559–570.

155. Hermanto U, Zong CS, Li W, Wang LH. RACK1, an insulin-like growth factor I (IGF-I) receptor-interacting protein, modulates IGF-I-dependent integrin signaling and promotes cell spreading and contact with extracellular matrix. Mol Cell Biol 2002;22(7):2345–2365.

156. Zhang D, Samani AA, Brodt P. The role of the IGF-I receptor in the regulation of matrix metalloproteinases, tumor invasion and metastasis. Horm Metab Res 2003;35(11–12):802–808.

157. Thompson JE, Thompson CB. Putting the rap on Akt. J Clin Oncol 2004;22(20):4217–4226.

158. Pollak MN, Schernhammer ES, Hankinson SE. Insulin-like growth factors and neoplasia. Nat Rev Cancer 2004;4(7):505–518.

159. Yakar S, Liu JL, Stannard B, Butler A, Accili D, Sauer B, LeRoith D. Normal growth and development in the absence of hepatic insulin-like growth factor I. Proc Natl Acad Sci U S A 1999;96(13):7324–7329.

160. Liu JP, Baker J, Perkins AS, Robertson EJ, Efstratiadis A. Mice carrying null mutations of the genes encoding insulin-like growth factor I (Igf-1) and type 1 IGF receptor (Igf1r). Cell 1993;75(1):59–72.

161. Abuzzahab MJ, Schneider A, Goddard A, Grigorescu F, Lautier C, Keller E, Kiess W, Klammt J, Kratzsch J, Osgood D, Pfaffle R, Raile K, Seidel B, Smith RJ, Chernausek SD. IGF-I receptor mutations resulting in intrauterine and postnatal growth retardation. N Engl J Med 2003;349(23):2211–2222.

162. Okubo Y, Siddle K, Firth H, O'Rahilly S, Wilson LC, Willatt L, Fukushima T, Takahashi S, Petry CJ, Saukkonen T, Stanhope R, Dunger DB. Cell proliferation activities on skin fibroblasts from a short child with absence of one copy of the type 1 insulin-like growth factor receptor (IGF1R) gene and a tall child with three copies of the IGF1R gene. J Clin Endocrinol Metab 2003;88(12):5981–5988.

163. Baserga R. The IGF-I receptor in cancer research. Exp Cell Res 1999;253(1):1–6.

164. Kaleko M, Rutter WJ, Miller AD. Overexpression of the human insulinlike growth factor I receptor promotes ligand-dependent neoplastic transformation. Mol Cell Biol 1990;10(2):464–473.

165. Catrina SB, Lewitt M, Massambu C, Dricu A, Grunler J, Axelson M, Biberfeld P, Brismar K. Insulin-like growth factor-I receptor activity is essential for Kaposi's sarcoma growth and survival. Br J Cancer 2005;92(8):1467–1474.

166. Dunn SE, Ehrlich M, Sharp NJ, Reiss K, Solomon G, Hawkins R, Baserga R, Barrett JC. A dominant negative mutant of the insulin-like growth factor-I receptor inhibits the adhesion, invasion, and metastasis of breast cancer. Cancer Res 1998;58(15):3353–3361.

167. Hellawell GO, Turner GD, Davies DR, Poulsom R, Brewster SF, Macaulay VM. Expression of the type 1 insulin-like growth factor receptor is up-regulated in primary prostate cancer and commonly persists in metastatic disease. Cancer Res 2002;62(10):2942–2950.

168. Lahm H, Amstad P, Wyniger J, Yilmaz A, Fischer JR, Schreyer M, Givel JC. Blockade of the insulin-like growth-factor-I receptor inhibits growth of human colorectal cancer cells: evidence of a functional IGF-II-mediated autocrine loop. Int J Cancer 1994;58(3):452–459.

169. Lee CT, Park KH, Adachi Y, Seol JY, Yoo CG, Kim YW, Han SK, Shim YS, Coffee K, Dikov MM, Carbone DP. Recombinant adenoviruses expressing dominant negative insulin-like growth factor-I receptor demonstrate antitumor effects on lung cancer. Cancer Gene Ther 2003;10(1):57–63.

170. Mitsiades CS, Mitsiades NS, McMullan CJ, Poulaki V, Shringarpure R, Akiyama M, Hideshima T, Chauhan D, Joseph M, Libermann TA, Garcia-Echeverria C, Pearson MA, Hofmann F, Anderson KC, Kung AL. Inhibition of the insulin-like growth factor receptor-1 tyrosine kinase activity as a therapeutic strategy for multiple myeloma, other hematologic malignancies, and solid tumors. Cancer Cell 2004;5(3):221–230.

171. Kanter-Lewensohn L, Dricu A, Wang M, Wejde J, Kiessling R, Larsson O. Expression of the insulin-like growth factor-1 receptor and its anti-apoptotic effect in malignant melanoma: a potential therapeutic target. Melanoma Res 1998;8(5):389–397.

172. Ouban A, Muraca P, Yeatman T, Coppola D. Expression and distribution of insulin-like growth factor-1 receptor in human carcinomas. Hum Pathol 2003;34(8):803–808.

173. Grose R, Fantl V, Werner S, Chioni AM, Jarosz M, Rudling R, Cross B, Hart IR, Dickson C. The role of fibroblast growth factor receptor 2b in skin homeostasis and cancer development. EMBO J 2007;26(5):1268–1278.

174. Jerome L, Shiry L, Leyland-Jones B. Deregulation of the IGF axis in cancer: epidemiological evidence and potential therapeutic interventions. Endocr Relat Cancer 2003;10(4):561–578.

175. Renehan AG, Zwahlen M, Minder C, O'Dwyer ST, Shalet SM, Egger M. Insulin-like growth factor (IGF)-I, IGF binding protein-3, and cancer risk: systematic review and meta-regression analysis. Lancet 2004;363(9418):1346–1353.

176. Jenkins PJ. Acromegaly and cancer. Horm Res 2004;62 (Suppl 1): 108–115.

177. Oates AJ, Schumaker LM, Jenkins SB, Pearce AA, DaCosta SA, Arun B, Ellis MJ. The mannose 6-phosphate/insulin-like growth factor 2 receptor (M6P/IGF2R), a putative breast tumor suppressor gene. Breast Cancer Res Treat 1998;47(3):269–281.

178. De Souza AT, Hankins GR, Washington MK, Orton TC, Jirtle RL. M6P/IGF2R gene is mutated in human hepatocellular carcinomas with loss of heterozygosity. Nat Genet 1995;11(4):447–449.

179. Takano Y, Shiota G, Kawasaki H. Analysis of genomic imprinting of insulin-like growth factor 2 in colorectal cancer. Oncology 2000;59(3):210–216.

180. Suzuki H, Ueda R, Takahashi T. Altered imprinting in lung cancer. Nat Genet 1994;6(4):332–333.

181. Cui H, Cruz-Correa M, Giardiello FM, Hutcheon DF, Kafonek DR, Brandenburg S, Wu Y, He X, Powe NR, Feinberg AP. Loss of IGF2 imprinting: a potential marker of colorectal cancer risk. Science 2003;299(5613):1753–1755.

182. Renehan AG, Frystyk J, Flyvbjerg A. Obesity and cancer risk: the role of the insulin-IGF axis. Trends Endocrinol Metab 2006;17(8):328–336.

183. Dunn SE, Kari FW, French J, Leininger JR, Travlos G, Wilson R, Barrett JC. Dietary restriction reduces insulin-like growth factor I levels, which modulates apoptosis, cell proliferation, and tumor progression in p53-deficient mice. Cancer Res 1997;57(21):4667–4672.

184. Fontana L, Klein S. Aging, adiposity, and calorie restriction. JAMA 2007;297(9):986–994.

185. Nishii T, Kono S, Abe H, Eguchi H, Shimazaki K, Hatano B, Hamada H. Glucose intolerance, plasma insulin levels, and colon adenomas in Japanese men. Jpn J Cancer Res 2001;92(8):836–840.

186. Warburg O, Geissler AW, Lorenz S. [On growth of cancer cells in media in which glucose is replaced by galactose]. Hoppe Seylers Z Physiol Chem 1967;348(12):1686–1687.

187. Burfeind P, Chernicky CL, Rininsland F, Ilan J. Antisense RNA to the type I insulin-like growth factor receptor suppresses tumor growth and prevents invasion by rat prostate cancer cells in vivo. Proc Natl Acad Sci U S A 1996;93(14):7263–7268.

188. Burtrum D, Zhu Z, Lu D, Anderson DM, Prewett M, Pereira DS, Bassi R, Abdullah R, Hooper AT, Koo H, Jimenez X, Johnson D, Apblett R, Kussie P, Bohlen P, Witte L, Hicklin DJ, Ludwig DL. A fully human monoclonal antibody to the insulin-like growth factor I receptor blocks ligand-dependent signaling and inhibits human tumor growth in vivo. Cancer Res 2003;63(24):8912–8921.

189. Goetsch L, Gonzalez A, Leger O, Beck A, Pauwels PJ, Haeuw JF, Corvaia N. A recombinant humanized anti-insulin-like growth factor receptor type I antibody (h7C10) enhances the antitumor activity of vinorelbine and anti-epidermal growth factor receptor therapy against human cancer xenografts. Int J Cancer 2005;113(2):316–328.

190. Hailey J, Maxwell E, Koukouras K, Bishop WR, Pachter JA, Wang Y. Neutralizing anti-insulin-like growth factor receptor 1 antibodies inhibit receptor function and induce receptor degradation in tumor cells. Mol Cancer Ther 2002;1(14):1349–1353.

191. Tao Y, Pinzi V, Bourhis J, Deutsch E. Mechanisms of disease: signaling of the insulin-like growth factor 1 receptor pathway—therapeutic perspectives in cancer. Nat Clin Pract Oncol 2007;4(10):591–602.

192. Peretz S, Jensen R, Baserga R, Glazer PM. ATM-dependent expression of the insulin-like growth factor-I receptor in a pathway regulating radiation response. Proc Natl Acad Sci U S A 2001;98(4):1676–1681.

193. Turner BC, Haffty BG, Narayanan L, Yuan J, Havre PA, Gumbs AA, Kaplan L, Burgaud JL, Carter D, Baserga R, Glazer PM. Insulin-like growth factor-I receptor overexpression mediates cellular radioresistance and local breast cancer recurrence after lumpectomy and radiation. Cancer Res 1997;57(15):3079–3083.

194. Dunn SE, Hardman RA, Kari FW, Barrett JC. Insulin-like growth factor 1 (IGF-1) alters drug sensitivity of HBL100 human breast cancer cells by inhibition of apoptosis induced by diverse anticancer drugs. Cancer Res 1997;57(13):2687–2693.

195. Warshamana-Greene GS, Litz J, Buchdunger E, Garcia-Echeverria C, Hofmann F, Krystal GW. The insulin-like growth factor-I receptor kinase inhibitor, NVP-ADW742, sensitizes small cell lung cancer cell lines to the effects of chemotherapy. Clin Cancer Res 2005;11(4):1563–1571.

196. Chakravarti A, Loeffler JS, Dyson NJ. Insulin-like growth factor receptor I mediates resistance to anti-epidermal growth factor receptor therapy in primary human glioblastoma cells through continued activation of phosphoinositide 3-kinase signaling. Cancer Res 2002;62(1):200–207.

197. Jones HE, Goddard L, Gee JM, Hiscox S, Rubini M, Barrow D, Knowlden JM, Williams S, Wakeling AE, Nicholson RI. Insulin-like growth factor-I receptor signalling and acquired resistance to gefitinib (ZD1839; Iressa) in human breast and prostate cancer cells. Endocr Relat Cancer 2004;11(4):793–814.

198. Riggi N, Stamenkovic I. The biology of Ewing sarcoma. Cancer Lett 2007;254(1):1–10.

199. Prieur A, Tirode F, Cohen P, Delattre O. EWS/FLI-1 silencing and gene profiling of Ewing cells reveal downstream oncogenic pathways and a crucial role for repression of insulin-like growth factor binding protein 3. Mol Cell Biol 2004;24(16):7275–7283.

200. Yee D, Favoni RE, Lebovic GS, Lombana F, Powell DR, Reynolds CP, Rosen N. Insulin-like growth factor I expression by tumors of neuroectodermal origin with the t(11;22) chromosomal translocation. A potential autocrine growth factor. J Clin Invest 1990;86(6):1806–1814.

201. Manara MC, Landuzzi L, Nanni P, Nicoletti G, Zambelli D, Lollini PL, Nanni C, Hofmann F, Garcia-Echeverria C, Picci P, Scotlandi K. Preclinical in vivo study of new insulin-like growth factor-I receptor—specific inhibitor in Ewing's sarcoma. Clin Cancer Res 2007;13(4):1322–1330.

202. Martins AS, Mackintosh C, Martin DH, Campos M, Hernandez T, Ordonez JL, De Alava E. Insulin-like growth factor I receptor pathway inhibition by ADW742, alone or in combination with imatinib, doxorubicin, or vincristine, is a novel therapeutic approach in Ewing tumor. Clin Cancer Res 2006;12(11Pt 1):3532–3540.

203. Scotlandi K, Manara MC, Nicoletti G, Lollini PL, Lukas S, Benini S, Croci S, Perdichizzi S, Zambelli D, Serra M, Garcia-Echeverria C, Hofmann F, Picci P. Antitumor activity of the insulin-like growth factor-I receptor kinase inhibitor NVP-AEW541 in musculoskeletal tumors. Cancer Res 2005;65(9):3868–3876.

204. Tolcher AW, Rothenberg ML, Rodon J, Delbeke D, Patnaik A, Nguyen L, Young F, Hwang Y, Haqq C, Puzanov I. A phase I pharmacokinetic and pharmacodynamic study of AMG 479, a fully human monoclonal antibody against insulin-like growth factor type 1 receptor (IGF-1R), in advanced solid tumors. J Clin Oncol 2007;25(18S):118s.

205. Finkeltov I, Kuhn S, Glaser T, Idelman G, Wright JJ, Roberts CT Jr, Werner H. Transcriptional regulation of IGF-I receptor gene expression by novel isoforms of the EWS-WT1 fusion protein. Oncogene 2002;21(12):1890–1898.

206. Karnieli E, Werner H, Rauscher FJ 3rd, Benjamin LE, LeRoith D. The IGF-I receptor gene promoter is a molecular target for the Ewing's sarcoma–Wilms' tumor 1 fusion protein. J Biol Chem 1996;271(32):19304–19309.

207. Werner H, Re GG, Drummond IA, Sukhatme VP, Rauscher FJ 3rd, Sens DA, Garvin AJ, LeRoith D, Roberts CT Jr. Increased expression of the insulin-like growth factor I receptor gene, IGF1R, in Wilms tumor is correlated with modulation of IGF1R promoter activity by the WT1 Wilms tumor gene product. Proc Natl Acad Sci U S A 1993;90(12):5828–5832.

208. Steenman MJ, Rainier S, Dobry CJ, Grundy P, Horon IL, Feinberg AP. Loss of imprinting of IGF2 is linked to reduced expression and abnormal methylation of H19 in Wilms' tumour. Nat Genet 1994;7(3):433–439.

209. Taniguchi T, Schofield AE, Scarlett JL, Morison IM, Sullivan MJ, Reeve AE. Altered specificity of IGF2 promoter imprinting during fetal development and onset of Wilms tumour. Oncogene 1995;11(4):751–756.

210. Werner H, Idelman G, Rubinstein M, Pattee P, Nagalla SR, Roberts CT Jr. A novel EWS-WT1 gene fusion product in desmoplastic small round cell tumor is a potent transactivator of the insulin-like growth factor-I receptor (IGF-IR) gene. Cancer Lett 2007;247(1):84–90.

211. Kalebic T, Blakesley V, Slade C, Plasschaert S, Leroith D, Helman LJ. Expression of a kinase-deficient IGF-I-R suppresses tumorigenicity of rhabdomyosarcoma cells constitutively expressing a wild type IGF-I-R. Int J Cancer 1998;76(2):223–227.

212. Kalebic T, Tsokos M, Helman LJ. in vivo treatment with antibody against IGF-1 receptor suppresses growth of human rhabdomyosarcoma and down-regulates p34cdc2. Cancer Res 1994;54(21):5531–5534.

213. Shapiro DN, Jones BG, Shapiro LH, Dias P, Houghton PJ. Antisense-mediated reduction in insulin-like growth factor-I receptor expression suppresses the malignant phenotype of a human alveolar rhabdomyosarcoma. J Clin Invest 1994;94(3):1235–1242.

214. Kim B, Van Golen CM, Feldman EL. Insulin-like growth factor-I signaling in human neuroblastoma cells. Oncogene 2004;23(1):130–141.

215. Van Golen CM, Feldman EL. Insulin-like growth factor I is the key growth factor in serum that protects neuroblastoma cells from hyperosmotic-induced apoptosis. J Cell Physiol 2000;182(1):24–32.

216. Singleton JR, Randolph AE, Feldman EL. Insulin-like growth factor I receptor prevents apoptosis and enhances neuroblastoma tumorigenesis. Cancer Res 1996;56(19):4522–4529.

217. Riedemann J, Takiguchi M, Sohail M, Macaulay VM. The EGF receptor interacts with the type 1 IGF receptor and regulates its stability. Biochem Biophys Res Commun 2007;355(3):707–714.

218. Ahmad T, Farnie G, Bundred NJ, Anderson NG. The mitogenic action of insulin-like growth factor I in normal human mammary epithelial cells requires the epidermal growth factor receptor tyrosine kinase. J Biol Chem 2004;279(3):1713–1719.

219. Wang D, Patil S, Li W, Humphrey LE, Brattain MG, Howell GM. Activation of the TGF alpha autocrine loop is downstream of IGF-I receptor activation during mitogenesis in growth factor dependent human colon carcinoma cells. Oncogene 2002;21(18):2785–2796.

220. Coppola D, Ferber A, Miura M, Sell C, D'Ambrosio C, Rubin R, Baserga R. A functional insulin-like growth factor I receptor is required for the mitogenic and transforming activities of the epidermal growth factor receptor. Mol Cell Biol 1994;14(7):4588–4595.

221. Burgaud JL, Baserga R. Intracellular transactivation of the insulin-like growth factor I receptor by an epidermal growth factor receptor. Exp Cell Res 1996;223(2):412–419.

222. Steinbach JP, Eisenmann C, Klumpp A, Weller M. Co-inhibition of epidermal growth factor receptor and type 1 insulin-like growth factor receptor synergistically sensitizes human malignant glioma cells to CD95L-induced apoptosis. Biochem Biophys Res Commun 2004;321(3):524–530.

223. Cappuzzo F, Toschi L, Tallini G, Ceresoli GL, Domenichini I, Bartolini S, Finocchiaro G, Magrini E, Metro G, Cancellieri A, Trisolini R, Crino L, Bunn PA Jr, Santoro A, Franklin WA, Varella-Garcia M, Hirsch FR. Insulin-like growth factor receptor 1 (IGFR-1) is significantly associated with longer survival in non-small-cell lung cancer patients treated with gefitinib. Ann Oncol 2006;17(7):1120–1127.

224. Price JA, Kovach SJ, Johnson T, Koniaris LG, Cahill PA, Sitzmann JV, McKillop IH. Insulin-like growth factor I is a comitogen for hepatocyte growth factor in a rat model of hepatocellular carcinoma. Hepatology 2002;36(5):1089–1097.

225. Bauer TW, Somcio RJ, Fan F, Liu W, Johnson M, Lesslie DP, Evans DB, Gallick GE, Ellis LM. Regulatory role of c-Met in insulin-like growth factor-I receptor-mediated migration and invasion of human pancreatic carcinoma cells. Mol Cancer Ther 2006;5(7):1676–1682.

226. Surmacz E, Bartucci M. Role of estrogen receptor alpha in modulating IGF-I receptor signaling and function in breast cancer. J Exp Clin Cancer Res 2004;23(3):385–394.

227. Dupont J, Le Roith D. Insulin-like growth factor 1 and oestradiol promote cell proliferation of MCF-7 breast cancer cells: new insights into their synergistic effects. Mol Pathol 2001;54(3):149–154.

228. Wu JD, Haugk K, Woodke L, Nelson P, Coleman I, Plymate SR. Interaction of IGF signaling and the androgen receptor in prostate cancer progression. J Cell Biochem 2006;99(2):392–401.

229. Masaki T, Igarashi K, Tokuda M, Yukimasa S, Han F, Jin YJ, Li JQ, Yoneyama H, Uchida N, Fujita J, Yoshiji H, Watanabe S, Kurokohchi K, Kuriyama S. pp60c-src activation in lung adenocarcinoma. Eur J Cancer 2003;39(10):1447–1455.

230. Culig Z, Hobisch A, Cronauer MV, Radmayr C, Trapman J, Hittmair A, Bartsch G, Klocker H. Androgen receptor activation in prostatic tumor cell lines by insulin-like growth factor-I, keratinocyte growth factor and epidermal growth factor. Eur Urol 1995;27 (Suppl 2): 45–47.

231. Pandini G, Mineo R, Frasca F, Roberts CT, Jr., Marcelli M, Vigneri R, Belfiore A. Androgens up-regulate the insulin-like growth factor-I receptor in prostate cancer cells. Cancer Res 2005;65(5):1849–1857.

232. Gripp KW, Stolle CA, McDonald-McGinn DM, Markowitz RI, Bartlett SP, Katowitz JA, Muenke M, Zackai EH. Phenotype of the fibroblast growth factor receptor 2 Ser351Cys mutation: Pfeiffer syndrome type III. Am J Med Genet 1998;78(4):356–360.

233. Hamelers IH, Steenbergh PH. Interactions between estrogen and insulin-like growth factor signaling pathways in human breast tumor cells. Endocr Relat Cancer 2003;10(2):331–345.

234. Reinikainen P, Palvimo JJ, Janne OA. Effects of mitogens on androgen receptor-mediated transactivation. Endocrinology 1996;137(10):4351–4357.

235. Murphy LJ. Estrogen induction of insulin-like growth factors and myc proto-oncogene expression in the uterus. J Steroid Biochem Mol Biol 1991;40(1–3):223–230.

236. Stoica GE, Kuo A, Aigner A, Sunitha I, Souttou B, Malerczyk C, Caughey DJ, Wen D, Karavanov A, Riegel AT, Wellstein A. Identification of anaplastic lymphoma kinase as a receptor for the growth factor pleiotrophin. J Biol Chem 2001;276(20):16772–16779.

237. Bowden ET, Stoica GE, Wellstein A. Anti-apoptotic signaling of pleiotrophin through its receptor, anaplastic lymphoma kinase. J Biol Chem 2002;277(39):35862–35868.

238. Perez-Pinera P, Zhang W, Chang Y, Vega JA, Deuel TF. Anaplastic lymphoma kinase is activated through the pleiotrophin/receptor protein-tyrosine phosphatase beta/zeta signaling pathway: an alternative mechanism of receptor tyrosine kinase activation. J Biol Chem 2007;282(39):28683–28690.

239. Powers C, Aigner A, Stoica GE, McDonnell K, Wellstein A. Pleiotrophin signaling through anaplastic lymphoma kinase is rate-limiting for glioblastoma growth. J Biol Chem 2002;277(16):14153–14158.

240. Degoutin J, Vigny M, Gouzi JY. ALK activation induces Shc and FRS2 recruitment: signaling and phenotypic outcomes in PC12 cells differentiation. FEBS Lett 2007;581(4):727–734.

241. Vernersson E, Khoo NK, Henriksson ML, Roos G, Palmer RH, Hallberg B. Characterization of the expression of the ALK receptor tyrosine kinase in mice. Gene Expr Patterns 2006;6(5):448–461.

242. Englund C, Loren CE, Grabbe C, Varshney GK, Deleuil F, Hallberg B, Palmer RH. Jeb signals through the Alk receptor tyrosine kinase to drive visceral muscle fusion. Nature 2003;425(6957):512–516.

243. Lee HH, Norris A, Weiss JB, Frasch M. Jelly belly protein activates the receptor tyrosine kinase Alk to specify visceral muscle pioneers. Nature 2003;425(6957):507–512.

244. Yang HL, Eriksson T, Vernersson E, Vigny M, Hallberg B, Palmer RH. The ligand Jelly Belly (Jeb) activates the *Drosophila* Alk RTK to drive PC12 cell differentiation, but is unable to activate the mouse ALK RTK. J Exp Zoolog B Mol Dev Evol 2007;308(3):269–282.

245. Moog-Lutz C, Degoutin J, Gouzi JY, Frobert Y, Brunet-de Carvalho N, Bureau J, Creminon C, Vigny M. Activation and inhibition of anaplastic lymphoma kinase receptor tyrosine kinase by monoclonal antibodies and absence of agonist activity of pleiotrophin. J Biol Chem 2005;280(28):26039–26048.

246. Fischer P, Nacheva E, Mason DY, Sherrington PD, Hoyle C, Hayhoe FG, Karpas A. A Ki-1 (CD30)-positive human cell line (Karpas 299) established from a high-grade non-Hodgkin's lymphoma, showing a 2;5 translocation and rearrangement of the T-cell receptor beta-chain gene. Blood 1988;72(1):234–240.

247. Benz-Lemoine E, Brizard A, Huret JL, Babin P, Guilhot F, Couet D, Tanzer J. Malignant histiocytosis: a specific t(2;5)(p23;q35) translocation? Review of the literature. Blood 1988;72(3):1045–1047.

248. Mason DY, Bastard C, Rimokh R, Dastugue N, Huret JL, Kristoffersson U, Magaud JP, Nezelof C, Tilly H, Vannier JP, et al. CD30-positive large cell lymphomas ("Ki-1 lymphoma") are associated with a chromosomal translocation involving 5q35. Br J Haematol 1990;74(2):161–168.

249. Morris SW, Kirstein MN, Valentine MB, Dittmer KG, Shapiro DN, Saltman DL, Look AT. Fusion of a kinase gene, ALK, to a nucleolar protein gene, NPM, in non-Hodgkin's lymphoma. Science 1994;263(5151):1281–1284.

250. Chiarle R, Voena C, Ambrogio C, Piva R, Inghirami G. The anaplastic lymphoma kinase in the pathogenesis of cancer. Nat Rev Cancer 2008;8(1):11–23.

251. Hernandez L, Bea S, Bellosillo B, Pinyol M, Falini B, Carbone A, Ott G, Rosenwald A, Fernandez A, Pulford K, Mason D, Morris SW, Santos E, Campo E. Diversity of genomic breakpoints in TFG-ALK translocations in anaplastic large cell lymphomas: identification of a new TFG-ALK(XL) chimeric gene with transforming activity. Am J Pathol 2002;160(4):1487–1494.

252. Hernandez L, Pinyol M, Hernandez S, Bea S, Pulford K, Rosenwald A, Lamant L, Falini B, Ott G, Mason DY, Delsol G, Campo E. TRK-fused gene (TFG) is a new partner of ALK in anaplastic large cell lymphoma producing two structurally different TFG-ALK translocations. Blood 1999;94(9):3265–3268.

253. Colleoni GW, Bridge JA, Garicochea B, Liu J, Filippa DA, Ladanyi M. ATIC-ALK: a novel variant ALK gene fusion in anaplastic large cell lymphoma resulting from the recurrent cryptic chromosomal inversion, inv(2)(p23q35). Am J Pathol 2000; 156(3):781–789.

254. Touriol C, Greenland C, Lamant L, Pulford K, Bernard F, Rousset T, Mason DY, Delsol G. Further demonstration of the diversity of chromosomal changes involving 2p23 in ALK-positive lymphoma: 2 cases expressing ALK kinase fused to CLTCL (clathrin chain polypeptide-like). Blood 2000;95(10):3204–3207.

255. Bridge JA, Kanamori M, Ma Z, Pickering D, Hill DA, Lydiatt W, Lui MY, Colleoni GW, Antonescu CR, Ladanyi M, Morris SW. Fusion of the ALK gene to the clathrin heavy chain gene, CLTC, in inflammatory myofibroblastic tumor. Am J Pathol 2001;159(2):411–415.

256. Tort F, Pinyol M, Pulford K, Roncador G, Hernandez L, Nayach I, Kluin-Nelemans HC, Kluin P, Touriol C, Delsol G, Mason D, Campo E. Molecular characterization of a new ALK translocation involving moesin (MSN-ALK) in anaplastic large cell lymphoma. Lab Invest 2001;81(3):419–426.

257. Tort F, Campo E, Pohlman B, Hsi E. Heterogeneity of genomic breakpoints in MSN-ALK translocations in anaplastic large cell lymphoma. Hum Pathol 2004;35(8):1038–1041.

258. Lawrence B, Perez-Atayde A, Hibbard MK, Rubin BP, Dal Cin P, Pinkus JL, Pinkus GS, Xiao S, Yi ES, Fletcher CD, Fletcher JA. TPM3-ALK and TPM4-ALK oncogenes in inflammatory myofibroblastic tumors. Am J Pathol 2000;157(2):377–384.

259. Meech SJ, McGavran L, Odom LF, Liang X, Meltesen L, Gump J, Wei Q, Carlsen S, Hunger SP. Unusual childhood extramedullary hematologic malignancy with natural killer cell properties that contains tropomyosin 4–anaplastic lymphoma kinase gene fusion. Blood 2001;98(4):1209–1216.

260. Cools J, Wlodarska I, Somers R, Mentens N, Pedeutour F, Maes B, De Wolf-Peeters C, Pauwels P, Hagemeijer A, Marynen P. Identification of novel fusion partners of ALK, the anaplastic lymphoma kinase, in anaplastic large-cell lymphoma and inflammatory myofibroblastic tumor. Genes Chromosomes Cancer 2002;34(4):354–362.

261. Ma Z, Hill DA, Collins MH, Morris SW, Sumegi J, Zhou M, Zuppan C, Bridge JA. Fusion of ALK to the Ran-binding protein 2 (RANBP2) gene in inflammatory myofibroblastic tumor. Genes Chromosomes Cancer 2003;37(1):98–105.

262. Lamant L, Gascoyne RD, Duplantier MM, Armstrong F, Raghab A, Chhanabhai M, Rajcan-Separovic E, Raghab J, Delsol G, Espinos E. Non-muscle myosin heavy chain (MYH9): a new partner fused to ALK in anaplastic large cell lymphoma. Genes Chromosomes Cancer 2003;37(4):427–432.

263. Debelenko LV, Arthur DC, Pack SD, Helman LJ, Schrump DS, Tsokos M. Identification of CARS-ALK fusion in primary and metastatic lesions of an inflammatory myofibroblastic tumor. Lab Invest 2003;83(9):1255–1265.

264. Panagopoulos I, Nilsson T, Domanski HA, Isaksson M, Lindblom P, Mertens F, Mandahl N. Fusion of the SEC31L1 and ALK genes in an inflammatory myofibroblastic tumor. Int J Cancer 2006;118(5):1181–1186.

265. Soda M, Choi YL, Enomoto M, Takada S, Yamashita Y, Ishikawa S, Fujiwara S, Watanabe H, Kurashina K, Hatanaka H, Bando M, Ohno S, Ishikawa Y, Aburatani H, Niki T, Sohara Y,

Sugiyama Y, Mano H. Identification of the transforming EML4-ALK fusion gene in non-small-cell lung cancer. Nature 2007;448(7153):561–566.

266. Kowalska A, Brunner B, Bozsaky E, Chen QR, Stock C, Lorch T, Khan J, Ambros PF. Sequence based high resolution chromosomal CGH. Cytogenet Genome Res 2008;121(1):1–6.

267. Osajima-Hakomori Y, Miyake I, Ohira M, Nakagawara A, Nakagawa A, Sakai R. Biological role of anaplastic lymphoma kinase in neuroblastoma. Am J Pathol 2005;167(1):213–222.

268. Caren H, Abel F, Kogner P, Martinsson T. High incidence of DNA mutations and gene amplifications of the ALK gene in advanced sporadic neuroblastoma tumours. Biochem J 2008;416(2):153–159.

269. Chen Y, Takita J, Choi YL, Kato M, Ohira M, Sanada M, Wang L, Soda M, Kikuchi A, Igarashi T, Nakagawara A, Hayashi Y, Mano H, Ogawa S. Oncogenic mutations of ALK kinase in neuroblastoma. Nature 2008;455(7215):971–974.

270. George RE, Sanda T, Hanna M, Frohling S, Ii WL, Zhang J, Ahn Y, Zhou W, London WB, McGrady P, Xue L, Zozulya S, Gregor VE, Webb TR, Gray NS, Gilliland DG, Diller L, Greulich H, Morris SW, Meyerson M, Look AT. Activating mutations in ALK provide a therapeutic target in neuroblastoma. Nature 2008;455(7215):975–978.

271. Janoueix-Lerosey I, Lequin D, Brugieres L, Ribeiro A, De Pontual L, Combaret V, Raynal V, Puisieux A, Schleiermacher G, Pierron G, Valteau-Couanet D, Frebourg T, Michon J, Lyonnet S, Amiel J, Delattre O. Somatic and germline activating mutations of the ALK kinase receptor in neuroblastoma. Nature 2008;455(7215):967–970.

272. Mosse YP, Laudenslager M, Longo L, Cole KA, Wood A, Attiyeh EF, Laquaglia MJ, Sennett R, Lynch JE, Perri P, Laureys G, Speleman F, Kim C, Hou C, Hakonarson H, Torkamani A, Schork NJ, Brodeur GM, Tonini GP, Rappaport E, Devoto M, Maris JM. Identification of ALK as a major familial neuroblastoma predisposition gene. Nature 2008;455(7215):930–935.

273. Pillay K, Govender D, Chetty R. ALK protein expression in rhabdomyosarcomas. Histopathology 2002;41(5):461–467.

274. Lamant L, Pulford K, Bischof D, Morris SW, Mason DY, Delsol G, Mariame B. Expression of the ALK tyrosine kinase gene in neuroblastoma. Am J Pathol 2000;156(5):1711–1721.

275. Dirks WG, Fahnrich S, Lis Y, Becker E, MacLeod RA, Drexler HG. Expression and functional analysis of the anaplastic lymphoma kinase (ALK) gene in tumor cell lines. Int J Cancer 2002;100(1):49–56.

276. Perez-Pinera P, Chang Y, Astudillo A, Mortimer J, Deuel TF. Anaplastic lymphoma kinase is expressed in different subtypes of human breast cancer. Biochem Biophys Res Commun 2007;358(2):399–403.

277. Fang W, Hartmann N, Chow DT, Riegel AT, Wellstein A. Pleiotrophin stimulates fibroblasts and endothelial and epithelial cells and is expressed in human cancer. J Biol Chem 1992;267(36):25889–25897.

278. Zhang N, Zhong R, Wang ZY, Deuel TF. Human breast cancer growth inhibited in vivo by a dominant negative pleiotrophin mutant. J Biol Chem 1997;272(27):16733–16736.

279. Perner S, Wagner PL, Demichelis F, Mehra R, Lafargue CJ, Moss BJ, Arbogast S, Soltermann A, Weder W, Giordano TJ, Beer DG, Rickman DS, Chinnaiyan AM, Moch H, Rubin MA. EML4-ALK fusion lung cancer: a rare acquired event. Neoplasia 2008;10(3):298–302.

280. Olsson AK, Dimberg A, Kreuger J, Claesson-Welsh L. VEGF receptor signalling in control of vascular function. Nat Rev Mol Cell Biol 2006;7(5):359–371.

281. Carmeliet P, Ferreira V, Breier G, Pollefeyt S, Kieckens L, Gertsenstein M, Fahrig M, Vandenhoeck A, Harpal K, Eberhardt C, Declercq C, Pawling J, Moons L, Collen D, Risau W, Nagy A. Abnormal blood vessel development and lethality in embryos lacking a single VEGF allele. Nature 1996;380(6573):435–439.

282. Vincenti V, Cassano C, Rocchi M, Persico G. Assignment of the vascular endothelial growth factor gene to human chromosome 6p21.3. Circulation 1996;93(8):1493–1495.

283. Cohen T, Gitay-Goren H, Sharon R, Shibuya M, Halaban R, Levi BZ, Neufeld G. VEGF121, a vascular endothelial growth factor (VEGF) isoform lacking heparin binding ability, requires cell-surface heparan sulfates for efficient binding to the VEGF receptors of human melanoma cells. J Biol Chem 1995;270(19):11322–11326.

284. Neufeld G, Cohen T, Gitay-Goren H, Poltorak Z, Tessler S, Sharon R, Gengrinovitch S, Levi BZ. Similarities and differences between the vascular endothelial growth factor (VEGF) splice variants. Cancer Metastasis Rev 1996;15(2):153–158.

285. Gluzman-Poltorak Z, Cohen T, Herzog Y, Neufeld G. Neuropilin-2 is a receptor for the vascular endothelial growth factor (VEGF) forms VEGF-145 and VEGF-165 [corrected]. J Biol Chem 2000;275(24):18040–18045.

286. Poltorak Z, Cohen T, Neufeld G. The VEGF splice variants: properties, receptors, and usage for the treatment of ischemic diseases. Herz 2000;25(2):126–129.

287. Krussel JS, Behr B, Milki AA, Hirchenhain J, Wen Y, Bielfeld P, Lake Polan M. Vascular endothelial growth factor (VEGF) mRNA splice variants are differentially expressed in human blastocysts. Mol Hum Reprod 2001;7(1):57–63.

288. Robinson CJ, Stringer SE. The splice variants of vascular endothelial growth factor (VEGF) and their receptors. J Cell Sci 2001;114(Pt 5):853–865.

289. Kress W, Petersen B, Collmann H, Grimm T. An unusual FGFR1 mutation (fibroblast growth factor receptor 1 mutation) in a girl with non-syndromic trigonocephaly. Cytogenet Cell Genet 2000;91(1–4):138–140.

290. Woolard J, Wang WY, Bevan HS, Qiu Y, Morbidelli L, Pritchard-Jones RO, Cui TG, Sugiono M, Waine E, Perrin R, Foster R, Digby-Bell J, Shields JD, Whittles CE, Mushens RE, Gillatt DA, Ziche M, Harper SJ, Bates DO. VEGF165b, an inhibitory vascular endothelial growth factor splice variant: mechanism of action, in vivo effect on angiogenesis and endogenous protein expression. Cancer Res 2004;64(21):7822–7835.

291. Rennel ES, Waine E, Guan H, Schuler Y, Leenders W, Woolard J, Sugiono M, Gillatt D, Kleinerman ES, Bates DO, Harper SJ. The endogenous anti-angiogenic VEGF isoform, VEGF165b inhibits human tumour growth in mice. Br J Cancer 2008;98(7):1250–1257.

292. Bu R, Purushotham KR, Kerr M, Tao Z, Jonsson R, Olofsson J, Humphreys-Beher MG. Alterations in the level of phosphotyrosine signal transduction constituents in human parotid tumors. Proc Soc Exp Biol Med 1996;211(3):257–264.

293. Lagercrantz J, Farnebo F, Larsson C, Tvrdik T, Weber G, Piehl F. A comparative study of the expression patterns for vegf, vegf-b/vrf and vegf-c in the developing and adult mouse. Biochim Biophys Acta 1998;1398(2):157–163.

294. Aase K, Von Euler G, Li X, Ponten A, Thoren P, Cao R, Cao Y, Olofsson B, Gebre-Medhin S, Pekny M, Alitalo K, Betsholtz C, Eriksson U. Vascular endothelial growth factor-B-deficient mice display an atrial conduction defect. Circulation 2001;104(3):358–364.

295. Karkkainen MJ, Haiko P, Sainio K, Partanen J, Taipale J, Petrova TV, Jeltsch M, Jackson DG, Talikka M, Rauvala H, Betsholtz C, Alitalo K. Vascular endothelial growth factor C is required for sprouting of the first lymphatic vessels from embryonic veins. Nat Immunol 2004;5(1):74–80.

296. Baldwin ME, Halford MM, Roufail S, Williams RA, Hibbs ML, Grail D, Kubo H, Stacker SA, Achen MG. Vascular endothelial growth factor D is dispensable for development of the lymphatic system. Mol Cell Biol 2005;25(6):2441–2449.

297. Lee J, Gray A, Yuan J, Luoh SM, Avraham H, Wood WI. Vascular endothelial growth factor-related protein: a ligand and specific activator of the tyrosine kinase receptor Flt4. Proc Natl Acad Sci U S A 1996;93(5):1988–1992.

298. Stacker SA, Caesar C, Baldwin ME, Thornton GE, Williams RA, Prevo R, Jackson DG, Nishikawa S, Kubo H, Achen MG. VEGF-D promotes the metastatic spread of tumor cells via the lymphatics. Nat Med 2001;7(2):186–191.

299. Kukk E, Lymboussaki A, Taira S, Kaipainen A, Jeltsch M, Joukov V, Alitalo K. VEGF-C receptor binding and pattern of expression with VEGFR-3 suggests a role in lymphatic vascular development. Development 1996;122(12):3829–3837.

300. Kaipainen A, Korhonen J, Mustonen T, Van Hinsbergh VW, Fang GH, Dumont D, Breitman M, Alitalo K. Expression of the fms-like tyrosine kinase 4 gene becomes restricted to lymphatic endothelium during development. Proc Natl Acad Sci U S A 1995;92(8):3566–3570.

301. Skobe M, Hawighorst T, Jackson DG, Prevo R, Janes L, Velasco P, Riccardi L, Alitalo K, Claffey K, Detmar M. Induction of tumor lymphangiogenesis by VEGF-C promotes breast cancer metastasis. Nat Med 2001;7(2):192–198.

302. Makinen T, Veikkola T, Mustjoki S, Karpanen T, Catimel B, Nice EC, Wise L, Mercer A, Kowalski H, Kerjaschki D, Stacker SA, Achen MG, Alitalo K. Isolated lymphatic endothelial cells transduce growth, survival and migratory signals via the VEGF-C/D receptor VEGFR-3. EMBO J 2001;20(17):4762–4773.

303. Joukov V, Kaipainen A, Jeltsch M, Pajusola K, Olofsson B, Kumar V, Eriksson U, Alitalo K. Vascular endothelial growth factors VEGF-B and VEGF-C. J Cell Physiol 1997;173(2):211–215.

304. Joukov V, Sorsa T, Kumar V, Jeltsch M, Claesson-Welsh L, Cao Y, Saksela O, Kalkkinen N, Alitalo K. Proteolytic processing regulates receptor specificity and activity of VEGF-C. EMBO J 1997;16(13):3898–3911.

305. Autiero M, Waltenberger J, Communi D, Kranz A, Moons L, Lambrechts D, Kroll J, Plaisance S, De Mol M, Bono F, Kliche S, Fellbrich G, Ballmer-Hofer K, Maglione D, Mayr-Beyrle U, Dewerchin M, Dombrowski S, Stanimirovic D, Van Hummelen P, Dehio C, Hicklin DJ, Persico G, Herbert JM, Communi D, Shibuya M, Collen D, Conway EM, Carmeliet P. Role of PlGF in the intra- and intermolecular cross talk between the VEGF receptors Flt1 and Flk1. Nat Med 2003;9(7):936–943.

306. Kim IJ, Park JH, Kang HC, Shin Y, Lim SB, Ku JL, Yang HK, Lee KU, Park JG. A novel germline mutation in the MET extracellular domain in a Korean patient with the diffuse type of familial gastric cancer. J Med Genet 2003;40(8):e97.

307. Satoh H, Yoshida MC, Matsushime H, Shibuya M, Sasaki M. Regional localization of the human c-ros-1 on 6q22 and flt on 13q12. Jpn J Cancer Res 1987;78(8):772–775.

308. Fong GH, Rossant J, Gertsenstein M, Breitman ML. Role of the Flt-1 receptor tyrosine kinase in regulating the assembly of vascular endothelium. Nature 1995;376(6535):66–70.

309. Hiratsuka S, Minowa O, Kuno J, Noda T, Shibuya M. Flt-1 lacking the tyrosine kinase domain is sufficient for normal development and angiogenesis in mice. Proc Natl Acad Sci U S A 1998;95(16):9349–9354.

310. Pitteloud N, Acierno JS Jr, Meysing A, Eliseenkova AV, Ma J, Ibrahimi OA, Metzger DL, Hayes FJ, Dwyer AA, Hughes VA, Yialamas M, Hall JE, Grant E, Mohammadi M, Crowley WF Jr. Mutations in fibroblast growth factor receptor 1 cause both Kallmann syndrome and normosmic idiopathic hypogonadotropic hypogonadism. Proc Natl Acad Sci U S A 2006;103(16):6281–6286.

311. Zhao S, Zoller K, Masuko M, Rojnuckarin P, Yang XO, Parganas E, Kaushansky K, Ihle JN, Papayannopoulou T, Willerford DM, Clackson T, Blau CA. JAK2, complemented by a second signal from c-kit or flt-3, triggers extensive self-renewal of primary multipotential hemopoietic cells. EMBO J 2002;21(9):2159–2167.

312. Yang S, Xin X, Zlot C, Ingle G, Fuh G, Li B, Moffat B, De Vos AM, Gerritsen ME. Vascular endothelial cell growth factor-driven endothelial tube formation is mediated by vascular endothelial cell growth factor receptor-2, a kinase insert domain-containing receptor. Arterioscler Thromb Vasc Biol 2001;21(12):1934–1940.

313. Ferrara N, Gerber HP, LeCouter J. The biology of VEGF and its receptors. Nat Med 2003;9(6):669–676.

314. Shalaby F, Rossant J, Yamaguchi TP, Gertsenstein M, Wu XF, Breitman ML, Schuh AC. Failure of blood-island formation and vasculogenesis in Flk-1-deficient mice. Nature 1995;376(6535):62–66.

315. Bellamy WT, Richter L, Sirjani D, Roxas C, Glinsmann-Gibson B, Frutiger Y, Grogan TM, List AF. Vascular endothelial cell growth factor is an autocrine promoter of abnormal localized immature myeloid precursors and leukemia progenitor formation in myelodysplastic syndromes. Blood 2001;97(5):1427–1434.

316. Graeven U, Fiedler W, Karpinski S, Ergun S, Kilic N, Rodeck U, Schmiegel W, Hossfeld DK. Melanoma-associated expression of vascular endothelial growth factor and its receptors FLT-1 and KDR. J Cancer Res Clin Oncol 1999;125(11):621–629.

317. Lacal PM, Failla CM, Pagani E, Odorisio T, Schietroma C, Falcinelli S, Zambruno G, D'Atri S. Human melanoma cells secrete and respond to placenta growth factor and vascular endothelial growth factor. J Invest Dermatol 2000;115(6):1000–1007.

318. Takahashi M. The GDNF/RET signaling pathway and human diseases. Cytokine Growth Factor Rev 2001;12(4):361–373.

319. Holmqvist K, Cross MJ, Rolny C, Hagerkvist R, Rahimi N, Matsumoto T, Claesson-Welsh L, Welsh M. The adaptor protein shb binds to tyrosine 1175 in vascular endothelial

growth factor (VEGF) receptor-2 and regulates VEGF-dependent cellular migration. J Biol Chem 2004;279(21):22267–22275.

320. Warner AJ, Lopez-Dee J, Knight EL, Feramisco JR, Prigent SA. The Shc-related adaptor protein, Sck, forms a complex with the vascular-endothelial-growth-factor receptor KDR in transfected cells. Biochem J 2000;347(Pt 2):501–509.

321. Lamalice L, Houle F, Huot J. Phosphorylation of Tyr1214 within VEGFR-2 triggers the recruitment of Nck and activation of Fyn leading to SAPK2/p38 activation and endothelial cell migration in response to VEGF. J Biol Chem 2006;281(45):34009–34020.

322. Matsumoto T, Bohman S, Dixelius J, Berge T, Dimberg A, Magnusson P, Wang L, Wikner C, Qi JH, Wernstedt C, Wu J, Bruheim S, Mugishima H, Mukhopadhyay D, Spurkland A, Claesson-Welsh L. VEGF receptor-2 Y951 signaling and a role for the adapter molecule TSAd in tumor angiogenesis. EMBO J 2005;24(13):2342–2353.

323. Matsumoto T, Mugishima H. Signal transduction via vascular endothelial growth factor (VEGF) receptors and their roles in atherogenesis. J Atheroscler Thromb 2006;13(3):130–135.

324. Hunger-Glaser I, Fan RS, Perez-Salazar E, Rozengurt E. PDGF and FGF induce focal adhesion kinase (FAK) phosphorylation at Ser-910: dissociation from Tyr-397 phosphorylation and requirement for ERK activation. J Cell Physiol 2004;200(2):213–222.

325. Marks JL, McLellan MD, Zakowski MF, Lash AE, Kasai Y, Broderick S, Sarkaria IS, Pham D, Singh B, Miner TL, Fewell GA, Fulton LL, Mardis ER, Wilson RK, Kris MG, Rusch VW, Varmus H, Pao W. Mutational analysis of EGFR and related signaling pathway genes in lung adenocarcinomas identifies a novel somatic kinase domain mutation in FGFR4. PLoS ONE 2007;2(5):e426.

326. Singh AJ, Meyer RD, Band H, Rahimi N. The carboxyl terminus of VEGFR-2 is required for PKC-mediated down-regulation. Mol Biol Cell 2005;16(4):2106–2118.

327. Ferrell RE, Levinson KL, Esman JH, Kimak MA, Lawrence EC, Barmada MM, Finegold DN. Hereditary lymphedema: evidence for linkage and genetic heterogeneity. Hum Mol Genet 1998;7(13):2073–2078.

328. Irrthum A, Karkkainen MJ, Devriendt K, Alitalo K, Vikkula M. Congenital hereditary lymphedema caused by a mutation that inactivates VEGFR3 tyrosine kinase. Am J Hum Genet 2000;67(2):295–301.

329. Karkkainen MJ, Ferrell RE, Lawrence EC, Kimak MA, Levinson KL, McTigue MA, Alitalo K, Finegold DN. Missense mutations interfere with VEGFR-3 signalling in primary lymphoedema. Nat Genet 2000;25(2):153–159.

330. Dumont DJ, Jussila L, Taipale J, Lymboussaki A, Mustonen T, Pajusola K, Breitman M, Alitalo K. Cardiovascular failure in mouse embryos deficient in VEGF receptor-3. Science 1998;282(5390):946–949.

331. Fournier E, Dubreuil P, Birnbaum D, Borg JP. Mutation at tyrosine residue 1337 abrogates ligand-dependent transforming capacity of the FLT4 receptor. Oncogene 1995;11(5):921–931.

332. Dixelius J, Makinen T, Wirzenius M, Karkkainen MJ, Wernstedt C, Alitalo K, Claesson-Welsh L. Ligand-induced vascular endothelial growth factor receptor-3 (VEGFR-3) heterodimerization with VEGFR-2 in primary lymphatic endothelial cells regulates tyrosine phosphorylation sites. J Biol Chem 2003;278(42):40973–40979.

333. Yuan L, Moyon D, Pardanaud L, Breant C, Karkkainen MJ, Alitalo K, Eichmann A. Abnormal lymphatic vessel development in neuropilin 2 mutant mice. Development 2002;129(20):4797–4806.

334. Karpanen T, Egeblad M, Karkkainen MJ, Kubo H, Yla-Herttuala S, Jaattela M, Alitalo K. Vascular endothelial growth factor C promotes tumor lymphangiogenesis and intralymphatic tumor growth. Cancer Res 2001;61(5):1786–1790.

335. Mattila MM, Ruohola JK, Karpanen T, Jackson DG, Alitalo K, Harkonen PL. VEGF-C induced lymphangiogenesis is associated with lymph node metastasis in orthotopic MCF-7 tumors. Int J Cancer 2002;98(6):946–951.

336. Mandriota SJ, Jussila L, Jeltsch M, Compagni A, Baetens D, Prevo R, Banerji S, Huarte J, Montesano R, Jackson DG, Orci L, Alitalo K, Christofori G, Pepper MS. Vascular endothelial growth factor-C-mediated lymphangiogenesis promotes tumour metastasis. EMBO J 2001;20(4):672–682.

337. He Y, Kozaki K, Karpanen T, Koshikawa K, Yla-Herttuala S, Takahashi T, Alitalo K. Suppression of tumor lymphangiogenesis and lymph node metastasis by blocking vascular endothelial growth factor receptor 3 signaling. J Natl Cancer Inst 2002;94(11):819–825.

338. Krishnan J, Kirkin V, Steffen A, Hegen M, Weih D, Tomarev S, Wilting J, Sleeman JP. Differential in vivo and in vitro expression of vascular endothelial growth factor (VEGF)-C and VEGF-D in tumors and its relationship to lymphatic metastasis in immunocompetent rats. Cancer Res 2003;63(3):713–722.

339. Lin J, Lalani AS, Harding TC, Gonzalez M, Wu WW, Luan B, Tu GH, Koprivnikar K, VanRoey MJ, He Y, Alitalo K, Jooss K. Inhibition of lymphogenous metastasis using adeno-associated virus-mediated gene transfer of a soluble VEGFR-3 decoy receptor. Cancer Res 2005;65(15):6901–6909.

340. Laakkonen P, Waltari M, Holopainen T, Takahashi T, Pytowski B, Steiner P, Hicklin D, Persaud K, Tonra JR, Witte L, Alitalo K. Vascular endothelial growth factor receptor 3 is involved in tumor angiogenesis and growth. Cancer Res 2007;67(2):593–599.

341. Ostman A, Heldin CH. PDGF receptors as targets in tumor treatment. Adv Cancer Res 2007;97: 247–274.

342. Li X, Eriksson U. Novel PDGF family members: PDGF-C and PDGF-D. Cytokine Growth Factor Rev 2003;14(2):91–98.

343. Heldin CH, Ostman A, Ronnstrand L. Signal transduction via platelet-derived growth factor receptors. Biochim Biophys Acta 1998;1378(1): F79–113.

344. Miyake S, Lupher ML Jr, Druker B, Band H. The tyrosine kinase regulator Cbl enhances the ubiquitination and degradation of the platelet-derived growth factor receptor alpha. Proc Natl Acad Sci U S A 1998;95(14):7927–7932.

345. Corless CL, Fletcher JA, Heinrich MC. Biology of gastrointestinal stromal tumors. J Clin Oncol 2004;22(18):3813–3825.

346. Lasota J, Wozniak A, Sarlomo-Rikala M, Rys J, Kordek R, Nassar A, Sobin LH, Miettinen M. Mutations in exons 9 and 13 of KIT gene are rare events in gastrointestinal stromal tumors. A study of 200 cases. Am J Pathol 2000;157(4):1091–1095.

347. Lux ML, Rubin BP, Biase TL, Chen CJ, Maclure T, Demetri G, Xiao S, Singer S, Fletcher CD, Fletcher JA. KIT extracellular and kinase domain mutations in gastrointestinal stromal tumors. Am J Pathol 2000;156(3):791–795.

348. Lasota J, Jasinski M, Sarlomo-Rikala M, Miettinen M. Mutations in exon 11 of c-Kit occur preferentially in malignant versus benign gastrointestinal stromal tumors and do not occur in leiomyomas or leiomyosarcomas. Am J Pathol 1999;154(1):53–60.

349. Moskaluk CA, Tian Q, Marshall CR, Rumpel CA, Franquemont DW, Frierson HF Jr. Mutations of c-kit JM domain are found in a minority of human gastrointestinal stromal tumors. Oncogene 1999;18(10):1897–1902.

350. Taniguchi M, Nishida T, Hirota S, Isozaki K, Ito T, Nomura T, Matsuda H, Kitamura Y. Effect of c-kit mutation on prognosis of gastrointestinal stromal tumors. Cancer Res 1999;59(17):4297–4300.

351. Hirota S, Isozaki K, Moriyama Y, Hashimoto K, Nishida T, Ishiguro S, Kawano K, Hanada M, Kurata A, Takeda M, Muhammad Tunio G, Matsuzawa Y, Kanakura Y, Shinomura Y, Kitamura Y. Gain-of-function mutations of c-kit in human gastrointestinal stromal tumors. Science 1998;279(5350):577–580.

352. Buchdunger E, Zimmermann J, Mett H, Meyer T, Muller M, Druker BJ, Lydon NB. Inhibition of the Abl protein-tyrosine kinase in vitro and in vivo by a 2-phenylaminopyrimidine derivative. Cancer Res 1996;56(1):100–104.

353. Corless CL, McGreevey L, Haley A, Town A, Heinrich MC. KIT mutations are common in incidental gastrointestinal stromal tumors one centimeter or less in size. Am J Pathol 2002;160(5):1567–1572.

354. Heinrich MC, Corless CL, Duensing A, McGreevey L, Chen CJ, Joseph N, Singer S, Griffith DJ, Haley A, Town A, Demetri GD, Fletcher CD, Fletcher JA. PDGFRA activating mutations in gastrointestinal stromal tumors. Science 2003;299(5607):708–710.

355. Chompret A, Kannengiesser C, Barrois M, Terrier P, Dahan P, Tursz T, Lenoir GM, Bressac-De Paillerets B. PDGFRA germline mutation in a family with multiple cases of gastrointestinal stromal tumor. Gastroenterology 2004;126(1):318–321.

356. Hardy W, Anderson R. The hypereosinophilic syndromes. Ann Intern Med 1968;68: 1220–1229.

357. Bain B, Pierre R, Imbert M, Vardiman J, Brunning R, Flandrin G. Chronic eosinophilic leukaemia and the hypereosinophilic syndrome. In: Jaffe ES, Harris N, Stein H, Vardiman J, editors. World

Health Organization of Tumours: Tumours of Haematopoietic and Lymphoid Tissues. Lyon, France: IARC Press; 2001. pp 29–31.

358. Stover EH, Chen J, Folens C, Lee BH, Mentens N, Marynen P, Williams IR, Gilliland DG, Cools J. Activation of FIP1L1-PDGFRalpha requires disruption of the juxtamembrane domain of PDGFRalpha and is FIP1L1-independent. Proc Natl Acad Sci U S A 2006;103(21):8078–8083.

359. Gotlib J, Cools J, Malone JM 3rd, Schrier SL, Gilliland DG, Coutre SE. The FIP1L1-PDGFRalpha fusion tyrosine kinase in hypereosinophilic syndrome and chronic eosinophilic leukemia: implications for diagnosis, classification, and management. Blood 2004;103(8):2879–2891.

360. Baxter EJ, Hochhaus A, Bolufer P, Reiter A, Fernandez JM, Senent L, Cervera J, Moscardo F, Sanz MA, Cross NC. The t(4;22)(q12;q11) in atypical chronic myeloid leukaemia fuses BCR to PDGFRA. Hum Mol Genet 2002;11(12):1391–1397.

361. Safley AM, Sebastian S, Collins TS, Tirado CA, Stenzel TT, Gong JZ, Goodman BK. Molecular and cytogenetic characterization of a novel translocation t(4;22) involving the breakpoint cluster region and platelet-derived growth factor receptor-alpha genes in a patient with atypical chronic myeloid leukemia. Genes Chromosomes Cancer 2004;40(1):44–50.

362. Curtis CE, Grand FH, Musto P, Clark A, Murphy J, Perla G, Minervini MM, Stewart J, Reiter A, Cross NC. Two novel imatinib-responsive PDGFRA fusion genes in chronic eosinophilic leukaemia. Br J Haematol 2007;138(1):77–81.

363. Cools J, DeAngelo DJ, Gotlib J, Stover EH, Legare RD, Cortes J, Kutok J, Clark J, Galinsky I, Griffin JD, Cross NC, Tefferi A, Malone J, Alam R, Schrier SL, Schmid J, Rose M, Vandenberghe P, Verhoef G, Boogaerts M, Wlodarska I, Kantarjian H, Marynen P, Coutre SE, Stone R, Gilliland DG. A tyrosine kinase created by fusion of the PDGFRA and FIP1L1 genes as a therapeutic target of imatinib in idiopathic hypereosinophilic syndrome. N Engl J Med 2003;348(13):1201–1214.

364. Griffin JH, Leung J, Bruner RJ, Caligiuri MA, Briesewitz R. Discovery of a fusion kinase in EOL-1 cells and idiopathic hypereosinophilic syndrome. Proc Natl Acad Sci U S A 2003;100(13):7830–7835.

365. Score J, Curtis C, Waghorn K, Stalder M, Jotterand M, Grand FH, Cross NC. Identification of a novel imatinib responsive KIF5B-PDGFRA fusion gene following screening for PDGFRA overexpression in patients with hypereosinophilia. Leukemia 2006;20(5):827–832.

366. Guha A, Dashner K, Black PM, Wagner JA, Stiles CD. Expression of PDGF and PDGF receptors in human astrocytoma operation specimens supports the existence of an autocrine loop. Int J Cancer 1995;60(2):168–173.

367. Fleming TP, Saxena A, Clark WC, Robertson JT, Oldfield EH, Aaronson SA, Ali IU. Amplification and/or overexpression of platelet-derived growth factor receptors and epidermal growth factor receptor in human glial tumors. Cancer Res 1992;52(16):4550–4553.

368. Lokker NA, Sullivan CM, Hollenbach SJ, Israel MA, Giese NA. Platelet-derived growth factor (PDGF) autocrine signaling regulates survival and mitogenic pathways in glioblastoma cells: evidence that the novel PDGF-C and PDGF-D ligands may play a role in the development of brain tumors. Cancer Res 2002;62(13):3729–3735.

369. Holtkamp N, Mautner VF, Friedrich RE, Harder A, Hartmann C, Theallier-Janko A, Hoffmann KT, Von Deimling A. Differentially expressed genes in neurofibromatosis 1-associated neurofibromas and malignant peripheral nerve sheath tumors. Acta Neuropathol (Berl) 2004;107(2):159–168.

370. Holtkamp N, Okuducu AF, Mucha J, Afanasieva A, Hartmann C, Atallah I, Estevez-Schwarz L, Mawrin C, Friedrich RE, Mautner VF, Von Deimling A. Mutation and expression of PDGFRA and KIT in malignant peripheral nerve sheath tumors, and its implications for imatinib sensitivity. Carcinogenesis 2006;27(3):664–671.

371. Grand FH, Burgstaller S, Kuhr T, Baxter EJ, Webersinke G, Thaler J, Chase AJ, Cross NC. p53-Binding protein 1 is fused to the platelet-derived growth factor receptor beta in a patient with a t(5;15)(q33;q22) and an imatinib-responsive eosinophilic myeloproliferative disorder. Cancer Res 2004;64(20):7216–7219.

372. Abe A, Emi N, Tanimoto M, Terasaki H, Marunouchi T, Saito H. Fusion of the platelet-derived growth factor receptor beta to a novel gene CEV14 in acute myelogenous leukemia after clonal evolution. Blood 1997;90(11):4271–4277.

373. Simon MP, Navarro M, Roux D, Pouyssegur J. Structural and functional analysis of a chimeric protein COL1A1-PDGFB generated by the translocation t(17;22)(q22;q13.1) in dermatofibrosarcoma protuberans (DP). Oncogene 2001;20(23):2965–2975.

374. Walz C, Metzgeroth G, Haferlach C, Schmitt-Graeff A, Fabarius A, Hagen V, Prummer O, Rauh S, Hehlmann R, Hochhaus A, Cross NC, Reiter A. Characterization of three new imatinib-responsive fusion genes in chronic myeloproliferative disorders generated by disruption of the platelet-derived growth factor receptor beta gene. Haematologica 2007;92(2):163–169.

375. Schwaller J, Anastasiadou E, Cain D, Kutok J, Wojiski S, Williams IR, LaStarza R, Crescenzi B, Sternberg DW, Andreasson P, Schiavo R, Siena S, Mecucci C, Gilliland DG. H4(D10S170), a gene frequently rearranged in papillary thyroid carcinoma, is fused to the platelet-derived growth factor receptor beta gene in atypical chronic myeloid leukemia with t(5;10)(q33;q22). Blood 2001;97(12):3910–3918.

376. Ross TS, Bernard OA, Berger R, Gilliland DG. Fusion of Huntingtin interacting protein 1 to platelet-derived growth factor beta receptor (PDGFbetaR) in chronic myelomonocytic leukemia with t(5;7)(q33;q11.2). Blood 1998;91(12):4419–4426.

377. Morerio C, Acquila M, Rosanda C, Rapella A, Dufour C, Locatelli F, Maserati E, Pasquali F, Panarello C. HCMOGT-1 is a novel fusion partner to PDGFRB in juvenile myelomonocytic leukemia with t(5;17)(q33;p11.2). Cancer Res 2004;64(8):2649–2651.

378. Levine RL, Wadleigh M, Sternberg DW, Wlodarska I, Galinsky I, Stone RM, DeAngelo DJ, Gilliland DG, Cools J. KIAA1509 is a novel PDGFRB fusion partner in imatinib-responsive myeloproliferative disease associated with a t(5;14)(q33;q32). Leukemia 2005;19(1):27–30.

379. Wilkinson K, Velloso ER, Lopes LF, Lee C, Aster JC, Shipp MA, Aguiar RC. Cloning of the t(1;5)(q23;q33) in a myeloproliferative disorder associated with eosinophilia: involvement of PDGFRB and response to imatinib. Blood 2003;102(12):4187–4190.

380. Vizmanos JL, Novo FJ, Roman JP, Baxter EJ, Lahortiga I, Larrayoz MJ, Odero MD, Giraldo P, Calasanz MJ, Cross NC. NIN, a gene encoding a CEP110-like centrosomal protein, is fused to PDGFRB in a patient with a t(5;14)(q33;q24) and an imatinib-responsive myeloproliferative disorder. Cancer Res 2004;64(8):2673–2676.

381. Magnusson MK, Meade KE, Brown KE, Arthur DC, Krueger LA, Barrett AJ, Dunbar CE. Rabaptin-5 is a novel fusion partner to platelet-derived growth factor beta receptor in chronic myelomonocytic leukemia. Blood 2001;98(8):2518–2525.

382. Golub TR, Barker GF, Lovett M, Gilliland DG. Fusion of PDGF receptor beta to a novel ets-like gene, tel, in chronic myelomonocytic leukemia with t(5;12) chromosomal translocation. Cell 1994;77(2):307–316.

383. Ritchie KA, Aprikyan AA, Bowen-Pope DF, Norby-Slycord CJ, Conyers S, Bartelmez S, Sitnicka EH, Hickstein DD. The Tel-PDGFRbeta fusion gene produces a chronic myeloproliferative syndrome in transgenic mice. Leukemia 1999;13(11):1790–1803.

384. Tomasson MH, Sternberg DW, Williams IR, Carroll M, Cain D, Aster JC, Ilaria RL Jr, Van Etten RA, Gilliland DG. Fatal myeloproliferation, induced in mice by TEL/PDGFbetaR expression, depends on PDGFbetaR tyrosines 579/581. J Clin Invest 2000;105(4):423–432.

385. Brose M, Nellore A, Paziana K, Ransone K, Redlinger M, Flaherty K, Mandel S, Troxel A, Loevner L, Gupta-Abramson V. A phase II study of sorafenib in metastatic thyroid carcinoma. J Clin Oncol 2008;26(May 20 suppl):Abstract 6026.

386. Bergers G, Song S, Meyer-Morse N, Bergsland E, Hanahan D. Benefits of targeting both pericytes and endothelial cells in the tumor vasculature with kinase inhibitors. J Clin Invest 2003;111(9):1287–1295.

387. Itoh N. The Fgf families in humans, mice, and zebrafish: their evolutional processes and roles in development, metabolism, and disease. Biol Pharm Bull 2007;30(10):1819–1825.

388. Ornitz DM, Xu J, Colvin JS, McEwen DG, MacArthur CA, Coulier F, Gao G, Goldfarb M. Receptor specificity of the fibroblast growth factor family. J Biol Chem 1996;271(25):15292–15297.

389. Bikfalvi A, Klein S, Pintucci G, Rifkin D. Biological roles of fibroblast growth factor-2. Endocr Rev 1997;18: 26–45.

390. Burgess W, Maciag T. The heparin-binding (fibroblast) growth factor family of proteins. Annu Rev Biochem 1989;58: 575–606.

391. Imamura T, Engleka K, Zhan X, Tokita Y, Forough R, Roeder D, Jackson A, Maier J, Hla T, Maciag T. Recovery of mitogenic activity of a growth factor mutant with a nuclear translocation sequence. Science 1990;249: 1567–1570.

392. Bugler B, Amalric F, Prats H. Alternative initiation of translation determines cytoplasmic or nuclear localization of basic fibroblast growth factor. Mol Cell Biol 1991;11: 573–577.

393. Dono R, Texido G, Dussel R, Ehmke H, Zeller R. Impaired cerebral cortex development and blood pressure regulation in FGF-2-deficient mice. EMBO J 1998;17(15):4213–4225.

394. Ortega S, Ittmann M, Tsang S, Ehrlich M, Basilico C. Neuronal defects and delayed wound healing in mice lacking fibroblast growth factor 2. Proc Natl Acad Sci U S A 1998;95: 5672–5677.

395. Zhou M, Sutliff R, Paul R, Lorenz J, Hoying J, Haudenschild C, Yin M, Coffin J, Kong L, Kranias E, Luo W, Boivin G, Duffy J, Pawlowski S, Doetschman T. Fibroblast growth factor 2 control of vascular tone. Nat Med 1998;4: 201–207.

396. Miller DL, Ortega S, Bashayan O, Basch R, Basilico C. Compensation by fibroblast growth factor 1 (FGF1) does not account for the mild phenotypic defects observed in FGF2 null mice. Mol Cell Biol 2000;20(6):2260–2268.

397. Duchesne L, Tissot B, Rudd TR, Dell A, Fernig DG. N-glycosylation of fibroblast growth factor receptor 1 regulates ligand and heparan sulfate co-receptor binding. J Biol Chem 2006;281(37):27178–27189.

398. Sleeman M, Fraser J, McDonald M, Yuan S, White D, Grandison P, Kumble K, Watson JD, Murison JG. Identification of a new fibroblast growth factor receptor, FGFR5. Gene 2001;271(2):171–182.

399. Simons M, Horowitz A. Syndecan-4 mediated signaling. Cell Signal 2001;13: 855–862.

400. Tkachenko E, Lutgens E, Stan R-V, Simons M. Fibroblast growth factor 2 endocytosis in endothelial cells proceed via syndecan-4-dependent activation of Rac1 and a Cdc42 dependent macropinocytotic pathway. J Cell Sci 2004;117: 3189–3199.

401. Mohammadi M, Schlessinger J, Hubbard SR. Structure of the FGF receptor tyrosine kinase domain reveals a novel autoinhibitory mechanism. Cell 1996;86(4):577–587.

402. Mohammadi M, Honegger AM, Rotin D, Fischer R, Bellot F, Li W, Dionne CA, Jaye M, Rubinstein M, Schlessinger J. A tyrosine-phosphorylated carboxy-terminal peptide of the fibroblast growth factor receptor (Flg) is a binding site for the SH2 domain of phospholipase C-gamma 1. Mol Cell Biol 1991;11(10):5068–5078.

403. Larsson H, Klint P, Landgren E, Claesson-Welsh L. Fibroblast growth factor receptor-1-mediated endothelial cell proliferation is dependent on the Src homology (SH) 2/SH3 domain-containing adaptor protein Crk. J Biol Chem 1999;274(36):25726–25734.

404. Powers CJ, McLeskey SW, Wellstein A. Fibroblast growth factors, their receptors and signaling. Endocr Relat Cancer 2000;7(3):165–197.

405. Sahadevan K, Darby S, Leung HY, Mathers ME, Robson CN, Gnanapragasam VJ. Selective over-expression of fibroblast growth factor receptors 1 and 4 in clinical prostate cancer. J Pathol 2007;213(1):82–90.

406. Elbauomy Elsheikh S, Green AR, Lambros MB, Turner NC, Grainge MJ, Powe D, Ellis IO, Reis-Filho JS. FGFR1 amplification in breast carcinomas: a chromogenic *in situ* hybridisation analysis. Breast Cancer Res 2007;9(2):R23.

407. Letessier A, Sircoulomb F, Ginestier C, Cervera N, Monville F, Gelsi-Boyer V, Esterni B, Geneix J, Finetti P, Zemmour C, Viens P, Charafe-Jauffret E, Jacquemier J, Birnbaum D, Chaffanet M. Frequency, prognostic impact, and subtype association of 8p12, 8q24, 11q13, 12p13, 17q12, and 20q13 amplifications in breast cancers. BMC Cancer 2006;6: 245.

408. Cuny M, Kramar A, Courjal F, Johannsdottir V, Iacopetta B, Fontaine H, Grenier J, Culine S, Theillet C. Relating genotype and phenotype in breast cancer: an analysis of the prognostic significance of amplification at eight different genes or loci and of p53 mutations. Cancer Res 2000;60(4):1077–1083.

409. Ugolini F, Adelaide J, Charafe-Jauffret E, Nguyen C, Jacquemier J, Jordan B, Birnbaum D, Pebusque MJ. Differential expression assay of chromosome arm 8p genes identifies Frizzled-related (FRP1/FRZB) and fibroblast growth factor receptor 1 (FGFR1) as candidate breast cancer genes. Oncogene 1999;18(10):1903–1910.

410. Bautista S, Theillet C. CCND1 and FGFR1 coamplification results in the colocalization of 11q13 and 8p12 sequences in breast tumor nuclei. Genes Chromosomes Cancer 1998;22(4):268–277.

411. Dib A, Adelaide J, Chaffanet M, Imbert A, Le Paslier D, Jacquemier J, Gaudray P, Theillet C, Birnbaum D, Pebusque MJ. Characterization of the region of the short arm of chromosome 8 amplified in breast carcinoma. Oncogene 1995;10(5):995–1001.

412. Jacquemier J, Adelaide J, Parc P, Penault-Llorca F, Planche J, deLapeyriere O, Birnbaum D. Expression of the FGFR1 gene in human breast-carcinoma cells. Int J Cancer 1994;59(3):373–378.

413. Theillet C, Adelaide J, Louason G, Bonnet-Dorion F, Jacquemier J, Adnane J, Longy M, Katsaros D, Sismondi P, Gaudray P, et al. FGFRI and PLAT genes and DNA amplification at 8p12 in breast and ovarian cancers. Genes Chromosomes Cancer 1993;7(4):219–226.

414. Freier K, Schwaenen C, Sticht C, Flechtenmacher C, Muhling J, Hofele C, Radlwimmer B, Lichter P, Joos S. Recurrent FGFR1 amplification and high FGFR1 protein expression in oral squamous cell carcinoma (OSCC). Oral Oncol 2007;43(1):60–66.

415. Ishizuka T, Tanabe C, Sakamoto H, Aoyagi K, Maekawa M, Matsukura N, Tokunaga A, Tajiri T, Yoshida T, Terada M, Sasaki H. Gene amplification profiling of esophageal squamous cell carcinomas by DNA array CGH. Biochem Biophys Res Commun 2002;296(1):152–155.

416. Simon R, Richter J, Wagner U, Fijan A, Bruderer J, Schmid U, Ackermann D, Maurer R, Alund G, Knonagel H, Rist M, Wilber K, Anabitarte M, Hering F, Hardmeier T, Schonenberger A, Flury R, Jager P, Fehr JL, Schraml P, Moch H, Mihatsch MJ, Gasser T, Sauter G. High-throughput tissue microarray analysis of 3p25 (RAF1) and 8p12 (FGFR1) copy number alterations in urinary bladder cancer. Cancer Res 2001;61(11):4514–4519.

417. Gorringe KL, Jacobs S, Thompson ER, Sridhar A, Qiu W, Choong DY, Campbell IG. High-resolution single nucleotide polymorphism array analysis of epithelial ovarian cancer reveals numerous microdeletions and amplifications. Clin Cancer Res 2007;13(16):4731–4739.

418. Mayr D, Kanitz V, Anderegg B, Luthardt B, Engel J, Lohrs U, Amann G, Diebold J. Analysis of gene amplification and prognostic markers in ovarian cancer using comparative genomic hybridization for microarrays and immunohistochemical analysis for tissue microarrays. Am J Clin Pathol 2006;126(1):101–109.

419. Goldstein M, Meller I, Orr-Urtreger A. FGFR1 over-expression in primary rhabdomyosarcoma tumors is associated with hypomethylation of a 5′ CpG island and abnormal expression of the AKT1, NOG, and BMP4 genes. Genes Chromosomes Cancer 2007;46(11):1028–1038.

420. Zhao X, Weir BA, LaFramboise T, Lin M, Beroukhim R, Garraway L, Beheshti J, Lee JC, Naoki K, Richards WG, Sugarbaker D, Chen F, Rubin MA, Janne PA, Girard L, Minna J, Christiani D, Li C, Sellers WR, Meyerson M. Homozygous deletions and chromosome amplifications in human lung carcinomas revealed by single nucleotide polymorphism array analysis. Cancer Res 2005;65(13):5561–5570.

421. Mao X, Orchard G, Lillington DM, Russell-Jones R, Young BD, Whittaker S. Genetic alterations in primary cutaneous CD30+ anaplastic large cell lymphoma. Genes Chromosomes Cancer 2003;37(2):176–185.

422. Rand V, Huang J, Stockwell T, Ferriera S, Buzko O, Levy S, Busam D, Li K, Edwards JB, Eberhart C, Murphy KM, Tsiamouri A, Beeson K, Simpson AJ, Venter JC, Riggins GJ, Strausberg RL. Sequence survey of receptor tyrosine kinases reveals mutations in glioblastomas. Proc Natl Acad Sci U S A 2005;102(40):14344–14349.

423. Macdonald D, Reiter A, Cross NC. The 8p11 myeloproliferative syndrome: a distinct clinical entity caused by constitutive activation of FGFR1. Acta Haematol 2002;107(2):101–107.

424. Cho K, Ishiwata T, Uchida E, Nakazawa N, Korc M, Naito Z, Tajiri T. Enhanced expression of keratinocyte growth factor and its receptor correlates with venous invasion in pancreatic cancer. Am J Pathol 2007;170(6):1964–1974.

425. Nomura S, Yoshitomi H, Takano S, Shida T, Kobayashi S, Ohtsuka M, Kimura F, Shimizu H, Yoshidome H, Kato A, Miyazaki M. FGF10/FGFR2 signal induces cell migration and invasion in pancreatic cancer. Br J Cancer 2008;99(2):305–313.

426. Takeda M, Arao T, Yokote H, Komatsu T, Yanagihara K, Sasaki H, Yamada Y, Tamura T, Fukuoka K, Kimura H, Saijo N, Nishio K. AZD2171 shows potent antitumor activity against gastric cancer over-expressing fibroblast growth factor receptor 2/keratinocyte growth factor receptor. Clin Cancer Res 2007;13(10):3051–3057.

427. Cha JY, Lambert QT, Reuther GW, Der CJ. Involvement of fibroblast growth factor receptor 2 isoform switching in mammary oncogenesis. Mol Cancer Res 2008;6(3):435–445.

428. Park S, Kim JH, Jang JH. Aberrant hypermethylation of the FGFR2 gene in human gastric cancer cell lines. Biochem Biophys Res Commun 2007;357(4):1011–1015.

429. Zhu X, Lee K, Asa SL, Ezzat S. Epigenetic silencing through DNA and histone methylation of fibroblast growth factor receptor 2 in neoplastic pituitary cells. Am J Pathol 2007;170(5):1618–1628.

430. Finch PW, Rubin JS. Keratinocyte growth factor expression and activity in cancer: implications for use in patients with solid tumors. J Natl Cancer Inst 2006;98(12):812–824.

431. Easton DF, Pooley KA, Dunning AM, Pharoah PD, Thompson D, Ballinger DG, Struewing JP, Morrison J, Field H, Luben R, Wareham N, Ahmed S, Healey CS, Bowman R, Meyer KB, Haiman CA, Kolonel LK, Henderson BE, Le Marchand L, Brennan P, Sangrajrang S, Gaborieau V, Odefrey F, Shen CY, Wu PE, Wang HC, Eccles D, Evans DG, Peto J, Fletcher O, Johnson N, Seal S, Stratton MR, Rahman N, Chenevix-Trench G, Bojesen SE, Nordestgaard BG, Axelsson CK, Garcia-Closas M, Brinton L, Chanock S, Lissowska J, Peplonska B, Nevanlinna H, Fagerholm R, Eerola H, Kang D, Yoo KY, Noh DY, Ahn SH, Hunter DJ, Hankinson SE, Cox DG, Hall P, Wedren S, Liu J, Low YL, Bogdanova N, Schurmann P, Dork T, Tollenaar RA, Jacobi CE, Devilee P, Klijn JG, Sigurdson AJ, Doody MM, Alexander BH, Zhang J, Cox A, Brock IW, MacPherson G, Reed MW, Couch FJ, Goode EL, Olson JE, Meijers-Heijboer H, van den Ouweland A, Uitterlinden A, Rivadeneira F, Milne RL, Ribas G, Gonzalez-Neira A, Benitez J, Hopper JL, McCredie M, Southey M, Giles GG, Schroen C, Justenhoven C, Brauch H, Hamann U, Ko YD, Spurdle AB, Beesley J, Chen X, Mannermaa A, Kosma VM, Kataja V, Hartikainen J, Day NE, Cox DR, Ponder BA. Genome-wide association study identifies novel breast cancer susceptibility loci. Nature 2007;447(7148):1087–1093.

432. Garcia-Closas M, Hall P, Nevanlinna H, Pooley K, Morrison J, Richesson DA, Bojesen SE, Nordestgaard BG, Axelsson CK, Arias JI, Milne RL, Ribas G, Gonzalez-Neira A, Benitez J, Zamora P, Brauch H, Justenhoven C, Hamann U, Ko YD, Bruening T, Haas S, Dork T, Schurmann P, Hillemanns P, Bogdanova N, Bremer M, Karstens JH, Fagerholm R, Aaltonen K, Aittomaki K, Von Smitten K, Blomqvist C, Mannermaa A, Uusitupa M, Eskelinen M, Tengstrom M, Kosma VM, Kataja V, Chenevix-Trench G, Spurdle AB, Beesley J, Chen X, Australian Ovarian Cancer Management Group, Kathleen Cuningham Foundation Consortium for Research into Familial Breast Cancer, Devilee P, Van Asperen CJ, Jacobi CE, Tollenaar RA, Huijts PE, Klijn JG, Chang-Claude J, Kropp S, Slanger T, Flesch-Janys D, Mutschelknauss E, Salazar H, Wang-Gohrke S, Couch F, Goode EL, Olson JE, Vachon C, Fredericksen ZS, Giles GG, Baglietto L, Severi G, Hopper JL, English DR, Southey MC, Haiman CA, Henderson BE, Kolonel LN, Le Marchand L, Stram DO, Hunter DJ, Hankinson SE, Cox DG, Tamimi R, Kraft P, Sherman ME, Chanock SJ, Lissowska J, Brinton LA, Peplonska B, Klijn JG, Hooning MJ, Meijers-Heijboer H, Collee JM, Van den Ouweland A, Uitterlinden AG, Liu J, Lin LY, Yuqing L, Humphreys K, Czene K, Cox A, Balasubramanian SP, Cross SS, Reed MW, Blows F, Driver K, Dunning A, Tyrer J, Ponder BA, Sangrajrang S, Brennan P, McKay J, Odefrey F, Gabrieau V, Sigurdson A, Doody M, Struewing JP, Alexander B, Easton DF, Pharoah PD. Heterogeneity of breast cancer associations with five susceptibility loci by clinical and pathological characteristics. PLoS Genet 2008;4(4):e1000054.

433. Gold B, Kirchhoff T, Stefanov S, Lautenberger J, Viale A, Garber J, Friedman E, Narod S, Olshen AB, Gregersen P, Kosarin K, Olsh A, Bergeron J, Ellis NA, Klein RJ, Clark AG, Norton L, Dean M, Boyd J, Offit K. Genome-wide association study provides evidence for a breast cancer risk locus at 6q22.33. Proc Natl Acad Sci U S A 2008;105(11):4340–4345.

434. Hunter DJ, Kraft P, Jacobs KB, Cox DG, Yeager M, Hankinson SE, Wacholder S, Wang Z, Welch R, Hutchinson A, Wang J, Yu K, Chatterjee N, Orr N, Willett WC, Colditz GA, Ziegler RG, Berg CD, Buys SS, McCarty CA, Feigelson HS, Calle EE, Thun MJ, Hayes RB, Tucker M, Gerhard DS, Fraumeni JF Jr, Hoover RN, Thomas G, Chanock SJ. A genome-wide association study identifies alleles in FGFR2 associated with risk of sporadic postmenopausal breast cancer. Nat Genet 2007;39(7):870–874.

435. Katoh M. Cancer genomics and genetics of FGFR2 (Review). Int J Oncol 2008;33(2):233–237.

436. Meyer KB, Maia AT, O'Reilly M, Teschendorff AE, Chin SF, Caldas C, Ponder BA. Allele-specific up-regulation of FGFR2 increases susceptibility to breast cancer. PLoS Biol 2008;6(5):e108.

437. Raskin L, Pinchev M, Arad C, Lejbkowicz F, Tamir A, Rennert HS, Rennert G, Gruber SB. FGFR2 is a breast cancer susceptibility gene in Jewish and Arab Israeli populations. Cancer Epidemiol Biomarkers Prev 2008;17(5):1060–1065.

438. Stacey SN, Manolescu A, Sulem P, Thorlacius S, Gudjonsson SA, Jonsson GF, Jakobsdottir M, Bergthorsson JT, Gudmundsson J, Aben KK, Strobbe LJ, Swinkels DW, Van Engelenburg KC, Henderson BE, Kolonel LN, Le Marchand L, Millastre E, Andres R, Saez B, Lambea J, Godino J, Polo E, Tres A, Picelli S, Rantala J, Margolin S, Jonsson T, Sigurdsson H, Jonsdottir T, Hrafnkelsson J, Johannsson J, Sveinsson T, Myrdal G, Grimsson HN, Sveinsdottir SG, Alexiusdottir K, Saemundsdottir J, Sigurdsson A, Kostic J, Gudmundsson L, Kristjansson K, Masson G, Fackenthal JD, Adebamowo C, Ogundiran T, Olopade OI, Haiman CA, Lindblom A, Mayordomo JI, Kiemeney LA, Gulcher JR, Rafnar T, Thorsteinsdottir U, Johannsson OT, Kong A, Stefansson K. Common variants on chromosome 5p12 confer susceptibility to estrogen receptor-positive breast cancer. Nat Genet 2008;40(6):703–706.

439. Rouzier C, Soler C, Hofman P, Brennetot C, Bieth E, Pedeutour F. Ovarian dysgerminoma and Apert syndrome. Pediatr Blood Cancer 2007;50(3):696–698.

440. Pollock PM, Gartside MG, Dejeza LC, Powell MA, Mallon MA, Davies H, Mohammadi M, Futreal PA, Stratton MR, Trent JM, Goodfellow PJ. Frequent activating FGFR2 mutations in endometrial carcinomas parallel germline mutations associated with craniosynostosis and skeletal dysplasia syndromes. Oncogene 2007;26(50):7158–7162.

441. Keats JJ, Reiman T, Belch AR, Pilarski LM. Ten years and counting: so what do we know about t(4;14)(p16;q32) multiple myeloma. Leuk Lymphoma 2006;47(11):2289–2300.

442. Intini D, Baldini L, Fabris S, Lombardi L, Ciceri G, Maiolo AT, Neri A. Analysis of FGFR3 gene mutations in multiple myeloma patients with t(4;14). Br J Haematol 2001;114(2):362–364.

443. Tavormina PL, Shiang R, Thompson LM, Zhu YZ, Wilkin DJ, Lachman RS, Wilcox WR, Rimoin DL, Cohn DH, Wasmuth JJ. Thanatophoric dysplasia (types I and II) caused by distinct mutations in fibroblast growth factor receptor 3. Nat Genet 1995;9(3):321–328.

444. Sturla LM, Merrick AE, Burchill SA. FGFR3IIIS: a novel soluble FGFR3 spliced variant that modulates growth is frequently expressed in tumour cells. Br J Cancer 2003;89(7):1276–1284.

445. Penault-Llorca F, Bertucci F, Adelaide J, Parc P, Coulier F, Jacquemier J, Birnbaum D, deLapeyriere O. Expression of FGF and FGF receptor genes in human breast cancer. Int J Cancer 1995;61(2):170–176.

446. Gowardhan B, Douglas DA, Mathers ME, McKie AB, McCracken SR, Robson CN, Leung HY. Evaluation of the fibroblast growth factor system as a potential target for therapy in human prostate cancer. Br J Cancer 2005;92(2):320–327.

447. Shah RN, Ibbitt JC, Alitalo K, Hurst HC. FGFR4 overexpression in pancreatic cancer is mediated by an intronic enhancer activated by HNF1 alpha. Oncogene 2002;21(54):8251–8261.

448. Jaakkola S, Salmikangas P, Nylund S, Partanen J, Armstrong E, Pyrhonen S, Lehtovirta P, Nevanlinna H. Amplification of fgfr4 gene in human breast and gynecological cancers. Int J Cancer 1993;54(3):378–382.

449. Wang J, Stockton DW, Ittmann M. The fibroblast growth factor receptor-4 Arg388 allele is associated with prostate cancer initiation and progression. Clin Cancer Res 2004;10(18Pt 1):6169–6178.

450. Thussbas C, Nahrig J, Streit S, Bange J, Kriner M, Kates R, Ulm K, Kiechle M, Hoefler H, Ullrich A, Harbeck N. FGFR4 Arg388 allele is associated with resistance to adjuvant therapy in primary breast cancer. J Clin Oncol 2006;24(23):3747–3755.

451. Bange J, Prechtl D, Cheburkin Y, Specht K, Harbeck N, Schmitt M, Knyazeva T, Muller S, Gartner S, Sures I, Wang H, Imyanitov E, Haring HU, Knayzev P, Iacobelli S, Hofler H, Ullrich A. Cancer progression and tumor cell motility are associated with the FGFR4 Arg(388) allele. Cancer Res 2002; 62(3):840–847.

452. Morimoto Y, Ozaki T, Ouchida M, Umehara N, Ohata N, Yoshida A, Shimizu K, Inoue H. Single nucleotide polymorphism in fibroblast growth factor receptor 4 at codon 388 is associated with prognosis in high-grade soft tissue sarcoma. Cancer 2003;98(10):2245–2250.

453. Spinola M, Leoni V, Pignatiello C, Conti B, Ravagnani F, Pastorino U, Dragani TA. Functional FGFR4 Gly388Arg polymorphism predicts prognosis in lung adenocarcinoma patients. J Clin Oncol 2005;23(29):7307–7311.

454. Streit S, Bange J, Fichtner A, Ihrler S, Issing W, Ullrich A. Involvement of the FGFR4 Arg388 allele in head and neck squamous cell carcinoma. Int J Cancer 2004;111(2):213–217.

455. Spinola M, Leoni VP, Tanuma J, Pettinicchio A, Frattini M, Signoroni S, Agresti R, Giovanazzi R, Pilotti S, Bertario L, Ravagnani F, Dragani TA. FGFR4 Gly388Arg polymorphism and prognosis of breast and colorectal cancer. Oncol Rep 2005;14(2):415–419.

456. Matakidou A, El Galta R, Rudd MF, Webb EL, Bridle H, Eisen T, Houlston RS. Further observations on the relationship between the FGFR4 Gly388Arg polymorphism and lung cancer prognosis. Br J Cancer 2007;96(12):1904–1907.

457. Jezequel P, Campion L, Joalland MP, Millour M, Dravet F, Classe JM, Delecroix V, Deporte R, Fumoleau P, Ricolleau G. G388R mutation of the FGFR4 gene is not relevant to breast cancer prognosis. Br J Cancer 2004;90(1):189–193.

458. Yang YC, Lu ML, Rao JY, Wallerand H, Cai L, Cao W, Pantuck A, Dalbagni G, Reuter V, Figlin RA, Belldegrun A, Cordon-Cardo C, Zhang ZF. Joint association of polymorphism of the FGFR4 gene and mutation TP53 gene with bladder cancer prognosis. Br J Cancer 2006;95(11):1455–1458.

459. Mawrin C, Kirches E, Diete S, Wiedemann FR, Schneider T, Firsching R, Kropf S, Bogerts B, Vorwerk CK, Kruger S, Dietzmann K. Analysis of a single nucleotide polymorphism in codon 388 of the FGFR4 gene in malignant gliomas. Cancer Lett 2006;239(2):239–245.

460. Streit S, Mestel DS, Schmidt M, Ullrich A, Berking C. FGFR4 Arg388 allele correlates with tumour thickness and FGFR4 protein expression with survival of melanoma patients. Br J Cancer 2006;94(12):1879–1886.

461. Wang J, Yu W, Cai Y, Ren C, Ittmann MM. Altered fibroblast growth factor receptor 4 stability promotes prostate cancer progression. Neoplasia 2008;10(8):847–856.

462. St Bernard R, Zheng L, Liu W, Winer D, Asa SL, Ezzat S. Fibroblast growth factor receptors as molecular targets in thyroid carcinoma. Endocrinology 2005;146(3):1145–1153.

463. Ho HK, Pok S, Streit S, Ruhe JE, Hart S, Lim KS, Loo HL, Aung MO, Lim SG, Ullrich A. Fibroblast growth factor receptor 4 regulates proliferation, anti-apoptosis and alpha-fetoprotein secretion during hepatocellular carcinoma progression and represents a potential target for therapeutic intervention. J Hepatol 2009;50(1):118–127.

464. Desnoyers LR, Pai R, Ferrando RE, Hotzel K, Le T, Ross J, Carano R, D'Souza A, Qing J, Mohtashemi I, Ashkenazi A, French DM. Targeting FGF19 inhibits tumor growth in colon cancer xenograft and FGF19 transgenic hepatocellular carcinoma models. Oncogene 2008;27(1):85–97.

465. Davies H, Hunter C, Smith R, Stephens P, Greenman C, Bignell G, Teague J, Butler A, Edkins S, Stevens C, Parker A, O'Meara S, Avis T, Barthorpe S, Brackenbury L, Buck G, Clements J, Cole J, Dicks E, Edwards K, Forbes S, Gorton M, Gray K, Halliday K, Harrison R, Hills K, Hinton J, Jones D, Kosmidou V, Laman R, Lugg R, Menzies A, Perry J, Petty R, Raine K, Shepherd R, Small A, Solomon H, Stephens Y, Tofts C, Varian J, Webb A, West S, Widaa S, Yates A, Brasseur F, Cooper CS, Flanagan AM, Green A, Knowles M, Leung SY, Looijenga LH, Malkowicz B, Pierotti MA, Teh BT, Yuen ST, Lakhani SR, Easton DF, Weber BL, Goldstraw P, Nicholson AG, Wooster R, Stratton MR, Futreal PA. Somatic mutations of the protein kinase gene family in human lung cancer. Cancer Res 2005;65(17):7591–7595.

466. Besmer P, Murphy JE, George PC, Qiu FH, Bergold PJ, Lederman L, Snyder HW Jr, Brodeur D, Zuckerman EE, Hardy WD. A new acute transforming feline retrovirus and relationship of its oncogene v-kit with the protein kinase gene family. Nature 1986;320(6061):415–421.

467. Hayashi S, Kunisada T, Ogawa M, Yamaguchi K, Nishikawa S. Exon skipping by mutation of an authentic splice site of c-kit gene in W/W mouse. Nucleic Acids Res 1991;19(6):1267–1271.

468. Reith AD, Ellis C, Lyman SD, Anderson DM, Williams DE, Bernstein A, Pawson T. Signal transduction by normal isoforms and W mutant variants of the Kit receptor tyrosine kinase. EMBO J 1991;10(9):2451–2459.

469. Rossi P, Marziali G, Albanesi C, Charlesworth A, Geremia R, Sorrentino V. A novel c-kit transcript, potentially encoding a truncated receptor, originates within a kit gene intron in mouse spermatids. Dev Biol 1992;152(1):203–207.

470. Williams DE, De Vries P, Namen AE, Widmer MB, Lyman SD. The Steel factor. Dev Biol 1992;151(2):368–376.

471. Sattler M, Salgia R. Targeting c-Kit mutations: basic science to novel therapies. Leuk Res 2004;28 (Suppl 1): S11–20.

472. Kitamura Y, Go S, Hatanaka K. Decrease of mast cells in W/Wv mice and their increase by bone marrow transplantation. Blood 1978;52(2):447–452.

473. Kitamura Y, Go S. Decreased production of mast cells in Sl/Sld anemic mice. Blood 1979;53(3):492–497.

474. Kirshenbaum AS, Goff JP, Semere T, Foster B, Scott LM, Metcalfe DD. Demonstration that human mast cells arise from a progenitor cell population that is CD34(+), c-kit(+), and expresses aminopeptidase N (CD13). Blood 1999;94(7):2333–2342.

475. Okayama Y, Kawakami T. Development, migration, and survival of mast cells. Immunol Res 2006;34(2):97–115.

476. Miettinen M, Virolainen M, Maarit Sarlomo R. Gastrointestinal stromal tumors—value of CD34 antigen in their identification and separation from true leiomyomas and schwannomas. Am J Surg Pathol 1995;19(2):207–216.

477. van de Rijn M, Hendrickson MR, Rouse RV. CD34 expression by gastrointestinal tract stromal tumors. Hum Pathol 1994;25(8):766–771.

478. Sakurai S, Fukasawa T, Chong JM, Tanaka A, Fukayama M. Embryonic form of smooth muscle myosin heavy chain (SMemb/MHC-B) in gastrointestinal stromal tumor and interstitial cells of Cajal. Am J Pathol 1999;154(1):23–28.

479. Sarlomo-Rikala M, Tsujimura T, Lendahl U, Miettinen M. Patterns of nestin and other intermediate filament expression distinguish between gastrointestinal stromal tumors, leiomyomas and schwannomas. APMIS 2002;110(6):499–507.

480. Tsujimura T, Makiishi-Shimobayashi C, Lundkvist J, Lendahl U, Nakasho K, Sugihara A, Iwasaki T, Mano M, Yamada N, Yamashita K, Toyosaka A, Terada N. Expression of the intermediate filament nestin in gastrointestinal stromal tumors and interstitial cells of Cajal. Am J Pathol 2001;158(3):817–823.

481. Ward SM, Burns AJ, Torihashi S, Harney SC, Sanders KM. Impaired development of interstitial cells and intestinal electrical rhythmicity in steel mutants. Am J Physiol 1995;269(6Pt 1): C1577–1585.

482. Huizinga JD, Thuneberg L, Kluppel M, Malysz J, Mikkelsen HB, Bernstein A. W/kit gene required for interstitial cells of Cajal and for intestinal pacemaker activity. Nature 1995;373(6512):347–349.

483. Komuro T, Zhou DS. Anti-c-kit protein immunoreactive cells corresponding to the interstitial cells of Cajal in the guinea-pig small intestine. J Auton Nerv Syst 1996;61(2):169–174.

484. Seidal T, Edvardsson H. Expression of c-kit (CD117) and Ki67 provides information about the possible cell of origin and clinical course of gastrointestinal stromal tumours. Histopathology 1999;34(5):416–424.

485. Robinson TL, Sircar K, Hewlett BR, Chorneyko K, Riddell RH, Huizinga JD. Gastrointestinal stromal tumors may originate from a subset of CD34-positive interstitial cells of Cajal. Am J Pathol 2000;156(4):1157–1163.

486. Miettinen M, Sarlomo-Rikala M, Lasota J. Gastrointestinal stromal tumours. Ann Chir Gynaecol 1998;87(4):278–281.

487. Sarlomo-Rikala M, Kovatich AJ, Barusevicius A, Miettinen M. CD117: a sensitive marker for gastrointestinal stromal tumors that is more specific than CD34. Mod Pathol 1998;11(8):728–734.

488. Nishida T, Hirota S, Taniguchi M, Hashimoto K, Isozaki K, Nakamura H, Kanakura Y, Tanaka T, Takabayashi A, Matsuda H, Kitamura Y. Familial gastrointestinal stromal tumours with germline mutation of the KIT gene. Nat Genet 1998;19(4):323–324.

489. Beghini A, Tibiletti MG, Roversi G, Chiaravalli AM, Serio G, Capella C, Larizza L. Germline mutation in the juxtamembrane domain of the kit gene in a family with gastrointestinal stromal tumors and urticaria pigmentosa. Cancer 2001;92(3):657–662.

490. Maeyama H, Hidaka E, Ota H, Minami S, Kajiyama M, Kuraishi A, Mori H, Matsuda Y, Wada S, Sodeyama H, Nakata S, Kawamura N, Hata S, Watanabe M, Iijima Y, Katsuyama T. Familial gastrointestinal stromal tumor with hyperpigmentation: association with a germline mutation of the c-kit gene. Gastroenterology 2001;120(1):210–215.

491. Li FP, Fletcher JA, Heinrich MC, Garber JE, Sallan SE, Curiel-Lewandrowski C, Duensing A, Van de Rijn M, Schnipper LE, Demetri GD. Familial gastrointestinal stromal tumor syndrome: phenotypic and molecular features in a kindred. J Clin Oncol 2005;23(12):2735–2743.

492. Hirota S, Okazaki T, Kitamura Y, O'Brien P, Kapusta L, Dardick I. Cause of familial and multiple gastrointestinal autonomic nerve tumors with hyperplasia of interstitial cells of Cajal is germline mutation of the c-kit gene. Am J Surg Pathol 2000;24(2):326–327.

493. Isozaki K, Terris B, Belghiti J, Schiffmann S, Hirota S, Vanderwinden JM. Germline-activating mutation in the kinase domain of KIT gene in familial gastrointestinal stromal tumors. Am J Pathol 2000;157(5):1581–1585.

494. Akin C. Molecular diagnosis of mast cell disorders: a paper from the 2005 William Beaumont Hospital Symposium on Molecular Pathology. J Mol Diagn 2006;8(4):412–419.

495. Longley BJ, Reguera MJ, Ma Y. Classes of c-KIT activating mutations: proposed mechanisms of action and implications for disease classification and therapy. Leuk Res 2001;25(7):571–576.

496. de Paulis A, Minopoli G, Arbustini E, de Crescenzo G, Dal Piaz F, Pucci P, Russo T, Marone G. Stem cell factor is localized in, released from, and cleaved by human mast cells. J Immunol 1999;163(5):2799–2808.

497. Russell ES. Hereditary anemias of the mouse: a review for geneticists. Adv Genet 1979;20: 357–459.

498. Sekido Y, Obata Y, Ueda R, Hida T, Suyama M, Shimokata K, Ariyoshi Y, Takahashi T. Preferential expression of c-kit protooncogene transcripts in small cell lung cancer. Cancer Res 1991;51(9):2416–2419.

499. DiPaola RS, Kuczynski WI, Onodera K, Ratajczak MZ, Hijiya N, Moore J, Gewirtz AM. Evidence for a functional kit receptor in melanoma, breast, and lung carcinoma cells. Cancer Gene Ther 1997;4(3):176–182.

500. Hida T, Ueda R, Sekido Y, Hibi K, Matsuda R, Ariyoshi Y, Sugiura T, Takahashi T, Takahashi T. Ectopic expression of c-kit in small-cell lung cancer. Int J Cancer Suppl 1994;8: 108–109.

501. Lopez-Martin A, Ballestin C, Garcia-Carbonero R, Castano A, Lopez-Rios F, Lopez-Encuentra A, Sanchez-Cespedes M, Castellano D, Bartolome A, Cortes-Funes H, Paz-Ares L. Prognostic value of KIT expression in small cell lung cancer. Lung Cancer 2007;56(3):405–413.

502. Rehfeld N, Geddert H, Atamna A, Gabbert HE, Steidl U, Fenk R, Kronenwett R, Haas R, Rohr UP. Coexpression of fragile histidine triad and c-kit is relevant for prediction of survival in patients with small cell lung cancer. Cancer Epidemiol Biomarkers Prev 2006;15(11):2232–2238.

503. Camps C, Sirera R, Bremnes RM, Garde J, Safont MJ, Blasco A, Berrocal A, Sanchez JJ, Calabuig C, Martorell M. Analysis of c-kit expression in small cell lung cancer: prevalence and prognostic implications. Lung Cancer 2006;52(3):343–347.

504. Sekido Y, Takahashi T, Ueda R, Takahashi M, Suzuki H, Nishida K, Tsukamoto T, Hida T, Shimokata K, Zsebo KM, et al. Recombinant human stem cell factor mediates chemotaxis of small-cell lung cancer cell lines aberrantly expressing the c-kit protooncogene. Cancer Res 1993;53(7):1709–1714.

505. Nishikawa S, Kusakabe M, Yoshinaga K, Ogawa M, Hayashi S, Kunisada T, Era T, Sakakara T, Nishikawa S. In utero manipulation of coat color formation by a monoclonal anti-c-kit antibody: two distinct waves of c-kit-dependency during melanocyte development. EMBO J 1991;10: 2111–2118.

506. Besmer P. The kit ligand encoded at the murine Steel locus: a pleiotropic growth and differentiation factor. Curr Opin Cell Biol 1991;3: 939–946.

507. Geissler E, Ryan M, Housman D. The dominant-what spotting (W) locus of the mouse encodes the c-kit proto-oncogene. Cell 1988;55: 185–192.

508. Chabot B, Stephenson DA, Chapman VM, Besmer P, Bernstein A. The proto-oncogene c-kit encoding a transmembrane tyrosine kinase receptor maps to the mouse W locus. Nature 1988;335(6185):88–89.

509. Fleischman RA, Saltman DL, Stastny V, Zneimer S. Deletion of the c-kit protooncogene in the human developmental defect piebald trait. Proc Natl Acad Sci U S A 1991;88(23):10885–10889.

510. Montone KT, Van Belle P, Elenitsas R, Elder DE. Proto-oncogene c-kit expression in malignant melanoma: protein loss with tumor progression. Mod Pathol 1997;10(9):939–944.

511. Natali PG, Nicotra MR, Winkler AB, Cavaliere R, Bigotti A, Ullrich A. Progression of human cutaneous melanoma is associated with loss of expression of c-kit proto-oncogene receptor. Int J Cancer 1992;52(2):197–201.

512. Antonescu CR, Busam KJ, Francone TD, Wong GC, Guo T, Agaram NP, Besmer P, Jungbluth A, Gimbel M, Chen CT, Veach D, Clarkson BD, Paty PB, Weiser MR. L576P KIT mutation in anal melanomas correlates with KIT protein expression and is sensitive to specific kinase inhibition. Int J Cancer 2007;121(2):257–264.

513. Curtin JA, Busam K, Pinkel D, Bastian BC. Somatic activation of KIT in distinct subtypes of melanoma. J Clin Oncol 2006;24(26):4340–4346.

514. Gadd SJ, Ashman LK. A murine monoclonal antibody specific for a cell-surface antigen expressed by a subgroup of human myeloid leukaemias. Leuk Res 1985;9(11):1329–1336.

515. Reuss-Borst MA, Buhring HJ, Schmidt H, Muller CA. AML: immunophenotypic heterogeneity and prognostic significance of c-kit expression. Leukemia 1994;8(2):258–263.

516. Beghini A, Ripamonti CB, Cairoli R, Cazzaniga G, Colapietro P, Elice F, Nadali G, Grillo G, Haas OA, Biondi A, Morra E, Larizza L. KIT activating mutations: incidence in adult and pediatric acute myeloid leukemia, and identification of an internal tandem duplication. Haematologica 2004;89(8):920–925.

517. Beghini A, Peterlongo P, Ripamonti CB, Larizza L, Cairoli R, Morra E, Mecucci C. C-kit mutations in core binding factor leukemias. Blood 2000;95(2):726–727.

518. Wang YY, Zhou GB, Yin T, Chen B, Shi JY, Liang WX, Jin XL, You JH, Yang G, Shen ZX, Chen J, Xiong SM, Chen GQ, Xu F, Liu YW, Chen Z, Chen SJ. AML1-ETO and C-KIT mutation/overexpression in t(8;21) leukemia: implication in stepwise leukemogenesis and response to Gleevec. Proc Natl Acad Sci U S A 2005;102(4):1104–1109.

519. Hongyo T, Li T, Syaifudin M, Baskar R, Ikeda H, Kanakura Y, Aozasa K, Nomura T. Specific c-kit mutations in sinonasal natural killer/T-cell lymphoma in China and Japan. Cancer Res 2000;60(9):2345–2347.

520. Hongyo T, Hoshida Y, Nakatsuka S, Syaifudin M, Kojya S, Yang WI, Min YH, Chan H, Kim CH, Harabuchi Y, Himi T, Inuyama M, Aozasa K, Nomura T. p53, K-ras, c-kit and beta-catenin gene mutations in sinonasal NK/T-cell lymphoma in Korea and Japan. Oncol Rep 2005;13(2):265–271.

521. Kurniawan AN, Hongyo T, Hardjolukito ES, Ham MF, Takakuwa T, Kodariah R, Hoshida Y, Nomura T, Aozasa K. Gene mutation analysis of sinonasal lymphomas in Indonesia. Oncol Rep 2006;15(5):1257–1263.

522. Kemmer K, Corless CL, Fletcher JA, McGreevey L, Haley A, Griffith D, Cummings OW, Wait C, Town A, Heinrich MC. KIT mutations are common in testicular seminomas. Am J Pathol 2004;164(1):305–313.

523. Przygodzki RM, Hubbs AE, Zhao FQ, O'Leary TJ. Primary mediastinal seminomas: evidence of single and multiple KIT mutations. Lab Invest 2002;82(10):1369–1375.

524. Brasel K, Escobar S, Anderberg R, de Vries P, Gruss HJ, Lyman SD. Expression of the flt3 receptor and its ligand on hematopoietic cells. Leukemia 1995;9(7):1212–1218.

525. DaSilva N, Hu ZB, Ma W, Rosnet O, Birnbaum D, Drexler HG. Expression of the FLT3 gene in human leukemia-lymphoma cell lines. Leukemia 1994;8(5):885–888.

526. Meierhoff G, Dehmel U, Gruss HJ, Rosnet O, Birnbaum D, Quentmeier H, Dirks W, Drexler HG. Expression of FLT3 receptor and FLT3-ligand in human leukemia-lymphoma cell lines. Leukemia 1995;9(8):1368–1372.

527. Rosnet O, Mattei MG, Marchetto S, Birnbaum D. Isolation and chromosomal localization of a novel FMS-like tyrosine kinase gene. Genomics 1991;9(2):380–385.

528. Lyman SD, James L, Vanden Bos T, de Vries P, Brasel K, Gliniak B, Hollingsworth LT, Picha KS, McKenna HJ, Splett RR, et al. Molecular cloning of a ligand for the flt3/flk-2 tyrosine kinase receptor: a proliferative factor for primitive hematopoietic cells. Cell 1993;75(6):1157–1167.

529. Turner AM, Lin NL, Issarachai S, Lyman SD, Broudy VC. FLT3 receptor expression on the surface of normal and malignant human hematopoietic cells. Blood 1996;88(9):3383–3390.

530. Lyman SD, James L, Johnson L, Brasel K, de Vries P, Escobar SS, Downey H, Splett RR, Beckmann MP, McKenna HJ. Cloning of the human homologue of the murine flt3 ligand: a growth factor for early hematopoietic progenitor cells. Blood 1994;83(10):2795–2801.

531. Hannum C, Culpepper J, Campbell D, McClanahan T, Zurawski S, Bazan JF, Kastelein R, Hudak S, Wagner J, Mattson J, et al. Ligand for FLT3/FLK2 receptor tyrosine kinase regulates growth of haematopoietic stem cells and is encoded by variant RNAs. Nature 1994;368(6472):643–648.

532. Imbert A, Rosnet O, Marchetto S, Ollendorff V, Birnbaum D, Pebusque MJ. Characterization of a yeast artificial chromosome from human chromosome band 13q12 containing the FLT1 and FLT3 receptor-type tyrosine kinase genes. Cytogenet Cell Genet 1994;67(3):175–177.

533. Mackarehtschian K, Hardin JD, Moore KA, Boast S, Goff SP, Lemischka IR. Targeted disruption of the flk2/flt3 gene leads to deficiencies in primitive hematopoietic progenitors. Immunity 1995;3(1):147–161.

534. McKenna HJ, Stocking KL, Miller RE, Brasel K, De Smedt T, Maraskovsky E, Maliszewski CR, Lynch DH, Smith J, Pulendran B, Roux ER, Teepe M, Lyman SD, Peschon JJ. Mice lacking flt3 ligand have deficient hematopoiesis affecting hematopoietic progenitor cells, dendritic cells, and natural killer cells. Blood 2000;95(11):3489–3497.

535. Gabbianelli M, Pelosi E, Montesoro E, Valtieri M, Luchetti L, Samoggia P, Vitelli L, Barberi T, Testa U, Lyman S, et al. Multi-level effects of flt3 ligand on human hematopoiesis: expansion of putative stem cells and proliferation of granulomonocytic progenitors/monocytic precursors. Blood 1995;86(5):1661–1670.

536. Rusten LS, Lyman SD, Veiby OP, Jacobsen SE. The FLT3 ligand is a direct and potent stimulator of the growth of primitive and committed human CD34+ bone marrow progenitor cells in vitro. Blood 1996;87(4):1317–1325.

537. Shah AJ, Smogorzewska EM, Hannum C, Crooks GM. Flt3 ligand induces proliferation of quiescent human bone marrow CD34+CD38− cells and maintains progenitor cells in vitro. Blood 1996;87(9):3563–3570.

538. Ray RJ, Paige CJ, Furlonger C, Lyman SD, Rottapel R. Flt3 ligand supports the differentiation of early B cell progenitors in the presence of interleukin-11 and interleukin-7. Eur J Immunol 1996;26(7):1504–1510.

539. Moore TA, Zlotnik A. Differential effects of Flk-2/Flt-3 ligand and stem cell factor on murine thymic progenitor cells. J Immunol 1997;158(9):4187–4192.

540. Lyman SD, Jacobsen SE. c-kit ligand and Flt3 ligand: stem/progenitor cell factors with overlapping yet distinct activities. Blood 1998;91(4):1101–1134.

541. Horiike S, Yokota S, Nakao M, Iwai T, Sasai Y, Kaneko H, Taniwaki M, Kashima K, Fujii H, Abe T, Misawa S. Tandem duplications of the FLT3 receptor gene are associated with leukemic transformation of myelodysplasia. Leukemia 1997;11(9):1442–1446.

542. Nakao M, Yokota S, Iwai T, Kaneko H, Horiike S, Kashima K, Sonoda Y, Fujimoto T, Misawa S. Internal tandem duplication of the flt3 gene found in acute myeloid leukemia. Leukemia 1996;10(12):1911–1918.

543. Yokota S, Kiyoi H, Nakao M, Iwai T, Misawa S, Okuda T, Sonoda Y, Abe T, Kahsima K, Matsuo Y, Naoe T. Internal tandem duplication of the FLT3 gene is preferentially seen in acute myeloid leukemia and myelodysplastic syndrome among various hematological malignancies. A study on a large series of patients and cell lines. Leukemia 1997;11(10):1605–1609.

544. Yamamoto Y, Kiyoi H, Nakano Y, Suzuki R, Kodera Y, Miyawaki S, Asou N, Kuriyama K, Yagasaki F, Shimazaki C, Akiyama H, Saito K, Nishimura M, Motoji T, Shinagawa K, Takeshita A, Saito H, Ueda R, Ohno R, Naoe T. Activating mutation of D835 within the activation loop of FLT3 in human hematologic malignancies. Blood 2001;97(8):2434–2439.

545. Small D. FLT3 mutations: biology and treatment. Hematology Am Soc Hematol Educ Program 2006: 178–184.

546. Armstrong SA, Mabon ME, Silverman LB, Li A, Gribben JG, Fox EA, Sallan SE, Korsmeyer SJ. FLT3 mutations in childhood acute lymphoblastic leukemia. Blood 2004;103(9):3544–3546.

547. Meshinchi S, Woods WG, Stirewalt DL, Sweetser DA, Buckley JD, Tjoa TK, Bernstein ID, Radich JP. Prevalence and prognostic significance of Flt3 internal tandem duplication in pediatric acute myeloid leukemia. Blood 2001;97(1):89–94.

548. Yoo SJ, Park CJ, Jang S, Seo EJ, Lee KH, Chi HS. Inferior prognostic outcome in acute promyelocytic leukemia with alterations of FLT3 gene. Leuk Lymphoma 2006;47(9):1788–1793.

549. Cloos J, Goemans BF, Hess CJ, Van Oostveen JW, Waisfisz Q, Corthals S, de Lange D, Boeckx N, Hahlen K, Reinhardt D, Creutzig U, Schuurhuis GJ, Zwaan Ch M, Kaspers GJ. Stability and prognostic influence of FLT3 mutations in paired initial and relapsed AML samples. Leukemia 2006;20(7):1217–1220.

550. Georgiou G, Karali V, Zouvelou C, Kyriakou E, Dimou M, Chrisochoou S, Greka P, Dufexis D, Vervesou E, Dimitriadou E, Efthymiou A, Petrikkos L, Dima K, Lilakos K, Panayiotidis P. Serial determination of FLT3 mutations in myelodysplastic syndrome patients at diagnosis, follow up or acute myeloid leukaemia transformation: incidence and their prognostic significance. Br J Haematol 2006;134(3):302–306.

551. Myers SM, Eng C, Ponder BA, Mulligan LM. Characterization of RET proto-oncogene 3′ splicing variants and polyadenylation sites: a novel C-terminus for RET. Oncogene 1995;11(10):2039–2045.

552. Schuchardt A, D'Agati V, Larsson-Blomberg L, Costantini F, Pachnis V. Defects in the kidney and enteric nervous system of mice lacking the tyrosine kinase receptor Ret. Nature 1994;367(6461):380–383.

553. Jain S, Naughton CK, Yang M, Strickland A, Vij K, Encinas M, Golden J, Gupta A, Heuckeroth R, Johnson EM Jr, Milbrandt J. Mice expressing a dominant-negative Ret mutation phenocopy human Hirschsprung disease and delineate a direct role of Ret in spermatogenesis. Development 2004;131(21):5503–5513.

554. Cacalano G, Farinas I, Wang LC, Hagler K, Forgie A, Moore M, Armanini M, Phillips H, Ryan AM, Reichardt LF, Hynes M, Davies A, Rosenthal A. GFR alpha1 is an essential receptor component for GDNF in the developing nervous system and kidney. Neuron 1998;21(1):53–62.

555. Bordeaux MC, Forcet C, Granger L, Corset V, Bidaud C, Billaud M, Bredesen DE, Edery P, Mehlen P. The RET proto-oncogene induces apoptosis: a novel mechanism for Hirschsprung disease. EMBO J 2000;19(15):4056–4063.

556. Veiga-Fernandes H, Coles MC, Foster KE, Patel A, Williams A, Natarajan D, Barlow A, Pachnis V, Kioussis D. Tyrosine kinase receptor RET is a key regulator of Peyer's patch organogenesis. Nature 2007;446(7135):547–551.

557. Airaksinen MS, Saarma M. The GDNF family: signalling, biological functions and therapeutic value. Nat Rev Neurosci 2002;3(5):383–394.

558. Jijiwa M, Fukuda T, Kawai K, Nakamura A, Kurokawa K, Murakumo Y, Ichihara M, Takahashi M. A targeting mutation of tyrosine 1062 in Ret causes a marked decrease of enteric neurons and renal hypoplasia. Mol Cell Biol 2004;24(18):8026–8036.

559. Wong A, Bogni S, Kotka P, de Graaff E, D'Agati V, Costantini F, Pachnis V. Phosphotyrosine 1062 is critical for the in vivo activity of the Ret9 receptor tyrosine kinase isoform. Mol Cell Biol 2005;25(21):9661–9673.

560. Drosten M, Putzer BM. Mechanisms of disease: cancer targeting and the impact of oncogenic RET for medullary thyroid carcinoma therapy. Nat Clin Pract Oncol 2006;3(10):564–574.

561. Besset V, Scott RP, Ibanez CF. Signaling complexes and protein–protein interactions involved in the activation of the Ras and phosphatidylinositol 3-kinase pathways by the c-Ret receptor tyrosine kinase. J Biol Chem 2000;275(50):39159–39166.

562. Hayashi H, Ichihara M, Iwashita T, Murakami H, Shimono Y, Kawai K, Kurokawa K, Murakumo Y, Imai T, Funahashi H, Nakao A, Takahashi M. Characterization of intracellular signals via tyrosine 1062 in RET activated by glial cell line-derived neurotrophic factor. Oncogene 2000;19(39):4469–4475.

563. Murakami H, Yamamura Y, Shimono Y, Kawai K, Kurokawa K, Takahashi M. Role of Dok1 in cell signaling mediated by RET tyrosine kinase. J Biol Chem 2002;277(36):32781–32790.

564. Shi N, Ye S, Bartlam M, Yang M, Wu J, Liu Y, Sun F, Han X, Peng X, Qiang B, Yuan J, Rao Z. Structural basis for the specific recognition of RET by the Dok1 phosphotyrosine binding domain. J Biol Chem 2004;279(6):4962–4969.

565. Schuringa JJ, Wojtachnio K, Hagens W, Vellenga E, Buys CH, Hofstra R, Kruijer W. MEN2A-RET-induced cellular transformation by activation of STAT3. Oncogene 2001;20(38):5350–5358.

566. Borrello MG, Alberti L, Arighi E, Bongarzone I, Battistini C, Bardelli A, Pasini B, Piutti C, Rizzetti MG, Mondellini P, Radice MT, Pierotti MA. The full oncogenic activity of Ret/ptc2 depends on tyrosine 539, a docking site for phospholipase C gamma. Mol Cell Biol 1996;16(5):2151–2163.

567. Bounacer A, Wicker R, Caillou B, Cailleux AF, Sarasin A, Schlumberger M, Suarez HG. High prevalence of activating ret proto-oncogene rearrangements, in thyroid tumors from patients who had received external radiation. Oncogene 1997;15(11):1263–1273.

568. Fugazzola L, Pilotti S, Pinchera A, Vorontsova TV, Mondellini P, Bongarzone I, Greco A, Astakhova L, Butti MG, Demidchik EP, et al. Oncogenic rearrangements of the RET proto-oncogene in papillary thyroid carcinomas from children exposed to the Chernobyl nuclear accident. Cancer Res 1995;55(23):5617–5620.

569. Ito T, Seyama T, Iwamoto KS, Mizuno T, Tronko ND, Komissarenko IV, Cherstovoy ED, Satow Y, Takeichi N, Dohi K, et al. Activated RET oncogene in thyroid cancers of children from areas contaminated by Chernobyl accident. Lancet 1994;344(8917):259.

570. Klugbauer S, Lengfelder E, Demidchik EP, Rabes HM. High prevalence of RET rearrangement in thyroid tumors of children from Belarus after the Chernobyl reactor accident. Oncogene 1995;11(12):2459–2467.

571. Mulligan LM, Kwok JB, Healey CS, Elsdon MJ, Eng C, Gardner E, Love DR, Mole SE, Moore JK, Papi L, et al. Germ-line mutations of the RET proto-oncogene in multiple endocrine neoplasia type 2A. Nature 1993;363(6428):458–460.

572. Hofstra RM, Landsvater RM, Ceccherini I, Stulp RP, Stelwagen T, Luo Y, Pasini B, Hoppener JW, Van Amstel HK, Romeo G, et al. A mutation in the RET proto-oncogene associated with multiple endocrine neoplasia type 2B and sporadic medullary thyroid carcinoma. Nature 1994;367(6461):375–376.

573. Eng C, Clayton D, Schuffenecker I, Lenoir G, Cote G, Gagel RF, Van Amstel HK, Lips CJ, Nishisho I, Takai SI, Marsh DJ, Robinson BG, Frank-Raue K, Raue F, Xue F, Noll WW, Romei C, Pacini F, Fink M, Niederle B, Zedenius J, Nordenskjold M, Komminoth P, Hendy GN, Mulligan LM, et al. The relationship between specific RET proto-oncogene mutations and disease phenotype in multiple endocrine neoplasia type 2. International RET mutation consortium analysis. JAMA 1996;276(19):1575–1579.

574. Asai N, Iwashita T, Matsuyama M, Takahashi M. Mechanism of activation of the ret proto-oncogene by multiple endocrine neoplasia 2A mutations. Mol Cell Biol 1995;15(3):1613–1619.

575. Bocciardi R, Mograbi B, Pasini B, Borrello MG, Pierotti MA, Bourget I, Fischer S, Romeo G, Rossi B. The multiple endocrine neoplasia type 2B point mutation switches the specificity of the Ret tyrosine kinase towards cellular substrates that are susceptible to interact with Crk and Nck. Oncogene 1997;15(19):2257–2265.

576. Santoro M, Carlomagno F, Romano A, Bottaro DP, Dathan NA, Grieco M, Fusco A, Vecchio G, Matoskova B, Kraus MH, et al. Activation of RET as a dominant transforming gene by germline mutations of MEN2A and MEN2B. Science 1995;267(5196):381–383.

577. Salvatore D, Melillo RM, Monaco C, Visconti R, Fenzi G, Vecchio G, Fusco A, Santoro M. Increased in vivo phosphorylation of ret tyrosine 1062 is a potential pathogenetic mechanism of multiple endocrine neoplasia type 2B. Cancer Res 2001;61(4):1426–1431.

578. Arighi E, Borrello MG, Sariola H. RET tyrosine kinase signaling in development and cancer. Cytokine Growth Factor Rev 2005;16(4–5):441–467.

579. Cooper CS, Park M, Blair DG, Tainsky MA, Huebner K, Croce CM, Vande Woude GF. Molecular cloning of a new transforming gene from a chemically transformed human cell line. Nature 1984;311(5981):29–33.

580. Liu Y. The human hepatocyte growth factor receptor gene: complete structural organization and promoter characterization. Gene 1998;215(1):159–169.

581. Sachs M, Weidner KM, Brinkmann V, Walther I, Obermeier A, Ullrich A, Birchmeier W. Motogenic and morphogenic activity of epithelial receptor tyrosine kinases. J Cell Biol 1996;133(5):1095–1107.

582. Sachs M, Brohmann H, Zechner D, Muller T, Hulsken J, Walther I, Schaeper U, Birchmeier C, Birchmeier W. Essential role of Gab1 for signaling by the c-Met receptor in vivo. J Cell Biol 2000;150(6):1375–1384.

583. Maroun CR, Holgado-Madruga M, Royal I, Naujokas MA, Fournier TM, Wong AJ, Park M. The Gab1PH domain is required for localization of Gab1 at sites of cell–cell contact and epithelial morphogenesis downstream from the met receptor tyrosine kinase. Mol Cell Biol 1999;19(3):1784–1799.

584. Birchmeier C, Birchmeier W, Gherardi E, Vande Woude GF. Met, metastasis, motility and more. Nat Rev Mol Cell Biol 2003;4(12):915–925.

585. Hammond DE, Urbe S, Vande Woude GF, Clague MJ. Down-regulation of MET, the receptor for hepatocyte growth factor. Oncogene 2001;20(22):2761–2770.

586. Jeffers M, Taylor GA, Weidner KM, Omura S, Vande Woude GF. Degradation of the Met tyrosine kinase receptor by the ubiquitin–proteasome pathway. Mol Cell Biol 1997;17(2):799–808.

587. Peschard P, Fournier TM, Lamorte L, Naujokas MA, Band H, Langdon WY, Park M. Mutation of the c-Cbl TKB domain binding site on the Met receptor tyrosine kinase converts it into a transforming protein. Mol Cell 2001;8(5):995–1004.

588. Potempa S, Ridley AJ. Activation of both MAP kinase and phosphatidylinositide 3-kinase by Ras is required for hepatocyte growth factor/scatter factor-induced adherens junction disassembly. Mol Biol Cell 1998;9(8):2185–2200.

589. Ridley AJ, Comoglio PM, Hall A. Regulation of scatter factor/hepatocyte growth factor responses by Ras, Rac, and Rho in MDCK cells. Mol Cell Biol 1995;15(2):1110–1122.

590. Lock LS, Royal I, Naujokas MA, Park M. Identification of an atypical Grb2 carboxyl-terminal SH3 domain binding site in Gab docking proteins reveals Grb2-dependent and -independent recruitment of Gab1 to receptor tyrosine kinases. J Biol Chem 2000;275(40):31536–31545.

591. Sakkab D, Lewitzky M, Posern G, Schaeper U, Sachs M, Birchmeier W, Feller SM. Signaling of hepatocyte growth factor/scatter factor (HGF) to the small GTPase Rap1 via the large docking protein Gab1 and the adapter protein CRKL. J Biol Chem 2000;275(15):10772–10778.

592. Lamorte L, Kamikura DM, Park M. A switch from p130Cas/Crk to Gab1/Crk signaling correlates with anchorage independent growth and JNK activation in cells transformed by the Met receptor oncoprotein. Oncogene 2000;19(52):5973–5981.

593. Di Renzo MF, Olivero M, Martone T, Maffe A, Maggiora P, Stefani AD, Valente G, Giordano S, Cortesina G, Comoglio PM. Somatic mutations of the MET oncogene are selected during metastatic spread of human HNSC carcinomas. Oncogene 2000;19(12):1547–1555.

594. Xiao GH, Jeffers M, Bellacosa A, Mitsuuchi Y, Vande Woude GF, Testa JR. Anti-apoptotic signaling by hepatocyte growth factor/Met via the phosphatidylinositol 3-kinase/Akt and mitogen-activated protein kinase pathways. Proc Natl Acad Sci U S A 2001;98(1):247–252.

595. Hartmann G, Weidner KM, Schwarz H, Birchmeier W. The motility signal of scatter factor/hepatocyte growth factor mediated through the receptor tyrosine kinase met requires intracellular action of Ras. J Biol Chem 1994;269(35):21936–21939.

596. Khwaja A, Lehmann K, Marte BM, Downward J. Phosphoinositide 3-kinase induces scattering and tubulogenesis in epithelial cells through a novel pathway. J Biol Chem 1998;273(30):18793–18801.

597. Royal I, Lamarche-Vane N, Lamorte L, Kaibuchi K, Park M. Activation of cdc42, rac, PAK, and rho-kinase in response to hepatocyte growth factor differentially regulates epithelial cell colony spreading and dissociation. Mol Biol Cell 2000;11(5):1709–1725.

598. Weidner KM, Di Cesare S, Sachs M, Brinkmann V, Behrens J, Birchmeier W. Interaction between Gab1 and the c-Met receptor tyrosine kinase is responsible for epithelial morphogenesis. Nature 1996;384(6605):173–176.

599. Schaeper U, Gehring NH, Fuchs KP, Sachs M, Kempkes B, Birchmeier W. Coupling of Gab1 to c-Met, Grb2, and Shp2 mediates biological responses. J Cell Biol 2000;149(7):1419–1432.

600. Longati P, Comoglio PM, Bardelli A. Receptor tyrosine kinases as therapeutic targets: the model of the MET oncogene. Curr Drug Targets 2001;2(1):41–55.

601. Pennacchietti S, Michieli P, Galluzzo M, Mazzone M, Giordano S, Comoglio PM. Hypoxia promotes invasive growth by transcriptional activation of the met protooncogene. Cancer Cell 2003;3(4):347–361.

602. Bottaro DP, Liotta LA. Cancer: out of air is not out of action. Nature 2003;423(6940):593–595.

603. Gerritsen ME, Tomlinson JE, Zlot C, Ziman M, Hwang S. Using gene expression profiling to identify the molecular basis of the synergistic actions of hepatocyte growth factor and vascular endothelial growth factor in human endothelial cells. Br J Pharmacol 2003;140(4):595–610.

604. Xin X, Yang S, Ingle G, Zlot C, Rangell L, Kowalski J, Schwall R, Ferrara N, Gerritsen ME. Hepatocyte growth factor enhances vascular endothelial growth factor-induced angiogenesis in vitro and in vivo. Am J Pathol 2001;158(3):1111–1120.

605. Cheng N, Bhowmick NA, Chytil A, Gorksa AE, Brown KA, Muraoka R, Arteaga CL, Neilson EG, Hayward SW, Moses HL. Loss of TGF-beta type II receptor in fibroblasts promotes mammary

carcinoma growth and invasion through upregulation of TGF-alpha-, MSP- and HGF-mediated signaling networks. Oncogene 2005;24(32):5053–5068.

606. Cheng N, Chytil A, Shyr Y, Joly A, Moses HL. Enhanced hepatocyte growth factor signaling by type II transforming growth factor-beta receptor knockout fibroblasts promotes mammary tumorigenesis. Cancer Res 2007;67(10):4869–4877.

607. Engelman JA, Zejnullahu K, Mitsudomi T, Song Y, Hyland C, Park JO, Lindeman N, Gale CM, Zhao X, Christensen J, Kosaka T, Holmes AJ, Rogers AM, Cappuzzo F, Mok T, Lee C, Johnson BE, Cantley LC, Janne PA. MET amplification leads to gefitinib resistance in lung cancer by activating ERBB3 signaling. Science 2007;316(5827):1039–1043.

608. Bean J, Brennan C, Shih JY, Riely G, Viale A, Wang L, Chitale D, Motoi N, Szoke J, Broderick S, Balak M, Chang WC, Yu CJ, Gazdar A, Pass H, Rusch V, Gerald W, Huang SF, Yang PC, Miller V, Ladanyi M, Yang CH, Pao W. MET amplification occurs with or without T790M mutations in EGFR mutant lung tumors with acquired resistance to gefitinib or erlotinib. Proc Natl Acad Sci U S A 2007;104(52):20932–20937.

609. Mak HH, Peschard P, Lin T, Naujokas MA, Zuo D, Park M. Oncogenic activation of the Met receptor tyrosine kinase fusion protein, Tpr-Met, involves exclusion from the endocytic degradative pathway. Oncogene 2007;26(51):7213–7221.

610. Heideman DA, Snijders PJ, Bloemena E, Meijer CJ, Offerhaus GJ, Meuwissen SG, Gerritsen WR, Craanen ME. Absence of tpr-met and expression of c-met in human gastric mucosa and carcinoma. J Pathol 2001;194(4):428–435.

611. Osaki M, Miyata H, Hayashi A, Gomyo Y, Tatebe S, Ito H. Lack of rearranged Tpr-met mRNA expression in human gastric cancer cell lines and gastric mucosa and carcinoma. Anticancer Res 1996;16(5A):2881–2884.

612. Soman NR, Correa P, Ruiz BA, Wogan GN. The TPR-MET oncogenic rearrangement is present and expressed in human gastric carcinoma and precursor lesions. Proc Natl Acad Sci U S A 1991;88(11):4892–4896.

613. Yu J, Miehlke S, Ebert MP, Hoffmann J, Breidert M, Alpen B, Starzynska T, Stolte PM, Malfertheiner P, Bayerdorffer E. Frequency of TPR-MET rearrangement in patients with gastric carcinoma and in first-degree relatives. Cancer 2000;88(8):1801–1806.

614. Kuniyasu H, Yasui W, Kitadai Y, Yokozaki H, Ito H, Tahara E. Frequent amplification of the c-met gene in scirrhous type stomach cancer. Biochem Biophys Res Commun 1992;189(1):227–232.

615. Tsujimoto H, Sugihara H, Hagiwara A, Hattori T. Amplification of growth factor receptor genes and DNA ploidy pattern in the progression of gastric cancer. Virchows Arch 1997;431(6):383–389.

616. Hara T, Ooi A, Kobayashi M, Mai M, Yanagihara K, Nakanishi I. Amplification of c-myc, K-sam, and c-met in gastric cancers: detection by fluorescence *in situ* hybridization. Lab Invest 1998;78(9):1143–1153.

617. Miller CT, Lin L, Casper AM, Lim J, Thomas DG, Orringer MB, Chang AC, Chambers AF, Giordano TJ, Glover TW, Beer DG. Genomic amplification of MET with boundaries within fragile site FRA7G and upregulation of MET pathways in esophageal adenocarcinoma. Oncogene 2006;25(3):409–418.

618. Schmidt L, Duh FM, Chen F, Kishida T, Glenn G, Choyke P, Scherer SW, Zhuang Z, Lubensky I, Dean M, Allikmets R, Chidambaram A, Bergerheim UR, Feltis JT, Casadevall C, Zamarron A, Bernues M, Richard S, Lips CJ, Walther MM, Tsui LC, Geil L, Orcutt ML, Stackhouse T, Lipan J, Slife L, Brauch H, Decker J, Niehans G, Hughson MD, Moch H, Storkel S, Lerman MI, Linehan WM, Zbar B. Germline and somatic mutations in the tyrosine kinase domain of the MET proto-oncogene in papillary renal carcinomas. Nat Genet 1997;16(1):68–73.

619. Park WS, Dong SM, Kim SY, Na EY, Shin MS, Pi JH, Kim BJ, Bae JH, Hong YK, Lee KS, Lee SH, Yoo NJ, Jang JJ, Pack S, Zhuang Z, Schmidt L, Zbar B, Lee JY. Somatic mutations in the kinase domain of the Met/hepatocyte growth factor receptor gene in childhood hepatocellular carcinomas. Cancer Res 1999;59(2):307–310.

620. Takaki Y, Furihata M, Yoshikawa C, Kishida T, Yao M, Shuin T. Sporadic bilateral papillary renal carcinoma exhibiting C-met mutation in the left kidney tumor. J Urol 2000;163(4):1241–1242.

621. Zhuang Z, Park WS, Pack S, Schmidt L, Vortmeyer AO, Pak E, Pham T, Weil RJ, Candidus S, Lubensky IA, Linehan WM, Zbar B, Weirich G. Trisomy 7-harbouring non-random duplication of the mutant MET allele in hereditary papillary renal carcinomas. Nat Genet 1998;20(1):66–69.

622. Ma PC, Kijima T, Maulik G, Fox EA, Sattler M, Griffin JD, Johnson BE, Salgia R. c-MET mutational analysis in small cell lung cancer: novel juxtamembrane domain mutations regulating cytoskeletal functions. Cancer Res 2003;63(19):6272–6281.

623. Ma PC, Jagadeeswaran R, Jagadeesh S, Tretiakova MS, Nallasura V, Fox EA, Hansen M, Schaefer E, Naoki K, Lader A, Richards W, Sugarbaker D, Husain AN, Christensen JG, Salgia R. Functional expression and mutations of c-Met and its therapeutic inhibition with SU11274 and small interfering RNA in non-small cell lung cancer. Cancer Res 2005;65(4):1479–1488.

624. Lee JH, Han SU, Cho H, Jennings B, Gerrard B, Dean M, Schmidt L, Zbar B, Vande Woude GF. A novel germ line juxtamembrane Met mutation in human gastric cancer. Oncogene 2000;19(43):4947–4953.

625. Tanyi J, Tory K, Rigo J Jr, Nagy B, Papp Z. Evaluation of the tyrosine kinase domain of the Met proto-oncogene in sporadic ovarian carcinomas. Pathol Oncol Res 1999;5(3):187–191.

626. Moon YW, Weil RJ, Pack SD, Park WS, Pak E, Pham T, Karkera JD, Kim HK, Vortmeyer AO, Fuller BG, Zhuang Z. Missense mutation of the MET gene detected in human glioma. Mod Pathol 2000;13(9):973–977.

627. Lorenzato A, Olivero M, Patane S, Rosso E, Oliaro A, Comoglio PM, Di Renzo MF. Novel somatic mutations of the MET oncogene in human carcinoma metastases activating cell motility and invasion. Cancer Res 2002;62(23):7025–7030.

628. Aebersold DM, Landt O, Berthou S, Gruber G, Beer KT, Greiner RH, Zimmer Y. Prevalence and clinical impact of Met Y1253D-activating point mutation in radiotherapy-treated squamous cell cancer of the oropharynx. Oncogene 2003;22(52):8519–8523.

629. Bieche I, Champeme MH, Lidereau R. Infrequent mutations of the MET gene in sporadic breast tumours. Int J Cancer 1999;82(6):908–910.

630. Puri N, Ahmed S, Janamanchi V, Tretiakova M, Zumba O, Krausz T, Jagadeeswaran R, Salgia R. c-Met is a potentially new therapeutic target for treatment of human melanoma. Clin Cancer Res 2007;13(7):2246–2253.

631. Jagadeeswaran R, Ma PC, Seiwert TY, Jagadeeswaran S, Zumba O, Nallasura V, Ahmed S, Filiberti R, Paganuzzi M, Puntoni R, Kratzke RA, Gordon GJ, Sugarbaker DJ, Bueno R, Janamanchi V, Bindokas VP, Kindler HL, Salgia R. Functional analysis of c-Met/hepatocyte growth factor pathway in malignant pleural mesothelioma. Cancer Res 2006;66(1):352–361.

632. Ronsin C, Muscatelli F, Mattei MG, Breathnach R. A novel putative receptor protein tyrosine kinase of the met family. Oncogene 1993;8(5):1195–1202.

633. Zabarovsky ER, Lerman MI, Minna JD. Tumor suppressor genes on chromosome 3p involved in the pathogenesis of lung and other cancers. Oncogene 2002;21(45):6915–6935.

634. Gaudino G, Follenzi A, Naldini L, Collesi C, Santoro M, Gallo KA, Godowski PJ, Comoglio PM. RON is a heterodimeric tyrosine kinase receptor activated by the HGF homologue MSP. EMBO J 1994;13(15):3524–3532.

635. Angeloni D, Danilkovitch-Miagkova A, Miagkov A, Leonard EJ, Lerman MI. The soluble sema domain of the RON receptor inhibits macrophage-stimulating protein-induced receptor activation. J Biol Chem 2004;279(5):3726–3732.

636. Comoglio PM, Tamagnone L, Boccaccio C. Plasminogen-related growth factor and semaphorin receptors: a gene superfamily controlling invasive growth. Exp Cell Res 1999;253(1):88–99.

637. Yoshimura T, Yuhki N, Wang MH, Skeel A, Leonard EJ. Cloning, sequencing, and expression of human macrophage stimulating protein (MSP, MST1) confirms MSP as a member of the family of kringle proteins and locates the MSP gene on chromosome 3. J Biol Chem 1993;268(21):15461–15468.

638. Wang MH, Ronsin C, Gesnel MC, Coupey L, Skeel A, Leonard EJ, Breathnach R. Identification of the ron gene product as the receptor for the human macrophage stimulating protein. Science 1994;266(5182):117–119.

639. Hughes AL. Modes of evolution in the protease and kringle domains of the plasminogen-prothrombin family. Mol Phylogenet Evol 2000;14(3):469–478.

640. Leonard EJ, Danilkovitch A. Macrophage stimulating protein. Adv Cancer Res 2000;77: 139–167.

641. Skeel A, Leonard EJ. Alpha 1-antichymotrypsin is the human plasma inhibitor of macrophage ectoenzymes that cleave pro-macrophage stimulating protein. J Biol Chem 2001;276(24):21932–21937.

642. Chen YQ, Fisher JH, Wang MH. Activation of the RON receptor tyrosine kinase inhibits inducible nitric oxide synthase (iNOS) expression by murine peritoneal exudate macrophages: phosphatidylinositol-3 kinase is required for RON-mediated inhibition of iNOS expression. J Immunol 1998;161(9):4950–4959.

643. Zhou YQ, Chen YQ, Fisher JH, Wang MH. Activation of the RON receptor tyrosine kinase by macrophage-stimulating protein inhibits inducible cyclooxygenase-2 expression in murine macrophages. J Biol Chem 2002;277(41):38104–38110.

644. Wang MH, Dlugosz AA, Sun Y, Suda T, Skeel A, Leonard EJ. Macrophage-stimulating protein induces proliferation and migration of murine keratinocytes. Exp Cell Res 1996;226(1):39–46.

645. Danilkovitch-Miagkova A. Oncogenic signaling pathways activated by RON receptor tyrosine kinase. Curr Cancer Drug Targets 2003;3(1):31–40.

646. Penengo L, Rubin C, Yarden Y, Gaudino G. c-Cbl is a critical modulator of the Ron tyrosine kinase receptor. Oncogene 2003;22(24):3669–3679.

647. Chan EL, Peace BE, Collins MH, Toney-Earley K, Waltz SE. Ron tyrosine kinase receptor regulates papilloma growth and malignant conversion in a murine model of skin carcinogenesis. Oncogene 2005;24(3):479–488.

648. Chen Q, Seol DW, Carr B, Zarnegar R. Co-expression and regulation of Met and Ron proto-oncogenes in human hepatocellular carcinoma tissues and cell lines. Hepatology 1997;26(1):59–66.

649. Cheng HL, Liu HS, Lin YJ, Chen HH, Hsu PY, Chang TY, Ho CL, Tzai TS, Chow NH. Co-expression of RON and MET is a prognostic indicator for patients with transitional-cell carcinoma of the bladder. Br J Cancer 2005;92(10):1906–1914.

650. Collesi C, Santoro MM, Gaudino G, Comoglio PM. A splicing variant of the RON transcript induces constitutive tyrosine kinase activity and an invasive phenotype. Mol Cell Biol 1996;16(10):5518–5526.

651. Leo C, Horn LC, Einenkel J, Hentschel B, Hockel M. Tumor hypoxia and expression of c-met in cervical cancer. Gynecol Oncol 2007;104(1):181–185.

652. Lin HS, Berry GJ, Fee WE Jr, Terris DJ, Sun Z. Identification of tyrosine kinases overexpressed in head and neck cancer. Arch Otolaryngol Head Neck Surg 2004;130(3):311–316.

653. Maggiora P, Lorenzato A, Fracchioli S, Costa B, Castagnaro M, Arisio R, Katsaros D, Massobrio M, Comoglio PM, Flavia Di Renzo M. The RON and MET oncogenes are co-expressed in human ovarian carcinomas and cooperate in activating invasiveness. Exp Cell Res 2003;288(2):382–389.

654. Maggiora P, Marchio S, Stella MC, Giai M, Belfiore A, De Bortoli M, Di Renzo MF, Costantino A, Sismondi P, Comoglio PM. Overexpression of the RON gene in human breast carcinoma. Oncogene 1998;16(22):2927–2933.

655. Rampino T, Gregorini M, Soccio G, Maggio M, Rosso R, Malvezzi P, Collesi C, Dal Canton A. The Ron proto-oncogene product is a phenotypic marker of renal oncocytoma. Am J Surg Pathol 2003;27(6):779–785.

656. Thomas RM, Toney K, Fenoglio-Preiser C, Revelo-Penafiel MP, Hingorani SR, Tuveson DA, Waltz SE, Lowy AM. The RON receptor tyrosine kinase mediates oncogenic phenotypes in pancreatic cancer cells and is increasingly expressed during pancreatic cancer progression. Cancer Res 2007;67(13):6075–6082.

657. Wang MH, Lee W, Luo YL, Weis MT, Yao HP. Altered expression of the RON receptor tyrosine kinase in various epithelial cancers and its contribution to tumourigenic phenotypes in thyroid cancer cells. J Pathol 2007;213(4):402–411.

658. Peace BE, Hughes MJ, Degen SJ, Waltz SE. Point mutations and overexpression of Ron induce transformation, tumor formation, and metastasis. Oncogene 2001;20(43):6142–6151.

659. Santoro MM, Penengo L, Minetto M, Orecchia S, Cilli M, Gaudino G. Point mutations in the tyrosine kinase domain release the oncogenic and metastatic potential of the Ron receptor. Oncogene 1998;17(6):741–749.

660. Okino T, Egami H, Ohmachi H, Takai E, Tamori Y, Nakagawa K, Nakano S, Akagi J, Sakamoto O, Suda T, Ogawa M. Presence of RON receptor tyrosine kinase and its splicing variant in malignant and non-malignant human colonic mucosa. Int J Oncol 1999;15(4):709–714.

661. Angeloni D, Danilkovitch-Miagkova A, Ivanov SV, Breathnach R, Johnson BE, Leonard EJ, Lerman MI. Gene structure of the human receptor tyrosine kinase RON and mutation analysis in lung cancer samples. Genes Chromosomes Cancer 2000;29(2):147–156.

662. Bardella C, Costa B, Maggiora P, Patane S, Olivero M, Ranzani GN, De Bortoli M, Comoglio PM, Di Renzo MF. Truncated RON tyrosine kinase drives tumor cell progression and abrogates cell–cell adhesion through E-cadherin transcriptional repression. Cancer Res 2004;64(15):5154–5161.

663. Wang MH, Wang D, Chen YQ. Oncogenic and invasive potentials of human macrophage-stimulating protein receptor, the RON receptor tyrosine kinase. Carcinogenesis 2003;24(8):1291–1300.

664. Chen YQ, Zhou YQ, Angeloni D, Kurtz AL, Qiang XZ, Wang MH. Overexpression and activation of the RON receptor tyrosine kinase in a panel of human colorectal carcinoma cell lines. Exp Cell Res 2000;261(1):229–238.

665. Wang MH, Kurtz AL, Chen Y. Identification of a novel splicing product of the RON receptor tyrosine kinase in human colorectal carcinoma cells. Carcinogenesis 2000;21(8):1507–1512.

666. Zhou YQ, He C, Chen YQ, Wang D, Wang MH. Altered expression of the RON receptor tyrosine kinase in primary human colorectal adenocarcinomas: generation of different splicing RON variants and their oncogenic potential. Oncogene 2003;22(2):186–197.

667. Peace BE, Toney-Earley K, Collins MH, Waltz SE. Ron receptor signaling augments mammary tumor formation and metastasis in a murine model of breast cancer. Cancer Res 2005;65(4):1285–1293.

668. O'Toole JM, Rabenau KE, Burns K, Lu D, Mangalampalli V, Balderes P, Covino N, Bassi R, Prewett M, Gottfredsen KJ, Thobe MN, Cheng Y, Li Y, Hicklin DJ, Zhu Z, Waltz SE, Hayman MJ, Ludwig DL, Pereira DS. Therapeutic implications of a human neutralizing antibody to the macrophage-stimulating protein receptor tyrosine kinase (RON), a c-MET family member. Cancer Res 2006;66(18):9162–9170.

NONRECEPTOR TYROSINE KINASES

THE NONRECEPTOR tyrosine kinases represent the second broad subdivision of the tyrosine kinase family. Although fewer in number than their membrane-bound cousins, these also fulfill important roles in intracellular signaling and their dysregulation underlies a number of pathologies, including multiple types of neoplasia. Indeed, the first targeted kinase inhibitor to achieve success in the clinic—imatinib mesylate (Gleevec®)—is an inhibitor of the ABL nonreceptor tyrosine kinase. Nonreceptor tyrosine kinases have no transmembrane or extracellular domains but are often closely associated with signaling at the plasma membrane. For example, SRC is associated with membrane lipids via myristoylation and signals in concert with many other plasma membrane receptors; JAK2 is a proximal effector of growth factor cytokine receptors, and FAK is an important mediator of integrin receptor signaling.

Members of the ABL family of kinases (ABL, ARG), the SRC family (SRC, YES, FYN, LYN, LCK, BLK, HCK, FGR, YRK), and the TEC family (BTK, ITK, TEC, BMX, TXK) have a similar domain organization (Figure 4.1). All of these proteins have a tyrosine kinase domain that is preceded by a SRC homology 2 (SH2) domain and a SH3 domain, conserved in both sequence identity and also in arrangement and spacing. SH2 domains are structurally conserved protein motifs that typically bind to a phosphorylated tyrosine residue. SH3 domains are conserved motifs of roughly 60 aa that usually play a role in the assembly of protein complexes. Classically, SH3 domains bind to proline-rich regions in their respective binding protein partners. In the case of ABL, the SH2 and SH3 domains assemble through intramolecular interactions and generate an autoinhibited conformation. The C-terminal region of ABL distinguishes it from the SRC and TEC family members and contains three nuclear localization signals (NLSs), a nuclear export signal (NES), as well as binding sites for G- and F-actin and a binding site for double stranded A/T-rich DNA. The last exon region encodes proline-rich motifs that function as binding sites for the SH3 domains of

Targeting Protein Kinases for Cancer Therapy, by David J. Matthews and Mary E. Gerritsen Copyright © 2010 John Wiley & Sons, Inc.

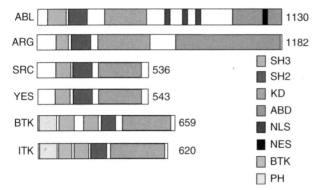

Figure 4.1 Domain organization of representative members of the ABL family (ABL, ARG) of kinases, the SRC family (SRC, YES) of kinases, and the TEC family (BTK and ITK). All of the proteins have a tyrosine kinase domain (cyan) preceded by an SH2 domain (pink) and a SH3 domain (green). Members of the ABL family have an actin binding domain (orange), and ABL is further distinguished by having NLS signals (blue rectangles) and nuclear export signals in the C-terminal domain. Members of the TEC family have a BTK (Bruton's tyrosine kinase) domain (brown) and a pleckstrin homology domain (yellow) in the N-terminal region.

the adaptor proteins CRK, GRB2, and NCK. There are also binding sites for ATM, p53, Rb, and the carboxy-terminal domain of RNA polymerase II.

4.1   ABL

ABL, an ubiquitiously expressed tyrosine kinase, plays a number of diverse roles in transducing cell extrinisic and intrinsic signals, including those from growth factors, integrins, inflammatory cytokines, oxidative stress, and DNA damage. When activated, ABL regulates cytoskeletal function, progression through the cell cycle, myogenic differentiation, and cell death. This enzyme is highly regulated, at the level of both activity and cellular localization. It is found in multiple cellular compartments, including the nucleus and cytoplasm and associated with the plasma membrane, and in each of these compartments it appears to play a distinct role.

The *ABL* gene is about 225 kb in length and is located on 9q34.1. It is expressed as either a 6- or 7-kb mRNA transcript. Two alternatively spliced forms occur, due to splicing variants in the first exon: exon 1b is found about 200 kb 5′ of exon 1a. Exons 2–11 are common to both forms. When the N-terminal region of ABL is encoded by exon 1a, the protein localizes to the nucleus. Alternatively, the 1b form results in a protein with an N-terminal glycine that can be myristoylated. This form is thought to localize to the plasma membrane.

The tyrosine kinase activity of ABL is very tightly controlled, probably because of its potentially deleterious effects. It is now generally accepted that the ABL kinase domain is under repression by an intramolecular mechanism. This inhibition is intrinsic and does not require any particular cellular inhibitor (1). ABL has an N-terminal cap that appears to bind at several regions across the molecule, stabilizing the regulated, inhibited conformation. Based on similarities to SRC (see later discussion) Pluk et al. (1) proposed that the KV/LV/LG motif, common to both the 1a and 1b exons of ABL and required for binding, undergoes strong interaction with the catalytic domain. The proximal portion of the common second exon interacts with the SH3 and/or SH2 domains, but not the catalytic domain. Pluk and co-workers further proposed that cellular proteins may regulate ABL activity by favoring or displacing any of the several intramolecular interactions. The first exon region of ABL is missing in all of the known fusion proteins formed with BCR or TEL (discussed later).

ABL is now known to shuttle between the cytoplasm and nucleus, using classical mechanisms that involve the NLS and NES sequences (2, 3). In fibroblasts, cell adhesion regulates the kinase activity and subcellular localization of ABL. When fibroblasts are detached from the extracellular matrix, kinase activity of both cytoplasmic and nuclear ABL decreases, but there is no detectable alteration in the subcellular distribution. Upon adhesion to the extracellular matrix protein fibronectin, there is a transient recruitment of a subset of ABL to early focal contacts coincident with ABL export from the nucleus to the cytoplasm. The cytoplasmic pool of ABL is reactivated within 5 minutes of adhesion, but the nuclear ABL is reactivated after 30 minutes, correlating closely with its return to the nucleus and suggesting that the active nuclear ABL originates in the cytoplasm (4). The NLSs appear to function differently in different cell types and also exhibit overlapping and redundant functions. In fibroblasts, the presence of any one of the NLS domains is sufficient to localize ABL to the nucleus. However, the accumulation of ABL in the nucleus is balanced by the NES, which interacts with CRM1/Exportin1, and mediates the translocation of ABL to the cytoplasm. Treatment of cells with LMB results in the nuclear accumulation of ABL (2). Vella and co-workers (5) generated ABL proteins that were exclusively cytoplasmic (NLS-mutated), exclusively nuclear (Nuk), or shuttling, using an inducible dimerization strategy to activate the ABL proteins. Previous work by this group had shown that when expressed in an appropriate cell context, dimerization of wild-type ABL or ABL-Nuk was sufficient to activate apoptosis; however, dimerization of cytoplasmic ABL does not initiate cell death, demonstrating the need for ABL nuclear import in the induction of apoptosis. Wild-type (shuttling) ABL was more efficient than the exclusively nuclear ABL in killing cells, suggesting that both nuclear import and export contribute to ABL-induced cell death, although ABL must be activated in the nucleus to stimulate cell death and nuclear export of activated ABL further enhances the death response. Thus ABL may activate cell death effectors in both the nucleus and cytoplasm.

Another mechanism that regulates ABL nuclear–cytoplasmic localization is acetylation by histone acetyltransferases (HATs). HATs, such as p300/CBP (CREB binding protein) and PCAF (p300/CBP associated factor), have recently been proposed to play roles in the modulation of subcellular localization. These enzymes trigger the transfer of an acetyl group from acetyl coenzyme A to the ε-amino group of a lysine residue: known substrates include core histones, but also transcription factors and other proteins (6). A recent report by di Bari and co-workers

(7) suggested that p300, CBP, and PCAF may trigger the acetylation of ABL, driving ABL accumulation in the cytoplasmic compartment and promoting myogenic differentiation mediated by ABL.

The precise molecular mechanism for the proapoptotic role of ABL remains to be determined. Ionizing radiation activates nuclear ABL in an ataxia-telangiectasia-mutated (ATM) dependent manner (8) through phosphorylation of S465. ATM is a nuclear member of the PIKK-like family of enzymes (Chapters 1 and 6), and it binds to the SH3 domain of ABL. Activation of death receptors (e.g., by tumor necrosis factor) also activates ABL in the nucleus through mechanisms involving both caspases and 14-3-3 proteins (9–11). It had been speculated that the tumor suppressor p53 might be a downstream and immediate effector (12–14). However, ABL can induce apoptosis regardless of p53 status (wild-type or null (5)) and p53–ABL interactions are only detectable in vitro. ABL does not appear to significantly phosphorylate p53, even when ABL is overexpressed (15). However, another p53 family member, p73, may play a role in apoptosis. p73 induces apoptosis in many cell lines and can support transcription from promoters with a p53 response element (16). Moreover, overexpression of p73 in concert with ABL is sufficient to induce apoptosis in fibroblasts. p73 interacts with the ABL SH3 domain through its PXXP motif, and p73 has been shown to be a direct substrate of ABL (16), and to accumulate in an ABL-dependent manner following induction of DNA damage with either cisplatin or ionizing radiation. Finally, p73 can support the transcription of downstream proapoptotic genes (15). When activated, ABL phosphorylates and negatively regulates the activity of a number of nuclear substrates, including DNA-PK (17), RAD51 (18), SHPTP1 (19), and the p85 subunit of PI3K (20).

In the nucleus, ABL is known to interact with a number of different proteins, including Rb, ATM, p73, BRCA1, and RNA pol II, and several nuclear functions of ABL have been delineated. One role appears to be in the regulation of the cell cycle. Some of the nuclear pool of ABL in cells in the G1 phase of the cell cycle is complexed with Rb; the C-terminal pocket of Rb binds to the ATP binding lobe of the ABL kinase domain, resulting in the inhibition of kinase activity (21). When cyclin D-CDK4/6 kinases phosphorylate Rb at the G1–S boundary (Chapter 6), ABL is released, and ABL kinase activity is activated during S phase. During S phase, ABL contributes to the phosphorylation of RNA pol II, perhaps playing a role in stimulating the transcription of S-phase genes. However, it is not clear whether ABL actually has a growth promoting function during S phase. One the one hand, transfection with *ABL* does abrogate Rb-dependent growth arrest in SAOS-2 cells that are Rb deficient (22). On the other hand, fibroblasts derived from $abl^{-/-}$ deficient mice do not have a defined defect in S-phase progression. Furthermore, while Rb can function as a stoichiometric inhibitor of nuclear ABL, the ABL SH3 domain is not required for Rb binding. Further confusion as to the role of ABL in cell growth is also provided by the observation that ABL can inhibit growth of cells in G1. Overexpression of ABL can induce cell cycle arrest in G1, resulting in apoptosis of many of the cells (3). This cytostatic and cytotoxic function requires the ABL SH2 domain as well as the kinase activity, in addition to the p53 and Rb gene products (3, 23). Furthermore, conditional expression of kinase dead ABL (predicted to act as a dominant-negative) or suppression of endogenous ABL with antisense oligodeoxynucleotides accelerates the onset of S phase and shortens G1. Taken together, these results suggest that endogenous ABL probably functions as a physiological regulator of the G1/S transition (reviewed in (24)).

ABL also has DNA binding activity that is mediated by three tandem DNA binding domains with homology to HMG (high mobility group-1) proteins (25); these domains are roughly coincident with the three ABL NLSs, perhaps suggesting duplication of the functional unit. However, the functional significance of the ABL DNA binding is unclear; there seems to be only a weak preference for AT-rich sequences, and ABL lacks intrinsic transcriptional activity. It has been proposed that the ABL:DNA interaction involves contacts within the minor groove of the double helix. The ABL DNA binding domain does recognize deformed DNA structures such as four-way junctions and bubble DNA containing a large single-stranded loop (26), possibly suggesting roles in recombination and DNA repair in addition to transcription. Both v-ABL and ABL have been shown to form complexes with other transcription factors (e.g., CREB and E2F-1) (27) and to modulate their transcriptional activity, although whether or not this coactivating function requires the ABL DNA binding domain has not been delineated. ABL does bind p53 in vitro and enhances p53-dependent transcription from a promoter containing p53 binding sites; this activity is lost in ABL mutants which lack p53 binding (23). Two other proteins that bind ABL, ABI1 and ABI2, also have putative DNA binding domains (28, 29).

ABL also plays an important role in modulation of the F-actin cytoskeleton. Cells that are deficient in ABL show a dramatic reduction in the ruffling response to PDGF, a defect that can be restored by physiological reexpression of ABL (30). As discussed previously, ABL contains actin binding domains, and moreover, ABL localizes to actin-containing cellular structures. ABL binds to ALP1/amphiphysin-2, inducing changes in the actin cytoskeleton (31). ABL can phosphorylate a number of proteins involved in the regulation of focal adhesions and F-actin structure and dynamics, including Mena, paxillin, SH3-SH2 containing adaptor proteins (e.g., CRK, p130^{CAS}, DISABLED), and CDK5 (24). Integrin clustering induced by proteins in the extracellular matrix activates ABL (4, 32) and promotes cell attachment and spreading. Mutating the F-actin binding domain of ABL results in a form that is active independent of integrins, and F-actin inhibits ABL enzymatic activity in in vitro assays (33). ABL also seems to play an important role in formation of F-actin microspikes and has been proposed to play a regulatory role in the extension and retraction of filopodia and lamellipodia (which requires F-actin assembly and disassembly and is critical in the the ability of cells to explore and migrate in response to extracellular stimuli) (34). A number of elegant genetic studies in *Drosophila* have demonstrated clear roles for the fly ortholog of ABL in axon guidance, and studies in mice also suggest roles in neurite outgrowth (for a review, see (35)).

The clinical importance of ABL emerged through discovery of the "Philadelphia chromosome," involving a translocation between chromosomes 22 and 9. This feature was readily recognized in a chromosome spread; the shortened chromosome 22 was the foundation of a highly sensitive test for chronic myelogenous leukemia (CML). The Philadelphia chromosome was identified in 1960 by Nowell and Hungerford (36) and was so named after the city in which it was discovered. The t(9;22) translocation occurs in greater than 90% of CML, 25–30% of adult and 2–10% of childhood acute ALL, and occasionally in AML. This translocation results in the head-to-tail fusion of the *BCR* and *ABL* genes (37), placing the gene under the control of the *BCR* promoter (Figure 4.2). The breakpoint in BCR can be quite variable, but when joined with ABL results in a hybrid M_r 210,000 ($p210^{BCR-ABL}$) or a M_r 190,000 ($p190^{BCR-ABL}$) protein. The larger p210 form is usually associated with CML. The $p190^{BCR-ABL}$ is associated with acute leukemia that is often of lymphoid (rather than myeloid) origin (38, 39) although it has also been demonstrated in Ph-positive AML (40), whereas the larger form is usually associated with CML. There are two common variants of the $p210^{BCR-ABL}$. In one form, the break (in an area of 5.8 kb known as M-BCR) is centromeric to exon 3 of

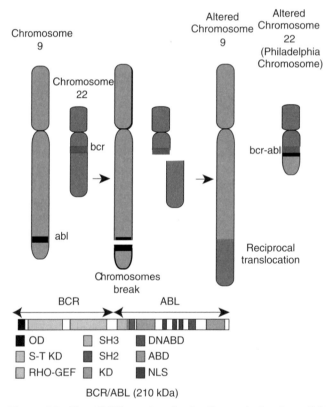

Figure 4.2 The t(9;22) translocation leading to the head-to-tail fusion of the BCR and ABL genes (upper) and generating the BCR-ABL fusion protein (lower figure). Domains shown in BCR-ABL are the oligomerization domain (black), serine–threonine kinase domain (light blue), RHO-GEF domain (orange), SH3 domain (green), SH2 domain (pink rectangle), tyrosine kinase domain (cyan), NLS signals (dark blue), DNA binding domain (dark green), and actin binding domain (orange).

M-BCR (b2a2) versus telomeric (b3a2); thus p210$^{BCR-ABL}$ may or may not contain a 25 amino acid sequence encoded by exon 3. All forms are constitutively active tyrosine kinases with higher levels of activity associated with the p190 subtype. An explosion of knowledge about BCR-ABL has now occurred: in particular, a series of important animal studies unequivocally demonstrated that this fusion protein is oncogenic and causes CML (41–44). Although BCR-ABL was originally considered to be just a dysregulated, constitutively active form of ABL, this is probably an oversimplification. The residues that confer imatinib resistance are identical to those that dysregulate ABL, suggesting that the mechanisms that govern BCR-ABL regulation may be similar to those of ABL and involve the same ABL, SRC-like, set of intramolecular interactions (for a recent review, see (45)).

The gene *BCR* (breakpoint cluster region) spans 130 kb and contains 23 exons. Two transcripts, one of 4.5 and one of 7.0 kb, have been found. These may correspond to the two major proteins encoded by the normal *BCR* gene; one is M$_r$ 160,000 and the other M$_r$ 130,000. *BCR* is ubiquitously expressed; however the aberrant *BCR-ABL* gene seems to specifically affect hematopoietic cells. Of possible relevance is the expression of BCR protein during the early stages of myeloid differentiation and the reduction in expression as cells mature to polymorphonuclear leukocytes (46). BCR protein was initially thought to be localized exclusively to the cytoplasm (46, 47), although electron microscopic evidence now suggests it associates with mitotic DNA and condensed heterochromatin in interphase cells (48). BCR has also been found to associate with XPB (xeroderma pigmentosum group B protein), a protein that plays a role in DNA repair, transcription initiation, and regulation of the cell cycle (49, 50). The first exon of *BCR* is of most significance since it is the one exon of *BCR* that is incorporated in all known BCR-ABL fusion proteins. Within this region of *BCR* reside a kinase domain, two serine-rich boxes containing SH2 domains, and an oligomerization domain. The BCR protein has serine/threonine kinase activity within the region encoded by the first exon (51) and is known to autophosphorylate on serine and threonine residues, as well as to phosphorylate casein and histones in in vitro kinase assays. BAP1 (BCR-associated protein), a member of the 14-3-3 family of proteins, is a substrate for the BCR serine–threonine kinase and is also phosphorylated on tyrosine by BCR-ABL but not by ABL (52). The oligomerization domain of BCR is characterized by a heptad repeat of hydrophobic residues, found between amino acids 28 and 68. This generates a coiled-coil domain, and disruption of the coiled coil by insertional mutagenesis inactivates the oligomerization function as well as the ability of BCR-ABL to transform Rat-1 fibroblasts or to abrogate IL3 dependence in lymphoid cells (53). Full-length BCR as well as BCR sequences retained in BCR-ABL bind specifically to the SH2 domain of ABL. The binding domain, essential for BCR-ABL-mediated transformation, has been localized within the first exon of *BCR* and consists of at least two SH2 binding sites (54).

In contrast to ABL, BCR-ABL exhibits a predominantly cytoplasmic localization, partly associated with the cytoskeleton through its C-terminal F-actin binding domain (46, 55, 56). The combination of the cytoplasmic localization and unregulated tyrosine kinase activity allows BCR-ABL to appropriate signaling pathways normally activated by growth factor receptor tyrosine kinases such as EGFR and PDGFR (as well as pathways activated by cytokine receptors that signal through nonreceptor tyrosine kinases such as SRC and JAK). The oligomerization domain of BCR seems to play a role in BCR-ABL localization in that deletion of this domain results in a decrease in binding of BCR-ABL to F-actin.

There are a number of cellular targets of BCR-ABL kinase whose tyrosine phosphorylation is upregulated in CML cells, including the E3 ubiquitin ligase (CBL), the SH2/SH3 adaptor proteins CRKL (CRK-like protein), CRK (v-SRC sarcoma virus CT (1) oncogene homolog), GRB2 (growth factor receptor bound protein 2), and VAV, as well as paxillin, STAT (signal transducer and activator of transcription) 5 and DOK1 (downstream of tyrosine kinase-1). Monitoring the phosphorylation status of these proteins in leukemic cells isolated from patients treated with the ABL inhibitor imatinib (or second generation compounds) has provided a convenient way to monitor pharmacodynamics. BCR-ABL also autophosphorylates (and thereby increases its activity) at several residues including Y1294 in the activation loop, and Y1127 in the SH2 catalytic domain. Autophosphorylation also occurs at Y177 in the BCR domain, an activity that promotes SH2-dependent binding of GRB2 and RAS/ERK signaling. RAS activation is necessary for transformation by both $p210^{BCR-ABL}$ and $p190^{BCR-ABL}$ (57–59); this may be mediated either through the GRB2 interaction (e.g., in fibroblasts) or alternatively through SHC proteins (in hematopoietic cells). The four PXXP motifs downstream of the catalytic domain interact with a number of SH3 domain signaling proteins, including the PI3K p85 regulatory subunit and NCK (noncatalytic region of tyrosine kinase).

Other activities that are stimulated by BCR-ABL include phosphorylation of the focal adhesion proteins FAK (focal adhesion kinase) and paxillin (60, 61), which may play a role in the increased expansion of committed myeloid progenitors and precursors and elevated levels of granulocytes. These features, characteristic of CML patients, have been attributed to defects in the adhesion properties of these cell populations due to disrupted focal adhesions and perturbed adhesion molecules such as β1 integrins.

Another proposed mechanism through which the oncogenic activity of BCR-ABL is mediated is the suppression of apoptosis; BCR-ABL can abrogate the dependence on growth factors in various hematopoietic cell lines. This is thought to be due to increased expression of the antiapoptotic protein BCL2, phosphorylation of the proapoptotic protein BAD, and possibly involves RAS-dependent pathways as well (62–64). The growth factor independence seen in BCR-ABL-positive cells is mediated at least in part through the constitutive activation of the STAT proteins, particularly STAT5 (65–70). Activation of STATs can occur through constitutive phosphorylation (and thus activation) of the upstream JAKs; alternatively, BCR-ABL can directly activate STATs, obviating the requirement for upstream activation of JAK (Section 4.5).

A fusion of *TEL* with *ABL* has been discovered in a small number of patients with leukemia (71–74). The *TEL* gene (also known as *ETS*-variant gene 6 *ETV6*), located on chromosome 12p13, encodes an ubiquitously expressed 452 amino acid protein with two regions of homology to the ETS family of transcription factors, the so-called PNT domain and DNA binding domain. The PNT (pointed) homology domain, or helix–loop–helix domain, mediates oligomerization and is required for the activation of the known TEL fusion tyrosine kinases (TEL-PDGFRβ, TEL-JAK2, and TEL-ABL). Two forms of TEL-ABL fusion proteins are known; in patients with B-ALL and atypical CML, the first four exons of *TEL* were fused to exon 2 of *ABL*, while in other patients exons 1–5 of *TEL* were fused to *ABL* exon 2. The resulting protein chimeras contain TEL amino acids 1–154 or 1–336, fused in frame to the same 1104 COOH-terminal amino acids of ABL that occur in the BCR-ABL fusion proteins. TEL-ABL fusion proteins have increased tyrosine kinase activity in vitro (71) and are constitutively tyrosine phosphorylated in vivo (72, 75). In contrast to TEL, which is a predominantly nuclear protein (76), TEL-ABL localizes to the cytoplasm where, similar to BCR–ABL, it interacts with F-actin (72). Also like BCR-ABL, TEL-ABL is capable of transforming Rat-1 fibroblasts (72), primary bone marrow B-lymphoid progenitor cells (72), and IL3-dependent BaF3 cells (75). Moreover, TEL-ABL and BCR-ABL appear to activate similar intracellular signaling pathways (77, 78).

4.2   ARG

The ABL family of kinases comprises ABL and ABL-related gene (ARG) proteins. ARG has considerable structural homology with ABL (Figure 4.1). At the amino acid sequence level, ARG exhibits a high degree of identity with ABL in the SH3, SH2, and kinase domains (89%, 90%, and 93% identity, respectively). However, the C terminus of ARG, while containing binding motifs for SH3 domains, F-actin, and G-actin, diverges from ABL with only 30% identity. *ARG* has been mapped to chromosome 1q24-q25. In contrast to ABL, ARG is localized predominantly to the cytoplasm (79). Similar to ABL, ARG is ubiquitously expressed, although during development, both ABL and ARG are highly expressed in the neural tube where they interact with bundles of apical actin filaments in neural epithelial cells (80). ARG is preferentially expressed in brain regions rich in axon and synapses, rather than neuronal cell bodies. Mice with targeted disruption of *ABL* are born runted with head and eye abnormalities and succumb shortly thereafter due to defective lymphopoiesis. $Arg^{-/-}$ mice, in contrast, develop normally but exhibit behavioral abnormalities. Double knockout ($abl^{-/-}$ and $arg^{-/-}$) mice die in utero before day 11, exhibiting severe defects in the nervous system, including malformations and incomplete closure of the neural tube (80).

Although the functions of ARG are much less well characterized than ABL, it is thought to play an important role in regulating cytoskeletal structure. ARG binds cooperatively to F-actin in vitro and can assemble F-actin into tight bundles, an activity that requires both the C-terminal F-actin binding domains and an internal F-actin binding domain (81). ARG is required for dynamic lamellipodial protrusion in fibroblasts after adhesion to fibronectin and is thought to mediate physical contact between F-actin and microtubules at the cell periphery (82). Other roles for ARG that have been reported include induction of apoptosis following oxidative stress through phosphorylation of the antiapoptotic protein SIVA-1 (83), and phosphorylation of RNA polymerase II (possibly associated with a role in regulation of transcription) (84). ARG activation has also been linked to PDGFR (85) and EPHB2 (86) signaling. ARG also associates with the proteasome subunit PSMA (prosteasome subunit) 7 and has been proposed to regulate proteasome degradation (87).

As discussed in Section 4.1, the *TEL* gene is fused to a number of different partners in many leukemia patients with rearrangements of 12p13. ARG was first identified as a new fusion partner of TEL in an AML patient with FAB M4eo (with eosinophilia), carrying t(1;12)(q25;p13) and inv (16) (88). Later studies also identified *TEL-ARG* fusion transcripts in a case of AML-M3 with a t(1;12)(q25;p13) in addition to t(15;17)(q22;q11.2) translocation (89) and in a TALL patient with t(1;10;12)(q25;p13;13) (90). All of the fusion transcripts contain the PNT domain of TEL, and most of the ARG protein, resulting in a constitutively active kinase. Two transcripts can occur, one with an alternative splice lacking part of an F-actin binding domain of Arg. However, transfection of 293T cells with either form demonstrated colocalization of the fusion protein with cellular β-actin, cell rounding, and detachment from tissue culture plastic. The aberrant kinase appears to phosphorylate the RHO inhibitor p190RHOGAP (91). When expressed in CHO cells, TEL-ARG induced the formation of filopodia, an activity requiring the C-terminal region and intact kinase activity (92). The expression of TEL-ARG transforms both BaF3 cells and Rat-1 cells (93).

4.3   SRC AND SRC FAMILY KINASES

The SRC family of tyrosine kinases (SFK) collectively has a number of cellular functions, including control of proliferation, survival, differentiation, and cell adhesion. Aberrant regulation of the SFKs has long been associated with malignant transformation: indeed, SRC was the first kinase shown to be an oncogene (94). The SFK family consists of nine members: LYN, HCK, LCK, BLK, SRC, FYN, YRK, YES, and FGR. All show similar levels of regulation but have been grouped into two subfamilies, LYN related (LYN, HCK, LCK, and BLK) and SRC related (SRC, YES, FYN, YRK, and FGR). A human homolog of YRK (originally identified in chicken) has not been identified. All of the family members share a related domain arrangement (95), with an N-terminal region of 50–70 residues that has considerable variability among the family members. All family members contain a SH4 membrane targeting region at the N terminus, which is myristoylated and sometimes palmitoylated (96, 97). This is followed by a ~50 aa SH3 domain and a ~100 aa SH2 domain. The SH2 domain also contains a unique region of 50–70 residues, which is quite divergent among SRC family members. The C-terminal kinase domain of ~300 residues is also known as the SH1 domain and accounts for the enzymatic activity. The substrate targeting and the activity of the SFKs are highly regulated and utilize both intramolecular interactions of the SH3 and SH2 domains and association with other molecules such as activators, inhibitors, and substrates. Three additional kinases, BRK, FRK, and SRM, are grouped with the

SFK family, although these kinases are not myristoylated; of these three, only BRK and FRK have potential regulatory C-terminal tyrosines.

The short C-terminal tail of the SFK is a hallmark property, bearing an autoinhibitory phosphorylation site (Y530 in human SRC, sometimes generically refered to as Y527 according to the chicken SRC sequence). Similar to many other protein kinases, SFKs require phosphorylation in the activation loop of the kinase domain to have full catalytic activity. In the case of SRC, this is Y419 (numbering for human SRC including the initiator methionine). Thus SRC is phosphorylated on Y419 in the active state, and Y530 in the inactive state. The inactivating phosphorylation on Y530 is mediated by the C-terminal SRC-specific kinase CSK (98) or its homolog CHK (99, 100). When the C-terminal tail is phosphorylated, it promotes the assembly of the SH2, SH3, and kinase domains into an inactive conformation (101–103) (Figure 4.3) by generating a binding site for the SH2 domain. The intramolecular binding between the SH2 domain and the C-terminal tail extends the linker region between the SH2 domain and the kinase domain in a polyproline type II helix, which forms an intramolecular binding site for the SH3 domain. The resulting quaternary complex of the SH2 and SH3 domains bound to the transverse side of the kinase domain inactivates kinase activity by restricting motion between the two lobes of the kinase domain. Structural features of SRC activation are discussed further in Chapter 2. Homozygous mice with targeted deletions of CSK exhibit a complex phenotype including defects in the neural tube and die between day 9 and day 10 of gestation. Cells derived from these embryos exhibit an order of magnitude increase in activity of SRC and the related FYN kinase (104).

SH2 and SH3 domains also play an important role in mediating interactions with other proteins, positively influencing SFK signaling. These domains are known to target tyrosine kinases to specific subcellular locations and further play a role in recognizing specific cellular substrates (105–107). A phenomenon known

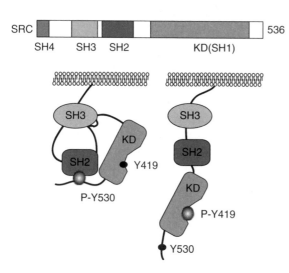

Figure 4.3 Activation of SRC kinase. The inactive form of SRC is phosphorylated at Y530, promoting interaction between the carboxyl-terminal tail and the SH2 domain. Dephosphorylation of Y530 results in structural rearrangement and activation of kinase activity. The dark circle denotes the nonphosphorylated tyrosine residue, the larger radiating circle, the phosphorylated form of the tyrosine residue.

as processive phosphorylation occurs when the catalytic domain of SRC phosphorylates a substrate, and this in turn creates a site that is recognized by the SH2 domain. Binding of the SH2 domain increases the local concentration of the substrate, allowing the catalytic domain to phosphorylate additional sites. An example of this is the focal adhesion protein p130^{CAS}. Binding of SRC to a SH2 domain near the C terminus of p130^{CAS} is thought to promote phosphorylation at multiple sites closer to the N terminus (108, 109). In another example, LCK phosphorylates several tyrosine residues in the ζ chain of the T-cell receptor. Each ζ chain contains three immunoreceptor tyrosine kinase-based activation motifs arranged in tandem. Mutation of amino acids in the SH2 domain of LCK that are important for phosphotyrosine recognition reduces receptor hyperphosphorylation and subsequent signal transduction (110, 111). Other studies have shown that molecules that bind with high affinity to the SH2 or SH3 domains of SFK can disrupt the relatively low affinity intramolecular interactions, leading to enzyme activation (112, 113).

SFK family members show a variety of expression patterns (Table 4.1). For example, SRC, FYN, YES, and LYN are expressed in a broad range of tissues in the mouse, although levels are higher in hematopoietic and neural cells. The expression patterns overlap, but not all of the kinases are coexpressed in a given cell type. However, most cells express at least one of these four kinases. Other SFKs (HCK, FGR, LCK, and BLK) are restricted to the hematopoietic cells but exhibit variability with lineage. For example, myeloid cells coexpress HCK, FGR, and LYN. T cells express predominantly LCK and FYN, whereas B cells express LYN, BLK, FYN, and FGR. To further complicate the expression pattern, different isoforms occur as a consequence of alternative splicing. For example, two neuronal forms of SRC are produced by alternative splicing of exons in the SH3 domain (114, 115), and FYN occurs in a hematopoietic-specific isoform FYN(T) and a so-called brain isoform FYN(B) as a consequence of alternative splicing of the seventh exon encoding the kinase domain (116). Additionally, LYN occurs in two forms, which result from alternative splicing of the "unique" domain at the N terminus (117, 118), and HCK has two isoforms produced as a result of alternative initiation sites (119).

Subcellular localization adds an additional layer to SFK regulation. Myristoylation of the second amino acid (glycine) is required to tether SFKs to membranes and association with membranes is required for SFK function (120). Some of the SFKs are also palmitoylated at cysteine residues within the SH4 region, and this is thought to further stabilize localization to the membrane (121). However, SFKs are found not only in association with the plasma membrane, but also with rough endoplasmic reticulum, secretory vesicles, and caveolae (121, 122). A major proportion of FGR is found in the nucleus of both bone marrow and peritoneal macrophages, but this distribution appears to be unique to FGR among the SFKs (123). In the context of the membrane, SFKs are thought to associate with the cytoplasmic tails of transmembrane receptors lacking kinase domains and, as such, to serve

TABLE 4.1 **Expression Patterns of SFK Family Members**

Kinase and MW protein product(s)	Chromosomal location	Expression	Phenotype of single deletion
SRC $p60^{c-src}$	20q12-q13	Broad, nearly ubiquitous	Osteopetrosis
YES $p62^{yes}$	18p11.3	Broad	None
FYN $p59^{fyn(B)}$ $p59^{fyn(T)}$	6q21	Broad FYN(B) in brain, fibroblasts, endothelial cells, keratinocytes, FYN(T) in T-cells, B cells	Abnormalities in brain development and function, defects in thymocyte signaling
FGR $p58^{c-fgr}$	1p36.2-p36.1	Hematopoietic–myeloid, mature B-cells	None
LYN $p53^{lyn}$ 56^{lyn}	8q13-qter	Broad, myeloid, B-cells	Impaired B-cell activity, autoimmunity
HCK $p59^{hck}$ $p61^{hck}$	20q11-q12	Hematopoietic–myeloid	None
LCK $p56^{lck}$	1p35-p34.3	Hematopoietic T-cells, NK cells	Block in T-cell development and impaired T-cell signaling
BLK $p56^{blk}$	8p23-p22	Hematopoietic B-cells	None

a role in the transduction of signals from these receptors. In addition, SFKs are activated by receptors with kinase domains. Binding of ligands to receptors for various tyrosine kinases (e.g., PDGF, EGF, VEGF, FGF, HGF), cytokines (e.g., IL2, IL3, IL6, endotoxin (LPS), TNF), antigens, antibodies (via Fc receptors), GPCRs (e.g., thrombin, chemokines), and adhesion receptors (integrins, ICAM) have all been reported to activate one or more SFKs. SFKs are also activated by UV treatment (probably due to oxidant stress) and during mitosis. Multiple combinations of SFKs are coexpressed in different cell types, and these combinations have been implicated in both overlapping and specific functions. For example, sucrose density gradient fractionation studies indicated that the subcellular distributions of SRC and LYN are different in HeLa cells (124). Follow-up time-lapse photobleaching studies demonstrated that SRC, a nonpalmitoylated SFK, rapidly exchanges between the plasma membrane and intracellular organelles (endosomes/lysosome). In contrast,

LYN, which is a palmitoylated SFK, is exocytosed to the plasma membrane via the Golgi apparatus (125). Mutations of LYN that result in a nonpalmitoylated form direct LYN away from exocytotic transport and to more of a SRC-like pattern, suggesting that palmitoylation and resulting distinct trafficking pathways are involved in dictating the specific function of SFKs (125).

Lipid rafts are specialized areas of the plasma membrane that are enriched in cholesterol, sphingolipids, glycolipids, and GPI (glycosylphosphatidylinositol)-linked proteins. Several types of receptors are associated with lipid rafts upon cell activation, among them KIT and EGFR. Additionally, SFKs and small GTP binding proteins of the RAS superfamily also localize to lipid rafts by virtue of lipid modification, and other signaling enzymes such as PI3K also localize to the rafts, although the mechanisms of their recruitment are poorly defined. Lipid rafts then are thought to create microdomains that facilitate signal transduction from membrane receptors. Mutation of the myristate or palmitate modification sites of SFKs prevents their partitioning into lipid rafts and also blocks downstream signaling (126).

Several signaling pathways are activated following activation of SFKs, including the RAS pathway, phosphatidylinositol kinases, STATs, and pathways involved in cytoskeletal reorganization and transcription factor activation. Cooperative interactions among SFKs may also be important. For example, PDGFRβ associates with SRC, FYN, and YES and interactions among these SFKs are thought to be important for the proliferative response to PDGF (127). However, elimination of one family member does not result in a failure to initiate a mitogenic response indicating that other SFKs can compensate.

4.3.1   SRC

v-SRC, the oncogene responsible for the transforming activity of Rous sarcoma virus, induces many of features of oncogenic growth including loss of contact inhibition, increased growth factor and anchorage independence, decreased anoikis, and the ability to induce tumors in animal models. Cells transformed by *v-SRC* exhibit marked changes in the organization of the actin cytoskeleton, namely, the loss of F-actin stress fibers and typical focal adhesion complexes, decreased adhesion to the extracellular matrix, and reduced cell:cell interactions, as well as an increase in several parameters of cellular motility (128, 129). The molecular mechanisms whereby v-SRC mediates cell transformation have been studied extensively, although still are not completely defined. SRC is thought to phosphorylate specific substrates including SHC, the small GTPase RAC, STAT3, the p85 subunit of PI3K, ABL, and ERK5 that in turn activate constitutive signaling that is required for cellular transformation. Table 4.2 summarizes the known substrates of SRC, and some of these substrates are discussed next.

SHC   SHC is an adaptor protein that contains both phosphotyrosine binding (PTB) and SH2 domains and becomes phosphorylated on tyrosine in response to many different extracellular stimuli. Y239 and Y240 of SHC are coordinately phosphorylated by SRC in vitro and in response to EGF or in *v-SRC*-transformed cells

TABLE 4.2   SFK Substrates

Protein	Cellular location	Reference
Vinculin	Focal adhesion, integrin signaling, actin binding	130, 131
Tubulin α-2		132
Tubulin β-5		132
Cortactin	Cortical actin binding	133–135
Cofilin	Actin depolymerization	136
Talin	Focal adhesions, integrin signaling, actin binding	137, 138
Paxillin	Focal adhesions, integrin signaling	139–141
FAK	Focal adhesions, integrin signaling	133, 142
Tensin	Focal adhesions, integrin signaling, actin binding	142, 143
p130^{cas}	Focal adhesions	108
SIN	Adaptor protein	113
Actin filament associated protein (AFAP)	Cytoskeleton; likely mechanical force sensor	105, 133, 144
β1- Integrin	Cell–substrate adhesion and signaling	145
CIP4	Cytoskeleton	146
WASP		147
WIP		147
ELMO		147
β-Catenin	Cell–cell junctions	148–150
γ-Catenin	Cell–cell junctions	149
Occludin	Cell–cell junctions (tight junctions)	151, 152
p120CTN	Cell–cell junctions	133, 144
Connexin 43	Cell–cell junctions (gap junctions)	153, 154
Nectin-2δ	Cell–cell junctions	155
PLCγ	Phospholipid metabolism	156
p85 (PI3K)	Phospholipid metabolism	157–159
p190RHOGAP	Phospholipid metabolism	160–162
p120RASGAP	Phospholipid metabolism	160, 161
EGFR	Phospholipid metabolism/growth factor signaling	163
EPS8	Phospholipid metabolism/growth factor signaling	164
SAM68	Mitosis	165–167
TKS14(PAN)	Adaptor protein: bind and cluster proteins with SH3 domains	167
DOK-1	Scaffold for adaptor proteins	160
GRUB	Likely guanine nucelotide exchange protein	167
TKS202	Unknown, ?protein trafficking, motor function	167
TKS5 (FISH)	Large adaptor protein; podosomes/invadopodia	168

(continued)

TABLE 4.2   SFK Substrates (*Continued*)

Protein	Cellular location	Reference
MEM3	Vesicle trafficking	167
SH3P7		167
VPS35P	Vesicle trafficking	167
SHPTP2/SYP	Protein tyrosine phosphatase	169
SHC	RAS pathway, binds GRB2	170
Caveolin	Caveolar structure/function	171, 172
Calpactin I/annexin II	Ca^{2+}/phospholipid signaling	173–176
Enolase	Glycolysis	177
STAT3		178–180
TIAM		181
VAV2		181
Calumenin	Endoplasmic reticulum	136
BIP	Endoplasmic reticulum	182
DAPK	Apoptosis	183

in vivo (170). This leads to GRB2/SOS recruitment to the membrane and subsequent activation of the RAS pathway. SOS is a nucleotide exchange factor and thus activates RAS by catalyzing the exchange of GDP for GTP. The activated RAS in turn recruits the serine/threonine kinase RAF to the membrane, leading to downstream signaling through MEK1/2 and ERK1/2 (Chapter 5). Mutagenesis studies indicate that Y239/240 make an important contribution to the association of SHC with GRB2 (184). However, active SRC only modestly activates ERK1/2 signaling.

RAC1   The small GTPase RAC1 of the RHO family has also been implicated in SRC-induced transformation. RAC1 is involved in the formation of membrane ruffles (lamellipodia) through formation of cortical actin fibers but also plays a role in activation of MAP kinase cascades. RAC1 appears to function through activation of JNK and p38 MAPK (185, 186), which in turn phosphorylate the transcription factors JUN and STAT3. A dominant-negative RAC1 mutant attenuated JNK activation by growth factors, v-SRC and HRAS. Cells transformed by *v-SRC* have high levels of GTP-bound RAC1, and interference with the activation of RAC1 or its induction of downstream pathways potently inhibits the focus-forming activity of v-SRC (181). This appears to involve v-SRC-mediated phosphophorylation of the nucleotide exchange factors VAV2 and TIAM1 (181).

PI3K   Class 1A PI3Ks are heterodimeric proteins composed of a noncatalytic p85 subunit and a catalytic p110 subunit (Chapter 5). The p85 subunit binds and integrates signals from a variety of cellular proteins, including RTKs, PKC, SHP1, RAC, RHO, hormonal receptors, mutated RAS, and SRC, thus providing an important integration point for the activation of p110 and downstream signaling. The SH3 domains of SFKs such as LYN, BLK, and FYN can bind to a proline-rich region in the p85 subunit, leading to an increase in PI3K activity.

STATs Another family of SFK substrates are STATs, a family of latent cytoplasmic transcription factors first identified as mediators of cellular responses to interferons. More recently, it has become evident that numerous cytokines and mitogenic growth factors (e.g., EGF and PDGF) also induce STAT signaling, resulting in downstream changes in diverse biological processes including cell differentiation, proliferation, and apoptosis (Section 4.5). Activation of STAT signaling is usually initiated by receptor aggregation and activation of Janus protein kinases (JAKs) that are associated with receptors. The STAT proteins are recruited to the receptor:JAK complex, become tyrosine phosphorylated, and then form homo- or heterodimers that translocate to the nucleus, where they bind to specific DNA response elements. There are at least seven genes that encode different STATs, and various combinations are activated in response to specific growth factors and cytokines. Transformation of mammalian fibroblasts by *v-SRC* induces constitutive activation of STAT3, and activation of STAT3 appears to be essential for transformation induced by *v-SRC* (179, 180, 187). Currently, it is thought that JAK1 recruits STAT3 to SRC, which in turn phosphorylates STAT3 on Y705 and directly activates STAT3. While there are multiple signaling pathways that are activated by SRC and involved in cellular transformation, it is intriguing that disruption of the STAT signaling pathway is sufficient to block cell transformation, suggesting that activated STAT3 signaling elicits some irreversible changes in the genetic program that are required either for the initiation or the maintenance of transformation.

ABL The tyrosine kinase ABL is also an important substrate for SRC signaling. ABL (as discussed earlier in this chapter) resembles SRC at its N terminus, while the C terminus differs considerably, bearing nuclear localization sequences and protein and DNA interaction domains. The functions of ABL are dependent on its cellular localization. Nuclear ABL plays a role in the cellular response to DNA damage whereas cytoplasmic ABL participates in downstream signaling events elicited by growth factors, cytokines, and integrins. The catalytic activity of ABL requires phosphorylation of Y245 and Y412 by SRC (45). ABL has also been shown to mediate SRC-induced MYC expression and cell cycle progression (188).

DAPK Another SRC substrate, death-associated protein kinase (DAPK), is a calmodulin-regulated serine/threonine kinase. It has a tumor suppressor function, inhibiting cell adhesion and migration and promoting apoptosis. DAPK expression is often reduced in tumor cell lines and tissues, and the degree of DAPK downregulation correlates with a poor prognostic outcome in several human cancers (189, 190). DAPK has been shown to suppress oncogenic transformation in vitro (191) and to block tumor metastasis in vivo (192). The proapoptotic function of DAPK has been ascribed to its role in integrin inactivation, in turn suppressing adhesion-mediated survival signals. DAPK also plays a role in the remodeling of the cytoskeleton by phosphorylating myosin light chain 2 (193) and in inhibiting cell migration (194). DAPK activity is regulated by two reciprocal modulators:

SRC and leukocyte common antigen related tyrosine phosphatase (LAR). SRC acts as an inhibitor of DAPK by phosphorylating Y491/492. LAR, in contrast, dephosphorylates DAPK at Y491/492. This reciprocal circuit is exemplified by the effects of EGF, which induces a concomitant SRC activation and LAR downregulation, and these two events act in synergy to promote DAPK inactivation (183).

4.3.2 Cellular Roles of SRC

During mitosis, SRC shows changes in activity and localization. Activity is increased in M phase and decreased in interphase (195). Treatment of cells with inhibitors of SFK blocks progression through metaphase (196) and also blocks cytokinesis (197). Cells injected with a neutralizing antibody for SRC, YES, FYN, or the SH2 domain of SRC or FYN fail to transit from G2/M and do not undergo cytokinesis (197–199). Coexpression studies with SRC, YES, and LYN demonstrate that these three SFKs are activated at different levels in the M phase, and that this activation is CDC2 dependent (200). SFKs are transiently activated at the transition from G2 to M and are required for entry into mitosis prior to breakdown of the nuclear envelope (196, 198). An equatorial domain enriched in ganglioside G_{M1}, cholesterol, and SFKs forms at the contractile ring in late anaphase and activation of SRC is required for progression of the cleavage furrow (197). Tyrosine phosphorylation of ERK1/2 occurs at the midbody, and this phosphorylation is dependent on SFK activity (201). MEK and ERK are known to be present on mitotic spindles and to regulate the assembly and maintenance of mitotic spindles in metaphase and anaphase. However, the mechanism of subsequent ERK1/2-regulated abscission is unclear and is an area of active investigation. Additionally, protein tyrosine phosphatase PTPα activity is also increased during M phase and is involved in SRC activation through dephosphorylation of the C-terminal Y530 (202). The precise mechanism of the CDC2 activation thus is unclear; it may activate SFK members directly, or act indirectly through the activation of PTPα. Mitotic activation of the chicken form of SRC also requires myristoylation and CDC2-mediated phosphorylation of S72, T34, and T46 (203–207). Through its SH2 and SH3 domains activated SRC binds to tyrosine phosphorylated p68 (SAM68, a protein related to the RNA binding protein p62 (165, 166, 208)).

The MEK5/ERK5 pathway is another MAP kinase pathway which, while much less extensively studied than the ERK1/2 pathway, is also thought to contribute to cellular proliferation (209, 210) and cell transformation (211). ERK5 has a unique C-terminal transcription factor domain that is activated through autophosphorylation and ERK is thus thought to signal both through itself (212) and via the phosphorylation of substrates such as SAP1A (213) and myocyte enhancer factor (MEF) (210, 214). Recent studies have demonstrated that activation of ERK5 can lead to loss of actin stress fibers, and ERK5 can be activated by oncogenic SRC, which leads to translocation of ERK5 from the cytoplasm to the nucleus where it then activates transcription (215). Moreover, ERK5 activation appears to be required for SRC-mediated transformation (215).

Another critical cellular activity regulated by SRC is cell migration. SFKs regulate cell migration in both normal and transformed cells by modifying cell:cell and cell:matrix interactions and by promoting the expression of various proteases that modify the extracellular matrix. Activated SRC localizes to focal adhesions, whereas nonactivated SRC is primarily perinuclear and in endosomes (122, 216–218). Upon cell adhesion, it has been reported that a fraction of total cellular SRC relocalizes to focal adhesions (219), although a conflicting report disagrees (220). Several important SRC substrates reside at focal adhesions, including focal adhesion kinase (FAK), p130^{CAS}, paxillin, and cortactin. As discussed later in this chapter, FAK is a cytoplasmic tyrosine kinase critically involved in integrin signaling networks (221). SRC directly binds FAK and promotes the phosphorylation of the C-terminal Y861 and Y925 in FAK and, in so doing, the activation of multiple intracellular signaling pathways. Cortactin is also a substrate of a number of kinases including SRC, which phosphorylates cortactin at Y421. Cortactin regulates actin polymerization and F-actin branching (222), thus influencing cell migration and the persistance of lamellipodia. Cortactin is localized to the sites of active "invadopodia," where it cooperates with activated SRC and MT1-MMP to degrade matrix (223). In addition to regulating cell migration, SFKs are required for the adhesion and spreading of many cell types on integrin ligands such as fibronectin and vitronectin. SFKs play a critical role in the regulation of podosomes, specialized, inducible adhesion structures with an extracellular matrix-degrading activity. Podosomes are typically found in invasive or tissue remodeling cell types such as monocytes, invasive tumor cells, and osteoclasts, as well as in activated endothelial and smooth muscle cells. Structurally, podosomes appear as small (~1 μm in diameter) dot-like structures on the ventral surface of cells and are enriched in F-actin and actin-regulating proteins such as N-WASP, WIP, ARP12/3 complex, dynamin, and the SRC substrate cortactin. The extracellular matrix-degrading activity associated with podosomes requires the local concentration of matrix metalloproteinases. SRC phosphorylation plays a major regulatory role in podosome development. A major clue to the role of SRC in podosome function came from studies with SRC knockout mice. These mice have severe osteopetrosis due to deficient osteoclast activity. Osteoclasts from $src^{-/-}$ mice do not adhere and spread properly and do not form mature sealing zones when plated on bone (224). Obversely, expression of the oncogenic SRC mutant, v-SRC, results in perturbed focal adhesions and induction of podosome formation in many cell types (225). Studies of the reorganization of podosomes during osteoclast polarization revealed that these structures undergo a transformation from a scattered distribution to the formation of clusters and ring-like superstructures, ultimately assembling a sealing zone at the cell periphery. The formation of the rings is associated with increased levels of podosome-associated actin. At the peripheral ring, levels of actin are high, whereas paxillin levels remain quite stable. SRC catalytic activity appears to be essential for podosome maturation and turnover and is inversely related to the local levels of the tyrosine–phosphorylated cortactin, a SRC substrate. While the precise molecular mechanism of SRC regulation of podosome formation is not entirely understood, it appears that SRC-mediated phosphorylation of the actin-nucleating protein cortactin results in a reduced ability of cortactin to enhance actin polymerization (226).

SRC and other SFKs show prominent accumulation at sites of cell–cell adhesion, although the signaling pathways and functional consequences of this localization remain to be fully elucidated. SRC is the target of E-cadherin activated cell signaling, stimulated by ligation of the cadherin. SRC is phosphorylated at Y419 as cells make contacts with one another, an effect blocked by E-cadherin-inhibitory antibodies (227). These antibodies also reduce the level of activated SRC detectable at contacts between cells in established monolayers, suggesting that ongoing cadherin ligation is necessary for the maintenance of active SRC at sites of cell–cell contact (227). The mechanism of E-cadherin activation of SRC is not fully characterized but requires the β-catenin binding region of the cadherin cytoplasmic tail. SFK signaling effects on cadherin function appear to be both positive and negative, possibly depending on the strength of the signal (228–230). SRC appears to be necessary for homophilic adhesive ligation to recruit PI3K into cadherin adhesions, indicating a critical role of SFK signaling in linking cell surface receptors with PI3K. Other potential SFK substrates including p120 catenin, β-catenin, and cortactin are also found at sites of cell–cell adhesion (227).

Anoikis, a process defined as apoptosis that occurs upon loss of attachment to the extracellular matrix, is a characteristic property of normal cells. However, as tumor cells begin to metastasize, they acquire resistance to anoikis, and this resistance is thought to involve aberrant integrin signaling independent of cell adhesion. Several integrins have an important role in cell survival (231), and both FAK and SRC have been shown to protect cells from anoikis (232). PI3K binds to phosphorylated Y397 of FAK, and Y397 of FAK is required for protection from apoptosis. Y397 is also the SFK binding site. Detachment of mammary epithelial cells from extracellular matrix results in a rapid, FAK-dependent translocation of the proapoptotic protein BAX to the mitochondria (233). A dominant-negative FAK construct induces the mitochondrial translocation of BAX, an effect that is overcome by overexpression of PI3K or SRC (233), leading to the hypothesis that a signal transmitted through the combination of FAK, SRC, and PI3K impairs mitochondrial translocation of BAX and thus blocks apoptosis when cells are adherent. Expression of activated SRC results in increased resistance to anoikis and is associated with altered AKT phosphorylation (234).

4.3.3 SRC and Cancer

SRC mutations are very rare, but elevated SRC expression and/or activation is associated with many tumor types. The increase in SRC activity in cancer can be the consequence of multiple perturbations, including tyrosine phosphatase-mediated dephosphorylation of the carboxy-terminal negative regulatory regions, an increase in overall protein expression (due to altered transcription, translation, and/or protein stability), an increase in upstream receptor tyrosine kinase activity, or the loss of critical regulatory proteins. SRC is expressed and activated in colon cancer cell lines (235), and SRC activity is higher in tumor tissue and adenomatous polyps than in normal colon mucosa (236–238).

Moreover, a correlation between the malignant potential of colon cancer lines in vitro and degree of SRC activation has been reported (239). The level of SRC activation has also been correlated with clinical parameters of advanced tumor status and poor prognosis (240). Human colon cancer cells transfected with SRC show enhanced tumor growth in vivo and increased resistance to detachment-induced apoptosis (241). Orally active SRC inhibitors have shown potent inhibitory activity on human colon cancer colony formation in vivo and xenograft tumor growth in vivo (242). Other SFKs are expressed in colon cancer, for example, YES expression has been correlated with poor prognosis (243), and LCK expression has been noted in a few cases of colon cancer (244) although the role of LCK in tumor growth and progression is poorly understood. Other cancers where SRC is also overexpressed (and often reported to be activated as well) include pancreatic carcinomas (245, 246), breast cancer (235, 247–250), non small cell lung cancer (251), human parotid tumors (252), hepatocellular carcinomas (253), ovarian cancer (254, 255), bladder cancer (256), gastric cancer (257), esophageal cancer (258, 259), brain cancer (260–262), and small cell lung cancer (263, 264).

4.4 FAK

Members of the integrin family of transmembrane receptors play important structural roles, linking extracellular matrix proteins with the cellular actin cytoskeleton and, in turn, regulate cell shape, motility, and tissue architecture. A variety of integrin-associated proteins (including nonreceptor tyrosine kinases) can be activated by integrin receptor clustering. Focal adhesion kinase (FAK), also known as protein tyrosine kinase, cytoplasmic 2 (PTK2) was identified in 1992 as a substrate of v-SRC and as a highly tyrosine phosphorylated protein localized to integrin-enriched cell adhesion sites known as focal contacts (265, 266). FAK associates with a number of intracellular signaling proteins, providing an important link between integrin receptors and downstream pathways such as the ERK and JNK MAPKs, and PI3K.

The gene for FAK maps to 8q24-qterm, a locus that is subject to amplification in human cancer cells (267). FAK has three well-defined domains: an N-terminal four-point-one, ezrin, radixin, moesin (FERM) domain, a central catalytic domain, and a C-terminal focal adhesion targeting (FAT) domain. The FERM and kinase domains are joined by a short linker containing a proline-rich motif (PR1, which binds to the SH3 domains of several proteins including SRC and TRIO), and the autophosphorylated Y397 (Figure 4.4). The kinase and FAT domains are joined by a longer and more poorly characterized region with two proline-rich motifs (PR2, PR3), which are involved in the many SH3-mediated protein:protein interactions of FAK.

FAK has six sites of tyrosine phosphorylation. Y397, the major site of autophosphorylation, lies just upstream of the kinase domain and is a docking site for SH2-containing proteins such as SFKs, PLCγ, SOCS, GRB7, SHC, p120^{RASGAP}, and the p85 subunit of PI3K (268–271). It is not clear whether these different signaling proteins bind differentially to unphosphorylated and

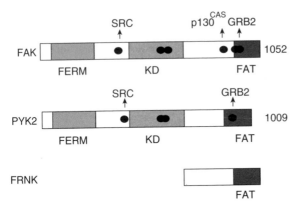

Figure 4.4 Domain structure of FAK, PYK3, and FRNK. Shown are the FERM (four-point-one, ezrin, radixin, moesin) domain (tan), the tyrosine kinase domain (cyan), and the focal adhesion targeting (FAT) domain (dark brown). Phosphorylation sites are denoted by the black circles.

Y397-phosphorylated FAK (e.g., in response to particular stimuli) or whether there are different complexes of activated FAK. One school of thought is that the binding of SRC to FAK initiates signaling, and the association of SOCS with FAK is a terminal event that leads to ubiquitin-mediated FAK degradation (272).

The activity of FAK is dependent on integrin-mediated cell adhesion, and one of the first events associated with FAK activation is the recruitment of SFKs into a signaling complex. When FAK is phosphorylated on Y397, this promotes SRC binding, which in turn leads to the conformational activation of SRC. SRC phosphorylates FAK at Y861, promoting the SH3 domain-mediated binding of p130^{CAS} to the FAK C-terminal PR2 and PR3 (273). Activated SRC also phosphorylates FAK Y925, in turn promoting binding of GRB2 and subsequent RAS/RAF/MEK/ERK activation (274). Maximal catalytic FAK activation occurs with SRC-mediated transphosphorylation of FAK within the kinase domain activation loop at Y576 and Y577 (270). The recruitment of SRC into a FAK/SRC signaling complex also facilitates the phosphorylation of various FAK-associated proteins. Many FAK targets are also independent binding partners and phosphorylation targets of SRC (e.g., p130^{CAS} and paxillin).

Although it was originally proposed that FAK might bind directly to the cytoplasmic tails of integrins (271), evidence now supports the concept that FAK is indirectly localized to sites of integrin clustering through protein:protein interactions of the C-terminal focal adhesion targeting (FAT) region. The FAT domain adopts a four-helix bundle structure that contains binding sites for the integrin-associated proteins paxillin and talin (275). The binding of paxillin to the FAT domain is mediated by two leucine-rich motifs (known as LD motifs), which interface with hydrophobic grooves on the FAT domain (276, 277). There is partial overlap of one of the two paxillin LD motif binding sites in the FAT domain with the SH2 binding site for GRB2 at FAK Y925 (276). There appears to be an important role of Y925 phosphorylation in the regulation of FAK localization (278). In vivo, the predominant state of Y925 is unphosphorylated. Although focal adhesions contain high levels of tyrosine phosphorylated proteins, nonphosphorylated or partially phosphorylated FAK appears to be the predominant form associated with matrix adhesion. Katz and co-workers (278) speculated that the reason hyperphosphory-lated FAK is excluded from focal adhesions could stem from a number of important interactions. Phosphorylation at Y925 and subsequent GRB2 binding might steri-cally block the focal adhesion targeting site, thus inhibiting the association of FAK with focal adhesions. Higher affinity associations of other molecular complexes with hyperphosphorylated FAK might compete with FAK binding at focal adhe-sions, or the hyperphosphorylated FAK could have a more restricted mobility in the plane of the membrane due to interactions with membrane lipoproteins. SRC-mediated phosphorylation of FAK at Y925 and subsequent GRB2 binding could lead to displacement of paxillin and then promote the dissociation of FAK from focal contacts. Another residue in the FAT domain that is phosphorylated is S910. This serine becomes phosphorylated by ERK2 during mitosis and also after growth factor stimulation and is associated with reduced paxillin binding to FAK (279).

Several different FAK isoforms can be produced as a consequence of use of an alternate promoter and also through alternative splicing. The alternative exons are short, coding for 3 to 28 amino acids. Exons 14 and 16 code for 6 and 7 residues (known as boxes 6 and 7, respectively) located on either side of the autophosphorylated tyrosine. FAK isoforms that include box 6 or 7 have dramat-ically increased autophosphorylation. This is thought to occur through alleviation of the inhibitory role exerted by the N-terminal domain of FAK as well as the ability of the alternatively spliced isoform to undergo intramolecular phosphoryla-tion. These alternately spliced forms also have higher levels of associated kinase activity compared to their wild-type counterparts. Additional variants of FAK have also been reported (280, 281). Many of these FAK isoforms are specific to neuronal tissues, suggesting possible unique properties of FAK in the brain. The mRNA for FRNK, an N-terminally truncated form of FAK, is generated from a promoter lying in an intron downstream of the catalytic domain (282). FRNK was first identified in chicken fibroblasts (282) but has subsequently been shown to be also expressed in the mouse (283). FRNK lacks the N-terminal and catalytic domains of FAK and acts in a dominant-negative manner, inhibiting many of FAK's functions (284, 285) (Figure 4.4).

The other member of the FAK family of cytoplasmic tyrosine kinases is PYK2 (also known as cell adhesion kinase β (CAKβ), CADTK, or RAFTK), which shares the structural features of FAK and has 45% sequence identity. The highest region of homology between the two kinases is in the catalytic domain (60% identity) and the extreme C terminus (which directs subcellular localization; 62% identity; for a review, see (286)). The two kinases both have molecular masses between 110 and 125 kDa. Like FAK, PYK2 possesses a central tyrosine kinase domain, flanked by an N-terminal FERM domain, and a multifunctional FAT domain. Four FAK tyrosine phosphorylation sites (Y397, Y576, Y577, and Y925) are conserved at analogous positions in PYK2 (Y402, Y579, Y580, and Y881) (Figure 4.4). PYK2 phosphorylation is much more dependent on increases in free Ca^{2+}, in contrast to FAK, which is controlled by integrin-mediated cell adhesion. While FAK is nearly ubiquitously expressed, PYK2 expression is restricted mainly to the brain and cells of the hematopoietic lineage. Moreover, the subcellular localization of PYK2 is cell-type specific. Depending on the cell type, PYK2 can be localized to focal adhesions, to specialized actin-containing structures such as podosomes of macrophages, to the sealing zone of osteoclasts, and to membrane ruffles and lamellipodia in some spreading and motile cells. FAK may also exhibit diffuse staining, either perinuclear or colocalized with the Golgi complex. Nuclear translocation of PYK2 has also been reported in fibroblasts (287, 288). Some cell types express both FAK and PYK2, while other cells express only one or the other. FAK, but not PYK2, binds talin; and PYK2, but not FAK, binds HIC-5 (289), NIRS (290), and PAP (291). Finally, although PYK can activate both ERK and JNK in response to a variety of stimuli, the precise function of PYK2 is poorly understood. Similar to FAK autophosphorylation at Y397, PYK2 is autophosphorylated at Y402, and this leads to the recruitment of SRC family kinases and ERK activation. The calcium-induced activation of PYK2 appears to be mediated by PKC. A number of ligands that signal through GPCRs have been shown to induce PYK2 phosphorylation, including bradykinin, lysophosphatidic acid, chemokine receptor 5 ligands, angiotensin II, and thrombin (292). PYK2 has a number of proposed roles including mediating cytoskeletal reorganization, cell migration, cell adhesion, and MAPK activation. Two spliced isoforms of PYK2 have been described, which are characterized by the presence or absence of an exon encoding for a 42 aa insert between the two proline-rich sequences of the C terminus. The variant without the exon is preferentially expressed in hematopoietic cells, while the unspliced form is predominant in the central nervous system (293).

4.4.1 FAK and Cancer

Several lines of evidence suggest roles for FAK in cancer. FAK expression is elevated in a number of human cancers including melanoma, sarcomas, head and neck squamous cell carcinomas, cervical carcinomas, prostate, colon, breast, and ovary (reviewed in (294)). There are a few instances of amplification of the region of 8q that encodes FAK and elevated FAK expression. FAK amplification has been described in a number of squamous cell carcinomas, as well as in the tumor cell lines Calu3 and HT29 (267). In breast cancers, elevated expression has been associated with poor prognostic indicators such as high mitotic index and HER2 overexpression (295). Targeting FAK may also interfere with angiogenesis. Mice with a targeted, endothelial-specific, conditional knockout of FAK demonstrated disrupted angiogenesis in late stage embryos (296) and overexpression of FAK in endothelial cells has been shown to promote angiogenesis (297).

4.5 JAK2

The JAK/STAT pathway is an essential, pleiotropic cascade that mediates the functions of a multitude of signals regulating growth, development, and homeostasis. In mammals, this pathway plays a central role in the signaling pathways for a wide array of cytokines and growth factors. There are four members of the Janus family of kinases: JAK1, JAK2, JAK3, and TYK2. With the exception of JAK3, which is selectively expressed in hematopoietic cells, the JAKs are widely expressed. The

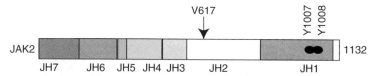

Figure 4.5 Domain structure of JAK2. Based on homology between JAKs, JAK homology domains have been identified (JH1–JH7). JAK2 contains an NH2-terminal FERM-like domain (JH4–7), a SH2 domain (JH3–4), a pseudokinase domain (JH2), and a tyrosine kinase domain (JH1, blue). The N terminus of JAKs, important for attachment to cytokine receptors' cytosolic domains, is important for JAK chaperone roles in cytokine receptor traffic. The pseudokinase domain has been suggested to inhibit the kinase domain and to be required for activation by cytokine receptors. The V617F mutation is located in the pseudokinase domain and leads to constitutive activation of JAK2. Phosphorylation sites in the JH1 domain are depicted by the black circles.

JAKs range in size from 120 to 140 kDa and have seven conserved JAK homology (JH) domains. The two carboxy-terminal JH regions feature a functional C-terminal kinase (JH1) and a pseudokinase domain (JH2, which is thought to regulate kinase activity). Similar to many other tyrosine kinases, activation is driven by phosphorylation of critical tyrosines in the activation loop. The four amino terminal JH domains (JH7–5 and half of JH4) comprise a FERM domain that mediates association with the proline-rich, membrane-proximal box1/box2 domains on cytokine receptors (Figure 4.5).

The JAK family kinases are activated by many cytokines (type 1 and 2 interferon, interleukins-2, 3, 4, 5, 6, 7, 10, 11, 12, 13) and growth factors (erythropoietin (EPO), granulocyte–macrophage colony stimulating factor (GM-CSF), granulocyte colony stimulating factor (G-CSF), thrombopoietin (TPO), growth hormone (GH), leptin, and prolactin (PRL)). However, growth factor signaling is almost exclusively mediated by JAK2. JAK2 can also mediate signaling stimulated by type 2 interferons, IL3, IL5, and IL6.

JAK2 signals via STAT proteins, principally STAT3 and STAT5, and promotes growth, survival, and angiogenesis. Intracellular activation of the JAKs occurs when ligand binding induces the multimerization of receptor subunits. For some ligands, such as erythropoietin and growth hormone, binding induces homodimers, whereas others such as the interferons and interleukins induce heterodimers or heteromultimers. The cytoplasmic domains of the receptor subunits are associated with the JAK kinases; when JAKs are brought into close proximity, transphosphorylation is facilitated. In the case of JAK2, the ligand-dependent tyrosine phosphosphorylation occurs principally on Y1007 (298). Activated JAK2 then phosphorylates specific tyrosine residues on the cytoplasmic domains of the receptors, which creates docking sites for SH2 domain–containing proteins such as the STATs; once bound to the receptors, the STATs are themselves phosphorylated by JAK2 on tyrosine residues. STATs are latent transcription factors that reside in the cytoplasm until activated by phosphorylation (Figure 4.6). All seven mammalian STAT proteins contain a conserved tyrosine residue near the C terminus that is phosphorylated by JAKs, resulting in STAT dimerization via SH2 domains. Phosphorylated STATs are

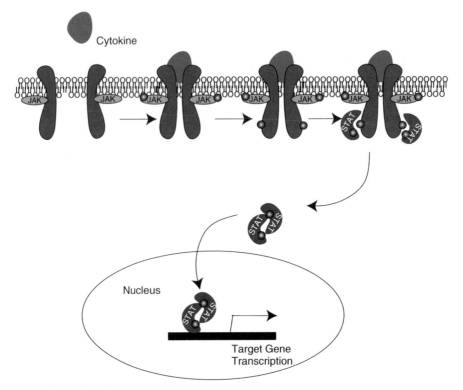

Figure 4.6 Activation of JAK2 phosphorylation and downstream signaling by cytokine ligand binding to the cytokine receptor. Cytokine ligands normally bind cytokine receptors, which results in Janus kinase 2 (JAK2) phosphorylation, recruitment of signal transducer and activator of transcription (STAT) signaling proteins, and phosphorylation and activation of downstream signaling pathways including STAT transcription factors, mitogen-activated protein kinase (MAPK) signaling proteins, and the phosphatidylinositol-3 kinase (PI3K)/AKT pathway. Following JAK-mediated phosphorylation, STAT proteins dimerize and are translocated to the nucleus, where they activate gene transcription.

translocated to the nucleus by a mechanism dependent on importin α5 and the RAN nuclear import pathway. In the nucleus, STAT dimers bind to specific regulatory sequences on the promoters of various genes, leading to the activation or repression of target genes. STAT3 is activated by tyrosine phosphorylation at residue 705 in response to growth factors, hormones, and cytokines. Tyrosine phosphorylation at residue 705 facilitates the dimerization of STAT3 and translocation to the nucleus. However, there is a second, serine phosphorylation site on STAT3, at residue 727, and phosphorylation of this site modulates the transcriptional activity of STAT3 and is required for maximal transcriptional activity.

The SOCS proteins are a family of at least eight members containing an SH2 domain and a SOCS box at the C terminus and can bind the phosphotyrosines on the C terminus of various receptors, blocking the recruitment of the STATs to the receptor. SOCS can also bind to JAKs directly or to the receptors, inhibiting

JAK kinase activity, and finally, SOCS proteins also interact with the elongin BC complex and cullin 2, facilitating the ubiquitination and subsequent degradation of the JAKs by the proteasome. For example, the phosphorylation of Y1007 of JAK results in SOCS1 binding via interactions of the SH2 domain of SOCS1 with the Y1007 of JAK2. When bound, SOCS1 inhibits JAK2 tyrosine kinase activity and downstream JAK2-dependent signaling (299).

JAKs also modulate other signaling pathways involved in malignant transformation. For instance, JAKs modulate activation of the RAS/RAF/MAPK pathway, regulate levels of the antiapoptotic proteins BCLXL, BCL2, BAX, MCL1, and survivin, and play a role in the regulation of p53-dependent cell-cycle arrest and apoptosis (reviewed in (300)). Both STAT3 and STAT5 signaling have been suggested to play roles in the regulation of MYC, a key transcription factor involved in cell transformation.

4.5.1 Activation and Known Mutations and Fusions of the JAK Family of Tyrosine Kinases

A number of mutations and translocations have been identified for the JAK family members, although most of literature has focused on activating mutations of JAK2 (Appendix XIII) and inactivating mutations of JAK3. In the case of JAK1, a number of inactivating somatic mutations were identified in prostate cancer cells (301), but to date, no mutations have been identified in primary tumors. Several IFNγ regulated genes, such as the proteasome subunits, low molecular weight proteins (LMP) 2, 7, and 10, and the "transporters associated with antigen processing" (TAP) 1 and 2, are thought to be obligatory for T-cell recognition of tumors but are often downregulated or inactivated in multiple tumor types, and this downregulation is associated with malignant transformation and disease progression (302). An inactivating G871E mutation in the ATP binding region of JAK1 was identified in cell lines from uterine leiomyosarcomas (303) and attributed to the defective TAP1 and LMP2 expression in these cells.

JAK3, as discussed earlier, is mainly found in lymphoid cells and appears to be only stimulated by activation of cytokine receptors that contain the γc subunit (e.g., IL2R, IL4R, IL7R, IL11R, IL13R), and therefore it would be predicted that JAK3 inhibition would result in immunosuppression by blocking the T-cell mitogenic signal mediated by IL2. Inactivating mutations in JAK3 result in autosomal recessive, severe combined immunodeficiency in both humans and mice (304–307).

Constitutive phosphorylation of STAT5 is found in approximately 70% of AML patients, although the presence of FLT3 or KIT mutations accounts for up to 35% of AML patients. A search for other possible tyrosine kinase mutations that might account for the STAT5 tyrosine phosphorylation in those patients without FLT3 or KIT mutations resulted in the identification of activating mutations in the JAK3 pseudokinase domain in the acute megakaryoblastic leukemia (AMKL) cell line CMK (A572K), and additional mutations V722I and P132T in cells from AMKL patients. All three mutations can transform BaF3 cells to factor-independent growth (308).

A role for TYK2 in infection and autoimmunity was first indicated from studies to identify the reason why B10.Q/J mice are susceptible to infection by *Toxoplasma gondii*. The phenotype was mapped to a single recessive locus on chromosome 9 and identified as *tyk2*. In this strain of mice, the *tyk2* gene contains a single missense mutation (E775K) in an invariant motif of the pseudokinase (JH2) domain. This mutation appeared to result in the absence of TYK2 protein, and B10.Q/J cells behaved similarly to TYK2-deficient cells with impaired signaling and biological responses to IL12, IL23, and type I IFNs (309). A later study identified a homozygous TYK2 mutation in a patient with hyper-IGE syndrome and unusual susceptibility to various microorganisms. Cells derived from this patient displayed defects in cyokine signaling, which were restored by transducing *TYK2* (310). In the Sanger COSMIC database, two mutations of TYK2 were identified in primary colon tumors: H732R and G763G (mutation without a change in coding). However, at present there is no information as to whether the H732R mutation results in any change in TYK2 activity.

JAK2 is constitutively active in tumor cells, contributing to the increased levels of activated STAT3 and STAT5. There are multiple mechanisms whereby JAK2 becomes activated in tumor cells, including activation of receptor tyrosine kinases, ectopic ligand production, gene amplification, or mutations. In addition, cytokines, released by tumor cells or tumor stroma (such as IL6), can lead to activation of JAK2. This is of particular relevance in multiple myeloma and prostate cancer, diseases in which the tumor cells release high levels of IL6. Another mechanism that results in upregulated JAK/STAT signaling is inhibition of negative regulators such as proteins of the SOCS family. SOCS proteins are downregulated in many cancers (311, 312). SOCS1 is frequently silenced by methylation in multiple myeloma (313), hepatocellular carcinoma (314), hepatoblastoma (315), pancreatic ductal neoplasms (316), pituitary adenomas (317), and primary gastric cancers (318). SOCS3 methylation occurs frequently in lung cancer (319), and in addition, SOCS1 mutations in Hodgkin's lymphoma occur quite often and are associated with nuclear pSTAT5 (320).

Activating mutations of JAK2 also occur. For example, there are translocations that occur in leukemias which result in constitutively activated fusion proteins including TEL-JAK2 (T-cell acute lymphoblastic leukemia (T-ALL), B-cell acute lymphoblastic leukemia (B-ALL and atypical chronic myelogenous leukemia (aCML) (321), BCR-JAK2 (aCML) (322), and PCM1-JAK2 (B-ALL, aCML) (323–325). Recently, a common point mutation of JAK2 (JAK2V617F) was identified in myeloproliferative disorders (326–328). The V617F mutation occurs in the autoinhibitory JH2 domain, leading to a constitutively activated form of JAK2. Although estimates of frequency vary between investigators, this mutation appears to occur in 65–97% of patients with polycythemia vera (PV), approximately 23–41% and 43–57% of patients with essential thrombcytosis (ET) and idiopathic myelofibrosis (IMF), respectively, 35% of patients with myelofibrosis with myeloid metaplasia (MMM), and roughly 8–20% of patients with chronic myelomonocytic leukemia (CMML) and aCML. Since the initial identification of the V617F mutation in JAK2, additional gain of function mutations have been described (Appendix XIII). In particular, novel mutations in JAK2 exon 12 (329) were identified in patients who had been diagnosed as V617F-negative PV patients.

4.5.2   Further Roles of JAK2 in Tumor Growth

In addition to the role of the JAK/STAT pathway in cytokine and growth factor signaling, this pathway also mediates diverse cellular responses to various forms of biological stress including hypoxia/reperfusion, endotoxin, ultraviolet light, and hyperosmolarity (330). Hypoxia, a common consequence of solid tumor growth, activates a cascade of molecular pathways that lead to the synthesis of proteins and key enzymes involved in angiogenesis, glycolysis, and cell-cycle control. Hypoxia results in increased phosphorylation of STAT1, 3, and 5 in breast cancer cells (331) and has been shown to upregulate JAK2/STAT1/STAT5 signaling, leading to induction of cyclin D1 (332). Hypoxia inducible factor-1 (HIF1) and STAT3 are the major transcription factors that regulate the expression of vascular endothelial cell growth factor (VEGF), a key regulator of tumor angiogenesis. Targeting STAT3 with a small-molecule inhibitor blocks HIF1 and VEGF expression in vitro and inhibits tumor growth and angiogenesis in vivo (333). Furthermore, induction of VEGF by diverse oncogenic growth stimuli, including IL6R, SRC, and ERBB2, is attenuated in cells without STAT3 signaling (333).

Erythropoietin (EPO), well known for its role in promoting erythropoiesis, signals through the JAK/STAT pathway. EPO is commonly used to treat anemia and fatigue in patients receiving radiation therapy and chemotherapy. However, recent data also suggest a role for EPO signaling in cancer. Numerous malignant cell lines express both EPO and its receptor (EPOR) (334). EPO/EPOR expression has been described in breast cancers, cervical carcinomas, head and neck squamous cell carcinomas, melanomas, glioblastomas, and neuroblastomas. Additionally, many cells upregulate EPO expression in response to hypoxia. In nude mice implanted with xenografts of EPO-expressing cell lines, intraperitoneal injection of an EPO antagonist inhibited angiogenesis and stimulated tumor destruction (334, 335). In uterine and cervical cancers, EPO and EPOR are widely expressed and the expression of EPOR increases with tumor grade (336). EPOR is also highly expressed in head and neck cancer, particularly in the regions of the tumors that are hypoxic or invasive (337). In head and neck squamous cell carcinoma, EPO contributes to tumor cell invasion through the JAK/STAT pathway (338). At least two clinical studies demonstrated worse tumor control in head and neck cancer patients treated with EPO. The Breast Cancer Erythropoietin Trial (BEST) in nonanemic patients was terminated early due to an increased mortality rate in patients given EPO compared to those receiving a placebo; the increase was mainly due to early disease progression (339). HNSCC patients receiving EPO concomitant with radiotherapy demonstrated increased locoregional recurrence and decreased survival (340). EPO may also play an important role in the resistance of tumors to radiation and chemotherapy. EPO increased the resistance of the glioblastoma cell line U87 and the primary cervical cancer cell line HT100 to ionizing radiation and cisplatin, an effect reversed by the JAK2 inhibitor AG490 (341). In addition to mediating EPOR signaling,

JAK2 also enhances the normally inefficient folding of EPOR by the endoplasmic reticulum, providing a further enhancement of EPOR signaling (342). In fact, the phenotype of the JAK2 null mouse is very similar to (although more severe than) that of the EPO and EPOR deficient mice. All three mutant mouse strains are embryonic lethal at day 12.5 due to the absence of definitive erythropoiesis (343, 344).

Prolactin, an important regulator of both breast and prostate tumor cell proliferation, also signals through the JAK/STAT pathway (345). Increased activation of STAT3 and STAT5 is associated with high histological grade and poor prognosis in prostate cancer (346). Constitutive activation of STAT3 is observed in prostate cancer cell lines (DU 145, PC-3, and LnCAP) (347, 348) and downregulation of STAT3 using siRNA inhibits their proliferation (349). Similarly, STAT3 single-stranded oligonucleotides that presumably block STAT3:DNA binding also inhibit prostate cancer cell line proliferation in vitro and tumor growth in vivo (350). Constitutive activation of STAT3 and STAT5 is frequently observed in breast cancer tissues and cell lines (351), and conversely, pharmacological or dominant-negative inhibition of STAT3 activity blocks the proliferation and survival of breast cancer cells in vitro (reviewed in (351)) and in vivo (352). Two other important regulators of breast tumor cell proliferation, growth hormone and leptin, also signal via the JAK/STAT pathway (345, 353, 354). Leptin also stimulates gastric cancer cell proliferation through a STAT3-dependent mechanism (355).

Germline mutations of the breast cancer susceptibility gene-1 (BRCA1) confer a high risk of breast and ovarian cancer in women and prostate cancer in men. In DU 145 prostate cancer cells, enhanced expression of BRCA1 resulted in constitutive activation of STAT3, as well as upstream activation of JAK1 and JAK2, and blocking STAT3 activation using antisense oligonucleotides significantly inhibited cell proliferation and triggered apoptosis in DU 145 cells with enhanced expression of BRCA1 (356).

Constitutive activation of STAT3 has also been reported in several human lung cancer lines (357) and in the majority of ovarian carcinomas (358) and about 50% of renal cell carcinomas (359). A role for activated STAT3 in promoting human melanoma brain metastases has been suggested (360). STAT3 is constitutively activated in nearly 50% of mantle cell lymphomas (361). Cell lines derived from malignant fibrous histiocytoma secrete high levels of IL6 and exhibit constitutive activation of STAT3, and their proliferation is inhibited by the JAK2 inhibitor AG490, SOCS3 overexpression, or introduction of dominant-negative STAT3 (362). Constitutive activation of STAT3 is observed in about 50% of the Ewing's sarcoma family of tumors, characterized by the fusion of the *EWS* gene with one of several ETS transcription factors, most commonly EWS-FLI1 (363). Constitutive activation of STAT3 is also observed in many colon cancers and is a predictor of poor prognosis (364, 365). Strong nuclear pSTAT3 staining was observed in 11/11 gastrointestinal stromal tumors (GISTs), and treatment of GIST-derived tumor cell lines with AG490 inhibits their proliferation (366). The activation of the JAK/STAT pathway has also been implicated in MEN-2, a disorder caused by activating RET mutations. Two of the RET mutations, Y791F and S891A, which both affect the tyrosine kinase domain, activate STAT3 by a mechanism involving SRC, JAK1, and JAK2 (367). Constitutive activation of STAT3 and STAT5 is observed in the majority of nasopharyngeal carcinomas (368). STAT3 is also constitutively activated in HNSCC, and a STAT3 decoy inhibits proliferation of HNSCC cells (369).

The JAK/STAT pathway has also been implicated in the pathogenesis of lymphomas, leukemias, and multiple myeloma. Many different cell lines derived from patients with Hodgkin's lymphoma exhibit constitutive activation of STAT3, and the JAK2 inhibitor AG490 inhibits proliferation of these cells. Constitutive activation of the JAK/STAT pathway has also been observed in EBV-infected spontaneous lymphoblastoid cell lines derived from patients with post-transplant lymphoproliferative disease, adult T-cell leukemia/lymphoma, Szerey syndrome, and mycosis fungoides (reviewed in (300)). Activated STAT3 is observed in HTLV-1-dependent leukemia, erythroleukemia, AML, CML, and large granular lymphocyte leukemia (370). In CML cells, the BCR-ABL kinase induces persistent activation of STAT5, which is blocked by BCR-ABL inhibitors (371). STAT5 is also activated by FLT3 in AML, an effect blocked by a FLT3 inhibitor (372). IL6 is the major growth and survival factor for many cell lines derived from bone marrow of multiple myeloma patients. In these cells, IL6 upregulates its own receptor (IL6Rα), a response that is inhibited by AG490 (373).

MPL (myeloproliferative leukemia virus oncogene homology) is the receptor for thrombopoietin and facilitates both global hematopoiesis and megakaryocyte growth and differentiation. Two somatic gain of function MPL mutations have been identified (MPLW515L and MPLW515K) in JAK2V617F-negative patients with primary myelofibrosis (PMF) and ET (374, 375). The frequency of both mutations was determined to be about 5% in PMF and 1% in ET. Additional mutations have been identified, including MPLW515S and MPLS505N (376). MPL signals through the JAK/STAT pathway; and the initial studies suggest that MPL mutations favor megakaryocytic/myeloid disease as opposed to the erythroid hyperproliferative diseases seen with JAK2 mutations. At present, it is thought that almost all patients with PV carry a JAK2 mutation (either V617F or an exon 12 mutation) and that JAK2V617F or a MPL mutation is found in the majority of patients with either ET or PMF (reviewed in (377)).

The JAK/STAT pathway also appears to play a role in the resistance of certain tumor cells to chemotherapeutics. For example, treatment of the IL10-dependent, AIDS-related non–Hodgkin's lymphoma cell line 2F7, and the IL6-dependent multiple myeloma cell line, U266, with JAK/STAT inhibitors (piceatannol or AG490) sensitizes the cells to a variety of chemotherapeutic agents including cisplatin, fludaribine, adriamycin, and vinblastine (378). Similarly, activated STAT3 is thought to contribute to the chemoresistance of estrogen-receptor-negative breast carcinoma cells; inhibition of STAT3 with JAK2 tyrosine kinase inhibitors or dominant-negative STAT3 increased sensitivity to chemotherapy-induced apoptosis (379). The chemoprotective effect of STAT3 is probably mediated through the induction of antiapoptotic proteins such as BCLXL and MCL1, both targets of STAT3 and STAT5 signaling.

REFERENCES

1. Pluk H, Dorey K, Superti-Furga G. Autoinhibition of c-Abl. Cell 2002;108(2):247–259.
2. Taagepera S, McDonald D, Loeb JE, Whitaker LL, McElroy AK, Wang JY, Hope TJ. Nuclear-cytoplasmic shuttling of C-ABL tyrosine kinase. Proc Natl Acad Sci U S A 1998;95(13):7457–7462.
3. Wen ST, Jackson PK, Van Etten RA. The cytostatic function of c-Abl is controlled by multiple nuclear localization signals and requires the p53 and Rb tumor suppressor gene products. EMBO J 1996;15(7):1583–1595.
4. Lewis JM, Baskaran R, Taagepera S, Schwartz MA, Wang JY. Integrin regulation of c-Abl tyrosine kinase activity and cytoplasmic-nuclear transport. Proc Natl Acad Sci U S A 1996;93(26):15174–15179.
5. Vella V, Zhu J, Frasca F, Li CY, Vigneri P, Vigneri R, Wang JY. Exclusion of c-Abl from the nucleus restrains the p73 tumor suppression function. J Biol Chem 2003;278(27):25151–25157.
6. Yang XJ. Lysine acetylation and the bromodomain: a new partnership for signaling. Bioessays 2004;26(10):1076–1087.
7. di Bari MG, Ciuffini L, Mingardi M, Testi R, Soddu S, Barila D. c-Abl acetylation by histone acetyltransferases regulates its nuclear-cytoplasmic localization. EMBO Rep 2006;7(7):727–733.
8. Shafman T, Khanna KK, Kedar P, Spring K, Kozlov S, Yen T, Hobson K, Gatei M, Zhang N, Watters D, Egerton M, Shiloh Y, Kharbanda S, Kufe D, Lavin MF. Interaction between ATM protein and c-Abl in response to DNA damage. Nature 1997;387(6632):520–523.
9. Dan S, Naito M, Seimiya H, Kizaki A, Mashima T, Tsuruo T. Activation of c-Abl tyrosine kinase requires caspase activation and is not involved in JNK/SAPK activation during apoptosis of human monocytic leukemia U937 cells. Oncogene 1999;18(6):1277–1283.
10. Chau BN, Chen TT, Wan YY, DeGregori J, Wang JY. Tumor necrosis factor alpha-induced apoptosis requires p73 and c-ABL activation downstream of RB degradation. Mol Cell Biol 2004;24(10):4438–4447.
11. Barila D, Rufini A, Condo I, Ventura N, Dorey K, Superti-Furga G, Testi R. Caspase-dependent cleavage of c-Abl contributes to apoptosis. Mol Cell Biol 2003;23(8):2790–2799.
12. Goldberg Z, Vogt Sionov R, Berger M, Zwang Y, Perets R, Van Etten RA, Oren M, Taya Y, Haupt Y. Tyrosine phosphorylation of Mdm2 by c-Abl: implications for p53 regulation. EMBO J 2002;21(14):3715–3727.
13. Sionov RV, Moallem E, Berger M, Kazaz A, Gerlitz O, Ben-Neriah Y, Oren M, Haupt Y. c-Abl neutralizes the inhibitory effect of Mdm2 on p53. J Biol Chem 1999;274(13):8371–8374.
14. Sawyers CL, McLaughlin J, Goga A, Havlik M, Witte O. The nuclear tyrosine kinase c-Abl negatively regulates cell growth. Cell 1994;77(1):121–131.
15. Ben-Yehoyada M, Ben-Dor I, Shaul Y. c-Abl tyrosine kinase selectively regulates p73 nuclear matrix association. J Biol Chem 2003;278(36):34475–34482.
16. White E, Prives C. DNA damage enables p73. Nature 1999;399(6738):734–735, 737.
17. Kharbanda S, Pandey P, Jin S, Inoue S, Bharti A, Yuan ZM, Weichselbaum R, Weaver D, Kufe D. Functional interaction between DNA-PK and c-Abl in response to DNA damage. Nature 1997;386(6626):732–735.
18. Yuan ZM, Huang Y, Ishiko T, Nakada S, Utsugisawa T, Kharbanda S, Wang R, Sung P, Shinohara A, Weichselbaum R, Kufe D. Regulation of Rad51 function by c-Abl in response to DNA damage. J Biol Chem 1998;273(7):3799–3802.
19. Kharbanda S, Bharti A, Pei D, Wang J, Pandey P, Ren R, Weichselbaum R, Walsh CT, Kufe D. The stress response to ionizing radiation involves c-Abl-dependent phosphorylation of SHPTP1. Proc Natl Acad Sci U S A 1996;93(14):6898–6901.
20. Yuan ZM, Utsugisawa T, Huang Y, Ishiko T, Nakada S, Kharbanda S, Weichselbaum R, Kufe D. Inhibition of phosphatidylinositol 3-kinase by c-Abl in the genotoxic stress response. J Biol Chem 1997;272(38):23485–23488.
21. Welch PJ, Wang JY. A C-terminal protein-binding domain in the retinoblastoma protein regulates nuclear c-Abl tyrosine kinase in the cell cycle. Cell 1993;75(4):779–790.

22. Welch PJ, Wang JY. Abrogation of retinoblastoma protein function by c-Abl through tyrosine kinase-dependent and -independent mechanisms. Mol Cell Biol 1995;15(10):5542–5551.

23. Goga A, Liu X, Hambuch TM, Senechal K, Major E, Berk AJ, Witte ON, Sawyers CL. p53 dependent growth suppression by the c-Abl nuclear tyrosine kinase. Oncogene 1995;11(4):791–799.

24. Van Etten RA. Cycling, stressed-out and nervous: cellular functions of c-Abl. Trends Cell Biol 1999;9(5):179–186.

25. Miao YJ, Wang JY. Binding of A/T-rich DNA by three high mobility group-like domains in c-Abl tyrosine kinase. J Biol Chem 1996;271(37):22823–22830.

26. David-Cordonnier MH, Hamdane M, Bailly C, D'Halluin JC. The DNA binding domain of the human c-Abl tyrosine kinase preferentially binds to DNA sequences containing an AAC motif and to distorted DNA structures. Biochemistry 1998;37(17):6065–6076.

27. Birchenall-Roberts MC, Yoo YD, Bertolette DC 3rd, Lee KH, Turley JM, Bang OS, Ruscetti FW, Kim SJ. The p120-v-Abl protein interacts with E2F-1 and regulates E2F-1 transcriptional activity. J Biol Chem 1997;272(14):8905–8911.

28. Shi Y, Alin K, Goff SP. Abl-interactor-1, a novel SH3 protein binding to the carboxy-terminal portion of the Abl protein, suppresses v-abl transforming activity. Genes Dev 1995;9(21):2583–2597.

29. Dai Z, Pendergast AM. Abi-2, a novel SH3-containing protein interacts with the c-Abl tyrosine kinase and modulates c-Abl transforming activity. Genes Dev 1995;9(21):2569–2582.

30. Plattner R, Kadlec L, DeMali KA, Kazlauskas A, Pendergast AM. c-Abl is activated by growth factors and Src family kinases and has a role in the cellular response to PDGF. Genes Dev 1999;13(18):2400–2411.

31. Kadlec L, Pendergast AM. The amphiphysin-like protein 1 (ALP1) interacts functionally with the cABL tyrosine kinase and may play a role in cytoskeletal regulation. Proc Natl Acad Sci U S A 1997;94(23):12390–12395.

32. Lewis JM, Schwartz MA. Integrins regulate the association and phosphorylation of paxillin by c-Abl. J Biol Chem 1998;273(23):14225–14230.

33. Woodring PJ, Hunter T, Wang JY. Inhibition of c-Abl tyrosine kinase activity by filamentous actin. J Biol Chem 2001;276(29):27104–27110.

34. Woodring PJ, Litwack ED, O'Leary DD, Lucero GR, Wang JY, Hunter T. Modulation of the F-actin cytoskeleton by c-Abl tyrosine kinase in cell spreading and neurite extension. J Cell Biol 2002;156(5):879–892.

35. Moresco EM, Koleske AJ. Regulation of neuronal morphogenesis and synaptic function by Abl family kinases. Curr Opin Neurobiol 2003;13(5):535–544.

36. Nowell P, Hungerford D. A minute chromosome in chronic granulocytic leukemia. Science 1960;132:1497.

37. Chissoe SL, Bodenteich A, Wang YF, Wang YP, Burian D, Clifton SW, Crabtree J, Freeman A, Iyer K, Jian L, et al. Sequence and analysis of the human ABL gene, the BCR gene, and regions involved in the Philadelphia chromosomal translocation. Genomics 1995;27(1):67–82.

38. Kurzrock R, Kloetzer WS, Talpaz M, Blick M, Walters R, Arlinghaus RB, Gutterman JU. Identification of molecular variants of p210bcr-abl in chronic myelogenous leukemia. Blood 1987;70(1):233–236.

39. Kurzrock R, Gutterman JU, Talpaz M. The molecular genetics of Philadelphia chromosome-positive leukemias. N Engl J Med 1988;319(15):990–998.

40. Kurzrock R, Shtalrid M, Talpaz M, Kloetzer WS, Gutterman JU. Expression of c-abl in Philadelphia-positive acute myelogenous leukemia. Blood 1987;70(5):1584–1588.

41. Daley GQ, Van Etten RA, Baltimore D. Induction of chronic myelogenous leukemia in mice by the P210bcr/abl gene of the Philadelphia chromosome. Science 1990;247(4944):824–830.

42. Elefanty AG, Hariharan IK, Cory S. bcr-abl, the hallmark of chronic myeloid leukaemia in man, induces multiple haemopoietic neoplasms in mice. EMBO J 1990;9(4):1069–1078.

43. Heisterkamp N, Jenster G, ten Hoeve J, Zovich D, Pattengale PK, Groffen J. Acute leukaemia in bcr/abl transgenic mice. Nature 1990;344(6263):251–253.

44. Kelliher MA, McLaughlin J, Witte ON, Rosenberg N. Induction of a chronic myelogenous leukemia-like syndrome in mice with v-abl and BCR/ABL. Proc Natl Acad Sci U S A 1990;87(17):6649–6653.

45. Hantschel O, Superti-Furga G. Regulation of the c-Abl and Bcr-Abl tyrosine kinases. Nat Rev Mol Cell Biol 2004;5(1):33–44.

46. Wetzler M, Talpaz M, Van Etten RA, Hirsh-Ginsberg C, Beran M, Kurzrock R. Subcellular localization of Bcr, Abl, and Bcr-Abl proteins in normal and leukemic cells and correlation of expression with myeloid differentiation. J Clin Invest 1993;92(4):1925–1939.

47. Dhut S, Dorey EL, Horton MA, Ganesan TS, Young BD. Identification of two normal bcr gene products in the cytoplasm. Oncogene 1988;3(5):561–566.

48. Wetzler M, Talpaz M, Yee G, Stass SA, Van Etten RA, Andreeff M, Goodacre AM, Kleine HD, Mahadevia RK, Kurzrock R. Cell cycle-related shifts in subcellular localization of BCR: association with mitotic chromosomes and with heterochromatin. Proc Natl Acad Sci U S A 1995;92(8):3488–3492.

49. Takeda N, Shibuya M, Maru Y. The BCR-ABL oncoprotein potentially interacts with the xeroderma pigmentosum group B protein. Proc Natl Acad Sci U S A 1999;96(1):203–207.

50. Maru Y, Kobayashi T, Tanaka K, Shibuya M. BCR binds to the xeroderma pigmentosum group B protein. Biochem Biophys Res Commun 1999;260(2):309–312.

51. Maru Y, Witte ON. The BCR gene encodes a novel serine/threonine kinase activity within a single exon. Cell 1991;67(3):459–468.

52. Reuther GW, Fu H, Cripe LD, Collier RJ, Pendergast AM. Association of the protein kinases c-Bcr and Bcr-Abl with proteins of the 14-3-3 family. Science 1994;266(5182):129–133.

53. McWhirter JR, Galasso DL, Wang JY. A coiled-coil oligomerization domain of Bcr is essential for the transforming function of Bcr-Abl oncoproteins. Mol Cell Biol 1993;13(12):7587–7595.

54. Pendergast AM, Muller AJ, Havlik MH, Maru Y, Witte ON. BCR sequences essential for transformation by the BCR-ABL oncogene bind to the ABL SH2 regulatory domain in a non-phosphotyrosine-dependent manner. Cell 1991;66(1):161–171.

55. McWhirter JR, Wang JY. Activation of tyrosinase kinase and microfilament-binding functions of c-abl by bcr sequences in bcr/abl fusion proteins. Mol Cell Biol 1991;11(3):1553–1565.

56. McWhirter JR, Wang JY. An actin-binding function contributes to transformation by the Bcr-Abl oncoprotein of Philadelphia chromosome-positive human leukemias. EMBO J 1993;12(4):1533–1546.

57. Sawyers CL, McLaughlin J, Witte ON. Genetic requirement for Ras in the transformation of fibroblasts and hematopoietic cells by the Bcr-Abl oncogene. J Exp Med 1995;181(1):307–313.

58. Mandanas RA, Leibowitz DS, Gharehbaghi K, Tauchi T, Burgess GS, Miyazawa K, Jayaram HN, Boswell HS. Role of p21 RAS in p210 bcr-abl transformation of murine myeloid cells. Blood 1993;82(6):1838–1847.

59. Tauchi T, Okabe S, Miyazawa K, Ohyashiki K. The tetramerization domain-independent Ras activation by BCR-ABL oncoprotein in hematopoietic cells. Int J Oncol 1998;12(6):1269–1276.

60. Salgia R, Li JL, Lo SH, Brunkhorst B, Kansas GS, Sobhany ES, Sun Y, Pisick E, Hallek M, Ernst T, et al. Molecular cloning of human paxillin, a focal adhesion protein phosphorylated by P210BCR/ABL. J Biol Chem 1995;270(10):5039–5047.

61. Gotoh A, Miyazawa K, Ohyashiki K, Tauchi T, Boswell HS, Broxmeyer HE, Toyama K. Tyrosine phosphorylation and activation of focal adhesion kinase (p125FAK) by BCR-ABL oncoprotein. Exp Hematol 1995;23(11):1153–1159.

62. Sanchez-Garcia I, Grutz G. Tumorigenic activity of the BCR-ABL oncogenes is mediated by BCL2. Proc Natl Acad Sci U S A 1995;92(12):5287–5291.

63. Cortez D, Stoica G, Pierce JH, Pendergast AM. The BCR-ABL tyrosine kinase inhibits apoptosis by activating a Ras-dependent signaling pathway. Oncogene 1996;13(12):2589–2594.

64. Sanchez-Garcia I, Martin-Zanca D. Regulation of Bcl-2 gene expression by BCR-ABL is mediated by Ras. J Mol Biol 1997;267(2):225–228.

65. Carlesso N, Frank DA, Griffin JD. Tyrosyl phosphorylation and DNA binding activity of signal transducers and activators of transcription (STAT) proteins in hematopoietic cell lines transformed by Bcr/Abl. J Exp Med 1996;183(3):811–820.

66. Frank DA, Varticovski L. BCR/abl leads to the constitutive activation of Stat proteins, and shares an epitope with tyrosine phosphorylated Stats. Leukemia 1996;10(11):1724–1730.

67. Ilaria RL Jr, Van Etten RA. P210 and P190(BCR/ABL) induce the tyrosine phosphorylation and DNA binding activity of multiple specific STAT family members. J Biol Chem 1996;271(49):31704–31710.

68. Shuai K, Halpern J, ten Hoeve J, Rao X, Sawyers CL. Constitutive activation of STAT5 by the BCR-ABL oncogene in chronic myelogenous leukemia. Oncogene 1996;13(2):247–254.

69. de Groot RP, Raaijmakers JA, Lammers JW, Jove R, Koenderman L. STAT5 activation by BCR-Abl contributes to transformation of K562 leukemia cells. Blood 1999;94(3):1108–1112.

70. Chai SK, Nichols GL, Rothman P. Constitutive activation of JAKs and STATs in BCR-Abl-expressing cell lines and peripheral blood cells derived from leukemic patients. J Immunol 1997;159(10):4720–4728.

71. Papadopoulos P, Ridge SA, Boucher CA, Stocking C, Wiedemann LM. The novel activation of ABL by fusion to an ets-related gene, TEL. Cancer Res 1995;55(1):34–38.

72. Golub TR, Goga A, Barker GF, Afar DE, McLaughlin J, Bohlander SK, Rowley JD, Witte ON, Gilliland DG. Oligomerization of the ABL tyrosine kinase by the Ets protein TEL in human leukemia. Mol Cell Biol 1996;16(8):4107–4116.

73. Van Limbergen H, Beverloo HB, van Drunen E, Janssens A, Hahlen K, Poppe B, Van Roy N, Marynen P, De Paepe A, Slater R, Speleman F. Molecular cytogenetic and clinical findings in ETV6/ABL1-positive leukemia. Genes Chromosomes Cancer 2001;30(3):274–282.

74. Andreasson P, Johansson B, Carlsson M, Jarlsfelt I, Fioretos T, Mitelman F, Hoglund M. BCR/ABL-negative chronic myeloid leukemia with ETV6/ABL fusion. Genes Chromosomes Cancer 1997;20(3):299–304.

75. Hannemann JR, McManus DM, Kabarowski JH, Wiedemann LM. Haemopoietic transformation by the TEL/ABL oncogene. Br J Haematol 1998;102(2):475–485.

76. Golub TR, Barker GF, Bohlander SK, Hiebert SW, Ward DC, Bray-Ward P, Morgan E, Raimondi SC, Rowley JD, Gilliland DG. Fusion of the TEL gene on 12p13 to the AML1 gene on 21q22 in acute lymphoblastic leukemia. Proc Natl Acad Sci U S A 1995;92(11):4917–4921.

77. Okuda K, Golub TR, Gilliland DG, Griffin JD. p210BCR/ABL, p190BCR/ABL, and TEL/ABL activate similar signal transduction pathways in hematopoietic cell lines. Oncogene 1996;13(6):1147–1152.

78. Voss J, Posern G, Hannemann JR, Wiedemann LM, Turhan AG, Poirel H, Bernard OA, Adermann K, Kardinal C, Feller SM. The leukaemic oncoproteins Bcr-Abl and Tel-Abl (ETV6/Abl) have altered substrate preferences and activate similar intracellular signalling pathways. Oncogene 2000;19(13):1684–1690.

79. Wang B, Kruh GD. Subcellular localization of the Arg protein tyrosine kinase. Oncogene 1996;13(1):193–197.

80. Koleske AJ, Gifford AM, Scott ML, Nee M, Bronson RT, Miczek KA, Baltimore D. Essential roles for the Abl and Arg tyrosine kinases in neurulation. Neuron 1998;21(6):1259–1272.

81. Wang Y, Miller AL, Mooseker MS, Koleske AJ. The Abl-related gene (Arg) nonreceptor tyrosine kinase uses two F-actin-binding domains to bundle F-actin. Proc Natl Acad Sci U S A 2001;98(26):14865–14870.

82. Miller AL, Wang Y, Mooseker MS, Koleske AJ. The Abl-related gene (Arg) requires its F-actin-microtubule cross-linking activity to regulate lamellipodial dynamics during fibroblast adhesion. J Cell Biol 2004;165(3):407–419.

83. Cao C, Ren X, Kharbanda S, Koleske A, Prasad KV, Kufe D. The ARG tyrosine kinase interacts with Siva-1 in the apoptotic response to oxidative stress. J Biol Chem 2001;276(15):11465–11468.

84. Baskaran R, Chiang GG, Mysliwiec T, Kruh GD, Wang JY. Tyrosine phosphorylation of RNA polymerase II carboxyl-terminal domain by the Abl-related gene product. J Biol Chem 1997;272(30):18905–18909.

85. Plattner R, Koleske AJ, Kazlauskas A, Pendergast AM. Bidirectional signaling links the Abelson kinases to the platelet-derived growth factor receptor. Mol Cell Biol 2004;24(6):2573–2583.

86. Yu HH, Zisch AH, Dodelet VC, Pasquale EB. Multiple signaling interactions of Abl and Arg kinases with the EphB2 receptor. Oncogene 2001;20(30):3995–4006.

87. Liu X, Huang W, Li C, Li P, Yuan J, Li X, Qiu XB, Ma Q, Cao C. Interaction between c-Abl and Arg tyrosine kinases and proteasome subunit PSMA7 regulates proteasome degradation. Mol Cell 2006;22(3):317–327.

88. Cazzaniga G, Tosi S, Aloisi A, Giudici G, Daniotti M, Pioltelli P, Kearney L, Biondi A. The tyrosine kinase abl-related gene ARG is fused to ETV6 in an AML-M4Eo patient with a t(1;12)(q25;p13): molecular cloning of both reciprocal transcripts. Blood 1999;94(12):4370–4373.

89. Iijima Y, Ito T, Oikawa T, Eguchi M, Eguchi-Ishimae M, Kamada N, Kishi K, Asano S, Sakaki Y, Sato Y. A new ETV6/TEL partner gene, ARG (ABL-related gene or ABL2), identified in an AML-M3 cell line with a t(1;12)(q25;p13) translocation. Blood 2000;95(6):2126–2131.

90. Griesinger F, Janke A, Podleschny M, Bohlander SK. Identification of an ETV6-ABL2 fusion transcript in combination with an ETV6 point mutation in a T-cell acute lymphoblastic leukaemia cell line. Br J Haematol 2002;119(2):454–458.

91. Palmi C, Fazio G, Cassetti A, Aloisi A, Villa A, Biondi A, Cazzaniga G. TEL/ARG induces cytoskeletal abnormalities in 293T cells. Cancer Lett 2006;241(1):79–86.

92. Okuda K, Oda A, Sato Y, Nakayama A, Fujita H, Sonoda Y, Griffin JD. Signal transduction and cellular functions of the TEL/ARG oncoprotein. Leukemia 2005;19(4):603–610.

93. Iijima Y, Okuda K, Tojo A, Tri NK, Setoyama M, Sakaki Y, Asano S, Tokunaga K, Kruh GD, Sato Y. Transformation of Ba/F3 cells and Rat-1 cells by ETV6/ARG. Oncogene 2002;21(28):4374–4383.

94. Levinson AD, Oppermann H, Levintow L, Varmus HE, Bishop JM. Evidence that the transforming gene of avian sarcoma virus encodes a protein kinase associated with a phosphoprotein. Cell 1978;15(2):561–572.

95. Boggon TJ, Eck MJ. Structure and regulation of Src family kinases. Oncogene 2004;23(48):7918–7927.

96. Koegl M, Zlatkine P, Ley SC, Courtneidge SA, Magee AI. Palmitoylation of multiple Src-family kinases at a homologous N-terminal motif. Biochem J 1994;303(Pt 3):749–753.

97. Resh MD. Fatty acylation of proteins: new insights into membrane targeting of myristoylated and palmitoylated proteins. Biochim Biophys Acta 1999;1451(1):1–16.

98. Nada S, Okada M, MacAuley A, Cooper JA, Nakagawa H. Cloning of a complementary DNA for a protein-tyrosine kinase that specifically phosphorylates a negative regulatory site of p60c-src. Nature 1991;351(6321):69–72.

99. Hamaguchi I, Yamaguchi N, Suda J, Iwama A, Hirao A, Hashiyama M, Aizawa S, Suda T. Analysis of CSK homologous kinase (CHK/HYL) in hematopoiesis by utilizing gene knockout mice. Biochem Biophys Res Commun 1996;224(1):172–179.

100. Davidson D, Chow LM, Veillette A. Chk, a Csk family tyrosine protein kinase, exhibits Csk-like activity in fibroblasts, but not in an antigen-specific T-cell line. J Biol Chem 1997;272(2):1355–1362.

101. Sicheri F, Moarefi I, Kuriyan J. Crystal structure of the Src family tyrosine kinase Hck. Nature 1997;385(6617):602–609.

102. Williams JC, Weijland A, Gonfloni S, Thompson A, Courtneidge SA, Superti-Furga G, Wierenga RK. The 2.35 Å crystal structure of the inactivated form of chicken Src: a dynamic molecule with multiple regulatory interactions. J Mol Biol 1997;274(5):757–775.

103. Xu W, Harrison SC, Eck MJ. Three-dimensional structure of the tyrosine kinase c-Src. Nature 1997;385(6617):595–602.

104. Imamoto A, Soriano P. Disruption of the csk gene, encoding a negative regulator of Src family tyrosine kinases, leads to neural tube defects and embryonic lethality in mice. Cell 1993;73(6):1117–1124.

105. Flynn DC, Leu TH, Reynolds AB, Parsons JT. Identification and sequence analysis of cDNAs encoding a 110-kilodalton actin filament-associated pp60src substrate. Mol Cell Biol 1993;13(12):7892–7900.

106. Kypta RM, Goldberg Y, Ulug ET, Courtneidge SA. Association between the PDGF receptor and members of the src family of tyrosine kinases. Cell 1990;62(3):481–492.

107. Mayer BJ, Baltimore D. Mutagenic analysis of the roles of SH2 and SH3 domains in regulation of the Abl tyrosine kinase. Mol Cell Biol 1994;14(5):2883–2894.

108. Sakai R, Iwamatsu A, Hirano N, Ogawa S, Tanaka T, Mano H, Yazaki Y, Hirai H. A novel signaling molecule, p130, forms stable complexes in vivo with v-Crk and v-Src in a tyrosine phosphorylation-dependent manner. EMBO J 1994;13(16):3748–3756.

109. Nakamoto T, Sakai R, Ozawa K, Yazaki Y, Hirai H. Direct binding of C-terminal region of p130Cas to SH2 and SH3 domains of Src kinase. J Biol Chem 1996;271(15):8959–8965.

110. DeFranco AL. Transmembrane signaling by antigen receptors of B and T lymphocytes. Curr Opin Cell Biol 1995;7(2):163–175.

111. Lewis LA, Chung CD, Chen J, Parnes JR, Moran M, Patel VP, Miceli MC. The Lck SH2 phosphotyrosine binding site is critical for efficient TCR-induced processive tyrosine phosphorylation of the zeta-chain and IL-2 production. J Immunol 1997;159(5):2292–2300.

112. Moarefi I, LaFevre-Bernt M, Sicheri F, Huse M, Lee CH, Kuriyan J, Miller WT. Activation of the Src-family tyrosine kinase Hck by SH3 domain displacement. Nature 1997;385(6617):650–653.

113. Alexandropoulos K, Baltimore D. Coordinate activation of c-Src by SH3- and SH2-binding sites on a novel p130Cas-related protein, Sin. Genes Dev 1996;10(11):1341–1355.

114. Martinez R, Mathey-Prevot B, Bernards A, Baltimore D. Neuronal pp60c-src contains a six-amino acid insertion relative to its non-neuronal counterpart. Science 1987;237(4813):411–415.

115. Pyper JM, Bolen JB. Identification of a novel neuronal C-SRC exon expressed in human brain. Mol Cell Biol 1990;10(5):2035–2040.

116. Cooke MP, Perlmutter RM. Expression of a novel form of the fyn proto-oncogene in hematopoietic cells. New Biol 1989;1(1):66–74.

117. Stanley E, Ralph S, McEwen S, Boulet I, Holtzman DA, Lock P, Dunn AR. Alternatively spliced murine lyn mRNAs encode distinct proteins. Mol Cell Biol 1991;11(7):3399–3406.

118. Yi TL, Bolen JB, Ihle JN. Hematopoietic cells express two forms of lyn kinase differing by 21 amino acids in the amino terminus. Mol Cell Biol 1991;11(5):2391–2398.

119. Lock P, Ralph S, Stanley E, Boulet I, Ramsay R, Dunn AR. Two isoforms of murine hck, generated by utilization of alternative translational initiation codons, exhibit different patterns of subcellular localization. Mol Cell Biol 1991;11(9):4363–4370.

120. Resh MD. Myristoylation and palmitoylation of Src family members: the fats of the matter. Cell 1994;76(3):411–413.

121. Robbins SM, Quintrell NA, Bishop JM. Myristoylation and differential palmitoylation of the HCK protein-tyrosine kinases govern their attachment to membranes and association with caveolae. Mol Cell Biol 1995;15(7):3507–3515.

122. Kaplan KB, Swedlow JR, Varmus HE, Morgan DO. Association of p60c-src with endosomal membranes in mammalian fibroblasts. J Cell Biol 1992;118(2):321–333.

123. Lowell CA, Soriano P. Knockouts of Src-family kinases: stiff bones, wimpy T cells, and bad memories. Genes Dev 1996;10(15):1845–1857.

124. Matsuda D, Nakayama Y, Horimoto S, Kuga T, Ikeda K, Kasahara K, Yamaguchi N. Involvement of Golgi-associated Lyn tyrosine kinase in the translocation of annexin II to the endoplasmic reticulum under oxidative stress. Exp Cell Res 2006;312(7):1205–1217.

125. Kasahara K, Nakayama Y, Kihara A, Matsuda D, Ikeda K, Kuga T, Fukumoto Y, Igarashi Y, Yamaguchi N. Rapid trafficking of c-Src, a non-palmitoylated Src-family kinase, between the plasma membrane and late endosomes/lysosomes. Exp Cell Res 2007;313(12):2651–2666.

126. Galbiati F, Razani B, Lisanti MP. Emerging themes in lipid rafts and caveolae. Cell 2001;106(4):403–411.

127. Twamley-Stein GM, Pepperkok R, Ansorge W, Courtneidge SA. The Src family tyrosine kinases are required for platelet-derived growth factor-mediated signal transduction in NIH 3T3 cells. Proc Natl Acad Sci U S A 1993;90(16):7696–7700.

128. Jove R, Hanafusa H. Cell transformation by the viral src oncogene. Annu Rev Cell Biol 1987;3:31–56.

129. Frame MC, Fincham VJ, Carragher NO, Wyke JA. v-Src's hold over actin and cell adhesions. Nat Rev Mol Cell Biol 2002;3(4):233–245.

130. Sefton BM, Hunter T, Ball EH, Singer SJ. Vinculin: a cytoskeletal target of the transforming protein of Rous sarcoma virus. Cell 1981;24(1):165–174.

131. Maness PF, Levy BT. Highly purified pp60src induces the actin transformation in microinjected cells and phosphorylates selected cytoskeletal proteins in vitro. Mol Cell Biol 1983;3(1):102–112.

132. Matten WT, Aubry M, West J, Maness PF. Tubulin is phosphorylated at tyrosine by pp60c-src in nerve growth cone membranes. J Cell Biol 1990;111(5Pt 1):1959–1970.

133. Kanner SB, Reynolds AB, Vines RR, Parsons JT. Monoclonal antibodies to individual tyrosine-phosphorylated protein substrates of oncogene-encoded tyrosine kinases. Proc Natl Acad Sci U S A 1990;87(9):3328–3332.

134. Wu H, Parsons JT. Cortactin, an 80/85-kilodalton pp60src substrate, is a filamentous actin-binding protein enriched in the cell cortex. J Cell Biol 1993;120(6):1417–1426.

135. Okamura H, Resh MD. p80/85 cortactin associates with the Src SH2 domain and colocalizes with v-Src in transformed cells. J Biol Chem 1995;270(44):26613–26618.

136. Shah K, Shokat KM. A chemical genetic screen for direct v-Src substrates reveals ordered assembly of a retrograde signaling pathway. Chem Biol 2002;9(1):35–47.

137. Pasquale EB, Maher PA, Singer SJ. Talin is phosphorylated on tyrosine in chicken embryo fibroblasts transformed by Rous sarcoma virus. Proc Natl Acad Sci U S A 1986;83(15):5507–5511.

138. DeClue JE, Martin GS. Phosphorylation of talin at tyrosine in Rous sarcoma virus-transformed cells. Mol Cell Biol 1987;7(1):371–378.

139. Glenney JR Jr, Zokas L. Novel tyrosine kinase substrates from Rous sarcoma virus-transformed cells are present in the membrane skeleton. J Cell Biol 1989;108(6):2401–2408.

140. Thomas SM, Soriano P, Imamoto A. Specific and redundant roles of Src and Fyn in organizing the cytoskeleton. Nature 1995;376(6537):267–271.

141. Turner JM, Brodsky MH, Irving BA, Levin SD, Perlmutter RM, Littman DR. Interaction of the unique N-terminal region of tyrosine kinase p56lck with cytoplasmic domains of CD4 and CD8 is mediated by cysteine motifs. Cell 1990;60(5):755–765.

142. Schaller M, Bouton A, Flynn D, Parsons J. Identification and characterization of novel substrates for protein tyrosine kinases. Prog Nucleic Acid Res Mol Biol 1993;44:205–227.

143. Davis S, Lu ML, Lo SH, Lin S, Butler JA, Druker BJ, Roberts TM, An Q, Chen LB. Presence of an SH2 domain in the actin-binding protein tensin. Science 1991;252(5006):712–715.

144. Reynolds AB, Roesel DJ, Kanner SB, Parsons JT. Transformation-specific tyrosine phosphorylation of a novel cellular protein in chicken cells expressing oncogenic variants of the avian cellular src gene. Mol Cell Biol 1989;9(2):629–638.

145. Hirst R, Horwitz A, Buck C, Rohrschneider L. Phosphorylation of the fibronectin receptor complex in cells transformed by oncogenes that encode tyrosine kinases. Proc Natl Acad Sci U S A 1986;83(17):6470–6474.

146. Dombrosky-Ferlan P, Grishin A, Botelho RJ, Sampson M, Wang L, Rudert WA, Grinstein S, Corey SJ. Felic (CIP4b), a novel binding partner with the Src kinase Lyn and Cdc42, localizes to the phagocytic cup. Blood 2003;101(7):2804–2809.

147. Scott MP, Zappacosta F, Kim EY, Annan RS, Miller WT. Identification of novel SH3 domain ligands for the Src family kinase Hck. Wiskott–Aldrich syndrome protein (WASP), WASP-interacting protein (WIP), and ELMO1. J Biol Chem 2002;277(31):28238–28246.

148. Behrens J, Vakaet L, Friis R, Winterhager E, Van Roy F, Mareel MM, Birchmeier W. Loss of epithelial differentiation and gain of invasiveness correlates with tyrosine phosphorylation of the E-cadherin/beta-catenin complex in cells transformed with a temperature-sensitive v-SRC gene. J Cell Biol 1993;120(3):757–766.

149. Reynolds AB, Daniel J, McCrea PD, Wheelock MJ, Wu J, Zhang Z. Identification of a new catenin: the tyrosine kinase substrate p120cas associates with E-cadherin complexes. Mol Cell Biol 1994;14(12):8333–8342.

150. Matsuyoshi N, Hamaguchi M, Taniguchi S, Nagafuchi A, Tsukita S, Takeichi M. Cadherin-mediated cell–cell adhesion is perturbed by v-src tyrosine phosphorylation in metastatic fibroblasts. J Cell Biol 1992;118(3):703–714.

151. Chen YH, Lu Q, Goodenough DA, Jeansonne B. Nonreceptor tyrosine kinase c-Yes interacts with occludin during tight junction formation in canine kidney epithelial cells. Mol Biol Cell 2002;13(4):1227–1237.

152. Kale G, Naren AP, Sheth P, Rao RK. Tyrosine phosphorylation of occludin attenuates its interactions with ZO-1, ZO-2, and ZO-3. Biochem Biophys Res Commun 2003;302(2):324–329.

153. Filson AJ, Azarnia R, Beyer EC, Loewenstein WR, Brugge JS. Tyrosine phosphorylation of a gap junction protein correlates with inhibition of cell-to-cell communication. Cell Growth Differ 1990;1(12):661–668.

154. Crow DS, Beyer EC, Paul DL, Kobe SS, Lau AF. Phosphorylation of connexin43 gap junction protein in uninfected and Rous sarcoma virus-transformed mammalian fibroblasts. Mol Cell Biol 1990;10(4):1754–1763.

155. Kikyo M, Matozaki T, Kodama A, Kawabe H, Nakanishi H, Takai Y. Cell–cell adhesion-mediated tyrosine phosphorylation of nectin-2delta, an immunoglobulin-like cell adhesion molecule at adherens junctions. Oncogene 2000;19(35):4022–4028.

156. Nakanishi O, Shibasaki F, Hidaka M, Homma Y, Takenawa T. Phospholipase C-gamma 1 associates with viral and cellular src kinases. J Biol Chem 1993;268(15):10754–10759.

157. Liu X, Marengere LE, Koch CA, Pawson T. The v-Src SH3 domain binds phosphatidylinositol 3'-kinase. Mol Cell Biol 1993;13(9):5225–5232.

158. Fukui Y, Hanafusa H. Requirement of phosphatidylinositol-3 kinase modification for its association with p60src. Mol Cell Biol 1991;11(4):1972–1979.

159. Haefner B, Baxter R, Fincham VJ, Downes CP, Frame MC. Cooperation of Src homology domains in the regulated binding of phosphatidylinositol 3-kinase. A role for the Src homology 2 domain. J Biol Chem 1995;270(14):7937–7943.

160. Ellis C, Moran M, McCormick F, Pawson T. Phosphorylation of GAP and GAP-associated proteins by transforming and mitogenic tyrosine kinases. Nature 1990;343(6256):377–381.

161. Bouton AH, Kanner SB, Vines RR, Wang HC, Gibbs JB, Parsons JT. Transformation by pp60src or stimulation of cells with epidermal growth factor induces the stable association of tyrosine-phosphorylated cellular proteins with GTPase-activating protein. Mol Cell Biol 1991;11(2):945–953.

162. Chang JH, Wilson LK, Moyers JS, Zhang K, Parsons SJ. Increased levels of p21ras-GTP and enhanced DNA synthesis accompany elevated tyrosyl phosphorylation of GAP-associated proteins, p190 and p62, in c-src overexpressors. Oncogene 1993;8(4):959–967.

163. Lombardo CR, Consler TG, Kassel DB. In Vitro phosphorylation of the epidermal growth factor receptor autophosphorylation domain by c-src: identification of phosphorylation sites and c-src SH2 domain binding sites. Biochemistry 1995;34(50):16456–16466.

164. Gallo R, Provenzano C, Carbone R, Di Fiore PP, Castellani L, Falcone G, Alema S. Regulation of the tyrosine kinase substrate Eps8 expression by growth factors, v-Src and terminal differentiation. Oncogene 1997;15(16):1929–1936.

165. Taylor SJ, Shalloway D. An RNA-binding protein associated with Src through its SH2 and SH3 domains in mitosis. Nature 1994;368(6474):867–871.

166. Fumagalli S, Totty NF, Hsuan JJ, Courtneidge SA. A target for Src in mitosis. Nature 1994;368(6474):871–874.

167. Courtneidge SA. Isolation of novel Src substrates. Biochem Soc Trans 2003;31(Pt 1):25–28.

168. Lock P, Abram CL, Gibson T, Courtneidge SA. A new method for isolating tyrosine kinase substrates used to identify fish, an SH3 and PX domain-containing protein, and Src substrate. EMBO J 1998;17(15):4346–4357.

169. Feng GS, Hui CC, Pawson T. SH2-containing phosphotyrosine phosphatase as a target of protein-tyrosine kinases. Science 1993;259(5101):1607–1611.

170. McGlade J, Cheng A, Pelicci G, Pelicci PG, Pawson T. Shc proteins are phosphorylated and regulated by the v-Src and v-Fps protein-tyrosine kinases. Proc Natl Acad Sci U S A 1992;89(19):8869–8873.

171. Rothberg KG, Heuser JE, Donzell WC, Ying YS, Glenney JR, Anderson RG. Caveolin, a protein component of caveolae membrane coats. Cell 1992;68(4):673–682.

172. Glenney JR Jr. Tyrosine phosphorylation of a 22-kDa protein is correlated with transformation by Rous sarcoma virus. J Biol Chem 1989;264(34):20163–20166.

173. Radke K, Gilmore T, Martin G. Transformation by Rous sarcoma virus: a cellular substrate for transformation-specific protein phosphorylation contains phosphotyrosine. Cell 1980;21:821–828.

174. Erikson E, Erikson R. Identification of a cellular protein substrate phosphorylated by the avian sarcoma virus-transforming gene product. Cell 1980;21:829–836.

175. Glenney JR Jr, Tack BF. Amino-terminal sequence of p36 and associated p10: identification of the site of tyrosine phosphorylation and homology with S-100. Proc Natl Acad Sci U S A 1985;82(23):7884–7888.

176. Cance WG, Craven RJ, Bergman M, Xu L, Alitalo K, Liu ET. Rak, a novel nuclear tyrosine kinase expressed in epithelial cells. Cell Growth Differ 1994;5(12):1347–1355.

177. Cooper JA, Reiss NA, Schwartz RJ, Hunter T. Three glycolytic enzymes are phosphorylated at tyrosine in cells transformed by Rous sarcoma virus. Nature 1983;302(5905):218–223.

178. Lund TC, Coleman C, Horvath E, Sefton BM, Jove R, Medveczky MM, Medveczky PG. The Src-family kinase Lck can induce STAT3 phosphorylation and DNA binding activity. Cell Signal 1999;11(11):789–796.

179. Bromberg JF, Horvath CM, Besser D, Lathem WW, Darnell JE Jr. Stat3 activation is required for cellular transformation by v-src. Mol Cell Biol 1998;18(5):2553–2558.

180. Turkson J, Bowman T, Garcia R, Caldenhoven E, De Groot RP, Jove R. Stat3 activation by Src induces specific gene regulation and is required for cell transformation. Mol Cell Biol 1998;18(5):2545–2552.

181. Servitja JM, Marinissen MJ, Sodhi A, Bustelo XR, Gutkind JS. Rac1 function is required for Src-induced transformation. Evidence of a role for Tiam1 and Vav2 in Rac activation by Src. J Biol Chem 2003;278(36):34339–34346.

182. Carlino A, Toledo H, Vidal V, Redfield B, Strassman J, Abdel-Ghany M, Racker E, Weissbach H, Brot N. BiP is a substrate for src kinase in vitro. Biochem Biophys Res Commun 1994;201(3):1548–1553.

183. Wang WJ, Kuo JC, Ku W, Lee YR, Lin FC, Chang YL, Lin YM, Chen CH, Huang YP, Chiang MJ, Yeh SW, Wu PR, Shen CH, Wu CT, Chen RH. The tumor suppressor DAPK is reciprocally regulated by tyrosine kinase Src and phosphatase LAR. Mol Cell 2007;27(5):701–716.

184. van der Geer P, Wiley S, Gish GD, Pawson T. The Shc adaptor protein is highly phosphorylated at conserved, twin tyrosine residues (Y239/240) that mediate protein–protein interactions. Curr Biol 1996;6(11):1435–1444.

185. Coso OA, Chiariello M, Yu JC, Teramoto H, Crespo P, Xu N, Miki T, Gutkind JS. The small GTP-binding proteins Rac1 and Cdc42 regulate the activity of the JNK/SAPK signaling pathway. Cell 1995;81(7):1137–1146.

186. Minden A, Lin A, Claret FX, Abo A, Karin M. Selective activation of the JNK signaling cascade and c-Jun transcriptional activity by the small GTPases Rac and Cdc42Hs. Cell 1995;81(7):1147–1157.

187. Yu CL, Meyer DJ, Campbell GS, Larner AC, Carter-Su C, Schwartz J, Jove R. Enhanced DNA-binding activity of a Stat3-related protein in cells transformed by the Src oncoprotein. Science 1995;269(5220):81–83.

188. Boureux A, Furstoss O, Simon V, Roche S. Abl tyrosine kinase regulates a Rac/JNK and a Rac/Nox pathway for DNA synthesis and Myc expression induced by growth factors. J Cell Sci 2005;118(Pt 16):3717–3726.

189. Raveh T, Kimchi A. DAP kinase-a proapoptotic gene that functions as a tumor suppressor. Exp Cell Res 2001;264(1):185–192.

190. Bialik S, Kimchi A. DAP-kinase as a target for drug design in cancer and diseases associated with accelerated cell death. Semin Cancer Biol 2004;14(4):283–294.

191. Raveh T, Droguett G, Horwitz MS, DePinho RA, Kimchi A. DAP kinase activates a p19ARF/p53-mediated apoptotic checkpoint to suppress oncogenic transformation. Nat Cell Biol 2001;3(1):1–7.

192. Inbal B, Cohen O, Polak-Charcon S, Kopolovic J, Vadai E, Eisenbach L, Kimchi A. DAP kinase links the control of apoptosis to metastasis. Nature 1997;390(6656):180–184.

193. Kuo JC, Lin JR, Staddon JM, Hosoya H, Chen RH. Uncoordinated regulation of stress fibers and focal adhesions by DAP kinase. J Cell Sci 2003;116(Pt 23):4777–4790.

194. Kuo JC, Wang WJ, Yao CC, Wu PR, Chen RH. The tumor suppressor DAPK inhibits cell motility by blocking the integrin-mediated polarity pathway. J Cell Biol 2006;172(4):619–631.

195. Chackalaparampil I, Shalloway D. Altered phosphorylation and activation of pp60c-src during fibroblast mitosis. Cell 1988;52(6):801–810.

196. Moasser MM, Srethapakdi M, Sachar KS, Kraker AJ, Rosen N. Inhibition of Src kinases by a selective tyrosine kinase inhibitor causes mitotic arrest. Cancer Res 1999;59(24):6145–6152.

197. Ng MM, Chang F, Burgess DR. Movement of membrane domains and requirement of membrane signaling molecules for cytokinesis. Dev Cell 2005;9(6):781–790.

198. Roche S, Fumagalli S, Courtneidge SA. Requirement for Src family protein tyrosine kinases in G2 for fibroblast cell division. Science 1995;269(5230):1567–1569.

199. Tominaga T, Sahai E, Chardin P, McCormick F, Courtneidge SA, Alberts AS. Diaphanous-related formins bridge Rho GTPase and Src tyrosine kinase signaling. Mol Cell 2000;5(1):13–25.

200. Kuga T, Nakayama Y, Hoshino M, Higashiyama Y, Obata Y, Matsuda D, Kasahara K, Fukumoto Y, Yamaguchi N. Differential mitotic activation of endogenous c-Src, c-Yes, and Lyn in HeLa cells. Arch Biochem Biophys 2007;466(1):116–124.

201. Kasahara K, Nakayama Y, Nakazato Y, Ikeda K, Kuga T, Yamaguchi N. Src signaling regulates completion of abscission in cytokinesis through ERK/MAPK activation at the midbody. J Biol Chem 2007;282(8):5327–5339.

202. Zheng XM, Shalloway D. Two mechanisms activate PTPalpha during mitosis. EMBO J 2001;20(21):6037–6049.

203. Bagrodia S, Chackalaparampil I, Kmiecik TE, Shalloway D. Altered tyrosine 527 phosphorylation and mitotic activation of p60c-src. Nature 1991;349(6305):172–175.

204. Bagrodia S, Taylor SJ, Shalloway D. Myristoylation is required for Tyr-527 dephosphorylation and activation of pp60c-src in mitosis. Mol Cell Biol 1993;13(3):1464–1470.

205. Kaech S, Schnierle B, Wyss A, Ballmer-Hofer K. Myristylation and amino-terminal phosphorylation are required for activation of pp60c-src during mitosis. Oncogene 1993;8(3):575–581.

206. Morgan DO, Kaplan JM, Bishop JM, Varmus HE. Mitosis-specific phosphorylation of p60c-src by p34cdc2-associated protein kinase. Cell 1989;57(5):775–786.

207. Shenoy S, Chackalaparampil I, Bagrodia S, Lin PH, Shalloway D. Role of p34cdc2-mediated phosphorylations in two-step activation of pp60c-src during mitosis. Proc Natl Acad Sci U S A 1992;89(15):7237–7241.

208. Weng Z, Thomas SM, Rickles RJ, Taylor JA, Brauer AW, Seidel-Dugan C, Michael WM, Dreyfuss G, Brugge JS. Identification of Src, Fyn, and Lyn SH3-binding proteins: implications for a function of SH3 domains. Mol Cell Biol 1994;14(7):4509–4521.

209. Dong F, Gutkind JS, Larner AC. Granulocyte colony-stimulating factor induces ERK5 activation, which is differentially regulated by protein-tyrosine kinases and protein kinase C. Regulation of cell proliferation and survival. J Biol Chem 2001;276(14):10811–10816.

210. Kato Y, Tapping RI, Huang S, Watson MH, Ulevitch RJ, Lee JD. Bmk1/Erk5 is required for cell proliferation induced by epidermal growth factor. Nature 1998;395(6703):713–716.

211. Pearson G, English JM, White MA, Cobb MH. ERK5 and ERK2 cooperate to regulate NF-kappa B and cell transformation. J Biol Chem 2001;276(11):7927–7931.

212. Kasler HG, Victoria J, Duramad O, Winoto A. ERK5 is a novel type of mitogen-activated protein kinase containing a transcriptional activation domain. Mol Cell Biol 2000;20(22):8382–8389.

213. Kamakura S, Moriguchi T, Nishida E. Activation of the protein kinase ERK5/BMK1 by receptor tyrosine kinases. Identification and characterization of a signaling pathway to the nucleus. J Biol Chem 1999;274(37):26563–26571.

214. Yang CC, Ornatsky OI, McDermott JC, Cruz TF, Prody CA. Interaction of myocyte enhancer factor 2 (MEF2) with a mitogen-activated protein kinase, ERK5/BMK1. Nucleic Acids Res 1998;26(20):4771–4777.

215. Barros JC, Marshall CJ. Activation of either ERK1/2 or ERK5 MAP kinase pathways can lead to disruption of the actin cytoskeleton. J Cell Sci 2005;118(Pt 8):1663–1671.

216. Seidel-Dugan C, Meyer BE, Thomas SM, Brugge JS. Effects of SH2 and SH3 deletions on the functional activities of wild-type and transforming variants of c-Src. Mol Cell Biol 1992;12(4):1835–1845.

217. Schaller MD, Hildebrand JD, Parsons JT. Complex formation with focal adhesion kinase: a mechanism to regulate activity and subcellular localization of Src kinases. Mol Biol Cell 1999;10(10):3489–3505.

218. Timpson P, Jones GE, Frame MC, Brunton VG. Coordination of cell polarization and migration by the Rho family GTPases requires Src tyrosine kinase activity. Curr Biol 2001;11(23):1836–1846.

219. Kaplan KB, Swedlow JR, Morgan DO, Varmus HE. c-Src enhances the spreading of src−/− fibroblasts on fibronectin by a kinase-independent mechanism. Genes Dev 1995;9(12):1505–1517.

220. Cary LA, Klinghoffer RA, Sachsenmaier C, Cooper JA. SRC catalytic but not scaffolding function is needed for integrin-regulated tyrosine phosphorylation, cell migration, and cell spreading. Mol Cell Biol 2002;22(8):2427–2440.

221. Schlaepfer DD, Mitra SK, Ilic D. Control of motile and invasive cell phenotypes by focal adhesion kinase. Biochim Biophys Acta 2004;1692(2–3):77–102.

222. Cosen-Binker LI, Kapus A. Cortactin: the gray eminence of the cytoskeleton. Physiology (Bethesda) 2006;21:352–361.

223. Artym VV, Zhang Y, Seillier-Moiseiwitsch F, Yamada KM, Mueller SC. Dynamic interactions of cortactin and membrane type 1 matrix metalloproteinase at invadopodia: defining the stages of invadopodia formation and function. Cancer Res 2006;66(6):3034–3043.

224. Lakkakorpi PT, Nakamura I, Young M, Lipfert L, Rodan GA, Duong LT. Abnormal localisation and hyperclustering of (alpha)(V)(beta)(3) integrins and associated proteins in Src-deficient or tyrphostin A9-treated osteoclasts. J Cell Sci 2001; 114(Pt 1):149–160.

225. Tarone G, Cirillo D, Giancotti FG, Comoglio PM, Marchisio PC. Rous sarcoma virus-transformed fibroblasts adhere primarily at discrete protrusions of the ventral membrane called podosomes. Exp Cell Res 1985;159(1):141–157.

226. Luxenburg C, Parsons JT, Addadi L, Geiger B. Involvement of the Src-cortactin pathway in podosome formation and turnover during polarization of cultured osteoclasts. J Cell Sci 2006;119(Pt 23):4878–4888.

227. McLachlan RW, Kraemer A, Helwani FM, Kovacs EM, Yap AS. E-cadherin adhesion activates c-Src signaling at cell-cell contacts. Mol Biol Cell 2007;18(8):3214–3223.

228. Takahashi F, Endo S, Kojima T, Saigo K. Regulation of cell–cell contacts in developing *Drosophila* eyes by Dsrc41, a new, close relative of vertebrate c-src. Genes Dev 1996;10(13):1645–1656.

229. Takahashi M, Takahashi F, Ui-Tei K, Kojima T, Saigo K. Requirements of genetic interactions between Src42A, armadillo and shotgun, a gene encoding E-cadherin, for normal development in *Drosophila*. Development 2005;132(11):2547–2559.

230. Calautti E, Cabodi S, Stein PL, Hatzfeld M, Kedersha N, Paolo Dotto G. Tyrosine phosphorylation and src family kinases control keratinocyte cell-cell adhesion. J Cell Biol 1998;141(6):1449–1465.

231. Grossmann J. Molecular mechanisms of "detachment-induced apoptosis—anoikis." Apoptosis 2002;7(3):247–260.

232. Frisch SM, Vuori K, Ruoslahti E, Chan-Hui PY. Control of adhesion-dependent cell survival by focal adhesion kinase. J Cell Biol 1996;134(3):793–799.

233. Gilmore AP, Metcalfe AD, Romer LH, Streuli CH. Integrin-mediated survival signals regulate the apoptotic function of Bax through its conformation and subcellular localization. J Cell Biol 2000;149(2):431–446.

234. Windham TC, Parikh NU, Siwak DR, Summy JM, McConkey DJ, Kraker AJ, Gallick GE. Src activation regulates anoikis in human colon tumor cell lines. Oncogene 2002;21(51):7797–7807.

235. Rosen N, Bolen JB, Schwartz AM, Cohen P, DeSeau V, Israel MA. Analysis of pp60c-src protein kinase activity in human tumor cell lines and tissues. J Biol Chem 1986;261(29):13754–13759.

236. Bolen JB, Veillette A, Schwartz AM, Deseau V, Rosen N. Analysis of pp60c-src in human colon carcinoma and normal human colon mucosal cells. Oncogene Res 1987;1(2):149–168.

237. Bolen JB, Veillette A, Schwartz AM, DeSeau V, Rosen N. Activation of pp60c-src protein kinase activity in human colon carcinoma. Proc Natl Acad Sci U S A 1987;84(8):2251–2255.

238. Cartwright CA, Kamps MP, Meisler AI, Pipas JM, Eckhart W. pp60c-src activation in human colon carcinoma. J Clin Invest 1989;83(6):2025–2033.

239. Cartwright CA, Meisler AI, Eckhart W. Activation of the pp60c-src protein kinase is an early event in colonic carcinogenesis. Proc Natl Acad Sci U S A 1990;87(2):558–562.

240. Aligayer H, Boyd DD, Heiss MM, Abdalla EK, Curley SA, Gallick GE. Activation of Src kinase in primary colorectal carcinoma: an indicator of poor clinical prognosis. Cancer 2002;94(2):344–351.

241. Irby R, Mao W, Coppola D, Jove R, Gamero A, Cuthbertson D, Fujita DJ, Yeatman TJ. Overexpression of normal c-Src in poorly metastatic human colon cancer cells enhances primary tumor growth but not metastatic potential. Cell Growth Differ 1997;8(12):1287–1295.

242. Golas JM, Lucas J, Etienne C, Golas J, Discafani C, Sridharan L, Boghaert E, Arndt K, Ye F, Boschelli DH, Li F, Titsch C, Huselton C, Chaudhary I, Boschelli F. SKI-606, a Src/Abl inhibitor with in vivo activity in colon tumor xenograft models. Cancer Res 2005;65(12):5358–5364.

243. Park J, Meisler AI, Cartwright CA. c-Yes tyrosine kinase activity in human colon carcinoma. Oncogene 1993;8(10):2627–2635.

244. Veillette A, Foss FM, Sausville EA, Bolen JB, Rosen N. Expression of the lck tyrosine kinase gene in human colon carcinoma and other non-lymphoid human tumor cell lines. Oncogene Res 1987;1(4):357–374.

245. Lutz MP, Esser IB, Flossmann-Kast BB, Vogelmann R, Luhrs H, Friess H, Buchler MW, Adler G. Overexpression and activation of the tyrosine kinase Src in human pancreatic carcinoma. Biochem Biophys Res Commun 1998;243(2):503–508.

246. Hakam A, Fang Q, Karl R, Coppola D. Coexpression of IGF-1R and c-Src proteins in human pancreatic ductal adenocarcinoma. Dig Dis Sci 2003;48(10):1972–1978.

247. Jacobs C, Rubsamen H. Expression of pp60c-src protein kinase in adult and fetal human tissue: high activities in some sarcomas and mammary carcinomas. Cancer Res 1983;43(4):1696–1702.

248. Ottenhoff-Kalff AE, Rijksen G, van Beurden EA, Hennipman A, Michels AA, Staal GE. Characterization of protein tyrosine kinases from human breast cancer: involvement of the c-src oncogene product. Cancer Res 1992;52(17):4773–4778.

249. Verbeek BS, Vroom TM, Adriaansen-Slot SS, Ottenhoff-Kalff AE, Geertzema JG, Hennipman A, Rijksen G. c-Src protein expression is increased in human breast cancer. An immunohistochemical and biochemical analysis. J Pathol 1996;180(4):383–388.

250. Reissig D, Clement J, Sanger J, Berndt A, Kosmehl H, Bohmer FD. Elevated activity and expression of Src-family kinases in human breast carcinoma tissue versus matched non-tumor tissue. J Cancer Res Clin Oncol 2001;127(4):226–230.

251. Masaki T, Igarashi K, Tokuda M, Yukimasa S, Han F, Jin YJ, Li JQ, Yoneyama H, Uchida N, Fujita J, Yoshiji H, Watanabe S, Kurokohchi K, Kuriyama S. pp60c-src activation in lung adenocarcinoma. Eur J Cancer 2003;39(10):1447–1455.

252. Bu R, Purushotham KR, Kerr M, Tao Z, Jonsson R, Olofsson J, Humphreys-Beher MG. Alterations in the level of phosphotyrosine signal transduction constituents in human parotid tumors. Proc Soc Exp Biol Med 1996;211(3):257–264.

253. Ito Y, Kawakatsu H, Takeda T, Sakon M, Nagano H, Sakai T, Miyoshi E, Noda K, Tsujimoto M, Wakasa K, Monden M, Matsuura N. Activation of c-Src gene product in hepatocellular carcinoma is highly correlated with the indices of early stage phenotype. J Hepatol 2001;35(1):68–73.

254. Wiener JR, Windham TC, Estrella VC, Parikh NU, Thall PF, Deavers MT, Bast RC, Mills GB, Gallick GE. Activated SRC protein tyrosine kinase is overexpressed in late-stage human ovarian cancers. Gynecol Oncol 2003;88(1):73–79.

255. Bourguignon LY, Zhu H, Shao L, Chen YW. CD44 interaction with c-Src kinase promotes cortactin-mediated cytoskeleton function and hyaluronic acid-dependent ovarian tumor cell migration. J Biol Chem 2001;276(10):7327–7336.

256. Fanning P, Bulovas K, Saini KS, Libertino JA, Joyce AD, Summerhayes IC. Elevated expression of pp60c-src in low grade human bladder carcinoma. Cancer Res 1992;52(6):1457–1462.

257. Takekura N, Yasui W, Yoshida K, Tsujino T, Nakayama H, Kameda T, Yokozaki H, Nishimura Y, Ito H, Tahara E. pp60c-src protein kinase activity in human gastric carcinomas. Int J Cancer 1990;45(5):847–851.

258. Jankowski J, Coghill G, Hopwood D, Wormsley KG. Oncogenes and onco-suppressor gene in adenocarcinoma of the oesophagus. Gut 1992;33(8):1033–1038.

259. Kumble S, Omary MB, Cartwright CA, Triadafilopoulos G. Src activation in malignant and premalignant epithelia of Barrett's esophagus. Gastroenterology 1997;112(2):348–356.

260. Takenaka N, Mikoshiba K, Takamatsu K, Tsukada Y, Ohtani M, Toya S. Immunohistochemical detection of the gene product of Rous sarcoma virus in human brain tumors. Brain Res 1985;337(2):201–207.

261. Bolen JB, Rosen N, Israel MA. Increased pp60c-src tyrosyl kinase activity in human neuroblastomas is associated with amino-terminal tyrosine phosphorylation of the src gene product. Proc Natl Acad Sci U S A 1985;82(21):7275–7279.

262. O'Shaughnessy J, Deseau V, Amini S, Rosen N, Bolen JB. Analysis of the c-src gene product structure, abundance, and protein kinase activity in human neuroblastoma and glioblastoma cells. Oncogene Res 1987;2(1):1–18.

263. Mellstrom K, Bjelfman C, Hammerling U, Pahlman S. Expression of c-src in cultured human neuroblastoma and small-cell lung carcinoma cell lines correlates with neurocrine differentiation. Mol Cell Biol 1987;7(12):4178–4184.

264. Pahlman S, Hammerling U. src expression in small-cell lung carcinoma and other neuroendocrine malignancies. Am Rev Respir Dis 1990;142(6Pt 2): S54-56.

265. Schaller MD, Borgman CA, Cobb BS, Vines RR, Reynolds AB, Parsons JT. pp125FAK a structurally distinctive protein-tyrosine kinase associated with focal adhesions. Proc Natl Acad Sci U S A 1992;89(11):5192–5196.

266. Hanks SK, Calalb MB, Harper MC, Patel SK. Focal adhesion protein-tyrosine kinase phosphorylated in response to cell attachment to fibronectin. Proc Natl Acad Sci U S A 1992;89(18):8487–8491.

267. Agochiya M, Brunton VG, Owens DW, Parkinson EK, Paraskeva C, Keith WN, Frame MC. Increased dosage and amplification of the focal adhesion kinase gene in human cancer cells. Oncogene 1999;18(41):5646–5653.

268. Parsons JT. Focal adhesion kinase: the first ten years. J Cell Sci 2003;116(Pt 8):1409–1416.

269. Ren XD, Kiosses WB, Sieg DJ, Otey CA, Schlaepfer DD, Schwartz MA. Focal adhesion kinase suppresses Rho activity to promote focal adhesion turnover. J Cell Sci 2000;113 (Pt 20):3673–3678.

270. Hanks SK, Ryzhova L, Shin NY, Brabek J. Focal adhesion kinase signaling activities and their implications in the control of cell survival and motility. Front Biosci 2003;8:d982-996.

271. Schaller MD. Biochemical signals and biological responses elicited by the focal adhesion kinase. Biochim Biophys Acta 2001;1540(1):1–21.

272. Liu E, Cote JF, Vuori K. Negative regulation of FAK signaling by SOCS proteins. EMBO J 2003;22(19):5036–5046.

273. Lim Y, Han I, Jeon J, Park H, Bahk YY, Oh ES. Phosphorylation of focal adhesion kinase at tyrosine 861 is crucial for Ras transformation of fibroblasts. J Biol Chem 2004;279(28):29060–29065.

274. Schlaepfer DD, Hanks SK, Hunter T, van der Geer P. Integrin-mediated signal transduction linked to Ras pathway by GRB2 binding to focal adhesion kinase. Nature 1994;372(6508):786–791.

275. Hayashi I, Vuori K, Liddington RC. The focal adhesion targeting (FAT) region of focal adhesion kinase is a four-helix bundle that binds paxillin. Nat Struct Biol 2002;9(2):101–106.

276. Liu G, Guibao CD, Zheng J. Structural insight into the mechanisms of targeting and signaling of focal adhesion kinase. Mol Cell Biol 2002;22(8):2751–2760.

277. Gao G, Prutzman KC, King ML, Scheswohl DM, DeRose EF, London RE, Schaller MD, Campbell SL. NMR solution structure of the focal adhesion targeting domain of focal adhesion kinase in complex with a paxillin LD peptide: evidence for a two-site binding model. J Biol Chem 2004;279(9):8441–8451.

278. Katz BZ, Romer L, Miyamoto S, Volberg T, Matsumoto K, Cukierman E, Geiger B, Yamada KM. Targeting membrane-localized focal adhesion kinase to focal adhesions: roles of tyrosine phosphorylation and SRC family kinases. J Biol Chem 2003;278(31):29115–29120.

279. Hunger-Glaser I, Fan RS, Perez-Salazar E, Rozengurt E. PDGF and FGF induce focal adhesion kinase (FAK) phosphorylation at Ser-910: dissociation from Tyr-397 phosphorylation and requirement for ERK activation. J Cell Physiol 2004;200(2):213–222.

280. Andre E, Becker-Andre M. Expression of an N-terminally truncated form of human focal adhesion kinase in brain. Biochem Biophys Res Commun 1993;190(1):140–147.

281. Corsi JM, Rouer E, Girault JA, Enslen H. Organization and post-transcriptional processing of focal adhesion kinase gene. BMC Genomics 2006;7:198.

282. Schaller MD, Borgman CA, Parsons JT. Autonomous expression of a noncatalytic domain of the focal adhesion-associated protein tyrosine kinase pp125FAK. Mol Cell Biol 1993;13(2):785–791.

283. Nolan K, Lacoste J, Parsons JT. Regulated expression of focal adhesion kinase-related nonkinase, the autonomously expressed C-terminal domain of focal adhesion kinase. Mol Cell Biol 1999;19(9):6120–6129.

284. Zhao JH, Reiske H, Guan JL. Regulation of the cell cycle by focal adhesion kinase. J Cell Biol 1998;143(7):1997–2008.

285. Richardson A, Parsons T. A mechanism for regulation of the adhesion-associated proteintyrosine kinase pp125FAK. Nature 1996;380(6574):538–540.

286. Schlaepfer DD, Hauck CR, Sieg DJ. Signaling through focal adhesion kinase. Prog Biophys Mol Biol 1999;71(3–4):435–478.

287. Aoto H, Sasaki H, Ishino M, Sasaki T. Nuclear translocation of cell adhesion kinase beta/proline-rich tyrosine kinase 2. Cell Struct Funct 2002;27(1):47–61.

288. Farshori PQ, Shah BH, Arora KK, Martinez-Fuentes A, Catt KJ. Activation and nuclear translocation of PKC delta, Pyk2 and ERK1/2 by gonadotropin releasing hormone in HEK293 cells. J Steroid Biochem Mol Biol 2003;85(2–5):337–347.

289. Matsuya M, Sasaki H, Aoto H, Mitaka T, Nagura K, Ohba T, Ishino M, Takahashi S, Suzuki R, Sasaki T. Cell adhesion kinase beta forms a complex with a new member, Hic-5, of proteins localized at focal adhesions. J Biol Chem 1998;273(2):1003–1014.

290. Lev S, Hernandez J, Martinez R, Chen A, Plowman G, Schlessinger J. Identification of a novel family of targets of PYK2 related to *Drosophila* retinal degeneration B (rdgB) protein. Mol Cell Biol 1999;19(3):2278–2288.

291. Andreev J, Simon JP, Sabatini DD, Kam J, Plowman G, Randazzo PA, Schlessinger J. Identification of a new Pyk2 target protein with Arf-GAP activity. Mol Cell Biol 1999;19(3):2338–2350.

292. Avraham H, Park SY, Schinkmann K, Avraham S. RAFTK/Pyk2-mediated cellular signalling. Cell Signal 2000;12(3):123–133.

293. Dikic I, Dikic I, Schlessinger J. Identification of a new Pyk2 isoform implicated in chemokine and antigen receptor signaling. J Biol Chem 1998;273(23):14301–14308.

294. Han EK, McGonigal T. Role of focal adhesion kinase in human cancer: a potential target for drug discovery. Anticancer Agents Med Chem 2007;7(6):681–684.

295. Lark AL, Livasy CA, Dressler L, Moore DT, Millikan RC, Geradts J, Iacocca M, Cowan D, Little D, Craven RJ, Cance W. High focal adhesion kinase expression in invasive breast carcinomas is associated with an aggressive phenotype. Mod Pathol 2005;18(10):1289–1294.

296. Shen TL, Park AY, Alcaraz A, Peng X, Jang I, Koni P, Flavell RA, Gu H, Guan JL. Conditional knockout of focal adhesion kinase in endothelial cells reveals its role in angiogenesis and vascular development in late embryogenesis. J Cell Biol 2005;169(6):941–952.

297. Peng X, Ueda H, Zhou H, Stokol T, Shen TL, Alcaraz A, Nagy T, Vassalli JD, Guan JL. Overexpression of focal adhesion kinase in vascular endothelial cells promotes angiogenesis in transgenic mice. Cardiovasc Res 2004;64(3):421–430.

298. Feng J, Witthuhn BA, Matsuda T, Kohlhuber F, Kerr IM, Ihle JN. Activation of Jak2 catalytic activity requires phosphorylation of Y1007 in the kinase activation loop. Mol Cell Biol 1997;17(5):2497–2501.

299. Yasukawa H, Misawa H, Sakamoto H, Masuhara M, Sasaki A, Wakioka T, Ohtsuka S, Imaizumi T, Matsuda T, Ihle JN, Yoshimura A. The JAK-binding protein JAB inhibits Janus tyrosine kinase activity through binding in the activation loop. EMBO J 1999;18(5):1309–1320.

300. Verma A, Kambhampati S, Parmar S, Platanias LC. Jak family of kinases in cancer. Cancer Metastasis Rev 2003;22(4):423–434.

301. Rossi MR, Hawthorn L, Platt J, Burkhardt T, Cowell JK, Ionov Y. Identification of inactivating mutations in the JAK1, SYNJ2, and CLPTM1 genes in prostate cancer cells using inhibition of nonsense-mediated decay and microarray analysis. Cancer Genet Cytogenet 2005;161(2):97–103.

302. Dovhey SE, Ghosh NS, Wright KL. Loss of interferon-gamma inducibility of TAP1 and LMP2 in a renal cell carcinoma cell line. Cancer Res 2000;60(20):5789–5796.

303. Hayashi T, Kobayashi Y, Kohsaka S, Sano K. The mutation in the ATP-binding region of JAK1, identified in human uterine leiomyosarcomas, results in defective interferon-gamma inducibility of TAP1 and LMP2. Oncogene 2006;25(29):4016–4026.

304. Macchi P, Villa A, Giliani S, Sacco MG, Frattini A, Porta F, Ugazio AG, Johnston JA, Candotti F, O'Shea JJ, et al. Mutations of Jak-3 gene in patients with autosomal severe combined immune deficiency (SCID). Nature 1995;377(6544):65–68.

305. Russell SM, Tayebi N, Nakajima H, Riedy MC, Roberts JL, Aman MJ, Migone TS, Noguchi M, Markert ML, Buckley RH, O'Shea JJ, Leonard WJ. Mutation of Jak3 in a patient with SCID: essential role of Jak3 in lymphoid development. Science 1995;270(5237):797–800.

306. Nosaka T, van Deursen JM, Tripp RA, Thierfelder WE, Witthuhn BA, McMickle AP, Doherty PC, Grosveld GC, Ihle JN. Defective lymphoid development in mice lacking Jak3. Science 1995;270(5237):800–802.

307. Thomis DC, Gurniak CB, Tivol E, Sharpe AH, Berg LJ. Defects in B lymphocyte maturation and T lymphocyte activation in mice lacking Jak3. Science 1995;270(5237):794–797.

308. Walters DK, Mercher T, Gu TL, O'Hare T, Tyner JW, Loriaux M, Goss VL, Lee KA, Eide CA, Wong MJ, Stoffregen EP, McGreevey L, Nardone J, Moore SA, Crispino J, Boggon TJ, Heinrich MC, Deininger MW, Polakiewicz RD, Gilliland DG, Druker BJ. Activating alleles of JAK3 in acute megakaryoblastic leukemia. Cancer Cell 2006;10(1):65–75.

309. Shaw MH, Boyartchuk V, Wong S, Karaghiosoff M, Ragimbeau J, Pellegrini S, Muller M, Dietrich WF, Yap GS. A natural mutation in the Tyk2 pseudokinase domain underlies altered susceptibility of B10.Q/J mice to infection and autoimmunity. Proc Natl Acad Sci U S A 2003;100(20):11594–11599.

310. Minegishi Y, Saito M, Morio T, Watanabe K, Agematsu K, Tsuchiya S, Takada H, Hara T, Kawamura N, Ariga T, Kaneko H, Kondo N, Tsuge I, Yachie A, Sakiyama Y, Iwata T, Bessho F, Ohishi T, Joh K, Imai K, Kogawa K, Shinohara M, Fujieda M, Wakiguchi H, Pasic S, Abinun M, Ochs HD, Renner ED, Jansson A, Belohradsky BH, Metin A, Shimizu N, Mizutani S, Miyawaki T, Nonoyama S, Karasuyama H. Human tyrosine kinase 2 deficiency reveals its requisite roles in multiple cytokine signals involved in innate and acquired immunity. Immunity 2006;25(5):745–755.

311. Melzner I, Bucur AJ, Bruderlein S, Dorsch K, Hasel C, Barth TF, Leithauser F, Moller P. Biallelic mutation of SOCS-1 impairs JAK2 degradation and sustains phospho-JAK2 action in the MedB-1 mediastinal lymphoma line. Blood 2005;105(6):2535–2542.

312. Melzner I, Weniger MA, Bucur AJ, Bruderlein S, Dorsch K, Hasel C, Leithauser F, Ritz O, Dyer MJ, Barth TF, Moller P. Biallelic deletion within 16p13.13 including SOCS-1 in Karpas1106P mediastinal B-cell lymphoma line is associated with delayed degradation of JAK2 protein. Int J Cancer 2006;118(8):1941–1944.

313. Galm O, Yoshikawa H, Esteller M, Osieka R, Herman JG. SOCS-1, a negative regulator of cytokine signaling, is frequently silenced by methylation in multiple myeloma. Blood 2003;101(7):2784–2788.

314. Yoshikawa H, Matsubara K, Qian GS, Jackson P, Groopman JD, Manning JE, Harris CC, Herman JG. SOCS-1, a negative regulator of the JAK/STAT pathway, is silenced by methylation in human hepatocellular carcinoma and shows growth-suppression activity. Nat Genet 2001;28(1):29–35.

315. Nagai H, Naka T, Terada Y, Komazaki T, Yabe A, Jin E, Kawanami O, Kishimoto T, Konishi N, Nakamura M, Kobayashi Y, Emi M. Hypermethylation associated with inactivation of the SOCS-1 gene, a JAK/STAT inhibitor, in human hepatoblastomas. J Hum Genet 2003;48(2):65–69.

316. Fukushima N, Sato N, Sahin F, Su GH, Hruban RH, Goggins M. Aberrant methylation of suppressor of cytokine signalling-1 (SOCS-1) gene in pancreatic ductal neoplasms. Br J Cancer 2003;89(2):338–343.

317. Komazaki T, Nagai H, Emi M, Terada Y, Yabe A, Jin E, Kawanami O, Konishi N, Moriyama Y, Naka T, Kishimoto T. Hypermethylation-associated inactivation of the SOCS-1 gene, a JAK/STAT inhibitor, in human pancreatic cancers. Jpn J Clin Oncol 2004;34(4):191–194.

318. To KF, Chan MW, Leung WK, Ng EK, Yu J, Bai AH, Lo AW, Chu SH, Tong JH, Lo KW, Sung JJ, Chan FK. Constitutional activation of IL-6-mediated JAK/STAT pathway through hypermethylation of SOCS-1 in human gastric cancer cell line. Br J Cancer 2004;91(7):1335–1341.

319. He B, You L, Uematsu K, Zang K, Xu Z, Lee AY, Costello JF, McCormick F, Jablons DM. SOCS-3 is frequently silenced by hypermethylation and suppresses cell growth in human lung cancer. Proc Natl Acad Sci U S A 2003;100(24):14133–14138.

320. Weniger MA, Melzner I, Menz CK, Wegener S, Bucur AJ, Dorsch K, Mattfeldt T, Barth TF, Moller P. Mutations of the tumor suppressor gene SOCS-1 in classical Hodgkin lymphoma are frequent and associated with nuclear phospho-STAT5 accumulation. Oncogene 2006;25(18):2679–2684.

321. Lacronique V, Boureux A, Valle VD, Poirel H, Quang CT, Mauchauffe M, Berthou C, Lessard M, Berger R, Ghysdael J, Bernard OA. A TEL-JAK2 fusion protein with constitutive kinase activity in human leukemia. Science 1997;278(5341):1309–1312.

322. Griesinger F, Hennig H, Hillmer F, Podleschny M, Steffens R, Pies A, Wormann B, Haase D, Bohlander SK. A BCR-JAK2 fusion gene as the result of a t(9;22)(p24;q11.2) translocation in a patient with a clinically typical chronic myeloid leukemia. Genes Chromosomes Cancer 2005;44(3):329–333.

323. Bousquet M, Quelen C, De Mas V, Duchayne E, Roquefeuil B, Delsol G, Laurent G, Dastugue N, Brousset P. The t(8;9)(p22;p24) translocation in atypical chronic myeloid leukaemia yields a new PCM1-JAK2 fusion gene. Oncogene 2005;24(48):7248–7252.

324. Reiter A, Walz C, Watmore A, Schoch C, Blau I, Schlegelberger B, Berger U, Telford N, Aruliah S, Yin JA, Vanstraelen D, Barker HF, Taylor PC, O'Driscoll A, Benedetti F, Rudolph C, Kolb HJ, Hochhaus A, Hehlmann R, Chase A, Cross NC. The t(8;9)(p22;p24) is a recurrent abnormality in chronic and acute leukemia that fuses PCM1 to JAK2. Cancer Res 2005;65(7):2662–2667.

325. Murati A, Gelsi-Boyer V, Adelaide J, Perot C, Talmant P, Giraudier S, Lode L, Letessier A, Delaval B, Brunel V, Imbert M, Garand R, Xerri L, Birnbaum D, Mozziconacci MJ, Chaffanet M. PCM1-JAK2 fusion in myeloproliferative disorders and acute erythroid leukemia with t(8;9) translocation. Leukemia 2005;19(9):1692–1696.

326. Kralovics R, Passamonti F, Buser AS, Teo SS, Tiedt R, Passweg JR, Tichelli A, Cazzola M, Skoda RC. A gain-of-function mutation of JAK2 in myeloproliferative disorders. N Engl J Med 2005;352(17):1779–1790.

327. Jones AV, Kreil S, Zoi K, Waghorn K, Curtis C, Zhang L, Score J, Seear R, Chase AJ, Grand FH, White H, Zoi C, Loukopoulos D, Terpos E, Vervessou EC, Schultheis B, Emig M, Ernst T, Lengfelder E, Hehlmann R, Hochhaus A, Oscier D, Silver RT, Reiter A, Cross NC. Widespread occurrence of the JAK2 V617F mutation in chronic myeloproliferative disorders. Blood 2005;106(6):2162–2168.

328. Levine RL, Wadleigh M, Cools J, Ebert BL, Wernig G, Huntly BJ, Boggon TJ, Wlodarska I, Clark JJ, Moore S, Adelsperger J, Koo S, Lee JC, Gabriel S, Mercher T, D'Andrea A, Frohling S, Dohner K, Marynen P, Vandenberghe P, Mesa RA, Tefferi A, Griffin JD, Eck MJ, Sellers WR, Meyerson M, Golub TR, Lee SJ, Gilliland DG. Activating mutation in the tyrosine kinase JAK2 in polycythemia vera, essential thrombocythemia, and myeloid metaplasia with myelofibrosis. Cancer Cell 2005;7(4):387–397.

329. Scott LM, Tong W, Levine RL, Scott MA, Beer PA, Stratton MR, Futreal PA, Erber WN, McMullin MF, Harrison CN, Warren AJ, Gilliland DG, Lodish HF, Green AR. JAK2 exon 12 mutations in polycythemia vera and idiopathic erythrocytosis. N Engl J Med 2007;356(5):459–468.

330. Dudley AC, Thomas D, Best J, Jenkins A. The STATs in cell stress-type responses. Cell Commun Signal 2004;2(1): 8.

331. Lee MY, Joung YH, Lim EJ, Park JH, Ye SK, Park T, Zhang Z, Park DK, Lee KJ, Yang YM. Phosphorylation and activation of STAT proteins by hypoxia in breast cancer cells. Breast 2006;15(2):187–195.

332. Joung YH, Lim EJ, Lee MY, Park JH, Ye SK, Park EU, Kim SY, Zhang Z, Lee KJ, Park DK, Park T, Moon WK, Yang YM. Hypoxia activates the cyclin D1 promoter via the Jak2/STAT5b pathway in breast cancer cells. Exp Mol Med 2005;37(4):353–364.

333. Xu Q, Briggs J, Park S, Niu G, Kortylewski M, Zhang S, Gritsko T, Turkson J, Kay H, Semenza GL, Cheng JQ, Jove R, Yu H. Targeting Stat3 blocks both HIF-1 and VEGF expression induced by multiple oncogenic growth signaling pathways. Oncogene 2005;24(36):5552–5560.

334. Yasuda Y, Fujita Y, Matsuo T, Koinuma S, Hara S, Tazaki A, Onozaki M, Hashimoto M, Musha T, Ogawa K, Fujita H, Nakamura Y, Shiozaki H, Utsumi H. Erythropoietin regulates tumour growth of human malignancies. Carcinogenesis 2003;24(6):1021–1029.

335. Yasuda Y, Musha T, Tanaka H, Fujita Y, Fujita H, Utsumi H, Matsuo T, Masuda S, Nagao M, Sasaki R, Nakamura Y. Inhibition of erythropoietin signalling destroys xenografts of ovarian and uterine cancers in nude mice. Br J Cancer 2001;84(6):836–843.

336. Acs G, Xu X, Chu C, Acs P, Verma A. Prognostic significance of erythropoietin expression in human endometrial carcinoma. Cancer 2004;100(11):2376–2386.

337. Arcasoy MO, Harris KW, Forget BG. A human erythropoietin receptor gene mutant causing familial erythrocytosis is associated with deregulation of the rates of Jak2 and Stat5 inactivation. Exp Hematol 1999;27(1):63–74.

338. Lai SY, Childs EE, Xi S, Coppelli FM, Gooding WE, Wells A, Ferris RL, Grandis JR. Erythropoietin-mediated activation of JAK-STAT signaling contributes to cellular invasion in head and neck squamous cell carcinoma. Oncogene 2005;24(27):4442–4449.

339. BEST. Investigators and Study Group. Lancet Oncol 2003;4:459–460.

340. Henke M, Laszig R, Rube C, Schafer U, Haase KD, Schilcher B, Mose S, Beer KT, Burger U, Dougherty C, Frommhold H. Erythropoietin to treat head and neck cancer patients with anaemia undergoing radiotherapy: randomised, double-blind, placebo-controlled trial. Lancet 2003;362(9392):1255–1260.

341. Belenkov AI, Shenouda G, Rizhevskaya E, Cournoyer D, Belzile JP, Souhami L, Devic S, Chow TY. Erythropoietin induces cancer cell resistance to ionizing radiation and to cisplatin. Mol Cancer Ther 2004;3(12):1525–1532.

342. Huang LJ, Constantinescu SN, Lodish HF. The N-terminal domain of Janus kinase 2 is required for Golgi processing and cell surface expression of erythropoietin receptor. Mol Cell 2001;8(6):1327–1338.

343. Parganas E, Wang D, Stravopodis D, Topham DJ, Marine JC, Teglund S, Vanin EF, Bodner S, Colamonici OR, van Deursen JM, Grosveld G, Ihle JN. Jak2 is essential for signaling through a variety of cytokine receptors. Cell 1998;93(3):385–395.

344. Neubauer H, Cumano A, Muller M, Wu H, Huffstadt U, Pfeffer K. Jak2 deficiency defines an essential developmental checkpoint in definitive hematopoiesis. Cell 1998;93(3):397–409.

345. Canbay E, Norman M, Kilic E, Goffin V, Zachary I. Prolactin stimulates the JAK2 and focal adhesion kinase pathways in human breast carcinoma T47-D cells. Biochem J 1997;324 (Pt 1):231–236.

346. Horinaga M, Okita H, Nakashima J, Kanao K, Sakamoto M, Murai M. Clinical and pathologic significance of activation of signal transducer and activator of transcription 3 in prostate cancer. Urology 2005;66(3):671–675.

347. Mora LB, Buettner R, Seigne J, Diaz J, Ahmad N, Garcia R, Bowman T, Falcone R, Fairclough R, Cantor A, Muro-Cacho C, Livingston S, Karras J, Pow-Sang J, Jove R. Constitutive activation of Stat3 in human prostate tumors and cell lines: direct inhibition of Stat3 signaling induces apoptosis of prostate cancer cells. Cancer Res 2002;62(22):6659–6666.

348. Barton BE, Karras JG, Murphy TF, Barton A, Huang HF. Signal transducer and activator of transcription 3 (STAT3) activation in prostate cancer: direct STAT3 inhibition induces apoptosis in prostate cancer lines. Mol Cancer Ther 2004;3(1):11–20.

349. Gao L, Zhang L, Hu J, Li F, Shao Y, Zhao D, Kalvakolanu DV, Kopecko DJ, Zhao X, Xu DQ. Down-regulation of signal transducer and activator of transcription 3 expression using vector-based small interfering RNAs suppresses growth of human prostate tumor in vivo. Clin Cancer Res 2005;11(17):6333–6341.

350. Barton BE, Murphy TF, Shu P, Huang HF, Meyenhofer M, Barton A. Novel single-stranded oligonucleotides that inhibit signal transducer and activator of transcription 3 induce apoptosis in vitro and in vivo in prostate cancer cell lines. Mol Cancer Ther 2004;3(10):1183–1191.

351. Clevenger CV. Roles and regulation of stat family transcription factors in human breast cancer. Am J Pathol 2004;165(5):1449–1460.

352. Ling X, Arlinghaus RB. Knockdown of STAT3 expression by RNA interference inhibits the induction of breast tumors in immunocompetent mice. Cancer Res 2005;65(7):2532–2536.

353. Yin N, Wang D, Zhang H, Yi X, Sun X, Shi B, Wu H, Wu G, Wang X, Shang Y. Molecular mechanisms involved in the growth stimulation of breast cancer cells by leptin. Cancer Res 2004;64(16):5870–5875.

354. Hu X, Juneja SC, Maihle NJ, Cleary MP. Leptin—a growth factor in normal and malignant breast cells and for normal mammary gland development. J Natl Cancer Inst 2002;94(22):1704–1711.

355. Pai R, Lin C, Tran T, Tarnawski A. Leptin activates STAT and ERK2 pathways and induces gastric cancer cell proliferation. Biochem Biophys Res Commun 2005;331(4):984–992.

356. Gao B, Shen X, Kunos G, Meng Q, Goldberg ID, Rosen EM, Fan S. Constitutive activation of JAK-STAT3 signaling by BRCA1 in human prostate cancer cells. FEBS Lett 2001;488(3):179–184.

357. Yeh HH, Lai WW, Chen HH, Liu HS, Su WC. Autocrine IL-6-induced Stat3 activation contributes to the pathogenesis of lung adenocarcinoma and malignant pleural effusion. Oncogene 2006;25(31):4300–4309.

358. Savarese TM, Campbell CL, McQuain C, Mitchell K, Guardiani R, Quesenberry PJ, Nelson BE. Coexpression of oncostatin M and its receptors and evidence for STAT3 activation in human ovarian carcinomas. Cytokine 2002;17(6):324–334.

359. Horiguchi A, Oya M, Shimada T, Uchida A, Marumo K, Murai M. Activation of signal transducer and activator of transcription 3 in renal cell carcinoma: a study of incidence and its association with pathological features and clinical outcome. J Urol 2002;168(2):762–765.

360. Xie TX, Huang FJ, Aldape KD, Kang SH, Liu M, Gershenwald JE, Xie K, Sawaya R, Huang S. Activation of stat3 in human melanoma promotes brain metastasis. Cancer Res 2006;66(6):3188–3196.

361. Yared MA, Khoury JD, Medeiros LJ, Rassidakis GZ, Lai R. Activation status of the JAK/STAT3 pathway in mantle cell lymphoma. Arch Pathol Lab Med 2005;129(8):990–996.

362. Shouda T, Hiraoka K, Komiya S, Hamada T, Zenmyo M, Iwasaki H, Isayama T, Fukushima N, Nagata K, Yoshimura A. Suppression of IL-6 production and proliferation by blocking STAT3 activation in malignant soft tissue tumor cells. Cancer Lett 2006;231(2):176–184.

363. Lai R, Navid F, Rodriguez-Galindo C, Liu T, Fuller CE, Ganti R, Dien J, Dalton J, Billups C, Khoury JD. STAT3 is activated in a subset of the Ewing sarcoma family of tumours. J Pathol 2006;208(5):624–632.

364. Kusaba T, Nakayama T, Yamazumi K, Yakata Y, Yoshizaki A, Inoue K, Nagayasu T, Sekine I. Activation of STAT3 is a marker of poor prognosis in human colorectal cancer. Oncol Rep 2006;15(6):1445–1451.

365. Ma XT, Wang S, Ye YJ, Du RY, Cui ZR, Somsouk M. Constitutive activation of Stat3 signaling pathway in human colorectal carcinoma. World J Gastroenterol 2004;10(11):1569–1573.

366. Paner GP, Silberman S, Hartman G, Micetich KC, Aranha GV, Alkan S. Analysis of signal transducer and activator of transcription 3 (STAT3) in gastrointestinal stromal tumors. Anticancer Res 2003;23(3B):2253–2260.

367. Plaza Menacho I, Koster R, van der Sloot AM, Quax WJ, Osinga J, van der Sluis T, Hollema H, Burzynski GM, Gimm O, Buys CH, Eggen BJ, Hofstra RM. RET-familial medullary thyroid carcinoma mutants Y791F and S891A activate a Src/JAK/STAT3 pathway, independent of glial cell line-derived neurotrophic factor. Cancer Res 2005;65(5):1729–1737.

368. Hsiao JR, Jin YT, Tsai ST, Shiau AL, Wu CL, Su WC. Constitutive activation of STAT3 and STAT5 is present in the majority of nasopharyngeal carcinoma and correlates with better prognosis. Br J Cancer 2003;89(2):344–349.

369. Leong PL, Andrews GA, Johnson DE, Dyer KF, Xi S, Mai JC, Robbins PD, Gadiparthi S, Burke NA, Watkins SF, Grandis JR. Targeted inhibition of Stat3 with a decoy oligonucleotide abrogates head and neck cancer cell growth. Proc Natl Acad Sci U S A 2003;100(7):4138–4143.

370. Yu H, Jove R. The STATs of cancer—new molecular targets come of age. Nat Rev Cancer 2004;4(2):97–105.

371. Huang M, Dorsey JF, Epling-Burnette PK, Nimmanapalli R, Landowski TH, Mora LB, Niu G, Sinibaldi D, Bai F, Kraker A, Yu H, Moscinski L, Wei S, Djeu J, Dalton WS, Bhalla K, Loughran TP, Wu J, Jove R. Inhibition of Bcr-Abl kinase activity by PD180970 blocks constitutive activation of Stat5 and growth of CML cells. Oncogene 2002;21(57):8804–8816.

372. Levis M, Allebach J, Tse KF, Zheng R, Baldwin BR, Smith BD, Jones-Bolin S, Ruggeri B, Dionne C, Small D. A FLT3-targeted tyrosine kinase inhibitor is cytotoxic to leukemia cells in vitro and in vivo. Blood 2002;99(11):3885–3891.

373. Thabard W, Collette M, Mellerin MP, Puthier D, Barille S, Bataille R, Amiot M. IL-6 upregulates its own receptor on some human myeloma cell lines. Cytokine 2001;14(6):352–356.

374. Laurent C, Demas V, Delabesse E, Brousset P. Detection of the MPL W515L mutation in bone marrow core biopsy specimens with essential thrombocythemia using the TaqMan assay. Hum Pathol 2007;38(10):1581–1582.

375. Chaligne R, James C, Tonetti C, Besancenot R, Le Couedic JP, Fava F, Mazurier F, Godin I, Maloum K, Larbret F, Lecluse Y, Vainchenker W, Giraudier S. Evidence for MPL W515L/K mutations in hematopoietic stem cells in primitive myelofibrosis. Blood 2007;110(10):3735–3743.

376. Ding J, Komatsu H, Wakita A, Kato-Uranishi M, Ito M, Satoh A, Tsuboi K, Nitta M, Miyazaki H, Iida S, Ueda R. Familial essential thrombocythemia associated with a dominant-positive activating mutation of the c-MPL gene, which encodes for the receptor for thrombopoietin. Blood 2004;103(11):4198–4200.

377. Tefferi A. JAK and MPL mutations in myeloid malignancies. Leuk Lymphoma 2008;49(3):388–397.

378. Alas S, Bonavida B. Inhibition of constitutive STAT3 activity sensitizes resistant non-Hodgkin's lymphoma and multiple myeloma to chemotherapeutic drug-mediated apoptosis. Clin Cancer Res 2003;9(1):316–326.

379. Real PJ, Sierra A, De Juan A, Segovia JC, Lopez-Vega JM, Fernandez-Luna JL. Resistance to chemotherapy via Stat3-dependent overexpression of Bcl-2 in metastatic breast cancer cells. Oncogene 2002;21(50):7611–7618.

CHAPTER 5

INTRACELLULAR SIGNAL TRANSDUCTION CASCADES

I N CHAPTERS 3 and 4, we reviewed a wide range of tyrosine kinases that convey extracellular signals to cells, initiating a plethora of intracellular effects. In most cases, phosphorylation of cell surface receptors or receptor-associated kinases represents just the first step in a complex series of signaling cascades, resulting in subcellular translocation, activation/inactivation of intracellular effector molecules, and, ultimately, coordinated regulation of gene transcription and translation. These diverse signaling events are orchestrated by an equally diverse range of kinases. We focus mainly on two major kinase cascades that are of paramount importance in cancer biology: the PI3K/PTEN (phosphatidylinositol-3 kinase/phosphatase and tensin homolog on chromosome ten) pathway and the ERK/MAPK (extracellular regulated kinase/mitogen-activated protein kinase) pathway. In addition, we review the PIM kinases, which are implicated in several tumors including prostate cancer and hematological malignancies, and the protein kinase C (PKC) family—an important group of signal transduction proteins that collectively have diverse (and sometimes contradictory) effects on tumor initiation, progression, and survival. As we explore and dissect these signal transduction systems, it will be important to bear in mind that these pathways do not exist in isolation but form a complex network of interactions with each other and with many other intracellular signaling systems. These interdependencies vary depending on cell type, environment, and subcellular localization in a temporal fashion. Researchers have taken a reductionist approach in order to simplify these networks and draw concrete conclusions regarding individual kinases: however, the area of signaling networks (or systems biology) is emerging as an important complement to the study of individual proteins and there may be emergent properties of these networks that are not obvious from consideration of individual proteins and pathways.

5.1 THE PI3K/PTEN PATHWAY

The PI3K/PTEN pathway regulates key biological processes in the cell such as growth, survival, and proliferation (Figure 5.1). PI3K catalyzes the formation of the phosphoinositide second messenger phosphatidylinositol(3,4,5)trisphosphate (PIP_3) in response to stimulation by activated growth factor receptor tyrosine kinases (1), G-protein coupled receptors, or RAS GTPase and thereby initiates pathway signaling. Increasing PIP_3 levels result in the recruitment and activation of downstream effectors PDK1 and AKT, whereas pathway signaling is attenuated by PTEN, a tumor suppressor that dephosphorylates $3'$-phosphoinositides. Hyperactivated signaling due to dysregulation of PI3K/PTEN pathway components (including PI3K (2) and PTEN (3)) is observed in many cancers and correlates with tumor growth and survival (4, 5). Moreover, resistance to a variety of anticancer therapies including receptor tyrosine kinase inhibitors and genotoxic agents has been attributed to a failure to downregulate signaling along the PI3K/PTEN pathway (6, 7). In this section we discuss the key components of the PI3K pathway, with particular reference to their role in promoting and maintaining tumor growth.

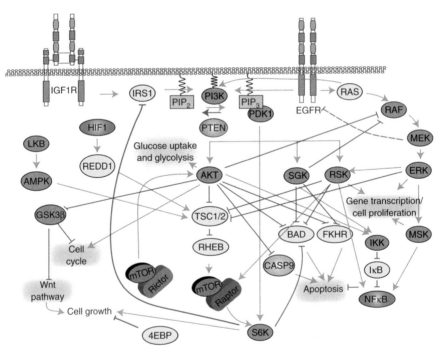

Figure 5.1 Overview of PI3K, mTOR, and RAS/ERK signaling pathways. The number of downstream effectors in these interconnected pathways is actually vastly greater than shown here. Of particular note are the complex interactions between the signaling pathways, the multiple mechanisms of upstream activation, and various feedback loops. For example, activation of p70S6 (S6K) promotes phosphorylation and inactivation of IRS1, which in turn can downregulate signaling through PI3K and its downstream effectors.

5.1.1 PI3K

PI3K (phosphatidylinositol-3 kinase) is a heterodimeric dual lipid/protein kinase with separate catalytic and regulatory subunits encoded by distinct genes. In mammals there are eight PI3Ks divided into three classes based on their primary sequence, domain structure, and substrate specificity (8). They share a common function in their ability to phosphorylate the 3'OH of second messenger phosphoinositide lipids (9). Class I PI3Ks preferentially convert phosphatidylinositol(4, 5)bisphosphate (PIP_2) to PIP_3 in response to external cell stimuli. These PI3Ks have historically been subdivided into Class I_A (PI3Kα/β/δ) and Class I_B (PI3Kγ), which are activated by receptor tyrosine kinases (RTKs) and G-protein coupled receptors (GPCRs), respectively (10, 11), although an increasing body of data suggests that PI3Kβ may also be an important mediator of GPCR signaling. Class I PI3Ks are composed of a catalytic subunit known as p110 and a regulatory subunit, typically described as p85 for Class I_A and p101 for Class I_B PI3Ks. To date, only Class I PI3Ks are known to activate PDK1 and AKT/PKB, which are important downstream effectors of the PI3K/PTEN pathway. These kinases bind to PIP_3 at the cell membrane and are subsequently activated by phosphorylation (9). This activation results in stimulation of growth pathways, inhibition of apoptotic signaling, and transition through the restriction point in the G1 phase of the cell cycle (12, 13). PI3K was first identified as a potential oncogene when its activity was associated with the ability of the Rous sarcoma virus gene product pp60v-src to transform chicken embryo fibroblasts (14, 15). The role of PI3K as an oncogene became more evident when it was found that *PIK3CA*, the gene that encodes the PI3Kα catalytic domain, p110α, was amplified in ovarian cancer (16).

The p110 catalytic subunits of the Class I PI3Ks are large, multidomain proteins of approximately 1100 residues (Figure 5.2). The four isoforms (α, β, δ, and γ) are homologous in primary sequence and order of individual domains (5, 8). The crystal structure of the PI3Kγ catalytic subunit has been solved (17, 18), and more recently the p110 subunit of PI3Kα was determined in complex with regulatory elements of the p85 subunit (19). All known p110 isoforms contain a RAS binding domain (RBD), a C2 domain, a helical domain (also called the PIK domain), and a C-terminal protein/lipid kinase domain. The Class I_A p110 proteins also contain an N-terminal adaptor binding domain (ABD), which contributes to heterodimerization with the p85 regulatory subunit. The domain structure of p85 comprises a single N-terminal SH3 domain and a RHO GTPase-activating domain, followed by two SH2 domains, which are separated by an intervening inter-SH2 (iSH2) region (Figure 5.2). The N-terminal SH2 domain and iSH2 region of p85 bind to and inhibit the p110 subunit, and PI3K activation is triggered by the interaction of the SH2 domains with phosphotyrosine residues in the cytoplasmic domains of upstream RTKs or adaptor proteins (20). For example, insulin or IGF1 receptor signaling is transduced via interactions of the SH2 domains with the adaptor proteins IRS1 and IRS2 (5). The first SH2 domain and iSH2 sequence appear to be particularly important for both regulating basal PI3K activity and promoting activation by interaction with upstream phosphotyrosine residues (21). Biochemical and

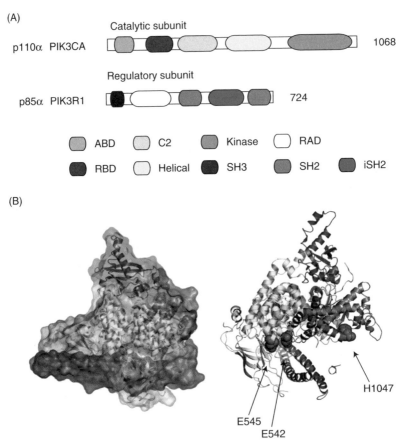

Figure 5.2 Structure of PI3K. (A) Domain structures of p110α (catalytic domain) and p85α (regulatory domain). (B) X-ray crystal structure of p110α in complex with the inter-SH2 domain of p85α. For p110α, the N-terminal ABD (adaptor binding domain) is in green, the RBD (RAS binding domain) is in blue; the C2 domain is in pale blue; the helical domain is in yellow; and the kinase domain is in teal. The p85 fragment is in red. The left panel shows the overall domain architecture: in this view, the kinase domain is somewhat obscured by the helical and ABD domains. The right panel view is looking toward the left face of the left panel and shows the location of several important activating mutations in p110α. See text for further details.

biophysical characterizations using truncated forms of p85 indicate that the N-terminal SH2 domain and iSH2 region of p85 are required for inhibition of the p110 catalytic activity (20–22). Interaction of the SH2 domains with upstream phosphotyrosines may then disrupt this interaction, promoting p110 activation. Consistent with this, oncogenic mutations such as E545K in the p110α helical domain inhibit the interaction with the p85 N-terminal SH2 domain, and this inhibition can be rescued by charge-reversal mutants of phosphotyrosine binding residues in the SH2 domain (23). The X-ray crystal structure of p110α in complex with a fragment of p85 (containing the N-terminal SH2 and iSH2 domains) has shed further light on the mechanism of p85/p110 regulation and the effects of oncogenic mutations (19). Although the SH2 domain was not well resolved in this structure, the iSH2 region was found to be tethered to the ABD and C2 domains of p110α. Modeling of the missing SH2 domain suggests that it directly contacts the helical domain, further supporting the rationale for the oncogenic mutations E542K and E545K. Another common oncogenic mutation, H1047R, lies in the C terminus of the kinase domain and may exert a direct effect of the activation loop (Figure 5.2). The structure of the p110/p85 complex also suggests that the p85 iSH2 domain and nearby regions of the C2 and kinase domains may present a positively charged surface to facilitate interaction with phospholipids in the plasma membrane.

Although all four isoforms of p110 have shown the potential to induce oncogenic transformation (24), focus has been placed on p110α due to the high frequency of cancer-specific point mutations identified in *PIK3CA* (2, 25) and its critical role in regulating growth factor and metabolic signaling (26). Missense mutations are observed throughout the *PIK3CA* gene from a variety of cancer cells, yet the majority (>85%) map to three distinct hot spots within the helical domain (E542K and E545K) and kinase domain (H1047R) (25). These findings suggest that the mutations provide a selective growth advantage to the cell (27), and functional analysis has shown that all three mutations increase PI3Kα activity in tumor models (28, 29). Recently, PI3Kβ/*PIK3CB* has also gained prominence as a mediator of oncogenic transformation: in particular, two independent studies have shown that in PTEN-deficient cell lines and tumors (discussed later), ablation of PIK3CB (but not PIK3CA) resulted in inhibition of downstream signaling and reduced cell growth and tumorigenesis (30, 31).

The RAS GTPase is another important signaling protein downstream of growth factor receptors that can promote PI3K activation. Phosphorylated RTKs signal to RAS via a series of adaptor proteins, and activated RAS can stabilize and activate the catalytic domain of PI3K (32, 33). RAS has been found to be mutated in over 20% of all human cancers (34, 35). There are three RAS genes: *HRAS, KRAS*, and *NRAS*, of which *KRAS* is the most frequently mutated. *KRAS* is mutated in about 22% of tumor samples examined, compared to 7.6% for *NRAS* and 3.7% for *HRAS* (34, 36). *KRAS* mutations are found in numerous tumor types, including pancreas (60%), biliary tract (33%), large intestine (31%), small intestine (26%), and lung (19%). The majority of *KRAS* mutations are localized to three amino acid residues: G12, G13, and Q61, the most prevalent of which is G12 (35). These mutations block GTPase activating proteins (GAPs) from promoting hydrolysis, allowing GTP-RAS to accumulate at the membrane. In addition to promoting PI3K/PTEN signaling, activated RAS alleles lead to dysregulation of multiple downstream signaling pathways including the RAF/MEK/ERK and PKC pathways (described later) and the RALGDS/RAL pathway (37, 38). Oncogenic forms of RAS may have a similar effect in the absence of RTK signaling, and PI3K activation is an important factor in mediating cellular transformation by RAS oncogenes (39). Indeed, recent transgenic mouse experiments have highlighted the particular importance of the physical interaction between RAS and PI3K p110α in promoting tumor formation (40). In this study, mice were engineered with a specific double mutation in p110α that blocks its interaction with RAS. Embryonic fibroblasts from homozygous mutant mice have normal ERK signaling but attenuated EGF- or FGF-dependent AKT signaling (although PDGF-dependent AKT signaling appears unaffected, possibly due to the fact that PDGF receptor can bind directly to the PI3K p85 subunit). The p110α mutation greatly reduces the transforming ability of oncogenic mutant KRAS, mutant EGFR, and NeuT in vitro, and crossing the p110α mutant mice with animals bearing mutationally activated KRAS showed that the resistance to KRAS-driven oncogenesis is recapitulated in vivo.

The tumor suppressor gene *PTEN* (also known as *MMAC1*, or mutated in multiple advanced cancers) is a critical negative regulator of PI3K signaling (41–43). Germline deletions of *PTEN* underlie several rare autosomal dominant disorders, including Cowden disease and Bannayan–Zonana syndrome (44). *PTEN* is a dual specificity protein and lipid phosphatase. Its principal function appears to be removal of the D3 phosphate from the inositol ring of phosphatidylinositol (3,4,5) trisphosphate. This attenuates the recruitment of the downstream effector proteins PDK1 and AKT/PKB to the plasma membrane (see later discussion), thus downregulating PDK1 and AKT-mediated signaling. The *PTEN* gene is one of the most frequently mutated in human cancers, perhaps second only to *P53* (45). Mutation or deletion of *PTEN* is found in many sporadic tumors and seems to be most prevalent in endometrial cancer (46), prostate cancer (47), and glioblastoma (48). *PTEN* gene silencing via promoter methylation has also been noted in several tumor types, including lung cancer (49). Loss of PTEN alone does not appear to be tumorigenic per se, but the resulting amplification of growth, proliferation, and survival pathways provides a cellular context that supports tumor development (43).

The major downstream effectors of PI3K are PDK1 and AKT, which phosphorylate a wide range of kinases and other effector proteins. Several of the key kinases involved are members of the AGC (PKA/PKG/PKC) family, including SGK (serum and glucocorticoid-inducible kinase), p90RSK, and protein kinase C (PKC). p90RSK is also discussed later in the context of ERK signaling and is a point of convergence between the RAS/RAF/MEK/ERK and PI3K/PTEN pathways; the diverse functions of PKC isozymes are discussed in Section 5.5. Although PI3K-dependent PIP$_3$ generation is predominantly associated with the PDK1/AKT axis, signaling can also proceed via different pathways. Notably, the small GTPases CDC42 and RAC1 are associated with PI3K/PTEN activity and may function to both promote cell migration and upregulate p70S6 kinase (50, 51). PI3K can also associate with PAK1 (p21-activated kinase), leading to cytoskeletal reorganization (52) and stimulation of RAF1 kinase activity (53).

5.1.2 PDK1

PDK1 is an important regulator of multiple signaling pathways downstream of PI3K (54). PDK1 has an N-terminal kinase domain and a C-terminal pleckstrin homology (PH) domain, which regulates its interaction with phosphoinositides, in particular, PIP$_3$ (Figure 5.3). Details of the structural basis for the activation of PDK1 and its substrates are discussed in Chapter 2. The principal target of PDK1 with regard to PI3K signaling is AKT/PKB, which modulates a wide range of effects in cell

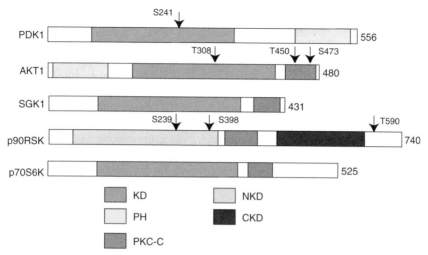

Figure 5.3 Domain structures of the AGC family kinases PDK1, AKT1, SGK1, p90RSK, and p70S6K. Abbreviations: KD, kinase domain; NKD, N-terminal kinase domain; CKD, C-terminal kinase domain; PH, pleckstrin homology domain; PKC-C, PKC C-terminal homology region.

cycle control, inhibition of apoptosis, and cell growth. PDK1 also phosphorylates other proteins in the AGC kinase family, including p70S6 kinase (55), p90RSK (56), serum and glucocorticoid-inducible kinase SGK (57), and various isoforms of PKC, described in Section 5.5 (58). The functional significance of AKT and other PDK1 substrate kinases downstream of PI3K is described next.

5.1.3 AKT

AKT (also known as PKB) is one of the major downstream effector kinases in the PI3K pathway and is known to phosphorylate a broad range of proteins involved in cell growth, proliferation, and survival (12, 59). There are three known isoforms: AKT1, AKT2, and AKT3. All AKT isoforms are highly homologous to each other but have somewhat distinct functions (60). AKT1 appears to be a regulator of placental development and animal growth, AKT2 is important for maintaining glucose homeostasis, and AKT3 appears to be involved in brain growth. Like PDK1, AKT contains a pleckstrin homology domain (involved in membrane localization) and a kinase domain, but the order is reversed: the PH domain of AKT is at the N terminus (Figure 5.3). An oncogenic mutation in the AKT1 PH domain (E17K) was recently identified in several breast, colorectal, and ovarian tumors and was shown to promote PI3K-independent membrane localization and activation (61).

AKT is activated by phosphorylation of two residues, T308 and S473. As described in Chapter 2, phosphorylation at S473 creates a site for PDK1 binding, and phosphorylation of T308 in the kinase activation loop by PDK1 promotes AKT activation. However, although S473 phosphorylation enhances AKT activity it is not obligatory, and T308 phosphorylation can still occur in the absence of S473 phosphorylation (62). The S473 kinase, hitherto known as PDK2, was identified as the mTOR:Rictor (mTORC2) protein complex (63), thus providing a positive feedback mechanism in PI3K/AKT/mTOR signaling. Integrin-linked kinase (ILK) may also play a role in promoting S473 phosphorylation (although this function is unlikely to directly involve kinase activity of ILK (64)), and in some cellular contexts the PI3K-related kinase DNAPK may be able to phosphorylate S473 (65, 66). A similar role has been proposed for PKCβII (67), and while these alternative activators may have limited or tissue-specific roles in normal homeostasis, it is possible that they may be important in the deregulated environment of tumor cells. A third regulatory phosphorylation site, termed the turn motif, is found at T450. This site was recently shown to be phosphorylated by the mTOR:Rictor complex and promotes folding and stabilization of the nascent protein during synthesis (68, 69). Once activated, AKT modulates a wide range of effects in cell cycle control, inhibition of apoptosis, and cell growth, summarized next.

Survival   AKT promotes cell survival via phosphorylation of a diverse range of substrates. For example, the proapoptotic protein BAD forms nonfunctional complexes with an antiapoptotic member of the BCL2 family, BCLXL (70); phosphorylation of BAD by AKT results in sequestration of BAD by 14-3-3 protein, thus restoring the antiapoptotic function of BCLXL. AKT also phosphorylates Forkhead transcription factors, preventing their nuclear translocation and subsequent activation of proapoptotic proteins (71). AKT may also directly phosphorylate and inhibit caspase 9 (72). As well as inhibiting apoptotic factors, AKT regulates cell survival via the NFκB transcription factor. Phosphorylation and activation of the IκB kinase (IKK) leads to degradation of IκB, an inhibitor of NFκB (73). Subsequent translocation of NFκB to the nucleus leads to activation of survival factors and many other genes involved in tumor cell proliferation, invasion, and metastasis (74, 75). Moreover, PTEN expression is downregulated by NFκB (76). Finally, AKT can phosphorylate the p53 regulator MDM2, leading to decreased p53 activity and downregulation of p53-dependent apoptosis (77).

Proliferation   The PI3K pathway is required for growth factor-dependent restriction point progression in the G1 phase of the cell cycle, and this activity appears to be largely mediated both directly and indirectly through AKT (13). Progression through G1 is highly dependent on the activity of the cyclin-dependent kinases CDK4 and CDK6 in complex with cyclin D1 (Chapter 6). However, GSK3β phosphorylates cyclin D1 and promotes its export from the nucleus and subsequent degradation, reducing CDK4:cyclin D1 activity. AKT phosphorylates and inactivates GSK3β, thereby upregulating cyclin D1 and driving cell cycle progression. The MYC transcription factor is downregulated by GSK3β in a similar manner to cyclin D1 (78): AKT activity inhibits GSK3β and thereby promotes the functions of MYC, which is implicated in the pathogenesis of many types of cancer (79, 80). GSK3β is also an integral component of WNT/β-catenin signaling, a pathway that is centrally involved in determining cell fate and neoplastic transformation (81). Inhibition of GSK3β by AKT promotes cytoplasmic accumulation and nuclear translocation of β-catenin. AKT has direct effects on cell cycle inhibitors p21$^{CIP1/WAF1}$ and p27^{KIP1}, preventing their interaction with nuclear cyclin:CDK complexes and thereby promoting cell cycle progression (82–85). In addition, p27 is transcriptionally downregulated through AKT-mediated inhibition of Forkhead transcription factors (71).

Growth AKT provides an important connection between PI3K and the mTORC1 complex, involving the key growth regulatory kinase mTOR (Section 5.2). Although AKT can directly phosphorylate mTOR (86), the functional significance of this is unclear and two alternative routes of activation appear to predominate. In the first of these, AKT phosphorylates and inactivates TSC2 (tuberin), which, together with TSC1 (hamartin), forms the tuberous sclerosis complex (87). This heterodimeric complex inhibits cell growth, and germline mutations in either protein are associated with tuberous sclerosis, an autosomal dominant syndrome associated with hamartoma formation (88). TSC2 contains a GTPase-activating protein (GAP) domain and can activate the small GTPase RHEB (89, 90). Genetic studies have indicated that RHEB is an upstream regulator of mTOR activity, and biochemical data indicate that RHEB directly binds to and activates mTOR (91). A second mechanism whereby AKT can promote mTORC1 activity involves PRAS40 (proline-rich AKT substrate, molecular weight 40 kDa). This protein associates with and inhibits mTORC1 in cells, possibly by competition with other substrates (92, 93). Phosphorylation of PRAS40 by AKT relieves this inhibition, thus promoting mTORC1 activity (94, 95).

Many additional activities appear to be regulated at least in part by AKT (12, 59). AKT-mediated phosphorylation of GSK3β (discussed earlier) is a key regulator of glycogen synthesis in response to insulin. However, AKT can also regulate glucose uptake, hexokinase activity, phosphofructokinase activity, and glycolysis (96). Enhanced glycolytic metabolism has been associated with tumor cells for almost 80 years (97) and may contribute to tumor cell survival and apoptotic resistance (98). Additional AKT substrates implicated in tumor progression include androgen receptor (99), estrogen receptor-α (100), and telomerase (101). AKT signaling is important for VEGF-mediated endothelial cell survival (102) and may also promote tumor vascularization via phosphorylation of eNOS (103). AKT was also shown to play a role in cell cycle checkpoint control via phosphorylation and inhibition of CHK1 kinase (104, 105), and tumor cells with upregulated AKT signaling may thereby promote their own genetic instability (106). Finally, AKT can directly phosphorylate and inactivate RAF kinase (107). This activity appears contrary to the proliferative and antiapoptotic effects of AKT signaling described earlier but may serve as a regulatory mechanism to inhibit uncontrolled growth or apoptosis, depending on cellular context.

5.1.4 Other AGC Kinases

In addition to the canonical PI3K/PDK1/AKT pathway described previously, a number of other AGC kinases are regulated by PDK1. In contrast to AKT, activation of these kinases is contingent on phosphorylation in the C-terminal tail of the kinase domain, which recruits PDK1 binding and leads to phosphorylation of the activation loop (108). Their functions overlap somewhat with those of AKT, in that they variously contribute to cellular growth, proliferation, and survival.

The serum and glucocorticoid-inducible kinases (SGKs, Figure 5.3) have several functional similarities with AKT. There are three mammalian SGK isoforms: SGK1, 2, and 3, of which SGK1 is the most widely studied (109). SGKs are activated by PDK1 (and potentially PDK2/mTOR:Rictor as well) and have been implicated in regulation of cell cycle progression and apoptosis. SGK1 has a similar phosphorylation consensus sequence to AKT (110) and phosphorylates the CDK inhibitor p27 at the same site as AKT (111). It can also phosphorylate the Forkhead transcription factor FKHRL1, though with different phosphorylation site specificity compared to AKT (112). SGK1 was also shown to elicit antiapoptotic effects by phosphorylation of the IkB kinase IKKβ (113); other putative SGK targets include RAF kinase (114), GSK3β (115), the cAMP-responsive element binding protein CREB (116), and BAD (117). SGK3 is unique among the SGK family in having a PX domain. This domain has high affinity for phosphatidylinositol-3-phosphate and targets SGK3 to endosomes, in contrast to the largely cytoplasmic localization of SGK1 and SGK2.

p90RSK (RSK1) is a ribosomal kinase that contains two distinct catalytic (kinase) domains (Figure 5.3). There are four members of the RSK family: RSK1, 2, 3, and 4. The N-terminal domain is homologous to the AGC kinases and is involved in phosphorylation of exogenous substrates, while the C-terminal domain is related to the mitogen and stress-activated kinases MNK1 and MNK2 and is involved in autophosphorylation. Activation of p90RSK involves constitutive phosphorylation by PDK1 at S227 in the N-terminal domain and mitogen-induced phosphorylation by ERK in the C-terminal domain, which leads to autophosphorylation and activation of the N-terminal kinase (56). p90RSK signaling therefore integrates signals from both the PI3K/PTEN and ERK/MAPK pathways. It phosphorylates both cytoplasmic and nuclear substrates and can translocate to the nucleus in response to mitogenic stimuli (118). In addition to ribosomal proteins, p90RSK substrates include GSK3β (119), BAD (120), CREB (121), NFκB p65 (122), and TSC1 (123). Recently, RSK1 and the closely related RSK2 were shown to phosphorylate and activate the mTOR regulatory protein Raptor, thus providing a direct conduit between the ERK/MAPK pathway and the integration of cellular growth signals by mTOR (124). RSK2 was also reported to allosterically activate estrogen receptor-α (125) and may also be implicated in osteosarcoma formation (126). Both RSK1 and RSK2 can phosphorylate and inactivate the proapoptotic kinase DAPK, which may promote survival in both normal cells and in cancer cells with aberrant activation of RAS, PI3K, and/or ERK/MAPK pathways (127). The C-terminal domain of RSK2 is also a direct substrate for FGFR3, which primes the kinase for subsequent binding of and activation by ERK (128). This mechanism may be particularly relevant to the pathogenesis of multiple myeloma, since FGFR3 is activated by the t(4;14) translocation in up to 25% of multiple myeloma cases (129).

p70S6 kinase is phosphorylated in a coordinated manner by at least two kinases: PDK1 and mTOR. p70S6K plays a critical role in mTOR-mediated control of cellular growth and translational control, and its role in this context is described in Section 5.2. In addition, p70S6K phosphorylates many other substrates including

GSK3β (119), the transcription factor CREM-τ (130), and the proapoptotic factor BAD (131). Importantly, p70S6K has also been shown to directly phosphorylate and inactivate IRS-1 and IRS-2, adaptor proteins that modulate the downstream effects of insulin and IGF1 receptor signaling through PI3K (132). Thus p70S6K signaling acts as a negative feedback mechanism for growth factor-mediated signaling, and so inhibition of p70S6K may actually upregulate PI3K pathway activity (Figure 5.1). Inhibition of IRS proteins and subsequent decoupling of insulin receptor signaling from the PI3K pathway has been implicated as a mechanism of insulin resistance, and p70S6K-deficient mice are both hypersensitive to insulin and resistant to diet-induced obesity (133). As well as affecting AKT signaling downstream of PI3K, this negative feedback mechanism can also affect RAS/RAF/MEK/ERK signaling, as recently demonstrated both in vitro and in samples from patients treated with mTOR inhibitors (134).

5.1.5   PI3K Pathway Activation in Cancer

Upregulation of PI3K signaling is prevalent in many tumor types (5, 12, 135). At the molecular level, this dysregulation may be caused by activating mutations in PI3K itself, by negative regulation of the PTEN phosphatase, or by a variety of factors both upstream and downstream of PI3K. Usually, disruptions in PTEN and PI3K are mutually exclusive, with the recently disclosed exception of endometrial cancer (136). Taken together, these data imply that there are many clinical settings where the majority of patients have tumors with elevated PI3K pathway signaling, and where a specific PI3K inhibitor might be expected to show therapeutic benefit. In addition to therapeutic utility based on the underlying biology of the tumor, activation of the PI3K pathway has been broadly associated with resistance to both targeted and genotoxic drugs, and so pathway inhibitors may have utility both as single agents and in combination with other therapeutic modalities. It should be noted that PI3K and mTOR signaling pathways share a particularly intimate interdependence, and the following discussion of indications for PI3K pathway inhibitors should be considered in parallel with the discussion of mTOR inhibitor indications in Section 5.2.

Breast Cancer   Dysregulation of the EGFR/HER family receptor tyrosine kinases is a major factor in proliferation of breast tumors. In particular, approximately 20% of breast tumors overexpress the HER2 (ERBB2) protein, correlating with decreased survival (137, 138). Inhibition of PI3K signaling is critical for the activity of EGFR family inhibitors such as the anti-HER2 antibody trastuzumab (7), and loss of PTEN correlates with trastuzumab resistance (139, 140). Therefore inhibitors of PI3K signaling may be particularly useful in HER2-positive tumors that either fail to respond or become resistant to trastuzumab. Loss of PTEN function is a common occurrence in breast tumors, either by mutation, deletion, or promoter methylation (141–145). Also, dysregulation of PI3K occurs frequently, with up to 30% of breast tumors bearing activating PI3K mutations (146–150) (Appendix XIV) or amplification of *PIK3CA* (151). In addition, multiple factors downstream of PI3K signaling have been found to be upregulated in breast tumors, including AKT, p70S6K, p90RSK, and PDK1. PI3K signaling has been implicated in resistance to various chemotherapy drugs, and there is strong preclinical support for combining PI3K pathway inhibitors with chemotherapy in breast tumors (152, 153).

Colorectal Cancer   PI3K is mutated in 13–32% of colorectal tumors (25, 154) (Appendix XIV), and loss of PTEN is observed in a high proportion of colorectal tumors, particularly those that display microsatellite instability (155, 156). Additionally, KRAS (which can also lead to upregulation of PI3K signaling) is the most frequently mutated oncogene in colorectal tumors (35, 157). PI3K pathway dysregulation has also been implicated in impaired response to the anti-EGFR antibody cetuximab and, as in the case of breast tumors, may also be of use in augmenting the response to chemotherapy (158).

Endometrial Cancer   Both PTEN loss and PI3K mutation (Appendix XIV) or amplification are common in endometrial tumors, with PTEN mutations found in up to 80% of the endometrioid subtype of endometrial carcinomas. Curiously, however, PTEN mutation was found to correlate with more favorable pathological features (159). In contrast to most other tumor types, PTEN and PI3K mutations are not always mutually exclusive; about 26% of endometrial tumors contained both PI3K and PTEN mutations (136). mTOR activation is also quite common in endometrial tumors, promoted by downregulation of the LKB1 and/or TSC2 tumor suppressors, and dual inhibition of both the PI3K and mTOR axes may be a particularly useful strategy (160).

Gastric Carcinoma   PTEN expression was found to be abnormally low in 36% of gastric carcinomas, and a similar proportion of tumors were found to have genomic amplifications of PIK3CA (161). Furthermore, PIK3CA amplification and PTEN loss of function were mostly mutually exclusive, so a large percentage of gastric tumors have dysregulated PI3K signaling. Estimates of the prevalence of PIK3CA mutation in gastric carcinomas range from ~4% to ~12% (154, 162, 163) (Appendix XIV). EGFR phosphorylation is also a prognostic factor for gastric tumors, and autocrine/juxtacrine secretion of EGFR ligands (particularly TGFα) may contribute to EGFR activation in these tumors (164–166).

Glioblastoma   Glioblastoma multiforme (GBM) is the most common and the most malignant glial tumor, and the EGF receptor gene represents the most prevalent genetic alteration in GBM (167). The constitutively active EGFRvIII variant is the most prevalent mutation (168, 169), and coexpression of EGFRvIII together with PTEN correlates with response to EGFR inhibitors (170, 171). However, PTEN mutation, deletion, or silencing is found in up to 30% of gliomas (172–174); hence PI3K inhibition (either alone or in combination with EGFR inhibitors) may be an effective strategy in GBM patients. In addition, PI3K mutation is found in GBM with estimates of incidence ranging from 7% (175) to 27% (25) (Appendix XIV). PI3K pathway activation is correlated with poor prognosis and confers resistance to radiation and chemotherapy in glioblastoma (176, 177). However, inhibition of PI3K signaling alone may not be sufficient, and there is preclinical evidence for enhanced efficacy by combining inhibitors of both PI3K and mTOR in order to achieve optimal antitumor activity (178–180).

Hepatocellular Carcinoma PI3K-activating mutations were reported to be found at high frequency in hepatocellular tumors (162) (Appendix XIV). Furthermore, PTEN protein levels are decreased in up to 40% of liver tumors and correlate inversely with pathological grade and disease progression (181, 182). Hepatitis B has been positively associated with hepatocellular carcinoma, and a recent report indicates that the HBx viral protein can disrupt p53-mediated PTEN transcription, perhaps contributing to tumorigenesis (183).

Lung Cancer PI3K signaling may play an important role in many lung tumors; a recent study found overexpression of AKT and loss of PTEN in 41% and 46% of non small cell lung carcinoma (NSCLC) samples, respectively (184). These factors also correlate with poor differentiation, lymph node involvement, distant metastasis, and late disease stages. Another recent analysis found 74% of NSCLC tumors with reduced or absent PTEN expression (185). PTEN mutation appears to be relatively rare in NSCLC but is more common in small cell lung carcinoma (SCLC) (186–188). Frequent amplification of PIK3CA has also been demonstrated in various subtypes of lung cancer, including small cell (67%), squamous (70%), large cell (38%), and adenocarcinoma (19%) (189). Notably, resistance to the EGFR inhibitor gefitinib correlates with failure to downregulate AKT signaling and loss of PTEN (190), and KRAS status may also play an important role in determining response to EGFR inhibitors (191).

Melanoma Loss of PTEN protein expression occurs in 18–19% of primary melanomas and 29–38% of melanoma cell lines and is associated with increased tumor thickness (192–195). Moreover, most PTEN-deficient melanomas also have activating mutations in BRAF or NRAS and it is likely that RAS/RAF and PTEN lesions act cooperatively to promote tumor growth and invasion (192, 196).

Ovarian Carcinoma Amplification of *PIK3CA* in ovarian cancer was one of the first indications that PI3Kα functions as a human oncogene (16). *PIK3CA* mutations are also found in ovarian tumors, with estimates of incidence ranging from 4% to 20% depending on tumor subtype and between studies (147, 197, 198) (Appendix XIV). PTEN loss of heterozygosity was observed in endometrioid (43%) and serous (28%) tumors but was infrequent among the other histological subtypes (199). *KRAS* mutations also occur in ovarian tumors, and KRAS activation combined with deletion of PTEN in a mouse model leads to highly invasive, metastatic, and aggressive endometrioid ovarian adenocarcinomas (200). Both *PIK3CA* amplification and loss of PTEN have been associated with resistance to cisplatin in ovarian tumors (201). Preclinical data in an intraperitoneal OVCAR3 xenograft model has shown that the PI3K inhibitor LY294002 suppresses tumor growth, decreases ascites formation, and inhibits tumor vascularization (202–204).

Pancreatic Cancer   Pancreatic tumors have a very high incidence of *KRAS* mutation, which elicits downstream activation of the PI3K pathway. In addition, decreased PTEN function has been reported in pancreatic cancer cell lines and tumor specimens, resulting in activated NFκB and stabilization of MYC (205). The decrease in PTEN activity may be due to either loss of heterozygosity or aberrant subcellular compartmentalization (206).

Prostate Carcinoma   Prostate cancer is characterized by frequent loss of PTEN function (47, 207–209), and PI3K inhibitors might have particular utility in this disease (210). Recent data suggests that PTEN loss may play a fundamental role in expansion of a tumor stem cell-like population (211). Studies with hypomorphic PTEN alleles in mice indicate that PTEN gene dose correlates with onset and severity of prostate neoplasia (212). There is also extensive crosstalk between androgen receptor (AR) and PI3K pathway signaling, and PI3K/AKT or mTOR inhibition has shown promise in both androgen-dependent and independent preclinical models of prostate cancer (213–217).

Thyroid Carcinoma   *PIK3CA* is frequently mutated in thyroid carcinoma, particularly in the anaplastic subtype (218). In a separate study, *PIK3CA* mutations were found to be relatively rare in thyroid carcinomas, but *PIK3CA* amplification was frequently found in follicular thyroid carcinoma (219).

Hematological Malignancies   PI3K is activated in blasts from acute myelogenous leukemia (AML) patients and may contribute not only to the pathophysiology of the disease but also to chemotherapy resistance. PI3K pathway activation may occur via mutations in *NRAS* or *KRAS*, mutations in upstream receptors such as FLT3 and KIT, or overexpression of PI3K (220). In particular, AML cells consistently express the p110δ isoform, and inhibition of PI3Kδ reduces proliferation and survival of AML cells without affecting normal hematopoietic progenitors (221, 222). However, caution may be warranted since, somewhat surprisingly, PI3K pathway activation has been associated with improved overall and relapse-free survival in newly diagnosed AML patients (223). In chronic myelogenous leukemia (CML), the *BCR-ABL* oncogene signals through the p85 subunit of PI3K, mediating leukemogenesis, cell growth, and cell survival (224). A similar mechanism may be involved in growth and survival of NPM-ALK-transformed anaplastic large cell lymphoma cells (225). In addition, the p110γ subunit may be transcriptionally upregulated by BCR-ABL, and as such, PI3Kγ, which is preferentially expressed in hematopoietic cells, may be an important target in drug-resistant CML (226). The PI3K pathway was also found to be activated in diffuse large B-cell lymphoma (DLBCL) cell lines and tumor samples, and PI3K inhibition led to apoptosis in several DLBCL cell lines (227). Mutations of *PIK3CA* have also been found in DLBCL, including H1047L/R in the kinase domain: notably, these mutations were mostly found in samples with normal expression of PTEN (228). In multiple myeloma, approximately 50% of samples overexpress AKT and are sensitive to AKT inhibition (229). mTOR inhibition may also be a viable strategy in myeloma cells: however, these tumors often involve IGF1R signaling in the bone marrow microenvironment, which may be exacerbated by mTOR inhibition due to the p70S6K-IRS1 negative feedback loop (Section 5.1.4 and Figure 5.1) (230–232). For this reason, combined PI3K/mTOR (or IGF1R/mTOR) inhibition may be required for robust effects on myeloma cell growth and survival.

5.2   mTOR SIGNALING

mTOR (mammalian target of rapamycin, also called FRAP) is a ancient protein kinase (found in all eukaryotes, including yeast) that integrates cellular responses to nutrients, energy levels, and oxygenation with PI3K pathway-dependent growth factor signaling (233, 234). mTOR signaling is important for cell growth and cell cycle progression and is frequently dysregulated in cancer and other diseases (135, 235, 236). Two distinct multiprotein complexes containing mTOR have been identified: mTORC1 (mTOR:Raptor) and mTORC2 (mTOR:Rictor). These complexes have distinct substrate specificities and have correspondingly distinct roles in regulation of intracellular signaling (Figure 5.1).

5.2.1   mTOR

mTOR is a member of the PIKK (PI3K-related kinase) family of atypical kinases that includes ATM, ATR, and DNAPK, and its catalytic domain is homologous to that of PI3K. Human mTOR is a protein of 2549 amino acids and contains multiple functional domains in addition to the kinase domain (Figure 5.4). The N-terminal region contains 20 HEAT (Huntington-elongation factor 1A-protein phosphatase 2A subunit-TOR) motifs, which likely form a stacked alpha-helical array. This extended domain promotes mTOR multimerization in a nutrient-dependent manner (237).

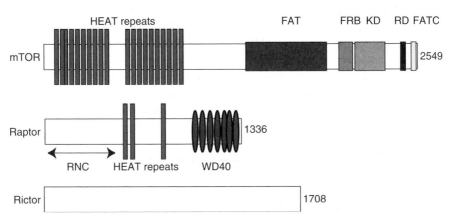

Figure 5.4   Domain structures of mTOR, Rictor, and Raptor. Abbreviations: KD—kinase domain; FAT—FRAP, ATM, and TRRAP; HEAT—Huntington elongation factor 3, PR65/A, and TOR; FRB—FKBP12–rapamycin binding domain; FATC—FRAP, ATM, TRRAP C-terminal domain; RNC—Raptor N-terminal conserved domain.

Following this are the FAT (FRAP, ATM, TRAPP2) and FRB (FKBP12–rapamycin binding) domains, the latter of which may modulate interactions with the regulatory GTPase RHEB (238, 239). The kinase domain follows, and at the C terminus are the RD (regulatory domain) and FATC (FAT domain, C terminus) sequences.

In cells, mTOR signaling occurs in complex with several additional proteins. The Raptor protein (regulatory associated protein of TOR; Figure 5.4) was discovered both to regulate the kinase activity of TOR and to confer sensitivity to amino acid availability, specifically leucine (240, 241). This regulation may be positive or negative, depending on the nutrient status of the cell, and involves an additional protein called GβL (LST8) (242). The resulting complex, typically referred to as mTORC1, is a key regulator of protein synthesis (243, 244). The AKT substrate PRAS40 is also involved in the mTORC1 complex, and as discussed earlier, phosphorylation of PRAS40 relieves its inhibitory effects on mTOR. Growth factor stimulation of mTOR activity also occurs via AKT-mediated inhibition of TSC1/2 and subsequent liberation of the G-protein RHEB, which directly stimulates the activity of mTORC1 (238). Once stimulated, mTORC1 recruits the substrates 4E-BP (eIF4E binding protein) and p70S6K to the signaling complex (245), which results in upregulating cellular protein synthesis (246). mTORC1 was also recently reported to bind and activate SGK1, which, in concert with AKT, leads to phosphorylation and mislocalization/inactivation of the CDK inhibitor p27 (111). The mTOR:Raptor complex is sensitive to inhibition by the macrolide immunosuppressant rapamycin (240, 244, 247). Rapamycin forms a complex with the peptidyl-prolyl cis–trans isomerase FKBP12, and this complex binds to a region in mTOR just N-terminal to the kinase domain, perturbing the Raptor:mTOR interaction. A second mTOR partner was subsequently discovered and named Rictor (rapamycin-insensitive companion of TOR; Figure 5.4), which is neither inhibited by rapamycin nor modulated by amino acid availability (248). However, although mTORC2 is not inhibited by rapamycin, chronic treatment with rapamycin has been proposed to sequester free mTOR and diminish cellular levels of mTORC2 in some, but not all, cell types (249). The mTOR:Rictor complex, or mTORC2, also involves at least three additional proteins: GβL, mSIN1 (62, 250), and PRO-TOR (251). mTORC2 functions in actin cytoskeletal remodeling via PKCα (248) and more recently was identified as the kinase that phosphorylates AKT at the S473 site (252). The upstream regulators of mTORC2 activity remain unclear, although, like mTORC1, its activity appears to be promoted by growth factor receptors.

mTOR:Raptor (mTORC1) regulates protein translation and cell growth by integrating mitogenic signals with sensors of cellular nutrients, energy (ATP) levels, and oxygenation. Understanding the mechanisms of the mTOR response to these factors is particularly relevant to tumor biology, since the rapid growth of tumor cells and the tortuous, malformed nature of tumor vasculature frequently lead to hypoxia and nutritional deficiency. Hence cell-autonomous regulation of mTOR signaling may be particularly critical in the solid tumor environment. As discussed previously, in response to extracellular mitogenic signals, mTORC1 is activated via AKT-mediated phosphorylation of PRAS40 and the TSC1:TSC2 complex. The activity of the TSC1:TSC2 complex can also be modulated by p90RSK, linking mTORC1 activation to the RAF/MEK/ERK pathway as well. Furthermore, TSC1:TSC2 integrates these growth factor signals with a sensor of cellular energy (ATP) levels, via the AMP-activated protein kinase AMPK (253) and its upstream kinase regulator LKB1 (254, 255). When ATP levels decrease relative to AMP, AMPK is activated and phosphorylates TSC2, leading to suppression of mTORC1 activity; this effect may also be indirectly mediated by AKT (256). *LKB1* has been identified as a tumor suppressor gene that may be mutated in a significant proportion of lung adenocarcinomas (257), and its dysregulation can uncouple mTORC1 signaling from the AMPK cellular energy-sensing mechanism. Of particular interest, *LKB1* mutations almost always occur in subsets of NSCLC patients who are not predisposed to have EGFR mutations, that is, in Caucasians rather than Asians and smokers rather than nonsmokers (see Chapter 3). Furthermore, a significant subset of tumors with *LKB1* mutations have concurrent *KRAS* mutations (258). Although initially identified as a tumor suppressor gene, LKB1 was recently shown also to promote AKT-mediated phosphorylation and inactivation of proapoptotic proteins and so may have a tumorigenic function in cells with constitutively active AKT (259). It is not clear, however, if this reflects a direct interaction with AKT or a response to downstream mTOR inhibition and subsequent upstream PI3K pathway activation via the p70S6 kinase-IRS1 feedback mechanism (Section 5.1.4 and Figure 5.1). mTORC1 can also be regulated by cellular amino acid levels. In particular, the Class III PI3K (VPS34) regulates mTORC1 in a nutrient-dependent manner, which, during amino acid limitation, results in the downregulation of protein synthesis independent of TSC1/2 regulation (260–262). VPS34 also appears to be important for triggering autophagy, a catabolic process whereby cells under stress can sequester and utilize their own cytoplasm and organelles as a source of nutrients and energy (263). Curiously, nutrient-driven activation of mTOR appears to suppress autophagy, while VPS34 promotes both mTOR signaling and autophagy. This interplay between growth and autophagy has important implications for cancer therapy, since tumor cells may rely on autophagy for short-term survival in nutrient-poor and hypoxic environments.

The regulation of mTOR activity under hypoxic conditions is somewhat complex. Hypoxia induces the synthesis and stabilization of the transcription factor HIF1α (hypoxia-inducible factor) in an mTOR-dependent manner and results in the expression of HIF1-responsive genes such as *VEGFA* (264). Nevertheless, hypoxia ultimately results in the inhibition of mTOR and overall downregulation of protein translation (265, 266). This occurs either by negative feedback via the HIF-dependent stress-induced proteins REDD1/2, which act upstream of TSC2 (267), or by activation of the AMPK-TSC1/2-RHEB pathway due to stress on energy levels in the cell (268). Mutations to the tumor suppressors PTEN and TSC2 allow for sustained mTOR activity and protein translation under hypoxic conditions (269) and may relate to the sporadic activity of rapamycin analogs, such as CCI-779 (temsirolimus), in cancer trials (270). Loss of the von Hippel–Lindau tumor suppressor gene (*VHL*), which functions in the turnover of HIF1α, correlates with sensitization of cancer cells to CCI-779 in mouse xenograft models (271) and may underlie the clinical activity of CCI-779 in advanced renal cell carcinoma (Chapter 10). Intriguingly, the expression of HIF2α in renal cancer cells was recently shown to be dependent on phospholipase D activity and phosphatidic acid (PA) (272). The role of PA in regulating mTORC1 activity is less well characterized than that of the PIP$_3$/PI3K pathway, but this phospholipid may be particularly relevant to maintaining mTOR activation in tumors (273). PA is generated from PIP$_2$ in perinuclear and plasma membranes by phospholipase D1 (PLD1) and PLD2, respectively, and elevated PLD activity has been noted in human tumor cells, particularly under conditions of metabolic stress (274). PA binds to the FRB domain of mTOR, stimulating phosphorylation of downstream targets (275); notably, this binding site overlaps with that of the rapamycin:FKBP12 complex, and elevated PA levels may therefore promote rapamycin resistance in tumor cells (276). Furthermore, PLD2 may directly bind to and contribute to activation of mTORC1 (277).

5.2.2 p70S6 Kinase

As mentioned earlier, p70S6 kinase (p70S6K, S6K) is a key regulator of cell growth and is phosphorylated and activated by mTOR, PDK1, and potentially other kinases. There are two isoforms of p70S6K: S6K1 and S6K2. Both isoforms are comprised of approximately 500 amino acids (S6K1 is slightly longer) and contain an N-terminal TOS (TOR-signaling) sequence, an AGC kinase domain, and a C-terminal regulatory sequence that is also involved in mTOR-dependent regulation. PDK1 phosphorylates p70S6K in the activation loop of the kinase domain (55), and mTOR activity is also indispensable for p70S6K activation (278, 279). In turn, p70S6K also phosphorylates and regulates mTOR activity (280). p70S6K promotes biogenesis by several mechanisms, and its substrates include the 40S ribosomal protein S6 (281, 282), eIF4B (a stimulator of eIF4A helicase (283)), and the eIF4A inhibitor PDCD4 (284). The choreography of mTOR/p70S6K-mediated translation has been elegantly elucidated (285). Under conditions of nutrient deprivation, S6K1 associates with a complex involving eIF3, eIF4E, and 4E-BP. When growth factors/nutrients are added, mTOR:Raptor associates with eIF3, phosphorylating 4E-BP and S6K1, promoting the dissociation of S6K1 and 4E-BP. The resulting preinitiation complex recruits the eIF4G scaffold complex, eIF4A helicase and the 40S ribosome. In parallel, PDK1 phosphorylates the dissociated S6K1, which phosphorylates 40S, eIF4B, and PDCD4 (Figure 5.5).

Accumulated evidence from biochemical and transgenic animal studies indicates that the two isoforms S6K1 and S6K2 have overlapping but distinct functions. Somewhat surprisingly, *s6k1* $^{-/-}$ mice were found to have relatively normal levels of S6 protein phosphorylation whereas S6 phosphorylation was impaired in *s6k2* $^{-/-}$ animals, suggesting that S6K2 may either be the major S6 kinase or be able to compensate for the lack of S6K1 in these animals (286). When both S6K1 and S6K2 were knocked out, extensive perinatal lethality was observed: however, phosphorylation of S6 was still observed in *s6k1* $^{-/-}$/*s6k2* $^{-/-}$ cells, suggesting further redundancy (perhaps involving p90RSK). Curiously, *s6k1* $^{-/-}$ mice were found to be smaller than their wild-type littermates, whereas *s6k2* $^{-/-}$ mice were slightly

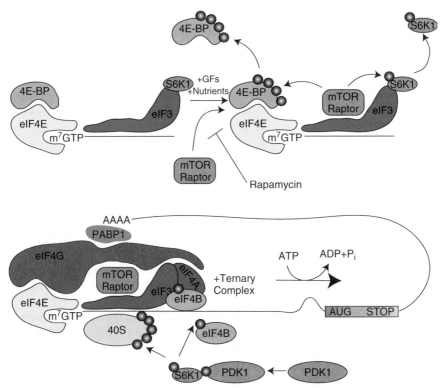

Figure 5.5 mTOR and S6K signaling. The eIF3 preinitiation complex associates with the ribosome and eIF4E and plays a key role in regulating translation. Following mitogenic stimulation, mTOR:Raptor is recruited to eIF3, where it phosphorylates S6K1 and 4E-BP. S6K1 then dissociates from the complex and is further activated by PDK1, promoting S6K1-mediated phosphorylation of ribosomal S6 protein and eIF4B, which form part of the translation initiation complex. Phosphorylated 4E-BP also dissociates from the complex, allowing recruitment of eIF4G, assembly of the eIF4F complex (comprising eIF4A, eIF4E, and eIF4G), and initiation of translation. Adapted from (285) with permission. Copyright © 2005 Elsevier.

larger than wild-type (286, 287). Together, these data suggested that the effects of S6K1 on growth are at least partly mediated by pathways other than ribosomal phosphorylation and translation initiation. One intriguing explanation has recently been uncovered, with the discovery that S6K1 (but not S6K2) enhances translation efficiency of spliced mRNAs during their initial encounter with ribosomes (288), via its binding partner and substrate SKAR (289).

5.2.3 mTOR Pathway Activation in Cancer

In general, mTOR inhibition may be considered as a strategy in many of the tumor types in which PI3K signaling is implicated and has already been discussed to some extent in Section 5.1.5. Some additional diseases where mTOR is particularly implicated are discussed next.

Breast Cancer   The rationale for PI3K pathway inhibition is discussed in Section 5.1.5 and supports the evaluation of mTOR pathway inhibitors as well as PI3K pathway inhibitors in breast cancer. In particular, hormone-positive breast tumors may be particularly suited to mTOR inhibitor treatment: both estrogen receptor (ER) and mTOR signaling promote cyclin D1 expression, and the crosstalk between ER and growth factor signaling may contribute to endocrine resistance (290, 291). mTOR inhibitors may therefore have utility in combination with estrogen receptor modulators and aromatase inhibitors (292–294).

Mantle Cell Lymphoma   Mantle cell lymphoma (MCL) is usually characterized by hyperactivation of cyclin D and subsequent cell cycle dysregulation. Transcription of cyclin D is largely mediated by mTOR signaling, and rapamycin has been reported to downregulate cyclin D levels in MCL cell lines in vitro (295). However, mTOR inhibition may also have other effects on MCL cells that may contribute to clinical activity, including induction of autophagy (296).

Renal Cell Carcinoma   mTOR promotes the translation of the hypoxia-inducible transcription factor HIF1α—which in turn enhances the expression of vascular growth factors. This may be particularly relevant in the case of tumors bearing loss of function mutations in the von Hippel–Lindau (VHL) protein, which serves to block proteasome-mediated destruction of HIF and thereby causes constitutive expression of proangiogenic growth factors (271). Such mutations are particularly prevalent in renal cell carcinoma and may underlie the promising clinical activity seen with mTOR inhibitors in this disease (Chapter 10).

Sarcoma   Activation of the IGF1R receptor and downstream PI3K–mTOR pathway signaling is implicated in the genesis and progression of several subtypes of sarcoma (297, 298). Dual inhibition of PI3K and mTOR is effective in a preclinical model of Kaposi sarcoma (299).

5.3   MAPK SIGNALING PATHWAYS

MAPK (mitogen-activated protein kinase) signaling has been highly conserved during evolution from yeast to humans. In multicellular organisms, there are four characterized MAPK pathway modules: extracellular signal regulated kinase (ERK), c-JUN NH$_2$-terminal kinase (JNK), p38 kinase, and ERK5 (300). Each pathway responds to different extracellular signals, which stimulate an intracellular pathway activator. This activator initiates a phospho-relay system composed of three sequentially activated kinases: a MAPK kinase kinase (MKKK), a MAPK kinase (MKK), and finally the MAPK for which the pathway is named. Of primary importance in cancer biology is the ERK/MAPK signaling cascade, which, depending on cellular context, can transduce proliferative, survival, apoptotic, and differentiation

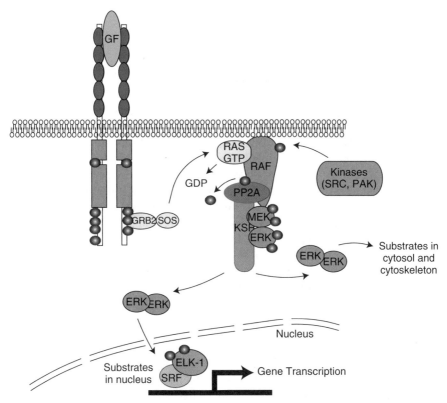

Figure 5.6   The RAS/RAF/MEK/ERK signaling complex. Receptor tyrosine kinase signaling leads to activation of RAS, which binds to and mediates activation of RAF kinases. Additional scaffolding proteins, including KSR, help to recruit the downstream effector kinases MEK and ERK. ERK has multiple cytoplasmic and nuclear substrates that promote mitogenic and prosurvival signals.

signals within the cell. ERK/MAPK signaling is initiated by activation of RAS GTPase and subsequent sequential activation of the RAF, MEK, and ERK kinases (Figure 5.6).

5.3.1   ERK/MAPK Signaling

The RAS/RAF/MEK/ERK pathway is activated by growth factors, hormones, and cytokines, resulting in RAS-induced localization of RAF to the plasma membrane and subsequent RAF activation. Activated RAF phosphorylates MEK, which in turn activates ERK. ERK then mediates a vast array of both cytoplasmic and nuclear signaling events that are critical for cellular functions such as proliferation, differentiation, and apoptosis. Some of these functions are contradictory (e.g., ERK/MAPK signaling can elicit both pro- and anti apoptotic effects) and signaling is likely to depend on multiple factors including binding of various partner proteins, crosstalk with other signaling pathways, and subcellular localization. Dysregulation of this pathway in tumors contributes to many hallmarks of cancer cells, including immortalization, uncontrolled proliferation (due to cell cycle activation and autocrine signaling), invasion, metastasis, angiogenesis, and evasion of apoptosis (36). The RAS/RAF/MEK/ERK pathway is stimulated by most growth factor ligands and associated receptor tyrosine kinases, so dysregulation of RTKs (discussed in Chapter 3) may lead to aberrant RAS/RAF/MEK/ERK signaling. These hyperactivated kinases include VEGFR2, PDGFRβ, EGFR, ERBB2 (HER2), and MET: as a result, the ERK pathway is upregulated in approximately 30% of all cancers (301). In addition to RTK dysregulation, RAS gene mutations (described in Section 5.1.1) occur in a diverse range of tumors and may also activate RAF/MEK/ERK signaling. However, different forms of RAS may have distinct effects on pathway activation and tumor progression. In mice engineered to express mutationally activated KRAS or NRAS in the colonic epithelium, only the KRAS mutant mice showed widespread hyperproliferation via activation of RAF and MEK kinases, although ERK signaling was not upregulated. In contrast, mice expressing mutant NRAS (but not KRAS) were found to be resistant to apoptosis. When combined with an additional (APC) tumorigenic mutation, tumor formation was more pronounced in KRAS mutant mice: however, downstream signaling was found to involve RAF but not MEK (302).

5.3.2   RAF Family Kinases

There are three distinct isoforms of human RAF kinase: ARAF, BRAF, and CRAF. Although CRAF (also known as RAF1) was the first of the human genes to be isolated (303), it is likely that BRAF represents the founder gene, as it is more closely related to the *Drosophila* gene (*d-raf*) and the *C. elegans* homolog lin-45 (304). The three RAF proteins share a common domain structure, with the kinase domain in the C-terminal half of the protein and two additional conserved sequences (CR1 and CR2) in the N-terminal half. ARAF and CRAF contain 606 and 648 amino acids, respectively, resulting in proteins of ~68 and ~72 kDa; BRAF has an extended N-terminal region and is further subject to alternative splicing, yielding proteins ranging from ~75 to 100 kDa. All forms are fairly ubiquitously expressed, although ARAF is particularly found in the genitourinary tract and BRAF is associated with neuronal tissue.

Regulation of RAF activity is complex and is accomplished by both activating and inhibitory phosphorylation as well as association with various partner/scaffolding proteins. Binding of RAS to RAF is mediated through two motifs in the RAF N-terminal CR1: the RAS binding domain (RBD) and a zinc binding, cysteine-rich domain (CRD) (305, 306). The RBD binds directly to the GTP-bound "switch" region of RAS (307), whereas CRD binding is associated with binding to the farnesylated C terminus of RAS (308). This lipid dependence is generally thought to be important for the membrane localization and activation of RAF: however, recent data suggest that the extended N-terminal region of BRAF may enable it to bind to cytoplasmic, nonfarnesylated RAS (309). The significance of this finding with respect to RAF activation remains obscure.

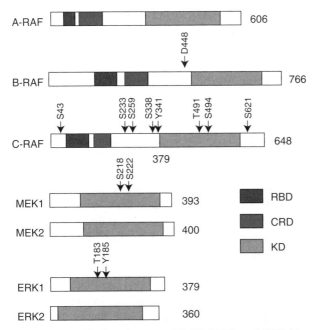

Figure 5.7 Domain structures of RAF, MEK, and ERK kinases. Key regulatory phosphorylation sites are shown for C-RAF; homologous sites exist in A-RAF and B-RAF. Abbreviations: RBD, Ras binding domain; CRD, cysteine-rich domain; KD, kinase domain.

RAF activity is regulated by multiple phosphorylation events, the details of which are still being determined (Figure 5.7). Three inhibitory sites are phosphorylated by PKA in response to high cellular levels of cAMP: S43, S233, and S259 (CRAF numbering, although these sites are conserved across all three isoforms). Phosphorylation at S43 directly inhibits the RAS binding interaction (310). S259 phosphorylation promotes recruitment of 14-3-3 proteins, which may also modulate the interaction with RAS (311). This site is also phosphorylated by AKT (312) and dephosphorylated by the PP2A phosphatase (313). Phosphorylation at S259 promotes phosphorylation (possibly by RAF itself *in trans*) at S621, another 14-3-3 binding site in the C terminus of CRAF (314), and phosphorylation of S233 forms a third 14-3-3 binding site. In contrast to the S259 and S233 sites, phosphorylation at S621 and subsequent 14-3-3 engagement leads to RAF activation. Intriguingly, 14-3-3 binding (possibly at the S621 site) may stimulate RAF activity by heterodimerization of RAF family proteins. In a recent study, BRAF and CRAF were found to form heterodimers in cell extracts. The heterodimers displayed higher activity than either monomers or homodimers, and dimeric 14-3-3 proteins were found to enhance the heterodimerization. Moreover, catalytically inactive BRAF mutants were found to stimulate the activity of CRAF in heterodimeric complexes, suggesting an allosteric mechanism for regulation of enzyme activity in the heterodimer (315). BRAF also has two inhibitory AKT phosphorylation sites (S428) that are not found in ARAF or CRAF (316).

Two phosphorylation sites just N-terminal of the kinase domain have a particularly important role in activation and may explain why activating oncogenic mutations are almost exclusively found in BRAF and not the two other isoforms. In CRAF, S338 and Y341 are located in the so-called negatively charged region, and their phosphorylation appears essential for activation. Y341 is a substrate for SRC family kinases, and phosphotyrosine is required in this position for subsequent phosphorylation at S338, most likely by CK2 in complex with kinase suppressor of RAS (KSR, discussed later) (317). Notably, the homologous residue to Y341 in BRAF is aspartate (D448), which eliminates the requirement for SRC kinase phosphorylation; furthermore, BRAF S445 (corresponding to CRAF S338) is constitutively phosphorylated. Therefore BRAF is primed for activation, such that an additional activating mutation has a much more profound effect compared to the analogous mutation in CRAF (318). Finally, two phosphorylation sites in the kinase domain activation segment (T491 and S494 in CRAF) provide an additional level of regulation. Activated BRAF also has higher kinase activity than CRAF or ARAF, further supporting its role as the most important proto-oncogene among the RAF kinases. RAF kinases may also have cellular activities that are independent of its catalytic function. For example, CRAF can exert prosurvival signals by binding to and inhibiting proapoptotic kinases (ASK1 and MST2), and this inhibition appears not to require RAF kinase activity (319, 320). There is also evidence that CRAF can promote cell migration in a kinase-independent manner via interaction with the RHO GTPase pathway (321).

In addition to RAS and 14-3-3 proteins, RAF activation is regulated by several scaffolding proteins that also mediate the engagement of RAF with downstream signaling proteins (322, 323). Of particular importance is KSR (kinase suppressor of RAS), which can bind to RAF, MEK, and ERK and has been implicated in oncogenic RAS/RAF signaling (324). KSR was first identified by genetic screening in *Drosophila* and *C. elegans*, and two mammalian isoforms are known: KSR1 and KSR2 (325, 326). Human KSR1 consists of 762 amino acids, with four N-terminal homology regions (KSR-specific, proline-rich, cysteine-rich, serine/threonine-rich) and a C-terminal kinase homology domain. Like RAF kinases, KSR is a member of the TLK family but it is debatable whether or not it possesses bona fide kinase activity. Several studies have ascribed a catalytic function to KSR, although others have reported no activity and the kinase domain has a Lys → Arg substitution at the highly conserved Glu-Lys salt bridge in the ATP binding site (322, 323). Currently, the majority of data support a model where KSR acts as a scaffold for assembly of ERK/MAPK signaling components and is regulated by changes in subcellular localization. The CDC25-associated kinase C-TAK1 (also known as MARK3) phosphorylates KSR and (in another interesting parallel to RAF) generates a 14-3-3 protein binding site, which promotes cytoplasmic localization. Growth factor stimulation leads to dephosphorylation of this site and promotes recruitment to the plasma membrane, where it acts as a platform for the RAF/MEK/ERK phosphorylation cascade (317, 327). Another scaffolding protein, connector-enhancer of KSR (CNK), can also bind to and activate RAF (322, 323). There are three human isoforms: the widely expressed CNK1, neuronal CNK2, and less well characterized CNK3. CNK1 contains 720 amino acids and several distinct regions, including

SAM (sterile alpha motif), CRIC (conserved region in CNK), PDZ, proline-rich (SH3 binding), and PH (pleckstrin homology) domains (328). CNK binds to both BRAF and CRAF and may mediate SRC-dependent RAF activation (329). In addition, CNK is implicated in several non-RAS GTPase pathways including RHO, RAC, and RAL (328, 330).

5.3.3 MEK and ERK Kinases

The primary (although not exclusive) substrates of the RAF kinases are MEK1 and MEK2, which are activated by phosphorylation on two serine residues in their respective activation loops (Ser218 and Ser222 of MEK1 and Ser222 and Ser226 of MEK2; Figure 5.7). Phosphorylation at these serine residues is necessary and sufficient for activation of MEK1 and MEK2, enhancing activity ∼7000-fold (331, 332) and enabling them to phosphorylate ERK1/2. MEK1 and MEK2 mediate their effects on cell differentiation and proliferation through activation of ERK1 and ERK2, the primary substrates for MEK proteins (Figure 5.7). MEK1 and MEK2 are dual-specificity tyrosine/threonine protein kinases and, as such, can phosphorylate ERK1 and ERK2 on both a threonine and a tyrosine residue in a specific motif (Thr-X-Tyr) in their activation loops (333, 334). Activation of ERK1/2 leads to the phosphorylation of over 150 cytosolic and nuclear proteins, depending on cellular context. The substrates can be categorized into several groups: (i) transcription factors, (ii) protein kinases and phosphatases, (iii) cytoskeletal and scaffold proteins, (iv) receptors and signaling molecules, and (v) apoptosis-related proteins. To regulate cellular proliferation, activated ERKs translocate to the nucleus and regulate gene expression through the activation of several key transcription factors. Specifically, ERK phosphorylates ETS family transcription factors including ELK1, which regulates expression of the FOS transcriptional activator in response to serum. FOS forms heterodimers with JUN to make up the AP1 transcription factor. ERK then activates AP1 through phosphorylation of JUN. Activated AP1 drives expression of key cell cycle proteins, such as the cyclin D family, which enable the cell to move from G1 phase into S and begin cell cycle progression (36, 335).

In addition, MAPK-activated protein kinases such as the p90RSK family (RSK1–4) (335) are phosphorylated and activated by ERK (56). As discussed in Section 5.1.4, RSK kinases represent a point of convergence between RAS/ERK and PI3K/mTOR pathways. Activated RSK1 promotes cell survival through at least two mechanisms. First, RSK1 inhibits apoptosis directly through phosphorylation and inactivation of multiple cytoplasmic and nuclear substrates, including the proapoptotic protein BAD and the p65 subunit of NFκB (120, 122). Second, RSK1 mediates crosstalk with the PI3K/AKT pathway through phosphorylation of TSC2 (tuberous sclerosis complex protein 2) and inactivation of the TSC1/2 complex, an inhibitor of the mTOR:Raptor complex (see previous discussion). RSK also directly phosphorylates Raptor, thus providing a second input to PI3K/mTOR signaling (124). mTOR:Raptor is thus able to phosphorylate and activate S6K, driving cell growth. Notably, since S6K mediates a negative feedback loop on PI3K/AKT signaling through inhibition of IRS1 (Figure 5.1), downregulation of S6K can lead to upregulation of the prosurvival PI3K/AKT pathway through the negative feedback loop. This feedback mechanism may be important in determining the sensitivity of certain tumor types to MEK1 inhibition. The mitogen and stress-activated kinases (MSK1 and MSK2) are also substrates for ERK. MSK1 is the more widely studied of the two proteins; it regulates gene transcription by phosphorylating multiple substrates including transcription factors such as AP1, CREB, and NFκB (336, 337). Recent data shows that MSK1 and MSK2 also promote phosphorylation of histone H3 in response to mitogenic stimuli, and that this plays a critical role in neoplastic transformation (338, 339). In cancer cells, dysregulation of histone H3 phosphorylation leads to chromatin decondensation and expression of genes that support tumor growth, including the proto-oncogenes *c-FOS* and *c-JUN*. MSK1 (and potentially MSK2) has also been implicated in upregulating NFκB activity by direct phosphorylation (336). MAPK-interacting kinase (MNK) is another ERK effector kinase that may have a role in promoting tumor cell growth. There are two isoforms, MNK1 and MNK2, both of which have been placed downstream of p38 as well as ERK (340). Both MNK1 and MNK2 are essential for phosphorylation of the translation factor eIF4E at S209, providing another connection between the ERK and PI3K/mTOR pathways: however, mice with deletions of MNK1 and/or MNK2 develop normally (341). Nevertheless, the phosphorylation of eIF4E by MNK1/MNK2 appears to be important for its oncogenic activity. Mice with constitutively phosphorylated eIF4E S209 (either through a phosphomimetic S209D mutation or MNK1 activation) show accelerated tumor formation in a MYC-driven model of lymphomagenesis, and mice that lack S209 phosphorylation (via a S209A mutation) are substantially resistant to tumor formation (342). Furthermore, inhibition of mTOR signaling is reported to increase eIF4E phosphorylation in an MNK-dependent manner, suggesting that targeting these kinases may augment the activity of mTOR inhibitors in tumor cells (343). MNK1 and eIF4E were also recently shown to play a role in increased nuclear export of HDM2 mRNA, thus linking MEK/ERK/MNK1 signaling to regulation of the p53 tumor suppressor (344).

MEK1/ERK signaling has also been implicated in angiogenesis. This role was initially identified by analysis of the phenotype of *mek1* $^{-/-}$ mice, which die in utero at 10.5 days of gestation due to a failure to establish a functional placenta (345). Analysis of the placentas of *mek1* $^{-/-}$ embryos revealed that vascular endothelial cells are present, but they fail to migrate. Analysis of *mek1* $^{-/-}$ mouse embryonic fibroblasts using in vitro migration assays determined that this failure to migrate was due to a block in αvβ3-integrin signaling. αvβ3-integrin signaling upregulates pERK and this sustained activation is required for angiogenesis (345, 346). Additionally, in vivo overexpression of a dominant-negative MEK1 mutant (S218A) in mouse tumor vasculature using engineered retroviruses suppresses tumor vascularization and angiogenesis of implanted human xenografts, ultimately resulting in inhibition of tumor growth (347). These data support a role for MEKs in angiogenesis and suggest that inhibitors may affect tumor growth not only through an effect on cell cycle control but also through a block on angiogenesis.

Although somatic activating mutations in *RAS* and *BRAF* have been identified in numerous cancers, somatic mutations in *MEK1* or *MEK2* are apparently very rare: only one mutation (D67N, conferring increased kinase activity) has been described in ovarian cancer (348). However, germline activating mutations in *MEK1, MEK2*, and *BRAF* have been identified in patients with cardio-facio-cutaneous (CFC) syndrome. This complex developmental disorder comprises characteristic craniofacial features, atrial septal defects, hair and skin abnormalities, and postnatal growth and developmental delays. In vitro analysis of the three activating MEK alleles (MEK1:F53S, Y130C, MEK2:F57C) indicate they activate MEK1 and MEK2 compared to the wild-type enzyme, but much less so than the phospho-mimetic mutants S218E/S222E (349). The numerous defects characterized by CFC highlight the important role of MEK1/2 in the proper development and maintenance of numerous tissues.

5.3.4 ERK/MAPK Pathway Activation in Cancer

Upregulation of the ERK/MAPK pathway module occurs in approximately 30% of all human cancers, including a high percentage of pancreatic, colon, lung, ovarian, and kidney tumors (301). Constitutive activation of ERK is driven by multiple mechanisms, including overexpression of growth factor receptor tyrosine kinases (RTKs), activating mutations in growth factor RTKs, and activating mutations in RAS or BRAF. The importance of RAS mutations in driving tumorigenesis is discussed in Section 5.3.1. Inhibition of MEK or RAF activity will lead to a block of the ERK/MAPK module, but not the other effectors downstream of RAS. This may have significant therapeutic benefit in some RAS mutant tumors, since ERK signaling is an important factor in RAS-driven tumor growth. However, MEK inhibitors may be even more efficacious in tumors that are solely dependent on proliferative signals from the ERK/MAPK module to drive tumorigenesis. For example, the BRAF mutant V600E exhibits in vitro kinase activity ∼500-fold greater than that of the wild-type enzyme (350). Several independent studies have shown that ectopically expressed BRAF V600E stimulates constitutive ERK signaling, induces proliferation and transformation, and induces tumor growth in xenograft models in nude mice (350–355). Additionally, BRAF V600E activates NFκB, eliciting an antiapoptotic response (356, 357). Tumors bearing the activated BRAF mutant V600E are highly sensitive to growth inhibition by MEK inhibitors both in vitro and in vivo, suggesting that tumorigenesis of cells bearing the BRAF V600E mutant is driven mainly by the deregulated ERK/MAPK pathway signals (358). Activating somatic mutations in the *BRAF* oncogene have been identified in a number of malignancies, with the highest incidence in malignant melanoma (60–80% (351, 359–363)), papillary thyroid cancer (35–70% (364–368)), colorectal cancer (∼10% (351, 369–371)), and endometrial cancers (10–20% (372)) (Appendix XV). Mutations of KRAS or BRAF are also found in ovarian cancer but appear to be confined to low grade tumors (373, 374), possibly due to promotion of oncogene-induced senescence by hyperactivated KRAS/BRAF (375). The relative lack of KRAS or BRAF mutations in more aggressive tumors suggests that these neoplasms develop via distinct pathways from the low grade tumors (373, 376). Nevertheless, a few (4%) KRAS/BRAF mutations are found in more aggressive tumors, and the presence of these mutations renders ovarian cancer cells sensitive to a MEK kinase inhibitor in vitro (377).

Melanoma   The BRAF V600E mutation is of particular importance in driving tumorigenicity and tumor progression in melanoma. A high proportion of benign melanocytic lesions carry the BRAF V600E mutation, suggesting that mutation of BRAF is an early event in the genesis of melanoma. These data also suggest that the BRAF V600E mutation alone is not sufficient to drive formation and metastases of fully malignant melanoma and that additional genetic lesions are required (362). However, sustained activity of mutant BRAF is required for growth of melanoma cell line xenografts in vivo (378), and tumor cells bearing BRAF V600E mutations are highly sensitive to specific inhibitors of the downstream MEK kinase (358). In addition to mutations in BRAF, 10–20% of all melanomas harbor activating mutations in NRAS, further suggesting a role for deregulation of MAPK signaling in melanoma progression. In almost all cases, NRAS and BRAF mutations are mutually exclusive, increasing the number of melanomas with activating ERK/MAPK pathway mutations (192, 352). The clinical prognosis for patients with metastatic lesions that are positive for BRAF/NRAS mutations is significantly poorer than those with wild-type BRAF/NRAS (352, 360, 379).

Thyroid Cancer   BRAF V600E mutations also occur with significant frequency in thyroid cancer, in particular, anaplastic thyroid carcinoma (366, 367). Anaplastic thyroid carcinoma tumors are resistant to conventional radioiodine and chemotherapy treatments and therefore represent good clinical candidates for treatment with new molecular therapies targeting ERK/MAPK signaling. In addition to anaplastic thyroid carcinomas, BRAF V600E occurs in ~45% of papillary thyroid carcinomas (380). While the majority of these patients respond to standard therapy, the BRAF V600E mutation was frequently associated with patients who had lost iodine sensitivity, had metastases to the lymph nodes, or had a recurrence of papillary thyroid carcinoma (367, 380, 381).

Colorectal Cancer   Association of ERK/MAPK dysregulation with sporadic colorectal cancer has emerged from the numerous sequencing efforts to identify the molecular basis of this disease (351, 369–371, 382). Sequencing studies in colorectal tumor cell lines and patient samples have identified a significant occurrence of activating somatic mutations in the *KRAS* (30–50%) and *BRAF* (10%) oncogenes. The presence of either KRAS or BRAF V600E mutations is associated with poor clinical outcome, suggesting that deregulation of ERK/MAPK signaling plays a role in driving tumorigenesis. Over 90% of the BRAF mutations are the BRAF V600E activating mutation. As seen in melanoma, the BRAF V600E and KRAS mutations are mutually exclusive; thus approximately 60% of all colorectal samples are upregulated in ERK/MAPK signaling. Another hallmark of colorectal tumors is genomic instability, as characterized by microsatellite instability (MSI), which is caused by deficiencies in the mismatch repair genes *hMSH2* and *hMLH1* (383–385). Analysis of BRAF V600E mutations in sporadic colon cancers with respect to MSI/mismatch repair (MMR) deficiency indicates BRAF V600E mutations are found at a higher rate in MMR-deficient tumors (31%) than in MMR-proficient cancers (7%). BRAF V600E has also been associated with morphological features consistent of poor prognosis: infiltrating lymphocytes, mucinous and poor histological grade (386). The KRAS G12V activating mutant has also been associated with more aggressive colorectal cancers and poor clinical outcome (387, 388).

5.4 PIM KINASES

The PIM (provirus integration site for Moloney murine leukemia virus) kinases form a three-member subgroup of the CAMK (Ser/Thr kinase) family and have attracted recent attention for their potential role in tumorigenesis, tumor cell survival and resistance to antitumor agents. PIM1 was identified as a potentiator of the oncogenic MYC transcription factor in a mouse model of lymphomagenesis (389). The human PIM1 protein comprises 313 amino acids and is located on chromosome 6p21.2. PIM2 (334 amino acids) is found on chromosome Xp11.23 and can also potentiate MYC-induced lymphomagenesis in PIM1-deficient mice (390). A third homolog, PIM3 (326 amino acids), is found on chromosome 22q13 (391). Each PIM kinase is highly homologous to the other two (PIM2 and PIM3 are 61% and 71% identical to PIM1, respectively), but collectively they share <30% sequence identity with other kinases. Within the PIM family, most of the sequence divergence is in the C-terminal region. The kinase domains are very closely related and all contain a unique motif (ERPXPX) in the linker region, notable for the two proline residues that introduce a "bulge" in the linker peptide and the adjacent ATP binding site (392, 393). The phenotype of PIM deletion in mice is relatively mild: in fact, when PIM1, PIM2, and PIM3 knockout mice are crossbred, the homozygous triple knockouts are produced at the expected Mendelian frequency (394). These triple-knockout mice are 30% smaller than their wild-type or single knockout littermates due to an overall reduction in cell number: phenotypically, they are remarkably normal apart from some defects in lymphocyte proliferation. Together with other biochemical and cellular data (summarized later), these results support the view that PIM kinases are somewhat dispensable for most normal cellular functions but may play a more important role under conditions of stress.

PIM1 is expressed in most tissues but, consistent with its role in lymphoma-genesis, is most abundant in hematopoietic and lymphoid tissues. PIM1 expression is regulated by STAT transcription factors and can therefore be induced by many cytokines and growth factors through JAK/STAT signaling pathways (see Chapter 4). High PIM1 expression is observed in B-cell non Hodgkin's lymphoma, a subset of which has amplification of the PIM1 locus; within diffuse large B-cell lymphomas, PIM1 expression is correlated with poor patient outcome (395). PIM1 is also upregulated in AML cells (396), and the most notable nonhematological malignancy involving PIM1 overexpression is prostate cancer (397). In addition to the lymphomagenesis studies just mentioned, synergy between PIM1 and MYC has also been noted in a murine model of prostate cancer, and a cross-species comparison of gene expression signatures (using both human and mouse tumors) showed that *PIM1* was the most consistently coregulated gene in MYC-driven tumors (398). Several mechanisms have been proposed to explain the tumorigenic role of PIM1 in collaboration with MYC. First, PIM1 appears to act as a histone kinase and coactivator of MYC (399). Second, PIM1 has been reported to activate the cell cycle phosphatases CDC25A and CDC25C: since these proteins are transcriptional targets of MYC, this may represent a second point of convergence between PIM and MYC signaling (400–402). Third, expression of PIM1 (or PIM2) in prostate cancer cells may inhibit the activity of PP2A phosphatase, which normally dephosphorylates MYC and leads to its ubiquitinylation and degradation (403). PIM1 also has several antiapoptotic functions, including phosphorylation and inactivation of the proapoptotic BCL2 family protein BAD (404). However, most of the data supporting the antiapoptotic role of PIM kinases has been demonstrated using PIM2. PIM2 expression is dysregulated in a number of tumor types, including lymphoma, leukemias, multiple myeloma, and prostate cancer. PIM2 RNA and protein are both highly labile and the protein is rapidly induced in response to cytokine growth factors, resulting in apoptotic resistance (405). This apoptotic resistance is mediated by multiple substrates, including 4E-BP and BAD. The role of PIM3 in both normal cellular homeostasis and cancer has been somewhat less well characterized than that of the other two PIM proteins. PIM3 was first identified in neuroendocrine cells (391), and aberrant overexpression of PIM3 has been reported in hepatocellular and pancreatic carcinoma cells but not in corresponding normal tissues (406, 407).

As summarized previously, PIM proteins have been variously implicated in cell cycle regulation and protection from apoptosis. In this respect, they bear some functional similarity with AKT and related AGC family kinases, which also have prosurvival and promitogenic effects. However, PIM kinases appear to operate in a largely orthogonal fashion to the AGC kinases. For example, ectopic expression of either AKT1 or PIM2 proteins can promote growth and survival of hematopoietic cells from AKT/PIM-deficient mice, but only PIM2 expression is insensitive to treatment with rapamycin (which inhibits mTOR, downstream of AKT) (408). PIM1 and PIM2-mediated rapamycin resistance has also been demonstrated in T cells (409). Moreover, PIM1 and PIM2 kinases appear to play a role in mediating resistance to several oncogenic tyrosine kinases (particularly in hematopoietic malignancies), including FLT3 and BCR-ABL (410). As the clinical investigation and use of tyrosine kinase inhibitors increases, development of PIM inhibitors may be an attractive strategy to circumvent drug resistance and tumor cell survival in these settings.

5.5   PROTEIN KINASE C

The human protein kinase C (PKC) family is comprised of ten proteins in the AGC subgroup, which play diverse and important roles in regulating intracellular signaling. PKC activity was first associated with tumor biology almost 25 years ago, with the finding that tumorigenic phorbol esters bind to and promote the activity of these enzymes (411–413). Phorbol esters were subsequently found to mimic (and compete for binding with) the endogenous molecule diacylglycerol (DAG), which is important for membrane localization and activation of most of the PKC isozymes (414). Despite being the first kinase implicated in carcinogenesis, the large number of PKC isoforms and the complexity and diversity of their regulation and function have presented significant challenges to understanding their collective roles in cellular transformation and tumor progression. In many cases, both tumorigenic and tumor suppressor functions have been ascribed to the same PKC isoform, and tumor expression data can be similarly conflicting. Nevertheless, recent advances in PKC research have highlighted several isozymes in particular as potentially attractive targets for therapeutic intervention.

There are nine PKC genes encoding ten isozymes (PKCβ undergoes alternative splicing to generate two distinct proteins). These isozymes are typically classified into three groups: classical (PKCα, PKCβI, PKCβII, PKCγ), novel (PKCδ, PKCε, PKCη, PKCθ), and atypical (PKCζ, PKCι; the mouse homolog of PKCι is referred to as PKCλ). In addition, two closely related AGC kinases, the PKC-related kinases (PRK1/PRK2, also known as PKN1/PKN2), are often grouped together with the atypical PKCs. (Another kinase, initially called PKCμ, actually belongs to the CAMK kinase family. This kinase is more widely known as PKD, although it appears to be activated by PKCs (415).) This classification reflects both the sequence similarity of the kinase domains and the primary means of activation for the respective isozymes. Classical PKCs require both DAG and calcium for activation, novel PKCs require only DAG, and atypical PKCs (as well as PRK1/PRK2) require neither. In addition to the kinase domains (which are located at the C-terminal end of the proteins), several other sequence elements are conserved to various degrees within the PKC family (Figure 5.8). The classical and novel PKCs contain N-terminal tandem-duplicated C1 domains (C1A and C1B), which mediate binding to DAG and acidic phospholipids at the plasma membrane, and a C2 domain that confers calcium-dependent phospholipid binding. The C1 domains are zinc finger motifs, although they are structurally distinct from other zinc fingers (416). A pseudosubstrate region, which plays an important role in regulation of activity, is located at the N-terminal end of the C1 region. The C2 domain also interacts with RACK (receptor for activated C kinase) proteins, which are important regulators of PKC intracellular localization and function (417). In the novel PKCs a region with homology to the C2 domain is located at the N terminus of the protein, although it does not appear to be regulated by calcium. Atypical PKCs also have an N-terminal C2 homology domain followed by a single C1 domain. The N-terminal region of atypical PKCs also contains a PHOX-BEM1 (PB1) domain, a ubiquitin-like module that also modulates protein:protein interactions. The kinase domains contain three key phosphorylation sites in the activation loop, the C-terminal hydrophobic/"PIF" motif and the C-terminal "turn" motif (see Chapter 2). The atypical PKCs differ somewhat from the others in that the PIF peptide contains a phosphomimetic glutamate residue.

5.5.1 PKC Activation

Figure 5.9 depicts the multiple phospholipid signaling pathways that converge to activate PKCs. (We focus here on the activation of classical PKCs, which

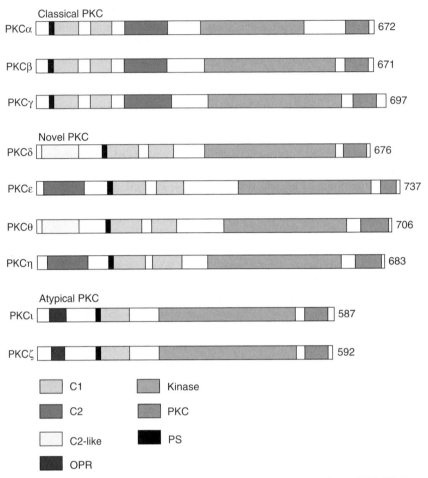

Figure 5.8 Domain structures of PKC family members. Abbreviations: PKC, PKC C-terminal extension; PS, pseudosubstrate sequence; OPR, octicosapeptide repeat domain.

are regulated by phosphorylation, phospholipid association, DAG, and calcium.) PKC activation is a complex process, involving multiple phosphorylation events, protein conformational states, and shuttling between the plasma membrane, cytoplasm, and other intracellular compartments (418) (Figure 5.10). Nascent PKC associates with plasma membranes via low affinity phospholipid interactions; in this state, the pseudosubstrate region is disengaged from the active site. The unphosphorylated hydrophobic motif/PIF sequence in the C-terminal tail of PKC (see Chapter 2) binds to PDK1, which phosphorylates the activation loop, stabilizes the protein, and primes PKC for activity. Stabilization of the active conformation leads to autophosphorylation (or phosphorylation by regulatory kinases) at the turn motif and PIF sites, disengaging PDK1 but allowing the pseudosubstrate to bind to and inactivate the catalytic domain. In this form, PKC is translocated to the

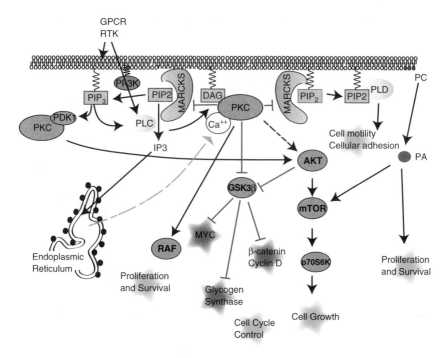

Figure 5.9 PKC signaling pathways. PKC elicits multiple effects on lipid and intracellular kinase signaling. As well as modulating the activity of multiple protein kinases (including RAF, AKT, GSK3β, and receptor tyrosine kinases), PKC affects plasma membrane phospholipid composition by regulation of MARCKS (myristoylated alanine-rich protein kinase C substrate). Phosphorylation of MARCKS blocks its sequestration of PIP₂, promoting mitogenic signaling via PI3K and PLD pathways.

cytosol where it remains, latent but phosphorylated and poised for activity. The PHLPP protein phosphatases provide an important negative regulatory function for PKCs, dephosphorylating the hydrophobic motif phosphopeptide and promoting protein degradation (419). Since atypical PKCs have a glutamate at the hydrophobic phospho-site, this mechanism is only likely to be relevant for the classical and novel isoforms.

Downstream of G-protein coupled receptors and RTKs, activation of phospholipase C results in generation of DAG and inositol trisphosphate (IP_3) from plasma membrane phospholipids (Figure 5.9). DAG recruits (classical and novel) PKCs to the membrane and promotes their activation. The role of IP_3 is more indirect, releasing intracellular calcium, which also serves as a coactivator for classical PKCs. At the same time, the conversion of PIP_2 to PIP_3 via PI3K results in activation of PDK1, which can phosphorylate and activate PKCs as described earlier (58). The activation mechanism for novel PKCs is similar to that of the classical isozymes, with the exception that there is no Ca^{2+} binding to promote phospholipid binding: hence the rate of membrane association and activation of these emzymes is generally slower. The regulation of atypical isozymes is not as clear: they are stimulated

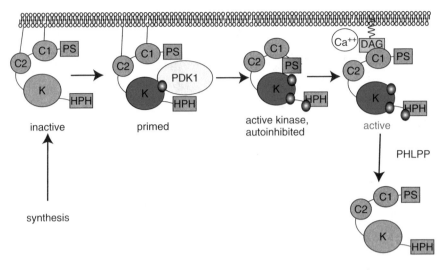

Figure 5.10 Activation of PKCs. Classical PKCs associate with the plasma membrane and are primed for activation by PDK1 binding and phosphorylation in the activation loop. This promotes phosphorylation at the turn motif and PIF sites, followed by engagement of the autoinhibitory pseudosubstrate sequence and translocation to the cytosol. Reassociation with the plasma membrane via DAG and calcium binding promotes full activation of the enzyme. PHLPP downregulates PKC by dephosphorylating the PIF sequence and promoting protein degradation.

by PDK1 phosphorylation and autoregulated by a pseudosubstrate sequence but are not dependent on DAG or calcium. The crosstalk between PKCs and plasma membrane phospholipids is also modulated by MARCKS (myristoylated alanine-rich protein kinase C substrate), a highly charged protein that sequesters and regulates the availability of PIP_2 in the plasma membrane (420). MARCKS is subject to phosphorylation by the novel and atypical PKC isozymes in a concerted, sequential manner (421). Phosphorylation of MARCKS results in its dissociation from the membrane and subsequent liberation of PIP_2, which in turn triggers the PI3K pathway and phospholipase activity. MARCKS also binds to actin and thus may link PKC to cytoskeleton signaling and cellular adhesion (422).

5.5.2 Classical PKCs

The classical PKC isoforms have long been implicated in tumor growth and survival, but the scientific literature is replete with conflicting data as to whether they promote or suppress the malignant phenotype. Here we focus on PKCα and PKCβ, which have been more widely studied and implicated in cancer than the mostly neuronal-specific PKCγ isoform. Immunohistochemical analysis has shown that PKCα is upregulated in certain tumors but can be downregulated in others. However, even within a given tumor type, these findings are by no means unambiguous:

for example, it has been reported that PKCα is downregulated in hepatocellular carcinomas and inversely correlated with tumor size (423), yet highly expressed in poorly differentiated hepatocellular cell lines (424). This inconsistency is also reflected in functional data. PKCα has been shown to have antiproliferative effects and in some cases it may have a bona fide tumor suppressor role: for example, PKCα knockout mice are predisposed to development of spontaneous intestinal tumors, and PKCα deficiency accelerates tumor formation in Apc$^{Min/+}$ mice (425). There are, however, many examples where PKCα expression and activity is linked to malignant phenotype. For example, in SK-Hep-1 hepatocellular carcinoma cells, PKCα silencing by siRNA was found to decrease growth, migration, and invasion via downregulation of p38 MAPK signaling (426). In breast cancer cells, PKCα promotes activity of the ETS1 transcription factor, which is widely linked to tumor invasion and poor prognosis (427); PKCα is also associated with hormone-independent growth and tamoxifen resistance in estrogen receptor positive cells (428) and regulation of HER2 receptor recycling in some HER2-positive tumors (429). PKCα (along with other PKC isoforms) has also been implicated in proliferation and survival of glioma cells (430).

Expression of PKCβ (in particular, PKCβII) is predictive of poor survival in diffuse large B-cell lymphoma (DLBCL) (431, 432). In addition, PKCβ is implicated in VEGF-induced angiogenesis, which has also been associated with poor prognosis in DLBCL (433, 434). Together, these findings present one of the most compelling rationales for inhibition of classical PKCs in cancer therapy. PKCβII is also overexpressed in murine colon tumors, compared to both PKCα and PKCβI, and may be an early driver of tumorigenesis, in collaboration with Ras and the atypical PKCι (435, 436). Nevertheless, PKCβII expression decreases with increasing grade in human colon tumors, so it is unclear if it plays a major role in the proliferation and survival of advanced tumors.

PKCβ phosphorylates and inactivates GSK3β, resulting in activation of multiple downstream effectors such as cyclin D, MYC, and β-catenin. In particular, the increase in cyclin D has been associated with PKCβ in breast cancer cell lines (437). However, as with PKCα, there are also examples where PKCβ may have an antitumor function. For example, PKCβ is expressed in melanocytes but frequently lost in melanoma cells (438, 439): overexpression of PKCβII in melanoma cells suppresses their invasive potential by interfering with HGF-PI3K signaling, suggesting that this loss of PKC activity enhances the metastatic potential of melanoma cells (440).

5.5.3 Novel PKCs

As with the classical isoforms, the activities of the novel PKCs appear to vary depending on cellular context. However, there is general consensus that PKCδ and PKCε have important and opposing activities relating to tumor growth, survival, and invasion. PKCδ mostly exhibits antiproliferative effects (via regulation of CDK inhibitors and cyclins) and proapoptotic effects (involving both intrinsic and extrinsic apoptotic pathways). Indeed, PKCδ catalytic activity may be an important mediator of the apoptotic effects of genotoxic anticancer drugs: several chemotherapy agents can induce proteolytic activation of PKCδ via caspase-3, and loss of PKCδ activity reduces the efficacy of these agents (441, 442). PKCδ has also been described in a proapoptotic effector in endometrial cancer and glioma cells, acting in opposition to PKCα in these models (430, 443). Similarly, overexpression of PKCδ in Caco-2 colon cancer cells leads to reduced proliferation and increased apoptosis, via downregulation of cyclins D1 and E, inhibition of cyclin-dependent kinases, and increased ratio of proapoptotic versus antiapoptotic BCL2 family proteins (444). Moreover, PKCδ may negatively regulate cell migration (445) and has been found to be suppressed in several tumor types (430, 446). Collectively, the evidence suggests that PKCδ acts to decrease cancer cell survival, so its inhibition should be avoided by anticancer drugs: nevertheless, PKCδ is not an unambiguous tumor suppressor and there are also reports of it having prosurvival and mitogenic activities (447, 448).

In contrast to PKCδ, the gene coding for PKCε is regarded as a transforming oncogene (449, 450), conferring anchorage-independent growth, enhanced survival, and an invasive phenotype (451). PKCε is overexpressed in breast (452) and brain (453) tumors, with increasing expression correlating with tumor grade. PKCε leads to increased RAF/MEK/ERK signaling and is likely to act downstream of RAS but upstream of RAF. Although PKCε has been shown to physically associate with RAF, it is unclear whether direct phosphorylation is involved. Signaling through PKCε is also linked to AKT activation in MCF7 breast cancer cells (through DNAPK; it is not clear if other "PDK2" enzymes are also involved (454)). Integrin signaling has also been indirectly linked to AKT activation via PKCε in prostate cancer cells (455).

5.5.4 Atypical PKCs

The atypical PKCs (PKCζ and PKCι) share 72% amino acid homology but have somewhat opposing functions (456). Both proteins appear to play a role in establishing cellular polarity and mediating proliferation and survival. However, in the context of tumor cells, PKCζ promotes adhesion, differentiation, and apoptosis (457, 458), whereas PKCι is proposed to be a bona fide oncogene that promotes RAS-mediated transformation, anchorage-independent growth, invasion, and resistance to chemotherapeutics. Multiple upstream signals can lead to oncogenic PKCι activation, including PDK1 (58), SRC (459), RAS (460), and phospholipase D (461).

Dissection of the PKCι signaling pathway in lung cancer cells revealed that transformation and invasion are mediated by interaction of the PB1 domain with the scaffolding protein PAR6 (partitioning-defective-6), a modulator of cellular polarity. This leads to activation of the small GTPase RAC1, and subsequent coupling to the MEK/ERK pathway via PAK1 kinase (462). Introduction of dominant-negative, kinase-inactivated PKCι or disruption of the PKCι:PAR6 interaction using the gold compounds aurothioglucose and aurothiomalate leads to inhibition of anchorage-independent growth in vitro and tumor growth inhibition in vivo (462, 463). In addition, PKCι promotes survival via the NFκB pathway (464, 465). The tumorigenic effects of PKCι have been demonstrated in several types of solid tumor and hematological malignancy, although the data supporting its role as a bona fide oncogene are derived from studies with non small cell lung carcinoma (NSCLC) and ovarian tumors (456). PKCι is highly expressed in NSCLC cells but not in normal lung or stromal tissue. In the squamous cell subtype of NSCLC, overexpression is related to amplification of the 3q26 locus; however, elevated expression in the absence of amplification is more widespread in adenocarcinoma (466). Moreover, high PKCι expression is correlated with poor prognosis irrespective of disease stage. Amplification and overexpression of PKCι is also prevalent in ovarian cancer, particularly the serous subtype, although in this case expression is correlated with stage of disease (467). In chronic myelogenous leukemia, PKCι is an effector of BCR-ABL-mediated transformation and is also implicated in chemoresistance (464, 468). Additional tumor types involving PKCι include pancreatic (469) and colon carcinoma (460): in the case of colon tumors, PKCι acts in collaboration with RAS and the classical PKC isoform PKCβII, again resulting in coupling to the MEK/ERK pathway (436).

REFERENCES

1. Arcaro A, Doepfner KT, Boller D, Guerreiro AS, Shalaby T, Jackson SP, Schoenwaelder SM, Delattre O, Grotzer MA, Fischer B. Novel role for insulin as an autocrine growth factor for malignant brain tumour cells. Biochem J 2007;406(1):57–66.
2. Karakas B, Bachman KE, Park BH. Mutation of the PIK3CA oncogene in human cancers. Br J Cancer 2006;94(4):455–459.
3. Bonneau D, Longy M. Mutations of the human PTEN gene. Hum Mutat 2000;16(2):109–122.
4. Cully M, You H, Levine AJ, Mak TW. Beyond PTEN mutations: the PI3K pathway as an integrator of multiple inputs during tumorigenesis. Nat Rev Cancer 2006;6(3):184–192.
5. Vivanco I, Sawyers CL. The phosphatidylinositol 3-kinase AKT pathway in human cancer. Nat Rev Cancer 2002;2(7):489–501.
6. Bianco R, Shin I, Ritter CA, Yakes FM, Basso A, Rosen N, Tsurutani J, Dennis PA, Mills GB, Arteaga CL. Loss of PTEN/MMAC1/TEP in EGF receptor-expressing tumor cells counteracts the antitumor action of EGFR tyrosine kinase inhibitors. Oncogene 2003;22(18):2812–2822.
7. Nagata Y, Lan KH, Zhou X, Tan M, Esteva FJ, Sahin AA, Klos KS, Li P, Monia BP, Nguyen NT, Hortobagyi GN, Hung MC, Yu D. PTEN activation contributes to tumor inhibition by trastuzumab, and loss of PTEN predicts trastuzumab resistance in patients. Cancer Cell 2004;6(2):117–127.
8. Domin J, Waterfield MD. Using structure to define the function of phosphoinositide 3-kinase family members. FEBS Lett 1997;410(1):91–95.
9. Rameh LE, Cantley LC. The role of phosphoinositide 3-kinase lipid products in cell function. J Biol Chem 1999;274(13):8347–8350.
10. Vanhaesebroeck B, Waterfield MD. Signaling by distinct classes of phosphoinositide 3-kinases. Exp Cell Res 1999;253(1):239–254.
11. Stoyanov B, Volinia S, Hanck T, Rubio I, Loubtchenkov M, Malek D, Stoyanova S, Vanhaesebroeck B, Dhand R, Nurnberg B, et al. Cloning and characterization of a G protein-activated human phosphoinositide-3 kinase. Science 1995;269(5224):690–693.
12. Mitsiades CS, Mitsiades N, Koutsilieris M. The Akt pathway: molecular targets for anti-cancer drug development. Curr Cancer Drug Targets 2004;4(3):235–256.
13. Liang J, Slingerland JM. Multiple roles of the PI3K/PKB (Akt) pathway in cell cycle progression. Cell Cycle 2003;2(4):339–345.
14. Sugimoto Y, Whitman M, Cantley LC, Erikson RL. Evidence that the Rous sarcoma virus transforming gene product phosphorylates phosphatidylinositol and diacylglycerol. Proc Natl Acad Sci USA 1984;81(7):2117–2121.

15. Whitman M, Kaplan DR, Schaffhausen B, Cantley L, Roberts TM. Association of phosphatidylinositol kinase activity with polyoma middle-T competent for transformation. Nature 1985;315(6016):239–242.

16. Shayesteh L, Lu Y, Kuo WL, Baldocchi R, Godfrey T, Collins C, Pinkel D, Powell B, Mills GB, Gray JW. PIK3CA is implicated as an oncogene in ovarian cancer. Nat Genet 1999;21(1):99–102.

17. Walker EH, Pacold ME, Perisic O, Stephens L, Hawkins PT, Wymann MP, Williams RL. Structural determinants of phosphoinositide 3-kinase inhibition by wortmannin, LY294002, quercetin, myricetin, and staurosporine. Mol Cell 2000;6(4):909–919.

18. Walker EH, Perisic O, Ried C, Stephens L, Williams RL. Structural insights into phosphoinositide 3-kinase catalysis and signalling. Nature 1999;402(6759):313–320.

19. Huang CH, Mandelker D, Schmidt-Kittler O, Samuels Y, Velculescu VE, Kinzler KW, Vogelstein B, Gabelli SB, Amzel LM. The structure of a human p110alpha/p85alpha complex elucidates the effects of oncogenic PI3K alpha mutations. Science 2007;318(5857):1744–1748.

20. Yu J, Zhang Y, McIlroy J, Rordorf-Nikolic T, Orr GA, Backer JM. Regulation of the p85/p110 phosphatidylinositol 3'-kinase: stabilization and inhibition of the p110 alpha catalytic subunit by the p85 regulatory subunit. Mol Cell Biol 1998;18(3):1379–1387.

21. Yu J, Wjasow C, Backer JM. Regulation of the p85/p110 alpha phosphatidylinositol 3'-kinase. Distinct roles for the N-terminal and C-terminal SH2 domains. J Biol Chem 1998;273(46):30199–30203.

22. Shekar SC, Wu H, Fu Z, Yip SC, Nagajyothi, Cahill SM, Girvin ME, Backer JM. Mechanism of constitutive phosphoinositide 3-kinase activation by oncogenic mutants of the p85 regulatory subunit. J Biol Chem 2005;280(30):27850–27855.

23. Miled N, Yan Y, Hon WC, Perisic O, Zvelebil M, Inbar Y, Schneidman-Duhovny D, Wolfson HJ, Backer JM, Williams RL. Mechanism of two classes of cancer mutations in the phosphoinositide 3-kinase catalytic subunit. Science 2007;317(5835):239–242.

24. Kang S, Denley A, Vanhaesebroeck B, Vogt PK. Oncogenic transformation induced by the p110-beta, -gamma, and -delta isoforms of class I phosphoinositide 3-kinase. Proc Natl Acad Sci USA 2006;103(5):1289–1294.

25. Samuels Y, Wang Z, Bardelli A, Silliman N, Ptak J, Szabo S, Yan H, Gazdar A, Powell SM, Riggins GJ, Willson JK, Markowitz S, Kinzler KW, Vogelstein B, Velculescu VE. High frequency of mutations of the PIK3CA gene in human cancers. Science 2004;304(5670): 554.

26. Foukas LC, Claret M, Pearce W, Okkenhaug K, Meek S, Peskett E, Sancho S, Smith AJ, Withers DJ, Vanhaesebroeck B. Critical role for the p110 alpha phosphoinositide-3-OH kinase in growth and metabolic regulation. Nature 2006;441(7091):366–370.

27. Vogt PK, Bader AG, Kang S. Phosphoinositide 3-kinase: from viral oncoprotein to drug target. Virology 2006;344(1):131–138.

28. Ikenoue T, Kanai F, Hikiba Y, Obata T, Tanaka Y, Imamura J, Ohta M, Jazag A, Guleng B, Tateishi K, Asaoka Y, Matsumura M, Kawabe T, Omata M. Functional analysis of PIK3CA gene mutations in human colorectal cancer. Cancer Res 2005;65(11):4562–4567.

29. Samuels Y, Diaz LA Jr, Schmidt-Kittler O, Cummins JM, Delong L, Cheong I, Rago C, Huso DL, Lengauer C, Kinzler KW, Vogelstein B, Velculescu VE. Mutant PIK3CA promotes cell growth and invasion of human cancer cells. Cancer Cell 2005;7(6):561–573.

30. Jia S, Liu Z, Zhang S, Liu P, Zhang L, Lee SH, Zhang J, Signoretti S, Loda M, Roberts TM, Zhao JJ. Essential roles of PI(3)K-p110 beta in cell growth, metabolism and tumorigenesis. Nature 2008; 454(7205):776–779.

31. Wee S, Wiederschain D, Maira SM, Loo A, Miller C, deBeaumont R, Stegmeier F, Yao YM, Lengauer C. PTEN-deficient cancers depend on PIK3CB. Proc Natl Acad Sci USA 2008;105(35):13057–13062.

32. Rodriguez-Viciana P, Warne PH, Dhand R, Vanhaesebroeck B, Gout I, Fry MJ, Waterfield MD, Downward J. Phosphatidylinositol-3-OH kinase as a direct target of Ras. Nature 1994;370(6490):527–532.

33. Rodriguez-Viciana P, Warne PH, Vanhaesebroeck B, Waterfield MD, Downward J. Activation of phosphoinositide 3-kinase by interaction with Ras and by point mutation. EMBO J 1996;15(10):2442–2451.

34. Bamford S, Dawson E, Forbes S, Clements J, Pettett R, Dogan A, Flanagan A, Teague J, Futreal PA, Stratton MR, Wooster R. The COSMIC (Catalogue of Somatic Mutations in Cancer) database and website. Br J Cancer 2004;91:355–358.

35. Bos JL. ras oncogenes in human cancer: a review. Cancer Res 1989;49(17):4682–4689.

36. Downward J. Targeting RAS signalling pathways in cancer therapy. Nat Rev Cancer 2003;3(1):11–22.

37. Peyssonnaux C, Provot S, Felder-Schmittbuhl MP, Calothy G, Eychene A. Induction of postmitotic neuroretina cell proliferation by distinct Ras downstream signaling pathways. Mol Cell Biol 2000;20(19):7068–7079.

38. Wolthuis RM, Bos JL. Ras caught in another affair: the exchange factors for Ral. Curr Opin Genet Dev 1999;9(1):112–117.

39. Rodriguez-Viciana P, Warne PH, Khwaja A, Marte BM, Pappin D, Das P, Waterfield MD, Ridley A, Downward J. Role of phosphoinositide 3-OH kinase in cell transformation and control of the actin cytoskeleton by Ras. Cell 1997;89(3):457–467.

40. Gupta S, Ramjaun AR, Haiko P, Wang Y, Warne PH, Nicke B, Nye E, Stamp G, Alitalo K, Downward J. Binding of ras to phosphoinositide 3-kinase p110 alpha is required for ras-driven tumorigenesis in mice. Cell 2007;129(5):957–968.

41. Wu X, Senechal K, Neshat MS, Whang YE, Sawyers CL. The PTEN/MMAC1 tumor suppressor phosphatase functions as a negative regulator of the phosphoinositide 3-kinase/Akt pathway. Proc Natl Acad Sci USA 1998;95(26):15587–15591.

42. Sansal I, Sellers WR. The biology and clinical relevance of the PTEN tumor suppressor pathway. J Clin Oncol 2004;22(14):2954–2963.

43. Sulis ML, Parsons R. PTEN: from pathology to biology. Trends Cell Biol 2003;13(9):478–483.

44. Marsh DJ, Coulon V, Lunetta KL, Rocca-Serra P, Dahia PL, Zheng Z, Liaw D, Caron S, Duboue B, Lin AY, Richardson AL, Bonnetblanc JM, Bressieux JM, Cabarrot-Moreau A, Chompret A, Demange L, Eeles RA, Yahanda AM, Fearon ER, Fricker JP, Gorlin RJ, Hodgson SV, Huson S, Lacombe D, Eng C, et al. Mutation spectrum and genotype-phenotype analyses in Cowden disease and Bannayan–Zonana syndrome, two hamartoma syndromes with germline PTEN mutation. Hum Mol Genet 1998;7(3):507–515.

45. Cantley LC, Neel BG. New insights into tumor suppression: PTEN suppresses tumor formation by restraining the phosphoinositide 3-kinase/AKT pathway. Proc Natl Acad Sci USA 1999;96(8):4240–4245.

46. Tashiro H, Blazes MS, Wu R, Cho KR, Bose S, Wang SI, Li J, Parsons R, Ellenson LH. Mutations in PTEN are frequent in endometrial carcinoma but rare in other common gynecological malignancies. Cancer Res 1997;57(18):3935–3940.

47. Cairns P, Okami K, Halachmi S, Halachmi N, Esteller M, Herman JG, Jen J, Isaacs WB, Bova GS, Sidransky D. Frequent inactivation of PTEN/MMAC1 in primary prostate cancer. Cancer Res 1997;57(22):4997–5000.

48. Wang SI, Puc J, Li J, Bruce JN, Cairns P, Sidransky D, Parsons R. Somatic mutations of PTEN in glioblastoma multiforme. Cancer Res 1997;57(19):4183–4186.

49. Soria JC, Lee HY, Lee JI, Wang L, Issa JP, Kemp BL, Liu DD, Kurie JM, Mao L, Khuri FR. Lack of PTEN expression in non-small cell lung cancer could be related to promoter methylation. Clin Cancer Res 2002;8(5):1178–1184.

50. Liliental J, Moon SY, Lesche R, Mamillapalli R, Li D, Zheng Y, Sun H, Wu H. Genetic deletion of the Pten tumor suppressor gene promotes cell motility by activation of Rac1 and Cdc42 GTPases. Curr Biol 2000;10(7):401–404.

51. Welch HC, Coadwell WJ, Stephens LR, Hawkins PT. Phosphoinositide 3-kinase-dependent activation of Rac. FEBS Lett 2003;546(1):93–97.

52. Papakonstanti EA, Stournaras C. Association of PI-3 kinase with PAK1 leads to actin phosphorylation and cytoskeletal reorganization. Mol Biol Cell 2002;13(8):2946–2962.

53. Chaudhary A, King WG, Mattaliano MD, Frost JA, Diaz B, Morrison DK, Cobb MH, Marshall MS, Brugge JS. Phosphatidylinositol 3-kinase regulates Raf1 through Pak phosphorylation of serine 338. Curr Biol 2000;10(9):551–554.

54. Mora A, Komander D, van Aalten DM, Alessi DR. PDK1, the master regulator of AGC kinase signal transduction. Semin Cell Dev Biol 2004;15(2):161–170.

55. Pullen N, Dennis PB, Andjelkovic M, Dufner A, Kozma SC, Hemmings BA, Thomas G. Phosphorylation and activation of p70s6k by PDK1. Science 1998;279(5351):707–710.

56. Richards SA, Fu J, Romanelli A, Shimamura A, Blenis J. Ribosomal S6 kinase 1 (RSK1) activation requires signals dependent on and independent of the MAP kinase ERK. Curr Biol 1999;9(15):810–820.

57. Park J, Leong ML, Buse P, Maiyar AC, Firestone GL, Hemmings BA. Serum and glucocorticoid-inducible kinase (SGK) is a target of the PI 3-kinase-stimulated signaling pathway. EMBO J 1999;18(11):3024–3033.

58. Le Good JA, Ziegler WH, Parekh DB, Alessi DR, Cohen P, Parker PJ. Protein kinase C isotypes controlled by phosphoinositide 3-kinase through the protein kinase PDK1. Science 1998;281(5385):2042–2045.

59. Manning BD, Cantley LC. AKT/PKB signaling: navigating downstream. Cell 2007;129(7):1261–1274.

60. Yang ZZ, Tschopp O, Baudry A, Dummler B, Hynx D, Hemmings BA. Physiological functions of protein kinase B/Akt. Biochem Soc Trans 2004;32(Pt 2):350–354.

61. Carpten JD, Faber AL, Horn C, Donoho GP, Briggs SL, Robbins CM, Hostetter G, Boguslawski S, Moses TY, Savage S, Uhlik M, Lin A, Du J, Qian YW, Zeckner DJ, Tucker-Kellogg G, Touchman J, Patel K, Mousses S, Bittner M, Schevitz R, Lai MH, Blanchard KL, Thomas JE. A transforming mutation in the pleckstrin homology domain of AKT1 in cancer. Nature 2007;448(7152):439–444.

62. Jacinto E, Facchinetti V, Liu D, Soto N, Wei S, Jung SY, Huang Q, Qin J, Su B. SIN1/MIP1 maintains rictor-mTOR complex integrity and regulates Akt phosphorylation and substrate specificity. Cell 2006;127(1):125–137.

63. Sarbassov D, Guertin DA, Ali SM, Sabatini DM. Phosphorylation and regulation of Akt/PKB by the rictor-mTOR complex. Science 2005;307(5712):1098–1101.

64. Lynch DK, Ellis CA, Edwards PA, Hiles ID. Integrin-linked kinase regulates phosphorylation of serine 473 of protein kinase B by an indirect mechanism. Oncogene 1999;18(56):8024–8032.

65. Dragoi AM, Fu X, Ivanov S, Zhang P, Sheng L, Wu D, Li GC, Chu WM. DNA-PKcs, but not TLR9, is required for activation of Akt by CpG-DNA. EMBO J 2005;24(4):779–789.

66. Feng J, Park J, Cron P, Hess D, Hemmings BA. Identification of a PKB/Akt hydrophobic motif Ser-473 kinase as DNA-dependent protein kinase. J Biol Chem 2004;279(39):41189–41196.

67. Kawakami Y, Nishimoto H, Kitaura J, Maeda-Yamamoto M, Kato RM, Littman DR, Leitges M, Rawlings DJ, Kawakami T. Protein kinase C betaII regulates Akt phosphorylation on Ser-473 in a cell type- and stimulus-specific fashion. J Biol Chem 2004;279(46):47720–47725.

68. Facchinetti V, Ouyang W, Wei H, Soto N, Lazorchak A, Gould C, Lowry C, Newton AC, Mao Y, Miao RQ, Sessa WC, Qin J, Zhang P, Su B, Jacinto E. The mammalian target of rapamycin complex 2 controls folding and stability of Akt and protein kinase C. EMBO J 2008;27(14):1932–1943.

69. Ikenoue T, Inoki K, Yang Q, Zhou X, Guan KL. Essential function of TORC2 in PKC and Akt turn motif phosphorylation, maturation and signalling. EMBO J 2008;27(14):1919–1931

70. Kelekar A, Chang BS, Harlan JE, Fesik SW, Thompson CB. Bad is a BH3 domain-containing protein that forms an inactivating dimer with Bcl-XL. Mol Cell Biol 1997;17(12):7040–7046.

71. Brunet A, Bonni A, Zigmond MJ, Lin MZ, Juo P, Hu LS, Anderson MJ, Arden KC, Blenis J, Greenberg ME. Akt promotes cell survival by phosphorylating and inhibiting a Forkhead transcription factor. Cell 1999;96(6):857–868.

72. Cardone MH, Roy N, Stennicke HR, Salvesen GS, Franke TF, Stanbridge E, Frisch S, Reed JC. Regulation of cell death protease caspase-9 by phosphorylation. Science 1998;282(5392):1318–1321.

73. Romashkova JA, Makarov SS. NF-kappaB is a target of AKT in anti-apoptotic PDGF signalling. Nature 1999;401(6748):86–90.

74. Karin M, Cao Y, Greten FR, Li ZW. NF-kappaB in cancer: from innocent bystander to major culprit. Nat Rev Cancer 2002;2(4):301–310.

75. Aggarwal BB. Nuclear factor-kappaB: the enemy within. Cancer Cell 2004;6(3):203–208.

76. Vasudevan KM, Gurumurthy S, Rangnekar VM. Suppression of PTEN expression by NF-kappa B prevents apoptosis. Mol Cell Biol 2004;24(3):1007–1021.

77. Mayo LD, Donner DB. A phosphatidylinositol 3-kinase/Akt pathway promotes translocation of Mdm2 from the cytoplasm to the nucleus. Proc Natl Acad Sci USA 2001;98(20):11598–11603.
78. Gregory MA, Qi Y, Hann Sr. Phosphorylation by glycogen synthase kinase-3 controls c-myc proteolysis and subnuclear localization. J Biol Chem 2003;278(51):51606–51612.
79. Nesbit CE, Tersak JM, Prochownik EV. MYC oncogenes and human neoplastic disease. Oncogene 1999;18(19):3004–3016.
80. Pelengaris S, Khan M, Evan G. c-MYC: more than just a matter of life and death. Nat Rev Cancer 2002;2(10):764–776.
81. Moon RT, Kohn AD, De Ferrari GV, Kaykas A. WNT and beta-catenin signalling: diseases and therapies. Nat Rev Genet 2004;5(9):691–701.
82. Liang J, Zubovitz J, Petrocelli T, Kotchetkov R, Connor MK, Han K, Lee JH, Ciarallo S, Catzavelos C, Beniston R, Franssen E, Slingerland JM. PKB/Akt phosphorylates p27, impairs nuclear import of p27 and opposes p27-mediated G1 arrest. Nat Med 2002;8(10):1153–1160.
83. Viglietto G, Motti ML, Bruni P, Melillo RM, D'Alessio A, Califano D, Vinci F, Chiappetta G, Tsichlis P, Bellacosa A, Fusco A, Santoro M. Cytoplasmic relocalization and inhibition of the cyclin-dependent kinase inhibitor p27(Kip1) by PKB/Akt-mediated phosphorylation in breast cancer. Nat Med 2002;8(10):1136–1144.
84. Zhou BP, Liao Y, Xia W, Spohn B, Lee MH, Hung MC. Cytoplasmic localization of p21Cip1/WAF1 by Akt-induced phosphorylation in HER-2/neu-overexpressing cells. Nat Cell Biol 2001;3(3):245–252.
85. Li Y, Dowbenko D, Lasky LA. AKT/PKB phosphorylation of p21Cip/WAF1 enhances protein stability of p21Cip/WAF1 and promotes cell survival. J Biol Chem 2002;277(13):11352–11361.
86. Sekulic A, Hudson CC, Homme JL, Yin P, Otterness DM, Karnitz LM, Abraham RT. A direct linkage between the phosphoinositide 3-kinase-AKT signaling pathway and the mammalian target of rapamycin in mitogen-stimulated and transformed cells. Cancer Res 2000;60(13):3504–3513.
87. Potter CJ, Pedraza LG, Xu T. Akt regulates growth by directly phosphorylating Tsc2. Nat Cell Biol 2002;4(9):658–665.
88. Kwiatkowski DJ. Tuberous sclerosis: from tubers to mTOR. Ann Hum Genet 2003;67(Pt 1):87–96.
89. Inoki K, Li Y, Xu T, Guan KL. Rheb GTPase is a direct target of TSC2 GAP activity and regulates mTOR signaling. Genes Dev 2003;17(15):1829–1834.
90. Li Y, Inoki K, Guan KL. Biochemical and functional characterizations of small GTPase Rheb and TSC2 GAP activity. Mol Cell Biol 2004;24(18):7965–7975.
91. Long X, Lin Y, Ortiz-Vega S, Yonezawa K, Avruch J. Rheb binds to and regulates the mTOR kinase. Curr Biol 2005;15:702–713.
92. Oshiro N, Takahashi R, Yoshino K, Tanimura K, Nakashima A, Eguchi S, Miyamoto T, Hara K, Takehana K, Avruch J, Kikkawa U, Yonezawa K. The proline-rich Akt substrate of 40kDa (PRAS40) is a physiological substrate of mammalian target of rapamycin complex 1. J Biol Chem 2007;282(28):20329–20339.
93. Wang L, Harris TE, Roth RA, Lawrence JC Jr. PRAS40 regulates mTORC1 kinase activity by functioning as a direct inhibitor of substrate binding. J Biol Chem 2007;282(27):20036–20044.
94. Sancak Y, Thoreen CC, Peterson TR, Lindquist RA, Kang SA, Spooner E, Carr SA, Sabatini DM. PRAS40 is an insulin-regulated inhibitor of the mTORC1 protein kinase. Mol Cell 2007;25(6):903–915.
95. Vander Haar E, Lee SI, Bandhakavi S, Griffin TJ, Kim DH. Insulin signalling to mTOR mediated by the Akt/PKB substrate PRAS40. Nat Cell Biol 2007;9(3):316–323.
96. Thompson JE, Thompson CB. Putting the rap on Akt. J Clin Oncol 2004;22(20):4217–4226.
97. Warburg O. On the origin of cancer cells. Science 1956;123:309–314.
98. Rathmell JC, Fox CJ, Plas DR, Hammerman PS, Cinalli RM, Thompson CB. Akt-directed glucose metabolism can prevent Bax conformation change and promote growth factor-independent survival. Mol Cell Biol 2003;23(20):7315–7328.
99. Lin HK, Yeh S, Kang HY, Chang C. Akt suppresses androgen-induced apoptosis by phosphorylating and inhibiting androgen receptor. Proc Natl Acad Sci USA 2001;98(13):7200–7205.

100. Campbell RA, Bhat-Nakshatri P, Patel NM, Constantinidou D, Ali S, Nakshatri H. Phosphatidyli-nositol 3-kinase/AKT-mediated activation of estrogen receptor alpha: a new model for anti-estrogen resistance. J Biol Chem 2001;276(13):9817–9824.

101. Kang SS, Kwon T, Kwon DY, Do SI. Akt protein kinase enhances human telomerase activity through phosphorylation of telomerase reverse transcriptase subunit. J Biol Chem 1999;274(19):13085–13090.

102. Gerber HP, McMurtrey A, Kowalski J, Yan M, Keyt BA, Dixit V, Ferrara N. Vascular endothelial growth factor regulates endothelial cell survival through the phosphatidylinositol 3'-kinase/Akt signal transduction pathway. Requirement for Flk-1/KDR activation. J Biol Chem 1998;273(46):30336–30343.

103. Michell BJ, Griffiths JE, Mitchelhill KI, Rodriguez-Crespo I, Tiganis T, Bozinovski S, de Montellano PR, Kemp BE, Pearson RB. The Akt kinase signals directly to endothelial nitric oxide synthase. Curr Biol 1999;9(15):845–848.

104. King FW, Skeen J, Hay N, Shtivelman E. Inhibition of Chk1 by activated PKB/Akt. Cell Cycle 2004;3(5):634–637.

105. Shtivelman E, Sussman J, Stokoe D. A role for PI 3-kinase and PKB activity in the G2/M phase of the cell cycle. Curr Biol 2002;12(11):919–924.

106. Puc J, Keniry M, Li HS, Pandita TK, Choudhury AD, Memeo L, Mansukhani M, Murty VV, Gaciong Z, Meek SE, Piwnica-Worms H, Hibshoosh H, Parsons R. Lack of PTEN sequesters CHK1 and initiates genetic instability. Cancer Cell 2005;7(2):193–204.

107. Jun T, Gjoerup O, Roberts TM. Tangled webs: evidence of cross-talk between c-Raf-1 and Akt. Sci STKE 1999;1999(13): PE1.

108. Biondi RM. Phosphoinositide-dependent protein kinase 1, a sensor of protein conformation. Trends Biochem Sci 2004;29(3):136–142.

109. Tessier M, Woodgett Jr. Serum and glucocorticoid-regulated protein kinases: variations on a theme. J Cell Biochem 2006;98(6):1391–1407.

110. Kobayashi T, Deak M, Morrice N, Cohen P. Characterization of the structure and regulation of two novel isoforms of serum- and glucocorticoid-induced protein kinase. Biochem J 1999;344 (Pt 1):189–197.

111. Hong F, Larrea MD, Doughty C, Kwiatkowski DJ, Squillace R, Slingerland JM. mTOR-raptor binds and activates SGK1 to regulate p27 phosphorylation. Mol Cell 2008;30(6):701–711.

112. Brunet A, Park J, Tran H, Hu LS, Hemmings BA, Greenberg ME. Protein kinase SGK mediates survival signals by phosphorylating the forkhead transcription factor FKHRL1 (FOXO3a). Mol Cell Biol 2001;21(3):952–965.

113. Zhang L, Cui R, Cheng X, Du J. Antiapoptotic effect of serum and glucocorticoid-inducible protein kinase is mediated by novel mechanism activating I{kappa}B kinase. Cancer Res 2005;65(2):457–464.

114. Zhang BH, Tang ED, Zhu T, Greenberg ME, Vojtek AB, Guan KL. Serum- and glucocorticoid-inducible kinase SGK phosphorylates and negatively regulates B-Raf. J Biol Chem 2001;276(34):31620–31626.

115. Sakoda H, Gotoh Y, Katagiri H, Kurokawa M, Ono H, Onishi Y, Anai M, Ogihara T, Fujishiro M, Fukushima Y, Abe M, Shojima N, Kikuchi M, Oka Y, Hirai H, Asano T. Differing roles of Akt and serum- and glucocorticoid-regulated kinase in glucose metabolism, DNA synthesis, and oncogenic activity. J Biol Chem 2003;278(28):25802–25807.

116. David S, Kalb RG. Serum/glucocorticoid-inducible kinase can phosphorylate the cyclic AMP response element binding protein, CREB. FEBS Lett 2005;579(6):1534–1538.

117. Liu D, Yang X, Songyang Z. Identification of CISK, a new member of the SGK kinase family that promotes IL-3-dependent survival. Curr Biol 2000;10(19):1233–1236.

118. Chen RH, Sarnecki C, Blenis J. Nuclear localization and regulation of erk- and rsk-encoded protein kinases. Mol Cell Biol 1992;12(3):915–927.

119. Frame S, Cohen P. GSK3 takes centre stage more than 20 years after its discovery. Biochem J 2001;359(Pt 1):1–16.

120. Shimamura A, Ballif BA, Richards SA, Blenis J. Rsk1 mediates a MEK-MAP kinase cell survival signal. Curr Biol 2000;10(3):127–135.

121. De Cesare D, Jacquot S, Hanauer A, Sassone-Corsi P. Rsk-2 activity is necessary for epidermal growth factor-induced phosphorylation of CREB protein and transcription of c-fos gene. Proc Natl Acad Sci USA 1998;95(21):12202–12207.

122. Bohuslav J, Chen LF, Kwon H, Mu Y, Greene WC. p53 induces NF-kappaB activation by an IkappaB kinase-independent mechanism involving phosphorylation of p65 by ribosomal S6 kinase 1. J Biol Chem 2004;279(25):26115–26125.

123. Roux PP, Ballif BA, Anjum R, Gygi SP, Blenis J. Tumor-promoting phorbol esters and activated Ras inactivate the tuberous sclerosis tumor suppressor complex via p90 ribosomal S6 kinase. Proc Natl Acad Sci USA 2004;101(37):13489–13494.

124. Carriere A, Cargnello M, Julien LA, Gao H, Bonneil E, Thibault P, Roux PP. Oncogenic MAPK signaling stimulates mTORC1 activity by promoting RSK-mediated raptor phosphorylation. Curr Biol 2008;18(17):1269–1277.

125. Clark DE, Poteet-Smith CE, Smith JA, Lannigan DA. Rsk2 allosterically activates estrogen receptor alpha by docking to the hormone-binding domain. EMBO J 2001;20(13):3484–3494.

126. David JP, Mehic D, Bakiri L, Schilling AF, Mandic V, Priemel M, Idarraga MH, Reschke MO, Hoffmann O, Amling M, Wagner EF. Essential role of RSK2 in c-Fos-dependent osteosarcoma development. J Clin Invest 2005;115(3):664–672

127. Anjum R, Roux PP, Ballif BA, Gygi SP, Blenis J. The tumor suppressor DAP kinase is a target of RSK-mediated survival signaling. Curr Biol 2005;15(19):1762–1767.

128. Kang S, Dong S, Gu TL, Guo A, Cohen MS, Lonial S, Khoury HJ, Fabbro D, Gilliland DG, Bergsagel PL, Taunton J, Polakiewicz RD, Chen J. FGFR3 activates RSK2 to mediate hematopoietic transformation through tyrosine phosphorylation of RSK2 and activation of the MEK/ERK pathway. Cancer Cell 2007;12(3):201–214.

129. Chesi M, Nardini E, Lim RS, Smith KD, Kuehl WM, Bergsagel PL. The t(4;14) translocation in myeloma dysregulates both FGFR3 and a novel gene, MMSET, resulting in IgH/MMSET hybrid transcripts. Blood 1998;92(9):3025–3034.

130. de Groot RP, Ballou LM, Sassone-Corsi P. Positive regulation of the cAMP-responsive activator CREM by the p70S6 kinase: an alternative route to mitogen-induced gene expression. Cell 1994;79(1):81–91.

131. Harada H, Andersen JS, Mann M, Terada N, Korsmeyer SJ. p70S6 kinase signals cell survival as well as growth, inactivating the pro-apoptotic molecule BAD. Proc Natl Acad Sci USA 2001;98(17):9666–9670.

132. Harrington LS, Findlay GM, Gray A, Tolkacheva T, Wigfield S, Rebholz H, Barnett J, Leslie NR, Cheng S, Shepherd PR, Gout I, Downes CP, Lamb RF. The TSC1-2 tumor suppressor controls insulin-PI3K signaling via regulation of IRS proteins. J Cell Biol 2004;166(2):213–223.

133. Um SH, Frigerio F, Watanabe M, Picard F, Joaquin M, Sticker M, Fumagalli S, Allegrini PR, Kozma SC, Auwerx J, Thomas G. Absence of S6K1 protects against age- and diet-induced obesity while enhancing insulin sensitivity. Nature 2004;431(7005):200–205.

134. Carracedo A, Ma L, Teruya-Feldstein J, Rojo F, Salmena L, Alimonti A, Egia A, Sasaki AT, Thomas G, Kozma SC, Papa A, Nardella C, Cantley LC, Baselga J, Pandolfi PP. Inhibition of mTORC1 leads to MAPK pathway activation through a PI3K-dependent feedback loop in human cancer. J Clin Invest 2008;118(9):3065–3074.

135. Bjornsti MA, Houghton PJ. The TOR pathway: a target for cancer therapy. Nat Rev Cancer 2004;4(5):335–348.

136. Oda K, Stokoe D, Taketani Y, McCormick F. High frequency of coexistent mutations of PIK3CA and PTEN genes in endometrial carcinoma. Cancer Res 2005;65(23):10669–10673.

137. Slamon DJ, Clark GM, Wong SG, Levin WJ, Ullrich A, McGuire WL. Human breast cancer: correlation of relapse and survival with amplification of the HER-2/neu oncogene. Science 1987;235(4785):177–182.

138. Slamon DJ, Godolphin W, Jones LA, Holt JA, Wong SG, Keith DE, Levin WJ, Stuart SG, Udove J, Ullrich A, et al. Studies of the HER-2/neu proto-oncogene in human breast and ovarian cancer. Science 1989;244(4905):707–712.

139. Nahta R, Yu D, Hung MC, Hortobagyi GN, Esteva FJ. Mechanisms of disease: understanding resistance to HER2-targeted therapy in human breast cancer. Nat Clin Pract Oncol 2006;3(5):269–280.

140. Pandolfi PP. Breast cancer—loss of PTEN predicts resistance to treatment. N Engl J Med 2004;351(22):2337–2338.

141. Engin H, Baltali E, Guler N, Guler G, Tekuzman G, Uner A. Expression of PTEN, cyclin D1, P27/KIP1 in invasive ductal carcinomas of the breast and correlation with clinicopathological parameters. Bull Cancer 2006;93(2): E21–26.

142. Tsutsui S, Inoue H, Yasuda K, Suzuki K, Tahara K, Higashi H, Era S, Mori M. Inactivation of PTEN is associated with a low p27Kip1 protein expression in breast carcinoma. Cancer 2005;104(10):2048–2053.

143. Tsutsui S, Inoue H, Yasuda K, Suzuki K, Higashi H, Era S, Mori M. Reduced expression of PTEN protein and its prognostic implications in invasive ductal carcinoma of the breast. Oncology 2005;68(4–6):398–404.

144. Di Vizio D, Cito L, Boccia A, Chieffi P, Insabato L, Pettinato G, Motti ML, Schepis F, D'Amico W, Fabiani F, Tavernise B, Venuta S, Fusco A, Viglietto G. Loss of the tumor suppressor gene PTEN marks the transition from intratubular germ cell neoplasias (ITGCN) to invasive germ cell tumors. Oncogene 2005;24(11):1882–1894.

145. Garcia JM, Silva J, Pena C, Garcia V, Rodriguez R, Cruz MA, Cantos B, Provencio M, Espana P, Bonilla F. Promoter methylation of the PTEN gene is a common molecular change in breast cancer. Genes Chromosomes Cancer 2004;41(2):117–124.

146. Li SY, Rong M, Grieu F, Iacopetta B. PIK3CA mutations in breast cancer are associated with poor outcome. Breast Cancer Res Treat 2006;96(1):91–95.

147. Levine DA, Bogomolniy F, Yee CJ, Lash A, Barakat RR, Borgen PI, Boyd J. Frequent mutation of the PIK3CA gene in ovarian and breast cancers. Clin Cancer Res 2005;11(8):2875–2878.

148. Saal LH, Holm K, Maurer M, Memeo L, Su T, Wang X, Yu JS, Malmstrom PO, Mansukhani M, Enoksson J, Hibshoosh H, Borg A, Parsons R. PIK3CA mutations correlate with hormone receptors, node metastasis, and ERBB2, and are mutually exclusive with PTEN loss in human breast carcinoma. Cancer Res 2005;65(7):2554–2559.

149. Samuels Y, Velculescu VE. Oncogenic mutations of PIK3CA in human cancers. Cell Cycle 2004;3(10):1221–1224.

150. Bachman KE, Argani P, Samuels Y, Silliman N, Ptak J, Szabo S, Konishi H, Karakas B, Blair BG, Lin C, Peters BA, Velculescu VE, Park BH. The PIK3CA gene is mutated with high frequency in human breast cancers. Cancer Biol Ther 2004;3(8):772–775.

151. Wu G, Xing M, Mambo E, Huang X, Liu J, Guo Z, Chatterjee A, Goldenberg D, Gollin SM, Sukumar S, Trink B, Sidransky D. Somatic mutation and gain of copy number of PIK3CA in human breast cancer. Breast Cancer Res 2005;7(5): R609–616.

152. Clark AS, West K, Streicher S, Dennis PA. Constitutive and inducible Akt activity promotes resistance to chemotherapy, trastuzumab, or tamoxifen in breast cancer cells. Mol Cancer Ther 2002;1(9):707–717.

153. Jin W, Wu L, Liang K, Liu B, Lu Y, Fan Z. Roles of the PI-3K and MEK pathways in Ras-mediated chemoresistance in breast cancer cells. Br J Cancer 2003;89(1):185–191.

154. Velho S, Oliveira C, Ferreira A, Ferreira AC, Suriano G, Schwartz S Jr, Duval A, Carneiro F, Machado JC, Hamelin R, Seruca R. The prevalence of PIK3CA mutations in gastric and colon cancer. Eur J Cancer 2005;41(11):1649–1654.

155. Nassif NT, Lobo GP, Wu X, Henderson CJ, Morrison CD, Eng C, Jalaludin B, Segelov E. PTEN mutations are common in sporadic microsatellite stable colorectal cancer. Oncogene 2004;23(2):617–628.

156. Goel A, Arnold CN, Niedzwiecki D, Carethers JM, Dowell JM, Wasserman L, Compton C, Mayer RJ, Bertagnolli MM, Boland CR. Frequent inactivation of PTEN by promoter hypermethylation in microsatellite instability-high sporadic colorectal cancers. Cancer Res 2004;64(9):3014–3021.

157. Fearon ER. Molecular genetics of colorectal cancer. Ann N Y Acad Sci 1995;768:101–110.

158. Perrone F, Lampis A, Orsenigo M, Di Bartolomeo M, Gevorgyan A, Losa M, Frattini M, Riva C, Andreola S, Bajetta E, Bertario L, Leo E, Pierotti MA, Pilotti S. PI3KCA/PTEN deregulation contributes to impaired responses to cetuximab in metastatic colorectal cancer patients. Ann Oncol 2008;20(1):84–90.

159. Risinger JI, Hayes K, Maxwell GL, Carney ME, Dodge RK, Barrett JC, Berchuck A. PTEN mutation in endometrial cancers is associated with favorable clinical and pathologic characteristics. Clin Cancer Res 1998;4(12):3005–3010.

160. Lu KH, Wu W, Dave B, Slomovitz BM, Burke TW, Munsell MF, Broaddus RR, Walker CL. Loss of tuberous sclerosis complex-2 function and activation of mammalian target of rapamycin signaling in endometrial carcinoma. Clin Cancer Res 2008;14(9):2543–2550.

161. Byun DS, Cho K, Ryu BK, Lee MG, Park JI, Chae KS, Kim HJ, Chi SG. Frequent monoallelic deletion of PTEN and its reciprocal association with PIK3CA amplification in gastric carcinoma. Int J Cancer 2003;104(3):318–327.

162. Lee JW, Soung YH, Kim SY, Lee HW, Park WS, Nam SW, Kim SH, Lee JY, Yoo NJ, Lee SH. PIK3CA gene is frequently mutated in breast carcinomas and hepatocellular carcinomas. Oncogene 2005;24(8):1477–1480.

163. Li VS, Wong CW, Chan TL, Chan AS, Zhao W, Chu KM, So S, Chen X, Yuen ST, Leung SY. Mutations of PIK3CA in gastric adenocarcinoma. BMC Cancer 2005;5:29.

164. Espinoza LA, Tone LG, Neto JB, Costa RS, Wang QJ, Ballejo G. Enhanced TGF alpha-EGFR expression and P53 gene alterations contributes to gastric tumors aggressiveness. Cancer Lett 2004;212(1):33–41.

165. Slesak B, Harlozinska A, Porebska I, Bojarowski T, Lapinska J, Rzeszutko M, Wojnar A. Expression of epidermal growth factor receptor family proteins (EGFR, c-erbB-2 and c-erbB-3) in gastric cancer and chronic gastritis. Anticancer Res 1998;18(4A):2727–2732.

166. Tanida S, Joh T, Itoh K, Kataoka H, Sasaki M, Ohara H, Nakazawa T, Nomura T, Kinugasa Y, Ohmoto H, Ishiguro H, Yoshino K, Higashiyama S, Itoh M. The mechanism of cleavage of EGFR ligands induced by inflammatory cytokines in gastric cancer cells. Gastroenterology 2004;127(2):559–569.

167. Ekstrand AJ, James CD, Cavenee WK, Seliger B, Pettersson RF, Collins VP. Genes for epidermal growth factor receptor, transforming growth factor alpha, and epidermal growth factor and their expression in human gliomas in vivo. Cancer Res 1991;51(8):2164–2172.

168. Ekstrand AJ, Longo N, Hamid ML, Olson JJ, Liu L, Collins VP, James CD. Functional characterization of an EGF receptor with a truncated extracellular domain expressed in glioblastomas with EGFR gene amplification. Oncogene 1994;9(8):2313–2320.

169. Wikstrand CJ, McLendon RE, Friedman AH, Bigner DD. Cell surface localization and density of the tumor-associated variant of the epidermal growth factor receptor, EGFRvIII. Cancer Res 1997;57(18):4130–4140.

170. Heimberger AB, Hlatky R, Suki D, Yang D, Weinberg J, Gilbert M, Sawaya R, Aldape K. Prognostic effect of epidermal growth factor receptor and EGFRvIII in glioblastoma multiforme patients. Clin Cancer Res 2005;11(4):1462–1466.

171. Mellinghoff IK, Wang MY, Vivanco I, Haas-Kogan DA, Zhu S, Dia EQ, Lu KV, Yoshimoto K, Huang JH, Chute DJ, Riggs BL, Horvath S, Liau LM, Cavenee WK, Rao PN, Beroukhim R, Peck TC, Lee JC, Sellers WR, Stokoe D, Prados M, Cloughesy TF, Sawyers CL, Mischel PS. Molecular determinants of the response of glioblastomas to EGFR kinase inhibitors. N Engl J Med 2005;353(19):2012–2024.

172. Knobbe CB, Reifenberger G. Genetic alterations and aberrant expression of genes related to the phosphatidyl-inositol-3'-kinase/protein kinase B (Akt) signal transduction pathway in glioblastomas. Brain Pathol 2003;13(4):507–518.

173. Baeza N, Weller M, Yonekawa Y, Kleihues P, Ohgaki H. PTEN methylation and expression in glioblastomas. Acta Neuropathol (Berl) 2003;106(5):479–485.

174. Rasheed BK, Stenzel TT, McLendon RE, Parsons R, Friedman AH, Friedman HS, Bigner DD, Bigner SH. PTEN gene mutations are seen in high-grade but not in low-grade gliomas. Cancer Res 1997;57(19);4187–4190.

175. Hartmann C, Bartels G, Gehlhaar C, Holtkamp N, von Deimling A. PIK3CA mutations in glioblastoma multiforme. Acta Neuropathol (Berl) 2005;109(6):639–642.

176. Chakravarti A, Zhai G, Suzuki Y, Sarkesh S, Black PM, Muzikansky A, Loeffler JS. The prognostic significance of phosphatidylinositol 3-kinase pathway activation in human gliomas. J Clin Oncol 2004;22(10):1926–1933.

177. Jiang Z, Pore N, Cerniglia GJ, Mick R, Georgescu MM, Bernhard EJ, Hahn SM, Gupta AK, Maity A. Phosphatase and tensin homologue deficiency in glioblastoma confers resistance to radiation and temozolomide that is reversed by the protease inhibitor nelfinavir. Cancer Res 2007;67(9):4467–4473.

178. Chen JS, Zhou LJ, Entin-Meer M, Yang X, Donker M, Knight ZA, Weiss W, Shokat KM, Haas-Kogan D, Stokoe D. Characterization of structurally distinct, isoform-selective phosphoinositide 3'-kinase inhibitors in combination with radiation in the treatment of glioblastoma. Mol Cancer Ther 2008;7(4):841–850.

179. Fan QW, Knight ZA, Goldenberg DD, Yu W, Mostov KE, Stokoe D, Shokat KM, Weiss WA. A dual PI3 kinase/mTOR inhibitor reveals emergent efficacy in glioma. Cancer Cell 2006;9(5):341–349.

180. Fan QW, Weiss WA. Isoform specific inhibitors of PI3 kinase in glioma. Cell Cycle 2006;5(20):2301–2305.

181. Hu TH, Huang CC, Lin PR, Chang HW, Ger LP, Lin YW, Changchien CS, Lee CM, Tai MH. Expression and prognostic role of tumor suppressor gene PTEN/MMAC1/TEP1 in hepatocellular carcinoma. Cancer 2003;97(8):1929–1940.

182. Wan XW, Jiang M, Cao HF, He YQ, Liu SQ, Qiu XH, Wu MC, Wang HY. The alteration of PTEN tumor suppressor expression and its association with the histopathological features of human primary hepatocellular carcinoma. J Cancer Res Clin Oncol 2003;129(2):100–106.

183. Chung TW, Lee YC, Ko JH, Kim CH. Hepatitis B virus X protein modulates the expression of PTEN by inhibiting the function of p53, a transcriptional activator in liver cells. Cancer Res 2003;63(13):3453–3458.

184. Tang JM, He QY, Guo RX, Chang XJ. Phosphorylated Akt overexpression and loss of PTEN expression in non-small cell lung cancer confers poor prognosis. Lung Cancer 2006;51(2):181–191.

185. Marsit CJ, Zheng S, Aldape K, Hinds PW, Nelson HH, Wiencke JK, Kelsey KT. PTEN expression in non-small-cell lung cancer: evaluating its relation to tumor characteristics, allelic loss, and epigenetic alteration. Hum Pathol 2005;36(7):768–776.

186. Forgacs E, Biesterveld EJ, Sekido Y, Fong K, Muneer S, Wistuba II, Milchgrub S, Brezinschek R, Virmani A, Gazdar AF, Minna JD. Mutation analysis of the PTEN/MMAC1 gene in lung cancer. Oncogene 1998;17(12):1557–1565.

187. Kohno T, Takahashi M, Manda R, Yokota J. Inactivation of the PTEN/MMAC1/TEP1 gene in human lung cancers. Genes Chromosomes Cancer 1998;22(2):152–156.

188. Yokomizo A, Tindall DJ, Drabkin H, Gemmill R, Franklin W, Yang P, Sugio K, Smith DI, Liu W. PTEN/MMAC1 mutations identified in small cell, but not in non-small cell lung cancers. Oncogene 1998;17(4):475–479.

189. Massion PP, Taflan PM, Shyr Y, Rahman SM, Yildiz P, Shakthour B, Edgerton ME, Ninan M, Andersen JJ, Gonzalez AL. Early involvement of the phosphatidylinositol 3-kinase/Akt pathway in lung cancer progression. Am J Respir Crit Care Med 2004;170(10):1088–1094.

190. Kokubo Y, Gemma A, Noro R, Seike M, Kataoka K, Matsuda K, Okano T, Minegishi Y, Yoshimura A, Shibuya M, Kudoh S. Reduction of PTEN protein and loss of epidermal growth factor receptor gene mutation in lung cancer with natural resistance to gefitinib (IRESSA). Br J Cancer 2005;92(9):1711–1719.

191. Pao W, Wang TY, Riely GJ, Miller VA, Pan Q, Ladanyi M, Zakowski MF, Heelan RT, Kris MG, Varmus HE. KRAS mutations and primary resistance of lung adenocarcinomas to gefitinib or erlotinib. PLoS Med 2005;2(1): e17.

192. Goel VK, Lazar AJ, Warneke CL, Redston MS, Haluska FG. Examination of mutations in BRAF, NRAS, and PTEN in primary cutaneous melanoma. J Invest Dermatol 2006;126(1):154–160.

193. Guldberg P, thor Straten P, Birck A, Ahrenkiel V, Kirkin AF, Zeuthen J. Disruption of the MMAC1/PTEN gene by deletion or mutation is a frequent event in malignant melanoma. Cancer Res 1997;57(17):3660–3663.

194. Tsao H, Zhang X, Benoit E, Haluska FG. Identification of PTEN/MMAC1 alterations in uncultured melanomas and melanoma cell lines. Oncogene 1998;16(26):3397–3402.

195. Whiteman DC, Zhou XP, Cummings MC, Pavey S, Hayward NK, Eng C. Nuclear PTEN expression and clinicopathologic features in a population-based series of primary cutaneous melanoma. Int J Cancer 2002;99(1):63–67.

196. Tsao H, Goel V, Wu H, Yang G, Haluska FG. Genetic interaction between NRAS and BRAF mutations and PTEN/MMAC1 inactivation in melanoma. J Invest Dermatol 2004;122(2):337–341.

197. Wang Y, Helland A, Holm R, Kristensen GB, Borresen-Dale AL. PIK3CA mutations in advanced ovarian carcinomas. Hum Mutat 2005;25(3): 322.

198. Campbell IG, Russell SE, Choong DY, Montgomery KG, Ciavarella ML, Hooi CS, Cristiano BE, Pearson RB, Phillips WA. Mutation of the PIK3CA gene in ovarian and breast cancer. Cancer Res 2004;64(21):7678–7681.

199. Obata K, Morland SJ, Watson RH, Hitchcock A, Chenevix-Trench G, Thomas EJ, Campbell IG. Frequent PTEN/MMAC mutations in endometrioid but not serous or mucinous epithelial ovarian tumors. Cancer Res 1998;58(10):2095–2097.

200. Dinulescu DM, Ince TA, Quade BJ, Shafer SA, Crowley D, Jacks T. Role of K-ras and Pten in the development of mouse models of endometriosis and endometrioid ovarian cancer. Nat Med 2005;11(1):63–70.

201. Lee S, Choi EJ, Jin C, Kim DH. Activation of PI3K/Akt pathway by PTEN reduction and PIK3CA mRNA amplification contributes to cisplatin resistance in an ovarian cancer cell line. Gynecol Oncol 2005;97(1):26–34.

202. Hu L, Hofmann J, Lu Y, Mills GB, Jaffe RB. Inhibition of phosphatidylinositol 3'-kinase increases efficacy of paclitaxel in in vitro and in vivo ovarian cancer models. Cancer Res 2002;62(4):1087–1092.

203. Hu L, Hofmann J, Jaffe RB. Phosphatidylinositol 3-kinase mediates angiogenesis and vascular permeability associated with ovarian carcinoma. Clin Cancer Res 2005;11(22):8208–8212.

204. Hu L, Zaloudek C, Mills GB, Gray J, Jaffe RB. In Vivo and in vitro ovarian carcinoma growth inhibition by a phosphatidylinositol 3-kinase inhibitor (LY294002). Clin Cancer Res 2000;6(3):880–886.

205. Asano T, Yao Y, Zhu J, Li D, Abbruzzese JL, Reddy SA. The PI 3-kinase/Akt signaling pathway is activated due to aberrant Pten expression and targets transcription factors NF-kappaB and c-Myc in pancreatic cancer cells. Oncogene 2004;23(53):8571–8580.

206. Perren A, Komminoth P, Saremaslani P, Matter C, Feurer S, Lees JA, Heitz PU, Eng C. Mutation and expression analyses reveal differential subcellular compartmentalization of PTEN in endocrine pancreatic tumors compared to normal islet cells. Am J Pathol 2000;157(4):1097–1103.

207. Gray IC, Stewart LM, Phillips SM, Hamilton JA, Gray NE, Watson GJ, Spurr NK, Snary D. Mutation and expression analysis of the putative prostate tumour-suppressor gene PTEN. Br J Cancer 1998;78(10):1296–1300.

208. Wang SI, Parsons R, Ittmann M. Homozygous deletion of the PTEN tumor suppressor gene in a subset of prostate adenocarcinomas. Clin Cancer Res 1998;4(3):811–815.

209. Whang YE, Wu X, Suzuki H, Reiter RE, Tran C, Vessella RL, Said JW, Isaacs WB, Sawyers CL. Inactivation of the tumor suppressor PTEN/MMAC1 in advanced human prostate cancer through loss of expression. Proc Natl Acad Sci USA 1998;95(9):5246–5250.

210. Majumder PK, Sellers WR. Akt-regulated pathways in prostate cancer. Oncogene 2005;24(50): 7465–7474.

211. Wang S, Garcia AJ, Wu M, Lawson DA, Witte ON, Wu H. Pten deletion leads to the expansion of a prostatic stem/progenitor cell subpopulation and tumor initiation. Proc Natl Acad Sci USA 2006;103(5):1480–1485.

212. Trotman LC, Niki M, Dotan ZA, Koutcher JA, Di Cristofano A, Xiao A, Khoo AS, Roy-Burman P, Greenberg NM, Van Dyke T, Cordon-Cardo C, Pandolfi PP. Pten dose dictates cancer progression in the prostate. PLoS Biol 2003;1(3): e59.

213. Mulholland DJ, Dedhar S, Wu H, Nelson CC. PTEN and GSK3beta: key regulators of progression to androgen-independent prostate cancer. Oncogene 2006;25(3):329–337.

214. Lu S, Ren C, Liu Y, Epner DE. PI3K-Akt signaling is involved in the regulation of p21(WAF/CIP) expression and androgen-independent growth in prostate cancer cells. Int J Oncol 2006;28(1):245–251.

215. Mikhailova M, Wang Y, Bedolla R, Lu XH, Kreisberg JI, Ghosh PM. AKT regulates androgen receptor-dependent growth and PSA expression in prostate cancer. Adv Exp Med Biol 2008;617:397–405.

216. Xin L, Teitell MA, Lawson DA, Kwon A, Mellinghoff IK, Witte ON. Progression of prostate cancer by synergy of AKT with genotropic and nongenotropic actions of the androgen receptor. Proc Natl Acad Sci USA 2006;103(20):7789–7794.

217. Wang Y, Mikhailova M, Bose S, Pan CX, White RW, Ghosh PM. Regulation of androgen receptor transcriptional activity by rapamycin in prostate cancer cell proliferation and survival. Oncogene 2008;27(56):7106–7117.

218. Garcia-Rostan G, Costa AM, Pereira-Castro I, Salvatore G, Hernandez R, Hermsem MJ, Herrero A, Fusco A, Cameselle-Teijeiro J, Santoro M. Mutation of the PIK3CA gene in anaplastic thyroid cancer. Cancer Res 2005;65(22):10199–10207.

219. Wu G, Mambo E, Guo Z, Hu S, Huang X, Gollin SM, Trink B, Ladenson PW, Sidransky D, Xing M. Uncommon mutation, but common amplifications, of the PIK3CA gene in thyroid tumors. J Clin Endocrinol Metab 2005;90(8):4688–4693.

220. Martelli AM, Nyakern M, Tabellini G, Bortul R, Tazzari PL, Evangelisti C, Cocco L. Phosphoinositide 3-kinase/Akt signaling pathway and its therapeutical implications for human acute myeloid leukemia. Leukemia 2006;20(6):911–928.

221. Billottet C, Grandage VL, Gale RE, Quattropani A, Rommel C, Vanhaesebroeck B, Khwaja A. A selective inhibitor of the p110 delta isoform of PI 3-kinase inhibits AML cell proliferation and survival and increases the cytotoxic effects of VP16. Oncogene 2006;25(50):6648–6659.

222. Sujobert P, Bardet V, Cornillet-Lefebvre P, Hayflick JS, Prie N, Verdier F, Vanhaesebroeck B, Muller O, Pesce F, Ifrah N, Hunault-Berger M, Berthou C, Villemagne B, Jourdan E, Audhuy B, Solary E, Witz B, Harousseau JL, Himberlin C, Lamy T, Lioure B, Cahn JY, Dreyfus F, Mayeux P, Lacombe C, Bouscary D. Essential role for the p110 delta isoform in phosphoinositide 3-kinase activation and cell proliferation in acute myeloid leukemia. Blood 2005;106(3):1063–1066.

223. Tamburini J, Elie C, Bardet V, Chapuis N, Park S, Broet P, Cornillet-Lefebvre P, Lioure B, Ugo V, Blanchet O, Ifrah N, Witz F, Dreyfus F, Mayeux P, Lacombe C, Bouscary D. Constitutive phosphoinositide 3-kinase/Akt activation represents a favorable prognostic factor in de novo acute myelogenous leukemia patients. Blood 2007;110(3):1025–1028.

224. Skorski T, Bellacosa A, Nieborowska-Skorska M, Majewski M, Martinez R, Choi JK, Trotta R, Wlodarski P, Perrotti D, Chan TO, Wasik MA, Tsichlis PN, Calabretta B. Transformation of hematopoietic cells by BCR/ABL requires activation of a PI-3k/Akt-dependent pathway. EMBO J 1997;16(20):6151–6161.

225. Bai RY, Ouyang T, Miething C, Morris SW, Peschel C, Duyster J. Nucleophosmin-anaplastic lymphoma kinase associated with anaplastic large-cell lymphoma activates the phosphatidylinositol 3-kinase/Akt antiapoptotic signaling pathway. Blood 2000;96(13):4319–4327.

226. Hickey FB, Cotter TG. BCR-ABL regulates phosphatidylinositol 3-kinase-p110 gamma transcription and activation and is required for proliferation and drug resistance. J Biol Chem 2006;281(5):2441–2450.

227. Uddin S, Hussain AR, Siraj AK, Manogaran PS, Al-Jomah NA, Moorji A, Atizado V, Al-Dayel F, Belgaumi A, El-Solh H, Ezzat A, Bavi P, Al-Kuraya KS. Role of phosphatidylinositol 3'-kinase/AKT pathway in diffuse large B-cell lymphoma survival. Blood 2006;108(13):4178–4186.

228. Abubaker J, Bavi PP, Al-Harbi S, Siraj AK, Al-Dayel F, Uddin S, Al-Kuraya K. PIK3CA mutations are mutually exclusive with PTEN loss in diffuse large B-cell lymphoma. Leukemia 2007;21(11):2368–2370.

229. Zollinger A, Stuhmer T, Chatterjee M, Gattenlohner S, Haralambieva E, Muller-Hermelink HK, Andrulis M, Greiner A, Wesemeier C, Rath JC, Einsele H, Bargou RC. Combined functional and molecular analysis of tumor cell signaling defines 2 distinct myeloma subgroups: Akt-dependent and Akt-independent multiple myeloma. Blood 2008;112(8):3403–3411.

230. Shi Y, Yan H, Frost P, Gera J, Lichtenstein A. Mammalian target of rapamycin inhibitors activate the AKT kinase in multiple myeloma cells by up-regulating the insulin-like growth factor receptor/insulin receptor substrate-1/phosphatidylinositol 3-kinase cascade. Mol Cancer Ther 2005;4(10):1533–1540.

231. Tai YT, Podar K, Catley L, Tseng YH, Akiyama M, Shringarpure R, Burger R, Hideshima T, Chauhan D, Mitsiades N, Richardson P, Munshi NC, Kahn CR, Mitsiades C, Anderson KC. Insulin-like growth factor-1 induces adhesion and migration in human multiple myeloma cells via activation of beta1-integrin and phosphatidylinositol 3'-kinase/AKT signaling. Cancer Res 2003;63(18):5850–5858.

232. Ge NL, Rudikoff S. Insulin-like growth factor I is a dual effector of multiple myeloma cell growth. Blood 2000;96(8):2856–2861.

233. Fingar DC, Blenis J. Target of rapamycin (TOR): an integrator of nutrient and growth factor signals and coordinator of cell growth and cell cycle progression. Oncogene 2004;23(18):3151–3171.

234. Harris TE, Lawrence JC Jr. TOR signaling. Sci STKE 2003;2003(212): re15.

235. Houghton PJ, Huang S. mTOR as a target for cancer therapy. Curr Top Microbiol Immunol 2004;279:339–359.

236. Inoki K, Corradetti MN, Guan KL. Dysregulation of the TSC-mTOR pathway in human disease. Nat Genet 2005;37(1):19–24.

237. Takahara T, Hara K, Yonezawa K, Sorimachi H, Maeda T. Nutrient-dependent multimerization of the mammalian target of rapamycin through the N-terminal HEAT repeat region. J Biol Chem 2006;281(39):28605–28614.

238. Long X, Lin Y, Ortiz-Vega S, Yonezawa K, Avruch J. Rheb binds and regulates the mTOR kinase. Curr Biol 2005;15(8):702–713.

239. Long X, Ortiz-Vega S, Lin Y, Avruch J. Rheb binding to mammalian target of rapamycin (mTOR) is regulated by amino acid sufficiency. J Biol Chem 2005;280(25):23433–23436.

240. Hara K, Maruki Y, Long X, Yoshino K, Oshiro N, Hidayat S, Tokunaga C, Avruch J, Yonezawa K. Raptor, a binding partner of target of rapamycin (TOR), mediates TOR action. Cell 2002;110(2):177–189.

241. Kim DH, Sarbassov DD, Ali SM, King JE, Latek RR, Erdjument-Bromage H, Tempst P, Sabatini DM. mTOR interacts with raptor to form a nutrient-sensitive complex that signals to the cell growth machinery. Cell 2002;110(2):163–175.

242. Kim DH, Sarbassov DD, Ali SM, Latek RR, Guntur KV, Erdjument-Bromage H, Tempst P, Sabatini DM. GbetaL, a positive regulator of the rapamycin-sensitive pathway required for the nutrient-sensitive interaction between raptor and mTOR. Mol Cell 2003;11(4):895–904.

243. Kunz J, Henriquez R, Schneider U, Deuter-Reinhard M, Movva NR, Hall MN. Target of rapamycin in yeast, TOR2, is an essential phosphatidylinositol kinase homolog required for G1 progression. Cell 1993;73(3):585–596.

244. Sabatini DM, Erdjument-Bromage H, Lui M, Tempst P, Snyder SH. RAFT1: a mammalian protein that binds to FKBP12 in a rapamycin-dependent fashion and is homologous to yeast TORs. Cell 1994;78(1):35–43.

245. Nojima H, Tokunaga C, Eguchi S, Oshiro N, Hidayat S, Yoshino K, Hara K, Tanaka N, Avruch J, Yonezawa K. The mammalian target of rapamycin (mTOR) partner, raptor, binds the mTOR substrates p70S6 kinase and 4E-BP1 through their TOR signaling (TOS) motif. J Biol Chem 2003;278(18):15461–15464.

246. Fingar DC, Richardson CJ, Tee AR, Cheatham L, Tsou C, Blenis J. mTOR controls cell cycle progression through its cell growth effectors S6K1 and 4E-BP1/eukaryotic translation initiation factor 4E. Mol Cell Biol 2004;24(1):200–216.

247. Oshiro N, Yoshino K, Hidayat S, Tokunaga C, Hara K, Eguchi S, Avruch J, Yonezawa K. Dissociation of raptor from mTOR is a mechanism of rapamycin-induced inhibition of mTOR function. Genes Cells 2004;9(4):359–366.

248. Sarbassov DD, Ali SM, Kim DH, Guertin DA, Latek RR, Erdjument-Bromage H, Tempst P, Sabatini DM. Rictor, a novel binding partner of mTOR, defines a rapamycin-insensitive and raptor-independent pathway that regulates the cytoskeleton. Curr Biol 2004;14(14):1296–1302.

249. Sarbassov DD, Ali SM, Sengupta S, Sheen JH, Hsu PP, Bagley AF, Markhard AL, Sabatini DM. Prolonged rapamycin treatment inhibits mTORC2 assembly and Akt/PKB. Mol Cell 2006;22(2):159–168.

250. Frias MA, Thoreen CC, Jaffe JD, Schroder W, Sculley T, Carr SA, Sabatini DM. mSin1 is necessary for Akt/PKB phosphorylation, and its isoforms define three distinct mTORC2s. Curr Biol 2006;16(18):1865–1870.

251. Pearce LR, Huang X, Boudeau J, Pawlowski R, Wullschleger S, Deak M, Ibrahim AF, Gourlay R, Magnuson MA, Alessi DR. Identification of Protor as a novel Rictor-binding component of mTOR complex-2. Biochem J 2007;405(3):513–522.

252. Sarbassov DD, Guertin DA, Ali SM, Sabatini DM. Phosphorylation and regulation of Akt/PKB by the rictor-mTOR complex. Science 2005;307(5712):1098–1101.

253. Inoki K, Zhu T, Guan KL. TSC2 mediates cellular energy response to control cell growth and survival. Cell 2003;115(5):577–590.

254. Shaw RJ, Bardeesy N, Manning BD, Lopez L, Kosmatka M, DePinho RA, Cantley LC. The LKB1 tumor suppressor negatively regulates mTOR signaling. Cancer Cell 2004;6(1):91–99.

255. Corradetti MN, Inoki K, Bardeesy N, DePinho RA, Guan KL. Regulation of the TSC pathway by LKB1: evidence of a molecular link between tuberous sclerosis complex and Peutz–Jeghers syndrome. Genes Dev 2004;18(13):1533–1538.

256. Hahn-Windgassen A, Nogueira V, Chen CC, Skeen JE, Sonenberg N, Hay N. Akt activates the mammalian target of rapamycin by regulating cellular ATP level and AMPK activity. J Biol Chem 2005;280(37):32081–32089.

257. Sanchez-Cespedes M, Parrella P, Esteller M, Nomoto S, Trink B, Engles JM, Westra WH, Herman JG, Sidransky D. Inactivation of LKB1/STK11 is a common event in adenocarcinomas of the lung. Cancer Res 2002;62(13):3659–3662.

258. Koivunen JP, Kim J, Lee J, Rogers AM, Park JO, Zhao X, Naoki K, Okamoto I, Nakagawa K, Yeap BY, Meyerson M, Wong KK, Richards WG, Sugarbaker DJ, Johnson BE, Janne PA. Mutations in the LKB1 tumour suppressor are frequently detected in tumours from Caucasian but not Asian lung cancer patients. Br J Cancer 2008;99(2):245–252.

259. Zhong D, Liu X, Khuri FR, Sun SY, Vertino PM, Zhou W. LKB1 is necessary for Akt-mediated phosphorylation of proapoptotic proteins. Cancer Res 2008;68(18):7270–7277.

260. Nobukuni T, Joaquin M, Roccio M, Dann SG, Kim SY, Gulati P, Byfield MP, Backer JM, Natt F, Bos JL, Zwartkruis FJ, Thomas G. Amino acids mediate mTOR/raptor signaling through activation of class 3 phosphatidylinositol 3OH-kinase. Proc Natl Acad Sci USA 2005;102(40):14238–14243.

261. Smith EM, Finn SG, Tee AR, Browne GJ, Proud CG. The tuberous sclerosis protein TSC2 is not required for the regulation of the mammalian target of rapamycin by amino acids and certain cellular stresses. J Biol Chem 2005;280(19):18717–18727.

262. Byfield MP, Murray JT, Backer JM. hVps34 is a nutrient-regulated lipid kinase required for activation of p70 S6 kinase. J Biol Chem 2005;280(38):33076–33082.

263. Klionsky DJ. Autophagy: from phenomenology to molecular understanding in less than a decade. Nat Rev Mol Cell Biol 2007;8(11):931–937.

264. Maxwell PH, Pugh CW, Ratcliffe PJ. Activation of the HIF pathway in cancer. Curr Opin Genet Dev 2001;11(3):293–299.

265. Arsham AM, Howell JJ, Simon MC. A novel hypoxia-inducible factor-independent hypoxic response regulating mammalian target of rapamycin and its targets. J Biol Chem 2003;278(32):29655–29660.

266. Hudson CC, Liu M, Chiang GG, Otterness DM, Loomis DC, Kaper F, Giaccia AJ, Abraham RT. Regulation of hypoxia-inducible factor 1alpha expression and function by the mammalian target of rapamycin. Mol Cell Biol 2002;22(20):7004–7014.

267. Brugarolas J, Lei K, Hurley RL, Manning BD, Reiling JH, Hafen E, Witters LA, Ellisen LW, Kaelin WG Jr. Regulation of mTOR function in response to hypoxia by REDD1 and the TSC1/TSC2 tumor suppressor complex. Genes Dev 2004;18(23):2893–2904.

268. Liu L, Cash TP, Jones RG, Keith B, Thompson CB, Simon MC. Hypoxia-induced energy stress regulates mRNA translation and cell growth. Mol Cell 2006;21(4):521–531.

269. Kaper F, Dornhoefer N, Giaccia AJ. Mutations in the PI3K/PTEN/TSC2 pathway contribute to mammalian target of rapamycin activity and increased translation under hypoxic conditions. Cancer Res 2006;66(3):1561–1569.

270. Atkins MB, Hidalgo M, Stadler WM, Logan TF, Dutcher JP, Hudes GR, Park Y, Liou SH, Marshall B, Boni JP, Dukart G, Sherman ML. Randomized phase II study of multiple dose levels of CCI-779, a novel mammalian target of rapamycin kinase inhibitor, in patients with advanced refractory renal cell carcinoma. J Clin Oncol 2004;22(5):909–918.

271. Thomas GV, Tran C, Mellinghoff IK, Welsbie DS, Chan E, Fueger B, Czernin J, Sawyers CL. Hypoxia-inducible factor determines sensitivity to inhibitors of mTOR in kidney cancer. Nat Med 2006;12(1):122–127.

272. Toschi A, Edelstein J, Rockwell P, Ohh M, Foster DA. HIF alpha expression in VHL-deficient renal cancer cells is dependent on phospholipase D. Oncogene 2007;27(19):2746–2753.

273. Foster DA. Regulation of mTOR by phosphatidic acid? Cancer Res 2007;67(1):1–4.

274. Zheng Y, Rodrik V, Toschi A, Shi M, Hui L, Shen Y, Foster DA. Phospholipase D couples survival and migration signals in stress response of human cancer cells. J Biol Chem 2006;281(23):15862–15868.

275. Fang Y, Vilella-Bach M, Bachmann R, Flanigan A, Chen J. Phosphatidic acid-mediated mitogenic activation of mTOR signaling. Science 2001;294(5548):1942–1945.

276. Chen Y, Zheng Y, Foster DA. Phospholipase D confers rapamycin resistance in human breast cancer cells. Oncogene 2003;22(25):3937–3942.

277. Ha SH, Kim DH, Kim IS, Kim JH, Lee MN, Lee HJ, Kim JH, Jang SK, Suh PG, Ryu SH. PLD2 forms a functional complex with mTOR/raptor to transduce mitogenic signals. Cell Signal 2006;18(12):2283–2291.

278. Weng QP, Kozlowski M, Belham C, Zhang A, Comb MJ, Avruch J. Regulation of the p70S6 kinase by phosphorylation in vivo. Analysis using site-specific anti-phosphopeptide antibodies. J Biol Chem 1998;273(26):16621–16629.

279. Pearson RB, Dennis PB, Han JW, Williamson NA, Kozma SC, Wettenhall RE, Thomas G. The principal target of rapamycin-induced p70s6k inactivation is a novel phosphorylation site within a conserved hydrophobic domain. EMBO J 1995;14(21):5279–5287.

280. Holz MK, Blenis J. Identification of S6 kinase 1 as a novel mammalian target of rapamycin (mTOR)-phosphorylating kinase. J Biol Chem 2005;280(28):26089–26093.

281. Krieg J, Hofsteenge J, Thomas G. Identification of the 40S ribosomal protein S6 phosphorylation sites induced by cycloheximide. J Biol Chem 1988;263(23):11473–11477.

282. Ferrari S, Bandi HR, Hofsteenge J, Bussian BM, Thomas G. Mitogen-activated 70K S6 kinase. Identification of in vitro 40S ribosomal S6 phosphorylation sites. J Biol Chem 1991;266(33):22770–22775.

283. Raught B, Peiretti F, Gingras AC, Livingstone M, Shahbazian D, Mayeur GL, Polakiewicz RD, Sonenberg N, Hershey JW. Phosphorylation of eucaryotic translation initiation factor 4B Ser422 is modulated by S6 kinases. EMBO J 2004;23(8):1761–1769.

284. Dorrello NV, Peschiaroli A, Guardavaccaro D, Colburn NH, Sherman NE, Pagano M. S6K1- and betaTRCP-mediated degradation of PDCD4 promotes protein translation and cell growth. Science 2006;314(5798):467–471.

285. Holz MK, Ballif BA, Gygi SP, Blenis J. mTOR and S6K1 mediate assembly of the translation preinitiation complex through dynamic protein interchange and ordered phosphorylation events. Cell 2005;123(4):569–580.

286. Pende M, Um SH, Mieulet V, Sticker M, Goss VL, Mestan J, Mueller M, Fumagalli S, Kozma SC, Thomas G. S6K1(-/-)/S6K2(-/-) mice exhibit perinatal lethality and rapamycin-sensitive 5'-terminal oligopyrimidine mRNA translation and reveal a mitogen-activated protein kinase-dependent S6 kinase pathway. Mol Cell Biol 2004;24(8):3112–3124.

287. Shima H, Pende M, Chen Y, Fumagalli S, Thomas G, Kozma SC. Disruption of the p70(s6k)/p85(s6k) gene reveals a small mouse phenotype and a new functional S6 kinase. EMBO J 1998;17(22):6649–6659.

288. Ma XM, Yoon SO, Richardson CJ, Julich K, Blenis J. SKAR links pre-mRNA splicing to mTOR/S6K1-mediated enhanced translation efficiency of spliced mRNAs. Cell 2008;133(2):303–313.

289. Richardson CJ, Broenstrup M, Fingar DC, Julich K, Ballif BA, Gygi S, Blenis J. SKAR is a specific target of S6 kinase 1 in cell growth control. Curr Biol 2004;14(17):1540–1549.

290. Schiff R, Massarweh SA, Shou J, Bharwani L, Mohsin SK, Osborne CK. Cross-talk between estrogen receptor and growth factor pathways as a molecular target for overcoming endocrine resistance. Clin Cancer Res 2004;10(1Pt 2): 331S-336S.

291. Yue W, Wang JP, Conaway MR, Li Y, Santen RJ. Adaptive hypersensitivity following long-term estrogen deprivation: involvement of multiple signal pathways. J Steroid Biochem Mol Biol 2003;86(3–5):265–274.

292. Sadler TM, Gavriil M, Annable T, Frost P, Greenberger LM, Zhang Y. Combination therapy for treating breast cancer using antiestrogen, ERA-923, and the mammalian target of rapamycin inhibitor, temsirolimus. Endocr Relat Cancer 2006;13(3):863–873.

293. Boulay A, Rudloff J, Ye J, Zumstein-Mecker S, O'Reilly T, Evans DB, Chen S, Lane HA. Dual inhibition of mTOR and estrogen receptor signaling in vitro induces cell death in models of breast cancer. Clin Cancer Res 2005;11(14):5319–5328.

294. deGraffenried LA, Friedrichs WE, Russell DH, Donzis EJ, Middleton AK, Silva JM, Roth RA, Hidalgo M. Inhibition of mTOR activity restores tamoxifen response in breast cancer cells with aberrant Akt Activity. Clin Cancer Res 2004;10(23):8059–8067.

295. Dal Col J, Zancai P, Terrin L, Guidoboni M, Ponzoni M, Pavan A, Spina M, Bergamin S, Rizzo S, Tirelli U, De Rossi A, Doglioni C, Dolcetti R. Distinct functional significance of Akt and mTOR constitutive activation in mantle cell lymphoma. Blood 2008;111(10):5142–5151.

296. Yazbeck VY, Buglio D, Georgakis GV, Li Y, Iwado E, Romaguera JE, Kondo S, Younes A. Temsirolimus downregulates p21 without altering cyclin D1 expression and induces autophagy and synergizes with vorinostat in mantle cell lymphoma. Exp Hematol 2008;36(4):443–450.

297. Wan X, Helman LJ. The biology behind mTOR inhibition in sarcoma. Oncologist 2007;12(8):1007–1018.

298. Hernando E, Charytonowicz E, Dudas ME, Menendez S, Matushansky I, Mills J, Socci ND, Behrendt N, Ma L, Maki RG, Pandolfi PP, Cordon-Cardo C. The AKT-mTOR pathway plays a critical role in the development of leiomyosarcomas. Nat Med 2007;13(6):748–753.

299. Chaisuparat R, Hu J, Jham BC, Knight ZA, Shokat KM, Montaner S. Dual inhibition of PI3K alpha and mTOR as an alternative treatment for Kaposi's sarcoma. Cancer Res 2008;68(20):8361–8368.

300. Johnson GL, Lapadat R. Mitogen-activated protein kinase pathways mediated by ERK, JNK, and p38 protein kinases. Science 2002;298(5600):1911–1912.

301. Hoshino R, Chatani Y, Yamori T, Tsuruo T, Oka H, Yoshida O, Shimada Y, Ari-i S, Wada H, Fujimoto J, Kohno M. Constitutive activation of the 41-/43-kDa mitogen-activated protein kinase signaling pathway in human tumors. Oncogene 1999;18(3):813–822.

302. Haigis KM, Kendall KR, Wang Y, Cheung A, Haigis MC, Glickman JN, Niwa-Kawakita M, Sweet-Cordero A, Sebolt-Leopold J, Shannon KM, Settleman J, Giovannini M, Jacks T. Differential effects of oncogenic K-Ras and N-Ras on proliferation, differentiation and tumor progression in the colon. Nat Genet 2008;40(5):600–608.

303. Bonner TI, Kerby SB, Sutrave P, Gunnell MA, Mark G, Rapp UR. Structure and biological activity of human homologs of the raf/mil oncogene. Mol Cell Biol 1985;5(6):1400–1407.

304. Marais R, Marshall CJ. Control of the ERK MAP kinase cascade by Ras and Raf. Cancer Surv 1996;27:101–125.

305. Brtva TR, Drugan JK, Ghosh S, Terrell RS, Campbell-Burk S, Bell RM, Der CJ. Two distinct Raf domains mediate interaction with Ras. J Biol Chem 1995;270(17):9809–9812.

306. Warne PH, Viciana PR, Downward J. Direct interaction of Ras and the amino-terminal region of Raf-1 in vitro. Nature 1993;364(6435):352–355.

307. Nassar N, Horn G, Herrmann C, Scherer A, McCormick F, Wittinghofer A. The 2.2 AA crystal structure of the Ras-binding domain of the serine/threonine kinase c-Raf1 in complex with Rap1A and a GTP analogue. Nature 1995;375(6532):554–560.

308. Thapar R, Williams JG, Campbell SL. NMR characterization of full-length farnesylated and non-farnesylated H-Ras and its implications for Raf activation. J Mol Biol 2004;343(5):1391–1408.

309. Fischer A, Hekman M, Kuhlmann J, Rubio I, Wiese S, Rapp UR. B- and C-RAF display essential differences in their binding to Ras: the isotype-specific N terminus of B-RAF facilitates Ras binding. J Biol Chem 2007;282(36):26503–26516.

310. Wu J, Dent P, Jelinek T, Wolfman A, Weber MJ, Sturgill TW. Inhibition of the EGF-activated MAP kinase signaling pathway by adenosine 3',5'-monophosphate. Science 1993;262(5136):1065–1069.

311. Light Y, Paterson H, Marais R. 14-3-3 antagonizes Ras-mediated Raf-1 recruitment to the plasma membrane to maintain signaling fidelity. Mol Cell Biol 2002;22(14):4984–4996.

312. Zimmermann S, Moelling K. Phosphorylation and regulation of Raf by Akt (protein kinase B). Science 1999;286(5445):1741–1744.

313. Ory S, Zhou M, Conrads TP, Veenstra TD, Morrison DK. Protein phosphatase 2A positively regulates Ras signaling by dephosphorylating KSR1 and Raf-1 on critical 14-3-3 binding sites. Curr Biol 2003;13(16):1356–1364.

314. Hekman M, Wiese S, Metz R, Albert S, Troppmair J, Nickel J, Sendtner M, Rapp UR. Dynamic changes in C-Raf phosphorylation and 14-3-3 protein binding in response to growth factor stimulation: differential roles of 14-3-3 protein binding sites. J Biol Chem 2004;279(14):14074–14086.

315. Rushworth LK, Hindley AD, O'Neill E, Kolch W. Regulation and role of Raf-1/B-Raf heterodimerization. Mol Cell Biol 2006;26(6):2262–2272.

316. Guan KL, Figueroa C, Brtva TR, Zhu T, Taylor J, Barber TD, Vojtek AB. Negative regulation of the serine/threonine kinase B-Raf by Akt. J Biol Chem 2000;275(35):27354–27359.

317. Ritt DA, Zhou M, Conrads TP, Veenstra TD, Copeland TD, Morrison DK. CK2 is a component of the KSR1 scaffold complex that contributes to Raf kinase activation. Curr Biol 2007;17(2):179–184.

318. Emuss V, Garnett M, Mason C, Marais R. Mutations of C-RAF are rare in human cancer because C-RAF has a low basal kinase activity compared with B-RAF. Cancer Res 2005;65(21):9719–9726.

319. Chen J, Fujii K, Zhang L, Roberts T, Fu H. Raf-1 promotes cell survival by antagonizing apoptosis signal-regulating kinase 1 through a MEK-ERK independent mechanism. Proc Natl Acad Sci USA 2001;98(14):7783–7788.

320. O'Neill E, Rushworth L, Baccarini M, Kolch W. Role of the kinase MST2 in suppression of apoptosis by the proto-oncogene product Raf-1. Science 2004;306(5705):2267–2270.

321. Ehrenreiter K, Piazzolla D, Velamoor V, Sobczak I, Small JV, Takeda J, Leung T, Baccarini M. Raf-1 regulates Rho signaling and cell migration. J Cell Biol 2005;168(6):955–964.

322. Claperon A, Therrien M. KSR and CNK: two scaffolds regulating RAS-mediated RAF activation. Oncogene 2007;26(22):3143–3158.

323. Kolch W. Coordinating ERK/MAPK signalling through scaffolds and inhibitors. Nat Rev Mol Cell Biol 2005;6(11):827–837.

324. Kortum RL, Lewis RE. The molecular scaffold KSR1 regulates the proliferative and oncogenic potential of cells. Mol Cell Biol 2004;24(10):4407–4416.

325. Channavajhala PL, Wu L, Cuozzo JW, Hall JP, Liu W, Lin LL, Zhang Y. Identification of a novel human kinase supporter of Ras (hKSR-2) that functions as a negative regulator of Cot (Tpl2) signaling. J Biol Chem 2003;278(47):47089–47097.

326. Therrien M, Chang HC, Solomon NM, Karim FD, Wassarman DA, Rubin GM. KSR, a novel protein kinase required for RAS signal transduction. Cell 1995;83(6):879–888.

327. Muller J, Ory S, Copeland T, Piwnica-Worms H, Morrison DK. C-TAK1 regulates Ras signaling by phosphorylating the MAPK scaffold, KSR1. Mol Cell 2001;8(5):983–993.

328. Jaffe AB, Aspenstrom P, Hall A. Human CNK1 acts as a scaffold protein, linking Rho and Ras signal transduction pathways. Mol Cell Biol 2004;24(4):1736–1746.

329. Ziogas A, Moelling K, Radziwill G. CNK1 is a scaffold protein that regulates Src-mediated Raf-1 activation. J Biol Chem 2005;280(25):24205–24211.

330. Jaffe AB, Hall A, Schmidt A. Association of CNK1 with Rho guanine nucleotide exchange factors controls signaling specificity downstream of Rho. Curr Biol 2005;15(5):405–412.

331. Alessi DR, Saito Y, Campbell DG, Cohen P, Sithanandam G, Rapp U, Ashworth A, Marshall CJ, Cowley S. Identification of the sites in MAP kinase kinase-1 phosphorylated by p74raf-1. EMBO J 1994;13(7):1610–1619.

332. Mansour M, Karmilowicz M, Hawrylik SJ, Nalcerio B, Angilly J, Conklyn MJ, Lilly CM, Drazen JM, Lee SE, Auperin DD, De Wet JR, Cohan VL, Showell HJ, Danley DE. Production and characterization of guinea pig IL-5 in baculovirus-infected insect cells. Am J Physiol 1996;270(6Pt 1): L1002–1007.

333. Crews CM, Alessandrini A, Erikson RL. The primary structure of MEK, a protein kinase that phosphorylates the ERK gene product. Science 1992;258(5081):478–480.

334. Zheng CF, Guan KL. Cloning and characterization of two distinct human extracellular signal-regulated kinase activator kinases, MEK1 and MEK2. J Biol Chem 1993;268(15):11435–11439.

335. Yoon S, Seger R. The extracellular signal-regulated kinase: multiple substrates regulate diverse cellular functions. Growth Factors 2006;24(1):21–44.

336. Vermeulen L, De Wilde G, Van Damme P, Vanden Berghe W, Haegeman G. Transcriptional activation of the NF-kappaB p65 subunit by mitogen- and stress-activated protein kinase-1 (MSK1). EMBO J 2003;22(6):1313–1324.

337. Wiggin GR, Soloaga A, Foster JM, Murray-Tait V, Cohen P, Arthur JS. MSK1 and MSK2 are required for the mitogen- and stress-induced phosphorylation of CREB and ATF1 in fibroblasts. Mol Cell Biol 2002;22(8):2871–2881.

338. Duncan EA, Anest V, Cogswell P, Baldwin AS. The kinases MSK1 and MSK2 are required for epidermal growth factor-induced, but not tumor necrosis factor-induced, histone H3 Ser10 phosphorylation. J Biol Chem 2006;281(18):12521–12525.

339. Kim HG, Lee KW, Cho YY, Kang NJ, Oh SM, Bode AM, Dong Z. Mitogen- and stress-activated kinase 1-mediated histone H3 phosphorylation is crucial for cell transformation. Cancer Res 2008;68(7):2538–2547.

340. Waskiewicz AJ, Flynn A, Proud CG, Cooper JA. Mitogen-activated protein kinases activate the serine/threonine kinases Mnk1 and Mnk2. EMBO J 1997;16(8):1909–1920.

341. Ueda T, Watanabe-Fukunaga R, Fukuyama H, Nagata S, Fukunaga R. Mnk2 and Mnk1 are essential for constitutive and inducible phosphorylation of eukaryotic initiation factor 4E but not for cell growth or development. Mol Cell Biol 2004;24(15):6539–6549.

342. Wendel HG, Silva RL, Malina A, Mills JR, Zhu H, Ueda T, Watanabe-Fukunaga R, Fukunaga R, Teruya-Feldstein J, Pelletier J, Lowe SW. Dissecting eIF4E action in tumorigenesis. Genes Dev 2007;21(24):3232–3237.

343. Wang X, Yue P, Chan CB, Ye K, Ueda T, Watanabe-Fukunaga R, Fukunaga R, Fu H, Khuri FR, Sun SY. Inhibition of mammalian target of rapamycin induces phosphatidylinositol 3-kinase-dependent and Mnk-mediated eukaryotic translation initiation factor 4E phosphorylation. Mol Cell Biol 2007;27(21):7405–7413.

344. Phillips A, Blaydes JP. MNK1 and EIF4E are downstream effectors of MEKs in the regulation of the nuclear export of HDM2 mRNA. Oncogene 2008;27(11):1645–1649.

345. Giroux S, Tremblay M, Bernard D, Cardin-Girard JF, Aubry S, Larouche L, Rousseau S, Huot J, Landry J, Jeannotte L, Charron J. Embryonic death of Mek1-deficient mice reveals a role for this kinase in angiogenesis in the labyrinthine region of the placenta. Curr Biol 1999;9(7):369–372.

346. Eliceiri BP, Klemke R, Stromblad S, Cheresh DA. Integrin alphavbeta3 requirement for sustained mitogen-activated protein kinase activity during angiogenesis. J Cell Biol 1998;140(5):1255–1263.

347. Mavria G, Vercoulen Y, Yeo M, Paterson H, Karasarides M, Marais R, Bird D, Marshall CJ. ERK-MAPK signaling opposes Rho-kinase to promote endothelial cell survival and sprouting during angiogenesis. Cancer Cell 2006;9(1):33–44.

348. Estep AL, Palmer C, McCormick F, Rauen KA. Mutation Analysis of BRAF, MEK1 and MEK2 in 15 ovarian cancer cell lines: implications for therapy. PLoS ONE 2007;2(12): e1279.

349. Rodriguez-Viciana P, Tetsu O, Tidyman WE, Estep AL, Conger BA, Cruz MS, McCormick F, Rauen KA. Germline mutations in genes within the MAPK pathway cause cardio-facio-cutaneous syndrome. Science 2006;311(5765):1287–1290.

350. Wan PT, Garnett MJ, Roe SM, Lee S, Niculescu-Duvaz D, Good VM, Jones CM, Marshall CJ, Springer CJ, Barford D, Marais R. Mechanism of activation of the RAF-ERK signaling pathway by oncogenic mutations of B-RAF. Cell 2004;116(6):855–867.

351. Davies H, Bignell GR, Cox C, Stephens P, Edkins S, Clegg S, Teague J, Woffendin H, Garnett MJ, Bottomley W, Davis N, Dicks E, Ewing R, Floyd Y, Gray K, Hall S, Hawes R, Hughes J, Kosmidou V, Menzies A, Mould C, Parker A, Stevens C, Watt S, Hooper S, Wilson R, Jayatilake H, Gusterson BA, Cooper C, Shipley J, Hargrave D, Pritchard-Jones K, Maitland N, Chenevix-Trench G, Riggins GJ, Bigner DD, Palmieri G, Cossu A, Flanagan A, Nicholson A, Ho JW, Leung SY, Yuen ST, Weber BL, Seigler HF, Darrow TL, Paterson H, Marais R, Marshall CJ, Wooster R, Stratton MR, Futreal PA. Mutations of the BRAF gene in human cancer. Nature 2002;417(6892):949–954.

352. Houben R, Becker JC, Kappel A, Terheyden P, Brocker EB, Goetz R, Rapp UR. Constitutive activation of the Ras-Raf signaling pathway in metastatic melanoma is associated with poor prognosis. J Carcinog 2004;3(1): 6.

353. Ikenoue T, Hikiba Y, Kanai F, Aragaki J, Tanaka Y, Imamura J, Imamura T, Ohta M, Ijichi H, Tateishi K, Kawakami T, Matsumura M, Kawabe T, Omata M. Different effects of point mutations within the B-Raf glycine-rich loop in colorectal tumors on mitogen-activated protein/extracellular signal-regulated kinase kinase/extracellular signal-regulated kinase and nuclear factor kappaB pathway and cellular transformation. Cancer Res 2004;64(10):3428–3435.

354. Ikenoue T, Hikiba Y, Kanai F, Tanaka Y, Imamura J, Imamura T, Ohta M, Ijichi H, Tateishi K, Kawakami T, Aragaki J, Matsumura M, Kawabe T, Omata M. Functional analysis of mutations within the kinase activation segment of B-Raf in human colorectal tumors. Cancer Res 2003;63(23):8132–8137.

355. Wellbrock C, Ogilvie L, Hedley D, Karasarides M, Martin J, Niculescu-Duvaz D, Springer CJ, Marais R. V599EB-RAF is an oncogene in melanocytes. Cancer Res 2004;64(7):2338–2342.

356. Liu J, Suresh Kumar KG, Yu D, Molton SA, McMahon M, Herlyn M, Thomas-Tikhonenko A, Fuchs SY. Oncogenic BRAF regulates beta-Trcp expression and NF-kappaB activity in human melanoma cells. Oncogene 2007;26(13):1954–1958.

357. Norris JL, Baldwin AS Jr. Oncogenic Ras enhances NF-kappaB transcriptional activity through Raf-dependent and Raf-independent mitogen-activated protein kinase signaling pathways. J Biol Chem 1999;274(20):13841–13846.

358. Solit DB, Garraway LA, Pratilas CA, Sawai A, Getz G, Basso A, Ye Q, Lobo JM, She Y, Osman I, Golub TR, Sebolt-Leopold J, Sellers WR, Rosen N. BRAF mutation predicts sensitivity to MEK inhibition. Nature 2006;439(7074):358–362.

359. Brose MS, Volpe P, Feldman M, Kumar M, Rishi I, Gerrero R, Einhorn E, Herlyn M, Minna J, Nicholson A, Roth JA, Albelda SM, Davies H, Cox C, Brignell G, Stephens P, Futreal PA, Wooster R, Stratton MR, Weber BL. BRAF and RAS mutations in human lung cancer and melanoma. Cancer Res 2002;62(23):6997–7000.

360. Dong J, Phelps RG, Qiao R, Yao S, Benard O, Ronai Z, Aaronson SA. BRAF oncogenic mutations correlate with progression rather than initiation of human melanoma. Cancer Res 2003;63(14):3883–3885.

361. Kumar R, Angelini S, Hemminki K. Activating BRAF and N-Ras mutations in sporadic primary melanomas: an inverse association with allelic loss on chromosome 9. Oncogene 2003;22(58):9217–9224.

362. Pollock PM, Harper UL, Hansen KS, Yudt LM, Stark M, Robbins CM, Moses TY, Hostetter G, Wagner U, Kakareka J, Salem G, Pohida T, Heenan P, Duray P, Kallioniemi O, Hayward NK, Trent JM, Meltzer PS. High frequency of BRAF mutations in nevi. Nat Genet 2003;33(1):19–20.

363. Satyamoorthy K, Li G, Gerrero MR, Brose MS, Volpe P, Weber BL, Van Belle P, Elder DE, Herlyn M. Constitutive mitogen-activated protein kinase activation in melanoma is mediated by both BRAF mutations and autocrine growth factor stimulation. Cancer Res 2003;63(4):756–759.

364. Cohen Y, Xing M, Mambo E, Guo Z, Wu G, Trink B, Beller U, Westra WH, Ladenson PW, Sidransky D. BRAF mutation in papillary thyroid carcinoma. J Natl Cancer Inst 2003;95(8):625–627.

365. Kimura ET, Nikiforova MN, Zhu Z, Knauf JA, Nikiforov YE, Fagin JA. High prevalence of BRAF mutations in thyroid cancer: genetic evidence for constitutive activation of the RET/PTC-RAS-BRAF signaling pathway in papillary thyroid carcinoma. Cancer Res 2003;63(7):1454–1457.

366. Nikiforova MN, Ciampi R, Salvatore G, Santoro M, Gandhi M, Knauf JA, Thomas GA, Jeremiah S, Bogdanova TI, Tronko MD, Fagin JA, Nikiforov YE. Low prevalence of BRAF mutations in radiation-induced thyroid tumors in contrast to sporadic papillary carcinomas. Cancer Lett 2004;209(1):1–6.

367. Nikiforova MN, Kimura ET, Gandhi M, Biddinger PW, Knauf JA, Basolo F, Zhu Z, Giannini R, Salvatore G, Fusco A, Santoro M, Fagin JA, Nikiforov YE. BRAF mutations in thyroid tumors are restricted to papillary carcinomas and anaplastic or poorly differentiated carcinomas arising from papillary carcinomas. J Clin Endocrinol Metab 2003;88(11):5399–5404.

368. Salvatore G, Giannini R, Faviana P, Caleo A, Migliaccio I, Fagin JA, Nikiforov YE, Troncone G, Palombini L, Basolo F, Santoro M. Analysis of BRAF point mutation and RET/PTC rearrangement

refines the fine-needle aspiration diagnosis of papillary thyroid carcinoma. J Clin Endocrinol Metab 2004;89(10):5175–5180.

369. Deng G, Bell I, Crawley S, Gum J, Terdiman JP, Allen BA, Truta B, Sleisenger MH, Kim YS. BRAF mutation is frequently present in sporadic colorectal cancer with methylated hMLH1, but not in hereditary nonpolyposis colorectal cancer. Clin Cancer Res 2004;10(1Pt 1):191–195.

370. Rajagopalan H, Bardelli A, Lengauer C, Kinzler KW, Vogelstein B, Velculescu VE. Tumorigenesis: RAF/RAS oncogenes and mismatch-repair status. Nature 2002;418(6901): 934.

371. Yuen ST, Davies H, Chan TL, Ho JW, Bignell GR, Cox C, Stephens P, Edkins S, Tsui WW, Chan AS, Futreal PA, Stratton MR, Wooster R, Leung SY. Similarity of the phenotypic patterns associated with BRAF and KRAS mutations in colorectal neoplasia. Cancer Res 2002;62(22):6451–6455.

372. Feng YZ, Shiozawa T, Miyamoto T, Kashima H, Kurai M, Suzuki A, Konishi I. BRAF mutation in endometrial carcinoma and hyperplasia: correlation with KRAS and p53 mutations and mismatch repair protein expression. Clin Cancer Res 2005;11(17):6133–6138.

373. Singer G, Oldt R 3rd, Cohen Y, Wang BG, Sidransky D, Kurman RJ, Shih Ie M. Mutations in BRAF and KRAS characterize the development of low-grade ovarian serous carcinoma. J Natl Cancer Inst 2003;95(6):484–486.

374. Ho CL, Kurman RJ, Dehari R, Wang TL, Shih Ie M. Mutations of BRAF and KRAS precede the development of ovarian serous borderline tumors. Cancer Res 2004;64(19):6915–6918.

375. Courtois-Cox S, Jones SL, Cichowski K. Many roads lead to oncogene-induced senescence. Oncogene 2008;27(20):2801–2809.

376. Sieben NL, Macropoulos P, Roemen GM, Kolkman-Uljee SM, Jan Fleuren G, Houmadi R, Diss T, Warren B, Al Adnani M, De Goeij AP, Krausz T, Flanagan AM. In ovarian neoplasms, BRAF, but not KRAS, mutations are restricted to low-grade serous tumours. J Pathol 2004;202(3):336–340.

377. Nakayama N, Nakayama K, Yeasmin S, Ishibashi M, Katagiri A, Iida K, Fukumoto M, Miyazaki K. KRAS or BRAF mutation status is a useful predictor of sensitivity to MEK inhibition in ovarian cancer. Br J Cancer 2008;99(12):2020–2028.

378. Hoeflich KP, Gray DC, Eby MT, Tien JY, Wong L, Bower J, Gogineni A, Zha J, Cole MJ, Stern HM, Murray LJ, Davis DP, Seshagiri S. Oncogenic BRAF is required for tumor growth and maintenance in melanoma models. Cancer Res 2006;66(2):999–1006.

379. Kumar R, Angelini S, Czene K, Sauroja I, Hahka-Kemppinen M, Pyrhonen S, Hemminki K. BRAF mutations in metastatic melanoma: a possible association with clinical outcome. Clin Cancer Res 2003;9(9):3362–3368.

380. Xing M. BRAF mutation in thyroid cancer. Endocr Relat Cancer 2005;12(2):245–262.

381. Xing M, Westra WH, Tufano RP, Cohen Y, Rosenbaum E, Rhoden KJ, Carson KA, Vasko V, Larin A, Tallini G, Tolaney S, Holt EH, Hui P, Umbricht CB, Basaria S, Ewertz M, Tufaro AP, Califano JA, Ringel MD, Zeiger MA, Sidransky D, Ladenson PW. BRAF mutation predicts a poorer clinical prognosis for papillary thyroid cancer. J Clin Endocrinol Metab 2005;90(12):6373–6379.

382. Chan TL, Zhao W, Leung SY, Yuen ST. BRAF and KRAS mutations in colorectal hyperplastic polyps and serrated adenomas. Cancer Res 2003;63(16):4878–4881.

383. Thibodeau SN, French AJ, Cunningham JM, Tester D, Burgart LJ, Roche PC, McDonnell SK, Schaid DJ, Vockley CW, Michels VV, Farr GH Jr, O'Connell MJ. Microsatellite instability in colorectal cancer: different mutator phenotypes and the principal involvement of hMLH1. Cancer Res 1998;58(8):1713–1718.

384. Herman JG, Umar A, Polyak K, Graff JR, Ahuja N, Issa JP, Markowitz S, Willson JK, Hamilton SR, Kinzler KW, Kane MF, Kolodner RD, Vogelstein B, Kunkel TA, Baylin SB. Incidence and functional consequences of hMLH1 promoter hypermethylation in colorectal carcinoma. Proc Natl Acad Sci USA 1998;95(12):6870–6875.

385. Cunningham JM, Christensen ER, Tester DJ, Kim CY, Roche PC, Burgart LJ, Thibodeau SN. Hypermethylation of the hMLH1 promoter in colon cancer with microsatellite instability. Cancer Res 1998;58(15):3455–3460.

386. Li WQ, Kawakami K, Ruszkiewicz A, Bennett G, Moore J, Iacopetta B. BRAF mutations are associated with distinctive clinical, pathological and molecular features of colorectal cancer independently of microsatellite instability status. Mol Cancer 2006;5:2.

387. Andreyev HJ, Norman AR, Cunningham D, Oates J, Dix BR, Iacopetta BJ, Young J, Walsh T, Ward R, Hawkins N, Beranek M, Jandik P, Benamouzig R, Jullian E, Laurent-Puig P, Olschwang S, Muller O, Hoffmann I, Rabes HM, Zietz C, Troungos C, Valavanis C, Yuen ST, Ho JW, Croke CT, O'Donoghue DP, Giaretti W, Rapallo A, Russo A, Bazan V, Tanaka M, Omura K, Azuma T, Ohkusa T, Fujimori T, Ono Y, Pauly M, Faber C, Glaesener R, de Goeij AF, Arends JW, Andersen SN, Lovig T, Breivik J, Gaudernack G, Clausen OP, De Angelis PD, Meling GI, Rognum TO, Smith R, Goh HS, Font A, Rosell R, Sun XF, Zhang H, Benhattar J, Losi L, Lee JQ, Wang ST, Clarke PA, Bell S, Quirke P, Bubb VJ, Piris J, Cruickshank NR, Morton D, Fox JC, Al-Mulla F, Lees N, Hall CN, Snary D, Wilkinson K, Dillon D, Costa J, Pricolo VE, Finkelstein SD, Thebo JS, Senagore AJ, Halter SA, Wadler S, Malik S, Krtolica K, Urosevic N. Kirsten ras mutations in patients with colorectal cancer: the "RASCAL II" study. Br J Cancer 2001;85(5):692–696.

388. Conlin A, Smith G, Carey FA, Wolf CR, Steele RJ. The prognostic significance of K-ras, p53, and APC mutations in colorectal carcinoma. Gut 2005;54(9):1283–1286.

389. van Lohuizen M, Verbeek S, Scheijen B, Wientjens E, van der Gulden H, Berns A. Identification of cooperating oncogenes in E mu-myc transgenic mice by provirus tagging. Cell 1991;65(5):737–752.

390. van der Lugt NM, Domen J, Verhoeven E, Linders K, van der Gulden H, Allen J, Berns A. Proviral tagging in E mu-myc transgenic mice lacking the Pim-1 proto-oncogene leads to compensatory activation of Pim-2. EMBO J 1995;14(11):2536–2544.

391. Feldman JD, Vician L, Crispino M, Tocco G, Marcheselli VL, Bazan NG, Baudry M, Herschman HR. KID-1, a protein kinase induced by depolarization in brain. J Biol Chem 1998;273(26):16535–16543.

392. Kumar A, Mandiyan V, Suzuki Y, Zhang C, Rice J, Tsai J, Artis DR, Ibrahim P, Bremer R. Crystal structures of proto-oncogene kinase Pim1: a target of aberrant somatic hypermutations in diffuse large cell lymphoma. J Mol Biol 2005;348(1):183–193.

393. Qian KC, Wang L, Hickey ER, Studts J, Barringer K, Peng C, Kronkaitis A, Li J, White A, Mische S, Farmer B. Structural basis of constitutive activity and a unique nucleotide binding mode of human Pim-1 kinase. J Biol Chem 2005;280(7):6130–6137.

394. Mikkers H, Nawijn M, Allen J, Brouwers C, Verhoeven E, Jonkers J, Berns A. Mice deficient for all PIM kinases display reduced body size and impaired responses to hematopoietic growth factors. Mol Cell Biol 2004;24(13):6104–6115.

395. Sivertsen EA, Galteland E, Mu D, Holte H, Meza-Zepeda L, Myklebost O, Patzke S, Smeland EB, Stokke T. Gain of chromosome 6p is an infrequent cause of increased PIM1 expression in B-cell non-Hodgkin's lymphomas. Leukemia 2006;20(3):539–542.

396. Kim KT, Baird K, Ahn JY, Meltzer P, Lilly M, Levis M, Small D. Pim-1 is up-regulated by constitutively activated FLT3 and plays a role in FLT3-mediated cell survival. Blood 2005;105(4):1759–1767.

397. Dhanasekaran SM, Barrette TR, Ghosh D, Shah R, Varambally S, Kurachi K, Pienta KJ, Rubin MA, Chinnaiyan AM. Delineation of prognostic biomarkers in prostate cancer. Nature 2001;412(6849):822–826.

398. Ellwood-Yen K, Graeber TG, Wongvipat J, Iruela-Arispe ML, Zhang J, Matusik R, Thomas GV, Sawyers CL. Myc-driven murine prostate cancer shares molecular features with human prostate tumors. Cancer Cell 2003;4(3):223–238.

399. Zippo A, De Robertis A, Serafini R, Oliviero S. PIM1-dependent phosphorylation of histone H3 at serine 10 is required for MYC-dependent transcriptional activation and oncogenic transformation. Nat Cell Biol 2007;9(8):932–944.

400. Bachmann M, Hennemann H, Xing PX, Hoffmann I, Moroy T. The oncogenic serine/threonine kinase Pim-1 phosphorylates and inhibits the activity of Cdc25C-associated kinase 1 (C-TAK1): a novel role for Pim-1 at the G2/M cell cycle checkpoint. J Biol Chem 2004;279(46):48319–48328.

401. Bachmann M, Kosan C, Xing PX, Montenarh M, Hoffmann I, Moroy T. The oncogenic serine/threonine kinase Pim-1 directly phosphorylates and activates the G2/M specific phosphatase Cdc25C. Int J Biochem Cell Biol 2006;38(3):430–443.

402. Mochizuki T, Kitanaka C, Noguchi K, Muramatsu T, Asai A, Kuchino Y. Physical and functional interactions between Pim-1 kinase and Cdc25A phosphatase. Implications for the Pim-1-mediated activation of the c-Myc signaling pathway. J Biol Chem 1999;274(26):18659–18666.

403. Chen WW, Chan DC, Donald C, Lilly MB, Kraft AS. Pim family kinases enhance tumor growth of prostate cancer cells. Mol Cancer Res 2005;3(8):443–451.

404. Macdonald A, Campbell DG, Toth R, McLauchlan H, Hastie CJ, Arthur JS. Pim kinases phosphorylate multiple sites on Bad and promote 14-3-3 binding and dissociation from Bcl-XL. BMC Cell Biol 2006;7:1.

405. Fox CJ, Hammerman PS, Cinalli RM, Master SR, Chodosh LA, Thompson CB. The serine/threonine kinase Pim-2 is a transcriptionally regulated apoptotic inhibitor. Genes Dev 2003;17(15):1841–1854.

406. Fujii C, Nakamoto Y, Lu P, Tsuneyama K, Popivanova BK, Kaneko S, Mukaida N. Aberrant expression of serine/threonine kinase Pim-3 in hepatocellular carcinoma development and its role in the proliferation of human hepatoma cell lines. Int J Cancer 2005;114(2):209–218.

407. Li YY, Popivanova BK, Nagai Y, Ishikura H, Fujii C, Mukaida N. Pim-3, a proto-oncogene with serine/threonine kinase activity, is aberrantly expressed in human pancreatic cancer and phosphorylates bad to block bad-mediated apoptosis in human pancreatic cancer cell lines. Cancer Res 2006;66(13):6741–6747.

408. Hammerman PS, Fox CJ, Birnbaum MJ, Thompson CB. Pim and Akt oncogenes are independent regulators of hematopoietic cell growth and survival. Blood 2005;105(11):4477–4483.

409. Fox CJ, Hammerman PS, Thompson CB. The Pim kinases control rapamycin-resistant T cell survival and activation. J Exp Med 2005;201(2):259–266.

410. Adam M, Pogacic V, Bendit M, Chappuis R, Nawijn MC, Duyster J, Fox CJ, Thompson CB, Cools J, Schwaller J. Targeting PIM kinases impairs survival of hematopoietic cells transformed by kinase inhibitor-sensitive and kinase inhibitor-resistant forms of Fms-like tyrosine kinase 3 and BCR/ABL. Cancer Res 2006;66(7):3828–3835.

411. Castagna M, Deleers M, Malaisse WJ. Ionophoretic effect of tumor promoter phorbol diester: a clue to its insulinotropic action? Carcinog Compr Surv 1982;7:555–559.

412. Kikkawa U, Takai Y, Tanaka Y, Miyake R, Nishizuka Y. Protein kinase C as a possible receptor protein of tumor-promoting phorbol esters. J Biol Chem 1983;258(19):11442–11445.

413. Leach KL, James ML, Blumberg PM. Characterization of a specific phorbol ester aporeceptor in mouse brain cytosol. Proc Natl Acad Sci USA 1983;80(14):4208–4212.

414. Sharkey NA, Leach KL, Blumberg PM. Competitive inhibition by diacylglycerol of specific phorbol ester binding. Proc Natl Acad Sci USA 1984;81(2):607–610.

415. Rozengurt E, Rey O, Waldron RT. Protein kinase D signaling. J Biol Chem 2005;280(14): 13205–13208.

416. Hommel U, Zurini M, Luyten M. Solution structure of a cysteine rich domain of rat protein kinase C. Nat Struct Biol 1994;1(6):383–387.

417. Schechtman D, Mochly-Rosen D. Adaptor proteins in protein kinase C-mediated signal transduction. Oncogene 2001;20(44):6339–6347.

418. Newton AC. Regulation of the ABC kinases by phosphorylation: protein kinase C as a paradigm. Biochem J 2003;370(Pt 2):361–371.

419. Gao T, Brognard J, Newton AC. The phosphatase PHLPP controls the cellular levels of protein kinase C. J Biol Chem 2007;283(10):6300–6311.

420. Arbuzova A, Schmitz AA, Vergeres G. Cross-talk unfolded: MARCKS proteins. Biochem J 2002;362(Pt 1):1–12.

421. Herget T, Oehrlein SA, Pappin DJ, Rozengurt E, Parker PJ. The myristoylated alanine-rich C-kinase substrate (MARCKS) is sequentially phosphorylated by conventional, novel and atypical isotypes of protein kinase C. Eur J Biochem 1995;233(2):448–457.

422. Myat MM, Anderson S, Allen LA, Aderem A. MARCKS regulates membrane ruffling and cell spreading. Curr Biol 1997;7(8):611–614.

423. Tsai JH, Hsieh YS, Kuo SJ, Chen ST, Yu SY, Huang CY, Chang AC, Wang YW, Tsai MT, Liu JY. Alteration in the expression of protein kinase C isoforms in human hepatocellular carcinoma. Cancer Lett 2000;161(2):171–175.

424. Hsieh YH, Wu TT, Tsai JH, Huang CY, Hsieh YS, Liu JY. PKC alpha expression regulated by Elk-1 and MZF-1 in human HCC cells. Biochem Biophys Res Commun 2006;339(1):217–225.

425. Oster H, Leitges M. Protein kinase C alpha but not PKC zeta suppresses intestinal tumor formation in ApcMin/+ mice. Cancer Res 2006;66(14):6955–6963.

426. Hsieh YH, Wu TT, Huang CY, Hsieh YS, Hwang JM, Liu JY. p38 mitogen-activated protein kinase pathway is involved in protein kinase C alpha-regulated invasion in human hepatocellular carcinoma cells. Cancer Res 2007;67(9):4320–4327.

427. Vetter M, Blumenthal SG, Lindemann RK, Manns J, Wesselborg S, Thomssen C, Dittmer J. Ets1 is an effector of protein kinase C alpha in cancer cells. Oncogene 2005;24(4):650–661.

428. Lin X, Yu Y, Zhao H, Zhang Y, Manela J, Tonetti DA. Overexpression of PKC alpha is required to impart estradiol inhibition and tamoxifen-resistance in a T47D human breast cancer tumor model. Carcinogenesis 2006;27(8):1538–1546.

429. Magnifico A, Albano L, Campaner S, Campiglio M, Pilotti S, Menard S, Tagliabue E. Protein kinase C alpha determines HER2 fate in breast carcinoma cells with HER2 protein overexpression without gene amplification. Cancer Res 2007;67(11):5308–5317.

430. Mandil R, Ashkenazi E, Blass M, Kronfeld I, Kazimirsky G, Rosenthal G, Umansky F, Lorenzo PS, Blumberg PM, Brodie C. Protein kinase C alpha and protein kinase C delta play opposite roles in the proliferation and apoptosis of glioma cells. Cancer Res 2001;61(11):4612–4619.

431. Hans CP, Weisenburger DD, Greiner TC, Chan WC, Aoun P, Cochran GT, Pan Z, Smith LM, Lynch JC, Bociek RG, Bierman PJ, Vose JM, Armitage JO. Expression of PKC-beta or cyclin D2 predicts for inferior survival in diffuse large B-cell lymphoma. Mod Pathol 2005;18(10):1377–1384.

432. Schaffel R, Morais JC, Biasoli I, Lima J, Scheliga A, Romano S, Milito C, Spector N. PKC-beta II expression has prognostic impact in nodal diffuse large B-cell lymphoma. Mod Pathol 2007;20(3):326–330.

433. Salven P, Teerenhovi L, Joensuu H. A high pretreatment serum vascular endothelial growth factor concentration is associated with poor outcome in non-Hodgkin's lymphoma. Blood 1997;90(8):3167–3172.

434. Yoshiji H, Kuriyama S, Ways DK, Yoshii J, Miyamoto Y, Kawata M, Ikenaka Y, Tsujinoue H, Nakatani T, Shibuya M, Fukui H. Protein kinase C lies on the signaling pathway for vascular endothelial growth factor-mediated tumor development and angiogenesis. Cancer Res 1999;59(17):4413–4418.

435. Gokmen-Polar Y, Murray NR, Velasco MA, Gatalica Z, Fields AP. Elevated protein kinase C betaII is an early promotive event in colon carcinogenesis. Cancer Res 2001;61(4):1375–1381.

436. Zhang J, Anastasiadis PZ, Liu Y, Thompson EA, Fields AP. Protein kinase C (PKC) betaII induces cell invasion through a Ras/Mek-, PKC iota/Rac 1-dependent signaling pathway. J Biol Chem 2004;279(21):22118–22123.

437. Li H, Weinstein IB. Protein kinase C beta enhances growth and expression of cyclin D1 in human breast cancer cells. Cancer Res 2006;66(23):11399–11408.

438. Krasagakis K, Fimmel S, Genten D, Eberle J, Quas P, Ziegler W, Haller H, Orfanos CE. Lack of protein kinase C (PKC)-beta and low PKC-alpha, -delta, -epsilon, and -zeta isozyme levels in proliferating human melanoma cells. Int J Oncol 2002;20(4):865–871.

439. Oka M, Ogita K, Ando H, Horikawa T, Hayashibe K, Saito N, Kikkawa U, Ichihashi M. Deletion of specific protein kinase C subspecies in human melanoma cells. J Cell Physiol 1996;167(3):406–412.

440. Oka M, Kikkawa U, Nishigori C. Protein kinase C-betaII represses hepatocyte growth factor-induced invasion by preventing the association of adapter protein Gab1 and phosphatidylinositol 3-kinase in melanoma cells. J Invest Dermatol 2008;128(1):188–195.

441. Persaud SD, Hoang V, Huang J, Basu A. Involvement of proteolytic activation of PKC delta in cisplatin-induced apoptosis in human small cell lung cancer H69 cells. Int J Oncol 2005;27(1):149–154.

442. Reyland ME, Anderson SM, Matassa AA, Barzen KA, Quissell DO. Protein kinase C delta is essential for etoposide-induced apoptosis in salivary gland acinar cells. J Biol Chem 1999;274(27):19115–19123.

443. Haughian JM, Jackson TA, Koterwas DM, Bradford AP. Endometrial cancer cell survival and apoptosis is regulated by protein kinase C alpha and delta. Endocr Relat Cancer 2006;13(4):1251–1267.

444. Cerda SR, Bissonnette M, Scaglione-Sewell B, Lyons MR, Khare S, Mustafi R, Brasitus TA. PKC-delta inhibits anchorage-dependent and -independent growth, enhances differentiation, and increases apoptosis in CaCo-2 cells. Gastroenterology 2001;120(7):1700–1712.

445. Jackson D, Zheng Y, Lyo D, Shen Y, Nakayama K, Nakayama KI, Humphries MJ, Reyland ME, Foster DA. Suppression of cell migration by protein kinase C delta. Oncogene 2005;24(18):3067–3072.

446. Perletti GP, Marras E, Concari P, Piccinini F, Tashjian AH Jr. PKC delta acts as a growth and tumor suppressor in rat colonic epithelial cells. Oncogene 1999;18(5):1251–1256.

447. Clark AS, West KA, Blumberg PM, Dennis PA. Altered protein kinase C (PKC) isoforms in non-small cell lung cancer cells: PKC delta promotes cellular survival and chemotherapeutic resistance. Cancer Res 2003;63(4):780–786.

448. Jackson DN, Foster DA. The enigmatic protein kinase C delta: complex roles in cell proliferation and survival. FASEB J 2004;18(6):627–636.

449. Cacace AM, Guadagno SN, Krauss RS, Fabbro D, Weinstein IB. The epsilon isoform of protein kinase C is an oncogene when overexpressed in rat fibroblasts. Oncogene 1993;8(8):2095–2104.

450. Mischak H, Goodnight JA, Kolch W, Martiny-Baron G, Schaechtle C, Kazanietz MG, Blumberg PM, Pierce JH, Mushinski JF. Overexpression of protein kinase C-delta and -epsilon in NIH 3T3 cells induces opposite effects on growth, morphology, anchorage dependence, and tumorigenicity. J Biol Chem 1993;268(9):6090–6096.

451. Basu A, Sivaprasad U. Protein kinase C epsilon makes the life and death decision. Cell Signal 2007;19(8):1633–1642.

452. Pan Q, Bao LW, Kleer CG, Sabel MS, Griffith KA, Teknos TN, Merajver SD. Protein kinase C epsilon is a predictive biomarker of aggressive breast cancer and a validated target for RNA interference anticancer therapy. Cancer Res 2005;65(18):8366–8371.

453. Sharif TR, Sharif M. Overexpression of protein kinase C epsilon in astroglial brain tumor derived cell lines and primary tumor samples. Int J Oncol 1999;15(2):237–243.

454. Lu D, Huang J, Basu A. Protein kinase C epsilon activates protein kinase B/Akt via DNA-PK to protect against tumor necrosis factor-alpha-induced cell death. J Biol Chem 2006;281(32):22799–22807.

455. Wu D, Thakore CU, Wescott GG, McCubrey JA, Terrian DM. Integrin signaling links protein kinase C epsilon to the protein kinase B/Akt survival pathway in recurrent prostate cancer cells. Oncogene 2004;23(53):8659–8672.

456. Fields AP, Regala RP. Protein kinase C iota: human oncogene, prognostic marker and therapeutic target. Pharmacol Res 2007;55(6):487–497.

457. de Vente J, Kiley S, Garris T, Bryant W, Hooker J, Posekany K, Parker P, Cook P, Fletcher D, Ways DK. Phorbol ester treatment of U937 cells with altered protein kinase C content and distribution induces cell death rather than differentiation. Cell Growth Differ 1995;6(4):371–382.

458. Ways DK, Posekany K, deVente J, Garris T, Chen J, Hooker J, Qin W, Cook P, Fletcher D, Parker P. Overexpression of protein kinase C-zeta stimulates leukemic cell differentiation. Cell Growth Differ 1994;5(11):1195–1203.

459. Wooten MW, Vandenplas ML, Seibenhener ML, Geetha T, Diaz-Meco MT. Nerve growth factor stimulates multisite tyrosine phosphorylation and activation of the atypical protein kinase C's via a src kinase pathway. Mol Cell Biol 2001;21(24):8414–8427.

460. Murray NR, Jamieson L, Yu W, Zhang J, Gokmen-Polar Y, Sier D, Anastasiadis P, Gatalica Z, Thompson EA, Fields AP. Protein kinase C iota is required for Ras transformation and colon carcinogenesis in vivo. J Cell Biol 2004;164(6):797–802.

461. Mwanjewe J, Spitaler M, Ebner M, Windegger M, Geiger M, Kampfer S, Hofmann J, Uberall F, Grunicke HH. Regulation of phospholipase D isoenzymes by transforming Ras and atypical protein kinase C-iota. Biochem J 2001;359(Pt 1):211–217.

462. Regala RP, Weems C, Jamieson L, Copland JA, Thompson EA, Fields AP. Atypical protein kinase C iota plays a critical role in human lung cancer cell growth and tumorigenicity. J Biol Chem 2005;280(35):31109–31115.

463. Stallings-Mann M, Jamieson L, Regala RP, Weems C, Murray NR, Fields AP. A novel small-molecule inhibitor of protein kinase C iota blocks transformed growth of non-small-cell lung cancer cells. Cancer Res 2006;66(3):1767–1774.

464. Lu Y, Jamieson L, Brasier AR, Fields AP. NF-kappaB/RelA transactivation is required for atypical protein kinase C iota-mediated cell survival. Oncogene 2001;20(35):4777–4792.

465. Sanz L, Sanchez P, Lallena MJ, Diaz-Meco MT, Moscat J. The interaction of p62 with RIP links the atypical PKCs to NF-kappaB activation. EMBO J 1999;18(11):3044–3053.

466. Regala RP, Weems C, Jamieson L, Khoor A, Edell ES, Lohse CM, Fields AP. Atypical protein kinase C iota is an oncogene in human non-small cell lung cancer. Cancer Res 2005;65(19):8905–8911.

467. Zhang L, Huang J, Yang N, Liang S, Barchetti A, Giannakakis A, Cadungog MG, O'Brien-Jenkins A, Massobrio M, Roby KF, Katsaros D, Gimotty P, Butzow R, Weber BL, Coukos G. Integrative genomic analysis of protein kinase C (PKC) family identifies PKC iota as a biomarker and potential oncogene in ovarian carcinoma. Cancer Res 2006;66(9):4627–4635.

468. Gustafson WC, Ray S, Jamieson L, Thompson EA, Brasier AR, Fields AP. Bcr-Abl regulates protein kinase C iota (PKC iota) transcription via an Elk1 site in the PKC iota promoter. J Biol Chem 2004;279(10):9400–9408.

469. Evans JD, Cornford PA, Dodson A, Neoptolemos JP, Foster CS. Expression patterns of protein kinase C isoenzymes are characteristically modulated in chronic pancreatitis and pancreatic cancer. Am J Clin Pathol 2003;119(3):392–402.

CHAPTER 6

CELL CYCLE CONTROL

T HE CELL division cycle is central to all organisms and consists of two sequential processes: interphase, during which the cell doubles its mass and duplicates its contents, and M (mitotic) phase, during which two daughter cells are formed, each with a complete set of chromosomes. Interphase is composed of successive G1 (Gap1), S (Synthesis), and G2 (Gap2) phases. During the G1 phase, cells resume a high rate of biosynthesis, especially those proteins needed for DNA replication. The S phase begins with the initiation of chromosomal DNA synthesis and ends when the DNA content of the nucleus has doubled with completion of chromosome replication. During G2 phase, cells synthesize proteins that are required for M phase, which consists of nuclear division (karyokinesis) and cytoplasmic division (cytokinesis). These complex events are under continuous surveillance by a series of coordinated cell cycle checkpoint mechanisms, which respond to aberrations in DNA replication or cell division by halting cell cycle progression, recruiting various repair mechanisms and, in the event of catastrophic damage, activating cell death pathways in order to prevent neoplastic growth. Protein kinases are central regulators of all of these aspects of cell cycle progression, DNA replication, cell division, and checkpoint control and, not surprisingly, tumor cells often hijack these pathways in order to fuel their unregulated growth. In this chapter, we review the biology of kinases that are prominently involved in cell cycle progression and consider their potential as cancer targets.

6.1 CYCLIN-DEPENDENT KINASES (CDKS) AND CELL CYCLE PROGRESSION

The cyclin-dependent kinases (CDKs) comprise a family of protein kinases characterized by a required association with regulatory cyclin proteins for functional kinase activity. CDKs, which typically are about 300 amino acids in length and have specific cyclin binding partners depending on their cellular function, phosphorylate diverse protein substrates to regulate vital steps in progression through the

Targeting Protein Kinases for Cancer Therapy, by David J. Matthews and Mary E. Gerritsen
Copyright © 2010 John Wiley & Sons, Inc.

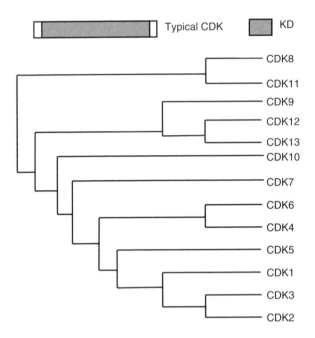

Figure 6.1 The CDK kinase family. Relationship between different CDKs is shown as a phylogenetic tree based on alignment of the human protein sequences. Typically, each protein is comprised of just the kinase domain with short N- and C-terminal flanking sequences.

cell division cycle, mRNA transcription, mRNA splicing, or neuronal cell development. CDK1, the prototypical CDK, was originally named CDC2. At the 1991 Cold Spring Harbor Symposium on the Cell Cycle, a consensus was established that CDC2-related kinases that bind to cyclins would be named "CDK" for cyclin-dependent kinase and numbered in order of their discovery. CDC2 was the first member of this family and renamed CDK1. To date, at least twelve CDKs and twelve cyclins have been identified in mammalian cells. Individual members of the CDK family associate with different cyclin partners, thereby serving as a central component of the control system that orders and coordinates the events of the cell-division cycle (e.g., CDKs 1, 2, 3, 4, and 6), transcriptional and post-transcriptional regulation (e.g., CDKs 7, 8, 9, 11, 12, and 13), and neuronal development (e.g., CDK5) (Figure 6.1). The composition and regulation of cyclin:CDK complexes varies according to cell type and environment. A diverse array of mechanisms that involve post-translational modification, subcellular localization, and protein interactions ensures tight control of the timing and extent of CDK activation. The various CDKs are discussed in two general groups based on their function: cell cycle regulation (this section) and mRNA production (Section 6.2).

6.1.1 Introduction

Progression through the cell-division cycle is regulated by the coordinated activities of cyclin:CDK complexes (Figure 6.2). Whereas CDK protein levels are constant throughout the cell cycle, cyclin protein levels are cell cycle regulated. Therefore cyclin expression restricts CDK function to distinct intervals within the cell cycle:

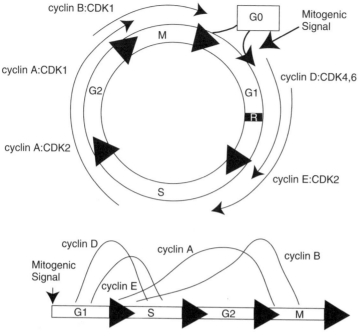

Figure 6.2 The cell cycle clock and CDKs/cyclins. The cell-division cycle consists of four sequential phases—G1, S, G2, and M—and the transition between these phases is regulated by the coordinated activities of cyclin:CDK complexes. Mitogenic signals are required for their activities and progression through the restriction point (R) of G1. When the signals are not strong enough to enhance CDK activity, cells exit the cell cycle and stay in the nonreplicative state (G0). The levels of cyclins, the regulatory subunits of CDKs, are cell cycle regulated, ensuring that CDKs are only functional during distinct intervals within the cell cycle. Adapted from (48) with permission. Copyright © 2008 Elsevier.

CDK2, CDK3, CDK4, and CDK6 activity allows cells to proceed through interphase, and CDK1 activity is required for cells to proceed through mitosis. CDK gene knockout studies in mice, including single, double, and triple gene deletion of interphase CDKs, have investigated the functional redundancy of cell cycle CDKs. These studies demonstrate that only CDK1 is essential for progression through the cell cycle. Deletion of CDK2, CDK3, CDK4, or CDK6 delays entry into S phase but does not prohibit cell cycle progression. Taken together, the results of genetic studies reveal functional plasticity among cell cycle CDKs and suggest that the existence of multiple interphase CDKs is critical for cell-type-specific activity (e.g., CDK4 and CDK6 in hematopoietic cells, CDK4 in pancreatic beta cells, CDK6 in erythroid cells, CDK2 and CDK4 in cardiomyocytes, and CDK2 in germ cells). The molecular events that control the cell cycle are ordered and each process occurs in a sequential fashion to ensure that genomic integrity is maintained.

Upon receiving a promitotic extracellular signal, G1-phase cyclin:CDK complexes (cyclin D:CDK4/6 and cyclin E:CDK2) become active to promote the expression of transcription factors for induction of enzymes required for DNA replication. The G1-phase cyclin:CDK complexes also promote the ubiquitin-proteasome-dependent degradation of S-phase inhibitors. Therefore their activities are required for transition through the later G1 phase of the cell cycle past the restriction point (R), where the cell cycle becomes independent from external mitogenic stimuli and the irreversible decision is made to enter into S phase and initiate DNA synthesis. When mitogenic signals in the G1 phase are not strong enough to promote CDK activity, cells cannot enter into S phase but eventually will exit the cell cycle and acquire a reversible nonreplicative state (termed quiescence, or G0). Active S phase cyclin:CDK complexes (cyclin A:CDK2) phosphorylate proteins that make up the prereplication complexes assembled on chromosomal DNA replication origins, thereby ensuring that the cell's genome will be replicated only once. Mitotic phase cyclin:CDK complexes (cyclin A:CDK1 and cyclin B:CDK1) promote the initiation of mitosis by stimulating downstream proteins involved in chromosome condensation and mitotic spindle assembly. Abrupt degradation of the mitotic cyclins, which deactivate CDK1, causes the cell to exit mitosis (Section 6.4).

The retinoblastoma gene (*RB*), which encodes a nuclear phosphoprotein (Rb) with a molecular weight of about 105 kDa, was the first tumor suppressor gene cloned. Repression of Rb activity occurs through phosphorylation on multiple serine and threonine sites by cyclin:CDK complexes in response to mitogenic stimuli. Loss of Rb function by gene deletion or mutation is involved in the development of many cancer types (1). Rb is essentially hypophosphorylated when cells are in G0 and becomes progressively phosphorylated by G1-phase cyclin:CDK complexes as cells enter G1, becoming hyperphosphorylated on a large number of serine and threonine residues as cells advance through the R point. After cells have passed through the R point, Rb remains hyperphosphorylated through the remainder of the cell cycle. The phosphate groups on Rb are removed by the protein phosphatase PP1 as cells exit mitosis. Rb plays a critical role in cell cycle progression as the molecular governor of the R-point transition.

In the hypophosphorylated form, Rb assembles transcriptional repressor complexes on the promoters of target genes that are required to initiate DNA replication (2–4). In the absence of Rb, many critical Rb target genes are primed for active transcription by residence of transcriptional activator E2F:DP1 complexes on the promoter regions; however, the transcriptional repressor complexes recruited by Rb, which include histone deacetylases, SWI:SNF chromatin remodeling complexes, and/or polycomb group proteins, act as potent inhibitors of transcriptional activation. Hence mitogenic stimuli balance Rb phosphorylation and function through modulation of cyclin:CDK complexes (5, 6) (Figure 6.3). Phosphorylation of Rb and the related p107 and p130 (collectively referred to as "pocket proteins") is initiated by CDK4/6, which leads to partial inhibition of the Rb transcriptional repressor function. CDK2 further phosphorylates Rb and thereby extinguishes its repressor function. The CDK2-associated cyclins (E and A) also are regulated via Rb-mediated transcriptional repression, and thereby inhibition of Rb amplifies CDK2 activity to further stimulate cell cycle progression. The positive feedback loop between Rb, CDK2, and cell cycle progression is attenuated through the activity of CDK inhibitor proteins that are expressed in response to Rb phosphorylation.

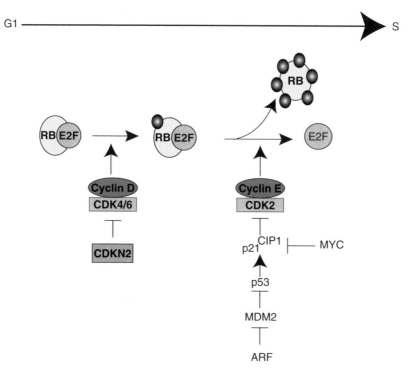

Figure 6.3 CDKs, tumor suppressors, and G1/S transition. Cyclin D:CDK4/6 and cyclin E:CDK2 phosphorylate the retinoblastoma protein (Rb) resulting in release of E2F, which is necessary for G1/S cell cycle progression. Members of the CDKN2 family of CDK inhibitors bind to and inactivate cyclin D:CDK4/6. ARF inhibits MDM2, resulting in p53 stabilization. p53 induces p21^{CIP1}, which inhibits cyclin E:CDK2. MYC blocks p21^{CIP1} induction by p53. The cyclin/CDK inhibitory pathways are often inactivated in tumor cells, which lead to hyperactivation of the cyclin:CDK complexes.

Disassociation of hyperphosphorylated Rb from E2F:DP1:Rb complexes activates E2F transcription factors (7, 8) and induces transcription of negative cell cycle regulators such as CDKN2 and ARF. The CDKN2/ARF locus on chromosome 9p21 is frequently deleted in human cancer, and CDKN2 and ARF play independent roles in tumor suppression (9, 10). CDKN2 (also known as INK4) family members are specific inhibitors of cyclin D:CDK4/6 complexes. ARF binds to and inactivates the MDM2 protein, an E3 ubiquitin ligase that targets the tumor suppressor p53 transcription factor for proteasomal degradation. As a result, p53 becomes stabilized and induces expression of the CDK2 inhibitor p21^{CIP1} (also known as CDKN1A or WAF1). The two major tumor-suppressor cascades mentioned earlier, the p16/CDK4/Rb and ARF/p53/p21/CDK2/Rb pathways, also are involved in control of senescence (a permanent nonreplicative state) (11), with cooperative signaling through these pathways. Therefore, in some tumor cells, the combined inhibition of CDK2 and CDK4 could lead to senescence and might be used as a possible therapeutic approach. The balance between mitogenic, antimitogenic, apoptotic, and stress response signals determines the ability of cells to proliferate by regulating CDK function.

6.1.2 CDK4 and CDK6

CDK4 was identified by screening a HeLa cell cDNA library with probes designed to recognize clones encoding protein–serine kinases (12) and was originally named PSK-J3. The CDK4 gene maps to chromosome 12q14 (13) and encodes a protein comprised of 303 amino acids with a molecular weight of 34 kDa. CDK6 was identified with degenerate primers corresponding to conserved regions of CDC2 including the PSTAIRE motif (a conserved sequence of amino acids in the C helix of the kinase domain) (14), and was originally named PLSTIRE. The gene for CDK6 maps to chromosome 7q21-q22, encoding a 326 amino acid protein with a molecular weight of 37 kDa. CDK4 and CDK6 are 70% identical with each other but only about 45% identical with other CDKs. CDK4 and CDK6 regulate progression through the G1 phase and entry into the S phase of the cell cycle. Both CDK4 and CDK6 are physiologic kinases of Rb and SMAD3, whose transcriptional activity and antiproliferative functions are inhibited by phosphorylation. CDK4 and CDK6 are activated early in G1 by binding to D-type cyclins (D1, D2, and D3), which share an average of 57% identity over their entire coding region and 78% within the cyclin box. The structure of an active CDK6 complex was solved by X-ray crystallography (15–17). The CDK6 structure, in common with other kinases, consists of two domains, with the smaller N-terminal domain rich in β-sheet structures (residues 1–100) and the larger C-terminal domain (residues 101–308) mostly α-helical. The ATP binding pocket is located between the two kinase domains. Cyclin:CDK binding induces a large conformational change of certain residues in the kinase ATP binding pocket, which leads to generation of an active CDK4/6 complex. The regulation of D-type cyclin:CDK complexes in vivo is complex and also involves various proteins that localize, fold, activate, export, and degrade the subunits. The activities of CDK4 and CDK6 also are regulated in a similar pattern as other cell cycle CDKs, by inhibitor protein binding and by protein phosphorylation. The CDK6 crystal structure indicates that the INK4 inhibitors bind next to the ATP binding site of the catalytic cleft, opposite the activating D-type cyclin binding site, and prevent cyclin binding indirectly by causing structural changes that propagate to the cyclin binding site. The INK4 inhibitors also distort the kinase catalytic cleft and interfere with ATP binding, which explains how they can also inhibit preassembled cyclin D:CDK4/6 complexes (15, 18). Stabilization of cyclin:CDK complex association requires phosphorylation at a threonine residue in the T-loop, an event that is mediated by the CDK activating kinase (CAK), which is a complex of CDK7, cyclin H, and MAT1 (19). Phosphorylation of threonine and tyrosine residues in the phosphate binding loop by tyrosine kinase WEE1 (20–22) and membrane-associated dual specificity kinase MYT1 (23) results in inactivation. This inactivation can be reversed by CDC25 phosphatases. Most cells express CDK4 and CDK6, although the activity of one often predominates in a particular cell type. For example, CDK4 is reported to be the main kinase activity in fibroblasts and macrophages, whereas CDK6 activity predominates in lymphocytes (24,

25). The ability to alter astrocyte morphology and to prevent terminal differentiation of erythrocytes is attributed specifically to CDK6 (26, 27).

Mouse genetic studies suggest that CDK4 and CDK6 might not completely compensate for each other. CDK4-null mice are viable but exhibit diabetes mellitus, growth retardation, and infertility (28). Embryonic fibroblasts from CDK4-null mice initially proliferate at normal rates, but they display a 4–5-hour delay in reentry into the cell cycle following quiescence (see Section 6.1.3). CDK6-null mice also are viable and develop normally, although hematopoiesis is slightly impaired (29). Embryos defective for both CDK4 and CDK6 die during the late stages of embryonic development due to severe anemia. However, these embryos display normal organogenesis, and most cell types proliferate normally. In vitro, embryonic fibroblasts lacking CDK4 and CDK6 proliferate and quiescent CDK4/CDK6-null cells respond to serum stimulation by entering S phase with normal kinetics, although with lower efficiency (29). Therefore D-type cyclin-dependent kinases are not essential for cell cycle entry upon mitogenic stimulation. Embryonic stem (ES) cells are consistently deficient in cyclin D-associated activity (30–32) and rely on CDK2 activity to drive the G1/S transition (33).

Cells lacking the CDK inhibitor $p21^{CIP1}/p27^{KIP1}$ have a substantial reduction in D-type cyclin/CDK activity, due in part to a function of the inhibitor that facilitates the assembly and import of cyclin:CDK complexes into the nucleus (28, 34). A cyclin-free form of CDK4/6, which binds to the cochaperone adaptor protein CDC37, is also found in cells (35, 36). CDC37 acts as a scaffold, simultaneously binding protein kinases and HSP90. The G15 and G18 residues of CDK4, which lie within the conserved GXGXXG motif that is required for ATP binding to the kinase, were identified as critical for CDC37:CDK4 complex formation (37). The crystal structure of a HSP90:CDC37:CDK4 complex reveals the binding locations of CDC37 and CDK4 and suggests a mechanism by which conformational changes in the kinase are coupled to the HSP90 ATPase cycle (38). CDC37 protein also specifically interacts with CDK6, but not with CDK1, CDK2, CDK3, CDK5, or any of a number of cyclins tested. CDC37 and the CDK inhibitor $p16^{INK4A}$ bind CDK4/6 competitively with each other (39). Whether CDC37 facilitates cyclin D1 binding independently of its role in CDK folding is unclear. An F-box protein, FBXO7 (F-box only protein 7), was determined to specifically enhance the activity of CDK6, but not CDK4 (40, 41). FBXO7 knockdown decreases CDK6 association with cyclin and its overexpression increases D-type cyclin/CDK6 activity and E2F activity. Transformed phenotypes due to FBXO7 overexpression are dependent on CDK6, as knockdown of CDK6 reverses the effect.

The INK4–cyclin D–CDK4/6–Rb pathway is frequently disrupted in human cancer. Although Rb loss occurs commonly in some tumor types, most tumors increase activity of cyclin D-dependent kinases by multiple mechanisms. Most commonly, the CDK inhibitor $p16^{INK4A}$ is inactivated by gene deletion, point mutation, or transcriptional silencing by methylation (42, 43). A $p18^{INK4C}$ mutant with a single amino acid substitution (A72 to P) is also found in human breast cancer cells (44). Another major increased activity of CDK4/6 can also occur by deregulation of D-type cyclins. Gene amplification or chromosomal translocation of cyclin D1 has been identified in the pathogenesis of parathyroid adenomas,

B-cell tumors, and a subset of breast and squamous cell cancers. Melanomas with wild-type BRAF or NRAS frequently have increased gene copy number for CDK4 and cyclin D1, which are downstream components of the RAS/BRAF pathway (Chapter 5). In fact, RAS-mediated tumorigenesis depends on signaling pathways that act preferentially through cyclin D1 (45–48). Cyclin D1 protein is stabilized by the chaperone HSPA8 (HSP73), and it was proposed that STAT5-mediated activation of HSPA8 induces nuclear translocation and activation of the cyclin D1:CDK4 complex, leading to increased proliferation of CML cells (49). Furthermore, cyclin D1 deficiency results in a dramatic reduction in the development of squamous tumors (50). Cells lacking D-type cyclins or CDK4/CDK6 exhibit resistance to transformation by known oncogenes, which further emphasizes the importance of this pathway in tumorigenesis (29, 51).

Mutations in the CDK4 locus are rare events, but R24C or H mutations with reduced affinity for p16^{INK4A} have been identified in malignant melanoma (52, 53). Indeed, tumor-derived mutations in INK4A and CDK4 map to interface contacts as confirmed by X-ray crystallography (15). Knockin mice expressing the CDK4 R24C mutant develop tumors with almost complete penetrance and melanoma with high frequency (54, 55). Alternatively, gene amplification of both wild-type CDK4 and R24C mutant CDK4 may also occur. CDK6 is overexpressed or disrupted by translocation in many cancers, for example, T-cell lymphoblastic lymphoma, T-cell ALL, natural killer/T-cell nasal lymphoma, glioblastoma multiforme, and B-cell splenic lymphomas with villous lymphocytes. However, no CDK6 mutations were identified within the p16^{INK4A} binding domain, and germline mutations in CDK6 do not make a significant contribution to melanoma predisposition. Rb loss, p16^{INK4A} inactivation, and CDK4 amplification/mutation are usually mutually exclusive events (56–59). Therefore, in cells that retain Rb, a CDK4/6 inhibitor would be expected to reduce Rb phosphorylation and induce G1 arrest (in the absence of CDK1 or CDK2 compensatory Rb phosphorylation); tumors lacking Rb, in which p16^{INK4A} is present at high levels and associated with CDK4/6, would not be responsive to such an agent (60).

6.1.3 CDK2

CDK2 was identified by screening a HeLa cell cDNA library for clones that can complement *CDC28* mutations of budding yeast *Saccharomyces cerevisiae* and was initially named cell division kinase 2 (61). The CDK2 gene maps to chromosome 12q13 (62) and encodes a protein of 298 amino acids with a molecular weight of 33 kDa. CDK2 shares 65% sequence identity with CDK1. After growth factor stimulation of normal human fibroblast cells, the mRNA for CDK2 appears late in G1 or in early S phase, slightly before CDK1 mRNA. Together with cyclin E, CDK2 is a key factor in the G1 checkpoint, promoting transition into S phase (63) and playing a role in the initiation of DNA replication (64). In complex with cyclin A, CDK2 promotes progression through S phase, and the active CDK2 complex persists in the nucleus through G2. CDK2 is positively regulated by phosphorylation of a conserved threonine residue (T160) that lies within the activation loop. CDK2 was proposed to be its own CAK (65), although the identity of the CAK that acts upon

CDK2 in cells remains unclear (see also Sections 6.1.7 and 6.2.2). CDK2 is also phosphorylated on T14 and Y15 during S and G2 phases and is dephosphorylated by CDC25 (66–69). Y15 phosphorylation by WEE1 significantly reduces CDK2 activity, primarily by reducing the affinity for protein substrate binding (70). Phosphorylation of CDK2 on T39 by AKT enhances cyclin A binding and causes the temporary cytoplasmic localization of the cyclin A:CDK2 complex (71). This CDK2 cytoplasmic redistribution is required for cell progression from S to G2-M phase, because the CDK2 T39A mutant, which lacks the phosphorylation site and is defective in cytoplasmic localization, severely affects cell cycle progression at the transition from S to G2-M. The structures of CDK2 in complex with cyclins A, B, and E have provided insight into the mechanism of cyclin:CDK activation and substrate recognition (72–78). Cyclin A binds to one side of the CDK2 catalytic cleft, inducing large conformational changes in the PSTAIRE helix and T-loop. These conformational changes activate the kinase through realignment of active site residues and alleviation of steric blockade at the catalytic cleft entrance (see Chapter 2).

CDK2 activity is regulated by binding of the protein inhibitor $p21^{CIP1}/p27^{KIP1}$. Activation of cyclin E:CDK2 is facilitated through sequestration of $p21^{CIP1}/p27^{KIP1}$ by cyclin D-dependent kinases as well as by D-type cyclins independently of CDK4, thus promoting G1–S progression (79–82). The underlying mechanism involves phosphorylation of $p27^{KIP1}$ on Y74, Y88, and/or Y89 by SRC, LYN, or ABL, which greatly decreases the ability of $p27^{KIP1}$ to inhibit CDK2 containing complexes. $p27^{KIP1}$ phosphorylation on Y88 and Y89 was reported to decrease its affinity for CDK2 while increasing affinity for CDK4 complexes (83). The S phase delay observed in $cdk4^{-/-}$ mouse embryonic fibroblasts is indirectly related to inhibition of CDK2 activity owing to the redistribution of $p27^{KIP1}$; the combined inactivation of CDK4 and $p27^{KIP1}$ restored CDK2 activity and S phase entry (84). Regulation of CDK2 activity by $p27^{KIP1}$ is influenced by degradation and localization of $p27^{KIP1}$. At physiologic levels of ATP the cyclin E:CDK2 complex phosphorylates $p27^{KIP1}$ at T187, which is then recognized by the ubiquitin-protein ligase SKP2, leading to the ubiquitination and degradation of $p27^{KIP1}$ (85, 86). Phosphorylation of $p27^{KIP1}$ by AKT at T157 within its nuclear localization motif, which impairs the nuclear import of $p27^{KIP1}$, relieves CDK2 from $p27^{KIP1}$-induced inhibition (87, 88). Cytoplasmic $p27^{KIP1}$ was seen in 41% of primary human breast cancers in conjunction with AKT activation and correlated with poor patient prognosis (89).

CDK2 in complex with cyclin E fully activates E2F by phosphorylation of Rb, thereby preventing Rb from binding E2F. However, this E2F transcriptional activation occurs only transiently to allow orderly S-phase progression. The attenuation of E2F activity also involves CDK2, although now in complex with cyclin A. The CDK2:cyclin A complex interacts with the N terminus of E2F1 and phosphorylates both E2F1 and its dimerization partner DP1. This phosphorylation event leads to inhibition of the DNA binding activity of the E2F1:DP1 dimer and the downregulation of E2F1 activity (90–93). An additional function of cyclin E:CDK2 is to couple the centrosome and DNA duplication cycles (94); however, in cells arrested in late G2 by the G2 DNA damage checkpoint response, cyclin A assumes an important role in centrosome amplification irrespective of the cyclin E status

(95). Centrosome amplification is commonly found in various types of cancers and is believed to contribute to chromosome instability in cancer cells (96–98).

CDK2 knockdown in cancer cell lines by siRNA has different effects depending on the cell lines tested. CDK2 siRNA does not interfere with proliferation of Rb-negative cervical cancer cell lines or U2OS osteosarcoma cells (99, 100). In contrast, CDK2 siRNA delays G1 progression in NCI-H1299 non small cell lung cancer cells (100) and induces G1 arrest in melanoma cells (101). $cdk2^{-/-}$ mice are viable and survive up to 2 years of age (102, 103), indicating that CDK2 is dispensable for proliferation and survival of most cell types. However, CDK2 is essential for completion of prophase I during meiotic cell division in male and female germ cells. In double knockouts of CDK2 and CDK4, Rb is initially phosphorylated but a negative feedback loop leads to concomitant decreases in Rb phosphorylation and transcription of E2F target genes (104, 105). Among these E2F-affected genes, CDK1 expression declines and further decreases Rb phosphorylation. $cdk2^{-/-}cdk4^{-/-}$ MEFs enter senescence prematurely, which contributes to their lack of proliferation at passage 4. In contrast, when CDK6 is deleted in a CDK2-null background, mice are viable and exhibit similar phenotypes to those that were observed in the respective single knockouts (29). CDK2 activity was found to increase in different types of human tumors, and correlations were found between the expression of CDK2 and its cyclin partners as well as progression and/or invasiveness of some cancers such as breast, leukemia, and melanoma (106) (see later discussion).

An oncogenic role for cyclin E has been suggested by studies of cyclin E-deficient cells, which are resistant to transformation by MYC alone or in combination with RAS, a dominant-negative p53, or adenovirus E1A, suggesting that cyclin E is a key component in oncogenic signaling (107). Perturbed downregulation of cyclin E:CDK2 activity might also contribute to tumorigenesis. Cyclin E is phosphorylated by GSK3β and CDK2; this modification is recognized by the SCF (FBW7) ubiquitin ligase, leading to ubiquitin-proteasome-dependent degradation (108–111). Following the G1/S-phase transition, downregulation of cyclin E:CDK2 kinase activity, but not D- or A-type cyclin-associated kinase activity, may be necessary for the maintenance of karyotypic stability in both immortalized rat embryo fibroblasts and human breast epithelial cells (112). Indeed, cyclin E-overexpressing transgenic mice develop mammary carcinomas (113), and the gene encoding FBW7 was found to be mutated in a cell line derived from breast cancer that expressed extremely high levels of cyclin E (108).

Cyclin A is synthesized and downregulated later than cyclin E but slightly earlier than cyclin B (114–116). Cyclin A1 is expressed at highest levels in the testis and certain myeloid leukemia cells (117), suggesting an important role of cyclin A1 in hematopoiesis and the etiology of myeloid leukemia. Cyclin A2 in cultured somatic cells is a rate-limiting component required for S- and M-phase progression (118), and targeted deletion of the murine gene is embryonically lethal (119). The important role of cyclin A2 in regulation of cell proliferation also is suggested by its transcriptional repression by promyelocytic leukemia zinc finger (PLZF) protein (120). PLZF is a negative regulator of cell cycle progression whose action ultimately leads to growth suppression, and which plays a role in maintaining the quiescent state in stem cells (121, 122). PLZF is phosphorylated by CDK2 at two consensus sites found within PEST domains present in the hinge region of the protein, which triggers the ubiquitination and subsequent degradation of PLZF (121). Therefore this CDK2-dpendent phosphorylation impairs PLZF transcriptional repression ability and increases the expression of cyclin A2, which in turn potentiates CDK2 activity, creating a positive feedback loop that antagonizes the growth inhibitory effects of PLZF.

6.1.4   CDK3

The CDK3 gene, like CDK1 and CDK2, was identified as a clone that can complement budding yeast kinase *CDC28* mutants (14). The gene for CDK3 has been mapped to chromosome 17q22-qter, telomeric to the BRCA1 and a locus that was shown to be frequently rearranged in breast cancer and other tumors (123). The CDK3 protein is comprised of 305 amino acids with a molecular weight of 36 kDa. CDK3 is closely related to CDK1 and CDK2 with 66% and 76% sequence identity, respectively, and shares the same PSTAIRE motif with them. CDK3 is expressed ubiquitously and binds to cyclin C, which was identified as a key regulator of cell cycle reentry in human cells (124). When mRNA levels of cyclin C peak during the G0/G1 transition, cyclin C/CDK3 stimulates Rb phosphorylation at S807/811, which is required for cells to exit G0 efficiently. CDK3 also binds to A- or E-type cyclins and phosphorylates $p70^{IK3-1}$ (interactor-1 with CDK3)/CABLES (connecting CDK5 with c-ABL) on S274 both in vitro and in vivo (125); however, the effect of CDK3-mediated phosphorylation on IK3-1 function is not clear.

CDK3-associated kinase activity is regulated by p27 but not by p16 or p21 and fluctuates throughout the cell cycle, peaking in mid-G1 and decreasing during G2 (126). CDK3 can bind to E2F complexes in vivo (127) and dominant-negative CDK3 inhibits E2F1, E2F2, and E2F3 but not E2F4 transcriptional activity in a phospho-Rb-independent manner, causing a G1 block that is specifically rescued by wild-type CDK3 but not by CDK2 (128). Constitutive ectopic expression of CDK3, but not CDK2, enhances MYC-induced proliferation and anchorage-independent growth, without any effect on cyclin D1, E, and A protein expression or kinase activities. However, in contrast to cyclin D- or E-associated kinase activities, CDK3 is unable to cooperate with RAS in fibroblast transformation, and it has no oncogenic potential (126).

Interestingly, there is a single point mutation in the *cdk3* gene of several *Mus musculus* strains commonly used in the laboratory but not in the gene of wild-mice species. This mutation results in truncation of the protein near the activation loop, thereby generating a null allele (129). Therefore CDK3 is not required for mouse development and any functional role played by CDK3 in the G1/S-phase transition is likely to be compensated by another CDK.

6.1.5   CDK1

CDK1 was identified as a cDNA clone that can complement a fission yeast temperature-sensitive *cdc2* mutation (130). The *CDK1* gene (initially named *p34 CDC2*) maps to chromosome 10q21.1 (131) and encodes a protein kinase comprised of 240 amino acids with a molecular weight of 34 kDa. CDK1 is transcriptionally and translationally regulated. Serum stimulation of fibroblasts results in a marked increase in *CDK1* transcription (132), and the eIF4G protein DAP5 mediates cap-independent translation through a functional internal ribosome entry site (IRES) in the 5′UTR (5′ untranslated region) of *CDK1*. The knockdown of endogenous DAP5 induced M-phase-specific caspase-dependent apoptosis, in part by attenuating translation of CDK1 (133). CDK1 is a catalytic subunit of a protein kinase complex, called the M-phase promoting factor, which induces entry into mitosis. It is activated by binding to A-type or B-type cyclins and by the removal of inhibitory phosphates from T14 and Y15 by the CDC25 dual function phosphatases. CDK1 contains the PSTAIRE C-helix sequence and requires activation loop phosphorylation at T161 by CAK (CDK7) for stable association with cyclins. Once active, the CDK1:cyclin complexes phosphorylate hundreds of substrate proteins, culminating with the successful transition into mitosis. Although there are no published crystallographic structures of CDK1, the homology model studies suggest that cyclin binding induces CDK1 conformational changes that reshape the ATP binding pocket's molecular volume (134, 135). Differences in the amino acid sequence and protein structure within and near the ATP pocket of CDK1, as compared to those of CDK2 and CDK5, might help the design of inhibitors with enhanced specificity for CDK1.

Cyclin A:CDK1 phosphorylates E2F-1 on S375 and promotes the formation of Rb:E2F1 complexes, contributing to the deactivation of E2F1 late in the cell cycle (136). Activation of cyclin A:CDK1 at the end of S phase also results in an inhibition of histone mRNA biosynthesis by phosphorylation of stem-loop binding protein (SLBP) on T61. SLBP binds the 3′ end of histone mRNAs, which is required for both histone pre-mRNA processing and histone mRNA translation (137). The CDK1 phosphorylation of SLBP primes phosphorylation on T60 by CK2 and is responsible for initiating SLBP degradation. This allows histone mRNAs to be cell cycle regulated, with their expression restricted to S phase (138).

In the normal cell cycle, mitotic cyclins accumulate during G2 and rapidly decline during mitotic exit. Cyclin B:CDK1 regulates assembly and activity of the DNA helicase MCM2–7 complex in late M and early G1 phases to prevent refiring of replication origins and ensure that replication of the genome occurs only once per cell division (139, 140). MCM2 can be phosphorylated by CDC7, CDK2, and CDK1. MCM3 was recently shown also to be phosphorylated by CDK1 (141). In Vivo, CDK1-dependent phosphorylation of MCM3 on S112 triggers its assembly with the remaining MCM subunits and subsequent chromatin loading of MCMs. Progression through mitosis requires the activation of cyclin B:CDK1 for successful nuclear envelope breakdown and chromosome condensation (142).

There are a number of interlinked positive and double-negative feedback loops in the cyclin B:CDK1 system (Figure 6.4). Active cyclin B:CDK1 phosphorylates and activates CDC25, which in turn activates cyclin B:CDK1. Active cyclin B:CDK1 phosphorylates and inactivates WEE1 and MYT1, which mediate inhibitory phosphorylation of CDK1 on T14 and Y15. In somatic cells, WEE1 becomes inactive at the onset of mitosis when active CDK1 phosphorylates it on

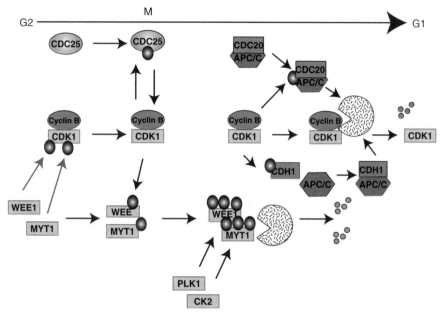

Figure 6.4 Feedback loops in the cyclin B:CDK1 system and G2/M/G1 transition. Active cyclin B:CDK1 kinase promotes the G2/M transition and M-phase progression through cyclin B/CDK1/CDC25/WEE1/MYT1 system. The activity of CDK1 is negatively controlled by WEE1/MYT1-dependent phosphorylation and positively regulated by CDC25-dependent dephosphorylation. The cyclin B:CDK1 complex remains active until cyclin B1 is polyubiquitinated and degraded by the E3-ubiquitin ligase APC/C^{CDC20} and APC/C^{CDH1} and the proteasome machinery, thereby resulting in the M/G1 transition.

S123 (143), thereby promoting the binding of WEE1 to the E3 ubiquitin ligase SKP1-cullin-Fbox (SCF), β-TrCP, and also priming phosphorylation of WEE1 by PLK1 and CK2 to generate additional β-TrCP binding sites. Subsequently, WEE1 is ubiquitinated and degraded by the proteasome machinery (144). This ensures rapid activation of CDK1 at the beginning of M phase assembly and activity of the DNA helicase MCM2–7 complex. The cyclin B:CDK1 complex remains active until cyclin B1 is degraded by the E3-ubiquitin ligase anaphase promoting complex/cyclosome (APC/C; see Section 6.4) (145).

Active CDK1 activates one form of the APC/C, APC/C^{CDC20} (146, 147), which catalyzes the polyubiquitination of the mitotic cyclins and results in the proteosome-mediated degradation of the cyclins, and hence the inactivation of CDK1. Both the CDK1/CDC25/WEE1/MYT1 system and the negative feedback loop (CDK1-APC/C^{CDC20}) are required for sustained, switch-like cell cycle oscillations in *Xenopus* egg extracts (148, 149). In somatic cells, another form of the APC/C, APC/C^{CDH1}, also promotes the ubiquitination and degradation of mitotic cyclins and other substrates at the end of mitosis and G1 (150, 151). With CDK1, APC/C^{CDH1} constitutes a double-negative feedback loop. During mitosis, active cyclin B:CDK1 inhibits CDH1 binding to APC/C. Subsequently, dephosphorylation of CDH1 allows the formation of active APC/C^{CDH1}, which continues to degrade cyclin B and inactivates CDK1. Studies in HeLa cells with a CDK1 mutant that cannot be phosphorylated by WEE1/MYT1 revealed the interplay between CDK1, WEE1/MYT1, and CDC25 that is required for the establishment of G1 phase, for the normal cell cycle period (~20 hours), and for the switch-like oscillations in cyclin B1 abundance characteristic of the somatic cell cycle (152).

Cdk1 knockout mouse embryos failed to develop to the morula and blastocyst stages (153). Conversely, mouse embryos lacking all interphase CDKs (CDK2, CDK3, CDK4, and CDK6) undergo organogenesis and develop to midgestation. In these embryos, CDK1 binds to all cyclins, resulting in the phosphorylation of Rb and the expression of genes that are regulated by E2F transcription factors. Mouse embryonic fibroblasts derived from these embryos proliferate in vitro and become immortal on continuous passage. Therefore CDK1 is the only essential cell cycle CDK and, in the absence of interphase CDKs, is capable of executing all the events required to drive cell division. Depletion of CDK1 in NCI-H1299 non small cell lung cancer or U2OS osteosarcoma cells results in an accumulation in G2/M and a moderate slowing of G2/M progression after release from synchronization (100), which might be due to compensation by CDK2. Combined depletion of CDK1 and CDK2 has a higher impact than the single knockdown, inducing apoptosis in U2OS and a strong G2/M block in NCI-H1299 cells. In MYC-overexpressing cells, inhibition of CDK1 leads to apoptosis instead of G2/M arrest (154). The cyclin B:CDK1 complex phosphorylates the inhibitor of apoptosis protein survivin on T34, resulting in protein stabilization (155). Inhibition of CDK1 rapidly downregulates survivin expression and induces MYC-dependent apoptosis. Furthermore, survivin depletion, like CDK1 inhibition, can cooperate with MYC overexpression to induce cell death. Therefore inhibition of CDK1 may have value in the treatment of human tumors that overexpress MYC. In a subset of AML, the NH_2-terminal region of the translocation liposarcoma (TLS) gene is fused to the COOH-terminal domain of ets-related gene (ERG) through a recurrent t(16; 21) translocation (156). The resultant TLS-ERG fusion protein is associated with poor clinical outcome (157). TLS-ERG transformation of L-G myeloid progenitor cells is accompanied by sustained expression of CDK1, and downregulation of CDK1 leads to restoration of terminal differentiation. Although it is unknown how TLS-ERG deregulates CDK1 expression in myeloid cells, CDK1 inhibitors or cell cycle blockers might provide new treatment strategies for acute myeloid leukemia characterized by the t(16; 21) chromosomal translocation (158). However, inhibition of CDK1 activity might result in resistance to chemotherapeutic drugs. For example, ERBB2 overexpression confers resistance to taxol-induced apoptosis in breast cancer cells by inhibiting CDK1 activation through ERBB2-mediated transcriptional upregulation of inhibitor p21^{CIP1} or through directly phosphorylating CDK1 Y15 (159, 160). A question regarding potential clinical utility of CDK1 inhibition is whether the tumor-cell benefit is adversely impacted by possible toxicities associated with loss of CDK1 activity in nontumor cells.

6.1.6   CDK10

CDK10 was identified by screening a HeLa cell cDNA library with probes designed to recognize clones encoding proteins containing regions conserved among CDK1-related proteins (161) and therefore was originally named PISSLRE based on the amino acid sequence of the region corresponding to the conserved CDK1 PSTAIRE motif. The CDK10 gene maps to chromosome 16q24, a region that is altered in several breast and prostate carcinomas (123), and encodes a protein comprised of 360 amino acids with a 33-kDa molecular weight. CDK10 shares 41% protein sequence identity with CDK1 including residues that are important regulatory sites in CDK1 and other CDKs, suggesting a similar regulation of its kinase activity. Both antisense and dominant-negative mutant constructs of CDK10 arrest cell cycle progression in G2-M and suppress cell growth, indicating that CDK10 is essential for cellular proliferation (162). Interestingly, no cyclin partner has yet been identified; however, CDK10 associates specifically with the N terminus of the ETS2 protein. ETS2 is a member of the ETS family of transcription factors, which are important regulators of gene expression during proliferation, differentiation, and development (163). CDK10 inhibits the transactivation capacity of ETS2 independently of its kinase activity. CDK10 silencing increases ETS2-driven transcription of RAF, resulting in MAPK pathway activation. In breast cancer patients treated with adjuvant tamoxifen, low CDK10 expression is associated with a statistically significant shorter time to distant relapse and poorer overall survival (164, 165), which appears to have no association with HER2 status or level of ERα expression. Low CDK10 expression is strongly associated with methylation of its promoter, suggesting an underlying mechanism of tamoxifen resistance. Therefore CDK10 may provide a new biomarker of endocrine responsiveness.

6.1.7   CCRK/CDCH/p42

Cell cycle-related kinase (CCRK)/cyclin-dependent protein kinase H (CDCH) was identified by using the BLAST search of lower eukaryotic genomes for the potential budding yeast CDK-activating kinase (CAK) ortholog and then comparing the resultant molecules to human and mouse genomes (166). The CCRK gene maps to chromosome 9q22.1 and encodes a protein comprised of 347 amino acids. CCRK was initially named p42 based on the relative mobility of its in vitro translated product. CCRK is a nuclear kinase with a PNQLARE C-helix motif and a threonine residue (T161) in the activation loop, in a position and sequence context identical to those of activating threonines in other CDKs. It is widely expressed in various cell lines and its expression level is similar across the cell cycle in HeLa cells. It shares 43% sequence identity with CDK7 but is distinct from CDK7 in terms of substrate specificity. CCRK is an activating T157 kinase for MRK/ICK (male germ cell-associated kinase-related kinase/intestinal cell kinase), whereas active CDK7:cyclin H:MAT1 complexes do not phosphorylate MRK/ICK (34). CCRK co-immunoprecipitates with CDK2 and phosphorylates and activates CDK2, and CCRK depletion reduces the level of phosphorylated T160 of CDK2 (166, 167).

However, the monomeric CCRK has been reported not to have an intrinsic CAK activity in cells, and it was proposed instead to be a potential negative regulator of apoptosis (19, 168). CCRK is essential for cell proliferation, and its inhibition promotes tumor cell death (19, 166, 167). Increased glioma cell proliferation and tumorigenicity were associated with the overexpression of CCRK and was dependent on its kinase activity. Suppression of CCRK expression was associated with the inhibition of glioma xenograft tumor growth. Therefore CCRK might be a potential therapeutic and diagnostic target for glioblastoma multiforme and other tumors.

6.2 CDKS AND mRNA PRODUCTION

6.2.1 Introduction

Eukaryotic mRNA transcription by RNA polymerase II (RNA Pol II) is an elaborate multistep process dependent on the interaction of a set of general transcription factors that regulate basal transcription, including core promoters and a wide range of gene-specific transcription factors that bind to distal regulatory elements. Assembly of a massive preinitiation complex (PIC) of more than 60 proteins on core promoters (169–171) is guided by a large multi-subunit complex, Mediator (MED). MED is comprised of up to 30 distinct subunits in mammals and serves as a modular interface bridging this RNA Pol II initiation machinery to diverse transcription factors arrayed on regulatory DNA regions, providing a regulatory link to proper expression of most RNAP II genes (172–175).

CDKs play numerous roles in transcriptional regulation including elongation, pre-mRNA processing, and export from the nucleus to the cytoplasm, as well as post-translational modification of histones (Figure 6.5). CDKs 7, 8, and 9 associate with the transcription cyclin family, which includes cyclins C, H, K, and T, and play roles in the regulation of transcriptional initiation and elongation by phosphorylating the RNA Pol II C-terminal domain (CTD). This group of protein kinases link various growth factor signaling pathways to transcription and RNA processing events and, by regulating the global expression of cellular mRNAs (and proteins), play an important role in the regulation of cell growth, proliferation, and survival. Therapeutic interventions targeting activity of these kinases may be of clinical value in cancer treatment. CDK12 (CRKRS) and CDK13 (CDK1L5) functions are related to pre-mRNA splicing. Interestingly, CDK11p110 plays roles in both transcription and splicing, suggesting that this CDK may link the two processes. CDK11, CDK12, and CDK13 associate with six cyclin L proteins. The combination of the cyclin L isoform and the CDK partner protein varies in a cell type-specific manner, and this affects splice site usage. Very little is known about regulation of cyclin L, CDK11, CDK12, and CDK13 expression during development, cell cycle, and differentiation by extracellular signals. Furthermore, substrates of these cyclin L:CDK complexes as well as genes regulated by cyclin L:CDK complexes remain to be identified. Estimates suggest that about 15% of disease-causing mutations in human genes involve misregulation of alternative splicing. Thus unraveling the pathways and the molecules involved in alternative splicing is crucial to an understanding

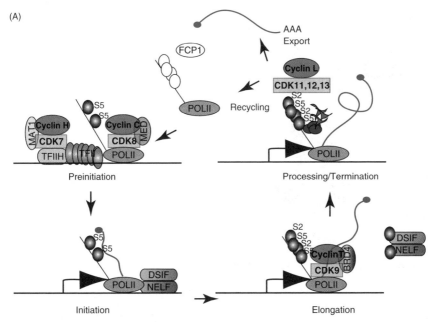

Figure 6.5   CDKs and mRNA production. (A) C-terminal domain (CTD) phosphorylation of the large subunit of RNA Pol II and the transcription cycle. The Pol II core enzyme assembles with coactivators such as the mediator complex (MED) including CDK8 complex to form a holoenzyme. The unphosphorylated Pol II core or holoenzyme assembles onto the promoter sequences with general transcription factors (TFII) including the TFIIH complex, thereby forming a transcription preinitiation complex. The CTD is phosphorylated on serines at position 5 (S5) of the consensus heptapeptide sequence by the CDK7 subunit of the TFIIH complex, and transcription initiation occurs. The phosphorylated CTD recruits the capping enzymes and the nascent transcript is capped at its 5′ end (represented by a red spot). Phosphorylation of the CTD on serine at position 2 (S2) by the cyclin T:CDK9 complex (also known as P-TEFb) relieves the block imposed by the DSIF/NELF factors and transcription elongation occurs. The phosphorylated CTD recruits the splicing factors and cyclin L:CDK complexes to remove introns and finally recruits the cleavage and polyadenylation factors that cleave the transcript and add a polyadenylic tail at its 3′ end. This step signals termination of transcription and Pol II falls off its DNA template. The resulting mRNA is then exported to the cytoplasm; Pol II is dephosphorylated by the FCP1 CTD phosphatase and recycled for another transcription round. (B) Transcriptional regulation by post-translational modification of histones. CDK8 subcomplex associates with the multisubunit Mediator complexes including TRRAP/GCN5L acetyltransferase, thereby increasing in tandem S10 phosphorylation and K14 acetylation of histone H3, which results in chromatin remodeling activities leading to transcription activation. The cyclin T:CDK9:BRD4 complex is recruited to phospho S10 of H3 and its binding is stabilized by acetylation of chromatin.

(B)

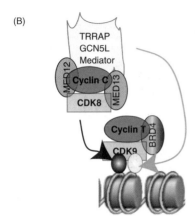

Figure 6.5 (*Continued*)

of various intricate cellular functions and for the management of human diseases including cancers.

6.2.2 CDK7

CDK7 was identified by molecular cloning of a human homolog of *Xenopus* CAK, p40^{MO15}, and was originally named (HS) CAK1 or STK1 for serine/threonine protein kinase (176–178). The *CDK7* gene maps to chromosome 5q12.1 and encodes a protein comprised of 346 amino acids with a molecular weight of 42 kDa. Both CDK7 transcript and protein level are constant throughout the cell cycle, and the CDK7 protein is localized predominantly to the nucleus (179). CDK7 contains a NRTALRE motif similar to the PSTAIRE motif found in prototypic CDK1 kinases, and its catalytic domain exhibits considerable homology with CDK1.

CDK7 forms the multi-subunit CDK-activating kinase or CAK complex with cyclin H and the RING finger protein MAT1, which phosphorylates and thus activates certain cyclin-dependent protein kinases in the regulation of cell cycle progression. Additionally, cyclin H:CDK7 phosphorylates S5 of the RNA Pol II CTD in the basal transcription machinery (180). In order to form a stable dimeric and active complex with cyclin H, CDK7 must be phosphorylated on a conserved T170 in the activation loop (181, 182). Unlike other CDKs, CDK7 has an additional phosphorylation site at S164 in the activation segment, whose phosphorylation enhances activity and cyclin binding. Cyclin H phosphorylation by CDK7 destabilizes the dimeric cyclin H:CDK7 complex. MAT1 binding counteracts the effects of cyclin H phosphorylation and provides additional stability to the trimeric complex (183). MAT1 also confers the change in substrate specificity. The crystal structure of CDK7 phosphorylated on T170 in the activation segment and in complex with ATP shows that the overall fold of the kinase is similar to that of inactive CDK2, as expected from their sequence similarity (183). Major differences occur in the activation segment, the C-terminal region, and the L14 loop. In contrast to T160-phosphorylated CDK2, where the phosphorylated activation segment is disordered, CDK7 shows an ordered activation segment. Several amino acid differences also create a hydrophobic pocket with greater nonpolar character in CDK7 than in CDK2, which might be exploited for the design of selective small molecule inhibitors.

CDK7 phosphorylates CDK1, CDK2, CDK4, and CDK6, but only CDK1 and CDK2 can also phosphorylate CDK7 on the activation segment (181). This specificity does not appear to be dictated by the sequences surrounding the phosphorylation sites but by structural determinants at remote sites (184). CDK7 functions in two mutually dependent steps of CDK1 activation: cyclin binding and activation loop phosphorylation (19). CDK1 requires activation loop phosphorylation for its stable association with cyclin A or cyclin B (19, 185). Inhibition of CDK7 in G2 phase disrupts cyclin B:CDK1 complex assembly and blocks entry into mitosis. In contrast, selective inhibition of CDK7 in G1 prevents activation (but not formation) of cyclin E:CDK2 complexes and delays S phase (19). However, whether CDK7 is the sole CAK for CDK2 in cells remains unclear (see also Sections 6.1.3 and 6.1.7).

CDK7 in complex with cyclin H also is present as a distinct component of the general RNA polymerase transcription factor IIH (TFIIH) multi-subunit protein complex. CDK7 participates in basal transcription by phosphorylating the CTD of the largest subunit of RNA Pol II. CDK7 preferentially phosphorylates the S5 sites of the consensus heptapeptide sequence of RNA Pol II CTD (186, 187). However, S5 of the RNA Pol II CTD is targeted by multiple kinases in vitro and in vivo (19, 188). Inactivation of CDK7 leads to an apparent increase in net phosphorylation by other S5 kinases but produces an RNA Pol II isoform of altered electrophoretic mobility, suggesting a derangement of normal CTD phosphorylation patterns. CDK7, as a kinase component of TFIIH, also influences cell cycle progression by phosphorylating E2F1 at S408 and T433, which is a prerequisite for ubiquitination and degradation (189) (see also Section 6.1.3). It also influences development and function of steroidogenic tissues by phosphorylating the steroidogenic factor-1 (SF1) at S203, which increases its transcriptional activity (190). The capacity of other transcriptional activators, including the nuclear receptors RARα, RARγ, and ERα, are also affected by CDK7. CDK7 phosphorylates serine residues located in a proline-rich motif within the N-terminal domain (NTD) of RARs at the promoter of target genes (191–194). CDK7 phosphorylation dissociates RARs from bound vinexin β, a cytoskeletal adaptor, and allows transcription initiation in response to retinoic acid (RA) (195). Interestingly, the efficiency of NTD phosphorylation by CDK7 relies on the docking of cyclin H at a specific site of the C-terminal ligand binding domain (LBD) of RARs, which determines the correct positioning of the CDK7 kinase (196). The importance of TFIIH-mediated phosphorylation of the NTD of RARs has been highlighted in studies using cells from patients suffering from photosensitive disorder xeroderma pigmentosum (XP). Cells from these patients have mutations in the helicase XPD (*ERCC2*) gene and are characterized by a hypophosphorylation of RAR and a deficient RA response (191). Recently, mutations of XPG (*ERCC5*) gene found in XP-associated Cockayne syndrome (XP-G/CS) patients have been reported to result in the dissociation of CAK and XPD from the core TFIIH, thereby affecting the transcriptional activation mediated by hormonal receptors and expression of the target genes (197).

The abundance of XPD in cells might dictate in part which CDK7 form (CAK vs. CTD kinase) is prominent. In the fruit fly *Drosophila*, excess XPD in the TFIIH complex titrates CAK activity, thereby decreasing CDK activation loop phosphorylation and increasing mitotic defects and lethality, whereas a decrease in XPD results in increased CAK activity and cell proliferation (198). At the beginning of mitosis, the downregulation of XPD might cause dissociation of the CAK complex from holo TFIIH, causing TFIIH to lose its CTD kinase activity concurrently with the loss of XPD. Both losses might then contribute to mitotic silencing of basal transcription. Simultaneously, XPD degradation may set the trimeric CAK complex free to phosphorylate its cell cycle target CDK1 and positively regulate mitotic progression. Because of dual functions in gene expression and cell proliferation, CDK7 could be an attractive anticancer drug target (180, 199); however, questions about possible toxicities associated with CDK7 inhibition may impact the clinical utility of CDK7 therapeutics.

6.2.3 CDK8

CDK8 was identified by screening a human testis cDNA library with K35, a partial cDNA from a promyelocytic leukemia cell line that was originally isolated from a PCR screen with degenerate oligonucleotides based on conserved motifs in the catalytic domain of the *Aspergillus nidulans* NIMA protein kinase (200, 201). The CDK8 gene maps to chromosome 13q12.13 (201), a locus that is associated with several human disease genes, including the breast cancer susceptibility gene BRCA2. The CDK8 protein is comprised of 464 amino acids with a molecular weight of 53 kDa and displays 36% sequence identity to CDK1. Like CDK1, CDK8 contains phosphorylation residues corresponding to T14 and Y15 in subdomain I. In contrast to CDK1, CDK8 contains a noncanonical DMG motif instead of a DFG motif at the start of the activation segment, and the sequence SMSACRE in the region corresponding to the PSTAIRE sequence of CDK1 in the C helix. CDK8 in complex with cyclin C associates functionally with the transcription apparatus. The mechanism of cyclin C:CDK8 activation may vary from that of other CDKs, since CDK8 has an extended activation loop and lacks an activation loop threonine residue in the position of CDK1 T161 (202). Because CDK8 can positively or negatively regulate transcription, precise control of CDK8 substrate specificity may be critical for regulating transcription initiation in humans.

The cyclin C:CDK8 complex is a component of the RNA Pol II holoenzyme complex, and it can phosphorylate the RNA Pol II CTD. The cyclin C:CDK8 complex also is found in a number of mammalian Mediator-like protein complexes that influence transcription independently of the CTD. Within the Mediator CDK8 subcomplex (consisting of CDK8, cyclin C, Med12, and Med13), CDK8 indirectly activates gene expression through association with the TRRAP polypeptide and GCN5L acetyltransferase (203). CDK8 phosphorylates S10 on histone H3, which in turn stimulates K14 acetylation by GCN5L. This tandem S10/K14 phosphoacetylation of histone H3 correlates strongly with active expression of certain human genes by altering chromatin structure and recruiting coactivators to specific genomic loci. Indeed, CDK8 knockdown causes substantial reduction of global H3 phospho-acetylation. CDK8 also functions as a stimulus-specific transcriptional coactivator within the p53 transcriptional apparatus (203). The levels of CDK8 occupancy at p53 target genes including *p21 CIP1* and *HDM2* correlate positively with gene activity. CDK8 also positively influences β-catenin/TCF activity by stabilizing the interaction of β-catenin with the target gene promoter, thereby facilitating transcription of the gene (204). Overexpression of CDK8 transforms normal mouse fibroblast cells, through a mechanism dependent on the functional β-catenin/TCF.

In contrast to its role as a positive regulator of transcription, CDK8 can also reversibly associate with the "core" Mediator, which strongly interacts with RNA Pol II to inhibit the coactivator function of the Mediator (195). CDK8 phosphorylates cyclin H at S5 and S304 and represses both the ability of TFIIH to activate transcription and the CDK7 kinase activity on the RNA Pol II CTD (205). Mimicking CDK8 phosphorylation of cyclin H in vivo has a dominant-negative effect on cell growth. CDK8 also directly phosphorylates E2F1 and negatively regulates E2F1-dependent transcription (206). Since E2F-1 is a negative regulator of β-catenin:TCF activity, CDK8 indirectly activates β-catenin-dependent transcription in addition to its direct interaction with β-catenin as mentioned earlier. Interestingly, significant CDK8 copy number increases were found in colorectal cancers. Therefore overexpressed CDK8 may increase β-catenin-dependent transcription and cause β-catenin-driven malignancies. Therapeutic interventions targeting CDK8 may confer a clinical benefit in cancers that are driven by deregulated β-catenin activity.

Deletion of CDK8 in cultured cells does not affect cell viability. Heterozygote $cdk8^{+/-}$ mice show no phenotype, but intercrossing these does not produce homozygous $cdk8^{-/-}$ offspring (207). This early embryonic lethality is due to preimplantation developmental arrest with fragmented blastomeres. Therefore CDK8 is not required for autonomous cell growth or survival but is essential for very early development prior to compaction, which is consistent with an induction of CDK8 transcription just prior to compaction (208).

6.2.4 CDK9

CDK9 was identified by screening a cDNA library with probes designed based on regions conserved among CDK1-related proteins and was initially named PITALRE, because it contains a motif similar to the PSTAIRE motif found in prototypic CDK1 kinases (209). The gene for CDK9 maps to chromosome 9q34.1 (123) and encodes a protein of 372 amino acids with a molecular weight of 43 kDa. CDK9 shares 41–43% amino acid sequence identity with CDK1, CDK2, CDK3, and CDK5 (209). CDK9 expression is ubiquitous but greatest in terminally differentiated tissues (210). A splice variant of CDK9, CDK9-55, originates from an upstream promoter region and has a 117 amino acid N-terminal extension containing a proline-rich region and a glycine-rich region (211). The shorter CDK9 isoform CDK9-42 is the predominant isoform in most cell types. Expression and activity of CDK9 do not appear to be regulated during the cell cycle (212).

The major role of CDK9 is to control the elongation phase of transcription by RNA Pol II by phosphorylation of the RNA Pol II CTD. CDK9 kinase activity is regulated by multiple mechanisms. CDK9 associates with various activator and suppressor proteins including T-type and K-type cyclins, 7SK small nuclear (sn) RNA, the hexamethylene bisacetamide-induced protein (HEXIM1), and a double bromodomain-containing protein BRD4. CDK9 also is modified by phosphorylation, acetylation, and ubiquitination.

CDK9 forms a heterodimer called positive transcription elongation factor b (P-TEFb) with one of four cyclin partners, K, T1, T2a, or T2b. Approximately 80% of cyclin T:CDK9 complexes contains cyclin T1. About half of cellular P-TEFb exists in an inactive complex with 7SK snRNA and HEXIM1 (213, 214), and the remaining half associates with BRD4 and displays high kinase activity (129). The balance of active and inactive P-TEFb, which functions as a global regulator of gene expression, is tightly controlled in cells. For example, in stress-induced HeLa cells, 7SK:HEXIM1-bound P-TEFb was converted into the BRD4-associated form. The bound BRD4 facilitates P-TEFb recruitment to promoters and its contact with the Mediator complex (215, 216). Acetylation of CDK9 enhances P-TEFb transcriptional elongation function (217). Lysine 44 was identified as a major acetylation site, and a single K44R mutation reduces CDK9 kinase activity.

The CDK9 structure exhibits a typical kinase fold. The structures of CDK9 and cyclin T1 in the cyclin T1:CDK9 complex are similar to previously determined structures for other CDKs and cyclins, with the exception that cyclin T1 exhibits a relative rotation of $26°$ with respect to CDK9, which decreases the cyclin T1:CDK9 interaction surface area relative to other cyclin:CDK complexes (218). Also in contrast to cell cycle CDKs, which are activated by CAK (CDK7:cyclin H:MAT1), CDK9 autophosphorylates on T186 in the activation segment (218, 219). This phosphorylation event promotes CDK9 kinase activity as well as its association with 7SK:HEXIM1 (214, 220). CDK9 also autophosphorylates three C-terminal sites (S347, T262, and T363), which ensures the nuclear localization of cyclin T1:CDK9 (221). Activation of the MEK1/ERK signaling pathway increases nuclear CDK9 levels (222), resulting either from increased cytoplasmic to nuclear translocation or increased stability due to interaction with the heat shock proteins HSP70 and HSP90 (223). Lastly, CDK9 degradation is initiated by its ubiquitination (212). Cyclin T1 is not ubiquitinated, but it functions as a scaffold connecting ubiquitinated CDK9 and the proteasome system (224).

P-TEFb phosphorylates two elongation repressors, the DRB (5,6-dichloro-benzimidazole1-*b*-D-ribofuranoside) sensitivity-inducing factor (DSIF) and the negative elongation factor (NELF) (225, 226). These elongation repressors provide a checkpoint to ensure the capping of pre-mRNAs. P-TEFb phosphorylation of the RNA Pol II CTD is required to release the repressor actions and allow productive transcription elongation. In the absence of P-TEFb activity, RNA Pol II complexes, which are phosphorylated at S5 of the CTD, stall following transcription initiation and accumulate 20–40 nucleotides downstream of the transcription start site. P-TEFb phosphorylates the RNA Pol II CTD on position S2 in the CTD heptad repeat sequence (YSPTSPS), which stimulates processive elongation of otherwise paused RNA Pol II transcripts (227, 228). P-TEFb also influences gene expression by integrating mRNA synthesis with histone modification, pre-mRNA processing, mRNA export, and even mRNA translation in the cytoplasm (229). Following transcription, P-TEFb itself accompanies the mature mRNA to the cytoplasm to promote translation elongation, and indeed, CDK9 has been detected on translating ribosomes (230).

Although amplification or mutation of the *CDK9* gene has not been observed in cancer cells, CDK9 is required for expression of proteins vital to cell proliferation and survival, and P-TEFb activity is more heavily involved in pathologic cellular processes than in normal cellular functions (231–235). Therefore targeting CDK9 might be a promising strategy in cancer and other diseases.

6.2.5 CDK11

CDK11 (also known as CDC2L for cell division cycle 2-like) contains a PIT-SLRE motif and is expressed as two major isoforms, CDK11p110 and CDK11p58. In humans, these two isoforms are encoded by two distinct but closely related genes, *CDC2L1* and *CDC2L2* (236). In contrast, a single CDK11p110/p58 gene, *cdcl*, is found in a syntenic region of mouse chromosome 4 (237). CDK11p110 is a 779 amino acid-containing protein. CDK11p58 is a polypeptide consisting of 440 amino acids, which maps to approximately amino acids 341 to 779 of CDK11p110 (includes the kinase domain). CDK11p58 lacks the N terminus, including the NLS sequences (238). The CDK11p110 isoform is produced by classic cap-dependent translation and its expression is ubiquitous and constant throughout the cell cycle (239). In contrast, CDK11p58 is expressed via an IRES located within the CDK11p110 mRNA (238, 240). CDK11p110 is associated with transcription and RNA processing, while CDK11p58 functions specifically in G2/M and affects cell cycle arrest and apoptosis in a kinase-dependent manner (241–244). During apoptosis, a third isoform, CDK11p46, is generated by caspase-dependent cleavage of CDK11p110 and CDK11p58, leaving the catalytic domain intact (241, 244, 245). All three CDK11 isoforms can form complexes with cyclin L (246).

CDK11p110 associates with multiple transcriptional elongation factors and RNA Pol II (242). Antibody-mediated inhibition of CDK11p110 specifically suppresses RNA Pol II-dependent in vitro transcription and can be rescued by addition of purified CDK11p110. CDK11 also plays a role in pre-mRNA splicing. CDK11p110 regulates alternative splicing and this regulation requires kinase activity (243, 246, 247). CDK11p110 and associated cyclin La/cyclin Lb proteins localize to splicing factor compartments within nucleoplasm and interact with the general splicing factor RNPS1 and serine- and arginine-rich (SR) proteins such as 9G8 (243, 248). In particular, CDK11p110 can phosphorylate 9G8 in vitro, and depletion of CDK11p110 by RNAi diminishes the amount of phosphorylated 9G8 in vivo (243).

CDK11p58 can function in both transcription and cell cycle control. In association with cyclin D3 it phosphorylates androgen receptor at S308, which negatively affects its transcriptional activity and inhibits androgen-dependent proliferation of prostate cancer cells (249). CDK11p58 localizes to mitotic centrosomes and plays a role in centrosome maturation and bipolar spindle morphogenesis (250).

Accordingly, CDK11 knockdown by RNAi in HeLa cells induces abnormal spindle assembly, mitotic arrest by checkpoint activation, and cell death (250, 251). Additional roles for CDK11 in mitotic progression and chromosome cohesion have been reported (251). Establishment of chromosome cohesion occurs during DNA synthesis in S phase, and the association of paired sister chromatids must be maintained until anaphase to ensure accurate chromosome segregation. Knockdown of CDK11 expression results in the premature loss of the chromosome cohesion complexes and a permanent mitotic arrest followed by cell death. This phenotype is rescued by CDK11p58 expression. Therefore the CDK11p58 kinase plays a crucial role in mitotic progression and is required for the maintenance of sister chromatid cohesion and completion of mitosis in human cells. Consistent with these findings, homozygous CDK11 knockout in mice results in early embryonic lethality; cells within CDK11-deficient mouse embryos exhibit both proliferative defects and mitotic arrest followed by apoptosis (252).

The human *CDC2L* genes encoding CDK11 variants are localized to human chromosome 1 band p36.3 (236). Since the chromosome 1 band p36 region is frequently deleted or translocated in a number of different human tumors, including neuroblastoma, breast cancer, melanoma, and lymphoma (253–256), *CDC2L* was proposed to be a tumor suppressor candidate gene. More recently, a much smaller consensus region of allelic loss of heterozygosity (LOH) associated with neuroblastoma was defined as 1p36.3-p36.2, excluding the *CDC2L* genes and indicating that *CDC2L* is not the neuroblastoma tumor suppressor gene (257). However, reduced CDK11 expression observed in several cancers suggests an association with carcinogenesis. Indeed, CDK11 haploinsufficient mice with a loss of one allele of *cdc2l* exhibit an increase in tumor size and number as compared to wild-type mice in a chemical-mediated skin cancer model system (258).

6.2.6 CDK12 (CDC2-Related Kinase CRKRS)

CDK12 was identified from a human cDNA library screen using a 270 nucleotide cDNA product encoding part of the CDK12 kinase domain, which was originally isolated in a PCR screen undertaken to identify the cyclin A-associated kinase (259). Human CDK12, which consists of 1490 amino acids and has a molecular weight of 164 kDa, is a significantly larger protein than prototypical CDKs. CDK12 contains an arginine/serine-rich (RS) domain, so it was initially named CRKRS for CDC2-related kinase with an RS domain. Subsequently, the CDK12 short isoform (CDK12S) was identified from the analysis of gene expression profiles of various protein kinases in rat cortical neurons and a cDNA screen using the conserved catalytic domain of all known kinases (260). CDK12S is an alternative splicing product of CDK12 (the long isoform is CDK12L) with the same 1249 amino acids at the amino termini. CDK12S and CDK12L have additional 9 and 235 distinct amino acid residues at the carboxyl termini, respectively. The CDK12 locus is on human chromosome 17q12, a locus associated with susceptibility to prostate and breast cancers and frequently amplified in gastrointestinal adenocarcinomas. CDK12 belongs to a new high molecular weight subfamily in the CDC2-like (CDC2L) protein kinase family with PITAI/VRE motifs shared by its closest homolog, CDK13 (261). The catalytic domain in the center of the protein (residues 719–984) has 42% identity to human CDK1. This CDK-homologous region includes the sequence PITAIRE, and the predicted ATP binding region of the kinase domain contains adjacent threonine and tyrosine residues in positions analogous to T14, Y15, and T161 residues of CDK1. It also has a bipartite nuclear localization signal and potential PEST sequences that correlate with protein degradation. Expression of CDK12 is ubiquitous and present at constant levels with some phosphorylation fluctuation throughout the cell cycle.

CDK12 associates with cyclin L1 and cyclin L2 (260) and is implicated in transcription and splicing roles. It localizes in nuclear speckles, the storage sites for splicing factors, and CDK12-immunoprecipitated complexes phosphorylate the RNA Pol II CTD and the splicing factor SF2/ASF in vitro (259). However, there is no direct phosphorylation of SF2/ASF in vitro by CDK12 (260). CDK12 alters the splicing pattern, an effect potentiated by the cyclin domain of cyclin L1 and counteracted by the splicing factors SF2/ASF and SC35. Knockdown of CDK12 isoforms by RNAi reverses their splicing choices. It is not clear whether there are functional differences between the CDK12S and CDK12L proteins.

6.2.7   CDK13 (CDC2L5)

CDK13 was originally identified serendipitously from a glioblastoma cDNA library screen with cholinesterase-specific oligodeoxynucleotide probes and was initially named CHED for cholinesterase-related cell division controller (262). Subsequently, the human cDNA encoding the full-length amino acid sequence of CHED was identified and named cell division cycle 2-like 5 (CDC2L5) (261). The CDK13 gene maps to chromosome 7p15 and encodes a 1512 amino acid protein with molecular weight ~170 kDa. CDK13 has a highly conserved kinase domain surrounded by extensive N and C termini that are greater than 400 amino acids in length. An alternatively spliced variant encodes a shortened protein lacking an internal 60 amino acid fragment. CDK13 is expressed ubiquitously in human tissues (261), several mouse fetal tissues, and tumor cell lines (262). It has 42% identity to human CDK1 and is very similar to CDK12 with 92% protein sequence identity in the kinase domain and 52% identity overall (261). CDK13, like CDK12, has the sequence PITAIRE, an RS domain, associates with L-type cyclins, and localizes in the nucleoplasmic speckles (263, 264). Moreover, like CDK12, CDK13 alters the splicing pattern, which is counteracted by SF2/ASF and SC35 (264). CDK13 directly interacts with the SF2/ASF-associated protein p32, a protein involved in splicing regulation (263). Overexpression of CDK13 disturbs constitutive splicing and switches alternative splice site selection in vivo. Taken together, CDK13 seems to play a functional role in splicing regulation. CDK13 also has been suggested to be involved in hematopoiesis (262). Mouse bone marrow cells treated with antisense oligonucleotides directed against the CDK13/CHED mRNA showed a reduction in the number of mature, polynuclear megakaryocytes and an increase in the number of early mononuclear cells.

6.3 OTHER CDK-RELATED KINASES

6.3.1 CDK5

CDK5 was identified by screening a cDNA library with probes designed to recognize regions conserved among CDK1-related proteins and was originally named PSSALRE, based on the amino acid sequence of the region corresponding to the conserved CDK1 PSTAIRE motif (14). The CDK5 gene maps to chromosome 7q36 (62) and encodes a protein comprised of 291 amino acids with a 31-kDa molecular weight. CDK5 shares 57% protein sequence identity with CDK1 and is expressed ubiquitously in all human tissues and cell lines tested. CDK5 is activated by binding to the noncyclin proteins p35 (CDK5R1; NCK5A), p39 (CDK5R2; NCK5AI), p25, and p29 (265–269). The p35 and p39 activators are homologous proteins with 57% amino acid identity to each other, while p25 and p29 are proteolytic fragments comprising the C-terminal portion of p35 and p39, respectively. The CDK5 activators have a limited sequence homology to cyclins and are most abundant in postmitotic neurons and brains rather than in proliferating cells. The X-ray crystal structure of CDK5:p25 indicates that CDK5 activation is distinct from the mechanism of other cellular CDKs (270, 271). To activate CDK5, p25 makes extensive contacts with the CDK5 activation loop and induces an active conformation, an interaction that is not observed in CDK:cyclin complexes. Additional p25:CDK5 interactions occur between PSSALRE helix region within the kinase domain small lobe and a highly divergent p25 cyclin box fold (CBF) domain. Phosphorylation of the activation loop at S159 (equivalent to T160 of CDK2) is not required to activate CDK5, and accordingly CDK5 is not phosphorylated by CAK. However, phosphorylation by ABL on Y15 increases CDK5 activity (272). Similar to other CDKs, active CDK5 is a proline-directed kinase that in vitro phosphorylates the amino acid sequence (S/T)PX(K/H/R) (X is any amino acid), a consensus sequence that is present in CDK5 substrates. CDK5 phosphorylates a diverse list of proteins including cytoskeletal, signaling, and regulatory proteins, which are associated with cell morphology, adhesion, motility, and cell–cell communication.

CDK5 is essential for brain development and is implicated in numerous complex functions in the central nervous system, including synaptic plasticity, dopaminergic neurotransmission, and drug addiction. CDK5 conditional knockout mice studies implicate CDK5 activity in numerous complex functions of the adult CNS (273), and deregulation of CDK5 has been implicated in neurodegenerative disorders including Alzheimer disease, amyotrophic lateral sclerosis, Parkinson disease, Huntington disease, and acute neuronal injury (274–277). CDK5 activity is associated with both neuronal cell survival and apoptosis. CDK5 contributes to neuronal cell survival by phosphorylation of BCL2 (278) and JNK3 (279); however, it also promotes neuronal cell apoptosis through phosphorylation of the tumor suppressor protein p53 (280, 281). In response to oxidative and genotoxic stresses, CDK5 activity leads to apoptosis in human neuroblastoma cells through a mechanism that involves phosphorylation of CDH1 and stabilization of cyclin B1 (282, 283).

Recently, roles of CDK5 in nonneuronal cells have been elucidated. CDK5 participates in a signaling cascade involved in the regulation of glucose-stimulated insulin secretion in pancreatic beta cells (284), and CDK5 activity is associated with apoptosis in nonneuronal normal and tumor cells. CDK5 activation is required for caspase-3 activation and subsequent cAMP-induced apoptosis in rat leukemia cells (285), and prostate cancer cells undergo apoptosis in response to digoxin through a CDK5-p35/p25-dependent pathway (286). CDK5-mediated MYC phosphorylation is implicated in the increased cyclin B1 expression and radiation sensitivity observed in association with cyclin G1 overexpression in various tumor tissues (see Section 6.3.2) (287). CDK5 also affects growth-signal-induced activation of phosphatidylinositol-3 kinase enhancer isoform A (PIKE-A) and AKT and induces tumor migration and invasion (288). CDK5 roles in DNA-damage response and cell cycle checkpoint activation have been shown by siRNA studies (289). Genomic loss of CDK5 has been observed in 5.5% (8/145) of breast cancers (289, 290). It remains to be determined if deletion of CDK5 plays a role in cancer predisposition, similar to germline mutations in other DNA-damage checkpoint genes that are linked to development of breast and other cancers (291).

6.3.2 GAK

GAK (cyclin G-associated kinase) was identified by cloning a rat cDNA that encodes a novel association partner of cyclin G identified by Western blotting (292), and subsequently by cloning of its human homolog (293). Cyclin G is a downstream transcriptional target and a negative regulator of the p53 tumor suppressor protein, and its expression is elevated in both breast and prostate cancer (294–296). GAK is expressed ubiquitously, with the highest level of expression in the testis. GAK expression oscillates slightly, peaking in G1 phase, although histone H_1 kinase activity remains constant throughout the cell cycle. GAK maps to chromosome 4p16 and encodes a protein comprised of 1311 amino acids with a molecular weight of 144 kDa. GAK harbors a S/T protein kinase catalytic domain at the N terminus, and the long C-terminal extension shares homology with tensin and auxilin and contains a leucine zipper region. GAK functions as auxilin 2, the ubiquitous form of the neuronal-specific protein auxilin 1, in receptor-mediated endocytosis and recruitment of both clathrin and clathrin adaptors (297). The Auxilin/Tensin homology domain of GAK has clathrin-binding motifs that allow for association with clathrin-coated vesicles (CCVs). The COOH-terminal J domain of GAK is known to interact with the molecular chaperone HSC70, which is the constitutively expressed form of HSP70. GAK is an essential cofactor for the HSC70-dependent uncoating of clathrin-coated vesicles, induces clathrin exchange on clathrin-coated pits, and mediates binding of clathrin and adaptors to the plasma membrane and the trans-Golgi network. Depletion of GAK by shRNA in HeLa cells causes a dramatic reduction in adaptor proteins on the plasma membrane and at the trans-Golgi network. A similar effect was caused by expression of a dominant-negative HSP70 mutant. GAK regulates lysosomal enzyme sorting by directly interacting with the adaptor protein 1 complex, and the kinase activity of GAK is essential for this process (298).

GAK is thought to be a negative regulator of EGFR signaling. Downregulation of GAK has pronounced effects on EGF receptor signaling by increasing the levels of EGF receptor expression and tyrosine kinase activity, producing outgrowth of cells in soft agar (299). Therefore loss of GAK function may promote tumorigenesis. Consistent with this, GAK is proposed to be involved in an undesirable effect of the clinical EGF receptor kinase inhibitor gefitinib that occurs downstream of the EGFR (300). Gefitinib inactivates GAK, which antagonizes the inhibitory effect of the drug on EGFR signaling in NSCLC cell lines. However, GAK is also proposed to be a positive regulator of tumor progression. GAK was identified as a novel androgen receptor (AR)-interacting transcriptional coactivator that enhances the transactivation function of AR even at low concentrations of androgens and allows for receptor activation and expression of AR-regulated growth and survival genes (301). Significantly increased GAK expression was associated with prostate cancer progression to androgen independence. High levels of GAK may amplify AR responses to low levels of circulating hormone and lead to AR transactivation in androgen-withdrawn conditions, and therefore GAK may play a prognostic role in advanced disease.

6.4 MITOTIC KINASES

Mitotic division is a complex, highly integrated cellular process that normally results in faithful division of a cell into two daughter cells. Not surprisingly, this process is frequently disrupted in cancer cells. First, disruption of normal mitosis can promote tumor formation by leading to aneuploidy, genetic instability, and unchecked proliferation, promoting tumor formation. Second, established tumors with aneuploid genomes may be critically dependent on the continued dysregulation of mitosis in order to productively proliferate in the face of genomic derangement. In order to provide context for discussion of the kinases that regulate various stages of mitosis, a brief overview of the process is shown in Figure 6.6. Generally, the transition from G2 phase to M phase is divided into five stages: prophase, prometaphase, metaphase, anaphase, and telophase. Cells enter mitosis with replicated chromosomes (pairs of sister chromatids) and duplicated centrosomes. During prophase, the chromosomes condense and the centrosomes migrate to opposite poles of the cell. Microtubules become increasingly more motile and form clusters (termed asters, or astral microtubules), which emanate from the polar centrosomes. In prometaphase, the nuclear membrane breaks down and the asters extend into the cellular milieu, where they attach to kinetochores at the center of the chromosomes. The details of this engagement process are critical: it is essential that the two sister chromatids are attached to microtubules emanating from centrosomes at opposite poles of the cell. Once attached to the microtubular mitotic apparatus, chromosomes migrate to the midzone of the cell, equidistant from each centrosome. During metaphase, the chromosomes align along the midzone of the cell and the anaphase-promoting complex (APC, a multiprotein assembly with ubiquitin ligase activity) is formed. Degradation of cell cycle regulators by the APC leads to anaphase, wherein the sister chromatids separate to the cellular poles

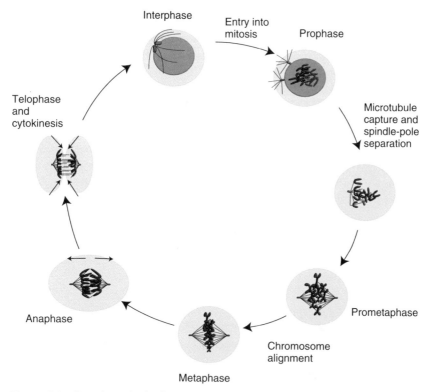

Figure 6.6 Overview of mitosis. At the start of mitosis, the cell has duplicated its chromosomes and centrosomes. In prophase, the chromosomes condense and the centrosomes begin to migrate to opposite poles of the cell, serving as nuclei for astral microtubules. In prometaphase, the nuclear envelope breaks down and the chromosomes attach to the mitotic spindle via the kinetochores. At metaphase, the chromosomes align at the cellular midzone, prior to initiation of anaphase, where the paired chromosomes separate and a microtubular bundle forms at the cellular midzone. In telophase, the nuclear envelope is reformed around each set of sister chromatids, and cytokinesis occurs, producing two separate daughter cells.

and the spindle midzone collapses to a cluster of microtubules. Telophase is the final step, wherein two nuclear envelopes are formed around the newly separated chromosomes and cellular division occurs.

Several clinically useful chemotherapy drugs target mitosis, notably the vinca alkaloids and taxanes, both of which interfere with tubulin polymerization/depolymerization and selectively inhibit the growth of rapidly dividing cells. However, although these agents have demonstrated clinical benefit, they also impact tubulin-dependent processes (such as molecular transport) in nonproliferating cells. Hence there has been significant interest in developing agents to specifically target alternative pathways and proteins (including several important kinases) that are specifically involved in regulating mitosis (302, 303).

6.4.1 PLKs

The PLK (polo-like kinase) family comprises four distinct mammalian homologs: PLK1, PLK2 (SNK), PLK3 (FNK), and PLK4 (SAK) (304). They are homologous to the kinases encoded by the *polo* gene in *Drosophila* (305) (from which they derive their name) and also to the yeast mitotic kinase CDC5. All of the polo kinases have an N-terminal Ser/Thr kinase domain of approximately 250 amino acids, and a C-terminal domain containing the eponymous Polo-box domain (Figure 6.7). PLK1, PLK2, and PLK3 have tandem polo box sequences of approximately 60–70 amino acids each, whereas PLK4 has only one polo box. The polo box domains bind to phosphoserine/phosphothreonine peptides with a preference for proline at the +1 position (306–308), and the resulting interactions are important for substrate interactions and directing subcellular localization. Furthermore, in the absence of phosphopeptide interactions the polo domains may negatively regulate the activity of the kinase domain (309). In *Drosophila*, polo was identified as a mitotic kinase, and this role is recapitulated by the human PLK1 isoform: however, the other PLK family members have distinct roles in regulating various aspects of cell cycle progression (304, 310).

PLK1 PLK1 is the most thoroughly characterized of the human polo kinases and is also the homolog most strongly linked to cancer (311). PLK1 is mainly found in proliferating cells and performs many functions relating to mitosis, including transit through the G2 checkpoint, centrosome maturation, chromosome segregation, spindle assembly, and cytokinesis (Figure 6.6). Among these functions, its role in mitotic spindle formation and mitotic exit is particularly important. Expression of PLK1 increases in late S phase and is sustained until late in mitosis, at which

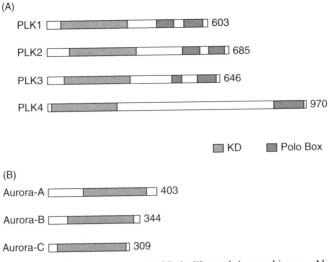

Figure 6.7 Domain structures of Polo-like and Aurora kinases. Abbreviation: KD, kinase domain.

point the protein is degraded by the APC:cyclosome complex. Immunofluorescence studies have shown PLK1 to be located at centrosomes, at the cellular midzone, and at kinetochores, consistent with its role in regulating multiple mitotic processes.

The initial function of PLK1 in regulating mitosis is to promote mitotic entry, although its role in this process appears to be at least partly dispensable (312). During the G2-M transition, PLK1 phosphorylates CDC25C and cyclin B1, promoting their nuclear accumulation and activation of CDK1:cyclin B (313). In addition, phosphorylation of the antimitotic kinases WEE1 and MYT1 kinases by PLK1 promotes mitotic entry (314, 315); furthermore, PLK1 also phosphorylates the mitotic regulator PIN1, a peptidyl-prolyl isomerase that in turn may modulate the activity of CDC25 and PLK1 (316). PLK1 also interacts with and/or phosphorylates several proteins involved in the G2 DNA damage checkpoint. Activation of the G2 checkpoint leads to PLK1 inhibition (317, 318), resulting in activation of p53 and CHK2 (319, 320). Moreover, PLK1 is required for reinitiation of mitosis following G2 arrest (321).

Centrosome maturation and microtubule nucleation were among the first functions ascribed to *Drosophila polo* and this is recapitulated in human cells (322–324). Following mitotic entry, PLK1 is also detected on chromosome arms and kinetochores and has been implicated in chromosome compaction and sister chromatid separation (325–327). PLK1 also plays a key role in regulating kinetochore attachment to mitotic spindles. It is recruited to kinetochores by INCENP (inner centromere protein) and helps to maintain the spindle assembly checkpoint by phosphorylating kinetochores that are not under tension, recruiting the spindle checkpoint kinases BUBR1 and MAD1/MAD2 (328, 329). Together with CDC20, these kinases prevent further mitotic transit until stable mitotic spindles are established. Following proper spindle attachment, PLK1 is displaced from the kinetochores, silencing the spindle checkpoint, and performs its next critical function, which helps to trigger its own destruction. In concert with CDK1 (which, as described earlier, is activated by PLK1 on mitotic entry), PLK1 contributes to activation of the APC:cyclosome complex and degradation of the APC:cyclosome inhibitor EMI1 (330–333). APC:cyclosome activation is essential for mitotic exit and results in degradation of multiple mitotic proteins including PLK1, CDC20, cyclin B1, and Aurora A (334). Although levels of PLK1 and other mitotic regulators are thereby decreased in late mitosis, PLK1 has also been implicated in phosphorylation of several proteins involved in cytokinesis and is found at the midbody between dividing cells.

Several lines of evidence have strongly implicated PLK1 in tumorigenesis and suggested that PLK1 inhibition may be a viable strategy for cancer therapy. Since PLK1 activity is largely confined to mitosis, it is not found in differentiated tissue. However, PLK1 overexpression is prevalent in many different tumor types (311). In some of these cases, notably non small cell lung cancer, colorectal cancer, esophageal and oropharyngeal carcinoma, hepatoblastoma, melanoma, and non Hodgkin's lymphoma, PLK1 overexpression is strongly correlated with tumor grade and/or negatively correlated with survival. As noted previously, PLK1 is silenced by the G2 DNA-damage checkpoint, so cells with aberrant PLK1 overexpression may be able to override the checkpoint and circumvent both intrinsic DNA damage (e.g., due to aneuploidy) and the effects of genotoxic drugs. In addition, the inhibitory effects of PLK1 on p53 may protect tumor cells from p53-dependent apoptosis (319). Consistent with this, overexpression of PLK1 in NIH3T3 cells leads to oncogenic transformation (335). PLK1 inhibition by intracellular antibody injection was shown to produce mitotic dysregulation in HeLa cells; interestingly, nonimmortalized cells did not enter mitosis, suggesting that they were protected from aberrant mitosis and that PLK1 inhibition may have some degree of selectivity for aneuploid tumor cells (323). Further validation of PLK1 inhibition as an antitumor strategy has been provided by the discovery of several selective small molecule inhibitors of the kinase, discussed further in Chapter 10.

PLK2   In contrast to PLK1, PLK2 is found in both proliferating and nonproliferating cells; in proliferating cells it is primarily active in G1 and early S phase. PLK2 is also expressed in postmitotic neurons and may play a role in modulating synaptic plasticity (336). PLK2 mRNA is upregulated in response to mitogenic signaling, and it is involved in duplication of centrioles during S phase (337). However, PLK2 appears to be somewhat functionally redundant since $plk2^{-/-}$ mice are viable, albeit with retarded growth (338). In contrast to the downregulation of PLK1 in response to G2 checkpoint signaling, PLK2 mRNA is induced following radiation (339). PLK2 expression is often downregulated in malignant B cells, and restoring PLK2 function to these cells promotes apoptosis, suggesting a tumor suppressor role for PLK2 in at least some cellular contexts (340). Conversely, PLK2 depletion has been reported to increase sensitivity of cancer cells to chemotherapy drugs (341, 342).

PLK3   PLK3 displays some functional similarities to PLK2: it is found in both proliferating and nonproliferating cells, is primarily active in G1 and early S phase, and is also expressed in postmitotic neurons. PLK3 expression is induced in response to mitogenic signaling and regulates entry into S phase, attenuating cyclin E activity via a post-transcriptional mechanism and also regulating CDC25A (343, 344). PLK3 is also functionally linked to the G2 checkpoint and is activated upon chemically mediated DNA damage (345). PLK3 is a positive regulator of p53 and may have a further role in promoting DNA repair via phosphorylation of DNA polymerase δ (346). In both lung and head and neck tumor cells, PLK3 is downregulated compared to matched normal tissue, and ectopic PLK3 expression has antiproliferative effects in fibroblasts (347, 348). Furthermore, $plk3$ knockout mice develop large tumors, mediated in part by deregulation of HIF1α expression (349). Hence PLK3 appears to have a tumor suppressor function and may not be an appropriate target for cancer therapy.

PLK4 (SAK)   PLK4 is structurally divergent from the other three family members in having only one polo box domain. It is expressed from late G1 through M phase and is essential for viability; $plk4^{-/-}$ mouse embryos die at E7.5 (350). $plk4^{+/-}$ mice are viable but display multiple signs of mitotic dysregulation including centrosome amplification and aneuploidy, thus suggesting a role for PLK4 in suppressing tumorigenesis (351). PLK4 is found at the nucleolus, centrosomes, and cleavage furrow in dividing cells and is required for centriole duplication in S phase (352, 353). Recent data implicates PLK4 in control of embryonic cellular differentiation, by promoting the nucleolar release of the Hand1 transcription factor (354, 355). However, the factors distinguishing the constitutive mitotic activity from the differentiating activity of PLK4 have not been clearly defined.

6.4.2 Aurora Kinases

There are three mammalian kinases in the Aurora family, usually designated Aurora-A, -B, and -C. All three have highly homologous kinase domains but differ in their sequences at the C terminus of the protein (Figure 6.7). The D-box regions in the C terminus, together with the A-box region at the N terminus, are implicated in protein degradation (356–358). Despite their similarities, each kinase plays a distinct spatial and temporal role in helping to orchestrate mitosis (359). Our discussion here focuses on Aurora-A and Aurora-B. Aurora-C has been somewhat less well studied: it is highly expressed in the testes and may play a role in meiotic cell division, although it also bears some functional similarities to the other Auroras. Its role in cancer has not been clearly defined, although it is overexpressed in some cancer cell lines and primary colorectal tumors (360, 361). Overexpression of Aurora-C in HeLa cells promotes centrosome duplication and polyploidy, although this effect appears to be independent of Aurora-C kinase activity and may represent a dominant-negative effect on Aurora-A and/or Aurora-B function (362).

Aurora-A *Aurora-A* bears many of the hallmarks of an oncogene: it is located in an amplicon (20q13) that is frequently amplified in primary tumors and cancer cell lines, and active Aurora-A confers tumorigenicity in NIH3T3 cells (363, 364). Inappropriate activation of Aurora-A may lead to bypass of the G2/M cell cycle checkpoint and cytokinetic failure resulting in centrosome amplification and polyploidy—a common feature of advanced tumor cells (365). It is also possible that cells lacking functional p53 may be particularly sensitive to the mitotic dysfunction promoted by Aurora overexpression and activation, since (i) p53 can bind to and inactivate Aurora-A and (ii) cells lacking p53 are defective in the G1 cell cycle checkpoint, so are unable to effectively arrest in the G1 phase following abnormal cell division. However, the relationship with p53 signaling is complex as Aurora-A can also phosphorylate and inhibit p53.

Aurora-A is expressed from the end of S phase to the beginning of G1 and, at the start of mitosis, is predominantly associated with centrosomes and with microtubules proximal to the centrosomes. During G2, Aurora-A becomes activated by the LIM protein Ajuba. This Aurora-A activation is essential for mitotic entry and appears to be critical for proper centrosome separation (366): more recent data indicates that it may also be involved in breakdown of the nuclear membrane (367). Aurora-A appears to perform multiple functions during mitosis. First, it is important for recruiting tubulin to the spindle poles and stabilizing the nascent mitotic microtubules. Second, some Aurora-A is found to be localized along the length of microtubules, where it helps to mediate spindle assembly. Activation of RAN GTPase by the GTPase exchange factor RCC1 results in release of spindle assembly factors such as TPX2 (368). TPX2 binds to the C-terminal domain of Aurora-A and targets it to the mitotic spindle, stimulating autophosphorylation and protecting it from degradation by the PP1 phosphatase (369, 370). As the dividing cell transitions to metaphase, the centrosomal Aurora-A relocalizes to the centromeres and can be found at the cellular midzone from anaphase until the end of cytokinesis (371). At the centromere, Aurora-A phosphorylates CENP-A (centrosomal protein A), a histone H3 variant that is involved in recruitment of Aurora-B (see below) and directing kinetochore-spindle interactions (372). During late mitosis, Aurora-A is degraded by the anaphase-promoting complex (APC) (373).

Aurora-B Unlike Aurora-A, Aurora-B is not found to be amplified in tumor cells although it is frequently overexpressed: however, it is not clear whether this overexpression is a cause of or response to mitotic dysregulation. Aurora-B is principally localized to the centromeres where, together with INCENP, survivin, and borealin, it is part of the so-called chromosomal passenger complex (374). Both INCENP and survivin are involved in activating Aurora-B, and this activity is important for appropriate attachment of microtubules to the kinetochores (375). Typically, one kinetochore first attaches to a microtubule emanating from one of the cellular poles (termed monotelic attachment). If the free chromatid then attaches to a microtubule from the opposite pole, amphitelic attachment occurs and the chromosomes can become appropriately positioned in the midzone and proceed to segregate. However, sometimes both chromatids become attached to the same pole (termed syntelic attachment), or one chromatid is attached to both poles (merotelic attachment). In these cases, Aurora-B regulates the activity of the microtubule depolymerase MCAK, promoting release of the improperly attached microtubules so that appropriate reengagement can occur and stabilizing correctly assembled mitotic spindles until all chromatids are correctly attached and anaphase can proceed (376, 377).

Aurora-B also provides a link between the structural integrity of microtubule:kinetochore interactions and the spindle checkpoint: in particular, Aurora-B kinase activity is required for recruitment of the spindle checkpoint proteins CENP-E, BUBR1 (BUB1B), and MAD2 to the kinetochore (378). Notably, overexpression of Aurora-A disrupts the localization of BUBR1 and MAD2, and the resulting abrogation of the spindle checkpoint may be important for mitotic competence in cancer cells. Furthermore, this mechanism may be important for resistance to antimitotic drugs such as paclitaxel in tumors that overexpress Aurora-A (379). In addition to its role in regulating spindle:chromatid interactions, Aurora-B has been associated with several other activities relating to mitosis. During mitotic entry, Aurora-B phosphorylates histone H3 and CENP-A (380, 381). Later in mitosis, Aurora-B localizes to the cellular midbody and, in concert with RHO GTPase, is essential for destabilizing intermediate filaments during cytokinesis (382). Like Aurora-A, Aurora-B is ubiquitinated and degraded by the APC following mitosis (383).

6.5   CELL CYCLE CHECKPOINT KINASES

Replicating cells may be subjected to various forms of genotoxic stress, including ionizing radiation, ultraviolet light, chemical mutagens, and reactive oxygen species. These mechanisms can cause extensive DNA damage, resulting in mutations, translocations, unequal nuclear divisions, and, ultimately, genomic instability—one of the hallmarks of neoplastic transformation. Accordingly, eukaryotic cells have evolved a complex DNA damage response signaling network, whose output is a series of interrelated cell cycle checkpoints (Figure 6.8). These checkpoints serve to detect DNA damage and activate DNA repair mechanisms at the sites of damage, while also propagating the DNA-damage signal throughout the cell in order to retard or block cell cycle progression. If the DNA lesion(s) can be repaired, the checkpoint signal is terminated and the cell cycle is reengaged: however, in the case of insurmountable damage, the checkpoint pathways initiate signaling programs leading to apoptosis or senescence. Several protein kinases are centrally involved in DNA-damage response signaling, and these proteins represent a double-edged sword with regard to the initiation, progression, and treatment of cancer. Tumorigenesis almost always involves defects in genomic integrity, and in early stages of carcinogenesis the DNA-damage response network acts as a barrier to tumor formation (384–386). In these nascent tumors, oncogene-induced replication stress leads to stalled replication forks and DNA breakage, activating DNA-damage checkpoint pathways and resulting in DNA repair, cell death, or senescence (387, 388). However, some cells may evade these checkpoints and develop into advanced tumors with widespread genetic defects.

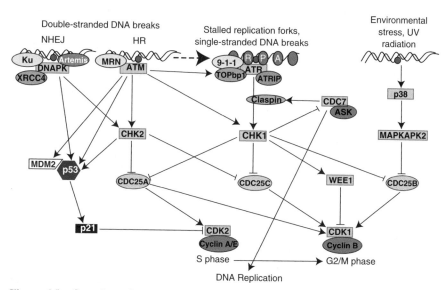

Figure 6.8   Overview of DNA checkpoint signaling in response to various DNA damage modalities. See text for further details.

In such cases, genomic instability may act as an intrinsic source of replication stress and cell cycle checkpoint mechanisms may turn from hero to villain, enabling the survival, DNA repair, and productive replication of cancer cells. Furthermore, these checkpoint pathways may play a significant role in protecting tumors against the damaging effects of genotoxic therapies, and inhibition of cell cycle checkpoint mechanisms has been proposed as a strategy for increasing the efficacy of radiotherapy and chemotherapy (389, 390). Research during the past few years has dramatically increased our knowledge of the spatial and temporal regulation of cell cycle checkpoint activation by different kinds of DNA damage. Next, we review some kinases that are important for cell cycle checkpoint control, and their potential as anticancer targets.

6.5.1 ATM, ATR, and DNAPK

The ATM (ataxia telangiectasia-mutated) and ATR (ataxia telangiectasia and Rad3-related) kinases are proximally involved in activating cell cycle checkpoint mechanisms in response to various kinds of DNA damage. As indicated by its name, ATM is mutated in ataxia telangiectasia (AT), a congenital disease characterized by multiple immunological and neurological defects. AT patients are also hypersensitive to ionizing radiation and predisposed to cancer, highlighting the role of ATM in modulating the cellular response to DNA damage. ATM and ATR are very large proteins, comprised of 3056 and 2644 amino acids, respectively, with the kinase domain located near the C terminus (Figure 6.9). They belong to the PI3K-related kinase (PIKK) family of atypical protein kinases, and their kinase domains are related in sequence to those of PI3K and mTOR. Collectively, ATM and ATR phosphorylate multiple proteins including the checkpoint kinases CHK1 and CHK2, promoting cell cycle arrest and DNA repair. Another PIKK family member, DNAPK, also responds to DNA damage by triggering the nonhomologous end joining (NHEJ) repair pathway and may also play a role in activating CHK2 (391). Although ATM, ATR, and DNAPK have distinct roles in responding to DNA damage, they are all recruited to sites of damaged DNA via interactions with specific partner proteins: NBS1 for ATM, ATRIP for ATR, and Ku for DNAPK (392, 393).

ATR is activated by DNA lesions resulting from stalled replication forks and other single-stranded DNA breaks, such as those induced by UV radiation, nucleotide depletion, and various cytotoxic agents (Figure 6.8). As such, activation of ATR plays a particularly important role during DNA replication in S phase, where aberrant progression of DNA synthesis can be particularly damaging. There may in fact be several related S-phase checkpoint mechanisms, resulting from stalled replication forks, double-stranded DNA breaks, and failure of the overall DNA replication process (394). In the case of stalled replication forks, persistent DNA helicase activity exposes a chain of single-stranded DNA (ssDNA), which becomes decorated with replication protein A (RPA). ATR is subsequently recruited to RPA-coated ssDNA via its association with ATRIP (395) and a multiprotein structure is formed, also involving the so-called 9-1-1 complex (RAD9:HUS1:RAD1). ATR activation involves several other factors, including TopBP1 (topoisomerase binding

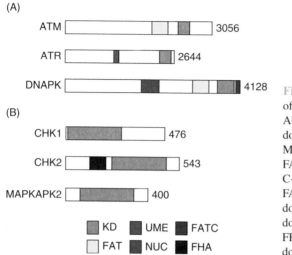

Figure 6.9   Domain structures of DNA checkpoint kinases. Abbreviations: KD—kinase domain; UME—UVSB PI3K, MEI-41, ESR1 domain; FATC—FRAP, ATM, TRRAP C-terminal domain; FAT—FRAP, ATM, and TRRAP domain; NUC—NUC194 domain; FHA—Forkhead-associated domain.

protein 1) (396). Once activated, ATR phosphorylates multiple targets at the DNA lesion, most notably the CHK1 kinase (discussed later). Phosphorylation of CHK1 downstream of ATR is dependent on phosphorylation of the chromatin-associated protein Claspin, which in turn is phosphorylated by the CDC7 kinase (397, 398). The concerted action of ATR/CHK1 signaling leads to stabilization of stalled replication forks. As well as being a critical transducer of DNA-damage signals, ATR appears to have a critical role in unperturbed cell cycles, since deletion of *atr* is embryonic lethal in mice (399, 400). In humans, partial loss of function mutations in ATR are found in Seckel syndrome, a severe human congenital defect characterized by growth and mental retardation, microcephaly, and "bird-like" facial features (401).

In contrast to ATR, ATM is primarily recruited to and activated by DNA double-strand breaks (DSBs), which are particularly damaging genetic lesions caused primarily by radiation and radiomimetic cytotoxic drugs (Figure 6.8) (392, 402). An ATM autophosphorylation site (Ser1981) is involved in its activation (403); activated ATM phosphorylates multiple substrates involved in the checkpoint/DNA-damage response including BRCA1, p53, Artemis, and CHK2. As noted earlier, ATM appears less critical than ATR in embryonic development, and both mice and humans with ATM deficiency survive (404). ATM is recruited to DSBs by the MRE11:RAD50:NBS1 (MRN) complex, which has nuclease activity and processes the ends of the breaks to generate ssDNA. This ssDNA subsequently associates with RPA and recruits ATR/ATRIP as described earlier: thus ATM also appears to help activate ATR (and hence CHK1) in response to ionizing radiation (405). ATM also phosphorylates TopBP1, enhancing its association with ATR (406). This process is cell cycle specific and occurs predominantly in S and G2 phases, where most DNA repair occurs by homologous recombination (involving the sister chromatid of the damaged region) rather than NHEJ. However, ATM may also participate in the NHEJ repair process via phosphorylation of Artemis, an exonuclease that forms part of the DNAPK DNA repair complex (discussed later) (407). The phosphorylation of Artemis by ATM in response to ionizing radiation may also be involved in recovery from the DNA checkpoint, although molecular details of this process are still unclear (408).

The DNAPK kinase (often referred to as DNAPK$_{cs}$, for catalytic subunit) is a 470-kDa protein containing 4128 amino acids. Like ATM, DNAPK responds to DSBs but activates the nonhomologous end joining pathway rather than homologous recombination. This pathway is most relevant in the G0 and G1 phases of the cell cycle; correspondingly activation of DNAPK does not promote S or G2/M cell cycle arrest. DNAPK is a complex consisting of DNAPK$_{cs}$ and the Ku heterodimer, consisting of Ku70 and Ku80. Ku is the sensor of DNA damage and recruits DNAPK$_{cs}$ to the lesion, where DNAPK is rapidly activated by autophosphorylation (409). DNAPK then phosphorylates the endonuclease Artemis, which promotes local unwinding of the DNA. The DNA ends are processed, possibly by the MRN complex and/or DNA polymerase μ. Finally, DNAPK phosphorylates and activates the XRCC4 DNA ligase, which religates the broken DNA. DNAPK also phosphorylates many additional substrates including p53, mediating an apoptotic tumor suppressor response following DNA damage. However, DNAPK may also promote resistance to radiation or chemotherapy by accelerating the repair of DSBs, and so DNAPK inhibition has been proposed as a therapeutic strategy in combination with genotoxic therapy (410). Further details can be found in several excellent reviews (411, 412).

6.5.2 CHK1, CHK2, and MAPKAPK2

Immediately downstream of ATM and ATR are the checkpoint kinases CHK1 and CHK2. ATM is regarded as the primary activator of CHK2 and ATR as the activator of CHK1, although there is likely to be substantial crosstalk between these pathways: indeed, as noted previously ATM can also indirectly activate CHK1 in response to DSBs. More recently, MAPKAPK2 has been shown to function also as a checkpoint kinase, and it responds to ultraviolet stress via p38 MAP kinase (413): this checkpoint may be particularly relevant in cells lacking p53 (414). CHK1, CHK2, and MAPKAPK2 are not particularly closely related by sequence, although all three fall within the CAMK family. One of the principal functions of these effector kinases is to retard or arrest cell cycle progression, in order to enable DNA repair to occur. This cell cycle arrest is achieved via multiple mechanisms. First, phosphorylation of CDC25 phosphatases leads to their degradation (CDC25A) or cytoplasmic sequestration (CDC25B/C) (415). Collectively, CDC25 phosphatases dephosphorylate and activate CDK1 and CDK2, promoting cell cycle progression: therefore checkpoint kinase-mediated CDC25 inhibition results in cell cycle arrest. CDC25A is active in S phase and may also play a role in the G2/M transition, whereas CDC25B and CDC25C function predominantly at the G2/M boundary. Second, CHK1 phosphorylates ASK, the cyclin-like regulator of CDC7, promoting its dissociation from chromatin and inactivation. CDC7-mediated phosphorylation of the MCM complex at DNA replication origins is essential for recruitment of CDC45 and subsequent initiation of replication (Chapter 1), so this provides an orthogonal mechanism for blockade of S-phase progression. Third, the ATM/ATR/CHK1/CHK2 pathways can promote the activity of p53 by various mechanisms, leading to upregulation of p53 transcriptional targets such as the CDK inhibitor p21. Fourth, CHK1 phosphorylates the CDK1 kinase WEE1, enhancing its activity toward CDK1 and contributing to the blockade of mitotic entry. Finally, CHK1 was recently shown to associate with chromatin and phosphorylate histone H3, promoting transcription of CDK1 and related cyclins. DNA damage leads to dissociation of CHK1 from chromatin, repressing CDK1/cyclin expression and causing cell cycle delay (416).

CHK1 contains an N-terminal kinase domain and a C-terminal regulatory region (Figure 6.9). Basal CHK1 activity is present in cells even in the absence of DNA damage: it is induced in late G1 phase and appears to be important for maintaining normal DNA synthesis (417) and mitotic entry (418, 419). The importance of CHK1 for regulation of unperturbed cell cycles is underscored by the fact that $chk1^{-/-}$ mice die early in embryogenesis (420, 421). Furthermore, mice that are haploinsufficient for CHK1 display defective cell cycle regulation, including premature entry into S phase and M phase and intrinsic DNA damage (422). Phosphorylation on the activation loop does not appear to be required for activation, but CHK1 activity is upregulated in response to DNA damage via phosphorylation (by ATM/ATR) at S317 and S345 in the C-terminal regulatory region, and mutational inactivation of these sites results in a significantly blunted DNA-damage response (423). These phosphorylation sites are also important for regulating the subcellular localization of CHK1. Under basal conditions, about 20% of CHK1 is associated with chromatin; in response to DNA damage, ATM/ATR-dependent phosphorylation of CHK1 results in rapid dissociation from chromatin at localized sites of DNA damage. This may enable mobilization of the checkpoint response throughout the nucleus, as well as further recruitment and activation of CHK1 from the nucleoplasm to the site of DNA damage (424). CHK1 is also found at centrosomes during interphase, where it regulates the timing of mitotic entry by inhibiting CDK1 activation (418). Phosphorylation at S345 promotes cytoplasmic localization of CHK1 (and possibly subsequent centrosomal accumulation) and appears to be critical for normal cell cycle function as well as checkpoint activation, whereas S317 phosphorylation was proposed to be the primary mediator of dissociation from chromatin in response to DNA damage (425). Intriguingly, CHK1 can also be phosphorylated by CDK1 at two different sites in the C-terminal domain (S286 and S381): the functional consequences of this are not yet clear, although it is notable that this phosphorylation can occur during mitosis whereas S317/S345 phosphorylation cannot occur (426).

Initial studies of the CHK1-mediated DNA-damage response focused on phosphorylation of CDC25C and regulation of the G2/M transition. CHK1 regulates CDC25C by phosphorylation on Ser216, resulting in its sequestration in the cytoplasm via binding to 14-3-3 proteins (427). This leads to hyperphosphorylation/inhibition of CDK1 function and blocking of the G2/M transition. CHK1 is also centrally involved in both normal and DNA-damaged cells during S phase, and this role is at least as important as, if not more so, than control of the G2/M transition (428). CHK1 phosphorylates CDC25A at Ser123 and other residues, leading to its ubiquitin-mediated degradation (429, 430). This activity is manifest in normal cell cycles and prevents excessive CDK2 activation during S phase. Following DNA damage, the CHK1-mediated degradation of CDC25A is accelerated, aided by the coordinated action of CHK2 (429). CHK1 performs several diverse functions apart from retarding and halting cell cycle progression. In addition to retarding or arresting cell cycle progression, CHK1 mediates the stabilization of stalled replication forks downstream of ATR as discussed previously. There is also evidence that CHK1 is required for DNA repair by homologous recombination via the recombination repair protein RAD51 (431). In addition to regulating S-phase progression and mitotic entry, CHK1 also promotes the mitotic spindle checkpoint via phosphorylation and activation of Aurora-B (432). In prometaphase (both in unperturbed cells and in response to antimitotic agents such as paclitaxel), CHK1 is found at kinetochores and regulates the activity of Aurora-B. Moreover, this relationship with Aurora-B may also be relevant in cytokinesis, when CHK1 colocalizes with Aurora-B at the midbody (432). CHK1 has also been associated with a mitotic exit checkpoint (433), which blocks cytokinesis in response to DNA damage and leads to mitotic catastrophe—a form of cell death resulting from premature mitotic entry and subsequent failure of mitosis (434). The increased genomic instability in CHK1-deficient cells may largely be due to its regulation of mitotic checkpoints, in addition to regulating S-phase progression and mitotic entry. More recently, it was shown that CHK1 represses a caspase2-dependent apoptotic pathway in p53-deficient zebrafish embryos and human cells (435). This pathway involves activation of ATM and ATR but is independent of the classical intrinsic and extrinsic apoptotic pathways and may represent an important mechanism of survival for tumor cells with loss of p53 and/or overexpression of antiapoptotic BCL2 family proteins.

In CHK2, the regulatory domains and ATM/ATR phosphorylation sites are at the N terminus of the kinase (Figure 6.9). The regulatory region of CHK2 is necessary for kinase activity and promotes the formation of CHK2 dimers in response to phosphorylation at T68 (436, 437); activation is subsequently achieved by CHK2 transphosphorylation (discussed in Chapter 2). CHK2 is rapidly activated in response to DNA damage (in particular, double-stranded breaks) and, like CHK1, phosphorylates CDC25 family phosphatases. However, many studies with diverse cancer cell lines and DNA-damaging agents have shown that deletion of CHK2 leaves S and G2 checkpoint mechanisms relatively intact, whereas deletion of CHK1 leads to checkpoint abrogation. In keeping with this (and in contrast to CHK1), $chk2^{-/-}$ mice are viable and relatively normal, apart from defects in their response to genotoxic insults (438, 439). Therefore, although CHK2 can phosphorylate many of the same substrates as CHK1, it appears to be less critical in the orchestration of checkpoint responses. The current evidence suggests that, at least with regard to blocking cell cycle progression, CHK1 is the "workhorse" kinase, with CHK2 acting as an amplifier of constitutive CHK1 activity under conditions where CHK1 is hyperactivated (440). Although CHK2 is specifically phosphorylated at sites of DNA damage, it subsequently migrates throughout the nucleus and may therefore help to convey the DNA checkpoint status from the area of DNA damage to other sites of DNA replication (394, 441).

Apart from its role in cell cycle progression, CHK2 has additional functions relating to various cell death pathways. These functions are highly dependent on cellular and environmental context, as different studies have indicated both a pro-survival and proapoptotic role for CHK2. CHK2 has been implicated in mediating p53-dependent apoptosis via multiple mechanisms, including direct phosphoryla-tion of p53 (442–444) and phosphorylation of the p53 regulator MDMX (445, 446). However, CHK2 seems to be at least partly dispensable in this role and its importance may depend on the type of DNA damage and the genetic background of the cell (447). CHK2 can also promote non-p53-dependent apoptosis via pathways involving E2F-1 (448), PML (449), and the release of survivin from mitochondria in response to DNA damage (450). $Chk2^{-/-}$ murine thymocytes are resistant to apop-tosis (444), and studies with $chk2^{-/-}$ mice indicate that they display significantly enhanced radioprotection compared to $chk2^{+/+}$ littermates, mediated through both ATM-dependent and ATM-independent pathways (439, 451). Notably, $chk2^{-/-}$ mice show little propensity for increased tumorigenesis, despite having defective DNA-damage-induced apoptosis. Activation of ATR and CHK2 in renal tissue has also recently been implicated in promoting apoptosis and nephrotoxicity associ-ated with cisplatin treatment (452). The radioprotective/chemoprotective activity of CHK2 inhibition raises the possibility that a CHK2 inhibitor may be able to increase the therapeutic index of genotoxic therapies by protecting normal cells rather than sensitizing tumor cells. Consistent with this, a specific 2-aryl benzim-idazole inhibitor of CHK2 was reported to protect human T cells from ionizing radiation (453). In contrast, CHK2 inhibition was reported to sensitize tumor cells to apoptosis following radiation or camptothecin treatment (454, 455). CHK2 is also a repressor of mitotic catastrophe: experiments with an artificial syncitia for-mation model and with tumor cells have shown that downregulation of CHK2 in the presence of catastrophic DNA damage can lead to premature mitotic pro-gression, formation of endopolyploid cells, and induction of apoptotic pathways (456, 457).

Which of the above kinases are the most promising targets for cancer ther-apy? The preponderance of evidence suggests that CHK1 is the primary driver of the DNA-damage response, and so it has perhaps received the most attention to date. Some caution may be warranted by the observation that CHK1 is important for normal cell cycles: however, CHK1 inhibition appears to be more toxic to tumor cells than to normal fibroblasts (458) and may be tolerable if administered intermittently in conjunction with chemotherapy or radiation. The potentiation of DNA-damage-induced cell death by CHK2 inhibition in tumor cells raises the pos-sibility that CHK2-targeted agents may be able to increase the activity of genotoxic agents in tumor cells while protecting normal cells from apoptosis. However, mul-tiple studies indicate that CHK2 may be dispensable for DNA-damage checkpoint function, and a specific small molecule CHK2 inhibitor did not affect the cytotoxic-ity of doxorubicin, paclitaxel, or cisplatin in cellular assays (459). It is also notable that CHK2 is a mediator of cellular senescence, in response to telomere erosion, DNA double-stranded breaks, or oncogene expression (387, 388, 460, 461), and

CHK2 activation has been proposed as a therapeutic strategy for driving tumor cells into senescence or apoptosis in the absence of DNA damage (462). Targeting all of the checkpoint kinases in parallel may appear to be an attractive strategy, although it has been reported that inhibition of other checkpoint pathways in addition to CHK1 may blunt the effect of CHK1 inhibition in the context of some cell lines and DNA-damage modalities (463). Furthermore, there may be additional as yet undiscovered checkpoint kinases: it was recently reported that, while S-phase checkpoint is dependent on CHK1, G2 arrest in response to topoisomerase inhibition could be triggered in the face of CHK1, CHK2, and MAPKAPK2 inhibition (464). In conclusion, the efficacy of checkpoint kinase inhibition depends on many complex genetic and environmental factors, and further empirical investigation of checkpoint kinase inhibitors in preclinical and clinical settings will ultimately determine which targets are appropriate for combination with selected genotoxic therapies and tumor types.

REFERENCES

1. Hanahan D, Weinberg RA. The hallmarks of cancer. Cell 2000;100(1):57–70.
2. Knudsen ES, Knudsen KE. Retinoblastoma tumor suppressor: where cancer meets the cell cycle. Exp Biol Med (Maywood) 2006;231(7):1271–1281.
3. Sears RC, Nevins JR. Signaling networks that link cell proliferation and cell fate. J Biol Chem 2002;277(14):11617–11620.
4. Stevaux O, Dyson NJ. A revised picture of the E2F transcriptional network and RB function. Curr Opin Cell Biol 2002;14(6):684–691.
5. Massague J. G1 cell-cycle control and cancer. Nature 2004;432(7015):298–306.
6. Mittnacht S. Control of pRB phosphorylation. Curr Opin Genet Dev 1998;8(1):21–27.
7. Johnson DG, Degregori J. Putting the oncogenic and tumor suppressive activities of E2F into context. Curr Mol Med 2006;6(7):731–738.
8. DeGregori J, Johnson DG. Distinct and overlapping roles for E2F family members in transcription, proliferation and apoptosis. Curr Mol Med 2006;6(7):739–748.
9. Kim WY, Sharpless NE. The regulation of INK4/ARF in cancer and aging. Cell 2006;127(2):265–275.
10. Sharpless NE. INK4a/ARF: a multifunctional tumor suppressor locus. Mutat Res 2005;576(1–2): 22–38.
11. Campisi J. Suppressing cancer: the importance of being senescent. Science 2005;309(5736): 886–887.
12. Hanks SK. Homology probing: identification of cDNA clones encoding members of the protein-serine kinase family. Proc Natl Acad Sci U S A 1987;84(2):388–392.
13. Mitchell C, Park MA, Zhang G, Yacoub A, Curiel DT, Fisher PB, Roberts JD, Grant S, Dent P. Extrinsic pathway- and cathepsin-dependent induction of mitochondrial dysfunction are essential for synergistic flavopiridol and vorinostat lethality in breast cancer cells. Mol Cancer Ther 2007;6(12Pt 1):3101–3112.
14. Meyerson M, Enders GH, Wu CL, Su LK, Gorka C, Nelson C, Harlow E, Tsai LH. A family of human cdc2-related protein kinases. EMBO J 1992;11(8):2909–2917.
15. Russo AA, Tong L, Lee JO, Jeffrey PD, Pavletich NP. Structural basis for inhibition of the cyclin-dependent kinase Cdk6 by the tumour suppressor p16INK4a. Nature 1998;395(6699):237–243.
16. Schulze-Gahmen U, Kim SH. Structural basis for CDK6 activation by a virus-encoded cyclin. Nat Struct Biol 2002;9(3):177–181.
17. Lu H, Chang DJ, Baratte B, Meijer L, Schulze-Gahmen U. Crystal structure of a human cyclin-dependent kinase 6 complex with a flavonol inhibitor, fisetin. J Med Chem 2005;48(3): 737–743.

18. Brotherton DH, Dhanaraj V, Wick S, Brizuela L, Domaille PJ, Volyanik E, Xu X, Parisini E, Smith BO, Archer SJ, Serrano M, Brenner SL, Blundell TL, Laue ED. Crystal structure of the complex of the cyclin D-dependent kinase Cdk6 bound to the cell-cycle inhibitor p19INK4d. Nature 1998;395(6699):244–250.

19. Larochelle S, Merrick KA, Terret ME, Wohlbold L, Barboza NM, Zhang C, Shokat KM, Jallepalli PV, Fisher RP. Requirements for Cdk7 in the assembly of Cdk1/cyclin B and activation of Cdk2 revealed by chemical genetics in human cells. Mol Cell 2007;25(6):839–850.

20. Igarashi M, Nagata A, Jinno S, Suto K, Okayama H. Wee1(+)-like gene in human cells. Nature 1991;353(6339):80–83.

21. Parker LL, Piwnica-Worms H. Inactivation of the p34cdc2-cyclin B complex by the human WEE1 tyrosine kinase. Science 1992;257(5078):1955–1957.

22. McGowan CH, Russell P. Human Wee1 kinase inhibits cell division by phosphorylating p34cdc2 exclusively on Tyr15. EMBO J 1993;12(1):75–85.

23. Liu F, Stanton JJ, Wu Z, Piwnica-Worms H. The human Myt1 kinase preferentially phosphorylates Cdc2 on threonine 14 and localizes to the endoplasmic reticulum and Golgi complex. Mol Cell Biol 1997;17(2):571–583.

24. Matsushime H, Quelle DE, Shurtleff SA, Shibuya M, Sherr CJ, Kato JY. D-type cyclin-dependent kinase activity in mammalian cells. Mol Cell Biol 1994;14(3):2066–2076.

25. Mahony D, Parry DA, Lees E. Active cdk6 complexes are predominantly nuclear and represent only a minority of the cdk6 in T cells. Oncogene 1998;16(5):603–611.

26. Ericson KK, Krull D, Slomiany P, Grossel MJ. Expression of cyclin-dependent kinase 6, but not cyclin-dependent kinase 4, alters morphology of cultured mouse astrocytes. Mol Cancer Res 2003;1(9):654–664.

27. Matushansky I, Radparvar F, Skoultchi AI. CDK6 blocks differentiation: coupling cell proliferation to the block to differentiation in leukemic cells. Oncogene 2003;22(27):4143–4149.

28. Schwartz GK, O'Reilly E, Ilson D, Saltz L, Sharma S, Tong W, Maslak P, Stoltz M, Eden L, Perkins P, Endres S, Barazzoul J, Spriggs D, Kelsen D. Phase I study of the cyclin-dependent kinase inhibitor flavopiridol in combination with paclitaxel in patients with advanced solid tumors. J Clin Oncol 2002;20(8):2157–2170.

29. Malumbres M, Sotillo R, Santamaria D, Galan J, Cerezo A, Ortega S, Dubus P, Barbacid M. Mammalian cells cycle without the D-type cyclin-dependent kinases Cdk4 and Cdk6. Cell 2004;118(4):493–504.

30. Savatier P, Lapillonne H, van Grunsven LA, Rudkin BB, Samarut J. Withdrawal of differentiation inhibitory activity/leukemia inhibitory factor up-regulates D-type cyclins and cyclin-dependent kinase inhibitors in mouse embryonic stem cells. Oncogene 1996;12(2):309–322.

31. Burdon T, Smith A, Savatier P. Signalling, cell cycle and pluripotency in embryonic stem cells. Trends Cell Biol 2002;12(9):432–438.

32. Jirmanova L, Afanassieff M, Gobert-Gosse S, Markossian S, Savatier P. Differential contributions of ERK and PI3-kinase to the regulation of cyclin D1 expression and to the control of the G1/S transition in mouse embryonic stem cells. Oncogene 2002;21(36):5515–5528.

33. Stead E, White J, Faast R, Conn S, Goldstone S, Rathjen J, Dhingra U, Rathjen P, Walker D, Dalton S. Pluripotent cell division cycles are driven by ectopic Cdk2, cyclin A/E and E2F activities. Oncogene 2002;21(54):8320–8333.

34. Miyashita K, Shiraki K, Fuke H, Inoue T, Yamanaka Y, Yamaguchi Y, Yamamoto N, Ito K, Sugimoto K, Nakano T. The cyclin-dependent kinase inhibitor flavopiridol sensitizes human hepatocellular carcinoma cells to TRAIL-induced apoptosis. Int J Mol Med 2006;18(2):249–256.

35. Stepanova L, Leng X, Parker SB, Harper JW. Mammalian p50Cdc37 is a protein kinase-targeting subunit of Hsp90 that binds and stabilizes Cdk4. Genes Dev 1996;10(12):1491–1502.

36. Wang X, Grammatikakis N, Hu J. Role of p50/CDC37 in hepadnavirus assembly and replication. J Biol Chem 2002;277(27):24361–24367.

37. Misra RN, Xiao HY, Kim KS, Lu S, Han WC, Barbosa SA, Hunt JT, Rawlins DB, Shan W, Ahmed SZ, Qian L, Chen BC, Zhao R, Bednarz MS, Kellar KA, Mulheron JG, Batorsky R, Roongta U, Kamath A, Marathe P, Ranadive SA, Sack JS, Tokarski JS, Pavletich NP, Lee FY, Webster KR, Kimball SD. N-(cycloalkylamino)acyl-2-aminothiazole inhibitors of

cyclin-dependent kinase 2. N-[5-[[[5-(1,1-dimethylethyl)-2-oxazolyl]methyl]thio]-2-thiazolyl]-4-piperidinecarboxamide (BMS-387032), a highly efficacious and selective antitumor agent. J Med Chem 2004;47(7):1719–1728.

38. Vaughan CK, Gohlke U, Sobott F, Good VM, Ali MM, Prodromou C, Robinson CV, Saibil HR, Pearl LH. Structure of an Hsp90-Cdc37-Cdk4 complex. Mol Cell 2006;23(5):697–707.

39. Lamphere L, Fiore F, Xu X, Brizuela L, Keezer S, Sardet C, Draetta GF, Gyuris J. Interaction between Cdc37 and Cdk4 in human cells. Oncogene 1997;14(16):1999–2004.

40. Laman H. Fbxo7 gets proactive with cyclin D/cdk6. Cell Cycle 2006;5(3):279–282.

41. Laman H, Funes JM, Ye H, Henderson S, Galinanes-Garcia L, Hara E, Knowles P, McDonald N, Boshoff C. Transforming activity of Fbxo7 is mediated specifically through regulation of cyclin D/cdk6. EMBO J 2005;24(17):3104–3116.

42. Shapiro GI, Park JE, Edwards CD, Mao L, Merlo A, Sidransky D, Ewen ME, Rollins BJ. Multiple mechanisms of p16INK4A inactivation in non-small cell lung cancer cell lines. Cancer Res 1995;55(24):6200–6209.

43. Ruas M, Peters G. The p16INK4a/CDKN2A tumor suppressor and its relatives. Biochim Biophys Acta 1998;1378(2):F115-177.

44. Lapointe J, Lachance Y, Labrie Y, Labrie C. A p18 mutant defective in CDK6 binding in human breast cancer cells. Cancer Res 1996;56(20):4586–4589.

45. Polakis P. Wnt signaling and cancer. Genes Dev 2000;14(15):1837–1851.

46. Reya T, Clevers H. Wnt signalling in stem cells and cancer. Nature 2005;434(7035):843–850.

47. Byrd JC, Shinn C, Waselenko JK, Fuchs EJ, Lehman TA, Nguyen PL, Flinn IW, Diehl LF, Sausville E, Grever MR. Flavopiridol induces apoptosis in chronic lymphocytic leukemia cells via activation of caspase-3 without evidence of bcl-2 modulation or dependence on functional p53. Blood 1998;92(10):3804–3816.

48. Takahashi-Yanaga F, Sasaguri T. GSK-3beta regulates cyclin D1 expression: a new target for chemotherapy. Cell Signal 2008;20(4):581–589.

49. Jose-Eneriz ES, Roman-Gomez J, Cordeu L, Ballestar E, Garate L, Andreu EJ, Isidro I, Guruceaga E, Jimenez-Velasco A, Heiniger A, Torres A, Calasanz MJ, Esteller M, Gutierrez NC, Rubio A, Perez-Roger I, Agirre X, Prosper F. BCR-ABL1-induced expression of HSPA8 promotes cell survival in chronic myeloid leukaemia. Br J Haematol 2008;142(4):571–582.

50. Robles AI, Rodriguez-Puebla ML, Glick AB, Trempus C, Hansen L, Sicinski P, Tennant RW, Weinberg RA, Yuspa SH, Conti CJ. Reduced skin tumor development in cyclin D1-deficient mice highlights the oncogenic ras pathway in vivo. Genes Dev 1998;12(16):2469–2474.

51. Kozar K, Ciemerych MA, Rebel VI, Shigematsu H, Zagozdzon A, Sicinska E, Geng Y, Yu Q, Bhattacharya S, Bronson RT, Akashi K, Sicinski P. Mouse development and cell proliferation in the absence of D-cyclins. Cell 2004;118(4):477–491.

52. Steitz J, Buchs S, Tormo D, Ferrer A, Wenzel J, Huber C, Wolfel T, Barbacid M, Malumbres M, Tuting T. Evaluation of genetic melanoma vaccines in cdk4-mutant mice provides evidence for immunological tolerance against authochthonous melanomas in the skin. Int J Cancer 2006;118(2):373–380.

53. Zuo L, Weger J, Yang Q, Goldstein AM, Tucker MA, Walker GJ, Hayward N, Dracopoli NC. Germline mutations in the p16INK4a binding domain of CDK4 in familial melanoma. Nat Genet 1996;12(1):97–99.

54. Sotillo R, Dubus P, Martin J, de la Cueva E, Ortega S, Malumbres M, Barbacid M. Wide spectrum of tumors in knock-in mice carrying a Cdk4 protein insensitive to INK4 inhibitors. EMBO J 2001;20(23):6637–6647.

55. Sotillo R, Garcia JF, Ortega S, Martin J, Dubus P, Barbacid M, Malumbres M. Invasive melanoma in Cdk4-targeted mice. Proc Natl Acad Sci U S A 2001;98(23):13312–13317.

56. He J, Allen JR, Collins VP, Allalunis-Turner MJ, Godbout R, Day RS 3rd, James CD. CDK4 amplification is an alternative mechanism to p16 gene homozygous deletion in glioma cell lines. Cancer Res 1994;54(22):5804–5807.

57. Otterson GA, Kratzke RA, Coxon A, Kim YW, Kaye FJ. Absence of p16INK4 protein is restricted to the subset of lung cancer lines that retains wildtype RB. Oncogene 1994;9(11):3375–3378.

58. Schmidt EE, Ichimura K, Reifenberger G, Collins VP. CDKN2 (p16/MTS1) gene deletion or CDK4 amplification occurs in the majority of glioblastomas. Cancer Res 1994;54(24):6321–6324.

59. Shapiro GI, Edwards CD, Kobzik L, Godleski J, Richards W, Sugarbaker DJ, Rollins BJ. Reciprocal Rb inactivation and p16INK4 expression in primary lung cancers and cell lines. Cancer Res 1995;55(3):505–509.

60. Shapiro GI. Cyclin-dependent kinase pathways as targets for cancer treatment. J Clin Oncol 2006;24(11):1770–1783.

61. Ninomiya-Tsuji J, Nomoto S, Yasuda H, Reed SI, Matsumoto K. Cloning of a human cDNA encoding a CDC2-related kinase by complementation of a budding yeast cdc28 mutation. Proc Natl Acad Sci U S A 1991;88(20):9006–9010.

62. Demetrick DJ, Zhang H, Beach DH. Chromosomal mapping of human CDK2, CDK4, and CDK5 cell cycle kinase genes. Cytogenet Cell Genet 1994;66(1):72–74.

63. Sherr CJ. G1 phase progression: cycling on cue. Cell 1994;79(4):551–555.

64. Krude T, Jackman M, Pines J, Laskey RA. Cyclin/Cdk-dependent initiation of DNA replication in a human cell-free system. Cell 1997;88(1):109–119.

65. Abbas T, Jha S, Sherman NE, Dutta A. Autocatalytic phosphorylation of CDK2 at the activating Thr160. Cell Cycle 2007;6(7):843–852.

66. Gu Y, Rosenblatt J, Morgan DO. Cell cycle regulation of CDK2 activity by phosphorylation of Thr160 and Tyr15. EMBO J 1992;11(11):3995–4005.

67. Hacker E, Muller HK, Irwin N, Gabrielli B, Lincoln D, Pavey S, Powell MB, Malumbres M, Barbacid M, Hayward N, Walker G. Spontaneous and UV radiation-induced multiple metastatic melanomas in Cdk4R24C/R24C/TPras mice. Cancer Res 2006;66(6):2946–2952.

68. Sebastian B, Kakizuka A, Hunter T. Cdc25M2 activation of cyclin-dependent kinases by dephosphorylation of threonine-14 and tyrosine-15. Proc Natl Acad Sci U S A 1993;90(8):3521–3524.

69. Blomberg I, Hoffmann I. Ectopic expression of Cdc25A accelerates the G(1)/S transition and leads to premature activation of cyclin E- and cyclin A-dependent kinases. Mol Cell Biol 1999;19(9):6183–6194.

70. Welburn JP, Tucker JA, Johnson T, Lindert L, Morgan M, Willis A, Noble ME, Endicott JA. How tyrosine 15 phosphorylation inhibits the activity of cyclin-dependent kinase 2-cyclin A. J Biol Chem 2007;282(5):3173–3181.

71. Maddika S, Ande SR, Panigrahi S, Paranjothy T, Weglarczyk K, Zuse A, Eshraghi M, Manda KD, Wiechec E, Los M. Cell survival, cell death and cell cycle pathways are interconnected: implications for cancer therapy. Drug Resist Updat 2007;10(1–2):13–29.

72. De Bondt HL, Rosenblatt J, Jancarik J, Jones HD, Morgan DO, Kim SH. Crystal structure of cyclin-dependent kinase 2. Nature 1993;363(6430):595–602.

73. Brown NR, Noble ME, Endicott JA, Johnson LN. The structural basis for specificity of substrate and recruitment peptides for cyclin-dependent kinases. Nat Cell Biol 1999;1(7):438–443.

74. Brown NR, Noble ME, Lawrie AM, Morris MC, Tunnah P, Divita G, Johnson LN, Endicott JA. Effects of phosphorylation of threonine 160 on cyclin-dependent kinase 2 structure and activity. J Biol Chem 1999;274(13):8746–8756.

75. Jeffrey PD, Russo AA, Polyak K, Gibbs E, Hurwitz J, Massague J, Pavletich NP. Mechanism of CDK activation revealed by the structure of a cyclinA-CDK2 complex. Nature 1995;376(6538):313–320.

76. Russo AA, Jeffrey PD, Patten AK, Massague J, Pavletich NP. Crystal structure of the p27Kip1 cyclin-dependent-kinase inhibitor bound to the cyclin A-Cdk2 complex. Nature 1996;382(6589):325–331.

77. Russo AA, Jeffrey PD, Pavletich NP. Structural basis of cyclin-dependent kinase activation by phosphorylation. Nat Struct Biol 1996;3(8):696–700.

78. Honda R, Lowe ED, Dubinina E, Skamnaki V, Cook A, Brown NR, Johnson LN. The structure of cyclin E1/CDK2: implications for CDK2 activation and CDK2-independent roles. EMBO J 2005;24(3):452–463.

79. Cheng M, Sexl V, Sherr CJ, Roussel MF. Assembly of cyclin D-dependent kinase and titration of p27Kip1 regulated by mitogen-activated protein kinase kinase (MEK1). Proc Natl Acad Sci U S A 1998;95(3):1091–1096.

80. Fischmann TO, Hruza A, Duca JS, Ramanathan L, Mayhood T, Windsor WT, Le HV, Guzi TJ, Dwyer MP, Paruch K, Doll RJ, Lees E, Parry D, Seghezzi W, Madison V. Structure-guided discovery of cyclin-dependent kinase inhibitors. Biopolymers 2008;89(5):372–379.

81. Perez-Roger I, Kim SH, Griffiths B, Sewing A, Land H. Cyclins D1 and D2 mediate myc-induced proliferation via sequestration of p27(Kip1) and p21(Cip1). EMBO J 1999;18(19):5310–5320.

82. Sherr CJ, Roberts JM. CDK inhibitors: positive and negative regulators of G1-phase progression. Genes Dev 1999;13(12):1501–1512.

83. Kardinal C, Dangers M, Kardinal A, Koch A, Brandt DT, Tamura T, Welte K. Tyrosine phosphorylation modulates binding preference to cyclin-dependent kinases and subcellular localization of p27Kip1 in the acute promyelocytic leukemia cell line NB4. Blood 2006;107(3):1133–1140.

84. Tsutsui T, Hesabi B, Moons DS, Pandolfi PP, Hansel KS, Koff A, Kiyokawa H. Targeted disruption of CDK4 delays cell cycle entry with enhanced p27(Kip1) activity. Mol Cell Biol 1999;19(10):7011–7019.

85. Bloom J, Pagano M. Deregulated degradation of the cdk inhibitor p27 and malignant transformation. Semin Cancer Biol 2003;13(1):41–47.

86. Nakayama KI, Nakayama K. Ubiquitin ligases: cell-cycle control and cancer. Nat Rev Cancer 2006;6(5):369–381.

87. Shin I, Yakes FM, Rojo F, Shin NY, Bakin AV, Baselga J, Arteaga CL. PKB/Akt mediates cell-cycle progression by phosphorylation of p27(Kip1) at threonine 157 and modulation of its cellular localization. Nat Med 2002;8(10):1145–1152.

88. Viglietto G, Motti ML, Bruni P, Melillo RM, D'Alessio A, Califano D, Vinci F, Chiappetta G, Tsichlis P, Bellacosa A, Fusco A, Santoro M. Cytoplasmic relocalization and inhibition of the cyclin-dependent kinase inhibitor p27(Kip1) by PKB/Akt-mediated phosphorylation in breast cancer. Nat Med 2002;8(10):1136–1144.

89. Liang J, Zubovitz J, Petrocelli T, Kotchetkov R, Connor MK, Han K, Lee JH, Ciarallo S, Catzavelos C, Beniston R, Franssen E, Slingerland JM. PKB/Akt phosphorylates p27, impairs nuclear import of p27 and opposes p27-mediated G1 arrest. Nat Med 2002;8(10):1153–1160.

90. Krek W, Ewen ME, Shirodkar S, Arany Z, Kaelin WG Jr, Livingston DM. Negative regulation of the growth-promoting transcription factor E2F-1 by a stably bound cyclin A-dependent protein kinase. Cell 1994;78(1):161–172.

91. Dynlacht BD, Flores O, Lees JA, Harlow E. Differential regulation of E2F transactivation by cyclin/cdk2 complexes. Genes Dev 1994;8(15):1772–1786.

92. Xu M, Sheppard KA, Peng CY, Yee AS, Piwnica-Worms H. Cyclin A/CDK2 binds directly to E2F-1 and inhibits the DNA-binding activity of E2F-1/DP-1 by phosphorylation. Mol Cell Biol 1994;14(12):8420–8431.

93. Kitagawa M, Higashi H, Suzuki-Takahashi I, Segawa K, Hanks SK, Taya Y, Nishimura S, Okuyama A. Phosphorylation of E2F-1 by cyclin A-cdk2. Oncogene 1995;10(2):229–236.

94. Lacey KR, Jackson PK, Stearns T. Cyclin-dependent kinase control of centrosome duplication. Proc Natl Acad Sci U S A 1999;96(6):2817–2822.

95. Hanashiro K, Kanai M, Geng Y, Sicinski P, Fukasawa K. Roles of cyclins A and E in induction of centrosome amplification in p53-compromised cells. Oncogene 2008;27(40):5288–5302.

96. Pihan GA, Purohit A, Wallace J, Knecht H, Woda B, Quesenberry P, Doxsey SJ. Centrosome defects and genetic instability in malignant tumors. Cancer Res 1998;58(17):3974–3985.

97. Carroll PE, Okuda M, Horn HF, Biddinger P, Stambrook PJ, Gleich LL, Li YQ, Tarapore P, Fukasawa K. Centrosome hyperamplification in human cancer: chromosome instability induced by p53 mutation and/or Mdm2 overexpression. Oncogene 1999;18(11):1935–1944.

98. Bennett RA, Izumi H, Fukasawa K. Induction of centrosome amplification and chromosome instability in p53-null cells by transient exposure to subtoxic levels of S-phase-targeting anticancer drugs. Oncogene 2004;23(40):6823–6829.

99. Tetsu O, McCormick F. Proliferation of cancer cells despite CDK2 inhibition. Cancer Cell 2003;3(3):233–245.

100. Cai D, Latham VM Jr, Zhang X, Shapiro GI. Combined depletion of cell cycle and transcriptional cyclin-dependent kinase activities induces apoptosis in cancer cells. Cancer Res 2006;66(18):9270–9280.

101. Du J, Widlund HR, Horstmann MA, Ramaswamy S, Ross K, Huber WE, Nishimura EK, Golub TR, Fisher DE. Critical role of CDK2 for melanoma growth linked to its melanocyte-specific transcriptional regulation by MITF. Cancer Cell 2004;6(6):565–576.

102. Ortega S, Prieto I, Odajima J, Martin A, Dubus P, Sotillo R, Barbero JL, Malumbres M, Barbacid M. Cyclin-dependent kinase 2 is essential for meiosis but not for mitotic cell division in mice. Nat Genet 2003;35(1):25–31.

103. Berthet C, Aleem E, Coppola V, Tessarollo L, Kaldis P. Cdk2 knockout mice are viable. Curr Biol 2003;13(20):1775–1785.

104. Berthet C, Kaldis P. Cdk2 and Cdk4 cooperatively control the expression of Cdc2. Cell Div 2006;1:10.

105. Berthet C, Klarmann KD, Hilton MB, Suh HC, Keller JR, Kiyokawa H, Kaldis P. Combined loss of Cdk2 and Cdk4 results in embryonic lethality and Rb hypophosphorylation. Dev Cell 2006;10(5):563–573.

106. Kuzbicki L, Aladowicz E, Chwirot BW. Cyclin-dependent kinase 2 expression in human melanomas and benign melanocytic skin lesions. Melanoma Res 2006;16(5):435–444.

107. Geng Y, Yu Q, Sicinska E, Das M, Schneider JE, Bhattacharya S, Rideout WM, Bronson RT, Gardner H, Sicinski P. Cyclin E ablation in the mouse. Cell 2003;114(4):431–443.

108. Strohmaier H, Spruck CH, Kaiser P, Won KA, Sangfelt O, Reed SI. Human F-box protein hCdc4 targets cyclin E for proteolysis and is mutated in a breast cancer cell line. Nature 2001;413(6853):316–322.

109. Koepp DM, Schaefer LK, Ye X, Keyomarsi K, Chu C, Harper JW, Elledge SJ. Phosphorylation-dependent ubiquitination of cyclin E by the SCFFbw7 ubiquitin ligase. Science 2001;294(5540):173–177.

110. Welcker M, Singer J, Loeb KR, Grim J, Bloecher A, Gurien-West M, Clurman BE, Roberts JM. Multisite phosphorylation by Cdk2 and GSK3 controls cyclin E degradation. Mol Cell 2003;12(2):381–392.

111. Grim JE, Gustafson MP, Hirata RK, Hagar AC, Swanger J, Welcker M, Hwang HC, Ericsson J, Russell DW, Clurman BE. Isoform- and cell cycle-dependent substrate degradation by the Fbw7 ubiquitin ligase. J Cell Biol 2008;181(6):913–920.

112. Spruck CH, Won KA, Reed SI. Deregulated cyclin E induces chromosome instability. Nature 1999;401(6750):297–300.

113. Bortner DM, Rosenberg MP. Induction of mammary gland hyperplasia and carcinomas in transgenic mice expressing human cyclin E. Mol Cell Biol 1997;17(1):453–459.

114. Henglein B, Chenivesse X, Wang J, Eick D, Brechot C. Structure and cell cycle-regulated transcription of the human cyclin A gene. Proc Natl Acad Sci U S A 1994;91(12):5490–5494.

115. Pines J, Hunter T. Human cyclin A is adenovirus E1A-associated protein p60 and behaves differently from cyclin B. Nature 1990;346(6286):760–763.

116. Erlandsson F, Linnman C, Ekholm S, Bengtsson E, Zetterberg A. A detailed analysis of cyclin A accumulation at the G(1)/S border in normal and transformed cells. Exp Cell Res 2000;259(1):86–95.

117. Yang R, Morosetti R, Koeffler HP. Characterization of a second human cyclin A that is highly expressed in testis and in several leukemic cell lines. Cancer Res 1997;57(5):913–920.

118. Furuno N, den Elzen N, Pines J. Human cyclin A is required for mitosis until mid prophase. J Cell Biol 1999;147(2):295–306.

119. Murphy M, Stinnakre MG, Senamaud-Beaufort C, Winston NJ, Sweeney C, Kubelka M, Carrington M, Brechot C, Sobczak-Thepot J. Delayed early embryonic lethality following disruption of the murine cyclin A2 gene. Nat Genet 1997;15(1):83–86.

120. Yeyati PL, Shaknovich R, Boterashvili S, Li J, Ball HJ, Waxman S, Nason-Burchenal K, Dmitrovsky E, Zelent A, Licht JD. Leukemia translocation protein PLZF inhibits cell growth and expression of cyclin A. Oncogene 1999;18(4):925–934.

121. Costoya JA, Hobbs RM, Pandolfi PP. Cyclin-dependent kinase antagonizes promyelocytic leukemia zinc-finger through phosphorylation. Oncogene 2008;27(27):3789–3796.

122. Costoya JA, Hobbs RM, Barna M, Cattoretti G, Manova K, Sukhwani M, Orwig KE, Wolgemuth DJ, Pandolfi PP. Essential role of Plzf in maintenance of spermatogonial stem cells. Nat Genet 2004;36(6):653–659.

123. Bullrich F, MacLachlan TK, Sang N, Druck T, Veronese ML, Allen SL, Chiorazzi N, Koff A, Heubner K, Croce CM, et al. Chromosomal mapping of members of the cdc2 family of protein

kinases, cdk3, cdk6, PISSLRE, and PITALRE, and a cdk inhibitor, p27Kip1, to regions involved in human cancer. Cancer Res 1995;55(6):1199–1205.

124. Newcomb EW, Tamasdan C, Entzminger Y, Arena E, Schnee T, Kim M, Crisan D, Lukyanov Y, Miller DC, Zagzag D. Flavopiridol inhibits the growth of GL261 gliomas in vivo: implications for malignant glioma therapy. Cell Cycle 2004;3(2):230–234.

125. Yamochi T, Semba K, Tsuji K, Mizumoto K, Sato H, Matsuura Y, Nishimoto I, Matsuoka M. ik3-1/Cables is a substrate for cyclin-dependent kinase 3 (cdk 3). Eur J Biochem 2001;268(23):6076–6082.

126. Braun K, Holzl G, Soucek T, Geisen C, Moroy T, Hengstschlager M. Investigation of the cell cycle regulation of cdk3-associated kinase activity and the role of cdk3 in proliferation and transformation. Oncogene 1998;17(17):2259–2269.

127. Hofmann F, Livingston DM. Differential effects of cdk2 and cdk3 on the control of pRb and E2F function during G1 exit. Genes Dev 1996;10(7):851–861.

128. van den Heuvel S, Harlow E. Distinct roles for cyclin-dependent kinases in cell cycle control. Science 1993;262(5142):2050–2054.

129. Nguyen VT, Kiss T, Michels AA, Bensaude O. 7SK small nuclear RNA binds to and inhibits the activity of CDK9/cyclin T complexes. Nature 2001;414(6861):322–325.

130. Lee MG, Nurse P. Complementation used to clone a human homologue of the fission yeast cell cycle control gene cdc2. Nature 1987;327(6117):31–35.

131. Nazarenko SA, Ostroverhova NV, Spurr NK. Regional assignment of the human cell cycle control gene CDC2 to chromosome 10q21 by in situ hybridization. Hum Genet 1991;87(5):621–622.

132. Lee MG, Norbury CJ, Spurr NK, Nurse P. Regulated expression and phosphorylation of a possible mammalian cell-cycle control protein. Nature 1988;333(6174):676–679.

133. Marash L, Liberman N, Henis-Korenblit S, Sivan G, Reem E, Elroy-Stein O, Kimchi A. DAP5 promotes cap-independent translation of Bcl-2 and CDK1 to facilitate cell survival during mitosis. Mol Cell 2008;30(4):447–459.

134. Benson C, White J, De Bono J, O'Donnell A, Raynaud F, Cruickshank C, McGrath H, Walton M, Workman P, Kaye S, Cassidy J, Gianella-Borradori A, Judson I, Twelves C. A phase I trial of the selective oral cyclin-dependent kinase inhibitor seliciclib (CYC202; R-Roscovitine), administered twice daily for 7 days every 21 days. Br J Cancer 2007;96(1):29–37.

135. Lacrima K, Valentini A, Lambertini C, Taborelli M, Rinaldi A, Zucca E, Catapano C, Cavalli F, Gianella-Borradori A, Maccallum DE, Bertoni F. In vitro activity of cyclin-dependent kinase inhibitor CYC202 (Seliciclib, R-roscovitine) in mantle cell lymphomas. Ann Oncol 2005;16(7):1169–1176.

136. Peeper DS, Keblusek P, Helin K, Toebes M, van der Eb AJ, Zantema A. Phosphorylation of a specific cdk site in E2F-1 affects its electrophoretic mobility and promotes pRB-binding In vitro. Oncogene 1995;10(1):39–48.

137. Marzluff WF. Metazoan replication-dependent histone mRNAs: a distinct set of RNA polymerase II transcripts. Curr Opin Cell Biol 2005;17(3):274–280.

138. Koseoglu MM, Graves LM, Marzluff WF. Phosphorylation of threonine 61 by cyclin a/Cdk1 triggers degradation of stem-loop binding protein at the end of S phase. Mol Cell Biol 2008;28(14):4469–4479.

139. Maiorano D, Moreau J, Mechali M. XCDT1 is required for the assembly of pre-replicative complexes in *Xenopus laevis*. Nature 2000;404(6778):622–625.

140. Forsburg SL. Eukaryotic MCM proteins: beyond replication initiation. Microbiol Mol Biol Rev 2004;68(1):109–131.

141. Lin DI, Aggarwal P, Diehl JA. Phosphorylation of MCM3 on Ser-112 regulates its incorporation into the MCM2-7 complex. Proc Natl Acad Sci U S A 2008;105(23):8079–8084.

142. Sanchez I, Dynlacht BD. New insights into cyclins, CDKs, and cell cycle control. Semin Cell Dev Biol 2005;16(3):311–321.

143. Watanabe N, Arai H, Nishihara Y, Taniguchi M, Hunter T, Osada H. M-phase kinases induce phospho-dependent ubiquitination of somatic Wee1 by SCFbeta-TrCP. Proc Natl Acad Sci U S A 2004;101(13):4419–4424.

144. Watanabe T, Yoshino A, Katayama Y. [Genetic analysis and individualized therapy for diffuse glioma]. No Shinkei Geka 2005;33(6):537–553.

145. Clute P, Pines J. Temporal and spatial control of cyclin B1 destruction in metaphase. Nat Cell Biol 1999;1(2):82–87.

146. King RW, Peters JM, Tugendreich S, Rolfe M, Hieter P, Kirschner MW. A 20S complex containing CDC27 and CDC16 catalyzes the mitosis-specific conjugation of ubiquitin to cyclin B. Cell 1995;81(2):279–288.

147. Sudakin V, Ganoth D, Dahan A, Heller H, Hershko J, Luca FC, Ruderman JV, Hershko A. The cyclosome, a large complex containing cyclin-selective ubiquitin ligase activity, targets cyclins for destruction at the end of mitosis. Mol Biol Cell 1995;6(2):185–197.

148. Pomerening JR, Sontag ED, Ferrell JE Jr. Building a cell cycle oscillator: hysteresis and bistability in the activation of Cdc2. Nat Cell Biol 2003;5(4):346–351.

149. Sha W, Moore J, Chen K, Lassaletta AD, Yi CS, Tyson JJ, Sible JC. Hysteresis drives cell-cycle transitions in *Xenopus laevis* egg extracts. Proc Natl Acad Sci U S A 2003;100(3):975–980.

150. Visintin R, Prinz S, Amon A. CDC20 and CDH1: a family of substrate-specific activators of APC-dependent proteolysis. Science 1997;278(5337):460–463.

151. Jaspersen SL, Charles JF, Morgan DO. Inhibitory phosphorylation of the APC regulator Hct1 is controlled by the kinase Cdc28 and the phosphatase Cdc14. Curr Biol 1999;9(5):227–236.

152. Pomerening JR, Ubersax JA, Ferrell JE Jr. Rapid cycling and precocious termination of G1 phase in cells expressing CDK1AF. Mol Biol Cell 2008;19(8):3426–3441.

153. Santamaria D, Barriere C, Cerqueira A, Hunt S, Tardy C, Newton K, Caceres JF, Dubus P, Malumbres M, Barbacid M. Cdk1 is sufficient to drive the mammalian cell cycle. Nature 2007;448(7155):811–815.

154. Goga A, Yang D, Tward AD, Morgan DO, Bishop JM. Inhibition of CDK1 as a potential therapy for tumors over-expressing MYC. Nat Med 2007;13(7):820–827.

155. Wall NR, O'Connor DS, Plescia J, Pommier Y, Altieri DC. Suppression of survivin phosphorylation on Thr34 by flavopiridol enhances tumor cell apoptosis. Cancer Res 2003;63(1):230–235.

156. Ichikawa H, Shimizu K, Hayashi Y, Ohki M. An RNA-binding protein gene, TLS/FUS, is fused to ERG in human myeloid leukemia with t(16;21) chromosomal translocation. Cancer Res 1994;54(11):2865–2868.

157. Kong XT, Ida K, Ichikawa H, Shimizu K, Ohki M, Maseki N, Kaneko Y, Sako M, Kobayashi Y, Tojou A, Miura I, Kakuda H, Funabiki T, Horibe K, Hamaguchi H, Akiyama Y, Bessho F, Yanagisawa M, Hayashi Y. Consistent detection of TLS/FUS-ERG chimeric transcripts in acute myeloid leukemia with t(16;21)(p11;q22) and identification of a novel transcript. Blood 1997;90(3):1192–1199.

158. Pan J, Zou J, Wu DY, Roberson RS, Hennings LJ, Ma X, Yared M, Blackburn ML, Chansky HA, Yang L. TLS-ERG leukemia fusion protein deregulates cyclin-dependent kinase 1 and blocks terminal differentiation of myeloid progenitor cells. Mol Cancer Res 2008;6(5):862–872.

159. Yu D, Jing T, Liu B, Yao J, Tan M, McDonnell TJ, Hung MC. Overexpression of ErbB2 blocks Taxol-induced apoptosis by upregulation of p21Cip1, which inhibits p34Cdc2 kinase. Mol Cell 1998;2(5):581–591.

160. Tan M, Jing T, Lan KH, Neal CL, Li P, Lee S, Fang D, Nagata Y, Liu J, Arlinghaus R, Hung MC, Yu D. Phosphorylation on tyrosine-15 of p34(Cdc2) by ErbB2 inhibits p34(Cdc2) activation and is involved in resistance to taxol-induced apoptosis. Mol Cell 2002;9(5):993–1004.

161. Brambilla R, Draetta G. Molecular cloning of PISSLRE, a novel putative member of the cdk family of protein serine/threonine kinases. Oncogene 1994;9(10):3037–3041.

162. Li S, MacLachlan TK, De Luca A, Claudio PP, Condorelli G, Giordano A. The cdc-2-related kinase, PISSLRE, is essential for cell growth and acts in G2 phase of the cell cycle. Cancer Res 1995;55(18):3992–3995.

163. Romano G, Kasten M, De Falco G, Micheli P, Khalili K, Giordano A. Regulatory functions of Cdk9 and of cyclin T1 in HIV tat transactivation pathway gene expression. J Cell Biochem 1999;75(3):357–368.

164. Iorns E, Turner NC, Elliott R, Syed N, Garrone O, Gasco M, Tutt AN, Crook T, Lord CJ, Ashworth A. Identification of CDK10 as an important determinant of resistance to endocrine therapy for breast cancer. Cancer Cell 2008;13(2):91–104.

165. Swanton C, Downward J. Unraveling the complexity of endocrine resistance in breast cancer by functional genomics. Cancer Cell 2008;13(2):83–85.

166. Liu G, Gandara DR, Lara PN Jr, Raghavan D, Doroshow JH, Twardowski P, Kantoff P, Oh W, Kim K, Wilding G. A Phase II trial of flavopiridol (NSC #649890) in patients with previously untreated metastatic androgen-independent prostate cancer. Clin Cancer Res 2004;10(3):924–928.

167. Ng SS, Cheung YT, An XM, Chen YC, Li M, Li GH, Cheung W, Sze J, Lai L, Peng Y, Xia HH, Wong BC, Leung SY, Xie D, He ML, Kung HF, Lin MC. Cell cycle-related kinase: a novel candidate oncogene in human glioblastoma. J Natl Cancer Inst 2007;99(12):936–948.

168. MacKeigan JP, Murphy LO, Blenis J. Sensitized RNAi screen of human kinases and phosphatases identifies new regulators of apoptosis and chemoresistance. Nat Cell Biol 2005;7(6):591–600.

169. Estable MC, Naghavi MH, Kato H, Xiao H, Qin J, Vahlne A, Roeder RG. MCEF, the newest member of the AF4 family of transcription factors involved in leukemia, is a positive transcription elongation factor-b-associated protein. J Biomed Sci 2002;9(3):234–245.

170. Woychik NA, Hampsey M. The RNA polymerase II machinery: structure illuminates function. Cell 2002;108(4):453–463.

171. Asturias FJ. RNA polymerase II structure, and organization of the preinitiation complex. Curr Opin Struct Biol 2004;14(2):121–129.

172. Conaway RC, Sato S, Tomomori-Sato C, Yao T, Conaway JW. The mammalian Mediator complex and its role in transcriptional regulation. Trends Biochem Sci 2005;30(5):250–255.

173. Kornberg RD. Mediator and the mechanism of transcriptional activation. Trends Biochem Sci 2005;30(5):235–239.

174. Malik S, Roeder RG. Dynamic regulation of pol II transcription by the mammalian Mediator complex. Trends Biochem Sci 2005;30(5):256–263.

175. Thomas MC, Chiang CM. The general transcription machinery and general cofactors. Crit Rev Biochem Mol Biol 2006;41(3):105–178.

176. Darbon JM, Devault A, Taviaux S, Fesquet D, Martinez AM, Galas S, Cavadore JC, Doree M, Blanchard JM. Cloning, expression and subcellular localization of the human homolog of p40MO15 catalytic subunit of cdk-activating kinase. Oncogene 1994;9(11):3127–3138.

177. Levedakou EN, He M, Baptist EW, Craven RJ, Cance WG, Welcsh PL, Simmons A, Naylor SL, Leach RJ, Lewis TB, et al. Two novel human serine/threonine kinases with homologies to the cell cycle regulating *Xenopus* MO15, and NIMA kinases: cloning and characterization of their expression pattern. Oncogene 1994;9(7):1977–1988.

178. Wu L, Yee A, Liu L, Carbonaro-Hall D, Venkatesan N, Tolo VT, Hall FL. Molecular cloning of the human CAK1 gene encoding a cyclin-dependent kinase-activating kinase. Oncogene 1994;9(7):2089–2096.

179. Tassan JP, Schultz SJ, Bartek J, Nigg EA. Cell cycle analysis of the activity, subcellular localization, and subunit composition of human CAK (CDK-activating kinase). J Cell Biol 1994;127(2):467–478.

180. Fisher RP. Secrets of a double agent: CDK7 in cell-cycle control and transcription. J Cell Sci 2005;118(Pt 22):5171–5180.

181. Fisher RP, Morgan DO. A novel cyclin associates with MO15/CDK7 to form the CDK-activating kinase. Cell 1994;78(4):713–724.

182. Martinez AM, Afshar M, Martin F, Cavadore JC, Labbe JC, Doree M. Dual phosphorylation of the T-loop in cdk7: its role in controlling cyclin H binding and CAK activity. EMBO J 1997;16(2):343–354.

183. Lolli G, Lowe ED, Brown NR, Johnson LN. The crystal structure of human CDK7 and its protein recognition properties. Structure 2004;12(11):2067–2079.

184. Lolli G, Johnson LN. Recognition of Cdk2 by Cdk7. Proteins 2007;67(4):1048–1059.

185. Desai D, Wessling HC, Fisher RP, Morgan DO. Effects of phosphorylation by CAK on cyclin binding by CDC2 and CDK2. Mol Cell Biol 1995;15(1):345–350.

186. Shiekhattar R, Mermelstein F, Fisher RP, Drapkin R, Dynlacht B, Wessling HC, Morgan DO, Reinberg D. Cdk-activating kinase complex is a component of human transcription factor TFIIH. Nature 1995;374(6519):283–287.

187. Meinhart A, Kamenski T, Hoeppner S, Baumli S, Cramer P. A structural perspective of CTD function. Genes Dev 2005;19(12):1401–1415.

188. Ramanathan Y, Rajpara SM, Reza SM, Lees E, Shuman S, Mathews MB, Pe'ery T. Three RNA polymerase II carboxyl-terminal domain kinases display distinct substrate preferences. J Biol Chem 2001;276(14):10913–10920.

189. Vandel L, Kouzarides T. Residues phosphorylated by TFIIH are required for E2F-1 degradation during S-phase. EMBO J 1999;18(15):4280–4291.

190. Lewis AE, Rusten M, Hoivik EA, Vikse EL, Hansson ML, Wallberg AE, Bakke M. Phosphorylation of steroidogenic factor 1 is mediated by cyclin-dependent kinase 7. Mol Endocrinol 2008;22(1):91–104.

191. Keriel A, Stary A, Sarasin A, Rochette-Egly C, Egly JM. XPD mutations prevent TFIIH-dependent transactivation by nuclear receptors and phosphorylation of RARalpha. Cell 2002;109(1):125–135.

192. Bastien J, Adam-Stitah S, Riedl T, Egly JM, Chambon P, Rochette-Egly C. TFIIH interacts with the retinoic acid receptor gamma and phosphorylates its AF-1-activating domain through cdk7. J Biol Chem 2000;275(29):21896–21904.

193. Gaillard E, Bruck N, Brelivet Y, Bour G, Lalevee S, Bauer A, Poch O, Moras D, Rochette-Egly C. Phosphorylation by PKA potentiates retinoic acid receptor alpha activity by means of increasing interaction with and phosphorylation by cyclin H/cdk7. Proc Natl Acad Sci U S A 2006;103(25):9548–9553.

194. Bour G, Lalevee S, Rochette-Egly C. Protein kinases and the proteasome join in the combinatorial control of transcription by nuclear retinoic acid receptors. Trends Cell Biol 2007;17(6):302–309.

195. Pavri R, Lewis B, Kim TK, Dilworth FJ, Erdjument-Bromage H, Tempst P, de Murcia G, Evans R, Chambon P, Reinberg D. PARP-1 determines specificity in a retinoid signaling pathway via direct modulation of mediator. Mol Cell 2005;18(1):83–96.

196. Kim YK, Bourgeois CF, Isel C, Churcher MJ, Karn J. Phosphorylation of the RNA polymerase II carboxyl-terminal domain by CDK9 is directly responsible for human immunodeficiency virus type 1 Tat-activated transcriptional elongation. Mol Cell Biol 2002;22(13):4622–4637.

197. Ito S, Kuraoka I, Chymkowitch P, Compe E, Takedachi A, Ishigami C, Coin F, Egly JM, Tanaka K. XPG stabilizes TFIIH, allowing transactivation of nuclear receptors: implications for Cockayne syndrome in XP-G/CS patients. Mol Cell 2007;26(2):231–243.

198. Chen J, Larochelle S, Li X, Suter B. Xpd/Ercc2 regulates CAK activity and mitotic progression. Nature 2003;424(6945):228–232.

199. Lolli G, Johnson LN. CAK-cyclin-dependent activating kinase: a key kinase in cell cycle control and a target for drugs? Cell Cycle 2005;4(4):572–577.

200. Schultz SJ, Nigg EA. Identification of 21 novel human protein kinases, including 3 members of a family related to the cell cycle regulator nimA of *Aspergillus nidulans*. Cell Growth Differ 1993;4(10):821–830.

201. Tassan JP, Jaquenoud M, Leopold P, Schultz SJ, Nigg EA. Identification of human cyclin-dependent kinase 8, a putative protein kinase partner for cyclin C. Proc Natl Acad Sci U S A 1995;92(19):8871–8875.

202. Hoeppner S, Baumli S, Cramer P. Structure of the mediator subunit cyclin C and its implications for CDK8 function. J Mol Biol 2005;350(5):833–842.

203. Meyer KD, Donner AJ, Knuesel MT, York AG, Espinosa JM, Taatjes DJ. Cooperative activity of cdk8 and GCN5L within Mediator directs tandem phosphoacetylation of histone H3. EMBO J 2008;27(10):1447–1457.

204. Firestein R, Bass AJ, Kim SY, Dunn IF, Silver SJ, Guney I, Freed E, Ligon AH, Vena N, Ogino S, Chheda MG, Tamayo P, Finn S, Shrestha Y, Boehm JS, Jain S, Bojarski E, Mermel C, Barretina J, Chan JA, Baselga J, Tabernero J, Root DE, Fuchs CS, Loda M, Shivdasani RA, Meyerson M, Hahn WC. CDK8 is a colorectal cancer oncogene that regulates beta-catenin activity. Nature 2008;455(7212):547–551.

205. Akoulitchev S, Chuikov S, Reinberg D. TFIIH is negatively regulated by cdk8-containing mediator complexes. Nature 2000;407(6800):102–106.

206. Echalier A, Bettayeb K, Ferandin Y, Lozach O, Clement M, Valette A, Liger F, Marquet B, Morris JC, Endicott JA, Joseph B, Meijer L. Meriolins (3-(pyrimidin-4-yl)-7-azaindoles): synthesis, kinase inhibitory activity, cellular effects, and structure of a CDK2/cyclin A/Meriolin complex. J Med Chem 2008;51(4):737–751.

207. Westerling T, Kuuluvainen E, Makela TP. Cdk8 is essential for preimplantation mouse development. Mol Cell Biol 2007;27(17):6177–6182.
208. Wang QT, Piotrowska K, Ciemerych MA, Milenkovic L, Scott MP, Davis RW, Zernicka-Goetz M. A genome-wide study of gene activity reveals developmental signaling pathways in the preimplantation mouse embryo. Dev Cell 2004;6(1):133–144.
209. Grana X, De Luca A, Sang N, Fu Y, Claudio PP, Rosenblatt J, Morgan DO, Giordano A. PITALRE, a nuclear CDC2-related protein kinase that phosphorylates the retinoblastoma protein In vitro. Proc Natl Acad Sci U S A 1994;91(9):3834–3838.
210. Bagella L, MacLachlan TK, Buono RJ, Pisano MM, Giordano A, De Luca A. Cloning of murine CDK9/PITALRE and its tissue-specific expression in development. J Cell Physiol 1998;177(2):206–213.
211. Shore SM, Byers SA, Maury W, Price DH. Identification of a novel isoform of Cdk9. Gene 2003;307:175–182.
212. Garriga J, Bhattacharya S, Calbo J, Marshall RM, Truongcao M, Haines DS, Grana X. CDK9 is constitutively expressed throughout the cell cycle, and its steady-state expression is independent of SKP2. Mol Cell Biol 2003;23(15):5165–5173.
213. Egloff S, Van Herreweghe E, Kiss T. Regulation of polymerase II transcription by 7SK snRNA: two distinct RNA elements direct P-TEFb and HEXIM1 binding. Mol Cell Biol 2006;26(2):630–642.
214. Li Q, Price JP, Byers SA, Cheng D, Peng J, Price DH. Analysis of the large inactive P-TEFb complex indicates that it contains one 7SK molecule, a dimer of HEXIM1 or HEXIM2, and two P-TEFb molecules containing Cdk9 phosphorylated at threonine 186. J Biol Chem 2005;280(31):28819–28826.
215. Jang MK, Mochizuki K, Zhou M, Jeong HS, Brady JN, Ozato K. The bromodomain protein Brd4 is a positive regulatory component of P-TEFb and stimulates RNA polymerase II-dependent transcription. Mol Cell 2005;19(4):523–534.
216. Yang H, Zheng S, Meijer L, Li SM, Leclerc S, Yu LL, Cheng JQ, Zhang SZ. Screening the active constituents of Chinese medicinal herbs as potent inhibitors of Cdc25 tyrosine phosphatase, an activator of the mitosis-inducing p34cdc2 kinase. J Zhejiang Univ Sci B 2005;6(7):656–663.
217. Fu J, Yoon HG, Qin J, Wong J. Regulation of P-TEFb elongation complex activity by CDK9 acetylation. Mol Cell Biol 2007;27(13):4641–4651.
218. Baumli S, Lolli G, Lowe ED, Troiani S, Rusconi L, Bullock AN, Debreczeni JE, Knapp S, Johnson LN. The structure of P-TEFb (CDK9/cyclin T1), its complex with flavopiridol and regulation by phosphorylation. EMBO J 2008;27(13):1907–1918.
219. Park KH, Seol JY, Kim TY, Yoo CG, Kim YW, Han SK, Shim YS, Lee CT. An adenovirus expressing mutant p27 showed more potent antitumor effects than adenovirus-p27 wild type. Cancer Res 2001;61(16):6163–6169.
220. Chen R, Yang Z, Zhou Q. Phosphorylated positive transcription elongation factor b (P-TEFb) is tagged for inhibition through association with 7SK snRNA. J Biol Chem 2004;279(6):4153–4160.
221. Napolitano G, Majello B, Lania L. Catalytic activity of Cdk9 is required for nuclear co-localization of the Cdk9/cyclin T1 (P-TEFb) complex. J Cell Physiol 2003;197(1):1–7.
222. Fujita T, Ryser S, Piuz I, Schlegel W. Up-regulation of P-TEFb by the MEK1-extracellular signal-regulated kinase signaling pathway contributes to stimulated transcription elongation of immediate early genes in neuroendocrine cells. Mol Cell Biol 2008;28(5):1630–1643.
223. O'Keeffe B, Fong Y, Chen D, Zhou S, Zhou Q. Requirement for a kinase-specific chaperone pathway in the production of a Cdk9/cyclin T1 heterodimer responsible for P-TEFb-mediated tat stimulation of HIV-1 transcription. J Biol Chem 2000;275(1):279–287.
224. Kiernan RE, Emiliani S, Nakayama K, Castro A, Labbe JC, Lorca T, Nakayama Ki K, Benkirane M. Interaction between cyclin T1 and SCF(SKP2) targets CDK9 for ubiquitination and degradation by the proteasome. Mol Cell Biol 2001;21(23):7956–7970.
225. Fujinaga K, Irwin D, Huang Y, Taube R, Kurosu T, Peterlin BM. Dynamics of human immunodeficiency virus transcription: P-TEFb phosphorylates RD and dissociates negative effectors from the transactivation response element. Mol Cell Biol 2004;24(2):787–795.
226. Oshita F, Kameda Y, Nishio K, Tanaka G, Yamada K, Nomura I, Nakayama H, Noda K. Increased expression levels of cyclin-dependent kinase inhibitor p27 correlate with good responses to platinum-based chemotherapy in non-small cell lung cancer. Oncol Rep 2000;7(3):491–495.

227. Marshall NF, Peng J, Xie Z, Price DH. Control of RNA polymerase II elongation potential by a novel carboxyl-terminal domain kinase. J Biol Chem 1996;271(43):27176–27183.

228. Palancade B, Bensaude O. Investigating RNA polymerase II carboxyl-terminal domain (CTD) phosphorylation. Eur J Biochem 2003;270(19):3859–3870.

229. Malumbres M, Pevarello P, Barbacid M, Bischoff JR. CDK inhibitors in cancer therapy: what is next? Trends Pharmacol Sci 2008;29(1):16–21.

230. Rother S, Strasser K. The RNA polymerase II CTD kinase Ctk1 functions in translation elongation. Genes Dev 2007;21(11):1409–1421.

231. Marshall RM, Grana X. Mechanisms controlling CDK9 activity. Front Biosci 2006;11: 2598–2613.

232. Cheok CF, Dey A, Lane DP. Cyclin-dependent kinase inhibitors sensitize tumor cells to nutlin-induced apoptosis: a potent drug combination. Mol Cancer Res 2007;5(11):1133–1145.

233. Hou T, Ray S, Brasier AR. The functional role of an interleukin 6-inducible CDK9.STAT3 complex in human gamma-fibrinogen gene expression. J Biol Chem 2007;282(51):37091–37102.

234. Salerno D, Hasham MG, Marshall R, Garriga J, Tsygankov AY, Grana X. Direct inhibition of CDK9 blocks HIV-1 replication without preventing T-cell activation in primary human peripheral blood lymphocytes. Gene 2007;405(1–2):65–78.

235. Wang S, Fischer PM. Cyclin-dependent kinase 9: a key transcriptional regulator and potential drug target in oncology, virology and cardiology. Trends Pharmacol Sci 2008;29(6):302–313.

236. Gururajanna B, Al-Katib AA, Li YW, Aranha O, Vaitkevicius VK, Sarkar FH. Molecular effects of taxol and caffeine on pancreatic cancer cells. Int J Mol Med 1999;4(5):501–507.

237. Mock BA, Padlan C, Kozak CA, Kidd V. The gene for mouse p58cdc2L1 (Cdc2l1) protein kinase maps to distal mouse chromosome 4. Mamm Genome 1994;5(3):191–192.

238. Cornelis S, Bruynooghe Y, Denecker G, Van Huffel S, Tinton S, Beyaert R. Identification and characterization of a novel cell cycle-regulated internal ribosome entry site. Mol Cell 2000;5(4):597–605.

239. Campbell I, Magliocco A, Moyana T, Zheng C, Xiang J. Adenovirus-mediated p16INK4 gene transfer significantly suppresses human breast cancer growth. Cancer Gene Ther 2000;7(9):1270–1278.

240. Sachs AB. Cell cycle-dependent translation initiation: IRES elements prevail. Cell 2000;101(3):243–245.

241. Lahti JM, Xiang J, Heath LS, Campana D, Kidd VJ. PITSLRE protein kinase activity is associated with apoptosis. Mol Cell Biol 1995;15(1):1–11.

242. Trembley JH, Hu D, Hsu LC, Yeung CY, Slaughter C, Lahti JM, Kidd VJ. PITSLRE p110 protein kinases associate with transcription complexes and affect their activity. J Biol Chem 2002;277(4):2589–2596.

243. Hu D, Mayeda A, Trembley JH, Lahti JM, Kidd VJ. CDK11 complexes promote pre-mRNA splicing. J Biol Chem 2003;278(10):8623–8629.

244. Lahti JM, Xiang J, Kidd VJ. The PITSLRE protein kinase family. Prog Cell Cycle Res 1995;1:329–338.

245. Beyaert R, Kidd VJ, Cornelis S, Van de Craen M, Denecker G, Lahti JM, Gururajan R, Vandenabeele P, Fiers W. Cleavage of PITSLRE kinases by ICE/CASP-1 and CPP32/CASP-3 during apoptosis induced by tumor necrosis factor. J Biol Chem 1997;272(18):11694–11697.

246. Loyer P, Trembley JH, Grenet JA, Busson A, Corlu A, Zhao W, Kocak M, Kidd VJ, Lahti JM. Characterization of cyclin L1 and L2 interactions with CDK11 and splicing factors: influence of cyclin L isoforms on splice site selection. J Biol Chem 2008;283(12):7721–7732.

247. Dickinson LA, Edgar AJ, Ehley J, Gottesfeld JM. Cyclin L is an RS domain protein involved in pre-mRNA splicing. J Biol Chem 2002;277(28):25465–25473.

248. Loyer P, Trembley JH, Lahti JM, Kidd VJ. The RNP protein, RNPS1, associates with specific isoforms of the p34cdc2-related PITSLRE protein kinase in vivo. J Cell Sci 1998;111(Pt 11):1495–1506.

249. Zong H, Chi Y, Wang Y, Yang Y, Zhang L, Chen H, Jiang J, Li Z, Hong Y, Wang H, Yun X, Gu J. Cyclin D3/CDK11p58 complex is involved in the repression of androgen receptor. Mol Cell Biol 2007;27(20):7125–7142.

250. Petretti C, Savoian M, Montembault E, Glover DM, Prigent C, Giet R. The PITSLRE/CDK11p58 protein kinase promotes centrosome maturation and bipolar spindle formation. EMBO Rep 2006;7(4):418–424.

251. Hu D, Valentine M, Kidd VJ, Lahti JM. CDK11(p58) is required for the maintenance of sister chromatid cohesion. J Cell Sci 2007;120(Pt 14):2424–2434.

252. Li T, Inoue A, Lahti JM, Kidd VJ. Failure to proliferate and mitotic arrest of CDK11(p110/p58)-null mutant mice at the blastocyst stage of embryonic cell development. Mol Cell Biol 2004;24(8):3188–3197.

253. Schwab M, Praml C, Amler LC. Genomic instability in 1p and human malignancies. Genes Chromosomes Cancer 1996;16(4):211–229.

254. Mori N, Morosetti R, Mizoguchi H, Koeffler HP. Progression of myelodysplastic syndrome: allelic loss on chromosomal arm 1p. Br J Haematol 2003;122(2):226–230.

255. Poetsch M, Dittberner T, Woenckhaus C. Microsatellite analysis at 1p36.3 in malignant melanoma of the skin: fine mapping in search of a possible tumour suppressor gene region. Melanoma Res 2003;13(1):29–33.

256. Barbashina V, Salazar P, Holland EC, Rosenblum MK, Ladanyi M. Allelic losses at 1p36 and 19q13 in gliomas: correlation with histologic classification, definition of a 150-kb minimal deleted region on 1p36, and evaluation of CAMTA1 as a candidate tumor suppressor gene. Clin Cancer Res 2005;11(3):1119–1128.

257. White PS, Maris JM, Beltinger C, Sulman E, Marshall HN, Fujimori M, Kaufman BA, Biegel JA, Allen C, Hilliard C, et al. A region of consistent deletion in neuroblastoma maps within human chromosome 1p36.2–36.3. Proc Natl Acad Sci U S A 1995;92(12):5520–5524.

258. Chandramouli A, Shi J, Feng Y, Holubec H, Shanas RM, Bhattacharyya AK, Zheng W, Nelson MA. Haploinsufficiency of the cdc2l gene contributes to skin cancer development in mice. Carcinogenesis 2007;28(9):2028–2035.

259. Ko TK, Kelly E, Pines J. CrkRS: a novel conserved Cdc2-related protein kinase that colocalises with SC35 speckles. J Cell Sci 2001;114(Pt 14):2591–2603.

260. Yao CJ, Lai GM, Chan CF, Cheng AL, Yang YY, Chuang SE. Dramatic synergistic anticancer effect of clinically achievable doses of lovastatin and troglitazone. Int J Cancer 2006;118(3):773–779.

261. Marques F, Moreau JL, Peaucellier G, Lozano JC, Schatt P, Picard A, Callebaut I, Perret E, Geneviere AM. A new subfamily of high molecular mass CDC2-related kinases with PITAI/VRE motifs. Biochem Biophys Res Commun 2000;279(3):832–837.

262. Lapidot-Lifson Y, Patinkin D, Prody CA, Ehrlich G, Seidman S, Ben-Aziz R, Benseler F, Eckstein F, Zakut H, Soreq H. Cloning and antisense oligodeoxynucleotide inhibition of a human homolog of cdc2 required in hematopoiesis. Proc Natl Acad Sci U S A 1992;89(2):579–583.

263. Chiu YL, Cao H, Jacque JM, Stevenson M, Rana TM. Inhibition of human immunodeficiency virus type 1 replication by RNA interference directed against human transcription elongation factor P-TEFb (CDK9/CyclinT1). J Virol 2004;78(5):2517–2529.

264. Chen HH, Wong YH, Geneviere AM, Fann MJ. CDK13/CDC2L5 interacts with L-type cyclins and regulates alternative splicing. Biochem Biophys Res Commun 2007;354(3):735–740.

265. Tsai LH, Delalle I, Caviness VS Jr, Chae T, Harlow E. p35 is a neural-specific regulatory subunit of cyclin-dependent kinase 5. Nature 1994;371(6496):419–423.

266. Kusakawa G, Saito T, Onuki R, Ishiguro K, Kishimoto T, Hisanaga S. Calpain-dependent proteolytic cleavage of the p35 cyclin-dependent kinase 5 activator to p25. J Biol Chem 2000;275(22):17166–17172.

267. Lew J, Huang QQ, Qi Z, Winkfein RJ, Aebersold R, Hunt T, Wang JH. A brain-specific activator of cyclin-dependent kinase 5. Nature 1994;371(6496):423–426.

268. Tang D, Yeung J, Lee KY, Matsushita M, Matsui H, Tomizawa K, Hatase O, Wang JH. An isoform of the neuronal cyclin-dependent kinase 5 (Cdk5) activator. J Biol Chem 1995;270(45):26897–26903.

269. Tang D, Chun AC, Zhang M, Wang JH. Cyclin-dependent kinase 5 (Cdk5) activation domain of neuronal Cdk5 activator. Evidence of the existence of cyclin fold in neuronal Cdk5a activator. J Biol Chem 1997;272(19):12318–12327.

270. Tarricone C, Dhavan R, Peng J, Areces LB, Tsai LH, Musacchio A. Structure and regulation of the CDK5-p25(nck5a) complex. Mol Cell 2001;8(3):657–669.

271. Mapelli M, Massimiliano L, Crovace C, Seeliger MA, Tsai LH, Meijer L, Musacchio A. Mechanism of CDK5/p25 binding by CDK inhibitors. J Med Chem 2005;48(3):671–679.

272. Zukerberg LR, Patrick GN, Nikolic M, Humbert S, Wu CL, Lanier LM, Gertler FB, Vidal M, Van Etten RA, Tsai LH. Cables links Cdk5 and c-Abl and facilitates Cdk5 tyrosine phosphorylation, kinase upregulation, and neurite outgrowth. Neuron 2000;26(3):633–646.

273. Hirasawa M, Ohshima T, Takahashi S, Longenecker G, Honjo Y, Veeranna, Pant HC, Mikoshiba K, Brady RO, Kulkarni AB. Perinatal abrogation of Cdk5 expression in brain results in neuronal migration defects. Proc Natl Acad Sci U S A 2004;101(16):6249–6254.

274. Dhariwala FA, Rajadhyaksha MS. An unusual member of the Cdk family: Cdk5. Cell Mol Neurobiol 2008;28(3):351–369.

275. Cruz JC, Tsai LH. Cdk5 deregulation in the pathogenesis of Alzheimer's disease. Trends Mol Med 2004;10(9):452–458.

276. Cruz JC, Tsai LH. A Jekyll and Hyde kinase: roles for Cdk5 in brain development and disease. Curr Opin Neurobiol 2004;14(3):390–394.

277. Dhavan R, Tsai LH. A decade of CDK5. Nat Rev Mol Cell Biol 2001;2(10):749–759.

278. Cheung ZH, Gong K, Ip NY. Cyclin-dependent kinase 5 supports neuronal survival through phosphorylation of Bcl-2. J Neurosci 2008;28(19):4872–4877.

279. Li BS, Zhang L, Takahashi S, Ma W, Jaffe H, Kulkarni AB, Pant HC. Cyclin-dependent kinase 5 prevents neuronal apoptosis by negative regulation of c-Jun N-terminal kinase 3. EMBO J 2002;21(3):324–333.

280. Gojo I, Zhang B, Fenton RG. The cyclin-dependent kinase inhibitor flavopiridol induces apoptosis in multiple myeloma cells through transcriptional repression and down-regulation of Mcl-1. Clin Cancer Res 2002;8(11):3527–3538.

281. Lee JH, Kim HS, Lee SJ, Kim KT. Stabilization and activation of p53 induced by Cdk5 contributes to neuronal cell death. J Cell Sci 2007;120(Pt 13):2259–2271.

282. Strocchi P, Pession A, Dozza B. Up-regulation of cDK5/p35 by oxidative stress in human neuroblastoma IMR-32 cells. J Cell Biochem 2003;88(4):758–765.

283. Lee JH, Kim KT. Regulation of cyclin-dependent kinase 5 and p53 by ERK1/2 pathway in the DNA damage-induced neuronal death. J Cell Physiol 2007;210(3):784–797.

284. Wei FY, Nagashima K, Ohshima T, Saheki Y, Lu YF, Matsushita M, Yamada Y, Mikoshiba K, Seino Y, Matsui H, Tomizawa K. Cdk5-dependent regulation of glucose-stimulated insulin secretion. Nat Med 2005;11(10):1104–1108.

285. Sandal T, Stapnes C, Kleivdal H, Hedin L, Doskeland SO. A novel, extraneuronal role for cyclin-dependent protein kinase 5 (CDK5): modulation of cAMP-induced apoptosis in rat leukemia cells. J Biol Chem 2002;277(23):20783–20793.

286. Lin H, Juang JL, Wang PS. Involvement of Cdk5/p25 in digoxin-triggered prostate cancer cell apoptosis. J Biol Chem 2004;279(28):29302–29307.

287. Seo HR, Kim J, Bae S, Soh JW, Lee YS. Cdk5-mediated phosphorylation of c-Myc on Ser-62 is essential in transcriptional activation of cyclin B1 by cyclin G1. J Biol Chem 2008;283(23):15601–15610.

288. Johnstone CN, Mongroo PS, Rich AS, Schupp M, Bowser MJ, Delemos AS, Tobias JW, Liu Y, Hannigan GE, Rustgi AK. Parvin-beta inhibits breast cancer tumorigenicity and promotes CDK9-mediated peroxisome proliferator-activated receptor gamma 1 phosphorylation. Mol Cell Biol 2008;28(2):687–704.

289. Kouroukis CT, Belch A, Crump M, Eisenhauer E, Gascoyne RD, Meyer R, Lohmann R, Lopez P, Powers J, Turner R, Connors JM. Flavopiridol in untreated or relapsed mantle-cell lymphoma: results of a phase II study of the National Cancer Institute of Canada Clinical Trials Group. J Clin Oncol 2003;21(9):1740–1745.

290. Chin K, DeVries S, Fridlyand J, Spellman PT, Roydasgupta R, Kuo WL, Lapuk A, Neve RM, Qian Z, Ryder T, Chen F, Feiler H, Tokuyasu T, Kingsley C, Dairkee S, Meng Z, Chew K, Pinkel D, Jain A, Ljung BM, Esserman L, Albertson DG, Waldman FM, Gray JW. Genomic and transcriptional aberrations linked to breast cancer pathophysiologies. Cancer Cell 2006;10(6):529–541.

291. Renwick A, Thompson D, Seal S, Kelly P, Chagtai T, Ahmed M, North B, Jayatilake H, Barfoot R, Spanova K, McGuffog L, Evans DG, Eccles D, Easton DF, Stratton MR, Rahman N. ATM mutations that cause ataxia-telangiectasia are breast cancer susceptibility alleles. Nat Genet 2006;38(8):873–875.

292. Kanaoka Y, Kimura SH, Okazaki I, Ikeda M, Nojima H. GAK: a cyclin G associated kinase contains a tensin/auxilin-like domain. FEBS Lett 1997;402(1):73–80.

293. Kimura SH, Tsuruga H, Yabuta N, Endo Y, Nojima H. Structure, expression, and chromosomal localization of human GAK. Genomics 1997;44(2):179–187.

294. Okamoto K, Beach D. Cyclin G is a transcriptional target of the p53 tumor suppressor protein. EMBO J 1994;13(20):4816–4822.

295. Ohtsuka T, Ryu H, Minamishima YA, Ryo A, Lee SW. Modulation of p53 and p73 levels by cyclin G: implication of a negative feedback regulation. Oncogene 2003;22(11):1678–1687.

296. Bates S, Rowan S, Vousden KH. Characterisation of human cyclin G1 and G2: DNA damage inducible genes. Oncogene 1996;13(5):1103–1109.

297. Bible KC, Lensing JL, Nelson SA, Lee YK, Reid JM, Ames MM, Isham CR, Piens J, Rubin SL, Rubin J, Kaufmann SH, Atherton PJ, Sloan JA, Daiss MK, Adjei AA, Erlichman C. Phase 1 trial of flavopiridol combined with cisplatin or carboplatin in patients with advanced malignancies with the assessment of pharmacokinetic and pharmacodynamic end points. Clin Cancer Res 2005;11(16):5935–5941.

298. Kametaka S, Moriyama K, Burgos PV, Eisenberg E, Greene LE, Mattera R, Bonifacino JS. Canonical interaction of cyclin G associated kinase with adaptor protein 1 regulates lysosomal enzyme sorting. Mol Biol Cell 2007;18(8):2991–3001.

299. Zhang L, Gjoerup O, Roberts TM. The serine/threonine kinase cyclin G-associated kinase regulates epidermal growth factor receptor signaling. Proc Natl Acad Sci USA 2004;101(28):10296–10301.

300. Brehmer D, Greff Z, Godl K, Blencke S, Kurtenbach A, Weber M, Muller S, Klebl B, Cotten M, Keri G, Wissing J, Daub H. Cellular targets of gefitinib. Cancer Res 2005;65(2):379–382.

301. El-Rayes BF, Gadgeel S, Parchment R, Lorusso P, Philip PA. A phase I study of flavopiridol and docetaxel. Invest New Drugs 2006;24(4):305–310.

302. Schmit TL, Ahmad N. Regulation of mitosis via mitotic kinases: new opportunities for cancer management. Mol Cancer Ther 2007;6(7):1920–1931.

303. Schmidt M, Bastians H. Mitotic drug targets and the development of novel anti-mitotic anticancer drugs. Drug Resist Updat 2007;10(4–5):162–181.

304. van de Weerdt BC, Medema RH. Polo-like kinases: a team in control of the division. Cell Cycle 2006;5(8):853–864.

305. Fenton B, Glover DM. A conserved mitotic kinase active at late anaphase-telophase in syncytial *Drosophila* embryos. Nature 1993;363(6430):637–640.

306. Cheng KY, Lowe ED, Sinclair J, Nigg EA, Johnson LN. The crystal structure of the human polo-like kinase-1 polo box domain and its phospho-peptide complex. EMBO J 2003;22(21):5757–5768.

307. Elia AE, Rellos P, Haire LF, Chao JW, Ivins FJ, Hoepker K, Mohammad D, Cantley LC, Smerdon SJ, Yaffe MB. The molecular basis for phosphodependent substrate targeting and regulation of Plks by the Polo-box domain. Cell 2003;115(1):83–95.

308. Elia AE, Cantley LC, Yaffe MB. Proteomic screen finds pSer/pThr-binding domain localizing Plk1 to mitotic substrates. Science 2003;299(5610):1228–1231.

309. Jang YJ, Lin CY, Ma S, Erikson RL. Functional studies on the role of the C-terminal domain of mammalian polo-like kinase. Proc Natl Acad Sci U S A 2002;99(4):1984–1989.

310. Winkles JA, Alberts GF. Differential regulation of polo-like kinase 1, 2, 3, and 4 gene expression in mammalian cells and tissues. Oncogene 2005;24(2):260–266.

311. Strebhardt K, Ullrich A. Targeting polo-like kinase 1 for cancer therapy. Nat Rev Cancer 2006;6(4):321–330.

312. van Vugt MA, van de Weerdt BC, Vader G, Janssen H, Calafat J, Klompmaker R, Wolthuis RM, Medema RH. Polo-like kinase-1 is required for bipolar spindle formation but is dispensable for anaphase promoting complex/Cdc20 activation and initiation of cytokinesis. J Biol Chem 2004;279(35):36841–36854.

313. Toyoshima-Morimoto F, Taniguchi E, Nishida E. Plk1 promotes nuclear translocation of human Cdc25C during prophase. EMBO Rep 2002;3(4):341–348.

314. Nakajima H, Toyoshima-Morimoto F, Taniguchi E, Nishida E. Identification of a consensus motif for Plk (Polo-like kinase) phosphorylation reveals Myt1 as a Plk1 substrate. J Biol Chem 2003;278(28):25277–25280.

315. Watanabe N, Arai H, Nishihara Y, Taniguchi M, Watanabe N, Hunter T, Osada H. M-phase kinases induce phospho-dependent ubiquitination of somatic Wee1 by SCFbeta-TrCP. Proc Natl Acad Sci U S A 2004;101(13):4419–4424.

316. Eckerdt F, Yuan J, Saxena K, Martin B, Kappel S, Lindenau C, Kramer A, Naumann S, Daum S, Fischer G, Dikic I, Kaufmann M, Strebhardt K. Polo-like kinase 1-mediated phosphorylation stabilizes Pin1 by inhibiting its ubiquitination in human cells. J Biol Chem 2005;280(44):36575–36583.

317. Smits VA, Klompmaker R, Arnaud L, Rijksen G, Nigg EA, Medema RH. Polo-like kinase-1 is a target of the DNA damage checkpoint. Nat Cell Biol 2000;2(9):672–676.

318. Tsvetkov L, Stern DF. Phosphorylation of Plk1 at S137 and T210 is inhibited in response to DNA damage. Cell Cycle 2005;4(1):166–171.

319. Ando K, Ozaki T, Yamamoto H, Furuya K, Hosoda M, Hayashi S, Fukuzawa M, Nakagawara A. Polo-like kinase 1 (Plk1) inhibits p53 function by physical interaction and phosphorylation. J Biol Chem 2004;279(24):25549–25561.

320. Tsvetkov LM, Tsekova RT, Xu X, Stern DF. The Plk1 Polo box domain mediates a cell cycle and DNA damage regulated interaction with Chk2. Cell Cycle 2005;4(4):609–617.

321. van Vugt MA, Medema RH. Getting in and out of mitosis with Polo-like kinase-1. Oncogene 2005;24(17):2844–2859.

322. Casenghi M, Meraldi P, Weinhart U, Duncan PI, Korner R, Nigg EA. Polo-like kinase 1 regulates Nlp, a centrosome protein involved in microtubule nucleation. Dev Cell 2003;5(1):113–125.

323. Lane HA, Nigg EA. Antibody microinjection reveals an essential role for human polo-like kinase 1 (Plk1) in the functional maturation of mitotic centrosomes. J Cell Biol 1996;135(6Pt 2):1701–1713.

324. Rapley J, Baxter JE, Blot J, Wattam SL, Casenghi M, Meraldi P, Nigg EA, Fry AM. Coordinate regulation of the mother centriole component nlp by nek2 and plk1 protein kinases. Mol Cell Biol 2005;25(4):1309–1324.

325. Leng M, Bessuso D, Jung SY, Wang Y, Qin J. Targeting Plk1 to chromosome arms and regulating chromosome compaction by the PICH ATPase. Cell Cycle 2008;7(10):1480–1489.

326. Hauf S, Roitinger E, Koch B, Dittrich CM, Mechtler K, Peters JM. Dissociation of cohesin from chromosome arms and loss of arm cohesion during early mitosis depends on phosphorylation of SA2. PLoS Biol 2005;3(3): e69.

327. Sumara I, Vorlaufer E, Stukenberg PT, Kelm O, Redemann N, Nigg EA, Peters JM. The dissociation of cohesin from chromosomes in prophase is regulated by Polo-like kinase. Mol Cell 2002;9(3):515–525.

328. Ahonen LJ, Kallio MJ, Daum JR, Bolton M, Manke IA, Yaffe MB, Stukenberg PT, Gorbsky GJ. Polo-like kinase 1 creates the tension-sensing 3F3/2 phosphoepitope and modulates the association of spindle-checkpoint proteins at kinetochores. Curr Biol 2005;15(12):1078–1089.

329. Goto H, Kiyono T, Tomono Y, Kawajiri A, Urano T, Furukawa K, Nigg EA, Inagaki M. Complex formation of Plk1 and INCENP required for metaphase-anaphase transition. Nat Cell Biol 2006;8(2):180–187.

330. Golan A, Yudkovsky Y, Hershko A. The cyclin-ubiquitin ligase activity of cyclosome/APC is jointly activated by protein kinases Cdk1-cyclin B and Plk. J Biol Chem 2002;277(18):15552–15557.

331. Moshe Y, Boulaire J, Pagano M, Hershko A. Role of Polo-like kinase in the degradation of early mitotic inhibitor 1, a regulator of the anaphase promoting complex/cyclosome. Proc Natl Acad Sci U S A 2004;101(21):7937–7942.

332. Hansen DV, Loktev AV, Ban KH, Jackson PK. Plk1 regulates activation of the anaphase promoting complex by phosphorylating and triggering SCFbetaTrCP-dependent destruction of the APC inhibitor Emi1. Mol Biol Cell 2004;15(12):5623–5634.

333. Kraft C, Herzog F, Gieffers C, Mechtler K, Hagting A, Pines J, Peters JM. Mitotic regulation of the human anaphase-promoting complex by phosphorylation. EMBO J 2003;22(24):6598–6609.

334. Eckerdt F, Strebhardt K. Polo-like kinase 1: target and regulator of anaphase-promoting complex/cyclosome-dependent proteolysis. Cancer Res 2006;66(14):6895–6898.

335. Smith MR, Wilson ML, Hamanaka R, Chase D, Kung H, Longo DL, Ferris DK. Malignant transformation of mammalian cells initiated by constitutive expression of the polo-like kinase. Biochem Biophys Res Commun 1997;234(2):397–405.

336. Kauselmann G, Weiler M, Wulff P, Jessberger S, Konietzko U, Scafidi J, Staubli U, Bereiter-Hahn J, Strebhardt K, Kuhl D. The polo-like protein kinases Fnk and Snk associate with a Ca(2+)- and integrin-binding protein and are regulated dynamically with synaptic plasticity. EMBO J 1999;18(20):5528–5539.

337. Warnke S, Kemmler S, Hames RS, Tsai HL, Hoffmann-Rohrer U, Fry AM, Hoffmann I. Polo-like kinase-2 is required for centriole duplication in mammalian cells. Curr Biol 2004;14(13):1200–1207.

338. Ma S, Charron J, Erikson RL. Role of Plk2 (Snk) in mouse development and cell proliferation. Mol Cell Biol 2003;23(19):6936–6943.

339. Shimizu-Yoshida Y, Sugiyama K, Rogounovitch T, Ohtsuru A, Namba H, Saenko V, Yamashita S. Radiation-inducible hSNK gene is transcriptionally regulated by p53 binding homology element in human thyroid cells. Biochem Biophys Res Commun 2001;289(2):491–498.

340. Syed N, Smith P, Sullivan A, Spender LC, Dyer M, Karran L, O'Nions J, Allday M, Hoffmann I, Crawford D, Griffin B, Farrell PJ, Crook T. Transcriptional silencing of Polo-like kinase 2 (SNK/PLK2) is a frequent event in B-cell malignancies. Blood 2006;107(1):250–256.

341. Matthew EM, Yen TJ, Dicker DT, Dorsey JF, Yang W, Navaraj A, El-Deiry WS. Replication stress, defective S-phase checkpoint and increased death in Plk2-deficient human cancer cells. Cell Cycle 2007;6(20):2571–2578.

342. Burns TF, Fei P, Scata KA, Dicker DT, El-Deiry WS. Silencing of the novel p53 target gene Snk/Plk2 leads to mitotic catastrophe in paclitaxel (taxol)-exposed cells. Mol Cell Biol 2003;23(16):5556–5571.

343. Myer DL, Bahassi el M, Stambrook PJ. The Plk3-Cdc25 circuit. Oncogene 2005;24(2):299–305.

344. Zimmerman WC, Erikson RL. Polo-like kinase 3 is required for entry into S phase. Proc Natl Acad Sci U S A 2007;104(6):1847–1852.

345. Xie S, Wu H, Wang Q, Cogswell JP, Husain I, Conn C, Stambrook P, Jhanwar-Uniyal M, Dai W. Plk3 functionally links DNA damage to cell cycle arrest and apoptosis at least in part via the p53 pathway. J Biol Chem 2001;276(46):43305–43312.

346. Xie S, Xie B, Lee MY, Dai W. Regulation of cell cycle checkpoints by polo-like kinases. Oncogene 2005;24(2):277–286.

347. Li B, Ouyang B, Pan H, Reissmann PT, Slamon DJ, Arceci R, Lu L, Dai W. Prk, a cytokine-inducible human protein serine/threonine kinase whose expression appears to be down-regulated in lung carcinomas. J Biol Chem 1996;271(32):19402–19408.

348. Dai W, Li Y, Ouyang B, Pan H, Reissmann P, Li J, Wiest J, Stambrook P, Gluckman JL, Noffsinger A, Bejarano P. PRK, a cell cycle gene localized to 8p21, is downregulated in head and neck cancer. Genes Chromosomes Cancer 2000;27(3):332–336.

349. Yang Y, Bai J, Shen R, Brown SA, Komissarova E, Huang Y, Jiang N, Alberts GF, Costa M, Lu L, Winkles JA, Dai W. Polo-like kinase 3 functions as a tumor suppressor and is a negative regulator of hypoxia-inducible factor-1 alpha under hypoxic conditions. Cancer Res 2008;68(11):4077–4085.

350. Hudson JW, Kozarova A, Cheung P, Macmillan JC, Swallow CJ, Cross JC, Dennis JW. Late mitotic failure in mice lacking Sak, a polo-like kinase. Curr Biol 2001;11(6):441–446.

351. Ko MA, Rosario CO, Hudson JW, Kulkarni S, Pollett A, Dennis JW, Swallow CJ. Plk4 haploinsufficiency causes mitotic infidelity and carcinogenesis. Nat Genet 2005;37(8):883–888.

352. Habedanck R, Stierhof YD, Wilkinson CJ, Nigg EA. The Polo kinase Plk4 functions in centriole duplication. Nat Cell Biol 2005;7(11):1140–1146.

353. Kleylein-Sohn J, Westendorf J, Le Clech M, Habedanck R, Stierhof YD, Nigg EA. Plk4-induced centriole biogenesis in human cells. Dev Cell 2007;13(2):190–202.

354. Tanenbaum ME, Medema RH. Cell fate in the Hand of Plk4. Nat Cell Biol 2007;9(10):1127–1129.

355. Martindill DM, Risebro CA, Smart N, Franco-Viseras Mdel M, Rosario CO, Swallow CJ, Dennis JW, Riley PR. Nucleolar release of Hand1 acts as a molecular switch to determine cell fate. Nat Cell Biol 2007;9(10):1131–1141.

356. Castro A, Vigneron S, Bernis C, Labbe JC, Prigent C, Lorca T. The D-box-activating domain (DAD) is a new proteolysis signal that stimulates the silent D-box sequence of Aurora-A. EMBO Rep 2002;3(12):1209–1214.

357. Crane R, Kloepfer A, Ruderman JV. Requirements for the destruction of human Aurora-A. J Cell Sci 2004;117(Pt 25):5975–5983.

358. Nguyen HG, Chinnappan D, Urano T, Ravid K. Mechanism of Aurora-B degradation and its dependency on intact KEN and A-boxes: identification of an aneuploidy-promoting property. Mol Cell Biol 2005;25(12):4977–4992.

359. Carmena M, Earnshaw WC. The cellular geography of aurora kinases. Nat Rev Mol Cell Biol 2003;4(11):842–854.

360. Takahashi T, Futamura M, Yoshimi N, Sano J, Katada M, Takagi Y, Kimura M, Yoshioka T, Okano Y, Saji S. Centrosomal kinases, HsAIRK1 and HsAIRK3, are overexpressed in primary colorectal cancers. Jpn J Cancer Res 2000;91(10):1007–1014.

361. Kimura M, Matsuda Y, Yoshioka T, Okano Y. Cell cycle-dependent expression and centrosome localization of a third human aurora/Ipl1-related protein kinase, AIK3. J Biol Chem 1999;274(11):7334–7340.

362. Dutertre S, Hamard-Peron E, Cremet JY, Thomas Y, Prigent C. The absence of p53 aggravates polyploidy and centrosome number abnormality induced by Aurora-C overexpression. Cell Cycle 2005;4(12):1783–1787.

363. Warner SL, Bearss DJ, Han H, Von Hoff DD. Targeting Aurora-2 kinase in cancer. Mol Cancer Ther 2003;2(6):589–595.

364. Marumoto T, Zhang D, Saya H. Aurora-A—a guardian of poles. Nat Rev Cancer 2005;5(1):42–50.

365. Meraldi P, Honda R, Nigg EA. Aurora-A overexpression reveals tetraploidization as a major route to centrosome amplification in p53−/− cells. EMBO J 2002;21(4):483–492.

366. Hirota T, Kunitoku N, Sasayama T, Marumoto T, Zhang D, Nitta M, Hatakeyama K, Saya H. Aurora-A and an interacting activator, the LIM protein Ajuba, are required for mitotic commitment in human cells. Cell 2003;114(5):585–598.

367. Portier N, Audhya A, Maddox PS, Green RA, Dammermann A, Desai A, Oegema K. A microtubule-independent role for centrosomes and Aurora A in nuclear envelope breakdown. Dev Cell 2007;12(4):515–529.

368. Gruss OJ, Vernos I. The mechanism of spindle assembly: functions of Ran and its target TPX2. J Cell Biol 2004;166(7):949–955.

369. Gruss OJ, Wittmann M, Yokoyama H, Pepperkok R, Kufer T, Sillje H, Karsenti E, Mattaj IW, Vernos I. Chromosome-induced microtubule assembly mediated by TPX2 is required for spindle formation in HeLa cells. Nat Cell Biol 2002;4(11):871–879.

370. Kufer TA, Sillje HH, Korner R, Gruss OJ, Meraldi P, Nigg EA. Human TPX2 is required for targeting Aurora-A kinase to the spindle. J Cell Biol 2002;158(4):617–623.

371. Marumoto T, Honda S, Hara T, Nitta M, Hirota T, Kohmura E, Saya H. Aurora-A kinase maintains the fidelity of early and late mitotic events in HeLa cells. J Biol Chem 2003;278(51):51786–51795.

372. Kunitoku N, Sasayama T, Marumoto T, Zhang D, Honda S, Kobayashi O, Hatakeyama K, Ushio Y, Saya H, Hirota T. CENP-A phosphorylation by Aurora-A in prophase is required for enrichment of Aurora-B at inner centromeres and for kinetochore function. Dev Cell 2003;5(6):853–864.

373. Honda K, Mihara H, Kato Y, Yamaguchi A, Tanaka H, Yasuda H, Furukawa K, Urano T. Degradation of human Aurora2 protein kinase by the anaphase-promoting complex-ubiquitin-proteasome pathway. Oncogene 2000;19(24):2812–2819.

374. Ruchaud S, Carmena M, Earnshaw WC. Chromosomal passengers: conducting cell division. Nat Rev Mol Cell Biol 2007;8(10):798–812.

375. Murata-Hori M, Wang YL. The kinase activity of Aurora B is required for kinetochore-microtubule interactions during mitosis. Curr Biol 2002;12(11):894–899.

376. Andrews PD, Ovechkina Y, Morrice N, Wagenbach M, Duncan K, Wordeman L, Swedlow JR. Aurora B regulates MCAK at the mitotic centromere. Dev Cell 2004;6(2):253–268.

377. Lan W, Zhang X, Kline-Smith SL, Rosasco SE, Barrett-Wilt GA, Shabanowitz J, Hunt DF, Walczak CE, Stukenberg PT. Aurora B phosphorylates centromeric MCAK and regulates its localization and microtubule depolymerization activity. Curr Biol 2004;14(4):273–286.

378. Ditchfield C, Johnson VL, Tighe A, Ellston R, Haworth C, Johnson T, Mortlock A, Keen N, Taylor SS. Aurora B couples chromosome alignment with anaphase by targeting BubR1, Mad2, and Cenp-E to kinetochores. J Cell Biol 2003;161(2):267–280.

379. Anand S, Penrhyn-Lowe S, Venkitaraman AR. AURORA-A amplification overrides the mitotic spindle assembly checkpoint, inducing resistance to taxol. Cancer Cell 2003;3(1):51–62.

380. Zeitlin SG, Shelby RD, Sullivan KF. CENP-A is phosphorylated by Aurora B kinase and plays an unexpected role in completion of cytokinesis. J Cell Biol 2001;155(7):1147–1157.

381. Crosio C, Fimia GM, Loury R, Kimura M, Okano Y, Zhou H, Sen S, Allis CD, Sassone-Corsi P. Mitotic phosphorylation of histone H3: spatio-temporal regulation by mammalian Aurora kinases. Mol Cell Biol 2002;22(3):874–885.

382. Mishima M, Glotzer M. Cytokinesis: a logical GAP. Curr Biol 2003;13(15): R589-591.

383. Stewart S, Fang G. Destruction box-dependent degradation of Aurora B is mediated by the anaphase-promoting complex/cyclosome and Cdh1. Cancer Res 2005;65(19):8730–8735.

384. Bartkova J, Horejsi Z, Koed K, Kramer A, Tort F, Zieger K, Guldberg P, Sehested M, Nesland JM, Lukas C, Orntoft T, Lukas J, Bartek J. DNA damage response as a candidate anti-cancer barrier in early human tumorigenesis. Nature 2005;434(7035):864–870.

385. Gorgoulis VG, Vassiliou LV, Karakaidos P, Zacharatos P, Kotsinas A, Liloglou T, Venere M, Ditullio RA Jr, Kastrinakis NG, Levy B, Kletsas D, Yoneta A, Herlyn M, Kittas C, Halazonetis TD. Activation of the DNA damage checkpoint and genomic instability in human precancerous lesions. Nature 2005;434(7035):907–913.

386. Bartek J, Bartkova J, Lukas J. DNA damage signalling guards against activated oncogenes and tumour progression. Oncogene 2007;26(56):7773–7779.

387. Bartkova J, Rezaei N, Liontos M, Karakaidos P, Kletsas D, Issaeva N, Vassiliou LV, Kolettas E, Niforou K, Zoumpourlis VC, Takaoka M, Nakagawa H, Tort F, Fugger K, Johansson F, Sehested M, Andersen CL, Dyrskjot L, Orntoft T, Lukas J, Kittas C, Helleday T, Halazonetis TD, Bartek J, Gorgoulis VG. Oncogene-induced senescence is part of the tumorigenesis barrier imposed by DNA damage checkpoints. Nature 2006;444(7119):633–637.

388. Di Micco R, Fumagalli M, Cicalese A, Piccinin S, Gasparini P, Luise C, Schurra C, Garre M, Nuciforo PG, Bensimon A, Maestro R, Pelicci PG, d'Adda di Fagagna F. Oncogene-induced senescence is a DNA damage response triggered by DNA hyper-replication. Nature 2006;444(7119):638–642.

389. Lord CJ, Garrett MD, Ashworth A. Targeting the double-strand DNA break repair pathway as a therapeutic strategy. Clin Cancer Res 2006;12(15):4463–4468.

390. Zhou BB, Bartek J. Targeting the checkpoint kinases: chemosensitization versus chemoprotection. Nat Rev Cancer 2004;4(3):216–225.

391. Li J, Stern DF. Regulation of CHK2 by DNA-dependent protein kinase. J Biol Chem 2005;280(12):12041–12050.

392. Falck J, Coates J, Jackson SP. Conserved modes of recruitment of ATM, ATR and DNA-PKcs to sites of DNA damage. Nature 2005;434(7033):605–611.

393. You Z, Chahwan C, Bailis J, Hunter T, Russell P. ATM activation and its recruitment to damaged DNA require binding to the C terminus of Nbs1. Mol Cell Biol 2005;25(13):5363–5379.

394. Bartek J, Lukas C, Lukas J. Checking on DNA damage in S phase. Nat Rev Mol Cell Biol 2004;5(10):792–804.

395. Zou L, Elledge SJ. Sensing DNA damage through ATRIP recognition of RPA-ssDNA complexes. Science 2003;300(5625):1542–1548.

396. Mordes DA, Glick GG, Zhao R, Cortez D. TopBP1 activates ATR through ATRIP and a PIKK regulatory domain. Genes Dev 2008;22(11):1478–1489.

397. Liu S, Bekker-Jensen S, Mailand N, Lukas C, Bartek J, Lukas J. Claspin operates downstream of TopBP1 to direct ATR signaling towards Chk1 activation. Mol Cell Biol 2006;26(16):6056–6064.

398. Kim JM, Kakusho N, Yamada M, Kanoh Y, Takemoto N, Masai H. Cdc7 kinase mediates Claspin phosphorylation in DNA replication checkpoint. Oncogene 2008;27(24):3475–3482.

399. Brown EJ, Baltimore D. ATR disruption leads to chromosomal fragmentation and early embryonic lethality. Genes Dev 2000;14(4):397–402.

400. de Klein A, Muijtjens M, van Os R, Verhoeven Y, Smit B, Carr AM, Lehmann AR, Hoeijmakers JH. Targeted disruption of the cell-cycle checkpoint gene ATR leads to early embryonic lethality in mice. Curr Biol 2000;10(8):479–482.

401. O'Driscoll M, Ruiz-Perez VL, Woods CG, Jeggo PA, Goodship JA. A splicing mutation affecting expression of ataxia-telangiectasia and Rad3-related protein (ATR) results in Seckel syndrome. Nat Genet 2003;33(4):497–501.

402. Lee JH, Paull TT. ATM activation by DNA double-strand breaks through the Mre11-Rad50-Nbs1 complex. Science 2005;308(5721):551–554.

403. Bakkenist CJ, Kastan MB. DNA damage activates ATM through intermolecular autophosphorylation and dimer dissociation. Nature 2003;421(6922):499–506.

404. Shiloh Y, Kastan MB. ATM: genome stability, neuronal development, and cancer cross paths. Adv Cancer Res 2001;83:209–254.

405. Jazayeri A, Falck J, Lukas C, Bartek J, Smith GC, Lukas J, Jackson SP. ATM- and cell cycle-dependent regulation of ATR in response to DNA double-strand breaks. Nat Cell Biol 2006;8(1):37–45.

406. Yoo HY, Kumagai A, Shevchenko A, Shevchenko A, Dunphy WG. Ataxia-telangiectasia mutated (ATM)-dependent activation of ATR occurs through phosphorylation of TopBP1 by ATM. J Biol Chem 2007;282(24):17501–17506.

407. Zhang X, Succi J, Feng Z, Prithivirajsingh S, Story MD, Legerski RJ. Artemis is a phosphorylation target of ATM and ATR and is involved in the G2/M DNA damage checkpoint response. Mol Cell Biol 2004;24(20):9207–9220.

408. Geng L, Zhang X, Zheng S, Legerski RJ. Artemis links ATM to G2/M checkpoint recovery via regulation of Cdk1-cyclin B. Mol Cell Biol 2007;27(7):2625–2635.

409. Chan DW, Chen BP, Prithivirajsingh S, Kurimasa A, Story MD, Qin J, Chen DJ. Autophosphorylation of the DNA-dependent protein kinase catalytic subunit is required for rejoining of DNA double-strand breaks. Genes Dev 2002;16(18):2333–2338.

410. Zhao Y, Thomas HD, Batey MA, Cowell IG, Richardson CJ, Griffin RJ, Calvert AH, Newell DR, Smith GC, Curtin NJ. Preclinical evaluation of a potent novel DNA-dependent protein kinase inhibitor NU7441. Cancer Res 2006;66(10):5354–5362.

411. Burma S, Chen BP, Chen DJ. Role of non-homologous end joining (NHEJ) in maintaining genomic integrity. DNA Repair (Amst) 2006;5(9–10):1042–1048.

412. Collis SJ, DeWeese TL, Jeggo PA, Parker AR. The life and death of DNA-PK. Oncogene 2005;24(6):949–961.

413. Manke IA, Nguyen A, Lim D, Stewart MQ, Elia AE, Yaffe MB. MAPKAP kinase-2 is a cell cycle checkpoint kinase that regulates the G2/M transition and S phase progression in response to UV irradiation. Mol Cell 2005;17(1):37–48.

414. Reinhardt HC, Aslanian AS, Lees JA, Yaffe MB. p53-deficient cells rely on ATM- and ATR-mediated checkpoint signaling through the p38MAPK/MK2 pathway for survival after DNA damage. Cancer Cell 2007;11(2):175–189.

415. Karlsson-Rosenthal C, Millar JB. Cdc25: mechanisms of checkpoint inhibition and recovery. Trends Cell Biol 2006;16(6):285–292.

416. Shimada M, Niida H, Zineldeen DH, Tagami H, Tanaka M, Saito H, Nakanishi M. Chk1 is a histone H3 threonine 11 kinase that regulates DNA damage-induced transcriptional repression. Cell 2008;132(2):221–232.

417. Petermann E, Maya-Mendoza A, Zachos G, Gillespie DA, Jackson DA, Caldecott KW. Chk1 requirement for high global rates of replication fork progression during normal vertebrate S phase. Mol Cell Biol 2006;26(8):3319–3326.

418. Kramer A, Mailand N, Lukas C, Syljuasen RG, Wilkinson CJ, Nigg EA, Bartek J, Lukas J. Centrosome-associated Chk1 prevents premature activation of cyclin-B-Cdk1 kinase. Nat Cell Biol 2004;6(9):884–891.

419. Schmitt E, Boutros R, Froment C, Monsarrat B, Ducommun B, Dozier C. CHK1 phosphorylates CDC25B during the cell cycle in the absence of DNA damage. J Cell Sci 2006;119(Pt 20):4269–4275.

420. Liu Q, Guntuku S, Cui XS, Matsuoka S, Cortez D, Tamai K, Luo G, Carattini-Rivera S, DeMayo F, Bradley A, Donehower LA, Elledge SJ. Chk1 is an essential kinase that is regulated by Atr and required for the G(2)/M DNA damage checkpoint. Genes Dev 2000;14(12):1448–1459.

421. Takai H, Tominaga K, Motoyama N, Minamishima YA, Nagahama H, Tsukiyama T, Ikeda K, Nakayama K, Nakanishi M. Aberrant cell cycle checkpoint function and early embryonic death in Chk1(−/−) mice. Genes Dev 2000;14(12):1439–1447.

422. Lam MH, Liu Q, Elledge SJ, Rosen JM. Chk1 is haploinsufficient for multiple functions critical to tumor suppression. Cancer Cell 2004;6(1):45–59.

423. Zhao H, Piwnica-Worms H. ATR-mediated checkpoint pathways regulate phosphorylation and activation of human Chk1. Mol Cell Biol 2001;21(13):4129–4139.

424. Smits VA, Reaper PM, Jackson SP. Rapid PIKK-dependent release of Chk1 from chromatin promotes the DNA-damage checkpoint response. Curr Biol 2006;16(2):150–159.

425. Niida H, Katsuno Y, Banerjee B, Hande MP, Nakanishi M. Specific role of Chk1 phosphorylations in cell survival and checkpoint activation. Mol Cell Biol 2007;27(7):2572–2581.

426. Shiromizu T, Goto H, Tomono Y, Bartek J, Totsukawa G, Inoko A, Nakanishi M, Matsumura F, Inagaki M. Regulation of mitotic function of Chk1 through phosphorylation at novel sites by cyclin-dependent kinase 1 (Cdk1). Genes Cells 2006;11(5):477–485.

427. Peng CY, Graves PR, Thoma RS, Wu Z, Shaw AS, Piwnica-Worms H. Mitotic and G2 checkpoint control: regulation of 14-3-3 protein binding by phosphorylation of Cdc25C on serine-216. Science 1997;277(5331):1501–1505.

428. Mailand N, Falck J, Lukas C, Syljuasen RG, Welcker M, Bartek J, Lukas J. Rapid destruction of human Cdc25A in response to DNA damage. Science 2000;288(5470):1425–1429.

429. Sorensen CS, Syljuasen RG, Falck J, Schroeder T, Ronnstrand L, Khanna KK, Zhou BB, Bartek J, Lukas J. Chk1 regulates the S phase checkpoint by coupling the physiological turnover and ionizing radiation-induced accelerated proteolysis of Cdc25A. Cancer Cell 2003;3(3):247–258.

430. Zhao H, Watkins JL, Piwnica-Worms H. Disruption of the checkpoint kinase 1/cell division cycle 25A pathway abrogates ionizing radiation-induced S and G2 checkpoints. Proc Natl Acad Sci U S A 2002;99(23):14795–14800.

431. Sorensen CS, Hansen LT, Dziegielewski J, Syljuasen RG, Lundin C, Bartek J, Helleday T. The cell-cycle checkpoint kinase Chk1 is required for mammalian homologous recombination repair. Nat Cell Biol 2005;7(2):195–201.

432. Zachos G, Black EJ, Walker M, Scott MT, Vagnarelli P, Earnshaw WC, Gillespie DA. Chk1 is required for spindle checkpoint function. Dev Cell 2007;12(2):247–260.

433. Huang X, Tran T, Zhang L, Hatcher R, Zhang P. DNA damage-induced mitotic catastrophe is mediated by the Chk1-dependent mitotic exit DNA damage checkpoint. Proc Natl Acad Sci U S A 2005;102(4):1065–1070.

434. Castedo M, Perfettini JL, Roumier T, Andreau K, Medema R, Kroemer G. Cell death by mitotic catastrophe: a molecular definition. Oncogene 2004;23(16):2825–2837.

435. Sidi S, Sanda T, Kennedy RD, Hagen AT, Jette CA, Hoffmans R, Pascual J, Imamura S, Kishi S, Amatruda JF, Kanki JP, Green DR, D'Andrea AA, Look AT. Chk1 suppresses a caspase-2 apoptotic response to DNA damage that bypasses p53, Bcl-2, and caspase-3. Cell 2008;133(5):864–877.

436. Ng CP, Lee HC, Ho CW, Arooz T, Siu WY, Lau A, Poon RY. Differential mode of regulation of the checkpoint kinases CHK1 and CHK2 by their regulatory domains. J Biol Chem 2004;279(10):8808–8819.

437. Xu X, Tsvetkov LM, Stern DF. Chk2 activation and phosphorylation-dependent oligomerization. Mol Cell Biol 2002;22(12):4419–4432.

438. Jack MT, Woo RA, Hirao A, Cheung A, Mak TW, Lee PW. Chk2 is dispensable for p53-mediated G1 arrest but is required for a latent p53-mediated apoptotic response. Proc Natl Acad Sci U S A 2002;99(15):9825–9829.

439. Takai H, Naka K, Okada Y, Watanabe M, Harada N, Saito S, Anderson CW, Appella E, Nakanishi M, Suzuki H, Nagashima K, Sawa H, Ikeda K, Motoyama N. Chk2-deficient mice exhibit radioresistance and defective p53-mediated transcription. EMBO J 2002;21(19):5195–5205.

440. Bartek J, Lukas J. Chk1 and Chk2 kinases in checkpoint control and cancer. Cancer Cell 2003;3(5):421–429.

441. Lukas C, Falck J, Bartkova J, Bartek J, Lukas J. Distinct spatiotemporal dynamics of mammalian checkpoint regulators induced by DNA damage. Nat Cell Biol 2003;5(3):255–260.

442. Chehab NH, Malikzay A, Appel M, Halazonetis TD. Chk2/hCds1 functions as a DNA damage checkpoint in G(1) by stabilizing p53. Genes Dev 2000;14(3):278–288.

443. Shieh SY, Ahn J, Tamai K, Taya Y, Prives C. The human homologs of checkpoint kinases Chk1 and Cds1 (Chk2) phosphorylate p53 at multiple DNA damage-inducible sites. Genes Dev 2000;14(3):289–300.

444. Hirao A, Kong YY, Matsuoka S, Wakeham A, Ruland J, Yoshida H, Liu D, Elledge SJ, Mak TW. DNA damage-induced activation of p53 by the checkpoint kinase Chk2. Science 2000;287(5459):1824–1827.

445. Chen L, Gilkes DM, Pan Y, Lane WS, Chen J. ATM and Chk2-dependent phosphorylation of MDMX contribute to p53 activation after DNA damage. EMBO J 2005;24(19):3411–3422.

446. LeBron C, Chen L, Gilkes DM, Chen J. Regulation of MDMX nuclear import and degradation by Chk2 and 14-3-3. EMBO J 2006;25(6):1196–1206.

447. Jallepalli PV, Lengauer C, Vogelstein B, Bunz F. The Chk2 tumor suppressor is not required for p53 responses in human cancer cells. J Biol Chem 2003;278(23):20475–20479.

448. Stevens C, Smith L, La Thangue NB. Chk2 activates E2F-1 in response to DNA damage. Nat Cell Biol 2003;5(5):401–409.

449. Yang S, Kuo C, Bisi JE, Kim MK. PML-dependent apoptosis after DNA damage is regulated by the checkpoint kinase hCds1/Chk2. Nat Cell Biol 2002;4(11):865–870.

450. Ghosh JC, Dohi T, Raskett CM, Kowalik TF, Altieri DC. Activated checkpoint kinase 2 provides a survival signal for tumor cells. Cancer Res 2006;66(24):11576–11579.

451. Hirao A, Cheung A, Duncan G, Girard PM, Elia AJ, Wakeham A, Okada H, Sarkissian T, Wong JA, Sakai T, De Stanchina E, Bristow RG, Suda T, Lowe SW, Jeggo PA, Elledge SJ, Mak TW. Chk2 is a tumor suppressor that regulates apoptosis in both an ataxia telangiectasia mutated (ATM)-dependent and an ATM-independent manner. Mol Cell Biol 2002;22(18):6521–6532.

452. Pabla N, Huang S, Mi QS, Daniel R, Dong Z. ATR-Chk2 signaling in p53 activation and DNA damage response during cisplatin-induced apoptosis. J Biol Chem 2008;283(10):6572–6583.

453. Arienti KL, Brunmark A, Axe FU, McClure K, Lee A, Blevitt J, Neff DK, Huang L, Crawford S, Pandit CR, Karlsson L, Breitenbucher JG. Checkpoint kinase inhibitors: SAR and radioprotective properties of a series of 2-arylbenzimidazoles. J Med Chem 2005;48(6):1873–1885.

454. Yu Q, Rose JH, Zhang H, Pommier Y. Antisense inhibition of Chk2/hCds1 expression attenuates DNA damage-induced S and G2 checkpoints and enhances apoptotic activity in HEK-293 cells. FEBS Lett 2001;505(1):7–12.

455. Huang M, Miao ZH, Zhu H, Cai YJ, Lu W, Ding J. Chk1 and Chk2 are differentially involved in homologous recombination repair and cell cycle arrest in response to DNA double-strand breaks induced by camptothecins. Mol Cancer Ther 2008;7(6):1440–1449.

456. Castedo M, Perfettini JL, Roumier T, Yakushijin K, Horne D, Medema R, Kroemer G. The cell cycle checkpoint kinase Chk2 is a negative regulator of mitotic catastrophe. Oncogene 2004;23(25):4353–4361.

457. Castedo M, Perfettini JL, Roumier T, Valent A, Raslova H, Yakushijin K, Horne D, Feunteun J, Lenoir G, Medema R, Vainchenker W, Kroemer G. Mitotic catastrophe constitutes a special case of apoptosis whose suppression entails aneuploidy. Oncogene 2004;23(25):4362–4370.

458. Cho SH, Tooulu CD, Fujii GH, Crain C, Parry D. Chk1 is essential for tumor cell viability following activation of the replication checkpoint. Cell Cycle 2005;4(1):131–139.

459. Carlessi L, Buscemi G, Larson G, Hong Z, Wu JZ, Delia D. Biochemical and cellular characterization of VRX0466617, a novel and selective inhibitor for the checkpoint kinase Chk2. Mol Cancer Ther 2007;6(3):935–944.

460. d'Adda di Fagagna F, Reaper PM, Clay-Farrace L, Fiegler H, Carr P, Von Zglinicki T, Saretzki G, Carter NP, Jackson SP. A DNA damage checkpoint response in telomere-initiated senescence. Nature 2003;426(6963):194–198.

461. Di Leonardo A, Linke SP, Clarkin K, Wahl GM. DNA damage triggers a prolonged p53-dependent G1 arrest and long-term induction of Cip1 in normal human fibroblasts. Genes Dev 1994;8(21):2540–2551.

462. Chen CR, Wang W, Rogoff HA, Li X, Mang W, Li CJ. Dual induction of apoptosis and senescence in cancer cells by Chk2 activation: checkpoint activation as a strategy against cancer. Cancer Res 2005;65(14):6017–6021.
463. Xiao Z, Xue J, Sowin TJ, Zhang H. Differential roles of checkpoint kinase 1, checkpoint kinase 2, and mitogen-activated protein kinase-activated protein kinase 2 in mediating DNA damage-induced cell cycle arrest: implications for cancer therapy. Mol Cancer Ther 2006;5(8):1935–1943.
464. Zhang WH, Poh A, Fanous AA, Eastman A. DNA damage-induced S phase arrest in human breast cancer depends on Chk1, but G2 arrest can occur independently of Chk1, Chk2 or MAPKAPK2. Cell Cycle 2008;7(11):1668–1677.

CHAPTER 7

STRUCTURAL BIOCHEMISTRY OF KINASE INHIBITORS

PROTEIN KINASES have received much attention as therapeutic targets for cancer and are also being developed for other indications, in particular, inflammatory diseases (for a historical perspective, see (1)). The fruits of these labors are beginning to be realized in the clinic: several structurally diverse small molecule kinase inhibitors are now approved for treatment of various malignancies, and many more are in various stages of clinical evaluation (reviewed in Chapters 8–10). Extensive medicinal chemistry structure–activity explorations, combined with X-ray crystal structures and molecular modeling, have provided insight into the structural features of kinases that can be exploited by small molecule inhibitors, and how to modulate potency and selectivity. More recently, as mutational resistance has emerged with some kinase inhibitor drugs in clinical studies (Chapter 11), we can start to formulate some rules regarding the structural features that give rise to resistance, and how to overcome these liabilities with second generation inhibitors.

In this chapter, we revisit the kinase catalytic site (described in Chapter 2), with particular reference to some key features that are exploited by various inhibitors. Our goal is not to provide an exhaustive catalog of kinase inhibitor structures but to outline some of the general principles that govern potency and specificity of binding, and to illustrate the diverse means by which small molecule kinase inhibitors can be accommodated within the ATP binding site and other regions of their target proteins. Kinase inhibitors may broadly be divided into two groups: those that inhibit the active, "DFG-in" form of the kinase (also referred to as Type I inhibitors) and those that bind preferentially (or even exclusively) to the "DFG-out," or inactive form (Type II inhibitors). Both classes of inhibitor have their merits and disadvantages, and it remains to be seen whether one strategy or the other consistently produces drugs with better clinical utility.

First, we review some of the salient features of the ATP binding site and consider how each feature plays a role in binding several diverse inhibitors, using

Targeting Protein Kinases for Cancer Therapy, by David J. Matthews and Mary E. Gerritsen
Copyright © 2010 John Wiley & Sons, Inc.

the example of the Ser/Thr kinase CHK1. The cyclin-dependent kinase CDK2 provides a second example of a Ser/Thr kinase that has been pursued extensively as a molecular target and presents the added complexity of two distinct structural forms: the inactive, monomeric CDK2 and the active, cyclin-bound conformation. We next review a different set of molecules that collectively inhibit SRC family tyrosine kinases, specifically SRC itself and ABL. The epidermal growth factor receptor (EGFR) provides a second example of a tyrosine kinase whose inhibitors have been structurally characterized. In particular, we describe the structures of three clinically approved quinazoline-based inhibitors (gefitinib, erlotinib, and lapatinib) as well as neratinib (HKI-272), one of several EGFR inhibitors in clinical testing that form a covalent adduct with the target protein. The somewhat distinct binding modes of neratinib and lapatinib will lead us to revisit the conformational differences between active and inactive kinases, and we discuss the structures of two clinically relevant inhibitors (imatinib and sorafenib) that bind to the inactive form of their respective cognate targets. We also discuss a unique mechanism of noncompetitive binding to MEK1 kinase, which has resulted in the advancement of several potent and specific MEK inhibitors into clinical trials. Finally, we discuss the relative merits of different strategies for inhibitor design and conclude with a review of the factors affecting selectivity for a given kinase, or subset of kinases. Additional details can be found in the primary references cited herein and in several comprehensive reviews that provide a structural and chemical perspective on kinase inhibitor design (2–6).

7.1 STRATEGIES FOR INHIBITOR DESIGN

The relative merits of antibodies, small molecule inhibitors, and other therapeutic modalities have been addressed in Chapter 1: here we discuss in more detail some of the issues specific to small molecules that target the kinase domain. There are several broad and somewhat overlapping issues to consider: whether the molecule targets the active or inactive form of the kinase, whether the molecule is ATP competitive, and whether the aim is to target one specific kinase or many. In practical terms, this may not be a completely free choice, since the chemical scaffolds selected for optimization (and their associated binding modes and promiscuities) may be dictated by the results of high-throughput screening or other lead discovery strategies. However, an appreciation of the relative merits of the above properties is of paramount importance.

7.1.1 Targeting the Active Versus Inactive Form

Kinases are typically tightly regulated and undergo an activation process in which the inactive state is converted to an active state (Chapter 2). Since these often represent structurally distinct conformations, it should often be possible to selectively target one form over another. Broadly speaking, active kinases have high structural homology whereas the inactive forms have much more structural diversity: hence if specific inhibitors are sought, it may seem preferable to seek inhibitors of the inactive form. The EGFR/ERBB2 inhibitor lapatinib (discussed in more detail later) is an example of a compound that targets an inactive-like conformation of EGFR and ERBB2 with very high specificity (7, 8). The structure of lapatinib in complex with EGFR also highlights the fact that ATP competition and inhibition of the inactive form are not necessarily mutually exclusive: lapatinib binds to an inactive-like conformation of the kinase but still occupies the ATP binding site (7). Nevertheless, high specificity is not the exclusive domain of inhibitors of the inactive conformation. Some inhibitors of the active kinase form (e.g., the EGFR inhibitors erlotinib and gefitinib) show quite high specificity for their cognate targets and, conversely, some inhibitors targeting the inactive conformation (e.g., the ABL inhibitor imatinib) show significant crossreactivity with other kinases. Compounds that specifically target the inactive form of the enzyme may also have different liabilities compared to active form inhibitors with respect to development of drug resistant mutations. Both classes of compound may be ineffective against kinase variants harboring mutations that sterically affect drug binding. However, compounds that target the inactive form may additionally be susceptible to mutations that do not directly impact protein:drug binding but instead destabilize the inactive form and promote kinase activation. Several such mutants in BCR-ABL have been shown to confer resistance to imatinib (see Chapter 11) and may be particularly problematic because they both abrogate inhibitor activity and increase the basal activity of the oncogenic kinase.

7.1.2 ATP-Competitive Versus Noncompetitive Inhibitors

Most of the kinase inhibitors discovered to date are ATP competitive although there are some intriguing exceptions, notably the noncompetitive MEK inhibitors discussed in Section 7.8. Competition with ATP was initially regarded as a liability for development of selective inhibitors, due to the high conservation of ATP binding features in the active sites of kinases and, potentially, of other ATP binding proteins. In addition, the high (millimolar) concentration of ATP in the intracellular milieu presents a challenge for ATP-competitive small molecules, in that potencies and/or intracellular concentrations of such molecules must be high in order to compete effectively with ATP for binding to the target (9). In contrast, the affinities of noncompetitive inhibitors are largely independent of ATP concentration and inhibitors that are uncompetitive with respect to ATP may benefit from having active intracellular kinases that are highly ATP-bound, since by definition they bind to the kinase:ATP complex. However, experience with development of kinase inhibitors has shown that, although the challenge of ATP competition is real, it is not insurmountable. Many ATP-competitive inhibitors have highly potent cellular activity: nevertheless, it may still be wise to find alternative strategies for inhibiting kinase targets for which the K_M for ATP is very low, since these will be intrinsically difficult to inhibit in cells (discussed in Chapter 1 and reference (9)).

ATP-competitive molecules may have varying susceptibility to mutations that enhance the binding affinity of ATP. For example, both the L858R and T790M mutants of EGFR are known to promote catalytic activity, but their impact on the efficacy of the EGFR inhibitors erlotinib and gefitinib is strikingly different: L858R confers enhanced sensitivity to erlotinib and gefitinib whereas T790M is associated with resistance (discussed later and in Chapter 8). Such mutants may be particularly prevalent in tumors since they enhance the catalytic activity of the oncogenic receptor. Nevertheless, for any given kinase the number of such mutants conferring resistance to ATP-competitive inhibitors may be quite restricted since it is necessary to preserve the residues within the ATP binding site that contribute to normal ATP binding and catalytic function—many of which are also employed in binding to ATP-competitive inhibitors. Molecules that bind at an allosteric site distal to the ATP binding site are not subject to such requirements, so it is theoretically possible for their binding to be disrupted by mutations that have little or no effect on catalytic activity. To date, there is insufficient clinical experience with such inhibitors to know if such resistance mutants represent a real problem.

7.1.3   Specific Versus Multitargeted Inhibitors

The issue of whether to target one or many kinases has received much attention since the advent of the first small molecule kinase inhibitors. From a purely academic point of view, highly specific inhibitors are of greater utility than nonspecific compounds, since they allow precise manipulation of intracellular signaling pathways and can be used to provide insight into the importance of specific targets and combinations of targets. A series of recent studies by Cohen and colleagues provide a broad survey of the specificities of many commonly used kinase inhibitors, with associated recommendations for or against their use in probing specific intracellular targets and pathways (10–12). Such molecules also have value in revealing any target-based toxicological liabilities, although even if a given inhibitor is highly specific for a single target kinase compared to a broad panel of other kinases, it should be noted that most if not all small molecule drugs can have activity against other pharmacologically relevant targets such as ion channels and G-protein coupled receptors. From a drug development point of view, a highly specific inhibitor affords more control over specific target/pathway modulation, which may be important for maximizing therapeutic index in cases where a specific target is known to be the primary driver of disease (e.g., BCR-ABL in CML). However, most cancers have many underlying aberrations in kinase signaling pathways and may require inhibition of multiple critical signaling nodes in order to achieve therapeutic benefit. In this regard, highly specific inhibitors may be more flexible than multitargeted inhibitors for use in combination therapies, where the relative timing and intensity of inhibiting one target/pathway relative to another may be important. One potential drawback, however, is that such multiple drug dosing schedules may be more challenging to administer from the point of view of drug:drug interactions and patient compliance.

Multitargeted inhibitors have the intrinsic benefit of acting on multiple signaling pathways so that many of the coexisting aberrations in tumors—for example, angiogenesis, cell cycle dysregulation, growth factor receptors, and downstream pathways—may be targeted simultaneously. Moreover, several studies have shown that resistance to kinase-targeted therapies can emerge by activation of alternative and/or downstream kinases (discussed in detail in Chapter 11), so multitargeted inhibitors may be able to reduce this liability—with the important assumption that they inhibit the appropriate subset of targets. There may also be unintentional but clinically useful off-target activity for multitargeted kinase inhibitors, perhaps the most commonly cited example being the inhibition of KIT by imatinib. Imatinib emerged from a high-throughput screening campaign against PDGF receptor, and although its initial utility was as an inhibitor of ABL kinase (in the treatment of chronic myelogenous leukemia), its crossreactivity with KIT has led to approval for use in treatment of gastrointestinal stromal tumors, which are frequently driven by KIT mutational activation. Also, as noted earlier, incorporating multiple functions into a single molecule avoids some complications due to drug:drug interactions and patient compliance. On the other hand, multitargeted inhibitors also have certain disadvantages. In general terms, inhibiting multiple kinases may be expected to produce more side effects than specific inhibition, so it may be more difficult to achieve maximum inhibition of a given kinase due to dose-limiting toxicities.

Multitargeted agents also offer less control over pharmacodynamics with respect to individual kinases. For example, both VEGF receptor and EGF receptor inhibition have been validated clinically as having therapeutic utility in various cancers and there is also evidence for interaction between the VEGFR and EGFR signaling pathways (13), so an agent combining inhibition of both of these targets may be attractive. In fact, several such agents are undergoing clinical testing, including vandetanib (ZD6474), and BMS-690514 (Chapter 8). However, potently inhibiting these targets with a single molecule results in less flexibility (compared to using two separate inhibitors) in optimizing the relative inhibition of EGF receptors with respect to VEGF receptors. Although one defensible strategy is to seek maximal continuous inhibition of both targets, there is at least some theoretical rationale for examining different dosing regimens that will result in differential inhibition profiles for different targets. Several studies have shown that inhibition of VEGF receptors produces upregulation of VEGF and downregulation of soluble VEGFR2 in plasma (14, 15), which may lead to a "rebound" in VEGF signaling if treatment is only administered intermittently—so durable inhibition may be important. In contrast, the "oncogenic shock" hypothesis suggests that pulsatile inhibition of receptor tyrosine kinases (including EGF receptors) may be a useful strategy. This stems from the observation that both prosurvival and proapoptotic pathways may be triggered by an oncogenic kinase, and kinase inhibition leads to downregulation of these pathways with different kinetics (16). In this case, intermittent inhibition may be required to take advantage of a "window of opportunity" during which prosurvival pathways are inhibited but proapoptotic pathways remain active.

7.2 ARCHITECTURE OF THE ATP BINDING SITE: DFG-in

The structural features of the protein kinase ATP binding site were discussed in Chapter 2: in this section we review specific features that are particularly important for the binding of ATP-competitive inhibitors. The ATP and substrate binding site of active kinases has historically been divided into several distinct regions (2, 3), although these all form one contiguous space that is accessible for inhibitor binding (Figure 7.1). The nomenclature for these regions is not consistent in the literature, although some common themes emerge in all descriptions of ATP-competitive kinase pharmacophores. Our description is focused on inhibitors of the "DFG-in," or active conformation of protein kinases (see Chapter 2), and largely follows an early analysis by Traxler and Furet (3) but with reference to the structure of CHK1 kinase in complex with ATP (Figure 7.2). Amino acid numbering refers to the CHK1 kinase sequence; corresponding residues in the other kinases discussed in this chapter are listed in Table 7.1. We use a consistent orientation of the kinase domain throughout this chapter: references to the front, back, top, and bottom of the kinase domain are consistent with the orientation depicted in Figure 7.2A.

Adenine Binding Site/Linker Region   The adenine moiety of ATP makes important contacts with the linker region—the short strand connecting the N- and C-terminal lobes of the kinase. In most (but not all) ATP-competitive inhibitors

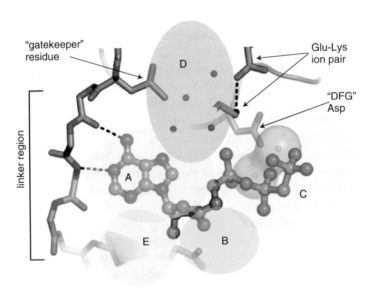

Figure 7.1   Overview of the kinase ATP binding site (active/"DFG-in" conformation), highlighting regions that are relevant for small molecule inhibitor binding: A, adenine binding site/linker region; B, ribose binding pocket; C, phosphate binding/catalytic aspartate/salt bridge region; D, back hydrophobic pocket; E, front specificity pocket. The kinase shown is CHK1; see text for further details.

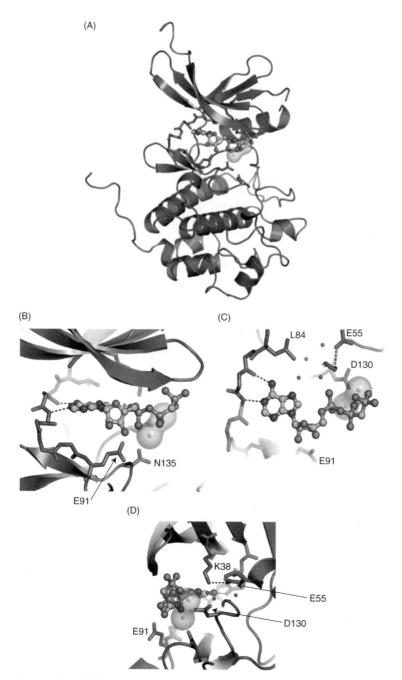

Figure 7.2   Different views of CHK1 ATP binding site. (A) Overview of the CHK1 kinase domain with non hydrolyzable ATP analog bound (green "ball and stick"). (B) Close view of the ATP binding pocket (same orientation as panel A), showing hydrogen bonds with the linker region and interactions of the ATP phosphate groups with magnesium ions (green). (C) Rotation of 90° around a horizontal axis compared to (B) (D) Rotation of 90° around a vertical axis compared to (B).

TABLE 7.1   Comparison of key active site residues in selected protein kinases

Description	CHK1	CDK2	SRC	ABL	EGFR	RAF	MEK
Ribose/hydrophobic pocket	L15	I10	L273	L248	L718	I463	L74
	G16	G11	G274	G249	G719	G464	G75
"Roof" of adenine pocket	V23	V18	V281	V256	V726	V471	V82
Glu-Lys ion pair	K38	K33	K295	K271	K745	K483	K97
	E55	E51	E310	E286	E762	E501	E114
Gatekeeper residue	L84	F80	T338	T315	T790	T529	M143
Linker region	E85	E81	E339	E316	Q791	Q530	E144
	Y86	F82	Y340	F317	L792	W531	H145
	C87	L83	M341	M318	M793	C532	M146
Front specificity pocket	G90	Q85	G344	G321	G796	S535	G149
Ribose pocket	E91	D86	S345	N322	C797	S536	S150
Catalytic aspartate	D130	D127	D386	D363	D837	D576	D190
Phosphate binding region	N135	N132	N391	N368	N842	N581	N195
"Floor" of adenine pocket	L137	L134	L393	L370	L844	F583	L197
Phosphate binding region (DFG)	D148	D145	D404	D381	D855	D594	D208
	F149	F146	F405	F382	F856	F595	F209
	G150	G147	G406	G383	G857	G596	G210

discovered to date, hydrogen bond interactions with the backbone amides (NH and C=O groups) of the linker region are an important component of the overall interaction. Apart from the polar linker interactions, the "floor" and "top" (as defined by the orientation in Figure 7.2A) of the cavity surrounding the adenosine moiety itself are somewhat hydrophobic in nature. These amino acid residues are derived from the glycine-rich loop (also referred to as the phosphate binding or P-loop) of the N-terminal domain (V23) and regions of the C-terminal domain including L137.

Ribose Binding Pocket   Since the ribose moiety is directly attached to the adenine of ATP, the ribose binding site overlaps with the adenine binding site described previously and is bounded by V23 and L137. In the glycine-rich loop, L15 and G16 also contribute, and E91 (just C-terminal to the linker region) makes important contacts with the ribose hydroxyl groups.

Phosphate Binding/Catalytic Aspartate/Salt Bridge Region   The phosphate binding site comprises the catalytic D130 and several other residues that are important for positioning the catalytic machinery and ATP phosphates, including D148, N135, and the conserved E55-K38 ion pair. The glycine-rich loop is a common motif in many ATP and GTP binding proteins and is an important determinant of the phosphate binding environment. This is another somewhat polar region of the active site that can accommodate various polar and charged moieties on inhibitors.

Back Hydrophobic Pocket   When ATP is bound to the active site, most kinases have a buried hydrophobic pocket that is blocked off by the ATP molecule, which we refer to here as the "back hydrophobic pocket." In many crystal structures, this pocket is occupied by several water molecules. The entry to and size of this pocket are largely defined by the side chain of the "gatekeeper" residue (L84 in CHK1), which resides on the N-terminal side of the linker region. In all kinases, the gatekeeper residue is a somewhat bulky amino acid, and in many cases the side chain of this residue is an important factor in determining the kinase specificity of a given inhibitor, as well as conferring resistance to inhibition. The lack of endogenous kinases with alanine or glycine at the gatekeeper position has been exploited to develop powerful and elegant tools for studying the function of individual kinases (17–21). In these studies, kinases were engineered to have A/G at the gatekeeper position and analogs of both ATP and kinase inhibitors were designed that impinged on the gatekeeper side chain position, with the result that only the engineered kinase could utilize the ATP analog or be inhibited by the designed inhibitor. These engineered kinases have proved to be useful tools for dissecting kinase activity in the context of the intracellular milieu.

Front Specificity Pocket   A relatively small hydrophobic region (featuring L15 from the glycine-rich loop and G90 from the C-terminal domain) serves as a transition zone between the ATP binding site and a hydrophilic, solvent-exposed region of the protein. This hydrophilic region is somewhat variable in sequence and structure between different kinases and may be a useful area to probe for gaining specificity, as well as for introducing "solubilizing" moieties that may help to confer favorable physicochemical properties to small molecule inhibitors. In PKA (and other kinases of the AGC family, including PKB/AKT), the C-terminal region of the kinase loops around this region and is anchored in the N-terminal domain, contributing another hydrophobic face to the pocket (F327 in PKA, F439 in AKT2; Figure 2.9C).

7.3   CASE STUDY: INHIBITORS OF CHK1

As an example of the structural features of kinase inhibitors and their interactions with the ATP binding site, we consider some of the diverse molecules whose three-dimensional X-ray crystal structures have been determined in complex with the cell cycle checkpoint kinase CHK1. The rationale for cell cycle checkpoint inhibition is reviewed in Chapter 6, and several CHK1 inhibitors are currently being evaluated in clinical studies (22). The molecules discussed next include natural products, initial leads, and optimized molecules (Figures 7.3–7.6). They span a broad range of potencies, with IC_{50} values ranging from subnanomolar to greater than 10 μM. Although our discussion is not exhaustive (and does not address the structures of the CHK1 inhibitors that have advanced into clinical development), it begins to illustrate the broad diversity of structures and binding interactions that can be employed by ATP-competitive kinase inhibitors.

The apo-CHK1 kinase domain structure was determined at high resolution (23) and displays the canonical two-lobe structure described in Chapter 2. Some disorder is present in the N-terminal lobe: however, the activation loop is stable, well-ordered, and in an active-like conformation, even in the absence of phosphorylation (Figure 7.2A). The characteristic kinase catalytic and structural elements described in Chapter 2 can be identified in this structure, including the catalytic aspartate D130; D148 and N135 (which chelate a Mg^{2+} ion), the E55-K38 ion pair, and the "gatekeeper" L84. Crystallographic analysis also reveals a rich solvent structure associated with the enzyme, which has been corroborated in subsequent studies. Of particular interest in the development of ATP-competitive inhibitors are the conserved water molecules located in the ATP binding site, particularly those in the "back hydrophobic pocket," which extends past the gatekeeper L84 side chain and is occupied by a channel of water molecules that lead out to the active site cleft (Figure 7.2C).

We consider first the structure of CHK1 in complex with staurosporine (CHK1 $K_I = 7.8$ nM; PDB accession code 1NVR (24)). Structures of two related analogs (UCN-01 and SB-218078) have also been solved in complex with CHK1 and display broadly similar interactions to those of staurosporine (24). Staurosporine is a highly promiscuous kinase inhibitor, displaying potent activity against a wide range of tyrosine and serine/threonine kinases. Compared to the complex with a nonhydrolyzable ATP analog (23), the staurosporine-bound kinase domain displays a slightly more open nucleotide binding cleft between the N- and C-terminal lobes. Overall, staurosporine makes extensive hydrophobic and electrostatic contacts with the extended ATP binding site (Figure 7.3B). The 6-amino group of the lactam ring makes a hydrogen bond with the main chain carbonyl of E85, and the 5-keto group accepts a hydrogen bond from the main chain —NH of Cys87. These donor–acceptor bonds with the kinase domain linker region are reminiscent of the interactions made by the ATP adenine moiety and represent some of the most prevalent binding interactions of ATP-competitive kinase inhibitors. Staurosporine also interacts with the ribose binding pocket via its tetrahydropyran moiety, which adopts an angular, "boat" conformation relative to the indolocarbazole plane. The 4′-N-methyl group of the tetrahydropyran makes hydrogen bond interactions with the E91 side chain and the E134 main chain carbonyl. Additional interactions are derived from the hydrophobic indolocarbazole core, which is in contact with both the N- and C-terminal lobes. Despite these extensive contacts, several important areas of the ATP binding site are not substantially occupied by staurosporine. These include the phosphate binding region, the Glu-Lys salt bridge, and the back hydrophobic pocket. In the staurosporine complex structure, the back hydrophobic pocket is occupied by three water molecules, which are also present in the apo and ATP-bound structures. The staurosporine analog UCN-01 has an additional —OH group at the 7-position of the lactam ring. In the CHK1:UCN-01 structure (PDB accession code 1NVQ), this —OH group interacts with one of the hydrophobic pocket water molecules and with the side chain of S147, contributing to its somewhat greater selectivity compared to staurosporine. These structural data provide some insight into why staurosporine is such a potent and nonselective kinase inhibitor. Its hydrogen bond interactions between the lactam moiety and the linker region mimic those of ATP and are highly conserved across all kinases; furthermore, there are extensive and relatively nonspecific hydrophobic interactions

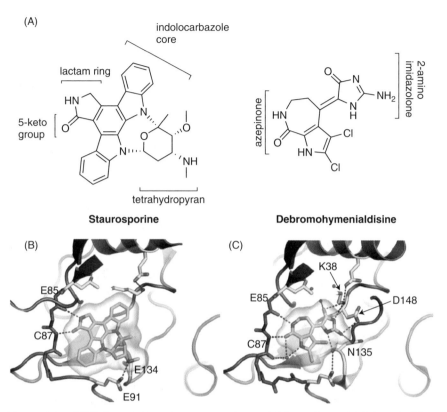

Figure 7.3 CHK1 in complex with staurosporine and debromohymenialdisine. (A) Line bond structures of staurosporine and debromohymenialdisine (DBH), showing structural elements involved in kinase interactions. Interactions of (B) staurosporine and (C) DBH with CHK1. Key amino acid residues are colored yellow and labeled; red spheres indicate conserved water molecules. See text for further details.

between the staurosporine core and the hydrophobic active site cavity of the kinase. Also, the other hydrogen bonds made by staurosporine are with conserved residues in the active site, and the molecule does not extend outside the highly conserved ATP binding pocket.

Debromohymenialdisine (DBH) is a natural marine product that inhibits CHK1 (CHK1 $K_I = 660$ nM (25); PDB accession codes 1ZLT, 2C3J). Despite the relatively weak binding affinity compared to staurosporine, DBH forms a rich hydrogen bonding network with various regions of the CHK1 active site, illustrating that the number of hydrogen bonds alone does not necessarily correlate with potency of inhibition (Figure 7.3C). First, the azepinone moiety interacts with the linker region via hydrogen bonds to the E85 main chain carbonyl and C87 —NH, in a similar manner to the lactam moiety of staurosporine. In addition, a third linker region hydrogen bond is made via a bridging water molecule, between the pyrrole nitrogen and the C87 main chain carbonyl. At the other end of the molecule in the ATP phosphate binding region, the 2-amino imidazolone exocyclic amine interacts with the side chains of D148 and N135, as well as with a water molecule. A nitrogen from the imidazolone is located near to K38 (which forms half of the conserved Glu-Lys ion pair), although the geometry and distance may not favor hydrogen bond formation. Due to the small size and polar nature of the molecule, hydrophobic interactions are relatively limited and the back hydrophobic pocket of CHK1 remains occupied by three water molecules, one of which interacts with the imidazolone carbonyl group. The imidazolone interaction is also reminiscent of a series of thiazolidinones that have been shown to inhibit CDK2 (Section 7.4). The thiazolidinone moieties of these inhibitors makes similar contacts with the analogous residues in CDK2, although there is no hydrogen bond with the linker region at the other side of the molecule (26).

We next consider several molecules that harbor some common chemical motifs but that occupy distinct regions of the catalytic site (Figure 7.4). In contrast to staurosporine and DBH, the first of these (an indazolo-benzimidazole inhibitor) makes extensive interactions with the back hydrophobic pocket (Figure 7.5A). This molecule is a potent CHK1 inhibitor (Compound 1 in (25), CHK1 $K_I = 26$ nM; PDB accession code 2C3K). Again, hydrogen bonds to the E85 and C87 main chains in the linker region help to anchor and orient the inhibitor, via the indazole nitrogens. An additional direct linker hydrogen bond is formed between the benzimidazole and the C87 carbonyl. The hydrophobic pocket is tightly occupied by the methoxyphenyl group, which extends past the L84 gatekeeper residue and displaces the water molecules observed in the above structures. The front specificity pocket is occupied by the phenyl ring of the benzimidazole. The benzimidazole-linker motif of Compound 1 is also present in a series of 3-benzimidazole quinolinones (ABIQ 11, CHK1 $IC_{50} = 0.32$ nM; PDB accession code 2GDO, reference (27)). Additional linker hydrogen bonds are provided by the carbonyl and amine from the quinolinone (Figure 7.5B). An (S)-3-aminoquinuclidine moiety at the benzimidazole 4-position was found to dramatically enhance potency, interacting with the side chain of E91 and the E134 main chain. A third acidic residue in the glycine-rich loop (E17) is also oriented toward this region, in contrast to its conformation in other structures. An independent quinolinone series, with an indolyl group in place of the benzimizadole, has also yielded compounds with subnanomolar potency (Compound 22, CHK1 $IC_{50} = 0.65$ nM; PDB accession code 2HY0). The linker region interactions for compounds in this series are broadly similar to those of the 3-benzimidazole quinolinones but displaced by approximately 1.5 Å (Figure 7.5C). These analogs lack the 4-position substitution of ABIQ 11 but gain binding affinity through a 6-position substitution (pyrazole in the case of Compound 22). The pyrazole group forms an extended hydrogen bond network with the three water molecules in the back hydrophobic pocket, as well as the neighboring D148 and E55 side chains.

Another variant on the quinolinone theme is demonstrated in a series of benzoisoquinolinones (28). Compound 54 in this series (CHK1 $IC_{50} = 1$ nM; PDB accession code 2R0U) shows similar core scaffold interactions with the linker region backbone compared to the molecules described previously, but due to the different positional isomerization (quinolinone versus isoquinolinone) the resulting orientation in the active site is quite different (Figure 7.5D). This molecule also

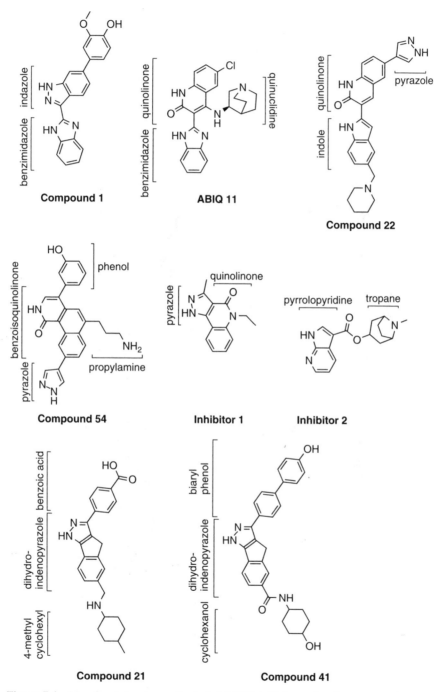

Figure 7.4 Line bond structures of selected CHK1 inhibitors, showing structural elements involved in kinase interactions. The orientations have been chosen to approximate those depicted in the crystal structure figures.

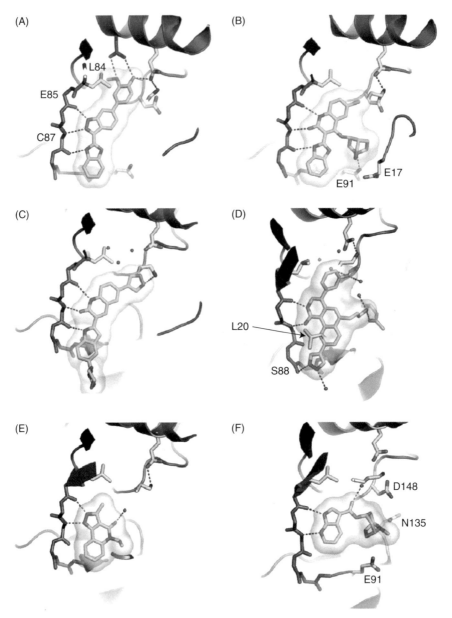

Figure 7.5 Crystal structures of small molecule CHK1 inhibitors I: (A) Compound 1, (B) ABIQ, (C) Compound 22, (D) Compound 54, (E) Inhibitor 1, and (F) Inhibitor 2. See text for further details.

incorporates a pyrazole group, but in contrast to the other pyrazoles discussed (Compound 22, above and Inhibitor 1, below) it binds in the front specificity pocket, making both electrostatic (S88) and hydrophobic (L20) interactions. The propylamine group in Compound 54 descends into the ribose pocket and also forms a coordinated hydrogen bond network with water molecules and the adjacent phenol group of the inhibitor.

The structure of a distinct quinolinone-based scaffold has recently been described. Inhibitor 1 (29) is a pyrazoloquinolinone (CHK1 IC_{50} 980 nM; PDB accession code 2QHN) and, in contrast to the quinolinones above it is the pyrazole moiety that forms the canonical linker hydrogen bonds (Figure 7.5E). Inhibitor 2 (CHK1 IC_{50} 660 nM; PDB accession code 2QHM) is a second lead compound based on a pyrrolopyridine core, with a tropane moiety that extends into the ribose binding pocket in the region of E91, N135, and D148 (although the tropane amine is rather too far from these polar side chains to form bona fide hydrogen bonds; Figure 7.5F). A propylamine group was incorporated at the quinolinone nitrogen of Inhibitor 1 in order to reach into the polar E91/N135/D148 binding pocket and, together with a cyclohexyl fusion to the pyrazoloquinolinone core, resulted in an inhibitor with 3-nM IC_{50} for CHK1, potent cellular activity, and good solubility (29).

The pyrazole-linker interaction is also employed by a series of dihydroindenopyrazoles, which adopt an elongated conformation extending from the E55-K38 salt bridge, through the front specificity pocket and into the solvent (30). Like Inhibitor 1 above, Compound 21 (CHK1 IC_{50} = 20 nM; PDB accession code 2E9O) is seen to donate an H-bond to E85 and accept an H-bond from C87 in the linker (Figure 7.6A). An additional hydrogen bond is formed between the carboxylic acid at one end of the molecule and the K38 amine; E55 and N59 also participate in this interaction via an intermediary water molecule. At the other end of the inhibitor, the terminal 4-methyl cyclohexyl moiety appears to wrap around the G-rich loop, perhaps minimizing solvent contact with this hydrophobic region of the molecule. A more potent analog in this series, Compound 41, has a biaryl phenol in place of the benzoic acid of Compound 21 (CHK1 IC_{50} 6.2 nM, PDB accession code 2E9N). The structure of this molecule in complex with CHK1 shows that the phenol group makes direct interactions with E55 and N59 (Figure 7.6B). In order to accommodate this extended biaryl phenol, the inhibitor is displaced by approximately 1 Å parallel to the linker region main chain, resulting in somewhat longer H-bonds between the pyrazole and the linker compared to Compound 21. The other end of the molecule extends through the front specificity pocket, making a polar contact with D94 and directing the cyclohexanol group out to solvent.

We conclude this survey of CHK1 inhibitors by briefly reviewing some much weaker-binding molecules. In contrast to the nanomolar binding affinities of the molecules described previously, the compounds shown in Figure 7.6 C–F are some of the initial hits from a virtual screening experiment and have CHK1 IC_{50} values between 10 and 20 μM (31). Despite these weak interactions, such molecules may serve as both starting points for optimization, as well as potentially providing insight into interactions that may be recruited using other scaffolds. These data also illustrate the point that, in at least some cases, well-ordered structures can be determined for relatively weak inhibitors. During the course of a drug lead

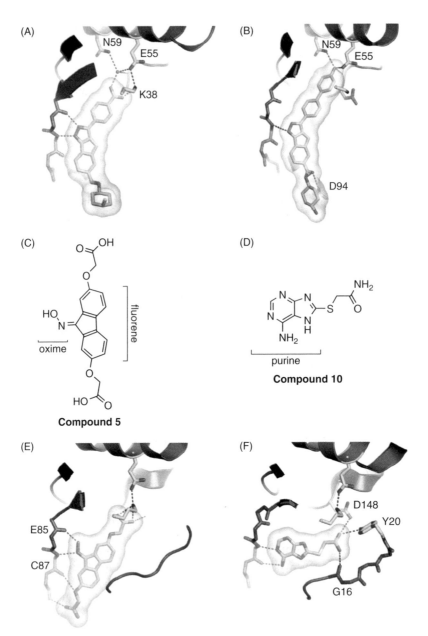

Figure 7.6 Crystal structures of small molecule CHK1 inhibitors II: (A) Compound 21, (B) Compound 41, (C, D) line bond structures of two weak inhibitors, (E) Compound 5, and (F) Compound 10. See text for further details.

optimization project, the data from such structures can be particularly helpful in that it may be equally useful to determine why a given molecule is a poor inhibitor and why another molecule is a potent inhibitor. Compound 5 (CHK1 IC_{50} = 13.4 μM; PDB accession code 2CGU) is a symmetrical fluorene derivative, containing an oxime moiety that interacts with E85 carbonyl and C87 main chain nitrogen of the linker region. Compound 10 (CHK1 IC_{50} = 15.6 μM; PDB accession code 2CGX) is a purine-based inhibitor that exhibits altered linker region interactions compared with the adenosine of ATP. In the ATP structure, the adenine ring is hydrogen bonded to the main chain nitrogen of C87 and the exocyclic amine is hydrogen bonded to the carbonyl oxygen of E85. The first of these interactions is conserved in Compound 10, but the purine ring is flipped 180° relative to the ATP adenine so that the exocyclic amine interacts with the carbonyl oxygen of C87. Of particular note in this structure is an interaction of the terminal amide of the compound with D148, and with G16 and Y20 in the glycine-rich loop.

7.4   CASE STUDY: INHIBITORS OF CDK2

Collectively, cell cycle regulatory kinases have attracted significant attention as cancer targets (Figure 7.7; Chapters 6 and 9). Several small molecule cell cycle inhibitors with varying specificities have entered clinical trials, and understanding the mode of binding and specificity with respect to the various cyclin-dependent kinases (and kinases in general) has been a key factor in the development of several of these drugs. The structure of CDK2 was reviewed in Chapter 2 and structural analysis of inhibitor binding to CDK2 presents an added layer of complexity compared to CHK1. The CHK1 crystal structures discussed earlier show the kinase to be in an active-like conformation, even in the absence of activation loop phosphorylation. However, CDK2 has been solved in two distinct activation states: an inactive monomeric form and an active complex with cyclin A (32, 33). Although some features of the ATP binding site are conserved between these two forms, there are differences that have significant implications for structure-based design of inhibitors. Most of the CDK2:inhibitor structures solved to date have been in complex with the inactive, monomeric form. This conformation is still competent to bind ATP, as indicated by the crystal structure in complex with Mg-ATP (PDB accession code 1HCK; Figure 7.8). Substituted purine analogs were among the earliest CDK2 inhibitors to be identified and structurally characterized, and one of these compounds (R-roscovitine; CYC202, or seliciclib) has been evaluated clinically. Notably, the purine ring of R-roscovitine adopts a distinct conformation compared to the adenine of ATP (PDB accession code 2A4L; Figure 7.8). The binding mode of selected purine analogs is discussed further in the next section, in the context of SRC family kinases.

There are several instructive examples where inhibitor structures have been determined with both monomeric CDK2 and the heterodimeric CDK2:cyclin A. Cyclin A binding promotes rotation of the C helix and formation of the E51-K33 ion pair interaction. The activation segment undergoes a substantial displacement, and the active site cleft becomes slightly wider and deeper in the active (cyclin-bound)

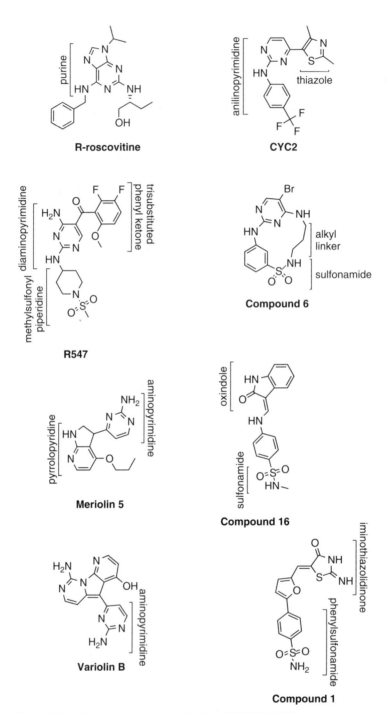

Figure 7.7 Line bond structures of selected CDK2 inhibitors, showing structural elements involved in kinase interactions. The orientations have been chosen to approximate those depicted in the crystal structure figures.

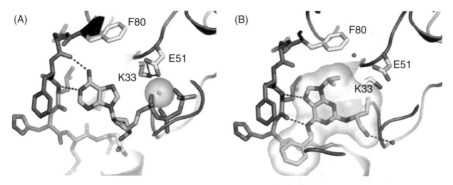

Figure 7.8   CDK2 in complex with (A) ATP and (B) R-roscovitine. The "gatekeeper" residue F80 and salt bridge residues E51/K33 are shown in yellow.

form (34). Although complexes with the inactive CDK2 may still be instructive, these differences indicate that caution is warranted when interpreting these structures in light of activity data generated with the active (cyclin-bound) kinase. Indeed, a comparison of calculated interaction energies for a series of pyrimidine-based inhibitors bound to both the active and inactive structures further supports this conclusion. Inhibitor IC_{50} values showed an excellent correlation with interaction energies calculated using the active CDK2:cyclin A structures, in contrast to a lack of correlation for the monomeric CDK2 interaction energies (35). The structures for one of these inhibitors in complex with active and inactive CDK2 (Compound 2 in (35), referred to as CYC2 in (36); $IC_{50} = 290$ nM, PDB accession codes 1PXL and 2C5V) are shown in Figure 7.9. The interactions between the anilinopyrimidine and the linker region are broadly conserved, although there is a ~1.6 Å displacement of the pyrimidine ring between the two structures that may contribute to the different binding energetics (for this molecule, the interaction with the active form of the enzyme is predicted to be more favorable). The thiazole portion of the ligand also makes favorable interactions with K33 and D145 in the CDK2:cyclin A structure; in contrast, an unfavorable interaction with D145 is found in the monomeric structure, which also has K33 displaced away from the thiazole.

R547 is a 2,4-diaminopyrimidine derivative with potent inhibitory activity against CDK1, CDK2, and CDK4 (IC_{50} values 2 nM, 3 nM, and 1 nM, respectively (37)). The structure (Figure 7.10A; PDB accession code 2FVD) was solved in complex with monomeric, unactivated CDK2 and shows that the two exocyclic amines of the diaminopyrimidine core donate hydrogen bonds to the main chain carbonyl groups of E81 and L83 in the linker region. The high resolution of this structure (1.85 Å) illustrates the rich water structure present in the active site, which often mediates interactions with small molecule ligands. In this structure, a pyrimidine nitrogen interacts with the water hydrogen bond network, indirectly coupling the compound binding to D86 and Q131. A methylsulfonyl piperidine group extends into the front specificity pocket, making both hydrophobic contacts via the piperidine and hydrogen bond interactions via the sulfonamide. A trisubstituted

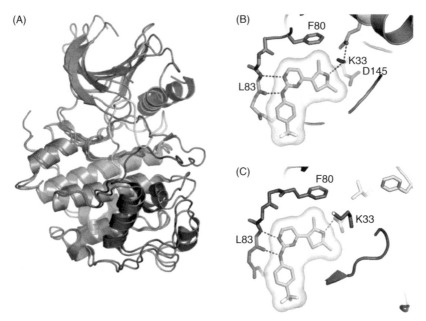

Figure 7.9 Structures of active and inactive CDK2 in complex with the inhibitor CYC2. (A) Comparison of active (brown; red activation loop) and inactive (teal; yellow activation loop) CDK2 structures. Although cyclin A is present in the active crystal structure, it has been removed from the figure for clarity. (B) CYC2 bound to active CDK2. (C) CYC2 bound to inactive CDK2. Interactions with K33 and D145 are shown.

phenyl ketone packs closely against the gatekeeper F80 side chain. A variation on the aminopyrimidine-sulfonamide theme has been further developed in a series of macrocyclic compounds that incorporate both binding motifs (Figure 7.10B; Compound 6 in (38), PDB accession code 2J9M). The sulfonamide occupies a somewhat distinct binding site relative to the sulfonamide of R547, forming hydrogen bonds with both the main chain and backbone of D86, and I10 from the glycine-rich loop. An alkyl linker is used to cyclize the molecule, and further elaboration of this series yielded molecules with potent activity against VEGFR2 as well as CDK2 (38).

A recently disclosed series of CDK inhibitors (3-(pyrimidin-4-yl)-7-azaindoles, termed "meriolins") is a hybrid between two series of marine natural products (meridianins and variolins) (39, 40). However, the structures of representative variolin and meriolin compounds in complex with CDK2:cyclin A indicate that they employ very different binding modes, underscoring the value of empirical structural analysis in kinase inhibitor optimization. Meriolin 5 (CDK2 $IC_{50} = 3$ nM; PDB accession code 3BHU) interacts with the kinase linker region via the nitrogens of the core pyrrolopyridine (Figure 7.10C). The aminopyrimidine moiety is directed toward the E51-K33 salt bridge; in particular, the exocyclic amino group is within hydrogen bonding distance of the E51 side chain. A second meriolin (meriolin 3; PDB accession code 3BHT) displays a very similar binding mode. By contrast, variolin B (CDK2 $IC_{50} = 80$ nM; PDB

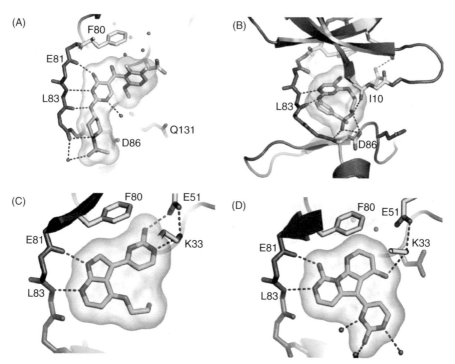

Figure 7.10   Small molecule inhibitors from Figure 7.7 bound to CDK2: (A) R547; (B) macrocyclic aminopyrimidine-based inhibitor; (C) meriolin 5, a pyrrolopyridine-based inhibitor; and (D) variolin B.

accession code 3BHV) has a pyridine-amine fused to the pyrrolopyridine core, and it is this pyridine-amine that interacts with the linker region (Figure 7.10D). Consequently, the molecule is rotated $180°$ with respect to meriolin 5, and the aminopyrimidine of variolin B is directed out toward solvent rather than toward the salt bridge region. (The salt bridge region is close to a hydroxyl group on the variolin B core, which may interact with K33.) There are also some structural differences in the glycine-rich loop, which appears to be stabilized more in the meriolin 5 structure compared to variolin B.

Oxindoles (indole-2-ones) represent another important class of kinase inhibitor: several derivatives of this scaffold have been shown to inhibit CDK2, and the core oxindole moiety forms the central scaffold for the clinically approved "angiokinase" inhibitor sunitinib. Figure 7.11A shows the lead compound for one series of oxindole inhibitors (Compound 16 in (41); $IC_{50} = 60$ nM) in complex with the inactive conformation of CDK2 (PDB accession code 1KE5). The oxindole forms the classic donor:acceptor hydrogen bond pair with E81 and L83 in the linker region: this mode of binding has also been observed for a series of oxindole inhibitors in complex with FGFR1 (42) and is reminiscent of the quinolinone CHK1 inhibitors described previously. This compound also features a sulfonamide group, the sulfonyl portion of which occupies a similar site to that of

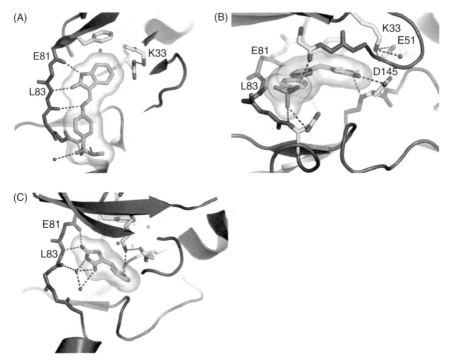

Figure 7.11 (A) Oxindole compound 16. (B, C) Two iminothiazolidinones with distinct binding modes in the CDK2 active site; in each figure the protein structure is rotated relative to (A) in order to show the interactions more clearly. In (B), the thiazolidinone moiety of Compound 1 interacts primarily with the water structure in the vicinity of D145, E51, and K33 (shown in yellow); at the other end of the molecule, a sulfonamide occupies a similar site to that of the aminopyrimidine R457 (Figure 7.10). There are no direct interactions with the linker region to the left of the figure. In (C), a smaller iminothiazolidinone shows interactions with the linker region as well as the neighboring water structure.

the aminopyrimidine compound described earlier (Figure 7.11). Substitution at the oxindole 5-position (Br in Compound 16) can be used to recruit interactions with the K33/D145 region of the protein (41). Several inhibitors with this core scaffold have also been solved in complex with FGFR (42).

All of the kinase inhibitors described previously are anchored by conserved interactions with the linker region: however, a series of iminothiazolidinones (discovered using a computational docking approach) were recently shown to interact primarily in the catalytic Asp/salt bridge region (26). One such molecule (Compound 1 from (26); $IC_{50} = 0.18$ μM, PDB accession code 2UZD) is shown in Figure 7.11B. The iminothiazolidinone binds to a site in the vicinity of D145, E51, and K33, in a manner akin to that of the imidazolone in the DBH:CHK1 structure described earlier. However, direct interactions are likely to be somewhat weak as only D145 is clearly within hydrogen bonding distance. At the other end of the molecule a phenylsulfonamide extends into the front specificity pocket: however, there are no hydrogen bonds to the linker region. Curiously, a smaller iminothiazolidinone fragment (PDB accession code 2V0D) was found to interact in a more canonical binding mode, the imino group acting as both hydrogen bond donor and acceptor with the E81 main chain carbonyl and the L83 main chain nitrogen (Figure 7.11C).

7.5 CASE STUDY: INHIBITORS OF SRC FAMILY KINASES

The SRC family kinases are an important group of nonreceptor tyrosine kinases, and several members of this group (including SRC itself) have attracted attention as targets for anticancer therapy (Chapter 4). Here we briefly review a diverse group of molecules that bind to the active form of SRC and/or ABL kinase, and for which X-ray structures are available (Figure 7.12). SRC kinase is subject to multiple intramolecular regulatory mechanisms (Chapter 2), and its structure has been solved in both active and inactive forms (43). Although several inhibitor structures have been solved in complex with full-length SRC protein, structural analysis of SRC:inhibitor complexes has been significantly aided by the expression of the isolated kinase domain (44), which adopts a more active-like conformation.

Several SRC family kinase domain structures have been determined in complex with small molecule purine and purine-like derivatives. Pyrazolopyrimidines were initially reported in the mid-1990s as specific SRC family kinase inhibitors; in particular, the inhibitors PP1 and PP2 were shown to be potent inhibitors of LCK and FYN (IC_{50} ~5 nM), with weak activity against EGFR and no crossreactivity with JAK2 or ZAP70 (45). Both mutagenesis (46) and structural studies with full-length SRC (PDB accession code 1QCF (47)) subsequently indicated that the selectivity of these inhibitors derived in part from interactions of the exocyclic amine with the hydroxyl group of the gatekeeper residue (T338, c-SRC numbering). The purine core of PP1 broadly mimics the orientation and linker interactions of the ATP adenine moiety. A t-butyl substituent occupies the ribose pocket, and several water molecules serve to bridge the inhibitor to other components of the active site, including the Glu-Lys salt bridge (Figure 7.13A). The pyrrolopyrimidine 4-amine derivative CGP77675 (PDB accession code 1YOL; SRC $IC_{50} = 5$–20 nM) also interacts with the linker region and gatekeeper residue (Figure 7.13B), with a phenyl group occupying the ribose binding pocket. However, not all purine analogs employ this binding mode (44). Purvalanol A (PDB accession code 1YOM; SRC $IC_{50} = 240$ nM) binds in approximately the same plane as the ATP adenine moiety but is rotated in that plane through almost 120°, such that the substitution at the exocyclic 4-position amine can be accommodated. A different adenine-linker hydrogen bond pattern is established, and an aminomethylbutanol group occupies that ribose binding pocket (Figure 7.13C). The trisubstituted purines AP23451 (PDB accession code 2BDF; SRC $IC_{50} = 67$ nM) and AP23464 (PDB accession code 2BDJ; SRC $IC_{50} = 6$ nM) also display variations on this theme. The purine core of AP23464 directs an ethylphenol group toward the back hydrophobic pocket

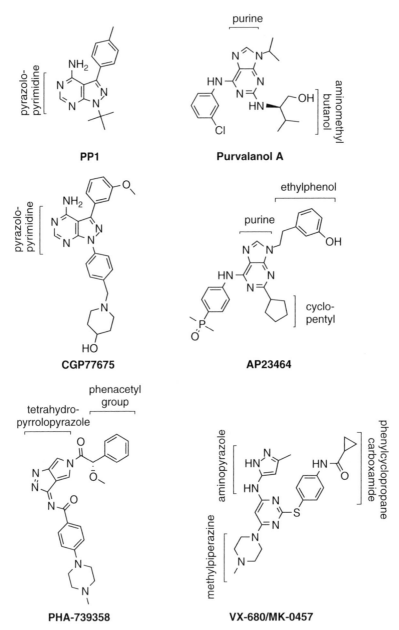

Figure 7.12 Line bond structures of selected SRC/ABL inhibitors, showing structural elements involved in kinase interactions. The orientations have been chosen to approximate those depicted in the crystal structure figures.

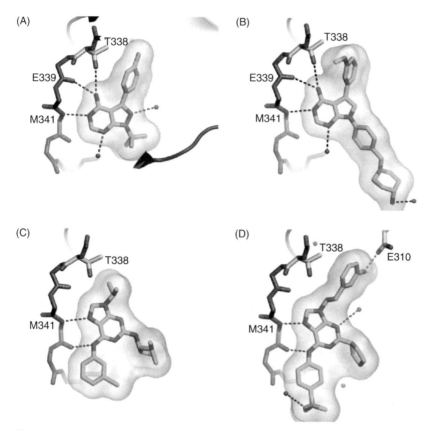

Figure 7.13   Selected purine derivatives in complex with SRC kinase: (A) PP1, (B) CGP77675, (C) purvalanol A, and (D) AP23464.

(with the hydroxyl group near the Glu-Lys salt bridge) and a cyclopentyl group occupying the ribose binding pocket. An additional substitution projects an aniline linker into the front specificity pocket, directing solubilizing phosphate groups to the hydrophilic solvent-exposed region outside of this pocket (48) (Figure 7.13D).

The structure of the clinically approved SRC/ABL inhibitor dasatinib (BMS-354825) has been solved in complex with ABL kinase (PDB accession code 2GQG; ABL $IC_{50} = 0.6$ nM) (49). This inhibitor resulted from optimization of a series of 2-aminothiazoles and is a potent pan-SRC family inhibitor, as well as an inhibitor of several other kinases including KIT and PDGFR (50). Dasatinib adopts an elongated conformation, anchored to the linker region via the central aminothiazole moiety (see Figure 7.18B). On one side of the aminothiazole core, a pyridine-piperazine moiety extends out through the front specificity pocket and into solvent. At the other end of the molecule, a 2-chloro 6-methylphenyl group is tightly packed into the back hydrophobic pocket; the close contact with the T315 gatekeeper residue clearly explains the inability of dasatinib to inhibit the T315I mutant protein with the more bulky isoleucine residue at this position.

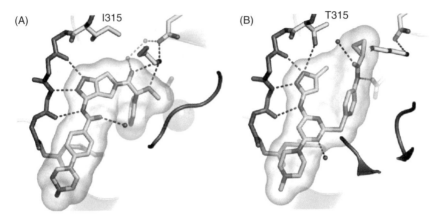

Figure 7.14 Structures of two ABL kinase inhibitors, PHA-739358 and VX-680. (A) PHA-739358 is shown in complex with the T315I mutant form of ABL. The tetrahydropyrrolopyrazole core makes hydrogen bond interactions with the linker region and directs the phenacetyl group toward the Glu-Lys salt bridge and the catalytic aspartate. The Mg^{2+} ion is represented by a solid sphere. (B) VX-680 couples to the linker region primarily via an aminopyrazole group: the cyclopropyl carboxamide extends toward the salt bridge and back hydrophobic pocket.

Several compounds have recently been demonstrated to inhibit the T315I mutant form of ABL. The structure of the tetrahydropyrrolopyrazole Aurora kinase inhibitor PHA-739358 in complex with the T315I mutant of ABL shows how the compound avoids the back hydrophobic pocket and gatekeeper residue entirely (PDB accession code 2V7A; ABL $IC_{50} = 25$ nM (51)). Like dasatinib, this molecule forms anchoring hydrogen bonds with the linker region and extends through the front specificity pocket into solvent, but instead of extending back past the gatekeeper residue, the tetrahydropyrrolopyrazole core directs the phenacetyl group toward the catalytic Asp and an associated Mg^{2+} ion (Figure 7.14A). Another Aurora kinase inhibitor, VX-680 (MK-0457), also inhibits the ABL T315I mutant, and its structure was solved in complex with ABL H396P, a clinically observed activation segment mutation that confers resistance to imatinib (PDB accession code 2F4J; ABL $IC_{50} = 10$ nM (52)). The compound is a trisubstituted pyrimidine, with the linker interaction being provided by an aminopyrazole group, and a methylpiperazine pointing toward the solvent. The third (phenylcyclopropane carboxamide) substituent occupies a region between the back hydrophobic pocket and the Glu-Lys salt bridge, avoiding direct contact with T315 (Figure 7.14B).

7.6 CASE STUDY: EGF RECEPTOR INHIBITORS

Quinazolines were identified as kinase inhibitors in the mid-1990s (53) and have since become an important and broadly explored structural class (Figure 7.15). Their kinase binding mode was first demonstrated experimentally in complex with CDK2 and p38 kinases (54), and two drugs from this structural class were

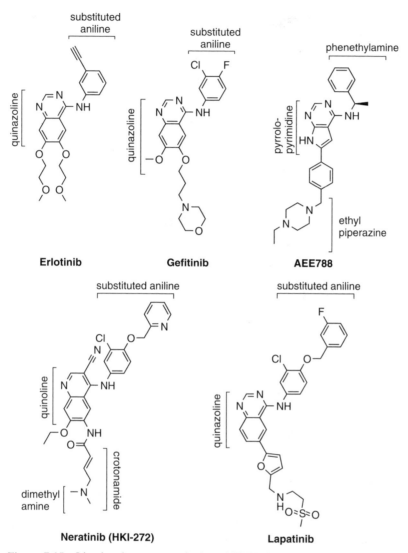

Figure 7.15 Line bond structures of selected ERBB inhibitors, showing structural elements involved in kinase interactions. The orientations have been chosen to approximate those depicted in the crystal structure figures.

among the first kinase inhibitors to gain clinical approval, namely, erlotinib (OSI-774; Tarceva®) and gefitinib (ZD1839; Iressa®). Both drugs have been solved in complex with EGF receptor kinase (55, 56) and are depicted in Figure 7.16A and B (PDB accession codes 1M17 and 2ITY). In both cases, the quinazoline 1-position nitrogen forms a kinase linker region interaction with the M793 main chain nitrogen, whereas the substituted aniline occupies the rear hydrophobic pocket, skirting around the T790 gatekeeper residue. The substituted aniline groups of

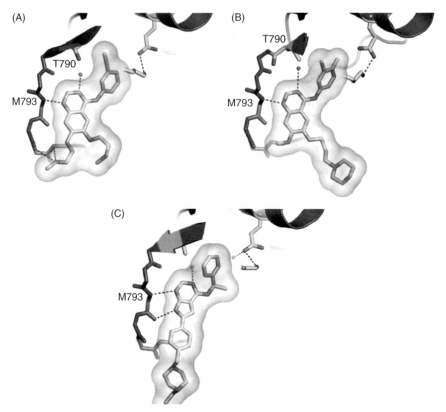

Figure 7.16 Crystal structures of ERBB inhibitors I: (A) erlotinib, (B) gefitinib, and (C) AEE788. T854 (mentioned in the main text) is hidden behind the inhibitor molecules.

both molecules pack tightly in this pocket; there is a small (~0.6 Å) displacement between the erlotinib/gefitinib aniline rings in order to accommodate the larger 3-ethynyl substituent of erlotinib. The quinazoline 3-position nitrogen interacts with a water molecule deep in the active site cavity and thereby makes an indirect hydrogen bond to the T790 and T854 side chains. In both inhibitors, the quinazoline 6- and 7-position substituents are ether-linked solubilizing groups, which extend through the front specificity pocket and ribose binding site toward solvent-exposed regions. The structure of a pyrrolopyrimidine inhibitor (AEE788; PDB accession code 2J6M, Figure 7.16C) has also been solved in complex with EGFR (56). In this case, nitrogens from both the pyrimidine and the pyrrole are hydrogen-bonded to the linker region. The 4-phenethylamine occupies the rear hydrophobic pocket in a manner similar (but not identical) to the quinazoline aniline groups, and a solubilizing ethylpiperazine moiety extends to solvent via the front specificity pocket (Figure 7.16C).

Several structures of EGFR:inhibitor complexes have been solved in complex with mutant forms of the kinase, affording insight into both the increased activity and transforming ability of the mutants and their increased sensitivity to EGFR

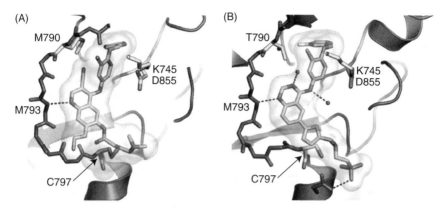

Figure 7.17   Crystal structures of ERBB inhibitors II: (A) neratinib (HKI-272) and (B) lapatinib. In (B), the helical region within the activation segment and the associated D855 residue are shown in blue.

inhibitors (56). The L858R (exon 21) mutation is located in the activation segment and confers increased catalytic activity (56, 57). The binding modes of gefitinib and AEE788 to this mutant kinase are essentially the same as in the wild-type kinase, indicating a more subtle explanation for their increased potency toward the mutant. In the inactive conformation of EGFR (Figure 7.17, described in more detail later), the leucine residue resides in a short helical region and plays a role in stabilizing the inactive conformation; mutation to arginine is incompatible with this arrangement, thereby favoring adoption of the active form of the kinase. The G719S (exon 18) mutation is somewhat less common and resides in the glycine-rich loop. Mutation to a nonglycine residue at this position restricts the available dihedral angles and alters the conformation and flexibility of the loop, resulting in weaker binding to ATP. Structurally, the binding modes of gefitinib and AEE788 are again similar in the G719S and wild-type structures, and gefitinib binding to G719S appears to be about twofold weaker than to wild-type kinase. However, both inhibitors bind more tightly to the G719S mutant relative to its affinity for ATP, resulting in a greater degree of cellular inhibition (56).

Recently, several EGFR inhibitors that bind irreversibly to the kinase domain have entered clinical trials including neratinib (HKI-272), the structure of which was solved in complex with the EGFR T790M mutant (58) (PDB accession code 2JIV, Figure 7.17A). These irreversible inhibitors capitalize on the fact that the EGFR kinase domain has a surface-accessible cysteine residue (C797) close to the ATP binding site; ERBB2 and ERBB4 also have cysteines at the homologous positions. The quinoline core of neratinib binds to EGFR in the canonical mode described earlier, and a crotonamide Michael acceptor in the 6-position substituent reacts with the C797 sulfydryl group to form a covalent adduct. It has been suggested that the terminal dimethylamino group of neratinib may act as an intramolecular catalyst to promote this covalent interaction (59). The methionine residue at the "gatekeeper" position does not sterically interfere with binding of neratinib. In fact, although this mutation causes profound resistance to gefitinib and erlotinib, it is unlikely that steric hindrance is the main reason for this effect. Instead, T790M appears to increase the affinity of ATP, thus making it more difficult for any ATP-competitive inhibitor to bind in the ATP-rich cellular environment (58).

Neratinib has a 4-position aniline substitution that results in the EGFR kinase domain adopting an inactive-like conformation in the complex. A similar moiety is also found in the quinazoline derivative lapatinib (GW572016; Tykerb®), which has also been solved in complex with EGFR (7). While the binding mode has some similarities with erlotinib and gefitinib, the structure of the kinase is substantially different (PDB accession code 1XKK; Figure 7.17B). Like erlotinib and gefitinib, lapatinib is anchored to the kinase domain linker region by an interaction between the quinazoline 1-position nitrogen and the M793 main chain nitrogen; the 3-position nitrogen:water interaction is also conserved, although the water molecule is substantially closer to T854 than T790. The 3-chloro aniline portion of the molecule is conserved between gefitinib and lapatinib and occupies a similar region in the binding pocket. However, the 4-position aniline substitution of lapatinib is incompatible with binding to the active conformation. Instead, the C helix is displaced to an inactive-like configuration, disrupting the Glu-Lys ion pair interaction and creating a larger binding pocket that can accommodate the 3-fluorylbenzyloxy group. The activation segment is also substantially different between the gefitinib and lapatinib structures. Although the aspartate of the "DFG" segment is in a similar position, there is a rotation of the adjacent phenylalanine side chain and the start of the activation loop is marked by a short helical segment that lies adjacent to the displaced C helix. (The short helical segment is the site of the L858R EGFR mutation described earlier.) Notably, this substantial rearrangement of the active site on binding of lapatinib may explain its relatively slow off-rate compared to erlotinib and gefitinib (7). Inhibitors that bind to inactive kinase conformations are further described in Section 7.7.

7.7   TARGETING THE INACTIVE CONFORMATION

As noted in Chapter 2, while the active conformations of kinase domains are relatively similar there is substantial variation between the unactivated forms. Consequently, drugs that specifically interact with the inactive conformation may be expected to be more specific than those targeting the active form. This is not a rigid rule: some highly specific molecules targeting the active form have been reported (e.g., the BRAF inhibitors XL281 and PLX4032, and the MET inhibitors JNJ38877605 and PF-4217903; see Chapters 8 and 10). On the other hand, cross-reactivity is observed with some of the DFG-out binding molecules, perhaps most notably the inhibition of KIT by the ABL kinase inhibitor imatinib. The situation is further complicated by the fact that a given inhibitor may interact with two different targets in distinctly different binding modes and may even bind to two distinctly different kinase conformations. Indeed, as well as targeting the inactive forms of ABL and KIT, imatinib adopts a completely different mode of interaction with the active form of the SRC family kinase SYK, albeit with relatively weak affinity

(60). The DFG-out inactive form is not employed by all kinases, so targeting this conformation is not possible in all cases. Nevertheless, there appear to be some common features to several of the DFG-out binding molecules identified so far, and it has been proposed that structures akin to imatinib (discussed next), wherein a "linker region binding" group is coupled to a "F pocket binding" group via an appropriate linker, may be a universal (or at least broadly generic) strategy to convert an inhibitor of the active form of a kinase to an inactive form inhibitor (61). We begin our exploration of inactive kinase inhibitors by comparing the structures of dasatinib and imatinib bound to ABL kinase.

7.7.1 Binding Mode of Imatinib

Figure 7.18 depicts the active conformation of ABL kinase bound to dasatinib and the inactive conformation bound to imatinib. (It should be noted that although we focus here on a recent structure of human ABL in complex with imatinib, the details of the imatinib:ABL interaction were first revealed in complex with murine ABL kinase (62).) The major rearrangement of the activation segment causes a dramatic shift in the binding pockets and structural features that are available for small molecule interactions. A rotation around the DFG aspartate N–C main chain bond displaces the aspartate side chain from the active site and causes occlusion of the substrate binding site by the activation segment. Of particular relevance is the disposition of the DFG phenyl group, which moves approximately 9 Å from a hydrophobic pocket in the N-terminal domain to a region close to (but not quite overlapping) the ATP binding site. This dramatically restructures the phosphate binding/catalytic Asp/salt bridge region and also opens up a "channel" between the adenosine pocket and the hydrophobic pocket hitherto occupied by the DFG Phe side chain. Imatinib binds in this channel and adopts an extended conformation that connects the linker region to the DFG phenylalanine hydrophobic pocket and beyond (Figure 7.18; PDB accession code 2HYY (63)). At one end of the molecule, the pyridine is anchored by a hydrogen bond with the linker region, and the glycine-rich loop also appears to wrap around the pyridine and pyrimidine groups. Next, the central portion of the molecule snakes through the channel behind the activation loop, with the aniline nitrogen adjacent to the pyrimidine making hydrogen bonds with the gatekeeper T315 hydroxyl. An amide bond within this central region interacts with E286 (of the Glu-Lys salt bridge) and also with the main chain backbone just N-terminal of the DFG sequence. At the other end of the molecule, a phenyl group is located near to the hydrophobic pocket that was vacated by the DFG phenylalanine, and the terminal N-methylpiperazine forms hydrogen bond interactions with main chain residues in the C-terminal domain. The structure also affords insight into how different mutations in the ABL kinase domain can give rise to imatinib resistance. In Figure 7.19, selected mutations are depicted according to their proposed mechanisms of imatinib resistance. Several prominent resistance mutations (including the T315I gatekeeper residue) impinge directly on the imatinib binding site, whereas others (notably residues in the glycine-rich loop and activation loop) are proposed to destabilize the inactive conformation, indirectly occluding the imatinib binding site by promoting kinase activation (64, 65).

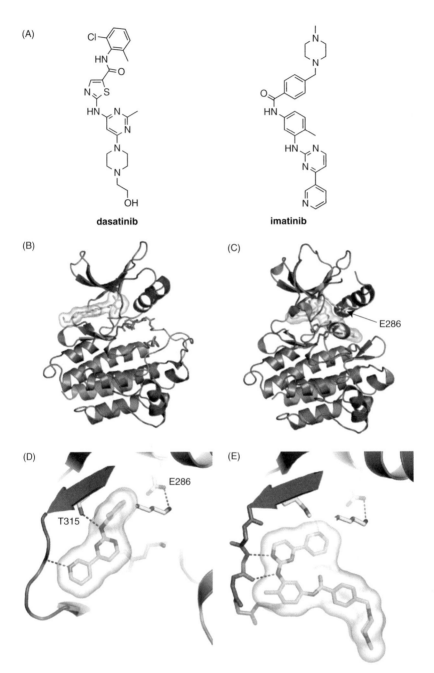

Figure 7.18 Interactions of dasatinib and imatinib with ABL kinase. (A) Line bond structures of dasatinib and imatinib. (B) Active form of ABL bound to dasatinib. (C) Inactive form of ABL bound to imatinib. In (B) and (C), the activation segment is shown in orange. (D) Detail of the imatinib interaction with the kinase linker region; the other half of the molecule extends back into the image and is hidden from view. (E) In complex with the active form of SYK kinase, imatinib adopts a distinctly different conformation compared to the inactive ABL structure.

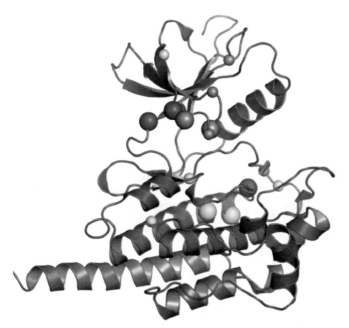

Figure 7.19 Location of prominent imatinib resistance mutations in ABL. Mutations that directly interfere with imatinib binding are shown in red; mutations that destabilize the inactive conformation (or stabilize the active conformation) are in orange, and mutations with other indirect effects are in yellow. Highly frequent mutations (residues Y253, T315, F317, M351, E355, and F359) are shown as large spheres: less common mutations are represented by smaller spheres.

The structure of imatinib has also been solved in complex with LCK and KIT (PDB accession codes 2PL0 and 1T46, respectively), revealing remarkably similar modes of binding compared to the ABL structure (66, 67). However, a crystallographic analysis of imatinib in complex with the active form of SYK kinase (PDB accession code 1XBB) revealed a completely novel binding mode (60). Although inhibition of SYK is relatively weak (K_i ~5 μM, on the same order as inhibition of phosphorylated ABL), the compound adopts a U shape, with the aminopyrimidine forming hydrogen bonds with the linker region and the benzylpiperazine moiety extending out to solvent under the glycine-rich loop (Figure 7.18E).

7.7.2 Binding of BAY-43-9006 (Sorafenib) to the Inactive BRAF Kinase

The X-ray crystal structure of sorafenib (BAY-43-9006) bound to BRAF shows that it also inhibits the inactive form, with some similarities to imatinib:ABL (Figure 7.20; PDB accession code 1UWH (68)). The pyridyl group of sorafenib interacts with the linker region and is sandwiched between three hydrophobic residues: W531 in the linker region, the DFG phenylalanine (F595), and another

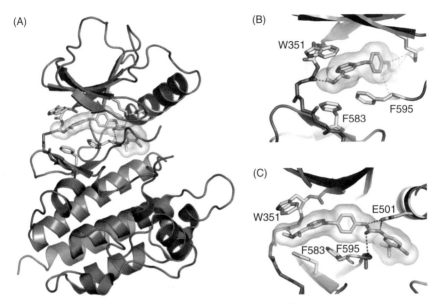

Figure 7.20 Structure of sorafenib in BRAF. (A) Overall structure, showing the conformation of the inhibitor in the inactive form of the kinase. (B) Line bond structure of sorafenib. (C) Interactions of the pyridyl group with the linker region. (D) Interactions of the central urea with E501 and D594. (Note that the numbering used in the PDB file 1UWH differs from the more commonly used numbering, so that, for example, E501 appears as E500.)

phenylalanine (F583) from the C-terminal lobe. The extended central portion of the molecule occupies a binding groove between the N-terminal lobe and the activation loop; a central urea group mimics some of the interactions of the central amide in imatinib, forming hydrogen bonds with E501 (from the Glu-Lys salt bridge) and the main chain backbone of D594 from the DFG motif. A trifluoromethylphenyl group anchors the inhibitor in the hydrophobic pocket vacated by F595. Although no suitable crystals have been obtained for apo-BRAF, there is also a structure of the active BRAF conformation in complex with an active form inhibitor (69): comparison with this structure shows that the sorafenib trifluoromethyl group closely overlaps with the phenyl ring of F595 in the active conformation.

7.8 NONCOMPETITIVE INHIBITION

In 1999, the discovery and characterization of a noncompetitive inhibitor of MEK1 and MEK2 kinases was reported (70), and subsequent X-ray crystallographic studies with MEK1 and MEK2 revealed an intriguing mode of binding for this series of molecules (71). Figure 7.21 shows the structure of MEK1 in complex with both ATP and the inhibitor PD318088 (PDB accession code 1S9J); the MEK2 structure

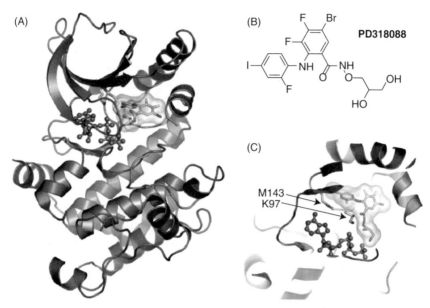

Figure 7.21 PD318088 bound to MEK kinase. (A) Overall structure, showing the relationship between ATP (ball and stick, colored teal) and the MEK inhibitor (stick figure, colored green). The activation loop (including a short helical segment shown in orange) displaces the C helix and forms one side of the inhibitor binding pocket. (B) Line bond structure of PD318088. (C) Close-up view of ATP and PD318088: the inhibitor extends into the back hydrophobic pocket, separated from the ATP adenine binding site by the side chains of M143 and K97, which are depicted in yellow.

is highly similar. MEK1 adopts a unique conformation with features of both active and inactive kinase structures. The lobes of the kinase domain adopt a relatively closed arrangement reminiscent of active kinases, and the activation loop does not occlude the active site, adopting a "DFG-in"-like conformation. However, the N-terminal portion of the activation loop forms a short helix, displacing the C helix and disrupting the Glu-Lys salt bridge (E114 and K97 become separated by over 15 Å). This rearrangement creates a unique binding pocket, which is occupied by the inhibitor molecule. A diaryl amine anchors the inhibitor in a largely hydrophobic binding site, which extends into the back hydrophobic pocket; the gatekeeper M143 and salt bridge K97 serve as a barrier between this diaryl amine and the adenosine moiety of ATP. At the other end of the inhibitor molecule, a diol moiety interacts with the K97 side chain and the ATP phosphates. Several clinical candidates have emerged from this series, including CI-1040 and PD0325901 (Chapter 9). Thermodynamic analysis of the interaction between PD0325901 and MEK1 indicate that, consistent with the structural data, the binding of inhibitor and nucleotide are synergistic; that is, the binding of each ligand with the protein enhances the affinity of the other. Furthermore, binding was found to be dependent on Mg^{2+} and to be enthalpically driven (72).

7.9 KINASE INHIBITOR SPECIFICITY

The design of kinase inhibitors with appropriate selectivity profile has received much attention and has important implications for both efficacy and safety. In particular, modulating the specificity of ATP-competitive inhibitors was initially viewed as being particularly challenging due to the high conservation of ATP binding determinants among family members (73). Nevertheless, as noted previously, it has been possible to derive ATP-competitive small molecule inhibitors with widely varying specificities, ranging from the highly specific to highly promiscuous. There are multiple questions to consider when reviewing the specificity of a given inhibitor, or series of inhibitors. For example, what amino acid residues and/or structural features of the kinase are the primary determinants of selectivity? What patterns of selectivity exist within the kinome—that is, are there certain kinases that are more promiscuous/easier to inhibit than others, and are certain kinases (and/or kinase sub-families) frequently coinhibited? Are there clearly demarked differences between the major kinase subfamilies, or at least between tyrosine kinases and serine/threonine kinases?

The advent of commercially available kinase specificity screens and novel assay technologies for high-throughput measurement of drug binding have enabled several broad sets of kinase inhibitor specificity profiles to be generated, providing some insight into these issues. In one such study, 156 kinase inhibitors were profiled against 60 diverse serine/threonine kinases using thermal stability shift binding assays, and the results correlated with structures of a subset of 23 kinases (74). Several notable conclusions emerged from this analysis. A wide range of selectivity was found, ranging from compounds like imatinib (which appears to only interact appreciably with tyrosine kinases) to the highly promiscuous staurosporine, for which binding to 44 kinases was detected. Conversely, some kinases appear to be more readily inhibited than others: SLK1 and ASK1 interacted with many compounds but others (PBK and ERK3) showed no interaction. Also, while sequence and structural homology can indicate a propensity for crossreactivity, this is not uniformly the case: for example, PAK family kinases showed broadly similar inhibition profiles but substantial differences were found in the CLK subfamily of CMGC kinases.

Another such study has illuminated the crossreactivity profile for 20 diverse kinase inhibitors, most of which have been evaluated clinically and several of which are approved for therapy (75). In this study, 113 distinct protein kinases were expressed as fusion proteins with T7 bacteriophage and captured using one of a number of immobilized ATP-competitive ligands. Phage plaque assays and quantitative PCR were used to measure kinase fusion proteins bound to the solid support, which could be depleted by competitive displacement with the kinase inhibitors of interest. In general, widely varying specificity profiles were observed, ranging from relatively specific inhibitors like lapatinib and vatalanib to the highly promiscuous kinase inhibitor staurosporine. Notably, molecules with the same core scaffold (e.g., quinazolines) were found to range broadly in specificity, as were inhibitors with the same primary target (e.g., EGFR inhibitors or VEGFR2 inhibitors). In addition, this study used several graphical methods for displaying potency and selectivity, and one of these methods in particular has been more widely adopted, presenting an intuitive view of the impact of a given inhibitor on the protein kinome (Figure 7.22A). A further study has expanded on this initial analysis and provided additional insight into the patterns of selectivity for 38 inhibitors and 287 distinct protein kinases (8). The kinase inhibitors (including many of those approved for clinical use in humans) display a wide range of selectivity, ranging from highly selective (e.g., lapatinib) to relatively promiscuous (e.g., sunitinib). Moreover, some of the inhibitors display clear preferences for certain classes of kinases: dasatinib, for example, is quite selective for tyrosine kinases compared to serine/threonine kinases. Indeed, one conclusion from this study is that molecules designed to target one or more tyrosine kinases tend to crossreact mainly with other tyrosine kinases, whereas molecules designed against Ser/Thr kinases frequently have many off-target tyrosine kinase activities.

Several metrics have been proposed for providing a quantitative measure of selectivity for a given inhibitor based on the results of profiling inhibitory activity against a broad panel of kinases. Perhaps the simplest descriptor is to specify just the difference in IC_{50} between the cognate target(s) of a given inhibitor and the most potent crossreacting kinase(s) among a selected panel—the "nearest neighbor." This value is perhaps the most widely used: one frequently encounters statements in the literature such as "inhibitor X is at least 20-fold specific against a panel of kinases." However, this provides no insight into the breadth of crossreactivity: there may be 100 kinases or only one with IC_{50} values $\sim 20-$fold above that of the cognate target(s). A slightly more sophisticated approach is to express the fraction of kinases tested that bind with a K_D/IC_{50} below a given cutoff value; furthermore, it may be somewhat more biologically relevant to calculate the fraction of kinases for which the K_D/IC_{50} is less than a given threshold above the corresponding value for the cognate target(s) of the inhibitor (8). An even more germane analysis might include the K_M^{ATP} for each kinase in the calculation, thus accounting for the fact that kinases with high affinity for ATP are more difficult to inhibit in the ATP-rich intracellular environment.

The above approach ideally requires evaluation of IC_{50} values or binding constants for each of the kinases in the specificity panel, although a similar value could probably be defined using percent inhibition values at a given test concentration. An intriguing alternative specificity score has recently been proposed, involving evaluation of single-point (percent inhibition) data using the Gini coefficient—a method previously used by economists to measure income disparity (76). The sum of all the percent inhibition values for a given inhibitor is calculated, and the cumulative fraction of this total inhibition value is calculated as a function of the cumulative fraction of kinases tested (in order of increasing potency). A completely unselective inhibitor (with equal potency against every kinase) would occupy a diagonal line on this diagram whereas a highly selective inhibitor would show a "hockey stick" profile, with little cumulative inhibition as the cumulative kinase fraction increases, then a dramatic increase in cumulative inhibition for the few kinases at the far right of the graph (Figure 7.22B). The Gini coefficient is the area under the diagonal curve divided by the area under the inhibitor curve.

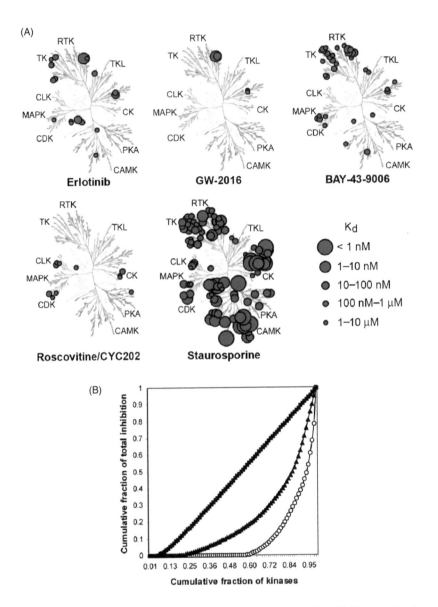

Figure 7.22 Graphical depictions of protein kinase specificity. (A) Kinome dendrogram diagrams provide an intuitive representation of specificity for different inhibitors: erlotinib, lapatinib (GW-2016), sorafenib (BAY-43-9006), R-roscovitine (CYC202), and staurosporine. The size of the red circle represents the potency toward a given target. Reproduced by permission from Macmillan Publishers Ltd (75); copyright © 2005. (B) Depiction of kinase specificity for three inhibitors using the Gini coefficient. The highly specific MEK inhibitor PD184352 (○) shows a "hockey stick" profile, whereas the highly promiscuous inhibitor staurosporine (■) yields a curve that approximates the diagonal. Another inhibitor, AG1024 (▲), lies between these two extremes. Reproduced with permission from (76); copyright © 2007 American Chemical Society.

The qualitative and quantitative methods just outlined have enabled selected drug development candidates to be broadly characterized. It would be helpful, however, if we could make educated guesses regarding the specificity of compounds in the absence of broad kinase profiling data, and to this end a recent computational and statistical analysis offers some useful insights into the relationship between sequence, structure, and specificity (77). In this study, the X-ray crystal structures of eight kinase inhibitors (each in complex with its cognate target) were analyzed to determine the energetic contributions of individual protein side chains to inhibitor binding, termed the "binding signature." All known kinases were subjected to a structure-guided sequence alignment and the binding signature for each inhibitor was mapped onto the aligned sequences. The results indicated that 7–16 residues in and around the active site were the primary determinants of inhibitor binding to the cognate target. Moreover, kinases that each had high affinity for a given inhibitor were found to be highly conserved at the binding signature residues, suggesting that this conservation is a necessary condition for the observed crossreactivity. However, this conservation of sequence is not a sufficient condition for inhibitor binding, since some kinases may have conserved sequences but divergent structures. For example, imatinib was shown to have a binding signature of 16 energetically important residues in the active site of ABL kinase: of 9 kinases with no nonconservative substitutions, 6 were found to bind imatinib with high affinity (within tenfold of that of ABL), while 3 differed substantially. This method was shown to have higher predictive power than simply comparing the overall kinase domain sequences, or even the sequences of residues within 4 Å of the inhibitor. Collectively, this study suggests that "binding signature" analysis may be one attractive strategy for predicting the crossreactivity profile of a given inhibitor, although it depends on the availability of a crystal structure of the inhibitor with at least one of its high affinity targets. The binding signature also indicates several key areas of the kinase active site that are particularly germane to modulating selectivity, most of which have been discussed in the previously mentioned case studies involving CHK1, CDK2, SRC, and EGFR. The concept of a binding signature was also explored in the structural genomics study of Ser/Thr kinases (74): compounds with unusual residues in the ATP binding site tended to produce low promiscuity scores, although no single residue is the predominant discriminator of inhibitor binding.

REFERENCES

1. Cohen P. Protein kinases—the major drug targets of the twenty-first century? Nat Rev Drug Discov 2002;1(4):309–315.
2. Liao JJ. Molecular recognition of protein kinase binding pockets for design of potent and selective kinase inhibitors. J Med Chem 2007;50(3):409–424.
3. Traxler P, Furet P. Strategies toward the design of novel and selective protein tyrosine kinase inhibitors. Pharmacol Ther 1999;82(2–3):195–206.
4. Fedorov O, Sundstrom M, Marsden B, Knapp S. Insights for the development of specific kinase inhibitors by targeted structural genomics. Drug Discov Today 2007;12(9–10):365–372.
5. Toledo LM, Lydon NB, Elbaum D. The structure-based design of ATP-site directed protein kinase inhibitors. Curr Med Chem 1999;6(9):775–805.

6. Ghose AK, Herbertz T, Pippin DA, Salvino JM, Mallamo JP. Knowledge based prediction of ligand binding modes and rational inhibitor design for kinase drug discovery. J Med Chem 2008;51(17):5149–5171

7. Wood ER, Truesdale AT, McDonald OB, Yuan D, Hassell A, Dickerson SH, Ellis B, Pennisi C, Horne E, Lackey K, Alligood KJ, Rusnak DW, Gilmer TM, Shewchuk L. A unique structure for epidermal growth factor receptor bound to GW572016 (lapatinib): relationships among protein conformation, inhibitor off-rate, and receptor activity in tumor cells. Cancer Res 2004;64(18):6652–6659.

8. Karaman MW, Herrgard S, Treiber DK, Gallant P, Atteridge CE, Campbell BT, Chan KW, Ciceri P, Davis MI, Edeen PT, Faraoni R, Floyd M, Hunt JP, Lockhart DJ, Milanov ZV, Morrison MJ, Pallares G, Patel HK, Pritchard S, Wodicka LM, Zarrinkar PP. A quantitative analysis of kinase inhibitor selectivity. Nat Biotechnol 2008;26(1):127–132.

9. Knight ZA, Shokat KM. Features of selective kinase inhibitors. Chem Biol 2005;12(6):621–637.

10. Davies SP, Reddy H, Caivano M, Cohen P. Specificity and mechanism of action of some commonly used protein kinase inhibitors. Biochem J 2000;351(Pt 1):95–105.

11. Bain J, Plater L, Elliott M, Shpiro N, Hastie CJ, McLauchlan H, Klevernic I, Arthur JS, Alessi DR, Cohen P. The selectivity of protein kinase inhibitors: a further update. Biochem J 2007;408(3):297–315.

12. Bain J, McLauchlan H, Elliott M, Cohen P. The specificities of protein kinase inhibitors: an update. Biochem J 2003;371(Pt 1):199–204.

13. Tabernero J. The role of VEGF and EGFR inhibition: implications for combining anti-VEGF and anti-EGFR agents. Mol Cancer Res 2007;5(3):203–220.

14. Deprimo SE, Bello CL, Smeraglia J, Baum CM, Spinella D, Rini BI, Michaelson MD, Motzer RJ. Circulating protein biomarkers of pharmacodynamic activity of sunitinib in patients with metastatic renal cell carcinoma: modulation of VEGF and VEGF-related proteins. J Transl Med 2007;5:32.

15. Norden-Zfoni A, Desai J, Manola J, Beaudry P, Force J, Maki R, Folkman J, Bello C, Baum C, DePrimo SE, Shalinsky DR, Demetri GD, Heymach JV. Blood-based biomarkers of SU11248 activity and clinical outcome in patients with metastatic imatinib-resistant gastrointestinal stromal tumor. Clin Cancer Res 2007;13(9):2643–2650.

16. Sharma SV, Fischbach MA, Haber DA, Settleman J. "Oncogenic shock": explaining oncogene addiction through differential signal attenuation. Clin Cancer Res 2006;12(14Pt 2): 4392s–4395s.

17. Bishop AC, Ubersax JA, Petsch DT, Matheos DP, Gray NS, Blethrow J, Shimizu E, Tsien JZ, Schultz PG, Rose MD, Wood JL, Morgan DO, Shokat KM. A chemical switch for inhibitor-sensitive alleles of any protein kinase. Nature 2000;407(6802):395–401.

18. Liu Y, Shah K, Yang F, Witucki L, Shokat KM. A molecular gate which controls unnatural ATP analogue recognition by the tyrosine kinase v-Src. Bioorg Med Chem 1998;6(8):1219–1226.

19. Bishop AC, Shah K, Liu Y, Witucki L, Kung C, Shokat KM. Design of allele-specific inhibitors to probe protein kinase signaling. Curr Biol 1998;8(5):257–266.

20. Liu Y, Shah K, Yang F, Witucki L, Shokat KM. Engineering Src family protein kinases with unnatural nucleotide specificity. Chem Biol 1998;5(2):91–101.

21. Shah K, Liu Y, Deirmengian C, Shokat KM. Engineering unnatural nucleotide specificity for Rous sarcoma virus tyrosine kinase to uniquely label its direct substrates. Proc Natl Acad Sci U S A 1997;94(8):3565–3570.

22. Janetka JW, Ashwell S, Zabludoff S, Lyne P. Inhibitors of checkpoint kinases: from discovery to the clinic. Curr Opin Drug Discov Dev 2007;10(4):473–486.

23. Chen P, Luo C, Deng Y, Ryan K, Register J, Margosiak S, Tempczyk-Russell A, Nguyen B, Myers P, Lundgren K, Kan CC, O'Connor PM. The 1.7 Å crystal structure of human cell cycle checkpoint kinase Chk1: implications for Chk1 regulation. Cell 2000;100(6):681–692.

24. Zhao B, Bower MJ, McDevitt PJ, Zhao H, Davis ST, Johanson KO, Green SM, Concha NO, Zhou BB. Structural basis for Chk1 inhibition by UCN-01. J Biol Chem 2002;277(48):46609–46615.

25. Foloppe N, Fisher LM, Francis G, Howes R, Kierstan P, Potter A. Identification of a buried pocket for potent and selective inhibition of Chk1: prediction and verification. Bioorg Med Chem 2006;14(6):1792–1804.

26. Richardson CM, Nunns CL, Williamson DS, Parratt MJ, Dokurno P, Howes R, Borgognoni J, Drysdale MJ, Finch H, Hubbard RE, Jackson PS, Kierstan P, Lentzen G, Moore JD, Murray JB, Simmonite H, Surgenor AE, Torrance CJ. Discovery of a potent CDK2 inhibitor with a novel

binding mode, using virtual screening and initial, structure-guided lead scoping. Bioorg Med Chem Lett 2007;17(14):3880–3885.

27. Ni ZJ, Barsanti P, Brammeier N, Diebes A, Poon DJ, Ng S, Pecchi S, Pfister K, Renhowe PA, Ramurthy S, Wagman AS, Bussiere DE, Le V, Zhou Y, Jansen JM, Ma S, Gesner TG. 4-(Aminoalkylamino)-3-benzimidazole-quinolinones as potent CHK-1 inhibitors. Bioorg Med Chem Lett 2006;16(12):3121–3124.

28. Garbaccio RM, Huang S, Tasber ES, Fraley ME, Yan Y, Munshi S, Ikuta M, Kuo L, Kreatsoulas C, Stirdivant S, Drakas B, Rickert K, Walsh ES, Hamilton KA, Buser CA, Hardwick J, Mao X, Beck SC, Abrams MT, Tao W, Lobell R, Sepp-Lorenzino L, Hartman GD. Synthesis and evaluation of substituted benzoisoquinolinones as potent inhibitors of Chk1 kinase. Bioorg Med Chem Lett 2007;17(22):6280–6285.

29. Brnardic EJ, Garbaccio RM, Fraley ME, Tasber ES, Steen JT, Arrington KL, Dudkin VY, Hartman GD, Stirdivant SM, Drakas BA, Rickert K, Walsh ES, Hamilton K, Buser CA, Hardwick J, Tao W, Beck SC, Mao X, Lobell RB, Sepp-Lorenzino L, Yan Y, Ikuta M, Munshi SK, Kuo LC, Kreatsoulas C. Optimization of a pyrazoloquinolinone class of Chk1 kinase inhibitors. Bioorg Med Chem Lett 2007;17(21):5989–5994.

30. Tong Y, Claiborne A, Stewart KD, Park C, Kovar P, Chen Z, Credo RB, Gu WZ, Gwaltney SL 2nd, Judge RA, Zhang H, Rosenberg SH, Sham HL, Sowin TJ, Lin NH. Discovery of 1,4-dihydroindeno[1,2-c]pyrazoles as a novel class of potent and selective checkpoint kinase 1 inhibitors. Bioorg Med Chem 2007;15(7):2759–2767.

31. Foloppe N, Fisher LM, Howes R, Potter A, Robertson AG, Surgenor AE. Identification of chemically diverse Chk1 inhibitors by receptor-based virtual screening. Bioorg Med Chem 2006;14(14):4792–4802.

32. Jeffrey PD, Russo AA, Polyak K, Gibbs E, Hurwitz J, Massague J, Pavletich NP. Mechanism of CDK activation revealed by the structure of a cyclin A–CDK2 complex. Nature 1995;376(6538):313–320.

33. De Bondt HL, Rosenblatt J, Jancarik J, Jones HD, Morgan DO, Kim SH. Crystal structure of cyclin-dependent kinase 2. Nature 1993;363(6430):595–602.

34. Davies TG, Pratt DJ, Endicott JA, Johnson LN, Noble ME. Structure-based design of cyclin-dependent kinase inhibitors. Pharmacol Ther 2002;93(2–3):125–133.

35. Kontopidis G, McInnes C, Pandalaneni SR, McNae I, Gibson D, Mezna M, Thomas M, Wood G, Wang S, Walkinshaw MD, Fischer PM. Differential binding of inhibitors to active and inactive CDK2 provides insights for drug design. Chem Biol 2006;13(2):201–211.

36. Wu SY, McNae I, Kontopidis G, McClue SJ, McInnes C, Stewart KJ, Wang S, Zheleva DI, Marriage H, Lane DP, Taylor P, Fischer PM, Walkinshaw MD. Discovery of a novel family of CDK inhibitors with the program LIDAEUS: structural basis for ligand-induced disordering of the activation loop. Structure 2003;11(4):399–410.

37. Chu XJ, DePinto W, Bartkovitz D, So SS, Vu BT, Packman K, Lukacs C, Ding Q, Jiang N, Wang K, Goelzer P, Yin X, Smith MA, Higgins BX, Chen Y, Xiang Q, Moliterni J, Kaplan G, Graves B, Lovey A, Fotouhi N. Discovery of [4-amino-2-(1-methanesulfonylpiperidin-4-ylamino)pyrimidin-5-yl](2,3-diflu oro-6- methoxyphenyl)methanone (R547), a potent and selective cyclin-dependent kinase inhibitor with significant in vivo antitumor activity. J Med Chem 2006;49(22):6549–6560.

38. Lucking U, Siemeister G, Schafer M, Briem H, Kruger M, Lienau P, Jautelat R. Macrocyclic aminopyrimidines as multitarget CDK and VEGF-R inhibitors with potent antiproliferative activities. ChemMedChem 2007;2(1):63–77.

39. Bettayeb K, Tirado OM, Marionneau-Lambot S, Ferandin Y, Lozach O, Morris JC, Mateo-Lozano S, Drueckes P, Schachtele C, Kubbutat MH, Liger F, Marquet B, Joseph B, Echalier A, Endicott JA, Notario V, Meijer L. Meriolins, a new class of cell death inducing kinase inhibitors with enhanced selectivity for cyclin-dependent kinases. Cancer Res 2007;67(17):8325–8334.

40. Echalier A, Bettayeb K, Ferandin Y, Lozach O, Clement M, Valette A, Liger F, Marquet B, Morris JC, Endicott JA, Joseph B, Meijer L. Meriolins (3-(pyrimidin-4-yl)-7-azaindoles): synthesis, kinase inhibitory activity, cellular effects, and structure of a CDK2/cyclin A/meriolin complex. J Med Chem 2008;51(4):737–751.

41. Bramson HN, Corona J, Davis ST, Dickerson SH, Edelstein M, Frye SV, Gampe RT Jr, Harris PA, Hassell A, Holmes WD, Hunter RN, Lackey KE, Lovejoy B, Luzzio MJ, Montana V, Rocque WJ,

Rusnak D, Shewchuk L, Veal JM, Walker DH, Kuyper LF. Oxindole-based inhibitors of cyclin-dependent kinase 2 (CDK2): design, synthesis, enzymatic activities, and X-ray crystallographic analysis. J Med Chem 2001;44(25):4339–4358.

42. Mohammadi M, McMahon G, Sun L, Tang C, Hirth P, Yeh BK, Hubbard SR, Schlessinger J. Structures of the tyrosine kinase domain of fibroblast growth factor receptor in complex with inhibitors. Science 1997;276(5314):955–960.

43. Xu W, Doshi A, Lei M, Eck MJ, Harrison SC. Crystal structures of c-Src reveal features of its autoinhibitory mechanism. Mol Cell 1999;3(5):629–638.

44. Breitenlechner CB, Kairies NA, Honold K, Scheiblich S, Koll H, Greiter E, Koch S, Schafer W, Huber R, Engh RA. Crystal structures of active SRC kinase domain complexes. J Mol Biol 2005;353(2):222–231.

45. Hanke JH, Gardner JP, Dow RL, Changelian PS, Brissette WH, Weringer EJ, Pollok BA, Connelly PA. Discovery of a novel, potent, and Src family-selective tyrosine kinase inhibitor. Study of Lck- and FynT-dependent T cell activation. J Biol Chem 1996;271(2):695–701.

46. Liu Y, Bishop A, Witucki L, Kraybill B, Shimizu E, Tsien J, Ubersax J, Blethrow J, Morgan DO, Shokat KM. Structural basis for selective inhibition of Src family kinases by PP1. Chem Biol 1999;6(9):671–678.

47. Schindler T, Sicheri F, Pico A, Gazit A, Levitzki A, Kuriyan J. Crystal structure of Hck in complex with a Src family-selective tyrosine kinase inhibitor. Mol Cell 1999;3(5):639–648.

48. Dalgarno D, Stehle T, Narula S, Schelling P, van Schravendijk MR, Adams S, Andrade L, Keats J, Ram M, Jin L, Grossman T, MacNeil I, Metcalf C 3rd, Shakespeare W, Wang Y, Keenan T, Sundaramoorthi R, Bohacek R, Weigele M, Sawyer T. Structural basis of Src tyrosine kinase inhibition with a new class of potent and selective trisubstituted purine-based compounds. Chem Biol Drug Des 2006;67(1):46–57.

49. Tokarski JS, Newitt JA, Chang CY, Cheng JD, Wittekind M, Kiefer SE, Kish K, Lee FY, Borzillerri R, Lombardo LJ, Xie D, Zhang Y, Klei HE. The structure of dasatinib (BMS-354825) bound to activated ABL kinase domain elucidates its inhibitory activity against imatinib-resistant ABL mutants. Cancer Res 2006;66(11):5790–5797.

50. Lombardo LJ, Lee FY, Chen P, Norris D, Barrish JC, Behnia K, Castaneda S, Cornelius LA, Das J, Doweyko AM, Fairchild C, Hunt JT, Inigo I, Johnston K, Kamath A, Kan D, Klei H, Marathe P, Pang S, Peterson R, Pitt S, Schieven GL, Schmidt RJ, Tokarski J, Wen ML, Wityak J, Borzilleri RM. Discovery of N-(2-chloro-6-methyl- phenyl)-2-(6-(4-(2-hydroxyethyl)- piperazin-1-yl)-2-methylpyrimidin-4- ylamino)thiazole-5-carboxamide (BMS-354825), a dual Src/Abl kinase inhibitor with potent antitumor activity in preclinical assays. J Med Chem 2004;47(27):6658–6661.

51. Modugno M, Casale E, Soncini C, Rosettani P, Colombo R, Lupi R, Rusconi L, Fancelli D, Carpinelli P, Cameron AD, Isacchi A, Moll J. Crystal structure of the T315I Abl mutant in complex with the aurora kinases inhibitor PHA-739358. Cancer Res 2007;67(17):7987–7990.

52. Young MA, Shah NP, Chao LH, Seeliger M, Milanov ZV, Biggs WH 3rd, Treiber DK, Patel HK, Zarrinkar PP, Lockhart DJ, Sawyers CL, Kuriyan J. Structure of the kinase domain of an imatinib-resistant Abl mutant in complex with the Aurora kinase inhibitor VX-680. Cancer Res 2006;66(2):1007–1014.

53. Ward WH, Cook PN, Slater AM, Davies DH, Holdgate GA, Green LR. Epidermal growth factor receptor tyrosine kinase. Investigation of catalytic mechanism, structure-based searching and discovery of a potent inhibitor. Biochem Pharmacol 1994;48(4):659–666.

54. Shewchuk L, Hassell A, Wisely B, Rocque W, Holmes W, Veal J, Kuyper LF. Binding mode of the 4-anilinoquinazoline class of protein kinase inhibitor: X-ray crystallographic studies of 4-anilinoquinazolines bound to cyclin-dependent kinase 2 and p38 kinase. J Med Chem 2000;43(1):133–138.

55. Stamos J, Sliwkowski MX, Eigenbrot C. Structure of the epidermal growth factor receptor kinase domain alone and in complex with a 4-anilinoquinazoline inhibitor. J Biol Chem 2002;277(48):46265–46272.

56. Yun CH, Boggon TJ, Li Y, Woo MS, Greulich H, Meyerson M, Eck MJ. Structures of lung cancer-derived EGFR mutants and inhibitor complexes: mechanism of activation and insights into differential inhibitor sensitivity. Cancer Cell 2007;11(3):217–227.

57. Zhang X, Gureasko J, Shen K, Cole PA, Kuriyan J. An allosteric mechanism for activation of the kinase domain of epidermal growth factor receptor. Cell 2006;125(6):1137–1149.

58. Yun CH, Mengwasser KE, Toms AV, Woo MS, Greulich H, Wong KK, Meyerson M, Eck MJ. The T790M mutation in EGFR kinase causes drug resistance by increasing the affinity for ATP. Proc Natl Acad Sci U S A 2008;105(6):2070–2075.

59. Tsou HR, Overbeek-Klumpers EG, Hallett WA, Reich MF, Floyd MB, Johnson BD, Michalak RS, Nilakantan R, Discafani C, Golas J, Rabindran SK, Shen R, Shi X, Wang YF, Upeslacis J, Wissner A. Optimization of 6,7-disubstituted-4-(arylamino)quinoline-3-carbonitriles as orally active, irreversible inhibitors of human epidermal growth factor receptor-2 kinase activity. J Med Chem 2005;48(4):1107–1131.

60. Atwell S, Adams JM, Badger J, Buchanan MD, Feil IK, Froning KJ, Gao X, Hendle J, Keegan K, Leon BC, Muller-Dieckmann HJ, Nienaber VL, Noland BW, Post K, Rajashankar KR, Ramos A, Russell M, Burley SK, Buchanan SG. A novel mode of Gleevec binding is revealed by the structure of spleen tyrosine kinase. J Biol Chem 2004;279(53):55827–55832.

61. Okram B, Nagle A, Adrian FJ, Lee C, Ren P, Wang X, Sim T, Xie Y, Wang X, Xia G, Spraggon G, Warmuth M, Liu Y, Gray NS. A general strategy for creating "inactive-conformation" abl inhibitors. Chem Biol 2006;13(7):779–786.

62. Schindler T, Bornmann W, Pellicena P, Miller WT, Clarkson B, Kuriyan J. Structural mechanism for STI-571 inhibition of abelson tyrosine kinase. Science 2000;289(5486):1938–1942.

63. Cowan-Jacob SW, Fendrich G, Floersheimer A, Furet P, Liebetanz J, Rummel G, Rheinberger P, Centeleghe M, Fabbro D, Manley PW. Structural biology contributions to the discovery of drugs to treat chronic myelogenous leukaemia. Acta Crystallogr D Biol Crystallogr 2007;63(Pt 1):80–93.

64. Roumiantsev S, Shah NP, Gorre ME, Nicoll J, Brasher BB, Sawyers CL, Van Etten RA. Clinical resistance to the kinase inhibitor STI-571 in chronic myeloid leukemia by mutation of Tyr-253 in the Abl kinase domain P-loop. Proc Natl Acad Sci U S A 2002;99(16):10700–10705.

65. Weisberg E, Manley PW, Cowan-Jacob SW, Hochhaus A, Griffin JD. Second generation inhibitors of BCR-ABL for the treatment of imatinib-resistant chronic myeloid leukaemia. Nat Rev Cancer 2007;7(5):345–356.

66. Mol CD, Dougan DR, Schneider TR, Skene RJ, Kraus ML, Scheibe DN, Snell GP, Zou H, Sang BC, Wilson KP. Structural basis for the autoinhibition and STI-571 inhibition of c-Kit tyrosine kinase. J Biol Chem 2004;279(30):31655–31663.

67. Jacobs MD, Caron PR, Hare BJ. Classifying protein kinase structures guides use of ligand-selectivity profiles to predict inactive conformations: structure of lck/imatinib complex. Proteins 2008;70(4):1451–1460.

68. Wan PT, Garnett MJ, Roe SM, Lee S, Niculescu-Duvaz D, Good VM, Jones CM, Marshall CJ, Springer CJ, Barford D, Marais R. Mechanism of activation of the RAF-ERK signaling pathway by oncogenic mutations of B-RAF. Cell 2004;116(6):855–867.

69. King AJ, Patrick DR, Batorsky RS, Ho ML, Do HT, Zhang SY, Kumar R, Rusnak DW, Takle AK, Wilson DM, Hugger E, Wang L, Karreth F, Lougheed JC, Lee J, Chau D, Stout TJ, May EW, Rominger CM, Schaber MD, Luo L, Lakdawala AS, Adams JL, Contractor RG, Smalley KS, Herlyn M, Morrissey MM, Tuveson DA, Huang PS. Demonstration of a genetic therapeutic index for tumors expressing oncogenic BRAF by the kinase inhibitor SB-590885. Cancer Res 2006;66(23):11100–11105.

70. Sebolt-Leopold JS, Dudley DT, Herrera R, Van Becelaere K, Wiland A, Gowan RC, Tecle H, Barrett SD, Bridges A, Przybranowski S, Leopold WR, Saltiel AR. Blockade of the MAP kinase pathway suppresses growth of colon tumors in vivo. Nat Med 1999;5(7):810–816.

71. Ohren JF, Chen H, Pavlovsky A, Whitehead C, Zhang E, Kuffa P, Yan C, McConnell P, Spessard C, Banotai C, Mueller WT, Delaney A, Omer C, Sebolt-Leopold J, Dudley DT, Leung IK, Flamme C, Warmus J, Kaufman M, Barrett S, Tecle H, Hasemann CA. Structures of human MAP kinase kinase 1 (MEK1) and MEK2 describe novel noncompetitive kinase inhibition. Nat Struct Mol Biol 2004;11(12):1192–1197.

72. Smith CK, Windsor WT. Thermodynamics of nucleotide and non-ATP-competitive inhibitor binding to MEK1 by circular dichroism and isothermal titration calorimetry. Biochemistry 2007;46(5):1358–1367.

73. Hanks SK, Quinn AM, Hunter T. The protein kinase family: conserved features and deduced phylogeny of the catalytic domains. Science 1988;241(4861):42–52.
74. Fedorov O, Marsden B, Pogacic V, Rellos P, Muller S, Bullock AN, Schwaller J, Sundstrom M, Knapp S. A systematic interaction map of validated kinase inhibitors with Ser/Thr kinases. Proc Natl Acad Sci U S A 2007;104(51):20523–20528.
75. Fabian MA, Biggs WH 3rd, Treiber DK, Atteridge CE, Azimioara MD, Benedetti MG, Carter TA, Ciceri P, Edeen PT, Floyd M, Ford JM, Galvin M, Gerlach JL, Grotzfeld RM, Herrgard S, Insko DE, Insko MA, Lai AG, Lelias JM, Mehta SA, Milanov ZV, Velasco AM, Wodicka LM, Patel HK, Zarrinkar PP, Lockhart DJ. A small molecule-kinase interaction map for clinical kinase inhibitors. Nat Biotechnol 2005;23(3):329–336.
76. Graczyk PP. Gini coefficient: a new way to express selectivity of kinase inhibitors against a family of kinases. J Med Chem 2007;50(23):5773–5779.
77. Sheinerman FB, Giraud E, Laoui A. High affinity targets of protein kinase inhibitors have similar residues at the positions energetically important for binding. J Mol Biol 2005;352(5):1134–1156.

CHAPTER 8

TYROSINE KINASE INHIBITORS

8.1 BCR-ABL INHIBITORS

Chronic myeloid leukemia (CML), a form of leukemia characterized by the increased and unregulated proliferation of myeloid cells, accounts for 15–20% of all adult leukemias in Western populations. In the United States, between 3500 and 5000 new cases are diagnosed per year. The disease is commonly diagnosed after leukocytosis is found on routine blood tests in otherwise asymptomatic patients, and most of these patients are diagnosed in the phase known as chronic phase CML. These patients have elevated white cell counts and circulating immature precursors and may also present with thrombocytosis and splenomegaly. Prior to the discovery of imatinib, this phase inevitably progressed to the more aggressive accelerated and blast phases, with characteristic increases in the number of leukemic blasts in the blood and bone marrow, as well as the development of constitutional symptoms. Once reaching blast phase, the median survival was less than 6 months. In CML, the underlying cause of the disease is a characteristic translocation between chromosomes 9 and 22, resulting in the recognizable cytogenetic feature known as the Philadelphia chromosome. The molecular product of this translocation is the chimeric gene, BCR-ABL (discussed in Chapter 4). The success of imatinib has spurred the discovery of many second and third generation BCR-ABL inhibitors (Table 8.1).

Imatinib   Imatinib (Gleevec®, Glivec®), an ABL kinase inhibitor that also inhibits KIT and PDGFR at physiologically relevant concentrations, was the first example of a targeted kinase inhibitor that dramatically altered the natural course of a disease. The compound (a 2-phenylaminopyridine derivative (Figure 8.1), initially known as CGP-57148 and later as STI-571) inhibits ABL and its activated derivatives v-ABL, BCR-ABL, and TEL-ABL with IC_{50} values in the range of 0.025 μM for protein autophosphorylation. Activity against both the PDGFR and KIT RTKs was found to be in a similar range. In contrast, the IC_{50} values for a large number of other RTKs and serine/threonine kinases were at least 100-fold higher. In cell-based assays, imatinib inhibited the v-ABL, PDGFR, and KIT tyrosine kinases with IC_{50} values of 0.25, 0.1, and 0.1 μM, respectively. Using cell lines dependent on *bcr-abl* for growth-factor-independent proliferation

TABLE 8.1 BCR-ABL Inhibitors

Drug	Company	Known targets	Structure[a]	Highest stage of development
Imatinib (STI-571; Gleevec®)	Novartis	ABL, KIT, PDGFR	Figure 8.1	Marketed
Dasatinib (BMS-354825; Sprycel®)	Bristol-Myers Squibb	ABL, EPH, FYN, LCK, SRC, PDGFR, p38	Figure 8.1	Marketed
Nilotinib (AMN107; Tasigna®)	Novartis	ABL, KIT, PDGFR, EPHB4, FGR, FYN, HCK, LCK, LYN, SRC, YES	Figure 8.1	Marketed
Bosutinib (SKI-606)	Wyeth	ABL, SRC, FGR, LYN	Figure 8.1	Phase III
Saracatinib (AZD0530)	AstraZeneca	ABL, SRC, KIT	Figure 8.1	Phase II
AT9283	Astex Therapeutics	Aurora-A, Aurora-B, TYK2, JAK2, JAK3, RSK2, RET, MER, YES, GSK3β	Figure 8.5	Phase II
PHA-739358	Pfizer/Nerviano Medical Sciences	ABL, Aurora, FGFR1, RET, TRKA	Figure 10.8	Phase II
Tozasertib (MK-0457; VX-680)	Merck	Aurora, FLT3, JAK2, ABL	Figure 10.8	Phase II (discontinued)
XL228	Exelixis	ABL, SRC, IGF1R, Aurora	ND	Phase I
INNO-406 (NS-187; CNS-9)	Innovive/Nippon Shinyaku	ABL, LYN, SRC	Figure 8.1	Phase I
LS-104 (AEG-41174)	Aegera Therapeutics	ABL, JAK2	Figure 8.1	Phase I
AP24534	Ariad Pharmaceuticals	ABL, SRC, LYN, VEGFR, FGFR, TIE2, FLT3	ND	Phase I
SGX393	SGX Pharmaceuticals	ABL, CSFR1, FLT3, LCK, TRKC	ND	Phase I

[a] ND, not disclosed.

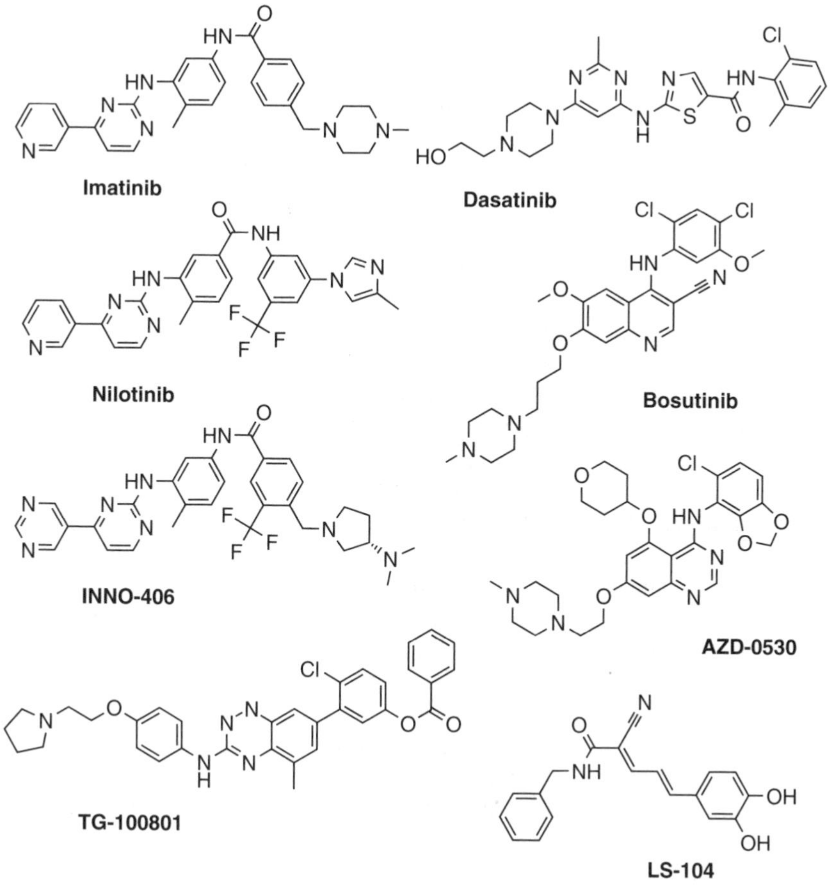

Figure 8.1   Structures of BCR-ABL and SRC inhibitors.

(MO7p210 and 32Dp210), imatinib at 1 or 10 μM completely inhibited proliferation. In contrast, imatinib had no effect on the growth of parental cells in the presence of exogenous growth factor (either GM-CSF or IL3), indicating that the compound was selectively toxic to cells expressing constitutively active BCR-ABL protein tyrosine kinase. The IC_{50} values for inhibition of proliferation correlated with those for inhibition of BCR-ABL tyrosine phosphorylation. Studies in primary cells derived from CML patients and normal volunteers demonstrated that imatinib selectively suppressed the growth of secondary colonies from CML patients. In animal models using the myeloid murine cell line 32D engineered to express BCR-ABL, imatinib (given intraperitoneally everyday) exhibited dose-dependent inhibition of tumor growth at doses ranging from 10 to 50 mg/kg. Similar promising preclinical data were obtained in other animal models of CML. In striking contrast, no effect was seen on tumor formation by *v-SRC*-transformed 32D cells, demonstrating the selective nature of this compound (for a review, see (6)).

Despite these promising preclinical data, there was considerable skepticism about whether this would be a useful therapy for CML patients. Arguments such as "kinase inhibitors won't work" and "kinase inhibitors will be toxic" were raised, as well as the concern that "the compound would never make enough money to justify its development" (http://www.ascb.org/iBioSeminars/druker/druker1.cfm). However, Brian Druker, a physician scientist at Oregon Health Sciences Center, convinced Novartis to begin a Phase I dose escalation trial in CML patients in the chronic phase who were resistant to or intolerant of interferon-α in 1998. Patients were dosed daily, with a starting dose of 25 mg. Hematological responses were seen with daily doses above 85 mg. At 300 mg/day and above, significant benefits were observed in CML patients, with 98% of those dosed achieving a complete hematological response (defined as a complete normalization of peripheral blood (PB) counts with white blood cells $<10 \times 10^9$/L and platelets $<450 \times 10^9$/L; no immature cells in PB, no signs/symptoms of disease and disappearance of splenomegaly). Within 2–3 weeks of dosing, the white blood cell count of the patients dropped and, for most patients, remained normal for the duration of therapy. These encouraging results in patients with CML in the chronic phase led to an expansion of the protocol to 58 patients in blast crisis or with Ph-positive acute lymphoblastic leukemia (ALL), with the minimal dose of 300 mg of imatinib every day (qd). Hematological responses were seen in 55% of patients with the myeloid phenotype and 70% of patients with the lymphoid phenotype, notably including four complete responses in each group. However, in contrast to patients treated in the chronic phase, this group had a higher relapse rate. Three multicenter Phase II studies were initiated in the second half of 1999. They enrolled patients with CML in blast crisis, relapsed Ph-positive ALL and CML in accelerated phase, and patients with CML who had failed interferon-α. All three trials strongly supported the clinical benefit of imatinib in all phases of CML and ALL, although the data also suggested that those patients treated earlier in the disease (i.e., prior to the accelerated phase or blast crisis) would have better outcomes. A randomized Phase III study was initiated in June 2000 with a total of 177 centers in 16 countries participating. Imatinib (400 mg) was compared to the best nontransplant therapy for CML (interferon-α and ARA-C (cytarabine)), with 553 patients in each group. This was one of the most rapidly accrued trials in clinical trial history and was highly successful. Ninety-seven percent of the imatinib-treated patients' white blood cell counts returned to normal compared to 6% in the interferon-α- and ARA-C-treated group, and 76% of the imatinib-treated patients demonstrated a complete cytogenetic response (CCR, no Ph+ cells). Moreover, imatinib was well tolerated, with only 3% of the patients discontinuing therapy versus 1/3 of the patients in the interferon-α and ARA-C group. Overall, imatinib showed clinically and statistically significantly better results for time to progression to accelerated phase or blast crisis, progression-free survival, complete hematological response rate, and cytogenetic response rate. Data from this trial were submitted to the FDA, and in an unprecedented move imatinib was approved within 6 weeks of the NDA submission (May 10, 2001). Since the drug was granted accelerated approval, Novartis agreed to provide follow-up reports on the imatinib study for the next 6 years as a Phase IV postmarketing commitment. At the time of approval, the impact of imatinib on overall survival had not been established, and the duration of follow-up was relatively short. As a consequence of this pivotal trial and FDA approval, imatinib has completely changed the outcome of CML with the 5-year survival of patients now exceeding 90%, and with only 6–7% of patients progressing to accelerated disease. The annual resistance rate to imatinib has been about 4% in the first 4 years, with the yearly risk of relapse appearing to decrease over time, with the biggest risk in the first two years. Overall, imatanib is very well tolerated, with mild side effects that only rarely lead to discontinuation of therapy. The nonhematological toxicities include edema and fluid retention (most frequently in the form of periorbital edema), mild nausea and abdominal pain, skin rashes, and bone joint and muscle pain. In patients with more advanced disease, severe neutropenia and thrombocytopenia frequently occur, requiring careful management of the aggressiveness of therapy versus the aggressive nature of the disease. Imatinib is well absorbed following oral administration, with minimal food effects. The half-life of the drug is about 18 h, and with once daily administration of a 400-mg oral dose, the median peak plasma concentrations at steady state are 5.4 μM and median trough levels are 1.43 μM. The compound is metabolized by the CYP3A4/5 enzyme system and thus inhibitors/inducers of this system are predicted to alter plasma concentrations.

A small percentage of patients with newly diagnosed CML in the chronic phase, as well as most patients with advanced phase CML and Ph+ ALL, relapse on imatinib therapy (1, 2). Several potential mechanisms for relapse have been reported, including point mutations within the ABL kinase domain, amplification of the BCR-ABL gene, overexpression of *BCR-ABL* mRNA, increased drug efflux by P-glycoprotein, and activation of the SRC-family protein LYN (3–11). There are also increasing reports of isolated central nervous system relapse, occurring mainly in patients with CML blast crisis and Ph+ ALL who continue to have complete cytogenetic responses (12–14). These patients develop an extramedullary blast crisis in the CNS. These cases of isolated CNS relapse may result from the low penetration of imatinib into the CNS, allowing the CNS to become a sanctuary site of relapse in patients on prolonged imatinib therapy.

Mutations that cause imatinib resistance are usually found in the kinase domain and result in a functional BCR-ABL fusion protein with abrogated or impaired drug binding. At the molecular level, these can be considered as direct or indirect in nature. Direct mutations occur in a region around the imatinib binding site, which partially overlaps with the ATP binding site, and result in reduced imatinib binding either as a consequence of changes to amino acid side chains (altering drug interactions with key lipophilic contacts or H-bonds) or as a result of topographical changes that sterically inhibit imatinib binding. Two common mutations of this type occur: T315 and F317. There are also a number of mutations that inhibit imatinib binding through an indirect mode. These mutations exploit the binding mode of imatinib to BCR-ABL. Imatinib binds to a catalytically inactive conformation of the ABL kinase, referred to as the DFG-out conformation. In this mode, the highly conserved Asp-Phe-Gly (DFG) loop is flipped out of its usual position in the active conformation (see Chapters 2, 7, and 11). Today, more than 50 different BCR-ABL mutations associated with imatinib resistance have been described, although many of these are quite rare. Sixty to seventy percent of the mutations affect residues G250, Y253, E255, T315, M351, and F359. The expansion of mutant clones in imatinib-treated patients often predicts relapse and disease progression, although different mutants have different transforming potency. Two of the most frequently seen mutants also seem to have the greatest transforming potential—Y253F and E255K. However, mutant clones do not necessarily have a proliferative advantage compared to the wild-type kinase. In retrospective studies, P-loop (e.g., Y253H and E255K) and "gatekeeper" (T315I) mutations are associated with a poor prognosis in terms of time to disease progression and overall survival. The origin of the mutations is still unclear. There may be a low-to-undetectable background level of BCR-ABL mutations that exist prior to imatinib treatment. Imatinib treatment exerts selective pressure, resulting in an increased prevalence of cells derived from the mutant clones. A second possibility is that the mutations are acquired due to point mutations that arise during drug treatment. A third hypothesis is that a population of leukemic stem cells remains viable on imatinib treatment, and these cells and their subsequent progeny are insensitive to imatinib. Recent data from an international, randomized study indicated that about 30% of 553 newly diagnosed patients with chronic phase CML treated with imatinib discontinued therapy after 5 years of follow-up, due either to unsatisfactory therapeutic effects or toxicity. Although increasing the dose of imatinib to 800 mg per day can overcome some cases of resistance, the resulting responses tend to be short in duration and tolerability of high-dose imatinib remains an important issue.

The discovery of imatinib-resistant mutations spurred the development of new compounds designed to overcome the resistance to imatinib. These second generation compounds include selective ABL inhibitors, inhibitors of ABL and SRC family kinases, Aurora kinase inhibitors, and non-ATP-competitive inhibitors of BCR-ABL. However, sequential emergence of ABL kinase mutations during targeted therapy of CML can also occur. In one case study, a 68-year-old patient with CML was treated with imatinib following failure of interferon-α therapy. The patient progressed to the accelerated phase of CML following 34 months of imatinib treatment. The V379I mutation was detected by denaturing gradient gel electrophoresis and sequencing. The unmutated BCR-ABL allele was replaced with the mutated allele. Imatinib treatment was stopped and the patient started on dasatinib treatment. However, after 7 months of treatment, although a minor cytogenic response was observed, mutational analysis revealed the progressive disappearance of the V379I allele, and its replacement by a novel BCR-ABL allele. Direct sequencing confirmed a double mutation at V379I and T315I. This study illustrated that the targeted therapy of CML led to clonal selection of BCR-ABL mutants. The initial imatinib treatment selected for imatinib-resistant cells carrying the V379I mutation, and dasatinib selected further among that population for those cells carrying the T315I mutation (15). Komarova and Wodarz (16) have suggested that the combination of three targeting drugs could overcome the problem or resistance in CML; alternatively, new compounds that inhibit all of the resistance mutations could have potential benefit in this patient population.

Dasatinib   Dasatinib (BMS-354825, Sprycel®; Figure 8.1) is an approved compound developed by Bristol-Myers Squibb for the treatment of patients with chronic, accelerated, or blast phases of CML or Ph+ ALL with resistance or intolerance to prior therapy, including imatinib (17). The drug is named after the chemist, Jagabundhu Das, who was one of the co-discoverers of the compound (18). This orally bioavailable inhibitor of BCR-ABL, SRC family kinases, KIT, EPHA2, and PDGFRβ kinases was discovered through the synthesis and testing of a thiazole-based series of compounds with activity against both SRC and ABL kinases. In contrast to imatinib, dasatinib can bind to both the active and inactive conformation of the ABL kinase domain, and because of these less stringent binding requirements, dasatinib is active against many imatinib-resistant kinase domain mutations of BCR-ABL. Dasatanib is active against all imatinib-resistant mutants tested except for the T315I gatekeeper mutant, due to steric hindrance caused by the side chain of the isoleucine (19, 20). In biochemical assays, dasatanib is a potent inhibitor of BCR-ABL, SRC, LCK, YES, and KIT, with IC_{50} values of $<1, 0.5$, 0.4, 0.5, and 5 nM, respectively. The compound also has significant activity against PDGFRβ, p38, and EGFR, with IC_{50} values of 28, 100, and 180 nM, respectively. Greater than 100-fold selectivity was observed for all other kinases evaluated. Preclinical studies also demonstrated that dasatinib possessed potent in vivo activity with a high safety margin in a K562 xenograft model of CML. Durable hematologic and cytogenic responses have been demonstrated for dasatinib in open-label Phase I and II clinical studies (21–23). Treatment with dasatinib was effective in patients who were clearly resistant to imatinib or nilotinib (24, 25), including patients who had progressed on high-dose imatinib and whose prognosis had been very poor (26). Dasatinib was associated with a greater degree of myelosuppression, particularly thrombocytopenia, an effect that may be attributable to both the greater potency of dasatinib and also possibly greater exposure of dasatinib to the hematopoietic progenitor cells. In those patients experiencing myelosuppression, dose interruptions or reductions were usually sufficient to result in recovery; other patients required transfusions (26). Another category of adverse events reported in patients treated with dasatinib is fluid retention. Fluid retention was also observed with imatinib, but in the case of dasatinib, the retention frequently occurs in the form of pleural effusion, pulmonary edema, and pericardial infusion. This occurs in about 8% of patients. Why this occurs is not clear, although inhibition of PDGFRβ by dasatinib may be a possibility (27). Initial studies with dasatinib employed a dose of 70 mg administered twice daily. This dose was established based on the relatively short half-life of the compound (3–5 h): however, it has recently been shown that a daily dose of 100 mg has similar efficacy to the twice-daily dose, but with improved tolerability (28). Indeed, preclinical studies have shown that transient exposure to 100 nM dasatinib for as little as 20 minutes is sufficient to induce substantial cell death (29). The major metabolic pathway of dasatinib is Cyp3A4, and clearance of the drug is predicted to increase in the presence of a Cyp3A4 inhibitor and decrease in the presence of a Cyp3A4 inducer. Antacids, H_2 histamine antagonists, and proton pump inhibitors may also decrease dasatinib absorption. The compound is also teratogenic and the product labeling cautions against its use in pregnant women. Ongoing clinical trials are evaluating dasatinib as first line therapy for CML.

Nilotinib   Nilotinib (AMN107, Tasigna®; Figure 8.1) was developed through rational modifications to the imatinib molecule; the result is a better topological fit that inhibits ABL with a 30-fold increase in potency compared to the parent compound. Sometimes called "imatinib's strong little brother," nilotinib inhibits ABL, KIT, and PDGFR with IC_{50} values of 25, 158, and 53 nM (compared to 658, 58, and 39 nM, respectively, for imatinib) (30). This activity profile also favors the primary therapeutic target (ABL) over KIT and PDGFR. Since fluid retention, a common side effect of imatinib, is thought to be due to the PDGFR inhibitory activity, it was thought that this might be clinically advantageous. Nilotinib shows inhibitory activity against most of the BCR-ABL mutants associated with imatinib resistance with the exception of T315I. Due to the increased potency of the drug, the inhibitory activity comes within the range of clinically achievable drug concentrations, although some mutations (e.g., Y253F and E255V) require quite high IC_{90} concentrations (1–2 μM). Similar to imatinib, nilotinib binds to the inactive conformation of ABL. Nilotinib is now approved for the treatment of patients with chronic and accelerated phase CML resistant or intolerant to prior therapy including imatinib. Nilotinib has also demonstrated significant activity in blast phase CML patients resistant to or intolerant of prior therapy, including imatinib. Importantly, nilotinib has an excellent tolerability profile with low rates of grade 3/4 myelosuppression and nonhematologic adverse events. However, nilotinib prolongs cardiac ventricular repolarization with a dose-dependent prolongation of the QT interval. In the registration trials as well as in the expanded access program, a 6% rate of sudden death was found, and thus may signal a cause for concern. Based on this, correction of serum potassium and magnesium levels before therapy, and periodic monitoring of serum electrolyte levels and EKG are mandatory. Consistent with the predictions from in vitro studies, patients with Y253F and E255V mutations tend to have less marked and less durable responses to nilotinib compared to patients with different imatinib-resistant mutations. Nilotinib is quite potent against the F317L mutation (which is relatively resistant to dasatinib). Thus the choice of second line therapy (currently nilotinib versus dasatinib) may be improved by drug selection based on the BCR-ABL genotype (recently reviewed in (31, 32)). Ongoing clinical trials are evaluating nilotinib as first line therapy for CML.

Bosutinib   Bosutinib (SKI-606), a 4-anilino-3-quinoline carbonitrile derivative (Figure 8.1), was developed by Wyeth as an inhibitor of SRC family kinases, but it also targets BCR-ABL. In biochemical assays, the compound has been shown to be a potent inhibitor (IC_{50} values in parentheses) of SRC (1.2 nM), FGR (0.17 nM), LYN (0.85 nM), and ABL (2.4 nM) (33–35) but has no significant inhibitory activity against PDGFR, FGFR, or IGF1R. Bosutinib is also very potent in a number of cell-based assays, including SRC-transformed fibroblasts and K562 CML cells. In HT29 cells, bosutinib inhibits SRC autophosphorylation with an IC_{50} of ∼0.25 μM (36). A molecular docking approach was used to investigate the propensity for bosutinib to bind the active and inactive forms of ABL, and its activity toward imatinib-resistant ABL mutants. These data predicted that, similar to imatinib, the interaction between bosutinib and ABL seems to be more stable when ABL is in its inactive conformation. Twenty-one ABL residues (including Y253, T315, F317, and F359) surround bosutinib and contribute H-bonds or van der Waals interactions. This suggests that bosutinib is likely to retain the ability to bind and inhibit the imatinib-resistant Y253H, M351T, F359V, F317L, and E255V ABL mutants, but binding to the E255K and T315I mutants is predicted to be less efficient (37).

Bosutinib is orally available and has been shown to be an effective tumor growth inhibitor in a number of xenograft models (33, 36). In the clinic, bosutinib was evaluated in a study of 69 patients with chronic phase CML or ALL who had relapsed or were resistant to imatinib. The first part of the study established that the appropriate dose was 500 mg/day. The Phase II part of the study included 51 patients. Nineteen patients had no prior exposure to imatinib, nilotinib, or dasatinib. The major cytogenetic response rate for these 19 patients was 52%. In 9 patients with advanced leukemia, 4 had a complete hematological response and 2 had a major cytogenetic response. Bosutinib was also found to be effective in patients with defined imatinib-resistant mutations. Side effects included diarrhea, nausea, vomiting, and abdominal pain. Grade 3/4 toxicities occurred in 5% of patients with chronic phase of CML. Dose reductions were made in 17 of the 69 patients studied (38). In 2008, Phase II data were presented demonstrating that the drug was effective in chronic phase CML patients resistant to or intolerant of imatinib and dasatinib (39). Bosutinib is also active in patients with advanced phase CML and blast phase CML with many different imatinib-resistant BCR-ABL mutations. Only patients harboring T315I were consistently resistant to bosutinib (40). Phase III trials in CML are ongoing.

INNO-406   INNO-406 (NS-187, CNS-9) is a small molecule inhibitor in development by Innovive, under license from Nippon Shinyaku. INNO-406 inhibits ABL, SRC, and LYN kinases with IC_{50} values of 5.8, 1700, and 19 nM, respectively. At a concentration of $0.1 \mu M$, the compound has no inhibitory activity on PDGFR, BLK, or YES tyrosine kinases. The compound is active in mouse xenograft models of CML, inclucing Balb/c nu/nu mice bearing stable BaF3 cell lines expressing BCR-ABL mutants M244V, G250E, Q252H, Y253F, M351T, or H396P. However, the compound is not active against the T315I mutation. Doses as low as 0.2 mg/kg/day were effective in the xenograft models (comparable to 200 mg/kg/day of imatinib). INNO-406 is a substrate for PGP (P-glycoprotein); however, it inhibits the growth of Ph+ leukemic cell lines in the murine CNS. Additionally, cyclosporin A, a PGP inhibitor, augmented the in vivo activity of INNO-406 against CNS Ph+ leukemia (41). Phase I trials indicated that the compound has clinical activity and is safe and well tolerated. The half-life of INNO-406 is 1.76 (30 mg qd) to 4.5 h (240 mg qd). Because of the relatively short half-life, twice-daily (bid) dosing was explored. A DLT of intrahepatic cholestasis was identified at 480 mg/bid. The 240-mg bid dose was selected based on efficacy and safety for the dose expansion part of the Phase I study. The patient population in the Phase I study was heavily pretreated, with the majority of patients having previously received two or more tyrosine kinase inhibitors. INNO-406 generated cytogenetic responses in CML patients who failed one or more TKIs. There was no evidence of fluid retention and a very low level of neutropenia. Drug-related grade 3/4 adverse events included reversible elevations of liver transaminases and bilirubin, thrombocytopenia, and acute renal failures (42). Minimal mean QTc effects were observed. Pivotal Phase II studies are planned.

AT9283 AT9283 is a multargeted kinase inhibitor in development by Astex Therapeutics for a number of indications. It inhibits a number of tyrosine and threonine/serine kinases with IC_{50} values of less than 10 nM including Aurora-A and -B, JAK2 and JAK3, TYK2, RSK2, RET, MER, YES, and GSK3β. It is also a potent inhibitor of wild-type and all of the common imatinib-resistant BCR-ABL mutations, including T315I. The compound was shown to be efficacious in subcutaneous xenograft tumor models using BaF3 cells transfected with either wild-type or T315I BCR-ABL. At 12.5 mg/kg tumor regression was observed, and 50% of the mice in this dose group remained tumor free for as long as 90 days, 78 days after administration of the final dose of AT9283. Preliminary Phase I data in leukemia patients have been presented. The compound was administered intravenously for 72 hours at doses ranging from 3 to 48 mg/m^2/ day; the MTD had not been identified. Following completion of the infusion the compound was rapidly cleared. Two patients at 12 mg/m^2/day $\times$ 3 developed tumor lysis syndrome and 6 of 20 patients (30%) exhibited evidence of anti-leukemia activity, with significant reductions in bone marrow blasts ($\geq$50%) observed at all dose levels (43). Phase II trials in leukemia patients are currently enrolling.

Saracatinib (AZD0530) Saracatinib (Figure 8.1) is an orally available anilinoquinazoline derivative that inhibits both SRC family kinases and ABL, in clinical development by AstraZeneca for a wide range of tumor types. Saracatinib is not currently being developed in hematological malignancies, but its activity as a SRC inhibitor is discussed further in Section 8.2.

PHA-739358 PHA-739358 (Figure 10.8) is a small molecule 3-aminopyrazole derivative originally identified from a series of Aurora kinase inhibitors at Nerviano Medical Sciences. In biochemical assays it has significant inhibitory activity against (IC_{50} values in parentheses) Aurora-A (13 nM), Aurora-B (79 nM), Aurora-C (61 nM), FGFR1 (47 nM), ABL (25 nM), RET (31 nM), and TRKA (31 nM). PHA-739358 is discussed further in Chapter 10 (Aurora kinase inhibitors).

XL228 XL228 is a small molecule inhibitor of multiple kinases in development by Exelixis for both CML and solid tumors. In biochemical assays, it inhibits all of the common imatinib- and dasatinib-resistant mutations (including T315I) with IC_{50} values <25 nM. XL228 has additional inhibitory activities that may contribute to clinical efficacy, including (IC_{50} values in parentheses) IGF1R (2 nM), Aurora-A (3 nM), and SRC (5 nM). In a Phase I study, CML and Ph+ ALL patients received a 4-hour infusion once weekly for 4 weeks. At the time of reporting, patients enrolled in the trial included CML patients in chronic phase (10 patients), accelerated phase (3 patients), blast crisis (2 patients), and Ph+ ALL (2 patients). All patients were either imatinib resistant or intolerant, and had also been treated with dasatinib and were resistant or intolerant to the second line therapy. A total of seven patients had the T315I BCR-ABL mutation. PK analysis showed that XL228 had a long terminal half-life ($t_{1/2} = 27$–55 h). All eight subjects dosed at ≥ 3.6 mg/kg have experienced prolonged stable disease, decreased leukocytosis, and/or decreased use of hydroxyurea while on study (44). In a recent update to this study, biomarker data demonstrated inhibition of BCR-ABL (including T315I), IGF1R, and SRC. Dose-limiting toxicities of hyperglycemia and syncope were observed in two patients treated at 10.8 mg/kg, which was the maximum administered dose. Two subjects demonstrated a major cytogenetic response including a subject with Ph+ ALL harboring the T315I BCR-ABL mutation. Promising clinical activity was also seen in additional patients (45). XL228 is also discussed under IGF1R inhibitors (Section 8.5).

LS-104 LS-104 (AEG-1174; LymphoSign) is a hydroxystyrylacrylonitrile compound that inhibits BCR-ABL and JAK2, but not SRC family kinases (46). It inhibits the growth and survival of both Ph+ and Ph− ALL and AML cells but does not affect the growth and differentiation of normal cells. The compound is now in Phase II clinical trials.

AP24534 AP24534 (Ariad Pharmaceuticals) is an orally bioavailable inhibitor of BCR-ABL, with IC_{50} values of 12 nM and 58 nM for wild-type and T315I mutant kinases, respectively. The compound also crossreacts with other SRC-family kinases (SRC and LYN, $IC_{50} = 2$ and 3 nM, respectively) and with a range of other tyrosine kinases including VEGFR1, VEGFR3, VEGFR3 ($IC_{50} = 3$, 24, and 58 nM, respectively), FGFR1, FGFR2, FGFR3, FGFR4 ($IC_{50} = 0.4$, 5, 18, and 58 nM, respectively), TIE2 ($IC_{50} = 3$ nM), and FLT3 ($IC_{50} = 26$ nM) (47). AP24534 inhibits proliferation of BaF3 cells expressing wild-type or mutant BCR-ABL, with IC_{50} values ranging from 0.5 to 36 nM, and was shown to potently inhibit cell growth after only transient (3-hour) exposure to the compound. In vivo, AP24534 induces durable regression of K562 CML tumors and is also active in a BCR-ABL T315I tumor model. A Phase I clinical study in CML and other hematological malignancies was initiated in 2008.

SGX393 SGX393 is an orally bioavailable, small molecule inhibitor of the BCR-ABL tyrosine kinase in development by SGX Pharmaceuticals. The compound is in Phase I development and has shown both potent in vitro blockade of the activity of BCR-ABL and in vivo activity against human leukemic cells that depend on BCR-ABL for their uncontrolled growth and proliferation. It is reported to be active against both wild-type and many drug-resistant forms of BCR-ABL including the T315I mutation (48). Since the acquisition of SGX Pharmaceuticals by Eli Lilly and Co. in 2008, the future develoment of SGX393 is unclear.

8.2 SRC INHIBITORS

SRC family kinases, and SRC in particular, play key integrative roles in cells, relaying signals from the cell surface to the nucleus. SRC activation is associated with many cellular activities intimately linked to cancer including proliferation, survival, differentiation, and motility. Although activating mutants of SRC have been described in a subset of colon and endometrial cancers, for the most part this seems to be a rare occurrence. More commonly, this oncogene is overexpressed and/or overactivated. High levels of SRC expression/activity have been observed in most of the major tumor types (see Chapter 4). Many of the SRC inhibitors in clinical development also crossreact with BCR-ABL (Table 8.2).

Dasatinib Dasatinib is a potent, orally active inhibitor of BCR-ABL, PDGFR, and SRC family kinases and is currently marketed for the treatment of patients with chronic, accelerated, or blast phases of CML or Ph+/− ALL with resistance or intolerance to prior therapy, including imatinib. In vitro assays have shown that dasatinib directly inhibits LYN and SRC kinase activity with IC_{50} values of 8.5 and 3 nM, respectively (49). In intact prostate cancer cell lines (DU 145 and LNCaP), dasatinib dramatically reduces autophosphorylated levels of p-LYN and p-SRC at 100 nM, with potent activity observed at concentrations as low as 1–10 nM. Dasatinib treatment inhibits the proliferation of prostate tumor cells in a dose-dependent manner, with significant effects observed above 100 nM. Dasatinib also inhibited downstream substrates of SRC, namely, p-FAK and p-p130^{CAS} (49), and these effects correlated with reduced cell adhesion and cell migration. In orthotopic nude mouse models, dasatinib inhibited both tumor growth and lymph node metastases in both androgen-sensitive and androgen-resistant prostate tumors. Dasatinib has also been reported to inhibit migration and invasion of sarcoma cell lines (50), to

TABLE 8.2 SRC Inhibitors

Drug	Company	Known targets	Structure[a]	Highest phase of development
Dasatinib (BMS-354825; Sprycel®)	Bristol Myers-Squibb	ABL, EPH, FYN, LCK, SRC, PDGFR, p38	Figure 8.1	Marketed
Bosutinib (SKI-606)	Wyeth	ABL, SRC, FGR, LYN	Figure 8.1	Phase III
Saracatinib (AZD-0530)	AstraZeneca	ABL, SRC, KIT	Figure 8.1	Phase II
TG-100801	TargeGen	SRC, VEGFR, EPHB4, FGFR	Figure 8.1	Phase II
XL228	Exelixis	ABL, SRC, IGF1R, Aurora	ND	Phase I
KX2-395	Kinex	SRC	ND	Phase I

[a] ND, not disclosed.

inhibit the proliferation of a subset of breast cancer cell lines ("triple negative") (51), and to also show significant inhibitory activity against a subset of colon (52), head and neck squamous cell carcinoma, and non small cell lung cancer cells (53).

Dasatinib has been evaluated in solid tumors in several Phase I and II clinical trials. In a Phase I dose escalation study evaluating safety, tolerability, pharmacokinetics, and biomarkers of dasatinib in solid tumors, 26 patients were treated with escalating dose levels. At the highest dose (180 mg), DLTs of pleural effusions were observed in 3/9 subjects. There were no objective responses by CT scan, although 6 patients had stable disease with continued study treatment for 2–10 months (54). In a Phase II trial in patients with hormone-refractory prostate cancer, preliminary evidence of clinical activity, as measured by tumor and prostate specific antigen (PSA) response, and levels of urinary N-telopeptide (a fragment of collagen released in osteoclast-mediated bone breakdown and used as biomarker of anti-osteoclastic activity) were observed (55). Dasatinib is also being evaluated in a Phase II trial in relapsed multiple myeloma. A subset of the patients enrolled in this trial had studies of bone metabolism performed. Dasatinib therapy was associated with decreased osteoclast function, but no change in osteoblast function. There are many ongoing single agent Phase I/II trials of dasatinib ongoing in various solid tumors (e.g., prostate, lung, breast, sarcoma, hepatocellular carcinoma, colorectal, pancreatic, mesothelioma), as well as combination studies with gemcitabine, cetuximab, erlotinib, capecitabine, bortezomib, and other regimens.

Bosutinib   Bosutinib (SKI-606) is a small molecule orally available inhibitor of SRC and ABL kinases in development by Wyeth to treat CML, Ph+ ALL, and also solid tumors. In in vitro biochemical assays, bosutinib inhibits SRC kinase activity with a reported IC_{50} of 1.2 nM. In cell-based assays, it blocks SRC autophosphorylation and the phosphorylation of downstream target proteins and submicromolar concentrations and, in addition, has antiproliferative activity against colon (HT29 and Colo205) tumor cell lines at somewhat higher (micromolar) concentrations (56). Bosutinib also demonstrated dose-dependent antitumor activity against HT29 tumor xenografts in nude mice over a dose range of 25–100 mg/kg/day (36).

Clinical trials have demonstrated that the compound has a favorable toxicity profile and clinical activity in patients with CML (see Section 8.1). Phase I data on bosutinib in patients with solid tumors showed that the compound was generally well tolerated with predominantly gastrointestinal adverse events. Evaluation of an expanded cohort restricted to patients with colorectal, pancreatic, and NSCLC tumors is ongoing. One patient with pancreatic cancer had stable disease >52 weeks (57). Phase II trials evaluating bosutinib in combination with exemestane, with capecitabine and with letrozole are ongoing.

Saracatinib (AZD0530)   Saracatinib (AZD0530) is an orally available SRC/ABL inhibitor in clinical development by AstraZeneca for a wide range of tumor types. The compound has an in vitro IC_{50} value in SRC enzyme assays of 2.5 nM, and in cell-based assays it inhibits SRC transformed NIH-3T3 cell proliferation with an IC_{50} value of 76 nM and A549 cell motility with an IC_{50} value of

140 nM. Other kinases inhibited in in vitro assays are CSK ($IC_{50} = 840$ nM), YES (4 nM), LCK (<4 nM), ABL (30 nM), and KIT (200 nM). Saracatinib also inhibits the tumor growth of SRC transformed NIH-3T3 fibroblasts, with >95% inhibition of tumor growth observed at oral doses of 6 mg/kg/day (58). Saracatinib also inhibits the invasion and migration of anti-hormone resistant and anti-growth factor receptor resistant breast tumor cells, although it has only modest inhibitory effects on their growth rate (59, 60). Saracatinib treatment led to cell cycle arrest, inhibition of migration, and apoptosis of several NSCLC cell lines with activating mutations in the kinase domain of EGFR. Saracatinib also inhibited growth and induced cell cycle arrest without inducing apoptosis in wild-type EGFR cell lines that are sensitive to the EGFR inhibitor gefitinib, as well as in the gefitinib-resistant H1703 cell line. Chronic dosing with saracatinib resulted in a moderate growth delay for 4/9 xenograft models screened (AsPc1, Calu6, BT474C, and MDA-MB-231T). In the remainder of the xenograft panel (ZR-75-1, Colo205, HT29, LoVo, and HPAC), saracatinib treatment failed to inhibit primary tumor growth (61). In prostate cancer cells, saracatinib treatment suppressed cell growth, induced cell cycle arrest, and reduced cell migration. In an orthotopically implanted DU 145 (prostate cancer) mouse xenograft model, saracatinib inhibited tumor growth (saracatinib treatment started shortly after implantation) (62). Saracatinib inhibits prostate (PC3) cell growth in a dose-dependent manner, as well as blocking the expression of IL8, urokinase plasminogen activator, and matrix metalloproteinase 9, suggesting that the compound many inhibit cancer cell invasion into bone matrix (63).

In a Phase I ascending single- and multiple-dose study to assess the safety, tolerability, and pharmacokinetics of saracatinib, the drug was well tolerated when administered in single doses up to 500 mg and multiple once-daily doses up to 250 mg. The principal adverse events were gastrointestinal (64). In a second Phase I trial paired tumor biopsies were acquired for investigation of SRC inhibition. Dose limiting toxicities occurred in 3 patients at the 250-mg dose, and in 2 patients at 200 mg; doses of 50, 125, and 175 mg were tolerated. Consistent modulation of the downstream mediators paxillin and FAK (phosphorylation and/or cellular localization) was observed, confirming inhibition of SRC in human cancers (65). Saracatinib is now being evaluated in a number of Phase II protocols on various solid tumors (e.g., head and neck, small cell lung, breast, prostate, stomach, ovarian, soft tissue sarcoma, melanoma, thymoma, and pancreatic).

8.3   JAK2 INHIBITORS

In just a little over a decade since the original cloning of JAK2 by Wilks and colleagues (66), this protein has distinguished itself as being far more than "just another kinase." The recent observations that the JAK2 V617F mutation was associated with several myeloproliferative diseases, rare cases of AML, and even rare cases of BCR-ABL negative CML elevated this kinase to one of the "hot new drug targets" of recent years. Within 3 years from the first description of the

TABLE 8.3   JAK2 Inhibitors

Drug	Company	Known targets	Structure[a]	Highest phase of development
Lestaurtinib (CEP-701)	Cephalon	FLT3, JAK2, JAK3, TRKA, RET	Figure 8.5	Phase II
INCB018424	Incyte	JAK1, JAK2	ND	Phase II
TG-101348	TargeGen	JAK2, FLT3, RET	Figure 8.2	Phase I
XL019	Exelixis	JAK2	ND	Phase I
LS-104 (AEG-41174)	Aegera	ABL, JAK-2	Figure 8.1	Phase I
AT-9283	Astex	Aurora-A, Aurora-B, TYK2, JAK2, JAK3, RSK2, RET, MER, YES, GSK3β	Figure 8.5	Phase II

[a] ND, not disclosed.

V617F mutation, several small molecule JAK2 inhibitors entered clinical trials (Table 8.3).

Lestaurtinib   Lestaurtinib (CEP-701, KT-5555) is an indolocarbazole derivative, derived from the microbial compound, broad specificity kinase inhibitor, K252. Lestaurtinib is described as an orally active FLT3, TRKA, and JAK2 inhibitor under development by Cephalon for the potential treatment of cancer. The parent compound, CEP-751 (lestaurtinib was later identified as an active metabolite), inhibits TRK family RTKs, inhibits the growth of SY5Y neuroblastoma xenografts expressing TRKB, and potentiates the effects of topotecan plus cyclophosphamide in this xenograft model (67, 68). In in vitro models with prostate cancer cells, lestaurtinib inhibits cell growth, cell migration, and invasion (69, 70) and also inhibits metastasis and enhances host survival in in vivo models using prostate cancer cells (71). Lestaurtinib also demonstrated significant antitumor activity in a number of pancreatic ductal adenocarcinoma xenografts (72, 73). Lestaurtinib was shown to be a potent inhibitor of FLT3 in BaF3/ITD cells, reverting the cells to IL3-dependent growth. The compound was also cytotoxic to FLT3-expressing leukemic cells such as MV-4-11 and EOL-1 (74). Lestaurtinib was selectively cytotoxic in pediatric AML cell preparations with FLT3-ITDs and pediatric ALL samples with overexpressed FLT3 or FLT3-ITDs (75). Reported in vitro IC_{50} values for tyrosine kinases are 3.7 nM for TRKA, 65 nM for VEGFR2, 218 nM for PKC, >500 nM for KIT, CSF1R, and PDGFRβ, and >1000 nM for IR and EGFR. Preclinical data indicate that lestaurtinib is a low nanomolar inhibitor of wild-type and V617F-mutated JAK2 in vitro and also inhibited the growth of cells from patients with PV, ET, and agnogenic myeloid metaplasia (76). Lestaurtinib also inhibits JAK3 in vitro, although human safety data to date has not indicated any significant immunosuppression (76). Lestaurtinib is also a low nanomolar inhibitor of the proto-oncogene RET and inhibits the growth of medullary thryoid cancers in culture (77, 78). Lestaurtinib inhibits the growth of HEL92.1.7 cells (which express the V617F JAK2 mutation) and also inhibits erythroid cell expansion from CD34$^+$ cells isolated from patients with myeloproliferative disease (76).

In April 2006, a Phase II/III trial for AML was initiated. The compound also was awarded orphan drug status from the FDA for this indication. Earlier trials in pancreatic and prostate cancer did not show promising efficacy (79, 80). However, in a Phase II trial of 42 relapsed AML patients, the compound was well tolerated, and 5 patients achieved complete responses (81). This activity is thought to be due to the FLT3 directed activity of the compound. In June 2007, a nonrandomized, uncontrolled open-label Phase II trial was initiated in myelofibrosis patients. Patients with primary myelofibrosis or myelofibrosis secondary to polycythemia vera or essential thrombocythemia with the JAK2 V617F mutation were enrolled. Clinical data presented in 2007 indicated that 5 of the 11 patients treated had shown disease stabilization (82). As of April 2008, Phase II trials of lestaurtinib in patients with polycythemia vera (PV) or essential thrombocytosis (ET) were initiated. A Phase II trial of lestaurtinib in combination with chemotherapy in infants with newly diagnosed ALL was also initiated in April 2008.

LS-104 LS-104 (Figure 8.1) is a small molecule kinase inhibitor of JAK2 and BCR-ABL, in development by Aegera Therapeutics for the treatment of leukemia and other hematological malignancies and MPDs. LS-104 inhibits its targets in a non-ATP-competitive manner and thus may be active on resistance mutations that have arisen due to mutations in the ATP binding site. LS-104 exhibits preferential induction of apoptosis of AML and ALL cells while being relatively nontoxic to normal bone marrow cells. LS-104 has demonstrated efficacy in animal models of leukemia. It is currently being tested in a Phase I, open-label, dose-escalating study in combination with cytarabine in patients with hematological malignancies and myeloproliferative disorders.

AT9283 AT9283 is a multitargeted inhibitor of JAK2 ($IC_{50} = 1.2$ nM), ABL (30 nM), T315I ABL (4 nM), Aurora-A (3 nM), and Aurora-B (3 nM) (83, 84). In vitro, AT9283 inhibited direct downstream substrates of JAK2 (STAT5) and BCR-ABL (CRKL) in HEL (erythroleukemia) and K562 (CML) cells, respectively. In Vivo, the compound also inhibited STAT5 phosphorylation in a HEL sc xenograft model. AT9283 has been shown to induce tumor growth arrest in a number of xenograft models. Patient dosing began in a Phase I/IIa clinical study in patients with hematological tumors including relapsed or refractory acute leukemias, chromic myeloid leukemia, or high-risk myelodysplastic syndromes in Q3 2006 in the United States and a Phase I clinical study in patients with solid tumors commenced at two sites in the United Kingdom in Q4 2006 and a further Phase I study in patients with solid tumors in Canada was initiated in Q1 2007. The compound was being administered as a 72-h continuous intravenous (IV) infusion at dose levels ranging from 3 to 49 mg/m^2. Two patients receiving the 12 mg/m^2 dose developed tumor lysis syndrome, and 30% of the patients (a total of 20 patients had been treated) exhibited anti-leukemic activity with significant reductions in bone marrow blasts. A 1-hour treatment with AT9283 was shown to inhibit substrates of Aurora-B and JAK2. The terminal $t_{1/2}$ was 6–13 h (84).

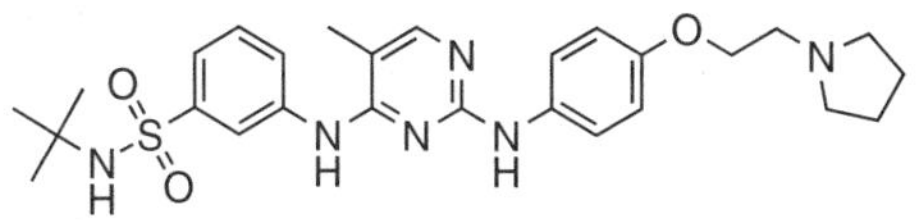

TG-101348

Figure 8.2 Structure of JAK2 inhibitor.

TG-101348 TG-101348 (Figure 8.2) is an orally available, potent, and selective inhibitor of JAK2, FLT3, and RET. In vitro, TG-101348 exhibits potent inhibitory activity against JAK2 ($IC_{50} = 3$ nM), FLT3 (15 nM), and RET (48 nM). Within the JAK family, it demonstrates 340-fold selectivity against JAK3, 135-fold selectivity against TYK2, and 35-fold selectivity against JAK1. In MV-4-11 cells, which have a FLT3-ITD, the compound exhibits a 57-nM IC_{50}, in HEL (JAK2 V617F) a 300-nM IC_{50}, in MOLM13 (FLT3-ITD) a 69-nM IC_{50}, and in Kasumi-1 cells (KIT mutation) a 266-nM IC_{50}. The compound induces tumor regression at 120 mg/kg given orally (po) in MV-4-11 xenograft models. In a mouse model of JAK2V617F-induced PV, TG-101348 showed therapeutic efficacy, including a statistically significant reduction in hematocrit, normalization of white blood cell count, a dose-dependent reduction in extramedullary hematopoiesis in the spleen and liver, and marked attenuation of myelofibrosis. There was no significant change in T-cell number in treated animals (85, 86). TG-101348 also inhibited ex vivo hematopoietic colony growth in cells derived from MPD patients (85, 87). TG-101348 also inhibits FLT3 autophosphorylation in MV-4-11 cells and exhibits potent antiproliferative effects in FLT3-ITD positive cell lines MV-4-11 (EC_{50} 57 nM) and MOLM13 (EC_{50} 69 nM)(88). In January 2008, a multicenter Phase I/II clinical trial of TG-101348 was initiated to evaluate the safety, tolerability, maximum tolerated dose, pharmacokinetics, pharmacodynamics, and preliminary clinical activity in patients with myelofibrosis. Patients received oral daily doses for 28-day cycles. Initial results from this study showed that the maximum tolerated dose was not reached at a daily dose of 800 mg and plasma pharmacokinetics was dose-proportional for doses between 30 and 520 mg/day, with a half-life of ~23–35 h. Adverse events included nausea/vomiting, diarrhea, abdominal pain, and grade 3/4 myelosuppression. Some early signs of clinical activity were seen, notably decreased splenomegaly (89).

INCB018424 INCB018424 is a small molecule JAK2 inhibitor in development by Incyte for the potential treatment of cancer, inflammation, and psoriasis. INCB018424 is a potent inhibitor of JAK1 ($IC_{50} = 2.7$ nM), JAK2 (4.5 nM), and TYK2 (19 nM) but not JAK3 (322 nM). The compound is also a potent inhibitor of BaF3 cells expressing JAK2V617F (IC_{50} 100–130 nM) and inhibits the cytokine-independent formation of erythroid progenitor colonies using cells harvested from JAK2V617F positive PV patients with an IC_{50} of 67 nM. In a mouse model of MPD, INCB018424 markedly reduced splenomegaly and eliminates neoplastic cells from the spleen, liver, and bone marrow, normalizing the histology of the affected organs and significantly prolonging survival (90). Initial data from the Phase I/II trial of INCB018424 given orally twice a day (bid) in patients with PPMF and post PV/ET MF were presented in December 2007. The initial oral dose of 25 mg bid resulted in a rapid and marked reduction in splenomegaly. PK/PD studies have shown the administered INCB018424 resulted in plasma drug concentrations sufficient to inhibit JAK2, as shown by the reduction in phosphorylated STAT3 in whole blood in the three patients in the first cohort (91). Inflammatory cytokines are elevated in the plasma of MF patients, and recent data from an ongoing Phase I/II trial in MF patients (dosed at 25–50 mg bid) showed that treatment with INCB018424 induced a rapid decrease in MF-associated plasma cytokines, in parallel with reductions in spleen size, reduction in constitutive JAK2 actvation in PBMC, and improvement in MF symptoms (fatigue, night sweats, pruritis). INCB018424 also improved the nutritional status of the patients and was associated with a modest, but significant, decrease in JAK2 V617F allele burden. Overall the compound was well tolerated, with a median duration of therapy of 7 months (92–94). Phase II trials in several indications (polycythemia vera, essential thrombocythemia, multiple myeloma, prostate cancer, psoriasis, and rheumatoid arthritis) are in progress.

XL019   XL019 is a potent and reversible inhibitor of JAK2, with a K_I of 2 nM. It is at least 50-fold selective against a panel of 120 other protein kinases, including other JAK family members, and inhibits STAT signaling in cell lines expressing both wild-type and V617FJAK2. The compound inhibits proliferation in cell lines with activity or overexpressed JAK2, with IC_{50} values ranging from 386 nM to 7 μM, and has shown antitumor efficacy in DU 145 and HEL xenograft models (95). In a Phase I dose escalation study, the compound demonstrated rapid and marked reductions in splenomegaly at all doses tested and reduction in erythropoietin-independent colony formation as well as a reduction in the number of cells with the JAK2V617F mutation. There was also a correlation between XL019 exposure and decreased STAT phosphorylation (95). Evaluation of safety data indicated that neuropathy was associated with compound treatment, and additional Phase I studies with lower doses were initiated. Updated Phase I data from 25 MF patients receiving either 25 mg or 50 mg of XL019 were recently presented. Evidence of clinical activity (reduction in spleen size, leukocytosis, relief of constitutional symptoms) was seen in patients with JAK2 V617F or MPL W515L mutations. XL019 was well tolerated with no drug-related hematologic adverse events. Mild neuropathy was seen in 1/16 patients at 25 mg and 2/5 patients at 50 mg. Of note, three of four preleukemic transformation patients showed a reduction in the levels of circulating blasts after the first cycle of XL019, and a duration on study of 2.5, 3+, and 7+ months (96). XL019 development has currently been discontinued.

8.4   EGFR/ERBB INHIBITORS

As outlined in Chapter 3, EGF receptor was one of the first kinases to be associated with cancer and, as a result, was among the first kinases to be targeted by both small molecule and antibody therapeutics. These efforts resulted in the approval of two antibodies (cetuximab and panitumumab) and two small molecules (gefitinib and erlotinib, although as discussed later gefitinib is no longer widely used outside Asia). However, the anti-ERBB2 antibody trastuzumab was the first agent targeting ERBB receptors to be approved by the FDA in 1998, for treatment of HER2-positive metastatic breast cancer in combination with paclitaxel. The selection of patients with HER2-positive tumors (and associated diagnostic assay) was of paramount importance in demonstrating therapeutic benefit in this population, and elucidation of the molecular and clinical determinants of response continues to be a major research interest for ERBB family kinase inhibitors. More recently, lapatinib—a small molecule targeting both EGFR and ERBB2—was also approved for treatment of metastatic breast cancer in combination with capecitabine, and as discussed in this chapter there are numerous additional small molecules with varying kinase specificities (both within and outside the ERBB receptor family) in various stages of clinical testing. Molecules that target multiple members of the ERBB receptor family, some of which bind irreversibly to the EGFR/ERBB2 kinase domain, are currently of particular interest (97).

Although our focus here is on small molecule inhibitors (Table 8.4), a brief summary of clinical results with anti-ERBB antibodies is warranted. Several antibodies targeting EGFR or ERBB2 have undergone clinical trials and three of these are FDA approved: cetuximab, panitumumab, and trastuzumab. There are currently no clinical data with antibodies targeting the ERBB3 or ERBB4 receptors, but an anti-ERBB3 antibody (MM-121) was recently advanced into clinical studies (Merrimack Pharmaceuticals press release).

Cetuximab is a human–mouse chimeric antibody that binds to and inhibits EGFR (98). Phase I studies showed that cetuximab is generally well tolerated, with some evidence of the acneiform rash common to most EGFR inhibitors (see later discussion) and a low incidence of allergic reaction (99). Clinical studies with this antibody have demonstrated modest single-agent activity in EGFR-expressing, chemotherapy-refractory colorectal cancer, with a response rate of approximately 10% (100, 101). However, a higher response rate was observed when cetuximab was coadministered with irinotecan, even though patients had previously progressed on irinotecan therapy: furthermore, median time to progression was significantly longer in the combination group (102). These studies led to the FDA approval of cetuximab, with or without concomitant irinotecan, in irinotecan-refractory colorectal cancer. Cetuximab has also demonstrated encouraging activity in combination with oxaliplatin-based therapies in colorectal cancer (103) and may also have utility when added to the FOLFIRI chemotherapy regimen in first line colorectal cancer patients with wild-type KRAS (104). Cetuximab was also approved by the FDA in combination with radiotherapy for treatment of head and neck squamous cell carcinoma, following demonstration that the combination treatment produced longer progression-free survival and overall survival compared to radiotherapy alone (105). Additional Phase II studies have shown clinical benefit in combining cetuximab with platinum-based chemotherapy in NSCLC (106). In a large randomized Phase III trial (FLEX), the effect of adding cetuximab to cisplatin/vinorelbine chemotherapy was evaluated in first line NSCLC, yielding a modest increase in overall survival (11.3 months vs. 10.1 months) (107).

TABLE 8.4   ERBB Inhibitors

Name	Company	Known targets	Structure	Highest phase of development
Gefitinib (ZD1839, Iressa®)	AstraZeneca	EGFR	Figure 8.3	Marketed
Erlotinib (OSI774; Tarceva®)	OSI/Genentech	EGFR	Figure 8.3	Marketed
Lapatinib (GW572016; Tykerb®)	GlaxoSmithKline	EGFR, ERBB2	Figure 8.3	Marketed
Vandetanib (ZD6474; Zactima®)	AstraZeneca	EGFR, VEGF, RET	Figure 9.1	Phase III
XL647	Exelixis	EGFR, ERBB2, VEGFR2, FLT4, EPHB4	ND	Phase II
PF-00299804	Pfizer	EGFR > ERBB2, ErbB4	ND	Phase II
BIBW 2992	Boehringer Ingelheim	EGFR, ERBB2	Figure 8.3	Phase II
Neratinib (HKI-272)	Wyeth	EGFR, ERBB2	Figure 8.3	Phase II
AV-412	AVEO	EGFR, ERBB2, ABL	Figure 8.3	Phase I
CP-724,714	Pfizer	ERBB2	Figure 8.3	Phase I
BMS-599626	Bristol-Myers Squibb	EGFR, ERBB2, ERBB4	ND	Phase I
BMS-690514	Bristol-Myers Squibb	EGFR > ERBB2, VEGFR	Figure 8.3	Phase I
ARRY-543	Array	EGFR, ERBB2, ERBB4	ND	Phase I
ARRY-380	Array	ERBB2	ND	Phase I
AZD-4769	AstraZeneca	EGFR?	ND	Phase I
AZD-8931	AstraZeneca	ERBB?	ND	Phase I
Pelitinib (EKB-569)	Wyeth	EGFR > ERBB2	Figure 8.3	Suspended
Canertinib (CI-1033)	Pfizer	EGFR, ERBB2	Figure 8.3	Suspended?
AEE788	Novartis	EGFR, ERBB2 > VEGFR1, VEGFR2, SRC, ABL	Figure 8.3	Suspended?

Another anti-EGFR antibody, panitumumab, has also been shown to have activity in chemotherapy-refractory colorectal cancer and was approved by the FDA for this indication in 2006 (108). Additional clinical studies with this agent are ongoing in patients with head and neck, esophageal, and lung tumors. Three additional anti-EGFR antibodies are in clinical trials. Nimotuzumab (YM Biosciences) is approved in India for treatment of head and neck cancer in combination with radiation and is also undergoing studies in glioma, pancreatic, and lung cancers. Zalutumumab (Medarex/Genmab) is in a Phase III trial for head and neck cancer and IMC-11F8 (Imclone) is in a Phase II study for colorectal carcinoma.

The anti-EGFR antibody matuzumab (EMD Pharmaceuticals/Takeda) blocks EGFR dimerization and has also been evaluated in early clinical studies: however, no recent development activity has been reported.

Trastuzumab is a humanized form of the mouse antibody 4D5 that targets the human ERBB2 receptor (109), although its precise mechanism of antitumor activity remains a source of debate. Trastuzumab binds to the juxtamembrane region of the ERBB2 extracellular domain (110) and may thereby impair efficient association with other ERBB family members and/or inhibit extracellular domain cleavage by disintegrin (ADAM) metalloproteinases. However, antibody binding may also downregulate ERBB2 in tumor cells, and the antibody Fc regions may contribute to antibody-dependent cell killing. Clinical studies have been conducted in breast cancer patients with overexpression of ERBB2 (as determined by immunohisto-chemistry and/or fluorescence in situ hybridization analysis (FISH)). Initial Phase I and II trials of trastuzumab established safety and preliminary activity, both as a single agent and in combination with chemotherapy (111). Initial approval was granted following a Phase III trial in which trastuzumab in combination with chemotherapy was compared to chemotherapy alone in previously untreated patients with HER2-positive metastatic breast cancer. Addition of trastuzumab to chemotherapy produced significant increases in time to progression, response rate, and overall survival (112). However, a study of single-agent trastuzumab in patients with ERBB2-overexpressing breast cancer who had received no prior chemotherapy showed a 26% response rate (35% in patients with strong ERBB2 overexpression), suggesting that trastuzumab alone may have utility in metastatic breast cancer (113). Multiple studies have shown potential benefit of adding trastuzumab to various chemotherapy regimens in adjuvant and neoadjuvant therapy of early stage breast cancer (reviewed in (114)): however, long-term follow-up of these studies is still in progress. In general, trastuzumab is well tolerated: the major toxicological concern is cardiac dysfunction, observed in a small fraction of patients treated with trastuzumab alone and a higher fraction of patients treated with a combination of trastuzumab and chemotherapy. Further details of safety and efficacy are summarized in a recent, comprehensive review of clinical experience with trastuzumab (114). More recently, a second anti-ERBB2 antibody, pertuzumab, has been evaluated clinically. The mechanism of action of this molecule differs from trastuzumab in that it binds to a region of the receptor that is critically involved in dimerization. Preliminary safety and clinical activity have been reported (115), and there are preclinical data supporting the combination of pertuzumab and trastuzumab in breast cancer (116). A Phase II study of pertuzumab and trastuzumab suggested that this combination may indeed have clinical benefit in ERBB2-positive metastatic breast cancer patients who have progressed on trastuzumab, although impaired cardiac function was also noted (117).

8.4.1 Determinants of Response and Resistance to ERBB Inhibitors

Multiple ERBB inhibitors—both antibodies and small molecules—have been shown to produce objective responses in cancer patients, although the response rates across broad populations are relatively modest. However, the growing body of data from multiple clinical trials is starting to reveal some of the factors that may predispose individuals to ERBB inhibitor sensitivity. In particular, clinical experience with the EGFR inhibitors erlotinib and gefitinib has highlighted the importance of mutations within the EGFR gene as well as other molecular factors as determinants of response to therapy. The best characterized disease setting is non small cell lung cancer (NSCLC); EGFR kinase domain mutations have been detected in other tumor types but they are relatively rare. Multiple studies with EGFR inhibitors in NSCLC have shown that although clinical benefit is observed, it is restricted to a relatively small (~10%) subset of patients. Subset analysis of clinical trials evaluating erlotinib and gefitinib in NSCLC showed that several factors were correlated with clinical activity: responders were more frequently found among women than men, in never-smokers compared to smokers, in patients of Asian ethnicity compared to other racial groups, and in patients whose tumors had histological features of adenocarcinoma (118–120). (These factors may not be completely independent: for example, never-smokers are more common among women than men.) It was subsequently determined that these subgroups of patients were more likely to have mutations in regions of the kinase domain encoded by exons 18–21, and that these mutations conferred sensitivity to gefitinib and erlotinib (121–123). Mutations are found in about 10% of lung adenocarcinomas in the United States and ~30% of lung adenocarcinomas in Asia. Several dozen mutations have been identified, but the vast majority fall into one of two classes: 45% have deletion of a short segment in exon 19 around amino acids 746–750, and 40–45% contain a point mutation in exon 21 (most frequently L858R), in a region encoding the activation segment of the kinase (124, 125). Two other regions of the protein are also known to harbor mutations associated with drug sensitivity: approximately 5% of tumors have mutations in the nucleotide binding loop (e.g., substitutions of G317C/S/A) encoded by exon 18, and a smaller fraction of mutations are scattered throughout exon 20 (Appendix I). The enhanced sensitivity conferred by these mutations is thought to be due to two related factors. First, mutations that increase the basal activity of the kinase may render tumors more dependent on EGFR signaling, and hence more sensitive to its inactivation: the "oncogene addiction" hypothesis (126). For example, the L858R mutation destabilizes the inactive form of the kinase and increases the second-order rate constant for kinase activity by 20-fold ((127); see also Chapter 7). Moreover, ERBB3, which can form a potent heterodimeric signaling complex with EGFR, may associate preferentially with mutant rather than wild-type receptors (128). Second, the same mutations that increase cellular EGFR kinase activity may also potentiate the interaction with small molecule inhibitors, thus increasing the fraction of kinase activity inhibited (relative to the wild-type protein) for a given dose of drug. Both the L858R and exon 19 deletion mutants bind more weakly to ATP but more tightly to erlotinib compared to wild-type EGFR (129).

Mutational status is a clear predictor of response: while the overall response rate in unselected patients is around 10%, retrospective analysis of multiple studies with gefitinib and erlotinib and subsequent prospective studies show a 75–80%

response rate in patients with mutations (reviewed in (125)). However, EGFR mutant tumors may be generally more sensitive to other therapeutic modalities as well as EGFR inhibitors. In a study comparing chemotherapy (carboplatin + paclitaxel) with and without concomitant erlotinib treatment in previously untreated NSCLC patients, improved survival was seen in patients with EGFR mutations irrespective of whether they received erlotinib or not (130). Also, different mutations appear to have different effects on outcome in response to EGFR inhibitors, with patients harboring exon 19 deletion mutations having significantly longer overall survival than patients with exon 21 point mutations (131, 132). Finally, it is also worth noting that although the response rate for patients without mutant receptors is low, it is not zero—indicating that there are likely to be other factors that can elicit sensitivity. Amplification of EGFR may be one such mechanism, since several studies show that patients with amplification or polysomy of EGFR have a higher response rate than those without: however, in most cases of NSCLC amplification is also associated with mutation (133). Increased EGFR copy number is also associated with response to cetuximab in combination with chemotherapy in NSCLC (134). Overexpression of ERBB2 may also impact sensitivity to EGFR inhibitors, even in the case of inhibitors like gefitinib that have no appreciable activity toward ERBB2 (135). ERBB2 mutations have also been found in NSCLC (Appendix II), although they are quite rare (136).

Several factors have been associated with resistance to EGFR inhibitors in NSCLC. The presence of KRAS mutations is perhaps the most clear molecular indicator of primary resistance: notably, mutations in KRAS tend to be mutually exclusive with mutations in EGFR and, consistent with this, are also more prevalent in smokers compared to nonsmokers (137, 138). The negative prognostic value of KRAS mutation has been found consistently in multiple studies with EGFR inhibitors (139–142). Acquired resistance to gefitinib or erlotinib—the resumption of tumor growth following an initial response—is seen in virtually all responding patients and is attributed in about 50% of cases to emergence of the EGFR T790M mutation (143). The effect of this mutation at the "gatekeeper" position in the kinase active site was initially thought to sterically hinder drug binding but is more likely to be due to increased affinity for ATP, thus making it more difficult for ATP-competitive drugs to compete for binding (144). A different resistance mutation, D761Y in exon 19, has also been found in a patient with acquired resistance to gefitinib (145). More recently, additional resistance mechanisms have been proposed, notably altered EGFR trafficking (146), IGF1R signaling (147, 148), and amplification of the MET tyrosine kinase receptor (149, 150).

The molecular determinants of response to erlotinib and gefitinib have also been examined in glioblastoma (GBM), wherein EGF receptor is frequently over-expressed and is often present as the truncated EGFRvIII form (Chapter 3). In one study, tumor tissue from patients treated with erlotinib or gefitinib was examined for the presence of EGFR/ERBB2 mutations and expression of EGFRvIII and PTEN (151). Both EGFRvIII and PTEN expression were more prevalent in responders than in nonresponders, and coexpression of both EGFRvIII and PTEN showed a particularly strong correlation with response. No kinase domain point mutations were found in either EGFR or ERBB2. In another Phase I study with erlotinib, EGFR overexpression and amplification were associated with response (although no responders were found to have EGFRvIII) and levels of phosphorylated AKT were inversely associated with response (152). As in the case of NSCLC the data are consistent with the "oncogene addiction" hypothesis; that is, tumors with constitutively activated EGF receptors may be more sensitive to inhibition of those receptors (126). Loss of PTEN may decouple EGFR from downstream PI3K signaling, leading to loss of sensitivity to EGFR inhibitors. In colorectal cancer, EGFR copy number has been explored as a potential determinant of sensitivity. A study of 31 colorectal cancer patients treated with cetuximab found that 8/9 responders, but only 1/15 nonresponders, had EGFR amplification as determined by FISH (153). These results were supported by a recent retrospective analysis of cetuximab (154) and with another anti-EGFR antibody, panitumumab (155). In contrast, a similar analysis of response to gefitinib in colorectal cancer showed that neither amplification nor overexpression of EGFR was associated with response (156). As with NSCLC, KRAS mutation is associated with primary resistance and poor outcome in colorectal carcinoma (157).

Molecular determinants of response have also been evaluated for the dual EGFR/ERBB2 inhibitor lapatinib in patients with inflammatory breast cancer (158). Responses were seen in 50% of patients whose tumors overexpressed ERBB2 (ERBB2+), but in only 1/15 patients with EGFR overexpression. Furthermore, within the ERBB2+ cohort, expression of ERBB3 and lack of p53 were significantly associated with response. ERBB3 and ERBB2 form particularly potent signaling heterodimers, and ERBB3 has been associated with loss of response to trastuzumab (159, 160). It is also notable that antitumor activity of lapatinib appears to be insensitive to loss of PTEN, which, along with mutational activation of PI3K, has been implicated in resistance to trastuzumab (161–163). Collectively, PTEN loss and PI3K mutation (which tend to be mutually exclusive in tumor samples) may be one of the main causes of intrinsic resistance to trastuzumab, which, although clinically useful, only produces objective responses in 50% of patients when combined with chemotherapy in previously untreated ERBB2+ breast cancer patients.

In general, EGFR inhibitors have been well tolerated clinically, with the main toxicities being diarrhea and acneiform rash. Diarrhea may be a target-related toxicity, since EGFR is known to be expressed on the basolateral side of the human gastrointestinal tract where it plays a role in repair of damaged tissue (164). Rash (along with other dermatological toxicities) is observed with both small molecule and antibody inhibitors and is also likely to be an EGFR-mediated response, reflecting the role of EGFR in the proliferation, differentiation, migration, and survival of keratinocytes and associated dermal cells (165, 166). Although frequently described as acneiform, the typical "EGFR rash" presents with different histological and clinical features compared to common acne, exhibiting no "blackheads" and frequently accompanied by pruritis. The rash is typically reversible, even in the presence of continuing EGFR inhibitor therapy, and can frequently be treated with anti-inflammatory agents. The appearance of rash in patients treated with EGFR inhibitors has been associated with a greater likelihood of response and longer survival, for both small molecule and antibody-based therapies and in multiple diseases including NSCLC, head and neck squamous cell carcinoma, colorectal cancer, and GBM (167). Experience with the dual EGFR/ERBB2 inhibitor lapatinib suggests that although dermatologic events are still observed, they are less frequent and not as severe as with single-targeted EGFR inhibitors (168).

Gefitinib Gefitinib (Iressa®, ZD1839; Figure 8.3) was the first small molecule inhibitor of EGFR to enter clinical trials. In preclinical studies, a K_I value of 2.1 nM was determined for binding to EGFR (169); the inhibition appears to be very specific, with only the cyclin G-associated kinase (GAK) showing crossreactivity (170). Inhibition of EGFR autophosphorylation was demonstrated in several cancer cell lines including DU 145, A549, HT29, and KB. This in vitro activity was recapitulated in vivo, with inhibition of EGFR phosphorylation and tumor growth inhibition in these cell lines grown as tumor xenografts (169). Further studies in vitro and in xenograft models have highlighted the potential for gefitinib to enhance the potency of chemotherapy agents (171, 172).

Phase I studies evaluated continual (173, 174) or 14 days on/14 days off (175, 176) dosing regimens and collectively indicated a maximum tolerated dose of 800–1000 mg daily. Steady state levels were achieved following 10 days of administration, and the elimination half-life was 48 h. The most prominent side effects were diarrhea and rash, and as outlined earlier, these toxicities have since been associated with other EGFR inhibitors. Several objective responses were noted, particularly in patients with NSCLC, prompting further evaluation of gefitinib in this disease. Daily doses of 250 and 500 mg were selected for evaluation in Phase II studies in patients with NSCLC who were refractory to chemotherapy (118, 119). In these trials (IDEAL 1 and 2), clinical benefit and objective responses were seen at both doses, leading to FDA approval in 2003.

However, the initial promise of this new mode of therapy was short lived. The Phase III ISEL trial, evaluating a 250-mg dose of gefitinib in patients with previously treated advanced NSCLC, failed to show a significant increase in median survival compared to placebo (177), although gefitinib-treated patients survived longer than placebo-treated patients in two specific patient subsets: patients of Asian origin and never-smokers. Gefitinib was also evaluated in combination with gemcitabine/cisplatin and carboplatin/paclitaxel in the INTACT 1 and INTACT 2 trials, respectively (178, 179). Despite acceptable tolerability for adding gefitinib to the chemotherapy regimens, no improvement in overall survival or response rate was seen in either case.

Gefitinib has also been evaluated in many other diseases apart from NSCLC (180). In squamous cell carcinoma of the head and neck (SCCHN), a response rate of ~10% was found, similar to that of cetuximab (181). This study enrolled patients with recurrent or metastatic SCCHN who had no more than one prior systemic therapy and no prior exposure to EGFR antagonists. Gefitinib was well tolerated, with acneiform rash and diarrhea being the major toxicities: notably, appearance of rash was strongly associated with longer progression-free survival and overall survival. In general, however, few objective responses have been observed with single-agent gefitinib in various other tumor types including breast, colon, brain, renal, gastric, and ovarian cancers. For example, a study of single-agent gefintinib (administered

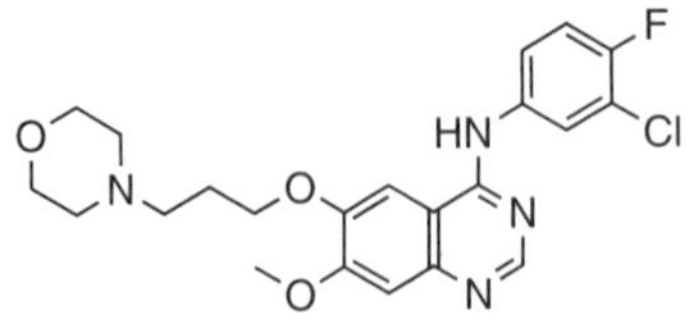

Gefitinib

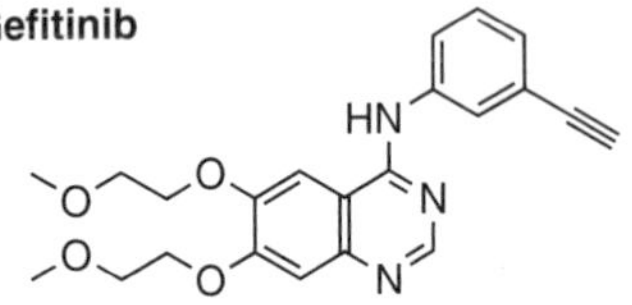

Erlotinib

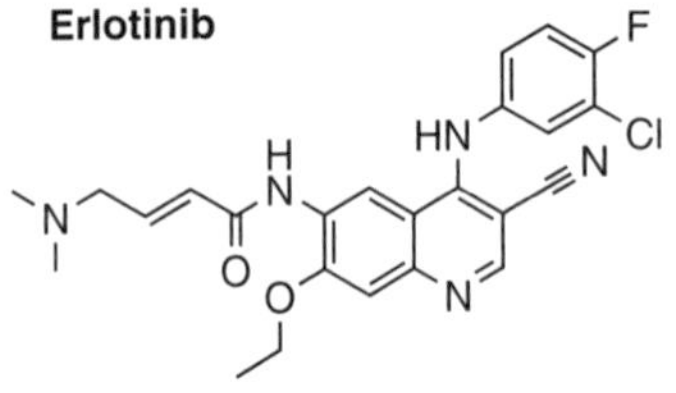

Pelitinib (EKB-569)

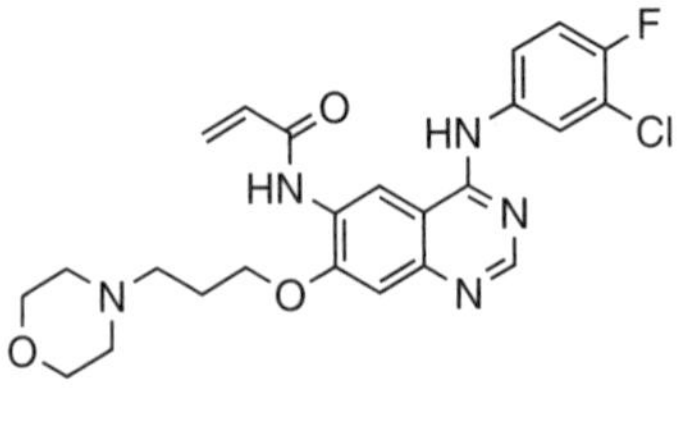

Canertinib (CI-1033)

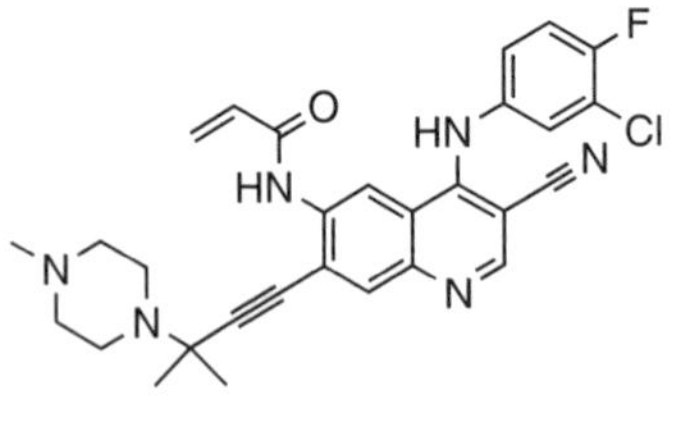

AV-412

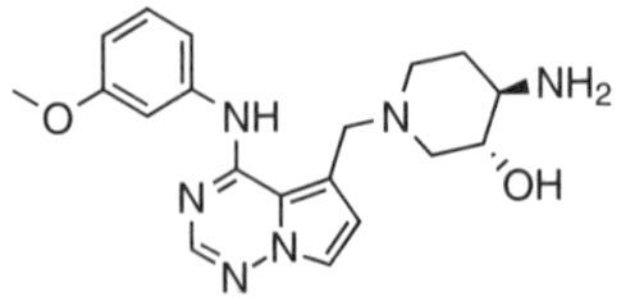

BMS-690514

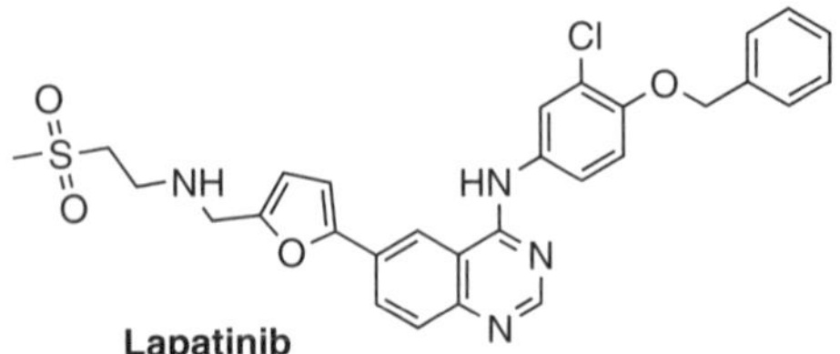

Lapatinib

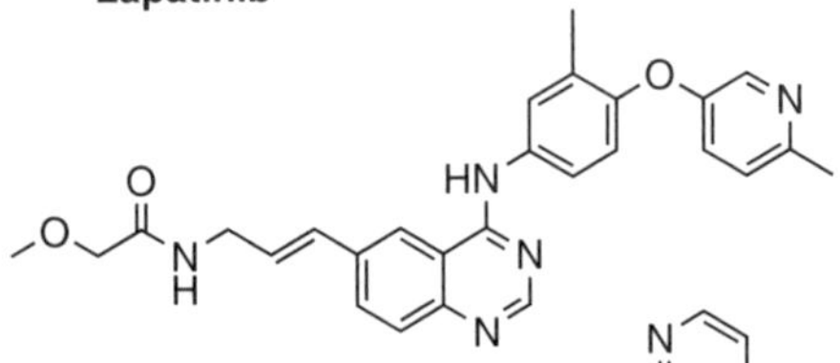

CP-724,714

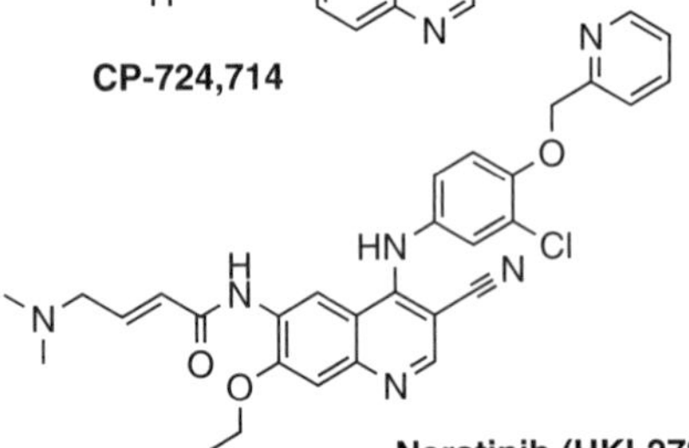

Neratinib (HKI-272)

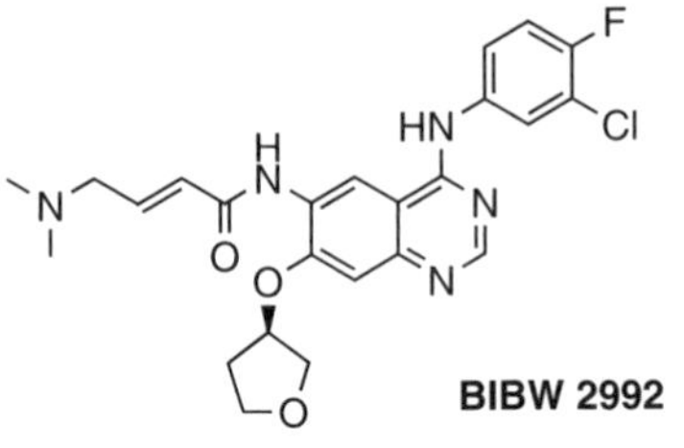

BIBW 2992

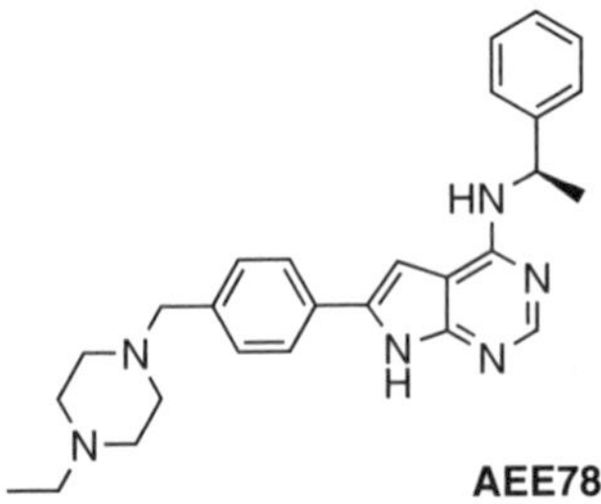

AEE788

Figure 8.3 Structures of EGFR/ERBB inhibitors.

daily at 250 or 500 mg) in colorectal carcinoma patients found only a ~1% response rate, and little modulation of EGFR pathway biomarkers was observed in tumor biopsies from treated patients (182). Any future therapeutic utility for gefitinib will most likely be focused on combinations with other anticancer therapies. In the case of colorectal cancer, a study of 500 mg daily gefitinib in combination with the FOLFOX4 chemotherapy regimen produced an encouraging response rate (33%) despite the fact that EGFR overexpression was not required for study entry. However, toxicity was also higher in cycles where gefitinib was administered, compared to the first cycle of FOLFOX4 alone (183).

Erlotinib   Erlotinib (OSI-774, CP-358,774; Tarceva®) is an EGFR inhibitor with the same quinazoline core scaffold as gefitinib (Figure 8.3). Erlotinib inhibits EGFR in vitro with $IC_{50} = 2$ nM and was initially reported to be selective against SRC, ABL, and IGF1R (184); more extensive specificity analysis has indicated that only a few kinases (GAK, LOK, and SLK) bind to erlotinib with K_D values <100 nM (170). In vitro, erlotinib inhibits EGF-induced mitogenesis and results in a G1 cell cycle blockade, accompanied in some cell lines by apoptosis (184). In preclinical in vivo studies, erlotinib inhibits EGFR phosphorylation in tumor cells and has antitumor activity in several xenograft models including HN5 and A431 tumors (185). Many studies also indicate the potential benefit of combining erlotinib with various other therapeutic modalities, including various chemotherapy agents, targeted therapies, antivascular agents, and anti-EGFR antibodies.

A Phase I clinical study established the maximum tolerated daily dose of erlotinib to be 150 mg: as with gefitinib, the main toxicities associated with erlotinib treatment were rash and diarrhea (186). Steady state levels are achieved following 7–8 days of administration, and the elimination half-life following a single dose is 36 h. The main clinical use of erlotinib is in previously treated NSCLC. In a Phase II study, erlotinib was evaluated in patients with NSCLC following failure of platinum-based chemotherapy (187). A response rate of 12% was found, with median overall survival of 8.4 months; toxicity was consistent with findings of the Phase I study, and rash and diarrhea were observed in 75% and 56% of patients, respectively. Single-agent activity of erlotinib was confirmed by the BR.21 Phase III trial (188), leading to its approval in 2004 for treatment of patients with locally advanced or metastatic non small cell lung cancer after failure of at least one prior chemotherapy regimen. In this study, 731 patients with stage IIIb or IV NSCLC who had failed one or two prior chemotherapy treatments were randomized to receive either erlotinib (150 mg/day) or placebo. The erlotinib-treated group showed a significant increase in response rate (8.9% vs.<1%), duration of response (7.9 months vs. 3.7 months), and progression-free survival (2.2 months vs. 1.8 months). As with other EGFR inhibitor studies, women, nonsmokers, and patients with adenocarcinoma histology had a higher incidence of objective responses: however, in marked contrast to the gefitinib ISEL trial, all subgroups analyzed showed clinical benefit. The reasons for the success of single-agent erlotinib and failure of gefitinib in NSCLC may be due to a combination of factors. Erlotinib was administered at the maximally tolerated dose of 150 mg/day, whereas gefitinib was dosed at 250 mg—approximately three-fold lower than the maximum tolerated dose.

Furthermore, the patient populations in these studies may have favored the BR.21 erlotinib study, since the ISEL study enrolled a much higher percentage of patients who were refractory to chemotherapy (180).

Erlotinib was also evaluated in NSCLC in combination with gemcitabine/cisplatin and with carboplatin/paclitaxel, in the TALENT and TRIBUTE trials, respectively (189, 190). These studies showed no survival advantage for adding erlotinib to chemotherapy. However, the patients enrolled in these studies were not preselected for factors predisposing them to sensitivity to EGFR inhibitors and retrospective subgroup analysis of both studies showed that some patients (such as those who had never smoked) had increased benefit from adding erlotinib to the chemotherapy regimen (189, 190).

Erlotinib is also approved by the FDA in combination with gemcitabine for treatment of pancreatic cancer. In a Phase III study, patients with locally advanced or metastatic pancreatic cancer all received gemcitabine and were randomized to receive either erlotinib (100 or 150 mg daily) or placebo (191). The improvement in survival was modest: median overall survival was 6.4 months for the combination compared to 5.9 months in the control group, and 1-year survival was also higher for gemcitabine plus erlotinib (23% vs. 17%). The increased survival was due to disease stabilization, since the partial response rate was similar in both treatment groups. Patients who developed a rash had improved outcomes (consistent with the therapeutic benefit of adding erlotinib treatment regimen) and the combination was well tolerated with the exception of increased diarrhea. Erlotinib has also shown activity in combination with capecitabine in patients with gemcitabine-refractory pancreatic cancer (192).

Many additional Phase II studies have been conducted with erlotinib, both as single-agent therapy and in combination with other agents (193). As with gefitinib and anti-EGFR antibodies, erlotinib has demonstrated activity as a single agent in head and neck cancer. In a Phase II trial of erlotinib in refractory, recurrent, and/or metastatic SCCHN, responses were only seen in 4% of patients treated, although 38% had stable disease for a median duration of over 16 weeks (194). Additional Phase II studies have evaluated combinations of erlotinib with cisplatin and cisplatin/docetaxel chemotherapy regimens in advanced SCCHN (195, 196). These combinations were well tolerated and the triple combination, in particular, produced encouraging signs of activity: a 21% response rate was seen in the cisplatin study (1 complete response, 8 partial responses) and a 67% response rate (4 complete responses, 25 partial responses) for the erlotinib/cisplatin/docetaxel combination. EGFR amplification was associated with response in combination with cisplatin, although these data were derived from a relatively small sample size (197).

Erlotinib has also demonstrated single-agent activity in glioma, although as with other agents the response rate is modest and patient selection is likely to be important for future use in this disease. A response rate of 8.4% was seen in a Phase II single-agent study in glioblastoma, with an additional 37.5% of patients showing disease stabilization (198). Several erlotinib combination regiment have also been evaluated in brain tumors, including platinum, radiation, temozolomide, and the combination of temozolomide and radiation (199–203). Additional clinical studies have demonstrated that erlotinib can produce significant disease control in other indications such as ovarian, colorectal, and hepatocellular cancers, although objective responses in these cases are rare (193).

Lapatinib   Lapatinib (GW-0572016; Tykerb®) is a dual inhibitor of EGFR and HER2 with in vitro IC_{50} values for both targets of approximately 10 nM. ERBB4 is inhibited to a lesser extent ($IC_{50} = 367$ nM), and little crossreactivity is observed with other kinases (204). Lapatinib inhibits EGFR and ERBB2 phosphorylation in cancer cells that overexpress EGFR or ERBB2, and this receptor inhibition translates into blockade of downstream ERK and AKT signaling, G1 cell cycle arrest, and apoptosis in vitro. Inhibition of receptor signaling and tumor growth inhibition are also observed in vivo (204–206). Of particular note, the combination of trastuzumab and lapatinib in ERBB2-positive breast cancer cells shows a greater reduction in cell viability compared to either agent alone (206). Lapatinib may also have utility in estrogen receptor positive tumors: preclinical studies suggest that EGFR/ERBB2 expression can contribute to antiestrogen resistance, and co-treatment with lapatinib and tamoxifen can inhibit the growth of tamoxifen-resistant ERBB2-positive mammary tumor xenografts (207).

Phase I studies in patients with advanced malignancies showed that lapatinib was well tolerated at doses up to 1800 mg qd or 900 mg bid, although further studies have employed doses of 1250–1500 mg qd or 500 mg bid (208, 209). Diarrhea and rash were the most common toxicities, although the incidence of rash appeared not to be dose dependent. In one study of 64 patients with advanced malignancies, one complete response was observed (head and neck cancer) and 22 patients had disease stabilization (209). In a separate study, 67 patients with advanced malignancies were treated. Notably, there were 4 partial responses in trastuzumab-resistant metastatic breast cancer, and 24 additional patients with various malignancies had disease stabilization (208). Lapatinib has also been reported to have activity in patients with previously untreated metastatic breast cancer (210). In this study, two dosing regimens (1500 mg qd or 500 mg bid) produced similar efficacy and toxicity, with response rates of 22% and 26%, respectively. A Phase II study of 1500 mg/day lapatinib in patients with relapsed or refractory inflammatory breast cancer found that 72% of patients with overexpression of ERBB2 had an objective response, and that ERBB2 (but not EGFR) overexpression predicted for sensitivity to lapatinib. High levels of ERBB2 phosphorylation and IGF1R expression were also associated with response (211). Although lapatinib has been pursued primarily as a breast cancer drug, additional studies have been performed in other solid tumors including head and neck and gastric cancers, for which Phase III trials are in progress.

Additional Phase I studies have explored various combination regimens, including trastuzumab, letrozole, docetaxel, capecitabine, and the FOLFOX4/FOLFIRI regimens (212–217). Of particular interest, lapatinib was evaluated in combination with trastuzumab in a dose escalation/pharmacokinetic study in 54 patients with ERBB2-positive metastatic breast cancer. The optimal lapatinib dose was determined to be 1000 mg qd; there were 8 objective responses (1 complete and 7 partial), all in patients who had previously received multiple chemotherapy regimens and trastuzumab (214). Phase II studies of single-agent lapatinib in trastuzumab-refractory patients provided further evidence for activity of lapatinib in this population, with 19 of 81 patients being progression-free at 16 weeks, 7 of whom had objective responses (218). More recently, a Phase III randomized trial in 296 trastuzumab and chemotherapy-refractory patients found that administration of lapatinib and trastuzumab produced significantly longer progression-free survival and clinical benefit rate than lapatinib alone, although objective responses were not significantly different between the two arms (219). The mechanism of lapatinib activity in trastuzumab-resistant patients may be due to several factors, particularly shedding of the ERBB2 extracellular domain, which produces a receptor that is resistant to trastuzumab but sensitive to lapatinib (220).

In a randomized double-blind Phase III study, lapatinib plus capecitabine was compared to capecitabine alone in patients with advanced metastatic breast cancer, following failure of anthracycline, taxane, and trastuzumab (221, 222). Lapatinib was administered at 1250 mg/day; capecitabine was administered on days 1–14 of a 21-day cycle at 2000 mg/m^2 for the combination arm and 2500 mg/m^2 for the single-agent arm. An interim analysis of 324 patients showed that the primary endpoint (time to progression, TTP) was superior for the combination group; updated results for 399 patients confirmed this early trend and showed that TTP was 27.1 weeks for the combination compared to 18.6 weeks for capecitabine alone. There was also an indication of lower CNS disease involvement in the lapatinib arm of the study. Lapatinib has generally been well tolerated across studies, and the concerns of cardiotoxicity with inhibition of HER2 (see earlier discussion) appear to be somewhat less of a concern for lapatinib than for trastuzumab (223). On March 13, 2007, the FDA approved lapatinib in combination with capecitabine for treatment of metastatic breast cancer following failure of anthracycline, taxane, and trastuzumab. Ongoing clinical studies are evaluating lapatinib in the breast cancer adjuvant setting. The TEACH trial will compare adjuvant lapatinib to placebo in patients with HER2+ breast cancer who have completed chemotherapy; the ALTTO study will compare trastuzumab with lapatinib in the adjuvant setting and also includes treatment arms to evaluate trastuzumab followed by lapatinib and concomitant administration of the two drugs.

Vandetanib   Vandetanib (ZD6474) is a relatively weak EGFR inhibitor with in vitro IC$_{50}$ = 500 nM. However, preclinical studies suggest that it can inhibit EGFR signaling at clinically achievable drug levels (224). Vandetanib is discussed in further detail in Chapter 9.

XL647   XL647 is a reversible, ATP-competitive inhibitor of EGFR and ERBB2 that also inhibits VEGFR signaling. In vitro, nanomolar IC$_{50}$ values were reported for inhibition of EGFR (0.3 nM), ERBB2 (16 nM), VEGFR2 (1.5 nM), VEGFR3 (8.7 nM), and EPHB4 (1.4 nM), with no crossreactivity toward 10 additional tyrosine kinases and 55 serine/threonine kinases (225). Inhibition of EGFR phosphorylation was demonstrated in various cell lines in vitro including the NCI-H1975 cell line, which has both the sensitizing L858R mutation and the T790M resistance mutation. XL647 also inhibits the L755S and T733I mutant forms of ERBB2 that have been found in breast and gastric tumors (226). Durable EGFR inhibition was shown in A431 tumors (at least 72 hours after a single dose), and tumor growth inhibition was seen in A431 and H1975 xenograft models (225). Phase I studies with XL647 initially employed an intermittent dosing schedule (5 days dosing followed by 9 days off (227)) and subsequently explored continuous dosing (228). Intermittent dose escalation yielded a maximum tolerated dose of 4.68 mg/kg, or a flat dose of 350 mg using the 5 on/9 off schedule. Out of 33 evaluable patients, one partial response was observed (NSCLC) and 14 additional patients had stable disease. Continuous dosing produced dose-proportional exposure and steady state drug levels by day 15, with accumulation of ~4.2−fold compared to a single dose. The MTD was established as 300 mg; rash and diarrhea were the main toxicities but were relatively mild across dose levels of 75−350 mg/day. Additional adverse events (mostly grade 1−2) included dry skin, fatigue, and dysgeusia; asymptomatic QTc prolongation was also observed in several patients. No objective responses were observed, though over half of the patients had stable disease for at least 3 months. Early Phase II data have been reported in selected populations of NSCLC patients. In one study, enrollment was restricted to patients with adenocarcinoma who either had a documented EGFR mutation or at least one of the following criteria: Asian, female, or minimal smoking history. XL647 was dosed at 350 mg for 5 consecutive days in 14-day cycles. Out of 38 subjects evaluated, 10 partial responses and 11 disease stabilizations were observed (229). In a second study, enrollment was limited to patients who had progressed on gefitinib or erlotinib therapy and XL647 was dosed at 300 mg daily. Approximately 50% of patients achieved disease control with XL647, although only 1 patient out of 39 had a partial response. Of note, median progression-free survival for 10 patients harboring the T790M mutation was only 1.9 months, suggesting that despite the encouraging activity in preclinical T790M models, clinical benefit was limited in this population (230).

AEE788   AEE788 is an oral tyrosine kinase inhibitor that was under development by Novartis, and inhibits EGFR, ERBB2, ERBB4, VEGFR1, and VEGFR2 with IC_{50} values of 2, 6, 160, 59, and 77 nM, respectively. The compound also inhibits ABL, SRC, and CSF1R with IC_{50} values of 52, 61, and 60 nM. The compound weakly inhibits PDGFRβ, FLT3, VEGFR3, RET, and KIT (IC_{50} values of 320, 720, 330, 740, and 790 nM, respectively) and does not inhibit IR, IGF1R, PKCα, or CDK1. In cell-based assays, the compound was shown to potently inhibit EGFR, VEGFR2, and ERBB2 phosphorylation in the submicromolar range; PDGF-induced phosphorylation of PDGFRβ was not inhibited. The compound also had potent antiproliferative activity, inhibiting the proliferation of cell lines that express or overexpress EGFR (e.g., NCI-H596) or ERBB2 (BT-474, SK-BR-3) with IC_{50} values ranging from 49 to 381 nM. In contrast, in cell lines such as T24 the IC_{50} was considerably higher ($IC_{50} = 4.5$ μM). In assays using human endothelial cells, AEE788 inhibited both EGF- and VEGF-driven proliferation in the nanomolar range (IC_{50} values of 43 and 155 nM, respectively) but did not inhibit FGF or serum-induced proliferation at concentrations up to 1 μM (231). In mouse models the compound had a favorable pharmacokinetic profile and demonstrated antitumor activity in a number of xenograft models. This inhibition was most likely due to a combination of both antitumor and antiangiogenic activities (231). Additive to synergistic antitumor activity of AEE788 with paclitaxel, gemcitabine, and the mTOR inhibitor RAD001 has been reported in a number of animal models (232–236).

A number of Phase I studies have been reported. The compound has shown dose-dependent inhibition of VEGFR2, EGFR2, and MAPK in skin and tumors but did not show significant clinical activity (237–240). However, elevated liver enzymes and impaired liver function tests were identified as a significant problem for this compound. Currently, no clinical trials are listed in the NCI clinical trial database, and it appears that further development has been discontinued.

CI-1033 and PF-00299804 CI-1033 (formerly PD-183805) was an early entrant in the field of irreversible ERBB inhibitors. These irreversible compounds all form a covalent interaction with a free cysteine residue near the active site of EGFR and/or ERBB2 (see Chapter 7), producing potent and durable inhibition. Inhibition of EGFR and ERBB2 autophosphorylation in cells is very potent ($IC_{50} = 7.4$ nM and 9.0 nM, respectively), and tumor growth inhibition was observed in multiple xenograft models (241, 242). Preclinically, CI-1033 also shows potential for enhanced activity in combination with various cytotoxic therapies, including cisplatin (243) and radiation (244). However, in combination with topoisomerase I poisons, the mechanism may not be EGFR pathway inhibition per se but inhibition of cytotoxic drug efflux by xenobiotic transporters in tumor cells (245).

Phase I studies with CI-1033 have evaluated several dosing schedules. Using a 7-day on/7-day off schedule, the MTD was 250 mg; higher doses produced unacceptable toxicities, which were as anticipated for EGFR inhibition (primarily rash and diarrhea) (246). When dosed for 14 days of a 21-day cycle, the MTD was established as 450 mg/day; dose-limiting toxicities were again rash, diarrhea, and/or anorexia (247). A dose of 650 mg was tolerated for 7 days of a 28-day cycle; using this regimen, emesis, persistent rash, and mouth ulcer were the dose-limiting toxicities (248). No objective responses were seen in these studies, but several heavily pretreated patients with advanced malignancies had stable disease as their best response. Additional studies have explored the combination of CI-1033 with other drugs including carboplatin/paclitaxel (249) and docetaxel (250).

A Phase II study in advanced NSCLC patients previously treated with platinum-based therapy compared three dosing regimens: 50 mg daily for 21 consecutive days, 150 mg daily for 21 consecutive days, and 450 mg daily for 14 days on followed by 7 days off (251). Although this last dosing schedule was established in a previous Phase I study, it was not well tolerated and enrollment of this arm was closed early. Response rates were low (2–4%, with stable disease in 16–24% of patients). The primary endpoint of 1-year survival was 26–29% depending on treatment arm; however, comparison to other studies is complicated by potential differences in factors known to associate with response to EGFR inhibitors. Of note, however, exploratory analysis suggested that both rash and baseline expression of ERBB2 were associated with prolonged survival in response to CI-1033 (251). No recent development activity has been reported for CI-1033, and it is likely that its progression has been suspended in favor of PF-00299804.

PF-00299804 is an irreversible, pan-ERBB inhibitor with in vitro IC_{50} values of 6 nM, 45.7 nM, and 73.7 nM toward EGFR, ERBB2, and ERBB4, respectively (252). PF-00299804 inhibited the proliferation of gefitinib-sensitive and gefitinib-resistant NSCLC cell lines in vitro, including cells with wild-type EGFR, gefitinib-sensitive EGFR mutants, and the T790M gefitinib resistance mutant. In vivo, both gefitinib and PF-00299804 caused regression of EGFR exon 19 mutant HCC827 tumors, but only PF-00299804 showed durable growth inhibition in HCC827 cells engineered to express T790M EGFR. Additional activity was observed in SKOV3, A431, and H125 xenograft models, with prolonged duration of action and increased antitumor activity compared to CI-1033. The increased activity with respect to CI-1033 is consistent with improved pharmacokinetic properties in rodent, dog, and monkey (253). Phase I clinical studies evaluated daily dosing, either continuously or for 2 weeks in a 3-week cycle. Using the continuous dosing regimen, an MTD of 45 mg was established. In 23 patients treated at this dose the most common toxicities were rash and diarrhea, although additional grade 3 (fatigue, deep vein thrombosis, nausea, acne, hypokalemia, diarrhea, hypoxia, and decreased appetite) and grade 4 (dyspnea, pulmonary embolism, and pain) toxicities were noted. Two partial responses and 8 stable diseases were reported among 29 evaluable patients (254, 255). Of note, the partial responses were long lasting (>200 days) and occurred in patients previously treated with multiple chemotherapy regimens and erlotinib/gefitinib.

EKB-569 and HKI-272   EKB-569 (pelitinib) is another compound in clinical development that was designed to irreversibly inhibit EGFR and/or ERBB2. Despite its reliance on covalent interaction with a conserved cysteine residue, EKB-569 is nevertheless somewhat selective for EGFR compared to ERBB2: although binding constants for irreversible inhibitors may not be directly comparable to those of reversible interactions, IC_{50} values of 80 nM and 1230 nM were reported for EGFR and ERBB2, respectively. The compound also inhibited in vitro cell proliferation and produced regression of EGFR-driven A431 xenograft tumors in nude mice (256). A Phase I study of EKB-569 was completed and showed dose-proportional exposure with a maximum tolerated dose of 75 mg qd. The dose-limiting toxicity was grade 3 diarrhea; rash, nausea, and asthenia were also noted. Additional Phase I/IIa studies were conducted in combination with FOLFOX4 and FOLFIRI chemotherapy regimens in patients with advanced colorectal carcinoma (257, 258). These studies showed acceptable tolerability and promising clinical activity: however, development of EKB-569 appears to have been suspended in favor of a more potent analog, HKI-272 (neratinib).

Like EKB-569, HKI-272 forms an irreversible adduct with its target proteins (Chapter 7), resulting in highly potent inhibition. HKI-272 is more potent toward ERBB2 than EKB-569, with IC_{50} values of 92 nM and 59 nM for EGFR and ERBB2, respectively (259). In vitro, HKI-272 inhibits the growth of NSCLC cells that are resistant to gefitinib, including the NCI-H1975 (L858R/T790M) cell line (146). The dual inhibition of both EGFR and ERBB2 translates into activity in xenograft models of EGFR-driven tumors (260, 261) as well as tumors bearing the ERBB2 G776insV_G/C mutation, which occurs at low frequency in NSCLC (262). Preliminary Phase I data were reported in 2006 (263). In this dose escalation study, entry was limited to patients with immunohistochemical evidence for tumor expression of EGFR and/or ERBB2. HKI-272 was administered as a single oral dose on day 1, then on days 8–28 of a 28-day cycle. A total of 72 patients were enrolled, including 29 with breast cancer and 16 with NSCLC. The maximum tolerated dose was 320 mg daily (corresponding to C_{max} ~89 ng/mL, AUC ~1434 ng · h/mL), although this was reduced to 240 mg in subsequent Phase II studies to control diarrhea. Dose-limiting toxicities included diarrhea, nausea, asthenia, and dyspnea, but interestingly, there was little or no evidence for rash. Of the 23 breast cancer patients, 7 had a confirmed partial response (6 of whom had progressed following trastuzumab) and one had stable disease for 24 weeks. There were no objective responses among the 16 NSCLC patients but 5 experienced disease stabilization. A three-arm Phase II study in stage IIIB/IV NSCLC has been initiated, enrolling (i) patients with EGFR mutations who have progressed on gefitinib or erlotinib, (ii) patients without EGFR who have progressed on gefitinib or erlotinib, and (iii) patients with no prior EGFR inhibitor therapy but with factors predisposing them to response (adenocarcinoma and light smoker) (264).

BIBW 2992 BIBW 2992 (Figure 8.3) is a specific, irreversible inhibitor of EGFR and ERBB2 with in vitro IC_{50} values of 0.5 nM and 14 nM, respectively (265). As with other irreversible inhibitors, BIBW 2992 also inhibits the T790M mutant of EGFR ($IC_{50} = 10$ nM) and inhibits survival of cell lines harboring both wild-type and L858R/T790M EGFR. In preclinical studies, antitumor activity was demonstrated in several xenograft models derived from A431, N87, and H1975 cancer cell lines (265). Multiple Phase I clinical studies have been conducted using different dosing schedules: continuous (266, 267), 2 weeks on/2 weeks off (268, 269), and 3 weeks on/1 week off (270). MTD values were established as 40 mg (continuous), 70 mg qd (2 weeks on/2 weeks off), and 40 mg qd (3 weeks on/1 week off). Dose-limiting toxicities of rash and diarrhea were consistent across all schedules and consistent with other EGFR inhibitors; mucositis and dyspnea were also observed (1 patient each) in the 3-weeks on/1-week off and continuous schedules, respectively. Two female lung adenocarcinoma patients treated with the continuous dosing schedule had partial responses, and stable disease was noted in several patients treated with each of the dosing regimens.

Based on the potential for irreversible inhibitors such as BIBW 2992 to inhibit mutant forms of EGFR, a single-arm Phase II study was initiated in lung adenocarcinoma patients with confirmed EGFR mutation in exons 18–21 and no prior treatment with EGFR inhibitors (271). A daily dose of 50 mg was used, and out of 24 patients evaluable for response there were 12 partial responses and a further 9 with stable disease. Adverse events included grade 3 diarrhea; grade 3 skin toxicity and stomatitis were also found, and the majority of patients had some skin disorder. Objective responses were observed in patients with both exon 19 deletions and L858R mutation; no T790M mutations were found in these EGFR inhibitor-naïve patients.

CP-724,714   CP-724,714 is a potent and specific ERBB2 inhibitor ($IC_{50} = 3$ nM) that has no appreciable activity toward EGFR ($IC_{50} = 6400$ nM) and is furthermore selective with respect to insulin receptor, IGF1R, PDGFRβ, VEGFR2, ABL, SRC, MET, JNK2, JNK3, ZAP-70, CDK2, and CDK5 (272). Consistent with this profile, CP-724,714 shows particularly potent growth inhibition of cell lines with amplification of ERBB2. Pharmacodynamic inhibition of ERBB2 autophosphorylation was also demonstrated in tumor xenografts in vivo, with concomitant effects on downstream signaling (pAKT, pERK) and tumor growth inhibition (272). The safety, tolerability, and pharmacokinetics of CP-724,714 were assessed in patients with advanced ERBB2-positive tumors (273). Oral administration of CP-724,714 was initiated at 250 mg daily in 21-day cycles and escalated in both dose and frequency. The MTD was determined to be 250 mg thrice daily with 250 mg bid as the recommended Phase II dose, yielding $C_{max} = 2740$ ng/mL, AUC $= 7360$ ng · h/mL, and $T_{1/2} = 4.8$ h. Dose-limiting toxicities were primarily hepatic, indicated by elevation of liver transaminases and bilirubin; additional adverse events included nausea, asthenia, abdominal pain, and rash. Of 28 patients evaluable for response, eight had stable disease after 2 cycles; no objective responses were observed.

BMS-599626   BMS-599626 is a pyrrolotriazine derivative that targets all EGFR family kinases, with in vitro activity against EGFR ($IC_{50} = 22$ nM) and ERBB2 ($IC_{50} = 32$ nM) and slightly lower potency toward ERBB4 ($IC_{50} = 190$ nM). Weak activity was found against VEGFR2, LCK, and MEK (IC_{50} values 2500–8800 nM) with no crossreactivity toward a panel of 110 additional kinases (274). Submicromolar antiproliferative activity was noted in cells expressing high levels of EGFR and/or ERBB2, and mechanistic cellular assays showed that BMS-599626 not only blocks EGFR and ERBB2 receptor autophosphorylation but inhibits receptor heterodimer formation. Inhibition of receptor signaling and antitumor activity were demonstrated in multiple xenograft models including Sal2, a mouse salivary gland cell line expressing a CD8-HER2 transgene (274). Phase I studies evaluated oral administration of BMS-599626, either continually or for 21 days out of a 28-day cycle; early results indicate that the drug was generally well tolerated, with only minor target-related toxicities at the dose levels reported (275, 276).

BMS-690514   BMS-690514 is another pan-ERBB inhibitor from Bristol-Myers Squibb that also has activity against VEGF receptors. The in vitro IC_{50} for EGFR is 5 nM; IC_{50} values for ERBB2, ERBB4, and VEGFR2 are somewhat higher (20 nM, 60 nM, and 50 nM, respectively) (277). In cellular proliferation assays, BMS-690514 was active against the erlotinib/gefitinib-resistant cell line H1975 and promoted G1 cell cycle arrest and apoptotic cell death. Antitumor activity in xenograft models was associated with inhibition of EGFR/ERBB2 signaling and antiangiogenic effects (278, 279). Phase I studies established the MTD for daily oral administration as 200 mg. Dose-limiting toxicities were grade 3–4 diarrhea and grade 3 reversible acute renal insufficiency: other adverse events included rash, nausea, vomiting, hypertension, dyspnea, and asthenia (280). Two objective responses were noted: one in a patient with esophageal cancer treated at 300 mg and the other in one of a MTD expansion cohort of 37 NSCLC patients.

ARRY-543   ARRY-543 is a quinazoline-based dual inhibitor of EGFR ($IC_{50} = 7$ nM) and ERBB2 ($IC_{50} = 2$ nM), with additional activity toward ERBB4 but little or no crossreactivity with over 100 additional kinases (281). ARRY-543 inhibits EGFR and ERBB2 receptor autophosphorylation in A431 and BT474 cells, respectively, and inhibits the growth of tumor xenografts following oral dosing (25–100 mg/kg twice daily) in mice. In Phase I studies, ARRY-543 was administered as a single dose on day 1 and continual dosing from days 8 to 22 (282). Exposure was dose dependent, with a consistent half-life across doses (∼6.6 h). Toxicities were generally as expected for this class of agent: rash, fatigue, nausea, diarrhea, and vomiting, with dose-limiting fatigue and diarrhea at 400 mg qd and similar tolerability at 400 mg bid. Stable disease was the best response noted. A second inhibitor from Array, ARRY-380, is specific for ERBB2 and also in Phase I.

AV-412   AV-412 (formerly MP-412) is another dual inhibitor of EGFR and ERBB2 with the potential to form a covalent bond with its target kinases (Figure 8.3). In addition to inhibiting EGFR and ERBB2 (IC_{50} values of 1.4 and 19 nM, respectively), AV-412 also inhibits ABL kinase with $IC_{50} = 41$ nM (283). AV-412 was also shown to inhibit receptor autophosphorylation in cells with IC_{50} values of 43 nM (EGFR) and 282 nM (ERBB2) and inhibited tumor growth in multiple tumor xenograft models (283). Phase I clinical trials are in progress.

8.5   IGF1R INHIBITORS

To date, only a few small molecule IGF1R inhibitors have advanced into clinical testing (Table 8.5). This may stem from the fact that IGF1R has high homology to the insulin receptor (IR), raising concerns that a small molecule kinase inhibitor is likely to inhibit both receptors and may have deleterious effects on the insulin signaling pathway. Many companies have consequently taken the approach of developing anti-IGF1R therapeutic antibodies, at least seven of which are in clinical trials: IMC-A12 (Imclone), SCH-717454 (Schering-Plough), CP-751871 (Pfizer), R1507 (Roche), AVE-1642 (Sanofi-Aventis), AMG479 (Amgen), and BIIB022 (Biogen-IDEC). Nevertheless, as discussed in Chapter 3, there may be substantial rationale for inhibiting insulin receptor in addition to IGF1R in tumors.

Clinical studies with the antibodies have provided the first insights into the effects of specifically inhibiting the IGF1R signaling pathway in humans. In general,

TABLE 8.5   IGF1R Inhibitors

Name	Company	Known targets	Structure	Highest phase of development
XL228	Exelixis	IGF1R, IR, SRC, ABL, FAK, Aurora	ND	Phase I
OSI-906 (PQIP)	OSI	IGF1R, IR	Figure 8.4	Phase I
AXL-1717	Axelar	IGF1R	ND	Phase I

administration of these agents has been well tolerated: however, despite specifically targeting IGF1R as opposed to IR, hyperglycemia has been reported as a relatively common adverse event with MK-0646 (284). Growth of Ewing's sarcoma is driven in many cases by deregulation of IGF1R signaling via the EWS-FLI translocation (Chapter 3), and some early signs of clinical activity have been noted in this disease with the antibodies AMG479, R1507, and MK0646 (284–286). Additional clinical studies with IGF1R antibodies are ongoing in multiple diseases: in addition to sarcoma, these include breast, pancreatic, lung, colorectal, prostate, liver, and neuroendocrine cancers.

OSI-906   Preclinical profiling of OSI-906 (Figure 8.4) indicates that it is a potent and specific inhibitor of IGF1R and IR, with biochemical IC_{50} values of 24 nM and 31 nM, respectively. However, in cellular assays OSI-906 appears to show 14-fold selectivity for IGF1R relative to IR (287). The reason for this remains obscure although it has also been noted with other small molecule IGF1R/IR inhibitors such as NVP-AEW541, which is also equipotent toward IGF1R and IR in biochemical assays but displays >20-fold selectivity for IGF1R inhibition in cellular assays (288). In vitro, OSI-906 inhibits proliferation and promotes apoptosis in GEO colon carcinoma cells, which have constitutive activation of IGF1R signaling via an IGF2-IGF1R autocrine loop. In preclinical in vivo studies in mice, OSI-906 was shown to have relatively modest effects on blood glucose levels, either following three consecutive daily doses or in an acute glucose tolerance test—despite the fact that mouse IR appears to be more potently inhibited in cells compared to human IR. Tumor growth inhibition has been demonstrated in several xenograft models including GEO colon carcinoma tumors (287). A Phase I dose escalation study of OSI-901 is in progress.

XL228   XL228 is a potent inhibitor of several kinases including IGF1R, IR, SRC, ABL, FAK, Aurora-A, Aurora-B, and FGF receptors 1, 2, and 3 (IC_{50} values 2, 4, 6, 6.5, 3, 1, 0.6, 8, 2, and 3 nM, respectively) (289–291). Potent inhibition of tumor cell proliferation has been reported (in vitro IC_{50} values ranging from 5 to 42 nM), and pharmacodynamic studies showed inhibition of target kinases in tumor tissue. Tumor growth inhibition was observed following oral dosing in several solid tumor xenografts, with regression in MCF7 and Colo205 models (289). Consistent with

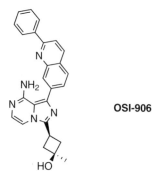

OSI-906

Figure 8.4   Structure of IGF1R inhibitor.

the target profile of XL228, significant inhibition of IGF1R and SRC signaling was observed in Colo205 tumors, with additional effects (decreased M phase and changes in cell size and shape) indicative of Aurora kinase inhibition. Two Phase I studies are being conducted using intravenous administration of XL228, one in patients with CML or Ph+ ALL (discussed in Section 8.1), and another in patients with advanced solid tumors. In the solid tumor study, intravenous weekly doses of 0.45–8.0 mg/kg were evaluated. The terminal half-life ranged from 27 to 55 h, with a volume of distribution of 6.2–34.8 L/kg. Adverse events were generally mild, and a dose-limiting toxicity of neutropenia was reported at the highest dose tested. Evidence for pharmacodynamic target modulation was reported, including decreased SRC and IGF1R pathway readouts in peripheral leukocytes, transient upregulation of plasma glucose and insulin, and decreased phospho-AKT/phospho-FAK in hair and skin. Seven patients experienced prolonged disease stabilization (291).

8.6   FLT3 INHIBITORS

Activating mutations in FLT3 are found in a significant proportion of adult (25–42%) and pediatric (18–26%) leukemias (292, 293). The most notable example is AML. In frame internal tandem duplications (ITDs) in the juxtamembrane domain (JMD) of FLT3 occur in 17–34% of adult AML patients and 10–17% in pediatric AML patients. ITDs are also found at lower frequencies in MDS. Point mutations, small in frame deletions, or insertions of the activation loop are also quite frequent, occurring in approximately 7–8% of AML patients and at a higher frequency in infant ALL patients with MLL rearrangements (294). A small number of patients may present with mutations in both the FLT3-ITD and FLT3-activation loop (295, 296). Patients with FLT3-ITDs are associated with poor prognosis in both pediatric and adult AML. The difference in outcome can be considerable. In one pediatric study, the event-free survival at 8 years for patients without a FLT3-ITD was 44% compared to only 7% for those patients with a FLT3-ITD mutation (297). Of particular poor prognosis are those patients with FLT3-ITD who have lost the wild-type FLT3 allele. Mutations in the tyrosine kinase domain of FLT3 are also found in AML; in most studies these mutations do not appear to have a worse prognosis. Additional studies have shown that constitutively active FLT3 mutations will transform hematopoietic cell lines (BaF3 and 32D), and that signaling through FLT3 contributes to enhanced proliferation and reduced differentiation. These and other observations made FLT3 an attractive target for new drug discovery.

AML is a disease with a high medical need. Although 70–80% of AML patients under the age of 60 years usually achieve complete remission with standard chemotherapy, only 40% of those who achieve remission can expect to achieve long-term disease-free survival. In older adults, up to 20% die during induction chemotherapy, and complete remissions are achievable in only 40–50%. Of the older adults, no more than 10–20% of those patients in initial remission live 3 years beyond their diagnosis (reviewed in (298)). Thus far, FLT3-TKIs used as single agents have reduced peripheral blood and bone marrow blasts in only a minority of AML patients, and the effect tends to be transient. This may be due to insufficient FLT3 inhibition (due in part to different sensitivities of the FLT3 mutations to different inhibitors), the selection of drug-resistant clones, and the independence of the cells on FLT3 signaling for proliferation and survival (due to activation of other signaling pathways such as RAS/MEK/MAPK or PI3K/AKT). Thus far, only 1 patient on FLT3 inhibitor trials has been shown to have acquired a FLT3 resistance mutation (299). FLT3 inhibitors in clinical trials are shown in Table 8.6.

Sorafenib   Sorafenib (Bay 43–9006, Nexavar®) was initially identified as a small molecule inhibitor of RAF but was found to be a potent inhibitor of several other kinases, including FLT3, VEGFR2, VEGFR3, PDGFR, and KIT. Additional activities of sorafenib are discussed in Sections 8.7 and 8.9 and Chapter 9. It is currently approved for the treatment of renal cell carcinoma and hepatocellular carcinoma and is in clinical trials for several other indications, including AML.

TABLE 8.6   FLT3 Inhibitors

Drug	Company	Known targets	Structure	Highest phase of development
Sorafenib (BAY43-9006; Nexavar®)	Bayer	RAF, VEGFR, FLT3, KIT, RET, PDGFRβ, p38	Figure 9.1	Launched (not approved for AML)
Sunitinib (SU11248; Sutent®)	Pfizer	FLT3, KIT, PDGFR, VEGFR, CSF1R, RET	Figure 9.1	Launched (not approved for AML)
Midostaurin (PKC412)	Novartis	FLT3, PDGFR, KIT, VEGFR, PKC	Figure 8.5	Phase III
Lestaurtinib (CEP-701)	Cephalon	FLT3, JAK2, TRKA	Figure 8.5	Phase III
Tandutinib (MLN518)	Takeda	PDGFR, FLT3, KIT	Figure 8.5	Phase II
AT9283	Astex	Aurora-A, Aurora-B, TYK2, JAK2, JAK3, RSK2, RET, MER, YES, GSK3β	Figure 8.5	Phase II
ABT-869	Abbott	FLT3, PDGFR, VEGFR, KIT	Figure 9.2	Phase II
TG-101348	TargeGen	FLT3, JAK2	Figure 8.2	Phase I
Dovitinib lactate (TKI258; CHIR258)	Chiron	FGFR, PDGFR, VEGFR, KIT, FLT3	Figure 9.3	Phase I
ENMD-2076	Miikana Therapeutics	FGFR, PDGFR, VEGFR, KIT, FLT3	Figure 10.8	Phase I

Sorafenib inhibits the proliferation of mouse BaF3 cells stably expressing wild-type human FLT3 or mutant FLT3 (FLT3-ITD, FLT3-D835G, FLT3-D835Y). Cells with FLT3-ITD (IC_{50} 1.2 nM) or D835G (IC_{50} 14.3 nM) mutations were 1000–3000-fold more sensitive to sorafenib than the FLT3-D835Y (IC_{50} 1593 nM) or FLT3 wild-type cells (300). Sorafenib induced cell death in those cells expressing the FLT3-ITD or the FLT3-D835G but did not elicit this response in the cells expressing the FLT3-D835Y mutation or the wild-type FLT3 receptor. The growth arrest induced by sorafenib could be rescued by IL3, providing evidence that sorafenib selectively kills FLT3-ITD mutant cells. In vitro studies showed that sorafenib inhibits the phosphorylation of tyrosine residues in the ITD mutant but does not inhibit tyrosine phosphorylation of the wild-type FLT3. Molecular modeling studies suggest that the amino-terminal region of the JMD of FLT3 is altered with the insertion of the ITD, resulting in an increased opening of the binding pocket, which may allow for more optimal interactions between FLT3-ITD and sorafenib (300).

In mouse models of leukemia using cells with the FLT3-ITD mutation, sorafenib treatment at 10 mg/kg qd on days 9–24 after leukemia cell injection significantly reduced the leukemic burden and prolonged survival 2.3 times over that of vehicle controls (300). In a Phase I clinical trial, patients with refractory or relapsed AML were randomized to one of two arms of sorafenib treatment: (i) receiving the drug in 21-day cycles of 5 days per week or (ii) a 14-day cycle. In both arms the starting dose level was 200 mg bid, with subsequent dose levels of 600, 800, and 1200 mg daily in cohorts of 3 subjects at two dose levels. The FLT3 mutation status was determined by PCR. Sorafenib induced apoptosis and/or the loss of mitochondrial membrane potential in peripheral blasts of AML patients carrying the FLT3-ITD mutation; these effects also correlated with decreases in pERK and pFLT3 occuring as early as 2 h after sorafenib. However, sorafenib had no significant effects on circulating or bone marrow blasts of AML patients with WT-FLT3 or an FLT3-D835 mutation. Sorafenib treatment resulted in at least a 50% reduction in the percentage of circulating blasts in all of the patients with the FLT3-ITD mutation (300). Two patients had circulating blasts drop to zero. A recent case report also describes a clinical case of molecular remission induced by sorafenib in a patient with FLT3-ITD and extramedullary disease after allogenic stem cell transplantation (301). The patient was treated with sorafenib at 400 mg bid starting on day 373 after transplantation. One week later all extramedullary chloromas had disappeared, and the patient became PCR negative for FLT3-ITD after 100 days of sorafenib therapy. The drug was well tolerated, although it induced asymptomatic tachycardia, grade II thrombocytopenia, and elevation of AST and ALT. The dose was reduced to 400 mg because of these toxicities. After 225 days of sorafenib treatment the patient remained PCR negative for the FLT3-ITD in the bone marrow but developed an isolated cerebellar chloroma, and died 6 days after the diagnosis of the CNS chloroma. The clinicians felt that the case was of particular significance because the patient had been refractory to all other treatments, including allogenic stem cell transplantation, and also felt that the reduction in the dose of sorafenib might have resulted in insufficient sorafenib exposure in the CNS, contributing to the development of the cerebellar chloroma (301). Phase I/II clinical trials are ongoing with sorafenib in combination with the standard chemotherapy for AML, idarubicin, and cytarabine.

Sunitinib In in vitro studies, sunitinib was shown to potently inhibit proliferation of FLT3-ITD expressing MV-4−11 cells (IC_{50} 25 nM). Sunitinib inhibited the autophosphorylation of FLT3 in MV-4-11 cells, as well as downregulating downstream effector signaling (pAKT, pERK, pSTAT). Sunitinib also induced the growth arrest of freshly isolated AML leukemic cells with either FLT3-ITD or FLT3-D835 mutation but was much less effective on the proliferation of leukemia cells with wild-type FLT3 (302). In vivo, sunitinib induced regression of subcutaneous FLT3-ITD xenografts and increased survival in a FLT3-ITD bone marrow engraftment model (303). PK/PD analysis of xenograft models showed that target plasma concentrations of 50−100 ng/mL and 30−50 ng/mL were required to markedly inhibit FLT3-WT and FLT3-ITD autophosphorylation, respectively (304).

In a single-arm Phase I study, sunitinib was evaluated to explore safety and target modulation in AML patients. Twenty-nine patients received a single dose of sunitinib, dosed at 50−350 mg, in increments of 50 mg, with 3−6 patients per cohort. FLT3 phosphorylation was determined and plasma PK evaluated, as well as the FLT3 genotype. Study-related adverse events were mainly grade 1−2 diarrhea and nausea, generally seen at high dose levels. The inhibition of FLT3 phosphorylation was seen in both wild-type and FLT3-ITD patients, although the FLT3-ITD patients showed increased sensitivity to sunitinib, in agreement with the preclinical studies. Doses of 200 mg and higher appeared to be required for strong inhibition of FLT3 phosphorylation in >50% of patients (305). In a second Phase I trial, various dosing regimens were explored. All patients with FLT3 mutations had morphologic or partial responses ($n = 4$) compared to only 2/10 evaluable patients with wild-type FLT3. However, responses were of short duration. The authors concluded that further evaluation in combination with chemotherapy was warranted (306). However, currently the NCI lists no open trials for sunitinib in AML.

Midostaurin Midostaurin (PKC412; N-benzoyl staurosporine) (Figure 8.5) inhibits the cytoplasmic kinase domain of FLT3 with an IC_{50} value of 528 nM. It also inhibits several other kinases, including protein kinase C, VEGFR2, PDGFRβ, and KIT with IC_{50} values of 22, 86, 80, and 300 nM (307). Midostaurin inhibits the proliferation of BaF3/FLT3-ITD cells, with IC_{50} values of less than 10 nM, but is relatively nontoxic against parental cells at concentrations up to 100 nM. The reduction in cell growth was due to both induction of apoptosis and cell cycle arrest. The IC_{50} for BaF3/FLT3-ITD cells treated with midostaurin was several orders of magnitude lower than the IC_{50} observed for the same cells cultured with IL3, indicating that the compound did not significantly inhibit signaling pathways used by the IL3 receptor. Midostaurin also inhibits the proliferation and reduces the viability of BaF3/FLT3-D835Y cells. Mice transplanted with bone marrow cells transduced with a FLT3-ITD retrovirus develop a myeloproliferative syndrome that is lethal in 30−90 days in 100% of recipients. Treatment with midostaurin (25−32 days after transplant) prevented the development of leukemia,

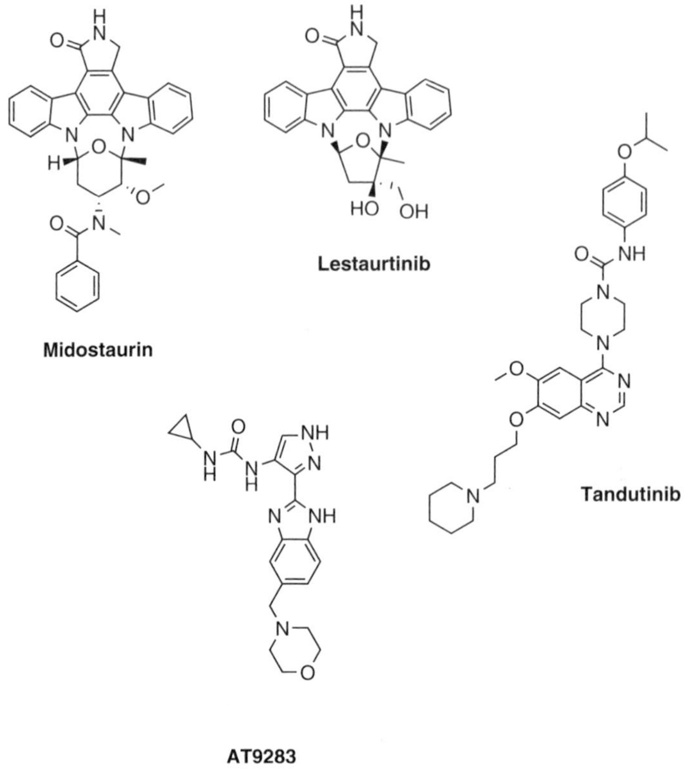

Figure 8.5 Structures of KIT/FLT3 inhibitors.

with all of the midostaurin-treated animals alive at the end of study (308). Barry et al. (309) tested the sensitivity of eight FLT3 activation loop mutants to midostaurin. Each mutant was shown to confer IL3-dependent proliferation to cells, resulting in the constitutive activation of FLT3 and downstream signaling (STAT5 and ERK). Midostaurin potently ($IC_{50} < 10$ nM) inhibited all of the mutants. In contrast, midostaurin did not inhibit cells stably transduced with FLT3-ITD and a G697R mutation (309).

Phase I clinical trials of midostaurin were conducted in patients with a variety of solid tumors and the results indicated that the drug could given up to 75 mg orally 3 times a day (310). In another Phase I/II trial in CLL patients, doses of 25–225 mg/day demonstrated a dose-dependent reduction in PKC activity in the malignant B cells (311). A Phase II trial of midostaurin was conducted in patients with advanced AML and MDS with documented activating mutations of FLT3 (312). Twenty patients were enrolled, of which ten had relapsed AML, seven had never achieved remission and were deemed refractory, and one had MDS. All patients had been heavily pretreated with a median of four prior regimens. A FLT3 mutation was confirmed in all patients. In 18 of 20 this was an ITD mutation and 2 patients had a D835Y mutation. All patients were treated with midostaurin

75 mg orally three times per day. In most patients the drug was very well tolerated. Twelve of the patients received more than 29 days of treatment; 8 discontinued the drug on or before day 29 due to adverse events, disease progression, or death from pulmonary complications. Six patients progressed after 72–330 days on treatment, and all six had an initial peripheral blood count response. In seven patients, a 2 log reduction in peripheral blast count lasting for at least 4 weeks was observed, and six patients achieved more than a 50% reduction in bone marrow blast count. PK studies showed that the plasma concentrations of midostaurin increased substantially during the first week but declined thereafter despite continued dosing. The declining concentrations of midostaurin were suggested to play an important role in the brief duration of blast remission and clinical efficacy. The mechanism for the decreases in plasma exposure is unknown. One of the AML FLT3-ITD patients who relapsed upon midostaurin treatment had a N676K mutation within the FLT3 kinase domain. Reconstitution studies expressing the N676K mutant in 32D cells demonstrated that this mutation, in the context of the FLT3-ITD, was sufficient to confer an intermediate level of resistance to midostaurin (299). A Phase III study is ongoing to determine if the addition of midostaurin to induction therapy comprising daunorubicin hydrochloride and cytarabine, consolidation therapy comprising high-dose cytarabine, and continuation therapy improves overall survival of patients with newly diagnosed acute myeloid leukemia with FLT3-ITD or FLT3 tyrosine kinase domain mutations.

Lestaurtinib   Lestaurtinib (CEP-701) is an orally available indolocarbazole alkaloid with in vitro kinase assay $IC_{50} = 2–3$ nM and similar IC_{50} for inhibition of FLT3 autophosphorylation in BaF3/FLT3-ITD cells. Cells transfected with FLT3 D835Y and D835H point mutants were also inhibited by lestaurtinib with similar IC_{50} values. In contrast, in cell-based assays, the compound inhibited PDGFRβ, CSF1R, and KIT expressing cells at concentrations of 500–1000 nM or higher. Lestaurtinib inhibited the proliferation of BaF3/FLT3-ITD cells with IC_{50} values of 5 nM and also inhibited cells expressing the FLT3 D835Y mutations with similar IC_{50} values. Much higher concentrations of lestaurtinib were required to inhibit parental cells (200 nM) and IL3 was shown to rescue the growth of BaF3/FLT3-ITD cells in the presence of lestaurtinib, an effect not mediated through any effect on FLT3 phosphorylation.. The compound is cytotoxic to several FLT3 expressing human leukemic cell lines (MV-4-11 and EOV-1) as well as to primary bone marrow AML blasts harboring FLT3 mutations. In Balb/c mice injected with cells expressing constitutively activated FLT3 (BaF3/FLT3-ITD), lestaurtinib inhibited FLT3 phosphorylation in vivo, lasting up to 8 hours after the last dose of compound. Lestaurtinib significantly prolonged survival in Balb/c mice injected with BaF3/FLT3-ITD cells (74).

Phase I studies showed that lestaurtinib had good exposure and a drug half-life of 6.8–9.2 hours in healthy volunteers and had similar profiles in patients with solid tumors. In a Phase I/II open-label, single-agent trial of lestaurtinib in patients with refractory, relapsed, or poor risk AML expressing FLT3-activating mutations, the compound was initially dosed at 40 mg bid. Intrapatient dose escalation to 60 mg bid at the completion of 28 days for patients without drug-related cytoxicity was planned, and patients with evidence of clinical activity (complete remission or hematologic response) were continued on monthly cycles of the compound until disease progression or DLT. Initial observations in the first three patients resulted in an amendment to the protocol to increase the starting dose to 60 mg bid, and intrapatient dose escalation to 80 mg bid. A total of 17 patients were enrolled. Eight patients did not complete the intial cycle of treatment (due to disease progression, death, or persistent nausea and poor oral intake); 12 patients were also treated with concurrent hydroxyurea due to elevated WBC counts. Commonly observed toxicities included mild nausea, mild emesis, and mild generalized weakness and fatigue. The grade or frequency of toxicity did not increase with the highest doses of drug administered. Clinical activity was seen in 5 of the 14 patients treated at an initial dose of 60 mg bid. These responses correlated with evidence of sustained FLT3 inhibition. Lestaurtinib effectively lowered peripheral blood blasts, and in some patients, there was evidence of stabilized, normal, hematopoiesis. These responses were also accompanied by decreased transfusion requirements in three patients. All responses were of short duration, ranging from 2 weeks to 3 months (81). A Phase II trial was conducted to determine the clinical effects of lestaurtinib in a population of previously untreated, older patients with AML who were not considered fit for conventional intensive chemotherapy. Twenty-nine patients were enrolled at 12 centers. Five patients harbored activating mutations of FLT3—two with ITDs and three with point mutations in the kinase domain. Lestaurtinib was well tolerated, with observed toxicities including mild nausea, emesis, constipation, diarrhea, and elevations in alkaline phosphatase. Clinical activity was observed in 8 (30% of evaluable patients), including 3 of 5 FLT3 mutant patients and 5 of 22 FLT3 WT patients; there was not a statistically significant difference in response rates between mutation groups. No patient attained either a CR or PR, although one patient did achieve more than 50% reduction in bone marrow blasts. This response was of short duration (14 days). A second patient had a more dramatic reduction in bone marrow blasts (to less than 5%). The majority of clinical responses were of short duration, and the median time until evidence of disease progression was 25 days. In two of the patients, a FLT3 point mutation and a FLT3 WT patient, prolonged delayed clinical responses to lestaurtinib were observed, peaking several weeks after study drug was withdrawn. These patients achieved blood count improvements and transfusion independence for 4 and 6 months, respectively, possibly implicating an effect on leukemic stem cells.

A Phase II study of lestaurtinib in combination with chemotherapy comprising cytarabine and idarubicin in younger patients with relapsed or refractory FLT3-mutant acute myeloid leukemia is ongoing, as is a Phase II study of lestaurtinib given in sequence with induction chemotherapy to determine if this regimen increases the proportion of patients with relapsed acute myeloid leukemia (AML) who achieve a second complete remission.

Tandutinib Tandutinib (MLN518) is an orally active, relatively selective RTK inhibitor, originally identified by COR Therapeutics as an inhibitor of PDGFR and currently in development by Takeda/Millennium. The compound was later shown also to inhibit FLT3, PDGFRβ, and KIT with IC_{50} values of 170, 200, and 220 nM, respectively. Tandutinib (Figure 8.5) is a 4-piperazinylquinazoline compound with no significant inhibition for a number of other receptor tyrosine kinases, including VEGFR2, EGFR, FGFR, and the IR (>30 μM). Tandutinib inhibits FLT3-ITD and FLT3 activation loop mutants. For example, in the FLT3-ITD+ MOLM13 and MOLM14 cell lines, tandutinib inhibits FLT3 phosphorylation and induces apoptosis with IC_{50} values around 10 nM. The responsiveness of FLT3 activation loop mutants was observed to vary greatly. In cells transformed with eight different FLT3 activation loop mutants, the IC_{50} values for tandutinib in proliferation assays ranged from <1 μM (I836del, D835E) to >10 μM (D835V) (313).

Tandutinib exhibited preferential inhibition of human AML cells harboring FLT3-ITD compared to normal human hematopoietic progenitor cells or AML cells with WT FLT3. In colony formation assays, tandutinib inhibited primary AML samples with FLT3-ITD with IC_{50} values ranging from 75 to 400 nM (314). The antileukemic activity of tandutinib was evaluated in athymic nude mice injected with stably transformed FLT3-ITD cells. Dosed orally at 120 mg/kg/day, tandutinib was shown to significantly delay disease progression compared to vehicle-treated controls (315). Tandutinib also prolonged survival in a nude mouse model of myeloproliferative disease (315) and demonstrated synergy when combined with retinoic acid in an acute promyelocytic leukemia model (315).

The first Phase I clinical trial with tandutinib was conducted in patients with relapsed or refractory AML, or in newly diagnosed AML patients considered unsuitable for treatment by chemotherapy. The FLT3-ITD status was determined by DNA sequencing but was not a prerequisite for enrollment in the study. In this dose escalation study, tandutinib was dosed orally at 50–700 mg bid to 40 patients with cohorts of 3–6 patients per group. No complete or partial remissions occurred in this clinical trial: however, in the two highest dose cohorts (525 and 700 mg bid) antileukemic activity was observed in two patients with FLT3-ITD. Both patients had a greater than 99% reduction in absolute blast counts, and there was also a marked reduction in bone marrow blasts in both patients. However, the effects were transient, and disease progression occurred in both patients after 1–2 months (316). A Phase I/II open-label, multicenter trial assessed the safety, tolerability, and response rates of tandutinib in combination with cytarabine and daunorubicin standard induction chemotherapy. The trial enrolled newly diagnosed patients, with or without FLT3-ITD. Tandutinib was administered at 200 mg twice daily during induction and consolidation therapy, and then for an additional 6 months. Of the 29 patients enrolled, 21 achieved complete remissions from the combination treatment (317). Currently, the NCI clinical trials website does not list any open trials for tandutinib in AML, although the Takeda/Millennium website still lists the compound as in development for AML. Single-agent clinical trials with tandutinib in glioblastoma and prostate cancer, and combination trials with bevacizumab in patients with recurrent high grade glioma are ongoing.

ABT-869   ABT-869 is a multitargeted, ATP-competitive RTK inhibitor with potent inhibitory activity against VEGFR2 (IC_{50} = 4 nM), VEGFR1 (3 nM), VEGFR3 (190 nM), PDGFRβ (66 nM), CSF1R (3 nM), KIT (14 nM), FLT3 (4 nM), and TIE2 (170 nM), but it has little or no inhibitory activity on many other nonrelated tyrosine and serine/threonine kinases (318). The drug was initially identified at Abbott, but licensed to Genentech.

Cell viability assays demonstrated that MV-4-11 cells (FLT3-ITD) were inhibited in a dose-dependent manner with an IC_{50} of approximately 10 nM. In contrast, other leukemic cell lines (HL60, NB4, KG1, and K562) were not responsive to ABT-869 at concentrations less than 10 μM. In the MV-4-11 cells and another cell line harboring the FLT3-ITD mutation (MOLM-13), ABT-869 induced an apoptotic response at doses between 10 and 100 nM. In the MV-4-11 tumor xenograft model, mice treated with 40 mg/kg/day ABT-869 showed complete regression of these tumors within 2 weeks of treatment; a lower dose (20 mg/kg/d) achieved the same response but required one month. ABT-869 also enhanced survival in a bone marrow engraftment model of leukemia (318).

ABT-869 was also evaluated in in vitro kinase assays against different activation loop mutants of FLT3. The D835H and D835Q mutants were about tenfold less sensitive to the compound (IC_{50} values of 52 and 64 nM, respectively) compared to WT-FLT3. The D835Y mutation was quite resistant (IC_{50} 4600 nM) as was the D835V mutant (IC_{50} 19800 nM) (318). Pretreatment of MV-4-11 and MOLM-4 cells with cytarabine or doxorubicin (standard chemotherapies for AML), followed by ABT-869, produced synergistic effects on inhibition of proliferation and induction of apoptosis. Adding ABT-869 concurrently with Ara-C resulted in at best an additive effect. Combining ABT-869 concurrently with doxorubicin was synergistic. The synergy of combination therapy was attributed to the downregulation of cell cycle related genes and genes in the MAPK pathway. In contrast, less than additive effects were observed when ABT-869 was administered prior to chemotherapy, suggesting an antagonism (319).

ABT-869 is currently in Phase I/II trials for hepatocellular (liver) carcinoma, metastatic breast cancer, metastatic colorectal cancer, non small cell lung cancer, and renal cell carcinoma. At present it is not in development for AML.

TG-101348   TargeGen is developing TG-101348 for the treatment of myeloproliferative disorders including polycythemia vera (PV), essential thrombocytopenia (ET), primary myelofibrosis (PMF) and AML. The compound inhibits JAK2 and FLT3 with IC_{50} values of 3 and 15 nM, respectively, and inhibits proliferation ($EC_{50} = 57$ nM) of the human myelomonocytic cell line MV-4-11. The compound also inhibits downstream signal transduction, further supporting the activity of this compound against JAK2 and FLT3. In human xenograft models in mice ($n = 8$), TG-101348 (120 mg/kg po, bid) caused the complete regression of MV-4-11 tumors after 22 days. TargeGen is currently focusing their development efforts on the JAK2 activity of the compound (see Section 8.3); no AML trials are currently listed on the NCI clinical trial website.

8.7   KIT INHIBITORS

Stromal tumors of the gastrointestinal tract (GIST) can affect patients over a wide age range, but they predominantly occur in middle-aged to elderly individuals and are slightly more common in females. In the United States, the incidence is between 3000 and 3500 new patients/year. The most common initial symptom is bleeding, and up to 20% of patients diagnosed with GIST present with anemia. These tumors are quite large, yet only a small proportion of them of them are palpable. The majority occur in the upper digestive tract. In 1998, the overall 5- and 10-year survival rates for malignant GISTs were estimated to be between 25% and 50%, with most patients dying from disseminated intra-abdominal disease with metastases to the omentum, mesentery, peritoneum, and liver, although more distant metastases can occur (mainly to the lungs and bone). Prior to the development of targeted therapies such as imatinib, treatment was essentially surgical. Surgical resection is still the traditional first-line treatment for GIST, with a 5-year survival of 48–54%, although with larger tumors (>10 cm) this figure is much lower (20%). Recurrence rates are variable, but it has been reported that up to 40% of tumors can recur within a 2-year period, and the response rate of recurrent tumors to conventional chemotherapy is extremely low (<5%); before the availability of imatinib the prognosis for recurrent GIST was dismal with a median survival of 15 months post-resection (320).

New insights into the biology of GIST triggered dramatic clinical progress. In 1998, a seminal paper by Hirota et al. (321) documented the presence of gain of function mutations in KIT in GIST patients. Studies from many laboratories around the world have confirmed this observation and it is now estimated that approximately 85% of patients with GIST have activating mutations of *KIT* (321–324), and another 5–7% have activating mutations of *PDGFR*α. These mutations occur early in GIST oncogenesis (325). The early and even initiating role of KIT (or PDGFRα) by constitutively active, gain of function mutations in GIST is evidenced by the observations of multiple kindreds where GISTs result, in an autosomal dominant manner, from germline *KIT* or *PDGFR*α mutations. The clinical manifestations that result from mutation depend on the KIT domain that is mutated. For example, mutations in the KIT juxtamembrane region have been associated with mastocytosis and hyperpigmentation in addition to the hyperplasia of the GIST progenitor interstitial cells of Cajal (ICC) that eventually progress to discrete GISTs. In contrast, mastocytosis and hyperpigmentation do not seem to occur (or at least not conspicuously) in patients with germline mutations that affect either of the split kinase domains (see Chapter 3 for further discussions of KIT mutations and GIST). (See Table 8.7.)

Imatinib Two important observations suggested that imatinib might be effective against GISTs. The first was the inhibitory activity of imatinib against wild-type and a common mutant KIT isoform in in vitro kinase assays (326); the second was the demonstration that imatinib had antiproliferative activity on a GIST cell line harboring a KIT gene mutation (327). In part, on the basis of these preclinical observations, the compassionate use of imatinib to treat a patient with GIST metastatic to the liver was granted in March 2000. Within a few weeks, metastases in this patient had shrunk by up to 75%, and 6 of 28 liver lesions were no longer detectable on MRI scans after 8 months of therapy. This correlated with a near complete inhibition of [^{18}F]fluorodeoxyglucose uptake on a PET scan (328). The

TABLE 8.7   KIT Inhibitors

Drug	Company	Known targets	Structure	Highest stage of development
Imatinib (STI-571; Gleevec®)	Novartis	ABL, KIT, PDGFR	Figure 8.1	Marketed
Sunitinib (SU-11248, Sutent®)	Pfizer	FLT3, KIT, PDGFRα, PDGFR,VEGFR, CSF1R, RET	Figure 9.1	Marketed
Sorafenib (BAY43-9006, Nexavar®)	Bayer	RAF, VEGFR, FLT3, KIT, RET, PDGFRβ, p38	Figure 9.1	Marketed
Dasatinib (BMS-354825, Sprycel®)	Bristol-Myers Squibb	ABL, EPH, FYN, LCK, SRC, PDGFR, p38	Figure 8.1	Phase II (marketed for CML)
Nilotinib (AMN107, Tasigna®)	Novartis	ABL, KIT, PDGFR, EPHB4, FGR, FYN, HCK, LCK, LYN, SRC, YES	Figure 8.1	Marketed
Motesanib diphosphate (AMG706)	Amgen/Takeda	Kit, PDGFR, VEGR1, VEGR2, VEGR3, RET	Figure 9.1	Phase III
Cediranib (AZD2171, Recentin®)	Astrazeneca	VEGR1,VEGR2, VEGR3, PDGFRα, PDGFRβ, FGFR1, SRC, ABL, CSF1R	Figure 9.1	Phase II
Masitinib (AB-1010)	AB Science	FGFR3, KIT, PDGFR	Figure 9.1	Phase II
Tandutinib (MLN518)	COR/Takeda	FLT3, PDGFR, KIT	Figure 8.5	Phase II
GSK-136089 (XL880)	GlaxoSmith Kline/Exelixis	MET, VEGFR1/2/3, KIT, TIE2	ND	Phase II
XL820	Exelixis	Kit, PDGFR, VEGFR	ND	Suspended
ABT-869	Abbott	VEGR1, VEGR2, VEGR3, FLT3, PDGFRβ, CSFR1, KIT	Figure 9.2	Phase II
Telatinib (BAY57−9352)	Bayer	KIT, VEGR2, VEGR3, PDGFR	Figure 9.2	Phase II
SU014813	Pfizer	PDGFR, VEGR1,VEGR2, KIT, FLT3	Figure 9.2	Phase II
Dovitinib (TKI258; CHIR258)	Chiron	FGFR, FLT3, VEGR, PDGFR, KIT	Figure 9.3	Phase I
BAY73−4506	Bayer	RAF, VEGR	ND	Phase I
E-7080	Eisai	KIT, VEGR2	Figure 9.3	Phase I

remarkable success of this treatment quickly led to a multicenter trial of patients with advanced, unresectable, KIT-positive GIST. In the Phase II trial, of the 147 patients in the trial (dosed at either 400 or 600 mg imatinib), 63% of the patients had a partial response and another 20% had stable disease (329). Disease progression was observed in only 14% of patients with initial follow-up. Similar exciting results were reported for the European Organization for Research and Treatment of Cancer Soft Tissue and Sarcoma group Phase I study of imatinib for soft tissue sarcomas, including GISTs (330). On the basis of these two trials, imatinib was approved by the FDA for the treatment of unresectable and metastatic GIST on February 1, 2002. Phase III data from both Europe and the United States confirmed the Phase II results. In patients with advanced disease, imatinib yields clinical improvement in 80% of patients. According to RECIST criteria this breaks down as 5% complete responses, 45–50% partial responses, and 25–30% with stable disease. The responses tend to be durable, with a median PFS of greater than 2 years and median overall survival time of 5 years (331, 332).

With the recognition that GISTs expressed KIT and frequently harbored activating mutations in KIT, and that many GIST patients were responsive to imatinib therapy, considerable interest developed among pathologists and oncologists to determine whether other tumor types might also express KIT and respond to imatinib. Initially there were many reports of immunoreactive KIT in a variety of tumors, although the results were highly variable due to the use of different reagents and methodologies, at least some of which resulted in artifactual reports of immunopositivity (333). Seminomas and systemic mastocyctosis express KIT and harbor KIT mutations; however, the KIT mutations in these tumor types most commonly occur in the kinase domain, and are not effectively inhibited by imatinib (see later discussion) (334). The most common mutation in systemic mastocytosis is the D816V mutation (335). Imatinib has minimal activity against KIT D816Y, D816F, or D816V mutant kinases (334). This is due to a steric clash between imatinib and the active ("open") conformation of the KIT activation loop. Gain of function mutations involving the KIT juxtamembrane domain also occur in some cases of AML (336). Other tumor types immunopositive for KIT include angiosarcoma, Ewing's sarcoma, and small cell carcinoma of the lung, although activating mutations have not been detected in these tumor types. Clinical trials of imatinib in small cell carcinoma did not show clinical benefit.

As discussed earlier, about 85% of GISTs harbor activating mutations in KIT, the majority of which occur in the juxtamembrane region (exon 11). However, a subset, approximately 15% of GISTs, have activating mutations in the extracellular domain (exon 9) or mutations in the split kinase domain (exon 13 or 17; <5%). Curiously, exon 9 mutations are found almost exclusively in the small intestine. A smaller subset (about 5%) of GISTs harbor mutations in *PDGFR*α, most of which occur in the second kinase domain (exon 18). The most frequent PDGFRα mutation is a single point mutation, D842V, which is resistant to imatinib (335). KIT expression in *PDGFR*α-mutant GISTs is quite often very low to undetectable. There are also so-called wild-type GISTs, which have neither *KIT* nor *PDGFR*α mutations. Recent clinical studies now indicate that the presence and location of mutations in *KIT* or *PDGFR*α show a strong correlation with the likelihood of a

TABLE 8.8   Response of KIT and PDGFRα Mutants to Imatinib

Genotype	Frequency	Responsive to imatinib
KIT exon 11 mutation	70%	85%
KIT exon 9 mutation	15%	45%
KIT exon 13 mutation	<5%	Some clinical responses
KIT exon 17 mutation	<5%	Some clinical responses
PDGFRα D842V	4%	No response
PDGFRα exon 12	1%	Some clinical responses
"Wild-type" GISTS	5–10%	Poor response

Source: Adapted from (333).

clinical response (Table 8.8). Thus it is now clear that GISTs are not a uniform group, but rather represent a group of closely related tumors. The molecular context of the tumor should be helpful in identifying patients in whom initial imatinib therapy is more likely to fail.

Despite the initial success of imatinib therapy, approximately 14% of patients are initially resistant and about 50% have tumor progression with the first two years. An additional 5% of patients are intolerant of imatinib therapy. Two kinds of progression are seen with GIST patients treated with imatinib: early and late. In progression-free survival curves, the early progressing subgroup is evidenced by a rapid decline in the first months of treatment ("initially resistant"); thereafter there is a more gradual decrease (late progression). Early progression (in general encountered within the first 6 months, frequently within 3 months on imatinib) is thought to be due to the initial mutational status (see Table 8.8) and also the occurrence of secondary KIT mutations. Some of the mutants (e.g., exon 9 mutations) may respond better to high-dose (800 mg) imatinib; for other mutants there is no difference in response to high or standard (400 mg) dose of imatinib. However, some patients with exon 9 mutations respond very well to imatinib at the standard dose. Moreover, in vitro studies have shown that imatinib inhibits wild-type KIT and exon 9 and exon 11 mutations at similar concentrations (323), suggesting that factors in addition to mutational status influence the initial sensitivity to imatinib therapy.

Patients progressing late on imatinib therapy are defined as those patients who initially had a response or PFS of 3 months or more (6 months in some studies) after initiation of imatinib therapy. This is thought to be due to occurrence of secondary *KIT* mutations, activation of alternative pathways, genomic amplification of *KIT*, upregulated expression of drug efflux pumps, or other pharmacological mechanisms that reduce exposure (e.g., increased clearance).

Secondary mutations have been found most often in exon 13, 14, 17, or 18 of *KIT*, all in regions near either the ATP binding site or the kinase activation loop. These mutations all cause changes in the conformation of KIT, resulting in reduced sensitivity to imatinib. Secondary mutations are more frequently found in tumors with mutated *KIT* in exon 11 than in exon 9 (337). Moreover, distinct secondary mutations can be found in distinct tumor lesions in a single patient (338–340), further illustrating both the heterogeneity and the genetic instability of GISTs. The most common KIT mutations associated with imatinib resistance are V654A, T670I (so-called gatekeeper mutation), S709F, D816V, D820Y, N822K, and Y823D (the latter four all activation loop mutations). Deletion of 559–560 VV in the juxtamembrane domain (exon 11) is also associated with imatinib resistance. Additionally, the D816V kinase domain mutation confers strong KIT activation.

Genomic amplification of *KIT* has been suggested as a potential mechanism to account for late progression. In this scenario, amplification would lead to an increased number of KIT molecules to inhibit, overwhelming the inhibitory capacity of imatinib. Whether or not this explanation is of clinical relevance remains to be demonstrated (338, 339). More classic mechanisms of drug resistance such as upregulation of efflux pumps and increased levels of the blood protein α1−glycoprotein (which binds imatinib, thus lowering the free-drug concentration) may also contribute to progression.

Management of progressive GIST has taken several approaches. One is to escalate the dose of imatinib, a strategy that has been beneficial with a subset of patients (e.g., those with exon 9 mutations, wild-type KIT, or genomic amplification). However, the maximum tolerated dose of imatinib in GIST patients is 800 mg (330). The alternative approach is to treat patients with another KIT-targeted tyrosine kinase inhibitor, either approved (e.g., sunitinib) or in clinical testing (see Table 8.7). These alternative compounds are discussed next.

Sunitinib   Sunitinib (SU11248; Sutent®) is a novel multitargeted tyrosine kinase inhibitor with activity against KIT, FLT3, PDGFR, and VEGFR (more detail on the in vitro and in vivo preclinical data on sunitinib is given in Chapter 9). For the treatment of GISTs, sunitinib offers two modes of therapy: antiangiogenic activity resulting in a reduction in tumor vessel density (via inhibition of VEGFRs and PDGFRs) and direct antitumor effects (through inhibition of KIT and PDGFRs). In a Phase I/II trial, 97 GIST patients who had failed imatinib therapy (due to resistance or drug intolerance) were randomized to receive 2 weeks of sunitinib at 25, 50, or 75 mg/d followed by 2 weeks off, 4 weeks of sunitnib (50 mg/d) followed by 2 weeks off, or 2 weeks of sunitinib 50 mg/d followed by 1 week off. Based on the early responses, the 4 weeks on/2 weeks off regimen was the most effective. Eight percent of the patients achieved a PR and 32% had stable disease of 6 weeks to 6 months, and 36% had stable disease for at least 6 months. Overall survival was 19.8 months, with considerable differences in survival based on initial KIT mutation status. The median survival was 29.2 months for those with wild-type KIT. A randomized, double-blind placebo controlled trial evaluating sunitinib as second-line therapy for GIST demonstrated a significantly increased median time to progression of nearly 30 weeks in the sunitinib arm versus 7 weeks in the placebo arm. In the Phase III trial, 312 GIST patients whose disease had failed imatinib therapy were assigned randomly to 50 mg qd of sunitinib or to a placebo. The primary endpoint was time to disease progression. Patients joined the trial at one of 56 sites in Europe, the United States, and elsewhere between December 2003 and May 2005. Sunitinib was given to 207 patients, while 105 received a placebo pill. The trial was designed to run for six treatment cycles, with patients receiving sunitinib or placebo for 4 weeks on/2 weeks off during each cycle. A planned interim analysis of the data was performed in January 2005 and revealed that patients taking sunitinib were living significantly longer without a recurrence of their disease. Following the recommendation of an independent review committee, patients in the placebo group were allowed to cross over to sunitinib for their final cycles. In the end, 88% of placebo patients crossed over to the sunitinib group. The updated analysis presented in June 2006 showed that disease progression was delayed for 27.3 weeks in those taking sunitinib, compared with 6.4 weeks for the placebo group. This means that patients taking sunitinib were 67% less likely to suffer a return of GIST than those taking a placebo. Overall survival was also extended by sunitinib. At 6 months, 13.4% of sunitinib patients had died, compared with 26.3% on placebo. On January 26, 2006, the FDA granted accelerated approval to sunitinib for the treatment of GIST patients whose disease has progressed after using imatinib or who were initially resistant to imatinib. This approval was based on the findings from the aforementioned trial. The approved dose of sunitinib is 50 mg/d given orally for 4 weeks, followed by a 2-week rest, with repetition of the cycle until tumor progression or intolerance develops. The most common adverse side effects are hypertension, diarrhea, mucositis/stomatitis, rash, and skin discoloration. Grade 3/4 toxicities, while relatively rare, include hypertension, diarrhea, fatigue, and hand–foot syndrome. Similar to the situation with imatinib, *KIT* mutation status seems to predict patient responsiveness to sunitinib.

Patients treated with sunitinib with wild-type or exon 9 mutations had significantly longer median time to progression than those patients with exon 11 mutations. However, this contrasts with the data for imatinib, where patients with exon 11 mutations had greater response rates and improved survival compared to wild-type or exon-9 mutated *KIT* (323). Sunitinib has no significant inhibitory effect on the kinase activity of the secondary imatinib-resistant mutations involving the KIT activation loop (exon 17, codons 815, 820, 822, and 823). Consistent with the in vitro studies, acquired imatinib-resistant mutations of these codons are associated with clinical resistance to both sunitinib and imatinib (341). Sunitinib also does not inhibit the imatinib-resistant PDGFRA-D842V mutant.

Hair depigmentation has been observed with several KIT inhibitors, including sunitinib, and appears to be a useful clinical biomarker for KIT inhibition. Changes in plasma levels of soluble KIT (sKIT) levels are being explored as a possible biomarker that could correlate with clinical benefit. Blackstein et al. (342) found that from the end of cycle 1 on, sunitinib treatment was associated with significant decreases in sKIT, and results from later time points (following cycle 2) suggested a predictive relationship between sKIT relative to baseline and clinical outcome. Most of the patients with increased sKIT relative to baseline had a poor prognosis, irrespective of treatment. In those patients with decreased levels relative to baseline, sunitinib treatment was associated with improved prognosis. The authors concluded the circulating sKIT may be a surrogate marker for time to progression in GIST patients and changes in sKIT could be predictive of time to progression and overall survival (343), although further studies are needed to confirm these findings.

Dasatinib   Dasatinib is a potent inhibitor of WT KIT and juxtamembrane domain mutant KIT autophosphorylation; it is also a potent inhibitor of imatinib-resistant KIT activation loop mutants (potency against KIT D816Y $\gg D816F > D816V$) and induces apoptosis in mast cell and leukemic cell lines expressing these mutations (344), although in cell-based assays, dasatinib is about tenfold more potent against wild-type and juxtamembrane domain mutant KIT isoforms than activation loop mutant isoforms (344). Since the most frequent gain of function KIT mutation in mast cell disorders, seminoma, and AML is the D816V mutation, it has been predicted that dasatinib would have biological and clinical activity against these human diseases, as well as against imatinib-resistant GIST (344). (See Table 8.9.)

In a Phase I study, 14 patients with GIST and other refractory solid tumors were treated with dasatinib at 35, 50, or 70 mg bid given orally, on a 5-day on/2-day off cycle for 5 days per week. There were no objective responses on CT, but activity was noted as mixed responses on FDG-PET, resolution of GIST-associated ascites (1 patient), and continued study treatment for ≥3 months in two GIST patients (345). In an update to this study, 18 patients with GIST were enrolled and the dose was escalated to 160 mg. Dose-limiting toxicities (rash and hypocalcemia) were observed in two of four patients at the 160-mg level. Patients were then enrolled into a continuous dosing schedule at 70 or 90 mg, where two of six patients experienced dose-limiting toxicities (rash, nausea, and lightheadedness). A dose of 100 mg bid continuously was being studied at that time. There was no significant myelosuppression, and nonhematological toxicities included fluid retention, gastrointestinal intolerance, headache, and bleeding causing dose reduction in 15% of patients. No objective responses were reported, although dasatinib treatment had been continued for ≥3 months in four GIST patients (346). Phase II studies evaluating dasatinib as first-line therapy in GIST patients are currently recruiting.

Sorafenib   Sorafenib (Nexavar®) inhibits KIT, VEGFR, RAF, and PDGFRβ. In cell-based assays using stable BaF3 cell lines harboring imatinib-resistant KIT

TABLE 8.9   Comparison of in Vitro Cell Proliferation Inhibition of KIT Single and Double Mutants Expressed in BaF3 Cells

Mutation	Imatinib	Dasatinib	Sorafenib	Nilotinib
V559D	63	27	66	44
Δ560V/V654A	3927	585	1074	192
Δ557 − 8WK/T670I	>10,000	>10,000	1063	>10,000
V559D/D820Y	3202	432	944	297
Δ557 − 8WK	460	58	211	83
502-503AY	509	74	400	671
T670I	>10,000	7543	918	>10,000
M822K	>10,000	868	3550	3083
AY502-3ins	509	74	400	671

Source: Adapted from (306).

mutations (V654A, T670I, D820Y, and N822K), sorafenib inhibited KIT activation (assessed by pKIT) and cell proliferation (347). In cell-based phosphorylation assays, however, sorafenib was less active against activation loop mutations (e.g., D816V) than the gatekeeper (T679I) mutants (348). In a randomized Phase II discontinuation trial of sorafenib, 2 patients with imatinib-resistant GIST developed partial responses lasting 11 months. In a preliminary report of a multicenter trial of sorafenib in patients with unresectable, KIT-expressing GIST that progressed either on imatinib or imatinib and sunitinib, 3 patients (13% of those evaluable) had partial responses, and 14 patients (58% of those evaluable) had stable disease (349). These data suggest that sorafenib may have clinical benefit in patients who have progressed on both imatinib and sunitinib therapies. This Phase II trial is continuing.

Nilotinib A Phase I study suggested that nilotinib has promising clinical activity in patients with GIST who are resistant to prior RTKs including imatinib. Fifty-three patients received nilotinib either alone ($n = 18$) or in combination with imatinib ($n = 35$), for a median of 134 days (range 8–430 days). Seventy-four percent of the patients had previously received second-line therapies including sunitinib, AMG706 (Motesanib diphosphate), dasatinib, or RAD001. One patient on nilotinib alone achieved partial response for >6 months and 36 patients (68%), 13 of which were on nilotinib alone, had stable disease ranging from 6 weeks to >6 months (350). As of July 2008, the NCI clinical trials website lists a Phase III evaluating nilotinib in patients who have failed both imatinib and sunitinib as currently recruiting.

Motesanib Diphosphate Motesanib diphosphate (AMG706) has inhibitory activity against VEGFR, PDGFR, and KIT and is currently being developed as an oral antiangiogenesis inhibitor (see Chapter 9). The compound was discovered by Amgen and was subsequently partnered with Takeda. Interim results from a Phase II study of motesanib diphosphate in Japanese patients with imatinib-resistant GIST were presented in January 2008. At the time of the abstract submission, 35 patients had been treated with at least one dose of motesanib diphosphate. One patient had a confirmed partial response, and seven patients had stable disease for ≥24 weeks. The patient with a confirmed partial response had a time to response of 28 days, and duration of response of 197 days. Common adverse events included hypertension, diarrhea, fatigue, headache, and weight loss. The authors concluded that in Japanese patients with advanced imatinib-resistant GIST, treatment with motesanib diphosphate was tolerable and showed an encouraging clinical benefit rate of 24% (351). Cholecystitis and enlargement of the gallbladder have been observed in 2–3% of patients who have received motesanib diphosphate (from patients treated with the compound in all indications). A Phase II study evaluating the efficacy of this compound in GIST is ongoing, but not actively recruiting.

Cediranib Cediranib (AZD2171) is an orally active anti-antiangiogenesis drug (Chapter 9) with potent KIT inhibitory activity from AstraZeneca that is being evaluated in GIST patients who are resistant or intolerant to imatinib. The drug is being dosed orally at 45 mg qd. A Phase II study to determine the antitumour activity and biological effects of Cediranib at a dose of 45 mg, primarily in GIST patients who are resistant to imatinib mesylate (current standard therapy) and also in patients with metastatic STS resistant to standard therapy, is ongoing but not actively recruiting.

Masitinib Masitinib (AB-1010) is a multikinase inhibitor that inhibits wild-type KIT and KIT-bearing juxtamembrane mutations. It also inhibits the PDGF and FGFR3 receptors. It is being developed by AB Science in France. In Phase I trials, a pathological complete response was observed in one patient who was intolerant of imatinib, leading to a multicenter Phase II trial in nontreated GIST patients. Twenty-six patients with advanced or metastatic GIST, naïve to imatinib treatment, were given masitinib orally at a dose of 7.5 mg/kg/d. Of the 21 evaluable patients, 52.4% of the patients had acheived a partial response, 38.1% were in stable disease, and 9.5% had progressed. The most frequent adverse events related to the study drug were asthenia, periorbital edema, muscle spasm, nausea, abdominal pain, rash, diarrhea, and vomiting (352). The compound had also been evaluated in mast cell tumors in dogs, but the Committee for Medicinal Products for Veterinary Use (CVMP) (London, UK) adopted a negative opinion and recommended the refusal of the granting of a marketing authorization for the veterinary medicinal product Masivet (50 mg and 150 mg film-coated tablets for dogs) based on tolerability problems and only a modest postponement in time to progression.

SU014813 SU014813 is an oral, multitargeted tyrosine kinase inhibitor that targets PDGFRs, VEGFRs, KIT, and FLT3 and is being developed by Pfizer. In a Phase I study evaluating the compound in combination with docetaxel in solid tumors, four GIST patients with TKI resistance were treated with SU014813. Prolonged stable disease was observed in one GIST patient who remained on study for more than 22 cycles, suggesting that the combination of 50 mg/d SU014813 with docetaxel 75 mg/m^2 might be active in treatment of refractory GIST and that Phase II studies were warranted (353). However, there do not appear to be any clinical trials with SU014813 in GIST currently ongoing.

XL820 XL820 (Exelixis) is an orally active, small molecule inhibitor of KIT, PDGFR, and VEGFR. In biochemical assays, XL820 exhibits IC$_{50}$ values of 0.9, 39.5, and 5.8 nM for KIT, PDGFRβ, and VEGFR2, respectively. In cellular phosphorylation assays, the compound inhibits the phosphorylation of wild-type receptors with IC$_{50}$ values of 110, 360, and 10 nM for c-KIT, PDGFRβ, and KDR, respectively. In HEK293 cells transiently expressing mutant KIT proteins, XL820 inhibits 26 of 27 mutated forms of KIT, with IC$_{50}$ values less than 300 nM. Only the D816V activation loop variant, which accounts for less than 10% of KIT mutations associated with sunitinib or imatinib GIST drug resistance, was substantially resistant to XL820 with IC$_{50}$ values >1000 nM (354).

In a Phase I clinical trial of XL820 in patients with metastatic or unresectable solid tumors, the compound was generally well tolerated with the most common treatment-related adverse events being nausea, fatigue, diarrhea, and vomiting (355). DLTs of grade 3 nausea and grade 3 fatigue were observed in one patient at 1600 mg qd and one patient at 300 mg bid. Modulation of biomarkers (VEGFR, VEGFA, PlGF, pERK, and pKIT in hair), consistent with VEGFR and KIT inhibition, was observed in some patients treated with XL820. Although two Phase II clinical trials with XL820 were initiated one as monotherapy in patients with solid tumors, and a second in advanced GIST patients with resistance to imatinib and/or sunitinib no further development has currently been reported.

ABT-869 ABT-869 is a small molecule RTK inhibitor identified by Abbott and licensed to Genentech (which is developing the compound) that inhibits VEGFR and PDGFR but has much less activity (IC_{50} values >1 μM) against unrelated RTKs, nonreceptor tyrosine kinases, or serine/threonine kinases. In cell-based assays, ABT-869 inhibits RTK phosphorylation with IC_{50} values of 2, 4, 7, and 31 nM against PDGFRβ, VEGFR2, CSFR1, and KIT, respectively. It is also a potent inhibitor of VEGF-stimulated endothelial proliferation ($IC_{50} = 0.2$ nM). This compound is discussed in more detail in Chapter 9. There are no ongoing clinical trials of ABT-869 in GIST.

E-7080 E-7080 is an inhibitor of the split kinase RTKs. In biochemical assays, the IC_{50} values for VEGFR1, VEGFR2, VEGFR3, FGFR1, PDGFRα, PDGFRβ, EGFR, and KIT are 4, 22, 5.2, 46, 51, 39, 6500, and 100 nM, respectively (356). In cell-based assays, E-7080 inhibits VEGF- and SCF-driven endothelial tube formation ($IC_{50} \approx 5$ nM) and also inhibits SCF-dependent H526 cell (small cell lung cancer) proliferation (356). E-7080 showed significant antitumor activity of H146 xenografts and caused tumor regression at 100 mg/kg (356). It has also shown activity in other xenograft models (lung, H460 and colorectal, Colo205).

E-7080 has now advanced into clinical studies. Results from a Phase I study were reported in 2008. The compound was administered once daily on a continuous dosing schedule in cycles of 4 weeks to patients with advanced solid tumors refractory to conventional therapies. A maximum tolerated dose of 25 mg/d was determined, with proteinuria and hypertension the most common adverse events. Other grade 3/4 toxicities included hemorrhage and thrombosis. Of the 52 treated patients, 39 were evaluable for response. The remaining 13 patients came off treatment prior to their first assessment due to disease progression, DLT, or other reasons. Of the remaining evaluable patients, 5 had a confirmed PR (1 sarcoma, 2 melanoma, 2 renal carcinoma), and 25 patients have had stable disease for a median of 16 weeks (range 8–88). Nine patients had disease progression. This promising indication of anticancer activity supported moving the compound into Phase II trials (357).

8.8 MET/RON INHIBITORS

Aberrant MET signaling is associated with many different cancer types, and the tumorgenic effects of sustained MET activation have been validated in many preclincial cancer models. In human malignancies, MET may be aberrantly activated as a consequence of activating mutations, translocations, or overexpression associated with or without gene amplification. Activation of MET promotes tumor cell invasiveness and triggers metastases, as well as playing an important role as a proangiogenic factor. A number of therapeutic strategies aimed at inhibition of HGF/MET signaling are currently being evaluated in clinical trials, including antibodies that directly inhibit HGF or its interaction with MET, antagonists of HGF, and small molecule MET tyrosine kinase inhibitors (Table 8.10).

Foretinib (GSK-136089/XL880) Foretinib (GSK-136089, formerly known as XL880) is being developed by GlaxoSmithKline (GSK) under license from Exelixis. This compound inhibits MET, VEGFR2, TIE2, PDGFRβ, FLT3, and KIT, with in vitro IC_{50} values of 0.4, 0.8, 1.1, 9.6, 3.6, and 6.7 nM, respectively (358). The compound is also very potent in cellular assays, inhibiting the autophosphorylation of the aforementioned receptors and concentrations ranging from 6.5 to 26 nM. In vivo, the compound was efficacious in a number of tumor xenograft models, and the efficacy was associated with rapid disruption of tumor vasculature and death of both tumor and vascular endothelial cells. In preclinical studies, the compound also demonstrated dose-dependent growth inhibition in tumor models of breast, colorectal, non small cell lung cancer, and glioblastoma and caused substantial tumor regression in all models tested. Significantly, in a glioma model a single dose of XL880 completely inhibited tumor growth for 21 days (358). Phase I data for XL880 were presented in 2007. The data presented were taken from two Phase I studies of XL880 in patients with advanced solid tumors. One study evaluated an intermittent, weight-based dosing regimen and the other a fixed (non-weight-based) daily dosing. Five partial responses (>30%

TABLE 8.10 MET Inhibitors

Drug	Developer	Known targets	Structure	Highest phase of development
BMS-907351/ XL184	Exelixis/Bristol-Myers Squibb	MET, RET, VEGFR, FLT3, KIT, TIE2	ND	Phase III
Foretinib (GSK-136089/XL880)	GlaxoSmith Kline/Exelixis	MET, VEGFR, KIT, TIE2	ND	Phase II
ARQ 197	Cyclis (ArQule)/ Kyowa Hakko Kogyo	MET	ND	Phase II
BMS-777607	Bristol-Myers Squibb	MET	Figure 8.6	Phase II
SGX-523	SGX Pharmaceuticals	MET	ND	Discontinued
JNJ-38877605	Ortho Biotech	MET	Figure 8.6	Phase I
MGCD-265	MethylGene	MET, RON, TIE2, VEGFR	ND	Phase I
PF-2341066	Pfizer	MET, ALK	Figure 8.6	Phase I
PF-4217903	Pfizer	MET	Figure 8.6	Phase I

tumor regression by RECIST) were observed, including three in papillary renal cell cancer, one in medullary thyroid cancer, and one in Hurthle cell thyroid cancer. Tumor shrinkage of less than 30% or prolonged stable disease of greater than 3 months was observed in an additional 20 patients. In a best response evaluation as determined by RECIST criteria, 39 of 45 patients in the combined Phase I studies had either tumor regression or stable disease. Histological analyses of tumor samples from four patients showed decreases in the phosphorylation of MET following administration of XL880. These decreases resulted in predicted downstream effects, including reduction of phosphorylated AKT levels and a marked increase in tumor cell death, effects not observed in control samples of normal tissue obtained from the same patients.

XL880 was generally well tolerated and reported side effects were treatable and reversible. DLTs included hypertension, dehydration, hand–foot syndrome, tumor hemorrhage, and elevation of liver enzymes and lipase. Most of the common reported side effects are consistent with previously identified effects associated with inhibition of VEGF signaling, such as hypertension and proteinuria. Elevations in liver function tests also were observed and considered possibly related to XL880. Interim data from an ongoing Phase II trial of XL880 in patients with papillary renal cell (PRC) carcinoma were reported in 2007. At the time of disclosure, a total of 21 patients had been enrolled in this ongoing study: five with activating MET mutations and 16 with wild-type MET. Of 19 patients with measurable disease evaluable for tumor responses, 15 (79%) had a decrease in tumor size (4–33%), including one patient with a partial response. All 19 evaluable patients with at least one post-baseline tumor assessment had stable disease for at least 3 months, including 12 patients with stable disease for 6 months to 15+ months. Results of preliminary analyses of plasma biomarkers and tumor samples were consistent with inhibition of angiogenesis and proliferation and an increase in apoptosis. Statistically significant changes in PIGF, VEGFA, sVEGFR2, and EPO, markers of antiangiogenic activity, were observed following administration of XL880. A potential plasma marker of MET inhibition, sMET, was statistically significantly increased in all 11 patients. Pre- and post-XL880 tumor biopsies from one patient with sporadic papillary renal cell carcinoma demonstrated decreased proliferation and induction of apoptosis following administration of XL880 (359). In December 2007, GSK exercised its option to exclusively license XL880, and the compound is now progressing into Phase III trial.

ARQ 197 ARQ 197 is described as a highly selective, non-ATP-competitive MET inhibitor. In cell-based assays, it inhibits HGF stimulated and constitutive MET phosphorylation in multiple cancer cell lines as well as reducing phosphorylation of downstream effectors including AKT, ERK1/2, and STAT3. The compound shows broad spectrum in vitro activity against multiple cell lines expressing MET, with highest activity on those cell types expressing constitutively active MET. ARQ 197 was relatively nontoxic to MET expressing primary CD34$^+$ bone marrow mononuclear cells (360). In vivo, oral administration of ARQ 197 inhibited the activity of MET, as well as inhibiting the growth of tumor xenografts (360). ARQ 197 also demonstrated significant inhibitory activity in tumor metastasis models

(361). In a Phase I dose escalation study in metastatic patients who had failed standard therapy, the compound was well tolerated and no DLT observed up to 180 mg bid of a total of 33 evaluable patients, 2 achieved a PR (1 confirmed) and 10 had stable disease from 10 to 34+ weeks. Additional Phase I data presented in November 2007 showed that 18 of 19 patients treated with ARQ 197 for 12 weeks or longer did not develop new metastatic lesions. Currently, ARQ 197 is in Phase II clinical trials in microphthalmia transcription factor-driven tumors (e.g., clear-cell sarcoma, alveolar soft parts sarcoma, and translocation-associated renal-cell carcinoma) and pancreatic cancer and NSCLC.

BMS-907351/XL184   BMS-907351/XL184 (Exelixis/Bristol-Myers Squibb) is a potent RTK inhibitor that targets primarily MET and VEGFR2 but also has significant activity against several other RTKs, including RET, KIT, FLT3, and TIE2. Reported in vitro IC_{50} values are 1.8 nM for MET, 0.035 nM for VEGFR2, 14.4 nM for FLT3, 14.3 nM for TIE2, and 4.6 nM for KIT. IC_{50} values for over 45 other serine/threonine kinases are all greater than 200 nM, and the IC_{50} values for PDGFR (234 nM) and IRK (1140 nM) are also quite high (362). In cells the compound is also very potent, with IC_{50} values under 10 nM for VEGFR2, MET, KIT, and FLT3-ITD mechanistic assays. In in vitro angiogenesis assays, the compound exhibits single-digit nanomolar potency (363). In mouse xenograft models, XL184, dosed orally, demonstrated dose-dependent inhibition of tumor growth and tumor regression, associated with disruption of the tumor vasculature and extensive tumor cell apoptosis (363). Interim results from two Phase I dose escalation studies were presented in 2007. The compound was generally well tolerated at all doses tested up to that date, with dose escalation ongoing to determine the daily dosing MTD. The compound has a terminal half-life of 59–136 hours, and preliminary analysis of biomarkers in plasma showed changes in VEGFA, sVEGFR2, and PlGF consistent with effects observed with other "angiokinase" inhibitors. Antitumor activity was observed in various cancers—4 PRs and 15 patients with stable disease. Of the seven patients with medullary thyroid cancer (MTC), six had tumor shrinkage and one had nonmeasurable disease. All seven assessable patients with MTC experienced a rapid decrease in plasma levels of calcitonin, a marker frequently elevated in MTC. Six of the seven patients had a decrease in the tumor marker carcinoembryonic antigen. At the time of reporting, all seven MTC patients remained on study. One patient with a neuroendocrine tumor has an unconfirmed partial response. In total, 15 patients with various malignancies have had stable disease lasting from 3 to 20 months, including nine patients with stable disease for more than 6 months. The compound is being evaluated in Phase II studies in NSCLC and glioblastoma, and a pivotal Phase III trial in MTC has also been initiated.

BMS-777607   Very little information is available in the public domain concerning BMS-777607, a MET inhibitor in Phase I/II clinical trials by Bristol-Myers Squibb. It is listed as being in a nonrandomized, open-label, dose-ranging trial in patients with advanced or metastatic tumors in the United States and Australia. BMS recently announced they have discontinued development of this drug.

SGX-523 SGX-523 (SGX Pharmaceuticals) is an orally available MET inhibitor for the potential treatment of solid tumors. SGX-523 exhibits low nanomolar IC_{50} values against the recombinant cytoplasmic domain of the kinase, and double-digit nanomolar IC_{50} values for proliferation in MET-driven cell lines. The compound was effective administered at 10 mg/kg bid in the GTL-16 and BaF3/TPR-MET xenograft models. SGX-523 was profiled against a panel of over 200 other kinases, and only significantly inhibited MET at concentrations <1 μM. The compound was orally available with good ADME properties. In January 2008, Phase I clinical trials were initiated with SGX-523; but in March 2008, unexpected dose-limiting toxicities were observed. A second MET inhibitor, SGX-126, was proposed as a development candidate, but its future is unclear following the acquisition of SGX pharmaceuticals by Eli Lilly and Co.

JNJ-38877605 JNJ-38877605 (Figure 8.6) is described as a small molecule that selectively and potently inhibits the MET pathway with promising preclinical properties and a clean toxicity profile. The compound inhibits MET with an IC_{50} of 4 nM; it is much less active on CSF1R (2650 nM), ARG (4070 nM), ABL (5950 nM), and TRKA (7120 nM) and exhibits an $IC_{50} > 10$ μM on 247 other kinases. The compound is also a potent inhibitor of cell proliferation in cell lines with activated or amplified MET (e.g., GTL16, SNU5, MKN45, and KATOIII; IC_{50} values <100 nM). The compound also demonstrated potent in vivo antitumor activity against KMN45 and U87 xenografts (364). A Phase I clinical trial was initiated in February 2008.

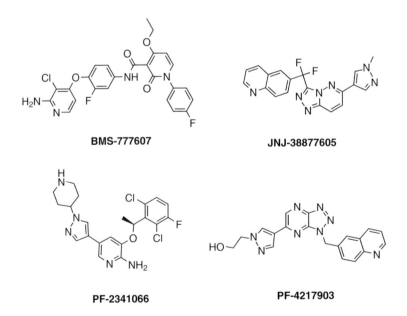

BMS-777607   JNJ-38877605

PF-2341066   PF-4217903

Figure 8.6 Structures of MET inhibitors.

MGCD-265   MGCD-265 is an orally active small molecule inhibitor of VEGFRs, MET, RON, and TIE2, currently in Phase I development by MethylGene. MGCD-265 inhibits the phosphorylation of wild-type and mutant forms of MET, TIE2, and VEGFR2 in cell-based assays with IC_{50} values in the nanomolar range. MGCD-265 also inhibited HGF-induced cell scattering and wound healing, and VEGF stimulated in vitro angiogenesis. The compound also inhibited tumor growth in multiple MET-dependent tumor xenografts, as well as other xenograft models using breast, kidney, pancreatic, and lung carcinoma cell lines (365).

PF-2341066   PF-2341066 (Figure 8.6) is an orally available, ATP-competitive, and selective small molecule inhibitor of MET and the NPM-ALK transgene product. It inhibits MET kinase activity with a mean K_I of 4 nM. In cell-based assays, the compound inhibits either ligand-induced WT and mutant (including those located at the ATP binding pocket, V1092I and H1094R), P-loop (M1250T), and juxtamembrane domain (R988C and T1010I)) MET phosphorylation or constitutive total tyrosine phosphorylation across a panel of cell lines with IC_{50} values ranging from 2 to 127 nM. PF-2341066 was less active against the Y1230C and Y1235D mutant variants of MET (these have mutations near the kinase domain activation loop). The compound was >100-fold selective for MET compared with the majority of kinases evaluated (with the notable exception of NPM-ALK). In cell-based assays the only two kinases with less than 20–30-fold higher IC_{50} values compared to MET were RON and AXL. PF-2341066 inhibits the NPM-ALK fusion variant of the ALK RTK expressed in KARPAS-299 cells with an IC_{50} value (24 nM) nearly equivalent to its MET activity. PF-2341066 inhibits growth of the GTL16 gastric carcinoma cell line with an IC_{50} of 9.7 nM and induced apoptosis in the same cell line with an IC_{50} of 8.4 nM. PF-2341066 also inhibits HGF-induced human NCI-H441 lung carcinoma cell migration and invasion at low nanomolar values. In endothelial cell assays, the compound showed potent inhibition of MET phosphorylation, cell survival, matrigel invasion, and branching tubulogenesis in fibrin gels. PF-2341066 was also a very potent inhibitor of GTL16 tumor xenograft growth, with 100% tumor growth inhibition at 50 mg/kg/day. The compound was also active in a number of other tumor xenograft models, including NCI-H441 NSCLC, CAKI-1 renal, and PC-3 prostate models (366).

In cell-based assays, PF-2341066 potently inhibits ALK phosphorylation and signal transduction resulting in G1-S phase cell cycle arrest and induction of apoptosis in NPM-ALK positive ALCL cells. Using KARPAS-299 ALCL tumor xenografts in SCID mice, the compound showed dose-dependent efficacy with complete tumor regression at 100 mg/kg qd (367). In addition, PD readouts of downstream NPM-ALK signaling mediators, including phospholipase Cγ, STAT3, ERK1/2, and AKT, were inhibited by PF-2341066 (367). The compound is currently in Phase I clinical trials in ALCL patients.

PF-4217903   PF-4217903 (Figure 8.6) is a small molecule, orally available inhibitor of MET ($K_I = 4.5$ nM). It is structurally unrelated to PF-2341066. The compound is ATP competitive and highly selective for MET, and inhibits MET-dependent cell proliferation, survival, migration, and invasion in tumor cells in vitro. Tumor growth inhibition was also observed in MET-dependent xenograft models. PF-4217903 is now in a Phase II clinical trial.

8.9 RET INHIBITORS

Medullary thyroid carcinoma (MTC) is a relatively uncommon malignancy that presents both in familial and sporadic forms. At present, there are no effective treatments for this disease other than total thyroidectomy (when applicable). The effects of external beam radiation are difficult to assess, and standard chemotherapeutic regimens for MTC are not therapeutically effective (368, 369). Germline and somatic mutations in RET are known to be causal of the familial form and greater than half of the sporadic cases of this cancer, respectively, suggesting that targeting RET may be a viable therapeutic strategy to treat this disease. RET germline mutations of MEN2A typically involve codons 634 and 618 and result in ligand-independent homodimerization resulting from covalent bonds of the cysteine-rich regions of the extracellular domain. MEN2B mutations most frequently involve codon 918 and apparently activate the RET receptor by increasing the level of Y1062 phosphorylation. The most frequent somatic mutation is M918T, which also results in constitutively activated RET. Several RET targeted agents are currently in various phases of development and have shown promising activity. (See Table 8.11.)

Sorafenib   Sorafenib, initially developed as a RAF inhibitor, was later found to inhibit other kinases including VEGFR, KIT, FLT3, PDGFR, and RET (see Chapter 9). In cell-based assays, sorafenib has IC_{50} values ranging from 20 to

TABLE 8.11   RET Inhibitors

Inhibitor	Developer	Known targets	Structure	Latest stage of development
Sunitinib (SU-11248, Sutent®)	Pfizer	FLT3, KIT, PDGFRα, PDGFR,VEGFR, CSF1R, RET	Figure 9.1	Launched
Sorafenib (BAY43-9006, Nexavar®)	Bayer	RAF, VEGFR, FLT3, KIT, RET, PDGFRβ, p38	Figure 9.1	Launched
BMS-907351/XL184	Exelixis/Bristol-Myers Squibb	MET, RET, VEGFR, FLT3, KIT, TIE2	ND	Phase III
Vandetanib (ZD6474; Zactima®)	AstraZeneca	EGFR, VEGF, RET	Figure 9.1	Phase III
AC-220	Ambit	CSF1R, KIT, FLT3, RET	ND	Phase I

50 nM on NIH-3T3 fibroblasts transfected with different activated RET mutants, with complete inhibition observed at 100 nM. The drug is active against C634R, M918T, V804L, and V804M RET mutations. Sorafenib also inhibited the proliferation of human TPC1 and TT thyroid carcinoma cells, which harbor activated RET mutations, as well as inhibiting the growth of TT xenografts (370). A Phase II study of sorafenib in metastatic thyroid carcinoma suggested that it may have significant activity in this indication. A total of 36 patients had been enrolled, and 34 patients were evaluable for response. A partial response was achieved in 7 patients with a duration of response of 23.7 to 82 weeks, and 20 patients had stable disease with a duration of response of 13.9 to 87.9 weeks. Among the patients who progressed, the median time to disease progression was 58.6 weeks (371). Phase II studies in MTC are ongoing.

Sunitinib Sunitinib is a small molecule, orally available inhibitor of VEGFR2, PDGFRβ, KIT, and FLT3, with modest activity against RET (see Chapter 9). Data from Phase II trials of sunitinib in thyroid cancer were presented in 2008. The compound showed modest activity in patients with MTC (of 10 patients treated, 1 PR and 2 with stable disease equal to or greater than 12 weeks) (372). Phase II studies evaluating sunitinib in MTC are ongoing.

BMS-907351/XL184 BMS-907351/XL184 is a potent inhibitor of MET, VEGFR2, and RET (see Section 8.8 and Chapter 9). In 2008, investigators presented Phase I data from an open-label, nonrandomized, dose escalation study of adult patients with solid tumors; the expanded MTD cohort included an additional 20 patients with MTC. The maximum tolerated dose was 175 mg qd. The drug was generally well tolerated, and antitumor activity was observed in various cancers. A partial response was observed in 10 patients (5 confirmed and 5 unconfirmed), 9 of which had MTC. Stable disease for 3 months or more was observed in 25 patients, 8 of whom had MTC. Many of the MTC patients had previously been treated with other RET inhibitors (vandetanib, motesanib, sorafenib, imatinib), as well as various other single-agent and combination chemotherapies. Response to XL184 was seen after failure of the other therapies. Genotyping studies of the responding MTC patients revealed mutations in RET (M918T, C620R, K808E, K821E, 629–630 del, C634Y, R982C, C634R, and C620W). The best overall response rate in MTC patients was 53%, and the disease control rate in MTC patients (partial response plus stable disease greater than 3 months) was 100% (373). An update on the activity of XL184 in MTC was presented in 2008. XL184 was generally well tolerated, with the most common drug-related adverse events being diarrhea, nausea, and fatigue. DLTs included AST, ALT, lipase activation, and mucositis. Evidence of clinical benefit was seen in various cancers with 13 PRs and 28 subjects with SD >3 months. The control rate in MTC was 84% (PR + SD >3 months). XL184 treatment in the MTD-expanded cohort was associated with statistically significant elevations in PlGF and VEGFa and decreases in sVEGFR2. Increased circulating sMET was also observed in some subjects (374). In July 2008, a pivotal Phase III study of XL184 in MTC was initiated.

Vandetanib   Vandetanib is a once-daily, orally active drug that targets VEGFR, EGFR, and RET (see Chapter 9). In in vitro assays, vandetanib inhibits RET enzymatic activity with an IC_{50} of 100 nM. It also blocks the in vivo phosphorylation and signaling of the RET/PTC3 and RET/MEN2B oncoproteins and of an epidermal growth factor (EGF)-activated EGF-receptor/RET chimeric receptor. Vandetanib inhibits the growth of papillary thyroid carcinoma cell lines that carry spontaneous RET/PTC1 rearrangements, and blocks anchorage-independent growth of RET/PTC3-transformed NIH-3T3 fibroblasts and the formation of tumors after injection of NIH-RET/PTC3 cells into nude mice (375). A methionine or leucine substitution for valine 804 (V804M and V804L) at the "gatekeeper residue" confers resistance to vandetanib (376). Data from Phase II open-label studies of vandetanib in patients with locally advanced or metastatic hereditary MTC were presented in 2007 and 2008. One trial dosed patients at 300 mg, and the second at 100 mg qd (377, 378). Both trials indicated that vandetanib demonstrated clinical activity and that the compound was well tolerated. These results suggest that vandetanib has clinical activity and a randomized, placebo-controlled, international Phase III study of vandetanib in MTC is ongoing.

Motesanib   Motesanib (AMG706) is a small molecule inhibitor of VEGFR, PDGFR, KIT, and RET currently in development by Amgen (see Chapter 9). Initial Phase II results from a trial of motesanib diphosphate in patients with thyroid cancer was presented in 2007. This multicenter open-label, single-arm study evaluated motesanib in patients with DTC and MTC. Patients received 125 mg motesanib daily until disease progression or unacceptable toxicity. This initial publication discussed the 93 patients with advanced, ^{131}I-resistant DTC that had been enrolled in the trial. After a median follow-up of 52 days, motesanib diphosphate showed some clinical activity (a low rate of objective responses, 12%, and a number of patients with durable ($\geq$24 weeks) stable disease, 24%) (379).

8.10   OTHER INHIBITORS

8.10.1   FAK

As of October 2008 there is only one small molecule focal adhesion kinase (FAK) inhibitor in clinical development (Figure 8.7). PF-00562271 is a selective, ATP-competitive inhibitor of FAK and PYK2 kinases, with in vitro IC_{50} values of 1.5 nM and 13 nM, respectively, and modest activity toward FLT3, GSK3α/β, and cyclin-dependent kinases CDK1, CDK2, CDK3, CDK5, and CDK7 (IC_{50} values 30–120 nM) (380). FAK is also potently inhibited by PF-00562271 in cellular assays and xenograft tumors and inhibits tumor growth in multiple models. Based on known mechanisms of FAK and immunohistochemical data, tumor growth inhibition may be due to induction of anoikis and/or antivascular effects: in addition, preclinical data support a role for FAK inhibitors such as PF-00562271 in metastatic bone tumors (381). PF-00562271 was evaluated in a Phase I dose escalation study given orally once or twice daily in 21-day cycles. Forty-seven patients received

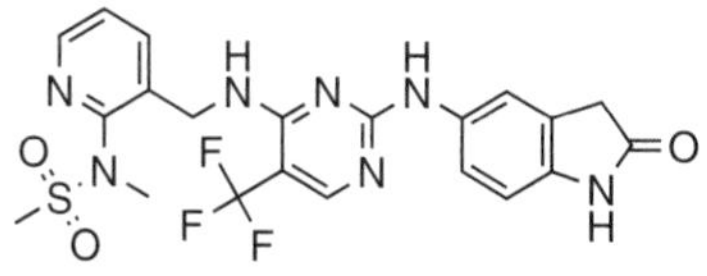

PF-00562271 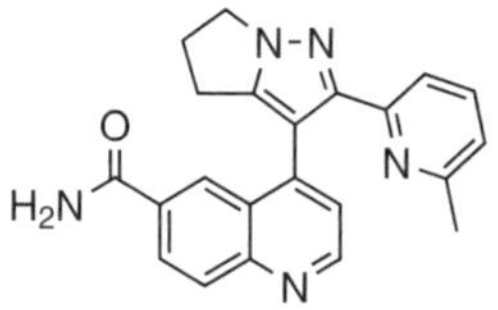   LY2157299

Figure 8.7   Structures of FAK and TGFβ receptor inhibitors.

doses ranging from 5 to 105 mg bid or qd. The maximal administered dose was 225 mg QD, and at that dose, DLT included nausea, vomiting, diarrhea, and orthostatic hypotension; all events reversed upon dose reduction or discontinuation. The compound displayed dose- and time-dependent nonlinearity of pharmacokinetics. The compound was tolerable with oral administration, and initial signs of clinical activity were observed in some patients who exhibited disease stabilization and in two patients who had improved tumor-related symptoms and central necrosis of metastatic or primary lesions (382).

8.10.2 TGFβ Receptor

Although the TGFβ receptor is a serine/threonine rather than a tyrosine kinase, we include it here in our discussion of receptor kinase inhibitors since it is a cell surface receptor protein. Transforming growth factor beta (TGFβ) is a pleiotrophic cytokine involved in the regulation of a number of physiological and pathological processes important to tumor growth, including angiogenesis, immune surveillance, and tissue remodeling. The activities of TGFβ can be both as a tumor suppressor and as a tumor promoter, depending on the stage of tumorigenesis and the response of the cancer cell (for a recent comprehensive review, see (383)). The actions of TGFβ are mediated by the binding of the cytokine to the type II TGFβ (TGFβRII) receptor, which in turn recruits a type I TGFβ (TGFβRI) receptor. The resulting heterotetramer enables the TGFβII receptor to phosphorylate the TGFβI receptor in the juxtamembrane domain, in a serine/threonine-rich region called the GS domain. The activated TGFβI receptor phosphorylates SMAD2 and SMAD3, which in turn form complexes with SMAD4. The SMAD complexes translocate to the nucleus and regulate gene transcription.

Currently, there is one small molecule TGFβ receptor kinase inhibitor in development, an ATP-competitive, dihydropyrrolopyrazole derivative, LY2157299 (Figure 8.7). This compound is an orally active, TGFβRI/II kinase dual inhibitor. In in vitro angiogenesis assays, LY2157299 dose-dependently potentiated VEGF- or bFGF-induced endothelial cell proliferation and VEGF-induced endothelial migration. The compound also neutralized TGFβ-induced inhibition of endothelial cord formation, resulting in a potentiation of angiogenesis in this model. In in vivo models, LY2157299 had some antitumor activity but did not show significant in vivo angiogenic effects (384). There is limited information available on the activity of this compound, but it has entered Phase I trials. Thus far two doses (40 and 80 mg) have been administered to patients with advanced/metastatic malignancies and who had exhausted all approved treatments. Daily oral administration of LY2157299 was safe and well tolerated at the two dose levels and the pharmacokinetic profile was consistent with the prediction derived from preclinical PK/PD models (385).

REFERENCES

1. Druker BJ, Sawyers CL, Kantarjian H, Resta DJ, Reese SF, Ford JM, Capdeville R, Talpaz M. Activity of a specific inhibitor of the BCR-ABL tyrosine kinase in the blast crisis of chronic myeloid leukemia and acute lymphoblastic leukemia with the Philadelphia chromosome. N Engl J Med 2001;344(14):1038–1042.
2. Ottmann OG, Druker BJ, Sawyers CL, Goldman JM, Reiffers J, Silver RT, Tura S, Fischer T, Deininger MW, Schiffer CA, Baccarani M, Gratwohl A, Hochhaus A, Hoelzer D, Fernandes-Reese S, Gathmann I, Capdeville R, O'Brien SG. A phase 2 study of imatinib in patients with relapsed or refractory Philadelphia chromosome-positive acute lymphoid leukemias. Blood 2002;100(6):1965–1971.
3. Gorre ME, Mohammed M, Ellwood K, Hsu N, Paquette R, Rao PN, Sawyers CL. Clinical resistance to STI-571 cancer therapy caused by BCR-ABL gene mutation or amplification. Science 2001;293(5531):876–880.
4. Hofmann WK, Jones LC, Lemp NA, de Vos S, Gschaidmeier H, Hoelzer D, Ottmann OG, Koeffler HP. Ph(+) acute lymphoblastic leukemia resistant to the tyrosine kinase inhibitor STI571 has a unique BCR-ABL gene mutation. Blood 2002;99(5):1860–1862.
5. Nardi V, Azam M, Daley GQ. Mechanisms and implications of imatinib resistance mutations in BCR-ABL. Curr Opin Hematol 2004;11(1):35–43.
6. Deininger M, Buchdunger E, Druker BJ. The development of imatinib as a therapeutic agent for chronic myeloid leukemia. Blood 2005;105(7):2640–2653.
7. Hegedus T, Orfi L, Seprodi A, Varadi A, Sarkadi B, Keri G. Interaction of tyrosine kinase inhibitors with the human multidrug transporter proteins, MDR1 and MRP1. Biochim Biophys Acta 2002;1587(2–3):318–325.
8. Donato NJ, Wu JY, Stapley J, Gallick G, Lin H, Arlinghaus R, Talpaz M. BCR-ABL independence and LYN kinase overexpression in chronic myelogenous leukemia cells selected for resistance to STI571. Blood 2003;101(2):690–698.
9. Dai Y, Rahmani M, Corey SJ, Dent P, Grant S. A Bcr/Abl-independent, Lyn-dependent form of imatinib mesylate (STI-571) resistance is associated with altered expression of Bcl-2. J Biol Chem 2004;279(33):34227–34239.
10. Ptasznik A, Nakata Y, Kalota A, Emerson SG, Gewirtz AM. Short interfering RNA (siRNA) targeting the Lyn kinase induces apoptosis in primary, and drug-resistant, BCR-ABL1(+) leukemia cells. Nat Med 2004;10(11):1187–1189.
11. Wu J, Meng F, Kong LY, Peng Z, Ying Y, Bornmann WG, Darnay BG, Lamothe B, Sun H, Talpaz M, Donato NJ. Association between imatinib-resistant BCR-ABL mutation-negative leukemia and persistent activation of LYN kinase. J Natl Cancer Inst 2008;100(13):926–939.
12. Rytting ME, Wierda WG. Central nervous system relapse in two patients with chronic myelogenous leukemia in myeloid blastic phase on imatinib mesylate therapy. Leuk Lymphoma 2004;45(8):1623–1626.
13. Rajappa S, Uppin SG, Raghunadharao D, Rao IS, Surath A. Isolated central nervous system blast crisis in chronic myeloid leukemia. Hematol Oncol 2004;22(4):179–181.
14. Matsuda M, Morita Y, Shimada T, Miyatake J, Hirase C, Tanaka M, Tatsumi Y, Maeda Y, Kanamaru A. Extramedullary blast crisis derived from 2 different clones in the central nervous system and neck during complete cytogenetic remission of chronic myelogenous leukemia treated with imatinib mesylate. Int J Hematol 2005;81(4):307–309.
15. Sorel N, Roy L, Martineau G, Guilhot F, Turhan AG, Chomel JC. Sequential emergence of ABL-kinase mutations with loss of unmutated BCR-ABL allele during targeted therapies of CML. Blood 2006;108(5):1782–1783.

16. Komarova NL, Wodarz D. Drug resistance in cancer: principles of emergence and prevention. Proc Natl Acad Sci U S A 2005;102(27):9714–9719.

17. Brave M, Goodman V, Kaminskas E, Farrell A, Timmer W, Pope S, Harapanhalli R, Saber H, Morse D, Bullock J, Men A, Noory C, Ramchandani R, Kenna L, Booth B, Gobburu J, Jiang X, Sridhara R, Justice R, Pazdur R. Sprycel for chronic myeloid leukemia and Philadelphia chromosome-positive acute lymphoblastic leukemia resistant to or intolerant of imatinib mesylate. Clin Cancer Res 2008;14(2):352–359.

18. Das J, Chen P, Norris D, Padmanabha R, Lin J, Moquin RV, Shen Z, Cook LS, Doweyko AM, Pitt S, Pang S, Shen DR, Fang Q, de Fex HF, McIntyre KW, Shuster DJ, Gillooly KM, Behnia K, Schieven GL, Wityak J, Barrish JC. 2-Aminothiazole as a novel kinase inhibitor template. Structure–activity relationship studies toward the discovery of N-(2-chloro-6-methylphenyl)-2-[[6-[4-(2-hydroxyethyl)-1- piperazinyl)]-2-methyl-4-pyrimidinyl]amino)]-1,3-thiazole-5-carbo-xamide (dasatinib, BMS-354825) as a potent pan-Src kinase inhibitor. J Med Chem 2006;49(23):6819–6832.

19. Shah NP, Tran C, Lee FY, Chen P, Norris D, Sawyers CL. Overriding imatinib resistance with a novel ABL kinase inhibitor. Science 2004;305(5682):399–401.

20. O'Hare T, Walters DK, Stoffregen EP, Jia T, Manley PW, Mestan J, Cowan-Jacob SW, Lee FY, Heinrich MC, Deininger MW, Druker BJ. In Vitro activity of Bcr-Abl inhibitors AMN107 and BMS-354825 against clinically relevant imatinib-resistant Abl kinase domain mutants. Cancer Res 2005;65(11):4500–4505.

21. Sawyers CL, Kantarjian H, Shah N, Cortes J, Paquette R, Donato N, Nicoll J, Bleickardt E, Chen TT, Talpaz M. Dasatinib (BMS-354825) in patients with chronic myeloid leukemia (CML) and Philadelphia-chromosome positive acute lymphoblastic leukemia (Ph+ ALL) who are resistant or intolerant to imatinib: update of a Phase I study. ASH Annual Meeting Abstracts 2005;106(11):Abstr 38.

22. Hochhaus A, Baccarani M, Sawyers C, Nagler A, Facon T, Goldberg SL, Cervantes F, Larson RA, Voi M, Ezzeddine R, Kantarjian H. Efficacy of dasatinib in patients with chronic phase Philadelphia chromosome-positive CML resistant or intolerant to imatinib: first results of the CA180013 "START-C" Phase II study. ASH Annual Meeting Abstracts 2005;106(11):Abstr 41.

23. Talpaz M, Shah NP, Kantarjian H, Donato N, Nicoll J, Paquette R, Cortes J, O'Brien S, Nicaise C, Bleickardt E, Blackwood-Chirchir MA, Iyer V, Chen TT, Huang F, Decillis AP, Sawyers CL. Dasatinib in imatinib-resistant Philadelphia chromosome-positive leukemias. N Engl J Med 2006;354(24):2531–2541.

24. Hochhaus A, Kantarjian HM, Baccarani M, Lipton JH, Apperley JF, Druker BJ, Facon T, Goldberg SL, Cervantes F, Niederwieser D, Silver RT, Stone RM, Hughes TP, Muller MC, Ezzeddine R, Countouriotis AM, Shah NP. Dasatinib induces notable hematologic and cytogenetic responses in chronic-phase chronic myeloid leukemia after failure of imatinib therapy. Blood 2007;109(6):2303–2309.

25. Quintas-Cardama A, Kantarjian H, Jones D, Nicaise C, O'Brien S, Giles F, Talpaz M, Cortes J. Dasatinib (BMS-354825) is active in Philadelphia chromosome-positive chronic myelogenous leukemia after imatinib and nilotinib (AMN107) therapy failure. Blood 2007;109(2):497–499.

26. Kantarjian H, Pasquini R, Hamerschlak N, Rousselot P, Holowiecki J, Jootar S, Robak T, Khoroshko N, Masszi T, Skotnicki A, Hellmann A, Zaritsky A, Golenkov A, Radich J, Hughes T, Countouriotis A, Shah N. Dasatinib or high-dose imatinib for chronic-phase chronic myeloid leukemia after failure of first-line imatinib: a randomized phase 2 trial. Blood 2007;109(12):5143–5150.

27. Jayson GC, Parker GJ, Mullamitha S, Valle JW, Saunders M, Broughton L, Lawrance J, Carrington B, Roberts C, Issa B, Buckley DL, Cheung S, Davies K, Watson Y, Zinkewich-Peotti K, Rolfe L, Jackson A. Blockade of platelet-derived growth factor receptor-beta by CDP860, a humanized, PEGylated di-Fab', leads to fluid accumulation and is associated with increased tumor vascularized volume. J Clin Oncol 2005;23(5):973–981.

28. Shah NP, Kantarjian HM, Kim DW, Rea D, Dorlhiac-Llacer PE, Milone JH, Vela-Ojeda J, Silver RT, Khoury HJ, Charbonnier A, Khoroshko N, Paquette RL, Deininger M, Collins RH, Otero I, Hughes T, Bleickardt E, Strauss L, Francis S, Hochhaus A. Intermittent target inhibition with

dasatinib 100mg once daily preserves efficacy and improves tolerability in imatinib-resistant and -intolerant chronic-phase chronic myeloid leukemia. J Clin Oncol 2008;26(19):3204–3212.

29. Shah NP, Kasap C, Weier C, Balbas M, Nicoll JM, Bleickardt E, Nicaise C, Sawyers CL. Transient potent BCR-ABL inhibition is sufficient to commit chronic myeloid leukemia cells irreversibly to apoptosis. Cancer Cell 2008;14(6):485–493.

30. Weisberg E, Manley PW, Breitenstein W, Bruggen J, Cowan-Jacob SW, Ray A, Huntly B, Fabbro D, Fendrich G, Hall-Meyers E, Kung AL, Mestan J, Daley GQ, Callahan L, Catley L, Cavazza C, Azam M, Neuberg D, Wright RD, Gilliland DG, Griffin JD. Characterization of AMN107, a selective inhibitor of native and mutant Bcr-Abl. Cancer Cell 2005;7(2):129–141.

31. Jabbour E, El Ahdab S, Cortes J, Kantarjian H. Nilotinib: a novel Bcr-Abl tyrosine kinase inhibitor for the treatment of leukemias. Expert Opin Investig Drugs 2008;17(7):1127–1136.

32. Deininger M. Nilotinib. Clin Cancer Res 2008;14: 4027–4031.

33. Golas JM, Arndt K, Etienne C, Lucas J, Nardin D, Gibbons J, Frost P, Ye F, Boschelli DH, Boschelli F. SKI-606, a 4-anilino-3-quinolinecarbonitrile dual inhibitor of Src and Abl kinases, is a potent antiproliferative agent against chronic myelogenous leukemia cells in culture and causes regression of K562 xenografts in nude mice. Cancer Res 2003;63(2):375–381.

34. Boschelli DH, Ye F, Wang YD, Dutia M, Johnson SL, Wu B, Miller K, Powell DW, Yaczko D, Young M, Tischler M, Arndt K, Discafani C, Etienne C, Gibbons J, Grod J, Lucas J, Weber JM, Boschelli F. Optimization of 4-phenylamino-3-quinolinecarbonitriles as potent inhibitors of Src kinase activity. J Med Chem 2001;44(23):3965–3977.

35. Puttini M, Coluccia AM, Boschelli F, Cleris L, Marchesi E, Donella-Deana A, Ahmed S, Redaelli S, Piazza R, Magistroni V, Andreoni F, Scapozza L, Formelli F, Gambacorti-Passerini C. In Vitro and in vivo activity of SKI-606, a novel Src-Abl inhibitor, against imatinib-resistant Bcr-Abl+ neoplastic cells. Cancer Res 2006;66(23):11314–11322.

36. Golas JM, Lucas J, Etienne C, Golas J, Discafani C, Sridharan L, Boghaert E, Arndt K, Ye F, Boschelli DH, Li F, Titsch C, Huselton C, Chaudhary I, Boschelli F. SKI-606, a Src/Abl inhibitor with in vivo activity in colon tumor xenograft models. Cancer Res 2005;65(12):5358–5364.

37. Soverini S, Tasco G, Grafone T, Colarossi S, Gnani A, Baccarani M, Casadio R, Martinelli G. Binding mode of the tyrosine kinase inhibitor bosutinib (SKI0606) to Abl kinase. J Clin Oncol (Meeting Abstracts) 2007;25(18 Suppl):Abstr 7049.

38. Gambacorti-Passerini C, Brummendorf TH, Kantarjian H, Martinelli G, Liu D, Fisher T, Hewes B, Volkert A, Abbas R, Cortes J. Bosutinib (SKI-606) exhibits clinical activity in patients with Philadelphia chromosome positive CML or AML who failed imatinib. J Clin Oncol (Meeting Abstracts) 2007;25(18 Suppl):Abstr 7006.

39. Bruemmendorf T, Cervantes F, Kim D, Chandy M, Fischer T, Hochhaus A, Liu D, Ossenkoppele G, Hewes B, Cortes J. Bosutinib is safe and active in patients (pts) with chronic phase (CP) chronic myeloid leukemia (CML) with resistance or intolerance to imatinib and other tyrosine kinase inhibitors. J Clin Oncol (Meeting Abstracts) 2008;26(15 Suppl):Abstr 2001.

40. Gambacorti-Passerini C, Kantarjian HM, Baccarani M, Porkka K, Turkina A, Zaritskey Y, Agarwal S, Hewes B, Khoury H. Activity and tolerance of bosutinib in patients with AP and BP CML and Ph+ALL. J Clin Oncol (Meeting Abstracts) 2008;26(15 Suppl):Abstr 7049.

41. Yokota A, Kimura S, Masuda S, Ashihara E, Kuroda J, Sato K, Kamitsuji Y, Kawata E, Deguchi Y, Urasaki Y, Terui Y, Ruthardt M, Ueda T, Hatake K, Inui K, Maekawa T. INNO-406, a novel BCR-ABL/Lyn dual tyrosine kinase inhibitor, suppresses the growth of Ph+ leukemia cells in the central nervous system, and cyclosporine A augments its in vivo activity. Blood 2007;109(1):306–314.

42. Pinilla-Ibarz J, Kantarjian HM, Cortes J, Nagler A, Hochhause A, Jones D, le Coutre P, Kimura S, Pima E, Gleich L, Ottman O. A phase I study of Inno-406 in patients with advanced Philadelphia chromosome-positive (Ph+) leukemias who are resistant or intolerant to imatinib and may have also failed second-generation tyrosine kinase inhibitors. J Clin Oncol (Meeting Abstracts) 2008;26(15 Suppl):Abstr 7018.

43. Ravandi F, Foran J, Verstovsek S, Cortes J, Wierda W, Boone P, Borthaku G, Sweeney T, Kantarjian H. A phase I trial of AT9283, a multitargeted kinase inhibitor, in patients with refractory hematological malignancies. Blood (ASH Annual Meeting Abstracts) 2007;110:Abstr 904.

44. Shah NP, Asatiani E, Cortes J, Paquette RL, Pinilla-Ibarz J, C. Kasap C, Bui LA, Yaron Y, Clary DO, Talpaz M. Interim results from a phase I clinical trial of the BCR-ABL inhibitor XL228 in drug-resistant PH+ leukemias. Haematologica 2008;93(s1): 47 Abstr 0120.

45. Cortes J, Paquette R, Talpaz M, Pinilla J, Asatiani E, Wetzler M, Lipton JH, Kasap C, Bui LA, Clary DO, Shah N. Preliminary clinical activity in a phase I trial of the BCR-ABL/IGF- 1R/Aurora kinase inhibitor XL228 in patients with Ph++ leukemias with either failure to multiple TKI therapies or with T315I mutation. ASH Annual Meeting Abstracts 2008;112(11): 3232.

46. Grunberger T, Demin P, Rounova O, Sharfe N, Cimpean L, Dadi H, Freywald A, Estrov Z, Roifman CM. Inhibition of acute lymphoblastic and myeloid leukemias by a novel kinase inhibitor. Blood 2003;102(12):4153–4158.

47. Rivera VM, Xu Q, Wang F, Snodgrass J, O'Hare T, Corbin AS, Keats J, Lamore S, Ning Y, Wardwell S, Russian K, Broudy M, Shakespeare WC, Druker BJ, Iuliucci JD, Clackson T. Potent antitumor activity of AP24534, an orally active inhibitor of Bcr-Abl variants including T315I, in in vitro and in vivo models of chronic myeloid leukemia (CML). ASH Annual Meeting Abstracts 2007;110(11):1032.

48. O'Hare T, Eide CA, Tyner JW, Corbin AS, Wong MJ, Buchanan S, Holme K, Jessen KA, Tang C, Lewis HA, Romero RD, Burley SK, Deininger MW. SGX393 inhibits the CML mutant Bcr-AblT315I and preempts in vitro resistance when combined with nilotinib or dasatinib. Proc Natl Acad Sci U S A 2008;105(14):5507–5512.

49. Nam S, Kim D, Cheng JQ, Zhang S, Lee JH, Buettner R, Mirosevich J, Lee FY, Jove R. Action of the Src family kinase inhibitor, dasatinib (BMS-354825), on human prostate cancer cells. Cancer Res 2005;65(20):9185–9189.

50. Shor AC, Keschman EA, Lee FY, Muro-Cacho C, Letson GD, Trent JC, Pledger WJ, Jove R. Dasatinib inhibits migration and invasion in diverse human sarcoma cell lines and induces apoptosis in bone sarcoma cells dependent on SRC kinase for survival. Cancer Res 2007;67(6):2800–2808.

51. Finn RS, Dering J, Ginther C, Wilson CA, Glaspy P, Tchekmedyian N, Slamon DJ. Dasatinib, an orally active small molecule inhibitor of both the src and abl kinases, selectively inhibits growth of basal-type/"triple-negative" breast cancer cell lines growing in vitro. Breast Cancer Res Treat 2007;105(3):319–326.

52. Serrels A, Macpherson IR, Evans TR, Lee FY, Clark EA, Sansom OJ, Ashton GH, Frame MC, Brunton VG. Identification of potential biomarkers for measuring inhibition of Src kinase activity in colon cancer cells following treatment with dasatinib. Mol Cancer Ther 2006;5(12):3014–3022.

53. Johnson FM, Saigal B, Talpaz M, Donato NJ. Dasatinib (BMS-354825) tyrosine kinase inhibitor suppresses invasion and induces cell cycle arrest and apoptosis of head and neck squamous cell carcinoma and non-small cell lung cancer cells. Clin Cancer Res 2005;11(19Pt 1):6924–6932.

54. Johnson F, Chiappori A, Burris HR, L, McCann B, Luo F, Mayfield S, Palme H, Platero J, Blackwood-Chirchir. A phase I study (CA 180021-Segment 2) of dasatinib in patients (pts) with advanced solid tumors. J Clin Oncol (Meeting Abstracts) 2007;25(18 Suppl):Abstr 14042.

55. Yu E, Wilding G, Posadas E, Gross M, Culine S, Massard C, GR H, Cheng S, Paliwal P, Sternberg C. Dasatinib in patients with hormone-refactory progressive prostate cancer: a phase II study. J Clin Oncol (Meeting Abstracts) 2008;26(15 Suppl):Abstr 5156.

56. Vultur A, Buettner R, Kowolik C, Liang W, Smith D, Boschelli F, Jove R. SKI-606 (bosutinib), a novel Src kinase inhibitor, suppresses migration and invasion of human breast cancer cells. Mol Cancer Ther 2008;7(5):1185–1194.

57. Messersmith W, Krishnamurthi S, Hewes B, Zacharchuck C, R A, Martins P, Dowling E, Volkert A, Martin A, Daud A. Bosutinib (SKI-606), a dual Src/Abl tyrosine kinase inhibitor: preliminary results from a phase I study in patients with advanced malignant solid tumors. J Clin Oncol (Meeting Abstracts) 2007;25(18 Suppl):Abstr 3552.

58. Hennequin LF, Allen J, Breed J, Curwen J, Fennell M, Green TP, Lambert-van der Brempt C, Morgentin R, Norman RA, Olivier A, Otterbein L, Ple PA, Warin N, Costello G. N-(5-chloro-1,3-benzodioxol-4-yl)-7-[2-(4-methylpiperazin-1-yl)ethoxy]-5- (tetrahydro-2H-pyran-4-yloxy)quinazolin-4-amine, a novel, highly selective, orally available, dual-specific c-Src/Abl kinase inhibitor. J Med Chem 2006;49(22):6465–6488.

59. Hiscox S, Morgan L, Green T, Nicholson RI. Src as a therapeutic target in anti-hormone/anti-growth factor-resistant breast cancer. Endocr Relat Cancer 2006;13 Suppl 1: S53-59.

60. Hiscox S, Morgan L, Green TP, Barrow D, Gee J, Nicholson RI. Elevated Src activity promotes cellular invasion and motility in tamoxifen resistant breast cancer cells. Breast Cancer Res Treat 2006;97(3):263–274.

61. Logie A, Jacobs M, Fennell M, Hargreaves J, Westwood R, Haupt N, Elvin P, Wilkinson R, Davies B, Green T. In Vivo evaluation of efficacy and pharmacodynamic biomarkers of AZD0530, a dual-specific Src/Abl kinase inhibitor, in preclinical, subcutaneous xenograft models. 18th EORTC-NCI-AACR Symposium on Molecular Targets and Cancer Therapeutics; 2006; Prague, Czech Republic. Abstr 617.

62. Chang YM, Bai L, Liu S, Yang JC, Kung HJ, Evans CP. Src family kinase oncogenic potential and pathways in prostate cancer as revealed by AZD0530. Oncogene 2008;27(49):6365–6375.

63. Evans C, Bi L, Hung K, Yang J. Effect of the specific Src kinase inhibitor AZD0530 on osteolytic lesions in prostate cancer. ASCO Genitourinary Cancers Symposium; 2008. Abstr 170.

64. Lockton J, Smethhurst D, McPherson M, Tootell R, Marshall A, Clack G, Gallagher N. Phase I ascending single and multiple dose studies to assess the safety, tolerability and pharmacokinetics of AZD0530, a highly selective, dual-specific Src-Abl inhibitor. J Clin Oncol (Meeting Abstracts) 2005;23(16 Suppl):Abstr 3125.

65. Tabernero J, Cervantes A, Hoekman K, Hurwitz H, Jodrell D, Hamberg P, Stuart M, Green T, Iacona R, Baselga J. Phase I study of AZD0530, an oral potent inhibitor of Src kinase: first demonstration of inhibition of Src activity in human cancers. J Clin Oncol (Meeting Abstracts) 2007;25(18 Suppl):Abstr 3520.

66. Harpur AG, Andres AC, Ziemiecki A, Aston RR, Wilks AF. JAK2, a third member of the JAK family of protein tyrosine kinases. Oncogene 1992;7(7):1347–1353.

67. Evans AE, Kisselbach KD, Liu X, Eggert A, Ikegaki N, Camoratto AM, Dionne C, Brodeur GM. Effect of CEP-751 (KT-6587) on neuroblastoma xenografts expressing TrkB. Med Pediatr Oncol 2001;36(1):181–184.

68. Evans AE, Kisselbach KD, Yamashiro DJ, Ikegaki N, Camoratto AM, Dionne CA, Brodeur GM. Antitumor activity of CEP-751 (KT-6587) on human neuroblastoma and medulloblastoma xenografts. Clin Cancer Res 1999;5(11):3594–3602.

69. Festuccia C, Muzi P, Gravina GL, Millimaggi D, Speca S, Dolo V, Ricevuto E, Vicentini C, Bologna M. Tyrosine kinase inhibitor CEP-701 blocks the NTRK1/NGF receptor and limits the invasive capability of prostate cancer cells in vitro. Int J Oncol 2007;30(1):193–200.

70. Miknyoczki SJ, Wan W, Chang H, Dobrzanski P, Ruggeri BA, Dionne CA, Buchkovich K. The neurotrophin-trk receptor axes are critical for the growth and progression of human prostatic carcinoma and pancreatic ductal adenocarcinoma xenografts in nude mice. Clin Cancer Res 2002;8(6):1924–1931.

71. Weeraratna AT, Dalrymple SL, Lamb JC, Denmeade SR, Miknyoczki S, Dionne CA, Isaacs JT. Pan-trk inhibition decreases metastasis and enhances host survival in experimental models as a result of its selective induction of apoptosis of prostate cancer cells. Clin Cancer Res 2001;7(8):2237–2245.

72. Miknyoczki SJ, Chang H, Klein-Szanto A, Dionne CA, Ruggeri BA. The Trk tyrosine kinase inhibitor CEP-701 (KT-5555) exhibits significant antitumor efficacy in preclinical xenograft models of human pancreatic ductal adenocarcinoma. Clin Cancer Res 1999;5(8):2205–2212.

73. Miknyoczki SJ, Dionne CA, Klein-Szanto AJ, Ruggeri BA. The novel Trk receptor tyrosine kinase inhibitor CEP-701 (KT-5555) exhibits antitumor efficacy against human pancreatic carcinoma (Panc1) xenograft growth and in vivo invasiveness. Ann N Y Acad Sci 1999;880: 252–262.

74. Levis M, Allebach J, Tse KF, Zheng R, Baldwin BR, Smith BD, Jones-Bolin S, Ruggeri B, Dionne C, Small D. A FLT3-targeted tyrosine kinase inhibitor is cytotoxic to leukemia cells in vitro and in vivo. Blood 2002;99(11):3885–3891.

75. Brown P, Levis M, Shurtleff S, Campana D, Downing J, Small D. FLT3 inhibition selectively kills childhood acute lymphoblastic leukemia cells with high levels of FLT3 expression. Blood 2005;105(2):812–820.

76. Hexner EO, Serdikoff C, Jan M, Swider CR, Robinson C, Yang S, Angeles T, Emerson SG, Carroll M, Ruggeri B, Dobrzanski P. Lestaurtinib (CEP701)is a JAK2 inhibitor that suppresses JAK2/STAT5 signaling and the proliferation of primary erythroid cells from patients with myeloproliferative disorders. Blood 2007.

77. Strock CJ, Park JI, Rosen DM, Ruggeri B, Denmeade SR, Ball DW, Nelkin BD. Activity of irinotecan and the tyrosine kinase inhibitor CEP-751 in medullary thyroid cancer. J Clin Endocrinol Metab 2006;91(1):79–84.

78. Strock CJ, Park JI, Rosen M, Dionne C, Ruggeri B, Jones-Bolin S, Denmeade SR, Ball DW, Nelkin BD. CEP-701 and CEP-751 inhibit constitutively activated RET tyrosine kinase activity and block medullary thyroid carcinoma cell growth. Cancer Res 2003;63(17):5559–5563.

79. Chan E, Mulkerin D, Rothenberg M, Holen KD, Lockhart AC, Thomas J, Berlin J. A phase I trial of CEP-701 + gemcitabine in patients with advanced adenocarcinoma of the pancreas. Invest New Drugs 2008;26(3):241–247.

80. Collins C, Carducci MA, Eisenberger MA, Isaacs JT, Partin AW, Pili R, Sinibaldi VJ, Walczak JS, Denmeade SR. Preclinical and clinical studies with the multi-kinase inhibitor CEP-701 as treatment for prostate cancer demonstrate the inadequacy of PSA response as a primary endpoint. Cancer Biol Ther 2007;6(9):1360–1367.

81. Smith BD, Levis M, Beran M, Giles F, Kantarjian H, Berg K, Murphy KM, Dauses T, Allebach J, Small D. Single-agent CEP-701, a novel FLT3 inhibitor, shows biologic and clinical activity in patients with relapsed or refractory acute myeloid leukemia. Blood 2004;103(10):3669–3676.

82. Verstovsek S, Tefferi A, Kornblau S, Thomas D, Cortes J, Ravandi-Kashani F, Garcia-Manero G, Kantarjian H. Phase II study of CEP701, an orally available JAK2 inhibitor, in patients with primary myelofibrosis and post polycythemia vera/essential thrombocythemia myelofibrosis. Blood (ASH Annual Meeting Abstracts) 2007;110(11): 3543.

83. Lyons J, Curry J, Mallet K, Miller D, Reule M, Sevears L, Tisi D, Wallis N. JAK2 and T315I Abl activity of clinical candidate, AT9283. AACR Annual Meeting; 2007 Apr 14–18; Los Angeles, CA. Abstr 5747.

84. Squires MS, Curry JE, Dawson MA, Scott MA, Barber K, Reule M, Smyth T, Wallis N, Yule M, Thompson NT, Lyons JF, Green AR. AT9283, a potent inhibitor of JAK2, is active in JAK2V617F myeloproliferative disease models. ASH Annual Meeting Abstracts 2007;110(11): 3537.

85. Wernig G, Kharas MG, Okabe R, Moore SA, Leeman DS, Cullen DE, Gozo M, McDowell EP, Levine RL, Doukas J, Mak CC, Noronha G, Martin M, Ko YD, Lee BH, Soll R, Tefferi A, Hood JD, Gilliland DG. Efficacy of TG101348, a selective JAK2 inhibitor, in treatment of a murine model of JAK2V617F-induced polycythemia vera. Blood (ASH Annual Meeting Abstracts) 2007;110(11): 556.

86. Wernig G, Kharas MG, Okabe R, Moore SA, Leeman DS, Cullen DE, Gozo M, McDowell EP, Levine RL, Doukas J, Mak CC, Noronha G, Martin M, Ko YD, Lee BH, Soll RM, Tefferi A, Hood JD, Gilliland DG. Efficacy of TG101348, a selective JAK2 inhibitor, in treatment of a murine model of JAK2V617F-induced polycythemia vera. Cancer Cell 2008;13(4):311–320.

87. Lasho TL, Tefferi A, Hood JD, Verstovsek S, Gilliland DG, Pardanani A. TG101348, a JAK2-selective antagonist, inhibits primary hematopoietic cells derived from myeloproliferative disorder patients with JAK2V617F, MPLW515K or JAK2 exon 12 mutations as well as mutation negative patients. Leukemia 2008;22(9):1790–1792.

88. Tam B, Mak CC, Stoughton S, Virata C, Lohse D, Hanna E, Alomia M, Jamieson C, Doukas J, Noronha G, Martin M, Soll R, Hood J. TG101348: a dual-acting JAK2/FLT3 small molecule kinase inhibitor for the treatment of AML. ASH Annual Meeting Abstracts 2007;110(11): 898.

89. Pardanani AD, Gotlib J, Jamieson C, Cortes J, Talpaz M, Stone RM, Silverman MH, Shorr J, Gilliland DG, Tefferi A. A phase I study of TG101348, an orally bioavailable JAK2-selective inhibitor, in patients with myelofibrosis. ASH Annual Meeting Abstracts 2008;112(11): 97.

90. Fridman J, Nussenzveig R, Liu P, Rodgers J, Burn T, Haley P, Scherle P, Newton R, Hollis G, Friedman S, Verstovsek S, Vaddi K. Discovery and preclinical characterization of INCB018424, a selective JAK2 inhibitor for the treatment of myeloproliferative disorders. Blood (ASH Annual Meeting Abstracts) 2007;110(11): 3538.

91. Verstovsek S, Kantarjian H, Pardanani A, Thomas D, Cortes J, Mesa R, Redman J, Staschen C-M, Fridman J, Vaddi K, Tefferi A. INCB018424, an oral, selective JAK2 inhibitor, shows significant clinical activity in a phase I/II study in patients with primary myelofibrosis (PMF) and post polycythemia vera/essential thrombocythemia myelofibrosis (post-PV/ET MF). Blood (ASH Annual Meeting Abstracts) 2007;110(11): 558.

92. Verstovsek S, Kantarjian HM, Pardanani AD, Thomas D, Cortes J, Mesa RA, Hogan WJ, Redman JR, Erickson-Viitanen S, Levy R, Vaddi K, Bradley E, Fridman J, Tefferi A. The JAK inhibitor, INCB018424, demonstrates durable and marked clinical responses in primary myelofibrosis (PMF) and post-polycythemia/essential thrombocythemia myelofibrosis (post PV/ETMF). Blood (ASH Annual Meeting Abstracts) 2008;112(11): 1762.

93. Mesa RA, Verstovsek S, Kantarjian HM, Pardanani AD, Friedman S, Newton R, Erickson-Viitanen S, Hunter D, Redman J, Yeleswaram S, Bradley E, Tefferi A. INCB018424, a selective JAK1/2 inhibitor, significantly improves the compromised nutritional status and frank cachexia in patients with myelofibrosis (MF). Blood (ASH Annual Meeting Abstracts) 2008;112(11): 1760.

94. Tefferi A, Kantarjian HM, Pardanani AD, Mesa RA, Newton RC, Scherle PA, Burn T, Verstovsek S. The clinical phenotype of myelofibrosis encompasses a chronic inflammatory state that is favorably altered by INCB018424, a selective inhibitor of JAK1/2. Blood (ASH Annual Meeting Abstracts) 2008;112(11): 2804.

95. Verstovsek S, Pardanani AD, Shah NP, Sokol L, Wadleigh M, Gilliland DG, List AF, Tefferi A, Kantarjian HM, Bui LA, Clary DO. A phase I study of XL019, a selective JAK2 inhibitor, in patients with primary myelofibrosis and post-polycythemia vera/essential thrombocythemia myelofibrosis. Blood (ASH Annual Meeting Abstracts) 2007;110(11): 553.

96. Shah NP, Olszynski P, Sokol L, Verstovsek S, Hoffman R, List AF, Cortes J, Kantarjian HM, Gilliland DG, Clary DO, Bui LA, Wadleigh M. A phase I study of XL019, a selective JAK2 inhibitor, in patients with primary myelofibrosis, post-polycythemia vera, or post-essential thrombocythemia myelofibrosis. Blood (ASH Annual Meeting Abstracts) 2008;112(11): 98.

97. Reid A, Vidal L, Shaw H, de Bono J. Dual inhibition of ErbB1 (EGFR/HER1) and ErbB2 (HER2/neu). Eur J Cancer 2007;43(3):481–489.

98. Goldstein NI, Prewett M, Zuklys K, Rockwell P, Mendelsohn J. Biological efficacy of a chimeric antibody to the epidermal growth factor receptor in a human tumor xenograft model. Clin Cancer Res 1995;1(11):1311–1318.

99. Baselga J, Pfister D, Cooper MR, Cohen R, Burtness B, Bos M, D'Andrea G, Seidman A, Norton L, Gunnett K, Falcey J, Anderson V, Waksal H, Mendelsohn J. Phase I studies of anti-epidermal growth factor receptor chimeric antibody C225 alone and in combination with cisplatin. J Clin Oncol 2000;18(4):904–914.

100. Saltz LB, Meropol NJ, Loehrer PJ Sr, Needle MN, Kopit J, Mayer RJ. Phase II trial of cetuximab in patients with refractory colorectal cancer that expresses the epidermal growth factor receptor. J Clin Oncol 2004;22(7):1201–1208.

101. Lenz HJ, Van Cutsem E, Khambata-Ford S, Mayer RJ, Gold P, Stella P, Mirtsching B, Cohn AL, Pippas AW, Azarnia N, Tsuchihashi Z, Mauro DJ, Rowinsky EK. Multicenter phase II and translational study of cetuximab in metastatic colorectal carcinoma refractory to irinotecan, oxaliplatin, and fluoropyrimidines. J Clin Oncol 2006;24(30):4914–4921.

102. Cunningham D, Humblet Y, Siena S, Khayat D, Bleiberg H, Santoro A, Bets D, Mueser M, Harstrick A, Verslype C, Chau I, Van Cutsem E. Cetuximab monotherapy and cetuximab plus irinotecan in irinotecan-refractory metastatic colorectal cancer. N Engl J Med 2004;351(4):337–345.

103. Moosmann N, Heinemann V. Cetuximab plus oxaliplatin-based chemotherapy in the treatment of colorectal cancer. Expert Rev Anticancer Ther 2008;8(3):319–329.

104. Van Cutsem E, Lang I, D'haens G, Moiseyenko V, Zaluski J, Folprecht G, Tejpar S, Kisker O, Stroh C, Rougier P. KRAS status and efficacy in the first-line treatment of patients with metastatic colorectal cancer (mCRC) treated with FOLFIRI with or without cetuximab: The CRYSTAL experience. J Clin Oncol 2008;26(15 Suppl):Abstr 2.

105. Bonner JA, Harari PM, Giralt J, Azarnia N, Shin DM, Cohen RB, Jones CU, Sur R, Raben D, Jassem J, Ove R, Kies MS, Baselga J, Youssoufian H, Amellal N, Rowinsky EK, Ang KK. Radiotherapy plus cetuximab for squamous-cell carcinoma of the head and neck. N Engl J Med 2006;354(6):567–578.

106. Rosell R, Robinet G, Szczesna A, Ramlau R, Constenla M, Mennecier BC, Pfeifer W, O'Byrne KJ, Welte T, Kolb R, Pirker R, Chemaissani A, Perol M, Ranson MR, Ellis PA, Pilz K, Reck M. Randomized phase II study of cetuximab plus cisplatin/vinorelbine compared with cisplatin/vinorelbine

alone as first-line therapy in EGFR-expressing advanced non-small-cell lung cancer. Ann Oncol 2008;19(2):362–369.

107. Pirker R, Szczesna A, von Pawel J, Krzakowski M, Ramlau R, Park K, Gatzemeier U, Bajeta E, Emig M, Pereira JR. FLEX: a randomized, multicenter, phase III study of cetuximab in combination with cisplatin/vinorelbine (CV) versus CV alone in the first-line treatment of patients with advanced non-small cell lung cancer (NSCLC). J Clin Oncol (Meeting Abstracts) 2008;26(15 Suppl):Abstr 3.

108. Van Cutsem E, Peeters M, Siena S, Humblet Y, Hendlisz A, Neyns B, Canon JL, Van Laethem JL, Maurel J, Richardson G, Wolf M, Amado RG. Open-label phase III trial of panitumumab plus best supportive care compared with best supportive care alone in patients with chemotherapy-refractory metastatic colorectal cancer. J Clin Oncol 2007;25(13):1658–1664.

109. Carter P, Presta L, Gorman CM, Ridgway JB, Henner D, Wong WL, Rowland AM, Kotts C, Carver ME, Shepard HM. Humanization of an anti-p185HER2 antibody for human cancer therapy. Proc Natl Acad Sci U S A 1992;89(10):4285–4289.

110. Cho HS, Mason K, Ramyar KX, Stanley AM, Gabelli SB, Denney DW Jr, Leahy DJ. Structure of the extracellular region of HER2 alone and in complex with the Herceptin Fab. Nature 2003;421(6924):756–760.

111. Baselga J. Phase I and II clinical trials of trastuzumab. Ann Oncol 2001;12 (Suppl 1): S49-55.

112. Slamon DJ, Leyland-Jones B, Shak S, Fuchs H, Paton V, Bajamonde A, Fleming T, Eiermann W, Wolter J, Pegram M, Baselga J, Norton L. Use of chemotherapy plus a monoclonal antibody against HER2 for metastatic breast cancer that overexpresses HER2. N Engl J Med 2001;344(11):783–792.

113. Vogel CL, Cobleigh MA, Tripathy D, Gutheil JC, Harris LN, Fehrenbacher L, Slamon DJ, Murphy M, Novotny WF, Burchmore M, Shak S, Stewart SJ, Press M. Efficacy and safety of trastuzumab as a single agent in first-line treatment of HER2-overexpressing metastatic breast cancer. J Clin Oncol 2002;20(3):719–726.

114. Hudis CA. Trastuzumab—mechanism of action and use in clinical practice. N Engl J Med 2007;357(1):39–51.

115. Agus DB, Gordon MS, Taylor C, Natale RB, Karlan B, Mendelson DS, Press MF, Allison DE, Sliwkowski MX, Lieberman G, Kelsey SM, Fyfe G. Phase I clinical study of pertuzumab, a novel HER dimerization inhibitor, in patients with advanced cancer. J Clin Oncol 2005;23(11):2534–2543.

116. Nahta R, Hung MC, Esteva FJ. The HER-2-targeting antibodies trastuzumab and pertuzumab synergistically inhibit the survival of breast cancer cells. Cancer Res 2004;64(7):2343–2346.

117. Portera CC, Walshe JM, Rosing DR, Denduluri N, Berman AW, Vatas U, Velarde M, Chow CK, Steinberg SM, Nguyen D, Yang SX, Swain SM. Cardiac toxicity and efficacy of trastuzumab combined with pertuzumab in patients with trastuzumab-insensitive human epidermal growth factor receptor 2-positive metastatic breast cancer. Clin Cancer Res 2008;14(9):2710–2716.

118. Fukuoka M, Yano S, Giaccone G, Tamura T, Nakagawa K, Douillard JY, Nishiwaki Y, Vansteenkiste J, Kudoh S, Rischin D, Eek R, Horai T, Noda K, Takata I, Smit E, Averbuch S, Macleod A, Feyereislova A, Dong RP, Baselga J. Multi-institutional randomized phase II trial of gefitinib for previously treated patients with advanced non-small-cell lung cancer (The IDEAL 1 Trial) [corrected]. J Clin Oncol 2003;21(12):2237–2246.

119. Kris MG, Natale RB, Herbst RS, Lynch TJ Jr, Prager D, Belani CP, Schiller JH, Kelly K, Spiridonidis H, Sandler A, Albain KS, Cella D, Wolf MK, Averbuch SD, Ochs JJ, Kay AC. Efficacy of gefitinib, an inhibitor of the epidermal growth factor receptor tyrosine kinase, in symptomatic patients with non-small cell lung cancer: a randomized trial. JAMA 2003;290(16):2149–2158.

120. Miller VA, Kris MG, Shah N, Patel J, Azzoli C, Gomez J, Krug LM, Pao W, Rizvi N, Pizzo B, Tyson L, Venkatraman E, Ben-Porat L, Memoli N, Zakowski M, Rusch V, Heelan RT. Bronchioloalveolar pathologic subtype and smoking history predict sensitivity to gefitinib in advanced non-small-cell lung cancer. J Clin Oncol 2004;22(6):1103–1109.

121. Lynch TJ, Bell DW, Sordella R, Gurubhagavatula S, Okimoto RA, Brannigan BW, Harris PL, Haserlat SM, Supko JG, Haluska FG, Louis DN, Christiani DC, Settleman J, Haber DA. Activating mutations in the epidermal growth factor receptor underlying responsiveness of non-small-cell lung cancer to gefitinib. N Engl J Med 2004;350(21):2129–2139.

122. Paez JG, Janne PA, Lee JC, Tracy S, Greulich H, Gabriel S, Herman P, Kaye FJ, Lindeman N, Boggon TJ, Naoki K, Sasaki H, Fujii Y, Eck MJ, Sellers WR, Johnson BE, Meyerson M. EGFR mutations in lung cancer: correlation with clinical response to gefitinib therapy. Science 2004;304(5676):1497–1500.

123. Pao W, Miller V, Zakowski M, Doherty J, Politi K, Sarkaria I, Singh B, Heelan R, Rusch V, Fulton L, Mardis E, Kupfer D, Wilson R, Kris M, Varmus H. EGF receptor gene mutations are common in lung cancers from "never smokers" and are associated with sensitivity of tumors to gefitinib and erlotinib. Proc Natl Acad Sci U S A 2004;101(36):13306–13311.

124. Sharma SV, Bell DW, Settleman J, Haber DA. Epidermal growth factor receptor mutations in lung cancer. Nat Rev Cancer 2007;7(3):169–181.

125. Riely GJ, Politi KA, Miller VA, Pao W. Update on epidermal growth factor receptor mutations in non-small cell lung cancer. Clin Cancer Res 2006;12(24):7232–7241.

126. Weinstein IB. Cancer. Addiction to oncogenes—the Achilles heal of cancer. Science 2002;297(5578):63–64.

127. Yun CH, Boggon TJ, Li Y, Woo MS, Greulich H, Meyerson M, Eck MJ. Structures of lung cancer-derived EGFR mutants and inhibitor complexes: mechanism of activation and insights into differential inhibitor sensitivity. Cancer Cell 2007;11(3):217–227.

128. Engelman JA, Janne PA, Mermel C, Pearlberg J, Mukohara T, Fleet C, Cichowski K, Johnson BE, Cantley LC. ErbB-3 mediates phosphoinositide 3-kinase activity in gefitinib-sensitive non-small cell lung cancer cell lines. Proc Natl Acad Sci U S A 2005;102(10):3788–3793.

129. Carey KD, Garton AJ, Romero MS, Kahler J, Thomson S, Ross S, Park F, Haley JD, Gibson N, Sliwkowski MX. Kinetic analysis of epidermal growth factor receptor somatic mutant proteins shows increased sensitivity to the epidermal growth factor receptor tyrosine kinase inhibitor, erlotinib. Cancer Res 2006;66(16):8163–8171.

130. Eberhard DA, Johnson BE, Amler LC, Goddard AD, Heldens SL, Herbst RS, Ince WL, Janne PA, Januario T, Johnson DH, Klein P, Miller VA, Ostland MA, Ramies DA, Sebisanovic D, Stinson JA, Zhang YR, Seshagiri S, Hillan KJ. Mutations in the epidermal growth factor receptor and in KRAS are predictive and prognostic indicators in patients with non-small-cell lung cancer treated with chemotherapy alone and in combination with erlotinib. J Clin Oncol 2005;23(25):5900–5909.

131. Jackman DM, Yeap BY, Sequist LV, Lindeman N, Holmes AJ, Joshi VA, Bell DW, Huberman MS, Halmos B, Rabin MS, Haber DA, Lynch TJ, Meyerson M, Johnson BE, Janne PA. Exon 19 deletion mutations of epidermal growth factor receptor are associated with prolonged survival in non-small cell lung cancer patients treated with gefitinib or erlotinib. Clin Cancer Res 2006;12(13):3908–3914.

132. Riely GJ, Pao W, Pham D, Li AR, Rizvi N, Venkatraman ES, Zakowski MF, Kris MG, Ladanyi M, Miller VA. Clinical course of patients with non-small cell lung cancer and epidermal growth factor receptor exon 19 and exon 21 mutations treated with gefitinib or erlotinib. Clin Cancer Res 2006;12(3Pt 1):839–844.

133. Cappuzzo F, Hirsch FR, Rossi E, Bartolini S, Ceresoli GL, Bemis L, Haney J, Witta S, Danenberg K, Domenichini I, Ludovini V, Magrini E, Gregorc V, Doglioni C, Sidoni A, Tonato M, Franklin WA, Crino L, Bunn PA Jr, Varella-Garcia M. Epidermal growth factor receptor gene and protein and gefitinib sensitivity in non-small-cell lung cancer. J Natl Cancer Inst 2005;97(9):643–655.

134. Hirsch FR, Herbst RS, Olsen C, Chansky K, Crowley J, Kelly K, Franklin WA, Bunn PA Jr, Varella-Garcia M, Gandara DR. Increased EGFR gene copy number detected by fluorescent in situ hybridization predicts outcome in non-small-cell lung cancer patients treated with cetuximab and chemotherapy. J Clin Oncol 2008;26(20):3351–3357.

135. Cappuzzo F, Varella-Garcia M, Shigematsu H, Domenichini I, Bartolini S, Ceresoli GL, Rossi E, Ludovini V, Gregorc V, Toschi L, Franklin WA, Crino L, Gazdar AF, Bunn PA Jr, Hirsch FR. Increased HER2 gene copy number is associated with response to gefitinib therapy in epidermal growth factor receptor-positive non-small-cell lung cancer patients. J Clin Oncol 2005;23(22):5007–5018.

136. Stephens P, Hunter C, Bignell G, Edkins S, Davies H, Teague J, Stevens C, O'Meara S, Smith R, Parker A, Barthorpe A, Blow M, Brackenbury L, Butler A, Clarke O, Cole J, Dicks E, Dike A, Drozd A, Edwards K, Forbes S, Foster R, Gray K, Greenman C, Halliday K, Hills K, Kosmidou V, Lugg R, Menzies A, Perry J, Petty R, Raine K, Ratford L, Shepherd R, Small A, Stephens

Y, Tofts C, Varian J, West S, Widaa S, Yates A, Brasseur F, Cooper CS, Flanagan AM, Knowles M, Leung SY, Louis DN, Looijenga LH, Malkowicz B, Pierotti MA, Teh B, Chenevix-Trench G, Weber BL, Yuen ST, Harris G, Goldstraw P, Nicholson AG, Futreal PA, Wooster R, Stratton MR. Lung cancer: intragenic ERBB2 kinase mutations in tumours. Nature 2004;431(7008):525–526.

137. Husgafvel-Pursiainen K, Hackman P, Ridanpaa M, Anttila S, Karjalainen A, Partanen T, Taikina-Aho O, Heikkila L, Vainio H. K-ras mutations in human adenocarcinoma of the lung: association with smoking and occupational exposure to asbestos. Int J Cancer 1993;53(2):250–256.

138. Ahrendt SA, Decker PA, Alawi EA, Zhu YR, Sanchez-Cespedes M, Yang SC, Haasler GB, Kajdacsy-Balla A, Demeure MJ, Sidransky D. Cigarette smoking is strongly associated with mutation of the K-ras gene in patients with primary adenocarcinoma of the lung. Cancer 2001;92(6):1525–1530.

139. Han SW, Kim TY, Jeon YK, Hwang PG, Im SA, Lee KH, Kim JH, Kim DW, Heo DS, Kim NK, Chung DH, Bang YJ. Optimization of patient selection for gefitinib in non-small cell lung cancer by combined analysis of epidermal growth factor receptor mutation, K-ras mutation, and Akt phosphorylation. Clin Cancer Res 2006;12(8):2538–2544.

140. Pao W, Wang TY, Riely GJ, Miller VA, Pan Q, Ladanyi M, Zakowski MF, Heelan RT, Kris MG, Varmus HE. KRAS mutations and primary resistance of lung adenocarcinomas to gefitinib or erlotinib. PLoS Med 2005;2(1): e17.

141. Giaccone G, Gallegos Ruiz M, Le Chevalier T, Thatcher N, Smit E, Rodriguez JA, Janne P, Oulid-Aissa D, Soria JC. Erlotinib for frontline treatment of advanced non-small cell lung cancer: a phase II study. Clin Cancer Res 2006;12(20Pt 1):6049–6055.

142. Jackman DM, Yeap BY, Lindeman NI, Fidias P, Rabin MS, Temel J, Skarin AT, Meyerson M, Holmes AJ, Borras AM, Freidlin B, Ostler PA, Lucca J, Lynch TJ, Johnson BE, Janne PA. Phase II clinical trial of chemotherapy-naive patients <or = 70 years of age treated with erlotinib for advanced non-small-cell lung cancer. J Clin Oncol 2007;25(7):760–766.

143. Pao W, Miller VA, Politi KA, Riely GJ, Somwar R, Zakowski MF, Kris MG, Varmus H. Acquired resistance of lung adenocarcinomas to gefitinib or erlotinib is associated with a second mutation in the EGFR kinase domain. PLoS Med 2005;2(3): e73.

144. Yun CH, Mengwasser KE, Toms AV, Woo MS, Greulich H, Wong KK, Meyerson M, Eck MJ. The T790M mutation in EGFR kinase causes drug resistance by increasing the affinity for ATP. Proc Natl Acad Sci U S A 2008;105(6):2070–2075.

145. Balak MN, Gong Y, Riely GJ, Somwar R, Li AR, Zakowski MF, Chiang A, Yang G, Ouerfelli O, Kris MG, Ladanyi M, Miller VA, Pao W. Novel D761Y and common secondary T790M mutations in epidermal growth factor receptor-mutant lung adenocarcinomas with acquired resistance to kinase inhibitors. Clin Cancer Res 2006;12(21):6494–6501.

146. Kwak EL, Sordella R, Bell DW, Godin-Heymann N, Okimoto RA, Brannigan BW, Harris PL, Driscoll DR, Fidias P, Lynch TJ, Rabindran SK, McGinnis JP, Wissner A, Sharma SV, Isselbacher KJ, Settleman J, Haber DA. Irreversible inhibitors of the EGF receptor may circumvent acquired resistance to gefitinib. Proc Natl Acad Sci U S A 2005;102(21):7665–7670.

147. Desbois-Mouthon C, Cacheux W, Blivet-Van Eggelpoel MJ, Barbu V, Fartoux L, Poupon R, Housset C, Rosmorduc O. Impact of IGF-1R/EGFR cross-talks on hepatoma cell sensitivity to gefitinib. Int J Cancer 2006;119(11):2557–2566.

148. Jones HE, Goddard L, Gee JM, Hiscox S, Rubini M, Barrow D, Knowlden JM, Williams S, Wakeling AE, Nicholson RI. Insulin-like growth factor-I receptor signalling and acquired resistance to gefitinib (ZD1839; Iressa) in human breast and prostate cancer cells. Endocr Relat Cancer 2004;11(4):793–814.

149. Bean J, Brennan C, Shih JY, Riely G, Viale A, Wang L, Chitale D, Motoi N, Szoke J, Broderick S, Balak M, Chang WC, Yu CJ, Gazdar A, Pass H, Rusch V, Gerald W, Huang SF, Yang PC, Miller V, Ladanyi M, Yang CH, Pao W. MET amplification occurs with or without T790M mutations in EGFR mutant lung tumors with acquired resistance to gefitinib or erlotinib. Proc Natl Acad Sci U S A 2007;104(52):20932–20937.

150. Engelman JA, Zejnullahu K, Mitsudomi T, Song Y, Hyland C, Park JO, Lindeman N, Gale CM, Zhao X, Christensen J, Kosaka T, Holmes AJ, Rogers AM, Cappuzzo F, Mok T, Lee C, Johnson BE, Cantley LC, Janne PA. MET amplification leads to gefitinib resistance in lung cancer by activating ERBB3 signaling. Science 2007;316(5827):1039–1043.

151. Mellinghoff IK, Wang MY, Vivanco I, Haas-Kogan DA, Zhu S, Dia EQ, Lu KV, Yoshimoto K, Huang JH, Chute DJ, Riggs BL, Horvath S, Liau LM, Cavenee WK, Rao PN, Beroukhim R, Peck TC, Lee JC, Sellers WR, Stokoe D, Prados M, Cloughesy TF, Sawyers CL, Mischel PS. Molecular determinants of the response of glioblastomas to EGFR kinase inhibitors. N Engl J Med 2005;353(19):2012–2024.

152. Haas-Kogan DA, Prados MD, Tihan T, Eberhard DA, Jelluma N, Arvold ND, Baumber R, Lamborn KR, Kapadia A, Malec M, Berger MS, Stokoe D. Epidermal growth factor receptor, protein kinase B/Akt, and glioma response to erlotinib. J Natl Cancer Inst 2005;97(12):880–887.

153. Moroni M, Veronese S, Benvenuti S, Marrapese G, Sartore-Bianchi A, Di Nicolantonio F, Gambacorta M, Siena S, Bardelli A. Gene copy number for epidermal growth factor receptor (EGFR) and clinical response to antiEGFR treatment in colorectal cancer: a cohort study. Lancet Oncol 2005;6(5):279–286.

154. Cappuzzo F, Finocchiaro G, Rossi E, Janne PA, Carnaghi C, Calandri C, Bencardino K, Ligorio C, Ciardiello F, Pressiani T, Destro A, Roncalli M, Crino L, Franklin WA, Santoro A, Varella-Garcia M. EGFR FISH assay predicts for response to cetuximab in chemotherapy refractory colorectal cancer patients. Ann Oncol 2008;19(4):717–723.

155. Sartore-Bianchi A, Moroni M, Veronese S, Carnaghi C, Bajetta E, Luppi G, Sobrero A, Barone C, Cascinu S, Colucci G, Cortesi E, Nichelatti M, Gambacorta M, Siena S. Epidermal growth factor receptor gene copy number and clinical outcome of metastatic colorectal cancer treated with panitumumab. J Clin Oncol 2007;25(22):3238–3245.

156. Italiano A, Follana P, Caroli FX, Badetti JL, Benchimol D, Garnier G, Gugenheim J, Haudebourg J, Keslair F, Lesbats G, Lledo G, Roussel JF, Pedeutour F, Francois E. Cetuximab shows activity in colorectal cancer patients with tumors for which FISH analysis does not detect an increase in EGFR gene copy number. Ann Surg Oncol 2008;15(2):649–654.

157. Cappuzzo F, Varella-Garcia M, Finocchiaro G, Skokan M, Gajapathy S, Carnaghi C, Rimassa L, Rossi E, Ligorio C, Di Tommaso L, Holmes AJ, Toschi L, Tallini G, Destro A, Roncalli M, Santoro A, Janne PA. Primary resistance to cetuximab therapy in EGFR FISH-positive colorectal cancer patients. Br J Cancer 2008;99(1):83–89.

158. Johnston S, Trudeau M, Kaufman B, Boussen H, Blackwell K, LoRusso P, Lombardi DP, Ben Ahmed S, Citrin DL, DeSilvio ML, Harris J, Westlund RE, Salazar V, Zaks TZ, Spector NL. Phase II study of predictive biomarker profiles for response targeting human epidermal growth factor receptor 2 (HER-2) in advanced inflammatory breast cancer with lapatinib monotherapy. J Clin Oncol 2008;26(7):1066–1072.

159. Holbro T, Beerli RR, Maurer F, Koziczak M, Barbas CF 3rd, Hynes NE. The ErbB2/ErbB3 heterodimer functions as an oncogenic unit: ErbB2 requires ErbB3 to drive breast tumor cell proliferation. Proc Natl Acad Sci U S A 2003;100(15):8933–8938.

160. Wehrman TS, Raab WJ, Casipit CL, Doyonnas R, Pomerantz JH, Blau HM. A system for quantifying dynamic protein interactions defines a role for Herceptin in modulating ErbB2 interactions. Proc Natl Acad Sci U S A 2006;103(50):19063–19068.

161. Xia W, Husain I, Liu L, Bacus S, Saini S, Spohn J, Pry K, Westlund R, Stein SH, Spector NL. Lapatinib antitumor activity is not dependent upon phosphatase and tensin homologue deleted on chromosome 10 in ErbB2-overexpressing breast cancers. Cancer Res 2007;67(3):1170–1175.

162. Berns K, Horlings HM, Hennessy BT, Madiredjo M, Hijmans EM, Beelen K, Linn SC, Gonzalez-Angulo AM, Stemke-Hale K, Hauptmann M, Beijersbergen RL, Mills GB, van de Vijver MJ, Bernards R. A functional genetic approach identifies the PI3K pathway as a major determinant of trastuzumab resistance in breast cancer. Cancer Cell 2007;12(4):395–402.

163. Nagata Y, Lan KH, Zhou X, Tan M, Esteva FJ, Sahin AA, Klos KS, Li P, Monia BP, Nguyen NT, Hortobagyi GN, Hung MC, Yu D. PTEN activation contributes to tumor inhibition by trastuzumab, and loss of PTEN predicts trastuzumab resistance in patients. Cancer Cell 2004;6(2):117–127.

164. Playford RJ, Hanby AM, Gschmeissner S, Peiffer LP, Wright NA, McGarrity T. The epidermal growth factor receptor (EGF-R) is present on the basolateral, but not the apical, surface of enterocytes in the human gastrointestinal tract. Gut 1996;39(2):262–266.

165. Galimont-Collen AF, Vos LE, Lavrijsen AP, Ouwerkerk J, Gelderblom H. Classification and management of skin, hair, nail and mucosal side-effects of epidermal growth factor receptor (EGFR) inhibitors. Eur J Cancer 2007;43(5):845–851.

166. Lacouture ME. Mechanisms of cutaneous toxicities to EGFR inhibitors. Nat Rev Cancer 2006;6(10):803–812.

167. Perez-Soler R, Saltz L. Cutaneous adverse effects with HER1/EGFR-targeted agents: is there a silver lining? J Clin Oncol 2005;23(22):5235–5246.

168. Lacouture ME, Laabs SM, Koehler M, Sweetman RW, Preston AJ, Di Leo A, Gomez HL, Salazar VM, Byrne JA, Koch KM, Blackwell KL. Analysis of dermatologic events in patients with cancer treated with lapatinib. Breast Cancer Res Treat 2009;114(3):485–493.

169. Wakeling AE, Guy SP, Woodburn JR, Ashton SE, Curry BJ, Barker AJ, Gibson KH. ZD1839 (Iressa): an orally active inhibitor of epidermal growth factor signaling with potential for cancer therapy. Cancer Res 2002;62(20):5749–5754.

170. Karaman MW, Herrgard S, Treiber DK, Gallant P, Atteridge CE, Campbell BT, Chan KW, Ciceri P, Davis MI, Edeen PT, Faraoni R, Floyd M, Hunt JP, Lockhart DJ, Milanov ZV, Morrison MJ, Pallares G, Patel HK, Pritchard S, Wodicka LM, Zarrinkar PP. A quantitative analysis of kinase inhibitor selectivity. Nat Biotechnol 2008;26(1):127–132.

171. Ciardiello F, Caputo R, Bianco R, Damiano V, Pomatico G, De Placido S, Bianco AR, Tortora G. Antitumor effect and potentiation of cytotoxic drugs activity in human cancer cells by ZD-1839 (Iressa), an epidermal growth factor receptor-selective tyrosine kinase inhibitor. Clin Cancer Res 2000;6(5):2053–2063.

172. Sirotnak FM, Zakowski MF, Miller VA, Scher HI, Kris MG. Efficacy of cytotoxic agents against human tumor xenografts is markedly enhanced by coadministration of ZD1839 (Iressa), an inhibitor of EGFR tyrosine kinase. Clin Cancer Res 2000;6(12):4885–4892.

173. Baselga J, Rischin D, Ranson M, Calvert H, Raymond E, Kieback DG, Kaye SB, Gianni L, Harris A, Bjork T, Averbuch SD, Feyereislova A, Swaisland H, Rojo F, Albanell J. Phase I safety, pharmacokinetic, and pharmacodynamic trial of ZD1839, a selective oral epidermal growth factor receptor tyrosine kinase inhibitor, in patients with five selected solid tumor types. J Clin Oncol 2002;20(21):4292–4302.

174. Herbst RS, Maddox AM, Rothenberg ML, Small EJ, Rubin EH, Baselga J, Rojo F, Hong WK, Swaisland H, Averbuch SD, Ochs J, LoRusso PM. Selective oral epidermal growth factor receptor tyrosine kinase inhibitor ZD1839 is generally well-tolerated and has activity in non-small-cell lung cancer and other solid tumors: results of a phase I trial. J Clin Oncol 2002;20(18):3815–3825.

175. Nakagawa K, Tamura T, Negoro S, Kudoh S, Yamamoto N, Yamamoto N, Takeda K, Swaisland H, Nakatani I, Hirose M, Dong RP, Fukuoka M. Phase I pharmacokinetic trial of the selective oral epidermal growth factor receptor tyrosine kinase inhibitor gefitinib ("Iressa," ZD1839) in Japanese patients with solid malignant tumors. Ann Oncol 2003;14(6):922–930.

176. Ranson M, Hammond LA, Ferry D, Kris M, Tullo A, Murray PI, Miller V, Averbuch S, Ochs J, Morris C, Feyereislova A, Swaisland H, Rowinsky EK. ZD1839, a selective oral epidermal growth factor receptor-tyrosine kinase inhibitor, is well tolerated and active in patients with solid, malignant tumors: results of a phase I trial. J Clin Oncol 2002;20(9):2240–2250.

177. Thatcher N, Chang A, Parikh P, Pemberton K, Archer V. Pr4 ISEL: a phase III survival study comparing gefitinib (IRESSA) plus best supportive care (BSC) with placebo plus BSC, in patients with advanced non-small-cell lung cancer (NSCLC) who had received one or two prior chemotherapy regimens. Lung Cancer (Amsterdam, Netherlands) 2005;49: S4.

178. Herbst RS, Giaccone G, Schiller JH, Natale RB, Miller V, Manegold C, Scagliotti G, Rosell R, Oliff I, Reeves JA, Wolf MK, Krebs AD, Averbuch SD, Ochs JS, Grous J, Fandi A, Johnson DH. Gefitinib in combination with paclitaxel and carboplatin in advanced non-small-cell lung cancer: a phase III trial—INTACT 2. J Clin Oncol 2004;22(5):785–794.

179. Giaccone G, Herbst RS, Manegold C, Scagliotti G, Rosell R, Miller V, Natale RB, Schiller JH, Von Pawel J, Pluzanska A, Gatzemeier U, Grous J, Ochs JS, Averbuch SD, Wolf MK, Rennie P, Fandi A, Johnson DH. Gefitinib in combination with gemcitabine and cisplatin in advanced non-small-cell lung cancer: a phase III trial—INTACT 1. J Clin Oncol 2004;22(5):777–784.

180. Cappuzzo F, Finocchiaro G, Metro G, Bartolini S, Magrini E, Cancellieri A, Trisolini R, Castaldini L, Tallini G, Crino L. Clinical experience with gefitinib: an update. Crit Rev Oncol Hematol 2006;58(1):31–45.

181. Cohen EE, Rosen F, Stadler WM, Recant W, Stenson K, Huo D, Vokes EE. Phase II trial of ZD1839 in recurrent or metastatic squamous cell carcinoma of the head and neck. J Clin Oncol 2003;21(10):1980–1987.
182. Rothenberg ML, LaFleur B, Levy DE, Washington MK, Morgan-Meadows SL, Ramanathan RK, Berlin JD, Benson AB 3rd, Coffey RJ. Randomized phase II trial of the clinical and biological effects of two dose levels of gefitinib in patients with recurrent colorectal adenocarcinoma. J Clin Oncol 2005;23(36):9265–9274.
183. Kuo T, Cho CD, Halsey J, Wakelee HA, Advani RH, Ford JM, Fisher GA, Sikic BI. Phase II study of gefitinib, fluorouracil, leucovorin, and oxaliplatin therapy in previously treated patients with metastatic colorectal cancer. J Clin Oncol 2005;23(24):5613–5619.
184. Moyer JD, Barbacci EG, Iwata KK, Arnold L, Boman B, Cunningham A, DiOrio C, Doty J, Morin MJ, Moyer MP, Neveu M, Pollack VA, Pustilnik LR, Reynolds MM, Sloan D, Theleman A, Miller P. Induction of apoptosis and cell cycle arrest by CP-358,774, an inhibitor of epidermal growth factor receptor tyrosine kinase. Cancer Res 1997;57(21):4838–4848.
185. Pollack VA, Savage DM, Baker DA, Tsaparikos KE, Sloan DE, Moyer JD, Barbacci EG, Pustilnik LR, Smolarek TA, Davis JA, Vaidya MP, Arnold LD, Doty JL, Iwata KK, Morin MJ. Inhibition of epidermal growth factor receptor-associated tyrosine phosphorylation in human carcinomas with CP-358,774: dynamics of receptor inhibition in situ and antitumor effects in athymic mice. J Pharmacol Exp Ther 1999;291(2):739–748.
186. Hidalgo M, Siu LL, Nemunaitis J, Rizzo J, Hammond LA, Takimoto C, Eckhardt SG, Tolcher A, Britten CD, Denis L, Ferrante K, Von Hoff DD, Silberman S, Rowinsky EK. Phase I and pharmacologic study of OSI-774, an epidermal growth factor receptor tyrosine kinase inhibitor, in patients with advanced solid malignancies. J Clin Oncol 2001;19(13):3267–3279.
187. Perez-Soler R, Chachoua A, Hammond LA, Rowinsky EK, Huberman M, Karp D, Rigas J, Clark GM, Santabarbara P, Bonomi P. Determinants of tumor response and survival with erlotinib in patients with non—small-cell lung cancer. J Clin Oncol 2004;22(16):3238–3247.
188. Shepherd FA, Rodrigues Pereira J, Ciuleanu T, Tan EH, Hirsh V, Thongprasert S, Campos D, Maoleekoonpiroj S, Smylie M, Martins R, van Kooten M, Dediu M, Findlay B, Tu D, Johnston D, Bezjak A, Clark G, Santabarbara P, Seymour L. Erlotinib in previously treated non-small-cell lung cancer. N Engl J Med 2005;353(2):123–132.
189. Gatzemeier U, Pluzanska A, Szczesna A, Kaukel E, Roubec J, De Rosa F, Milanowski J, Karnicka-Mlodkowski H, Pesek M, Serwatowski P, Ramlau R, Janaskova T, Vansteenkiste J, Strausz J, Manikhas GM, Von Pawel J. Phase III study of erlotinib in combination with cisplatin and gemcitabine in advanced non-small-cell lung cancer: the Tarceva Lung Cancer Investigation Trial. J Clin Oncol 2007;25(12):1545–1552.
190. Herbst RS, Prager D, Hermann R, Fehrenbacher L, Johnson BE, Sandler A, Kris MG, Tran HT, Klein P, Li X, Ramies D, Johnson DH, Miller VA. TRIBUTE: a phase III trial of erlotinib hydrochloride (OSI-774) combined with carboplatin and paclitaxel chemotherapy in advanced non-small-cell lung cancer. J Clin Oncol 2005;23(25):5892–5899.
191. Moore MJ, Goldstein D, Hamm J, Figer A, Hecht JR, Gallinger S, Au HJ, Murawa P, Walde D, Wolff RA, Campos D, Lim R, Ding K, Clark G, Voskoglou-Nomikos T, Ptasynski M, Parulekar W. Erlotinib plus gemcitabine compared with gemcitabine alone in patients with advanced pancreatic cancer: a phase III trial of the National Cancer Institute of Canada Clinical Trials Group. J Clin Oncol 2007;25(15):1960–1966.
192. Kulke MH, Blaszkowsky LS, Ryan DP, Clark JW, Meyerhardt JA, Zhu AX, Enzinger PC, Kwak EL, Muzikansky A, Lawrence C, Fuchs CS. Capecitabine plus erlotinib in gemcitabine-refractory advanced pancreatic cancer. J Clin Oncol 2007;25(30):4787–4792.
193. Bareschino MA, Schettino C, Troiani T, Martinelli E, Morgillo F, Ciardiello F. Erlotinib in cancer treatment. Ann Oncol 2007;18 (Suppl 6): vi35–41.
194. Soulieres D, Senzer NN, Vokes EE, Hidalgo M, Agarwala SS, Siu LL. Multicenter phase II study of erlotinib, an oral epidermal growth factor receptor tyrosine kinase inhibitor, in patients with recurrent or metastatic squamous cell cancer of the head and neck. J Clin Oncol 2004;22(1):77–85.
195. Siu LL, Soulieres D, Chen EX, Pond GR, Chin SF, Francis P, Harvey L, Klein M, Zhang W, Dancey J, Eisenhauer EA, Winquist E. Phase I/II trial of erlotinib and cisplatin in patients with recurrent or metastatic squamous cell carcinoma of the head and neck: a Princess Margaret Hospital

phase II consortium and National Cancer Institute of Canada Clinical Trials Group Study. J Clin Oncol 2007;25(16):2178–2183.

196. Kim ES, Kies MS, Glisson BS, Tsao A, Ginsberg LE, Holsinger FC, Burke BJ, Truong M, Papadimitrakopoulou VA, Lippman SM. Final results of a phase II study of erlotinib, docetaxel and cisplatin in patients with recurrent/metastatic head and neck cancer. J Clin Oncol (Meeting Abstracts) 2007;25(18 Suppl):Abstr 6013.

197. Agulnik M, da Cunha Santos G, Hedley D, Nicklee T, Dos Reis PP, Ho J, Pond GR, Chen H, Chen S, Shyr Y, Winquist E, Soulieres D, Chen EX, Squire JA, Marrano P, Kamel-Reid S, Dancey J, Siu LL, Tsao MS. Predictive and pharmacodynamic biomarker studies in tumor and skin tissue samples of patients with recurrent or metastatic squamous cell carcinoma of the head and neck treated with erlotinib. J Clin Oncol 2007;25(16):2184–2190.

198. Cloughesy T, Yung A, Vrendenberg J, Aldape K, Eberhard D, Prados M, Vandenberg S, Klencke B, Mischel P. Phase II study of erlotinib in recurrent GBM: molecular predictors of outcome. J Clin Oncol (Meeting Abstracts) 2005;23(16 Suppl): 1507.

199. Brewer CJ, Suh JH, Stevens GHJ, Barnett GH, Toms S, Vogelbaum MA, Weil R, Peereboom DM. Phase II trial of erlotinib with temozolomide and concurrent radiation therapy in patients with newly-diagnosed glioblastoma multiforme. J Clin Oncol (Meeting Abstracts) 2005;23(16 Suppl): 1567.

200. Brown PD, Krishnan S, Sarkaria J, Wu W, Mischel P, Yong WH, Arusell R, Jenkins RB, Buckner JC, Giannini C. A phase II trial (N0177) of erlotinib and temozolomide (TMZ) combined with radiation therapy (RT) in glioblastoma multiforme (GBM). J Clin Oncol (Meeting Abstracts) 2008;26(15 Suppl): 2016.

201. Groot JFD, Gilbert MR, Hess KR, Hanna T, Groves M, Conrad C, Aldape K, Colman H, Puduvalli V, Yung WA. Phase II study of combination carboplatin and erlotinib in patients with recurrent glioblastoma multiforme. J Clin Oncol (Meeting Abstracts) 2007;25(18 Suppl): 2024.

202. Krishnan S, Brown P, Ballman K, Fiveash J, Uhm J, Giannini C, Geoffroy F, Nabors L, Buckner J. Phase I trial of erlotinib with radiation therapy (RT) in patients with glioblastoma multiforme (GBM). J Clin Oncol (Meeting Abstracts) 2005;23(16 Suppl): 1513.

203. de Groot JF, Gilbert MR, Aldape K, Hess KR, Hanna TA, Ictech S, Groves MD, Conrad C, Colman H, Puduvalli VK, Levin V, Yung WK. Phase II study of carboplatin and erlotinib (Tarceva, OSI-774) in patients with recurrent glioblastoma. J Neurooncol 2008;90(1):89–97.

204. Rusnak DW, Lackey K, Affleck K, Wood ER, Alligood KJ, Rhodes N, Keith BR, Murray DM, Knight WB, Mullin RJ, Gilmer TM. The effects of the novel, reversible epidermal growth factor receptor/ErbB-2 tyrosine kinase inhibitor, GW2016, on the growth of human normal and tumor-derived cell lines in vitro and in vivo. Mol Cancer Ther 2001;1(2):85–94.

205. Xia W, Mullin RJ, Keith BR, Liu LH, Ma H, Rusnak DW, Owens G, Alligood KJ, Spector NL. Anti-tumor activity of GW572016: a dual tyrosine kinase inhibitor blocks EGF activation of EGFR/erbB2 and downstream Erk1/2 and AKT pathways. Oncogene 2002;21(41):6255–6263.

206. Konecny GE, Pegram MD, Venkatesan N, Finn R, Yang G, Rahmeh M, Untch M, Rusnak DW, Spehar G, Mullin RJ, Keith BR, Gilmer TM, Berger M, Podratz KC, Slamon DJ. Activity of the dual kinase inhibitor lapatinib (GW572016) against HER-2-overexpressing and trastuzumab-treated breast cancer cells. Cancer Res 2006;66(3):1630–1639.

207. Chu I, Blackwell K, Chen S, Slingerland J. The dual ErbB1/ErbB2 inhibitor, lapatinib (GW572016), cooperates with tamoxifen to inhibit both cell proliferation- and estrogen-dependent gene expression in antiestrogen-resistant breast cancer. Cancer Res 2005;65(1):18–25.

208. Burris HA 3rd, Hurwitz HI, Dees EC, Dowlati A, Blackwell KL, O'Neil B, Marcom PK, Ellis MJ, Overmoyer B, Jones SF, Harris JL, Smith DA, Koch KM, Stead A, Mangum S, Spector NL. Phase I safety, pharmacokinetics, and clinical activity study of lapatinib (GW572016), a reversible dual inhibitor of epidermal growth factor receptor tyrosine kinases, in heavily pretreated patients with metastatic carcinomas. J Clin Oncol 2005;23(23):5305–5313.

209. Versola M, Burris HA, Jones S, Wilding G, Taylor C, Pandite L, Smith DA, Stead A, Spector NL. Clinical activity of GW572016 in EGF10003 in patients with solid tumors. J Clin Oncol (Meeting Abstracts) 2004;22(14 Suppl):Abstr 3047.

210. Gomez HL, Doval DC, Chavez MA, Ang PC, Aziz Z, Nag S, Ng C, Franco SX, Chow LW, Arbushites MC, Casey MA, Berger MS, Stein SH, Sledge GW. Efficacy and safety of lapatinib as

first-line therapy for ErbB2-amplified locally advanced or metastatic breast cancer. J Clin Oncol 2008;26(18):2999–3005.

211. Spector NL, Blackwell K, Hurley J, Harris JL, Lombardi D, Bacus S, Ahmed SB, Boussen H, Frikha M, Ayed FB. EGF103009, a phase II trial of lapatinib monotherapy in patients with relapsed/refractory inflammatory breast cancer (IBC): clinical activity and biologic predictors of response. J Clin Oncol (Meeting Abstracts) 2006;24(18 Suppl):Abstr 502.

212. Chu QS, Cianfrocca ME, Goldstein LJ, Gale M, Murray N, Loftiss J, Arya N, Koch KM, Pandite L, Fleming RA, Paul E, Rowinsky EK. A phase I and pharmacokinetic study of lapatinib in combination with letrozole in patients with advanced cancer. Clin Cancer Res 2008;14(14):4484–4490.

213. LoRusso PM, Jones SF, Koch KM, Arya N, Fleming RA, Loftiss J, Pandite L, Gadgeel S, Weber BL, Burris HA 3rd. Phase I and pharmacokinetic study of lapatinib and docetaxel in patients with advanced cancer. J Clin Oncol 2008;26(18):3051–3056.

214. Storniolo AM, Pegram MD, Overmoyer B, Silverman P, Peacock NW, Jones SF, Loftiss J, Arya N, Koch KM, Paul E, Pandite L, Fleming RA, Lebowitz PF, Ho PT, Burris HA 3rd. Phase I dose escalation and pharmacokinetic study of lapatinib in combination with trastuzumab in patients with advanced ErbB2-positive breast cancer. J Clin Oncol 2008;26(20):3317–3323.

215. Midgley RS, Kerr DJ, Flaherty KT, Stevenson JP, Pratap SE, Koch KM, Smith DA, Versola M, Fleming RA, Ward C, O'Dwyer PJ, Middleton MR. A phase I and pharmacokinetic study of lapatinib in combination with infusional 5-fluorouracil, leucovorin and irinotecan. Ann Oncol 2007;18(12):2025–2029.

216. Chu QS, Schwartz G, de Bono J, Smith DA, Koch KM, Versola MJ, Pandite L, Arya N, Curtright J, Fleming RA, Ho PT, Rowinsky EK. Phase I and pharmacokinetic study of lapatinib in combination with capecitabine in patients with advanced solid malignancies. J Clin Oncol 2007;25(24):3753–3758.

217. Siegel-Lakhai WS, Beijnen JH, Vervenne WL, Boot H, Keessen M, Versola M, Koch KM, Smith DA, Pandite L, Richel DJ, Schellens JH. Phase I pharmacokinetic study of the safety and tolerability of lapatinib (GW572016) in combination with oxaliplatin/fluorouracil/leucovorin (FOLFOX4) in patients with solid tumors. Clin Cancer Res 2007;13(15Pt 1):4495–4502.

218. Blackwell KL, Burstein H, Pegram M, Storniolo AM, Salazar VM, Maleski JE, Lin X, Spector N, Stein SH, Berger MS. Determining relevant biomarkers from tissue and serum that may predict response to single agent lapatinib in trastuzumab refractory metastatic breast cancer. J Clin Oncol (Meeting Abstracts) 2005;23(16 Suppl):Abstr 3004.

219. O'Shaughnessy J, Blackwell KL, Burstein H, Storniolo AM, Sledge G, Baselga J, Koehler M, Laabs S, Florance A, Roychowdhury D. A randomized study of lapatinib alone or in combination with trastuzumab in heavily pretreated HER2+ metastatic breast cancer progressing on trastuzumab therapy. J Clin Oncol (Meeting Abstracts) 2008;26(15 Suppl):Abstr 1015.

220. Xia W, Liu LH, Ho P, Spector NL. Truncated ErbB2 receptor (p95ErbB2) is regulated by heregulin through heterodimer formation with ErbB3 yet remains sensitive to the dual EGFR/ErbB2 kinase inhibitor GW572016. Oncogene 2004;23(3):646–653.

221. Cameron D, Casey M, Press M, Lindquist D, Pienkowski T, Romieu CG, Chan S, Jagiello-Gruszfeld A, Kaufman B, Crown J, Chan A, Campone M, Viens P, Davidson N, Gorbounova V, Raats JI, Skarlos D, Newstat B, Roychowdhury D, Paoletti P, Oliva C, Rubin S, Stein S, Geyer CE. A phase III randomized comparison of lapatinib plus capecitabine versus capecitabine alone in women with advanced breast cancer that has progressed on trastuzumab: updated efficacy and biomarker analyses. Breast Cancer Res Treat 2008;112(3):533–543.

222. Geyer CE, Forster J, Lindquist D, Chan S, Romieu CG, Pienkowski T, Jagiello-Gruszfeld A, Crown J, Chan A, Kaufman B, Skarlos D, Campone M, Davidson N, Berger M, Oliva C, Rubin SD, Stein S, Cameron D. Lapatinib plus capecitabine for HER2-positive advanced breast cancer. N Engl J Med 2006;355(26):2733–2743.

223. Tuma RS. Lapatinib moves forward in inflammatory and early HER2-positive breast cancer trials. J Natl Cancer Inst 2007;99(5):348–349.

224. Brave S, Odedra R, Smith N, James N, Marshall G, Acheson N, Howard Z, Baker D, Jackson L, Hickinson M, Wilkinson R, Ratcliffe K, Walker M, Wainwright A, Barry S, Wedge S, Ryan

A. Vandetanib inhibits both pVEGFR2 and pEGFR at clinically achievable drug levels in pre-clinical models. AACR Meeting Abstracts 2007(Molecular Targets and Cancer Therapeutics, San Francisco, CA):Abstr A226.

225. Gendreau SB, Ventura R, Keast P, Laird AD, Yakes FM, Zhang W, Bentzien F, Cancilla B, Lutman J, Chu F, Jackman L, Shi Y, Yu P, Wang J, Aftab DT, Jaeger CT, Meyer SM, De Costa A, Engell K, Chen J, Martini JF, Joly AH. Inhibition of the T790M gatekeeper mutant of the epidermal growth factor receptor by EXEL-7647. Clin Cancer Res 2007;13(12):3713–3723.

226. Trowe T, Boukouvala S, Calkins K, Cutler RE Jr, Fong R, Funke R, Gendreau SB, Kim YD, Miller N, Woolfrey JR, Vysotskaia V, Yang JP, Gerritsen ME, Matthews DJ, Lamb P, Heuer TS. EXEL-7647 inhibits mutant forms of ErbB2 associated with lapatinib resistance and neoplastic transformation. Clin Cancer Res 2008;14(8):2465–2475.

227. Wakelee HA, Adjei AA, Halsey J, Lensing JL, Dugay JD, Hanson LJ, Reid JM, Piens JR, Sikic BI. A phase I dose-escalation and pharmacokinetic (PK) study of a novel spectrum selective kinase inhibitor, XL647, in patients with advanced solid malignancies (ASM). J Clin Oncol (Meeting Abstracts) 2006;24(18 Suppl):Abstr 3044.

228. Wakelee HA, Molina JR, Fehling JM, Lensing JL, Sikic BI. A phase I study with exploratory pharmacodynamic endpoints of XL647, a novel spectrum selective kinase inhibitor, administered orally daily to patients (pts) with advanced solid malignancies. J Clin Oncol (Meeting Abstracts) 2007;25(18 Suppl):Abstr 14044.

229. Rizvi NA, Kris MG, Miller VA, Krug LM, Bekele S, Dowlati A, Rowland KM, Salgia R, Aggarwal N, Gadgeel SM. Activity of XL647 in clinically selected NSCLC patients (pts) enriched for the presence of EGFR mutations: results from phase 2. J Clin Oncol (Meeting Abstracts) 2008;26(15 Suppl):Abstr 8053.

230. Miller VA, Wakelee HA, Lara PN, Cho J, Chowhan NM, Costa D, Vrindavanam N, Yanagihara R, Pennell N, Lynch TJ. Activity and tolerance of XL647 in NSCLC patients with acquired resistance to EGFR-TKIs: preliminary results of a phase II trial. J Clin Oncol (Meeting Abstracts) 2008;26(15 Suppl):Abstr 8028.

231. Traxler P, Allegrini PR, Brandt R, Brueggen J, Cozens R, Fabbro D, Grosios K, Lane HA, McSheehy P, Mestan J, Meyer T, Tang C, Wartmann M, Wood J, Caravatti G. AEE788: a dual family epidermal growth factor receptor/ErbB2 and vascular endothelial growth factor receptor tyrosine kinase inhibitor with antitumor and antiangiogenic activity. Cancer Res 2004;64(14):4931–4941.

232. Yu Z, Boggon TJ, Kobayashi S, Jin C, Ma PC, Dowlati A, Kern JA, Tenen DG, Halmos B. Resistance to an irreversible epidermal growth factor receptor (EGFR) inhibitor in EGFR-mutant lung cancer reveals novel treatment strategies. Cancer Res 2007;67(21):10417–10427.

233. Failly M, Korur S, Egler V, Boulay JL, Lino MM, Imber R, Merlo A. Combination of sublethal concentrations of epidermal growth factor receptor inhibitor and microtubule stabilizer induces apoptosis of glioblastoma cells. Mol Cancer Ther 2007;6(2):773–781.

234. Kamat AA, Kim TJ, Landen CN Jr, Lu C, Han LY, Lin YG, Merritt WM, Thaker PH, Gershenson DM, Bischoff FZ, Heymach JV, Jaffe RB, Coleman RL, Sood AK. Metronomic chemotherapy enhances the efficacy of antivascular therapy in ovarian cancer. Cancer Res 2007;67(1):281–288.

235. Goudar RK, Shi Q, Hjelmeland MD, Keir ST, McLendon RE, Wikstrand CJ, Reese ED, Conrad CA, Traxler P, Lane HA, Reardon DA, Cavenee WK, Wang XF, Bigner DD, Friedman HS, Rich JN. Combination therapy of inhibitors of epidermal growth factor receptor/vascular endothelial growth factor receptor 2 (AEE788) and the mammalian target of rapamycin (RAD001) offers improved glioblastoma tumor growth inhibition. Mol Cancer Ther 2005;4(1):101–112.

236. Yokoi K, Kim SJ, Thaker P, Yazici S, Nam DH, He J, Sasaki T, Chiao PJ, Sclabas GM, Abbruzzese JL, Hamilton SR, Fidler IJ. Induction of apoptosis in tumor-associated endothelial cells and therapy of orthotopic human pancreatic carcinoma in nude mice. Neoplasia 2005;7(7):696–704.

237. Xiong H, Takimoto CH, Rojo F, Davis DW, Huang J, Abbruzzese JL, Dugan M, Thomas A, Mita A, Steward W. A phase I study of AEE788, a multitargeted inhibitor of ErbB and VEGF receptor family tyrosine kinases, to determine safety, PK and PD in patients (pts) with advanced colorectal cancer (CRC) and liver metastases. J Clin Oncol (Meeting Abstracts) 2007;25(18 Suppl):Abstr 4065.

238. Baselga J, Rojo F, Dumez H, Mita A, Takimoto CH, Tabernero J, Dilea C, Parker K, Dugan M, Van Oosterom A. Phase I study of AEE788. a novel multitargeted inhibitor of ErbB and VEGF

receptor family tyrosine kinases: a pharmacokinetic (PK)-pharmacodynamic (PD) study to identify the optimal therapeutic dose regimen. J Clin Oncol 2005;23(16 Suppl):Abstr 3028.

239. Reardon D, Cloughesy T, Conrad C, Prados M, Xia J, Mietlowski W, Dugan D, Mischel P, Friedman H, Yung A. A phase I study of AEE788, a novel multitargeted inhibitor of ErbB and VEGF receptor family tyrosine kinases, in recurrent GBM patients. J Clin Oncol (Meeting Abstracts) 2005;23(16 Suppl):Abstr 3063.

240. Davis DW, Huang J, Liu W, Xiao L, Thomas A, Mita A, Steward W, Takimoto C, Mietlowski W, Xiong H. Pharmacodynamic analysis of receptor tyrosine kinase (RTK) activity reveals differential target inhibition in skin and tumor in a phase I study of advanced colorectal cancer patients treated with AEE788. J Clin Oncol (Meeting Abstracts) 2007;25(18 Suppl):Abstr 3601.

241. Smaill JB, Rewcastle GW, Loo JA, Greis KD, Chan OH, Reyner EL, Lipka E, Showalter HD, Vincent PW, Elliott WL, Denny WA. Tyrosine kinase inhibitors. 17. Irreversible inhibitors of the epidermal growth factor receptor: 4-(phenylamino)quinazoline- and 4-(phenylamino)pyrido[3,2-d]pyrimidine-6-acrylamides bearing additional solubilizing functions. J Med Chem 2000;43(7):1380–1397.

242. Slichenmyer WJ, Elliott WL, Fry DW. CI-1033, a pan-erbB tyrosine kinase inhibitor. Semin Oncol 2001;28(5 Suppl 16): 80–85.

243. Gieseg MA, de Bock C, Ferguson LR, Denny WA. Evidence for epidermal growth factor receptor-enhanced chemosensitivity in combinations of cisplatin and the new irreversible tyrosine kinase inhibitor CI-1033. Anticancer Drugs 2001;12(8):683–690.

244. Nyati MK, Maheshwari D, Hanasoge S, Sreekumar A, Rynkiewicz SD, Chinnaiyan AM, Leopold WR, Ethier SP, Lawrence TS. Radiosensitization by pan ErbB inhibitor CI-1033 in vitro and in vivo. Clin Cancer Res 2004;10(2):691–700.

245. Erlichman C, Boerner SA, Hallgren CG, Spieker R, Wang XY, James CD, Scheffer GL, Maliepaard M, Ross DD, Bible KC, Kaufmann SH. The HER tyrosine kinase inhibitor CI1033 enhances cytotoxicity of 7-ethyl-10-hydroxycamptothecin and topotecan by inhibiting breast cancer resistance protein-mediated drug efflux. Cancer Res 2001;61(2):739–748.

246. Calvo E, Tolcher AW, Hammond LA, Patnaik A, de Bono JS, Eiseman IA, Olson SC, Lenehan PF, McCreery H, Lorusso P, Rowinsky EK. Administration of CI-1033, an irreversible pan-erbB tyrosine kinase inhibitor, is feasible on a 7-day on, 7-day off schedule: a phase I pharmacokinetic and food effect study. Clin Cancer Res 2004;10(21):7112–7120.

247. Nemunaitis J, Eiseman I, Cunningham C, Senzer N, Williams A, Lenehan PF, Olson SC, Bycott P, Schlicht M, Zentgraff R, Shin DM, Zinner RG. Phase 1 clinical and pharmacokinetics evaluation of oral CI-1033 in patients with refractory cancer. Clin Cancer Res 2005;11(10):3846–3853.

248. Zinner RG, Nemunaitis J, Eiseman I, Shin HJ, Olson SC, Christensen J, Huang X, Lenehan PF, Donato NJ, Shin DM. Phase I clinical and pharmacodynamic evaluation of oral CI-1033 in patients with refractory cancer. Clin Cancer Res 2007;13(10):3006–3014.

249. Chiappori AA, Ellis PM, Hamm JT, Bitran JD, Eiseman I, Lovalvo J, Burnett D, Olson S, Lenehan P, Zinner RG. A phase I evaluation of oral CI-1033 in combination with paclitaxel and carboplatin as first-line chemotherapy in patients with advanced non-small cell lung cancer. J Thorac Oncol 2006;1(9):1010–1019.

250. Garland LL, Hidalgo M, Mendelson DS, Ryan DP, Arun BK, Lovalvo JL, Eiseman IA, Olson SC, Lenehan PF, Eder JP. A phase I clinical and pharmacokinetic study of oral CI-1033 in combination with docetaxel in patients with advanced solid tumors. Clin Cancer Res 2006;12(14Pt 1):4274–4282.

251. Janne PA, von Pawel J, Cohen RB, Crino L, Butts CA, Olson SS, Eiseman IA, Chiappori AA, Yeap BY, Lenehan PF, Dasse K, Sheeran M, Bonomi PD. Multicenter, randomized, phase II trial of CI-1033, an irreversible pan-ERBB inhibitor, for previously treated advanced non small-cell lung cancer. J Clin Oncol 2007;25(25):3936–3944.

252. Engelman JA, Zejnullahu K, Gale CM, Lifshits E, Gonzales AJ, Shimamura T, Zhao F, Vincent PW, Naumov GN, Bradner JE, Althaus IW, Gandhi L, Shapiro GI, Nelson JM, Heymach JV, Meyerson M, Wong KK, Janne PA. PF00299804, an irreversible pan-ERBB inhibitor, is effective in lung cancer models with EGFR and ERBB2 mutations that are resistant to gefitinib. Cancer Res 2007;67(24):11924–11932.

253. Gonzales AJ, Hook KE, Althaus IW, Ellis PA, Trachet E, Delaney AM, Harvey PJ, Ellis TA, Amato DM, Nelson JM, Fry DW, Zhu T, Loi CM, Fakhoury SA, Schlosser KM, Sexton KE, Winters RT, Reed JE, Bridges AJ, Lettiere DJ, Baker DA, Yang J, Lee HT, Tecle H, Vincent PW. Antitumor activity and pharmacokinetic properties of PF-00299804, a second-generation irreversible pan-erbB receptor tyrosine kinase inhibitor. Mol Cancer Ther 2008;7(7):1880–1889.

254. Schellens JH, Britten CD, Camidge DR, Boss D, Wong S, Diab S, Guo F, Maguire RP, Letret SP, Eckhardt SG. First-in-human study of the safety, tolerability, pharmacokinetics (PK), and pharmacodynamics (PD) of PF-00299804, a small molecule irreversible panHER inhibitor in patients with advanced cancer. J Clin Oncol (Meeting Abstracts) 2007;25(18 Suppl):Abstr 3599.

255. Janne PA, Schellens JH, Engelman JA, Eckhardt SG, Millham R, Denis LJ, Britten CD, Wong SG, Boss DS, Camidge DR. Preliminary activity and safety results from a phase I clinical trial of PF-00299804, an irreversible pan-HER inhibitor, in patients (pts) with NSCLC. J Clin Oncol 2008;26(May 20 Suppl):Abstr 8027.

256. Wissner A, Overbeek E, Reich MF, Floyd MB, Johnson BD, Mamuya N, Rosfjord EC, Discafani C, Davis R, Shi X, Rabindran SK, Gruber BC, Ye F, Hallett WA, Nilakantan R, Shen R, Wang YF, Greenberger LM, Tsou HR. Synthesis and structure–activity relationships of 6,7-disubstituted 4-anilinoquinoline-3-carbonitriles. The design of an orally active, irreversible inhibitor of the tyrosine kinase activity of the epidermal growth factor receptor (EGFR) and the human epidermal growth factor receptor-2 (HER-2). J Med Chem 2003;46(1):49–63.

257. Tejpar S, Van Cutsem E, Gamelin E, Machover D, Soulie P, Ulusakarya A, Laurent S, Vauthier JM, Quinn S, Zacharchuk C. Phase 1/2a study of EKB-569, an irreversible inhibitor of epidermal growth factor receptor, in combination with 5-fluorouracil, leucovorin, and oxaliplatin (FOLFOX-4) in patients with advanced colorectal cancer (CRC). J Clin Oncol (Meeting Abstracts) 2004;22(14 Suppl):Abstr 3579.

258. Casado E, Folprecht G, Paz-Ares L, Rojo F, Kohne CH, Cortes-Funes H, Vauthier JM, Zacharchuk C, Baselga J, Tabernero J. A phase I/IIA pharmacokinetic (PK) and serial skin and tumor pharmacodynamic (PD) study of the EGFR irreversible tyrosine kinase inhibitor EKB-569 in combination with 5-fluorouracil (5FU), leucovorin (LV) and irinotecan (CPT-11) (FOLFIRI regimen) in patients (pts) with advanced colorectal cancer (ACC). J Clin Oncol (Meeting Abstracts) 2004;22(14 Suppl):Abstr 3543.

259. Tsou HR, Overbeek-Klumpers EG, Hallett WA, Reich MF, Floyd MB, Johnson BD, Michalak RS, Nilakantan R, Discafani C, Golas J, Rabindran SK, Shen R, Shi X, Wang YF, Upeslacis J, Wissner A. Optimization of 6,7-disubstituted-4-(arylamino)quinoline-3-carbonitriles as orally active, irreversible inhibitors of human epidermal growth factor receptor-2 kinase activity. J Med Chem 2005;48(4):1107–1131.

260. Ji H, Li D, Chen L, Shimamura T, Kobayashi S, McNamara K, Mahmood U, Mitchell A, Sun Y, Al-Hashem R, Chirieac LR, Padera R, Bronson RT, Kim W, Janne PA, Shapiro GI, Tenen D, Johnson BE, Weissleder R, Sharpless NE, Wong KK. The impact of human EGFR kinase domain mutations on lung tumorigenesis and in vivo sensitivity to EGFR-targeted therapies. Cancer Cell 2006;9(6):485–495.

261. Ji H, Zhao X, Yuza Y, Shimamura T, Li D, Protopopov A, Jung BL, McNamara K, Xia H, Glatt KA, Thomas RK, Sasaki H, Horner JW, Eck M, Mitchell A, Sun Y, Al-Hashem R, Bronson RT, Rabindran SK, Discafani CM, Maher E, Shapiro GI, Meyerson M, Wong KK. Epidermal growth factor receptor variant III mutations in lung tumorigenesis and sensitivity to tyrosine kinase inhibitors. Proc Natl Acad Sci U S A 2006;103(20):7817–7822.

262. Shimamura T, Ji H, Minami Y, Thomas RK, Lowell AM, Shah K, Greulich H, Glatt KA, Meyerson M, Shapiro GI, Wong KK. Non-small-cell lung cancer and Ba/F3 transformed cells harboring the ERBB2 G776insV_G/C mutation are sensitive to the dual-specific epidermal growth factor receptor and ERBB2 inhibitor HKI-272. Cancer Res 2006;66(13):6487–6491.

263. Wong KK, Fracasso PM, Bukowski RM, Munster PN, Lynch T, Abbas R, Quinn SE, Zacharchuk C, Burris H. HKI-272, an irreversible pan erbB receptor tyrosine kinase inhibitor: preliminary phase 1 results in patients with solid tumors. J Clin Oncol (Meeting Abstracts) 2006;24(18 Suppl):Abstr 3018.

264. Wong KK. HKI-272 in non small cell lung cancer. Clin Cancer Res 2007;13(15Pt 2): s4593–4596.

265. Li D, Ambrogio L, Shimamura T, Kubo S, Takahashi M, Chirieac LR, Padera RF, Shapiro GI, Baum A, Himmelsbach F, Rettig WJ, Meyerson M, Solca F, Greulich H, Wong KK. BIBW2992, an irreversible EGFR/HER2 inhibitor highly effective in preclinical lung cancer models. Oncogene 2008;27(34):4702–4711.

266. Shaw H, Plummer R, Vidal L, Perrett R, Pilkington M, Temple G, Fong P, Amelsberg A, Calvert H, De Bono J. A phase I dose escalation study of BIBW 2992, an irreversible dual EGFR/HER2 receptor tyrosine kinase inhibitor, in patients with advanced solid tumours. ASCO Meeting Abstracts 2006;24(18 Suppl):Abstr 3027.

267. Agus DB, Terlizzi E, Stopfer P, Amelsberg A, Gordon MS. A phase I dose escalation study of BIBW 2992, an irreversible dual EGFR/HER2 receptor tyrosine kinase inhibitor, in a continuous schedule in patients with advanced solid tumours. J Clin Oncol (Meeting Abstracts) 2006;24(18 Suppl):Abstr 2074.

268. Mom CH, Eskens FA, Gietema JA, Nooter K, De Jonge MJ, Amelsberg A, Huisman H, Stopfer P, De Vries EG, Verweij J. Phase 1 study with BIBW 2992, an irreversible dual tyrosine kinase inhibitor of epidermal growth factor receptor 1 (EGFR) and 2 (HER2) in a 2 week on 2 week off schedule. J Clin Oncol (Meeting Abstracts) 2006;24(18 Suppl):Abstr 3025.

269. Eskens FA, Mom CH, Planting AS, Gietema JA, Amelsberg A, Huisman H, van Doorn L, Burger H, Stopfer P, Verweij J, de Vries EG. A phase I dose escalation study of BIBW 2992, an irreversible dual inhibitor of epidermal growth factor receptor 1 (EGFR) and 2 (HER2) tyrosine kinase in a 2-week on, 2-week off schedule in patients with advanced solid tumours. Br J Cancer 2008;98(1):80–85.

270. Lewis N, Marshall J, Amelsberg A, Cohen RB, Stopfer P, Hwang J, Malik S. A phase I dose escalation study of BIBW 2992, an irreversible dual EGFR/HER2 receptor tyrosine kinase inhibitor, in a 3 week on 1 week off schedule in patients with advanced solid tumors. J Clin Oncol (Meeting Abstracts) 2006;24(18 Suppl):Abstr 3091.

271. Yang C, Shih J, Chao T, Tsai C, Yu C, Yang P, Streit M, Shahidi M, Miller VA. Use of BIBW 2992, a novel irreversible EGFR/HER2 TKI, to induce regression in patients with adenocarcinoma of the lung and activating EGFR mutations: preliminary results of a single-arm phase II clinical trial. J Clin Oncol (Meeting Abstracts) 2008;26(15 Suppl):Abstr 8026.

272. Jani JP, Finn RS, Campbell M, Coleman KG, Connell RD, Currier N, Emerson EO, Floyd E, Harriman S, Kath JC, Morris J, Moyer JD, Pustilnik LR, Rafidi K, Ralston S, Rossi AM, Steyn SJ, Wagner L, Winter SM, Bhattacharya SK. Discovery and pharmacologic characterization of CP-724,714, a selective ErbB2 tyrosine kinase inhibitor. Cancer Res 2007;67(20):9887–9893.

273. Munster PN, Britten CD, Mita M, Gelmon K, Minton SE, Moulder S, Slamon DJ, Guo F, Letrent SP, Denis L, Tolcher AW. First study of the safety, tolerability, and pharmacokinetics of CP-724,714 in patients with advanced malignant solid HER2-expressing tumors. Clin Cancer Res 2007;13(4):1238–1245.

274. Wong TW, Lee FY, Yu C, Luo FR, Oppenheimer S, Zhang H, Smykla RA, Mastalerz H, Fink BE, Hunt JT, Gavai AV, Vite GD. Preclinical antitumor activity of BMS-599626, a pan-HER kinase inhibitor that inhibits HER1/HER2 homodimer and heterodimer signaling. Clin Cancer Res 2006;12(20Pt 1):6186–6193.

275. Garland LL, Pegram M, Song S, Mendelson D, Parker KE, Martell RE, Gordon MS. Phase I study of BMS-599626, an oral pan-HER tyrosine kinase inhibitor, in patients with advanced solid tumors. J Clin Oncol (Meeting Abstracts) 2005;23(16 Suppl):Abstr 3152.

276. Soria JC, Cortes J, Armand JP, Taleb A, van Bree L, Lopez E, Song S, Zeradib K, Vazquez F, Martell RE, Baselga J. Phase I pharmacokinetic profile and early clinical evaluation of the pan-HER inhibitor BMS-599626. J Clin Oncol (Meeting Abstracts) 2005;23(16 Suppl):Abstr 3109.

277. de La Motte Rouge T, Galluzzi L, Olaussen KA, Zermati Y, Tasdemir E, Robert T, Ripoche H, Lazar V, Dessen P, Harper F, Pierron G, Pinna G, Araujo N, Harel-Belan A, Armand JP, Wong TW, Soria JC, Kroemer G. A novel epidermal growth factor receptor inhibitor promotes apoptosis in non-small cell lung cancer cells resistant to erlotinib. Cancer Res 2007;67(13):6253–6262.

278. Malone H, Kukral D, Henley B, Zhang H, Fargnoli J, Wong T, Krishnan B. Dose dependent effects of pan HER/VEGFR2 inhibitor BMS-690514 on tumor micro circulation in tumor bearing mice measured by dynamic contrast enhanced magnetic resonance imaging (DCE-MRI). J Clin Oncol (Meeting Abstracts) 2007;25(18 Suppl):Abstr 4001.

279. Wong T, Ayers M, Emanuel S, Fargnoli J, Harbison C, Lee F, Oppenheimer S, Yu C, Krishnan B, Zhang H, Chen P, Fink B, Norris D, Vite G, Gavai A. Inhibition of EGFR/HER2 signaling in tumor cells and VEGFR2 activity in tumor endothelium contribute to the preclinical anti-tumor activity of BMS-690514. AACR Annual Meeting; 2007 Apr 14–18; Los Angeles, CA. Abstr 4007.

280. Bahleda R, Felip E, Herbst RS, Hanna NH, Laurie SA, Shepherd FA, Armand JP, Sweeney CJ, Calvo-Aller E, Soria JC. Phase I multicenter trial of BMS-690514: safety, pharmacokinetic profile, biological effects, and early clinical evaluation in patients with advanced solid tumors and non-small cell lung cancer. J Clin Oncol (Meeting Abstracts) 2008;26(15 Suppl):Abstr 2564.

281. Miknis G, Wallace E, Lyssikatos J, Lee P, Zhao Q, Hans J, Topalov G, Buckmelter A, Tarlton G, Ren L, Tullis J, Bernat B, Pieti Opie L, Von Carlowitz I, Parry J, Morales T, Perrier M, Woessner R, Pheneger T, Hoffman K, Winkler J, Koch K. ARRY-334543, a potent, orally active small molecule inhibitor of EGFR and ErbB-2. AACR Annual Meeting 2005;46:Abstr 3399.

282. Rothenberg M, Kane K, Kollmannsberger C, Berlin JD, Cooper W, Maloney L, Gordon GS, Litwiler K, D'Aloisio S, Gelmon K. A Phase 1 study of ARRY-543, a potent, selective, reversible inhibitor of ErbB receptors. AACR-NCI-EORTC Conference on Molecular Targets and Cancer Therapeutics; 2007 October 22; San Francisco, CA. Abstr B257.

283. Suzuki T, Fujii A, Ohya J, Amano Y, Kitano Y, Abe D, Nakamura H. Pharmacological characterization of MP-412 (AV-412), a dual epidermal growth factor receptor and ErbB2 tyrosine kinase inhibitor. Cancer Sci 2007;98(12):1977–1984.

284. Atzori F, Tabernero J, Cervantes A, Botero M, Hsu K, Brown H, Hanley W, Macarulla T, Rosello S, Baselga J. A phase I, pharmacokinetic (PK) and pharmacodynamic (PD) study of weekly (qW) MK-0646, an insulin-like growth factor-1 receptor (IGF1R) monoclonal antibody (MAb) in patients (pts) with advanced solid tumors. J Clin Oncol (Meeting Abstracts) 2008;26(15 Suppl):Abstr 3519.

285. Tolcher AW, Rothenberg ML, Rodon J, Delbeke D, Patnaik A, Nguyen L, Young F, Hwang Y, Haqq C, Puzanov I. A phase I pharmacokinetic and pharmacodynamic study of AMG 479, a fully human monoclonal antibody against insulin-like growth factor type 1 receptor (IGF-1R), in advanced solid tumors. J Clin Oncol (Meeting Abstracts) 2007;25(18 Suppl):Abstr 3002.

286. Leong S, Gore L, Benjamin R, Warren T, Eckhardt SG, Camidge DR, Dias C, Greig G, Frankel S, Kurzrock R. A phase I study of R1507, a human monoclonal antibody IGF-1R (insulin-like growth factor receptor) antagonist given weekly in patients with advanced solid tumors. AACR Meeting Abstracts 2007(Molecular Targets and Cancer Therapeutics, San Francisco, CA):Abstr A78.

287. Ji QS, Mulvihill MJ, Rosenfeld-Franklin M, Cooke A, Feng L, Mak G, O'Connor M, Yao Y, Pirritt C, Buck E, Eyzaguirre A, Arnold LD, Gibson NW, Pachter JA. A novel, potent, and selective insulin-like growth factor-I receptor kinase inhibitor blocks insulin-like growth factor-I receptor signaling in vitro and inhibits insulin-like growth factor-I receptor dependent tumor growth in vivo. Mol Cancer Ther 2007;6(8):2158–2167.

288. Garcia-Echeverria C, Pearson MA, Marti A, Meyer T, Mestan J, Zimmermann J, Gao J, Brueggen J, Capraro HG, Cozens R, Evans DB, Fabbro D, Furet P, Porta DG, Liebetanz J, Martiny-Baron G, Ruetz S, Hofmann F. In Vivo antitumor activity of NVP-AEW541—a novel, potent, and selective inhibitor of the IGF-IR kinase. Cancer Cell 2004;5(3):231–239.

289. Aftab DT. Simultaneous inhibition of IGF1R and Src family kinases causes tumor growth inhibition and tumor regression in xenograft models. Eur J Cancer Suppl 2006;4(12): 178.

290. Zhang W. Inhibition of the drug-resistant T315l mutant of BCR-Abl. Eur J Cancer Suppl 2006;4(12): 54.

291. Britten C, Smith DC, Bui LA, Clary DO, Hurwitz HI. A phase I dose-escalation study of XL228, a potent IGF-1R/SRC/Aurora inhibitor, in patients with advanced malignancies. 20th EORTC-NCI-AACR Symposium on Molecular Targets and Cancer Therapeutics. Volume Abstr 390. Geneva, Swizerland; 2008.

292. Brown P, Small D. FLT3 inhibitors: a paradigm for the development of targeted therapeutics for paediatric cancer. Eur J Cancer 2004;40(5):707–721, discussion 722–724.

293. Small D. FLT3 mutations: biology and treatment. Hematology Am Soc Hematol Educ Program 2006: 178–184.

294. Armstrong SA, Kung AL, Mabon ME, Silverman LB, Stam RW, Den Boer ML, Pieters R, Kersey JH, Sallan SE, Fletcher JA, Golub TR, Griffin JD, Korsmeyer SJ. Inhibition of FLT3 in MLL. Validation of a therapeutic target identified by gene expression based classification. Cancer Cell 2003;3(2):173–183.

295. Nakao M, Yokota S, Iwai T, Kaneko H, Horiike S, Kashima K, Sonoda Y, Fujimoto T, Misawa S. Internal tandem duplication of the flt3 gene found in acute myeloid leukemia. Leukemia 1996;10(12):1911–1918.

296. Abu-Duhier FM, Goodeve AC, Wilson GA, Care RS, Peake IR, Reilly JT. Identification of novel FLT-3 Asp835 mutations in adult acute myeloid leukaemia. Br J Haematol 2001;113(4):983–988.

297. Meshinchi S, Woods WG, Stirewalt DL, Sweetser DA, Buckley JD, Tjoa TK, Bernstein ID, Radich JP. Prevalence and prognostic significance of Flt3 internal tandem duplication in pediatric acute myeloid leukemia. Blood 2001;97(1):89–94.

298. Stone RM. Novel therapeutic agents in acute myeloid leukemia. Exp Hematol 2007;35(4 Suppl 1): 163–166.

299. Heidel F, Solem FK, Breitenbuecher F, Lipka DB, Kasper S, Thiede MH, Brandts C, Serve H, Roesel J, Giles F, Feldman E, Ehninger G, Schiller GJ, Nimer S, Stone RM, Wang Y, Kindler T, Cohen PS, Huber C, Fischer T. Clinical resistance to the kinase inhibitor PKC412 in acute myeloid leukemia by mutation of Asn-676 in the FLT3 tyrosine kinase domain. Blood 2006;107(1):293–300.

300. Zhang W, Konopleva M, Shi YX, McQueen T, Harris D, Ling X, Estrov Z, Quintas-Cardama A, Small D, Cortes J, Andreeff M. Mutant FLT3: a direct target of sorafenib in acute myelogenous leukemia. J Natl Cancer Inst 2008;100(3):184–198.

301. Safaian NN, Czibere A, Bruns I, Fenk R, Reinecke P, Dienst A, Haas R, Kobbe G. Sorafenib (Nexavar^register^) induces molecular remission and regression of extramedullary disease in a patient with FLT3-ITD(+) acute myeloid leukemia. Leuk Res 2009;33(2):348–350.

302. Ikezoe T, Nishioka C, Tasaka T, Yang Y, Komatsu N, Togitani K, Koeffler HP, Taguchi H. The antitumor effects of sunitinib (formerly SU11248) against a variety of human hematologic malignancies: enhancement of growth inhibition via inhibition of mammalian target of rapamycin signaling. Mol Cancer Ther 2006;5(10):2522–2530.

303. O'Farrell AM, Abrams TJ, Yuen HA, Ngai TJ, Louie SG, Yee KW, Wong LM, Hong W, Lee LB, Town A, Smolich BD, Manning WC, Murray LJ, Heinrich MC, Cherrington JM. SU11248 is a novel FLT3 tyrosine kinase inhibitor with potent activity in vitro and in vivo. Blood 2003;101(9):3597–3605.

304. Mendel DB, Laird AD, Xin X, Louie SG, Christensen JG, Li G, Schreck RE, Abrams TJ, Ngai TJ, Lee LB, Murray LJ, Carver J, Chan E, Moss KG, Haznedar JO, Sukbuntherng J, Blake RA, Sun L, Tang C, Miller T, Shirazian S, McMahon G, Cherrington JM. In Vivo antitumor activity of SU11248, a novel tyrosine kinase inhibitor targeting vascular endothelial growth factor and platelet-derived growth factor receptors: determination of a pharmacokinetic/pharmacodynamic relationship. Clin Cancer Res 2003;9(1):327–337.

305. O'Farrell AM, Foran JM, Fiedler W, Serve H, Paquette RL, Cooper MA, Yuen HA, Louie SG, Kim H, Nicholas S, Heinrich MC, Berdel WE, Bello C, Jacobs M, Scigalla P, Manning WC, Kelsey S, Cherrington JM. An innovative phase I clinical study demonstrates inhibition of FLT3 phosphorylation by SU11248 in acute myeloid leukemia patients. Clin Cancer Res 2003;9(15):5465–5476.

306. Fiedler W, Serve H, Dohner H, Schwittay M, Ottmann OG, O'Farrell AM, Bello CL, Allred R, Manning WC, Cherrington JM, Louie SG, Hong W, Brega NM, Massimini G, Scigalla P, Berdel WE, Hossfeld DK. A phase 1 study of SU11248 in the treatment of patients with refractory or resistant acute myeloid leukemia (AML) or not amenable to conventional therapy for the disease. Blood 2005;105(3):986–993.

307. Fabbro D, Buchdunger E, Wood J, Mestan J, Hofmann F, Ferrari S, Mett H, O'Reilly T, Meyer T. Inhibitors of protein kinases: CGP 41251, a protein kinase inhibitor with potential as an anticancer agent. Pharmacol Ther 1999;82(2–3):293–301.

308. Weisberg E, Boulton C, Kelly LM, Manley P, Fabbro D, Meyer T, Gilliland DG, Griffin JD. Inhibition of mutant FLT3 receptors in leukemia cells by the small molecule tyrosine kinase inhibitor PKC412. Cancer Cell 2002;1(5):433–443.

309. Barry EV, Clark JJ, Cools J, Roesel J, Gilliland DG. Uniform sensitivity of FLT3 activation loop mutants to the tyrosine kinase inhibitor midostaurin. Blood 2007;110(13):4476–4479.

310. Propper DJ, McDonald AC, Man A, Thavasu P, Balkwill F, Braybrooke JP, Caponigro F, Graf P, Dutreix C, Blackie R, Kaye SB, Ganesan TS, Talbot DC, Harris AL, Twelves C. Phase I and pharmacokinetic study of PKC412, an inhibitor of protein kinase C. J Clin Oncol 2001;19(5):1485–1492.

311. Ganeshaguru K, Wickremasinghe RG, Jones DT, Gordon M, Hart SM, Virchis AE, Prentice HG, Hoffbrand AV, Man A, Champain K, Csermak K, Mehta AB. Actions of the selective protein kinase C inhibitor PKC412 on B-chronic lymphocytic leukemia cells in vitro. Haematologica 2002;87(2):167–176.

312. Stone RM, DeAngelo DJ, Klimek V, Galinsky I, Estey E, Nimer SD, Grandin W, Lebwohl D, Wang Y, Cohen P, Fox EA, Neuberg D, Clark J, Gilliland DG, Griffin JD. Patients with acute myeloid leukemia and an activating mutation in FLT3 respond to a small-molecule FLT3 tyrosine kinase inhibitor, PKC412. Blood 2005;105(1):54–60.

313. Clark JJ, Cools J, Curley DP, Yu JC, Lokker NA, Giese NA, Gilliland DG. Variable sensitivity of FLT3 activation loop mutations to the small molecule tyrosine kinase inhibitor MLN518. Blood 2004;104(9):2867–2872.

314. Griswold IJ, Shen LJ, La Rosee P, Demehri S, Heinrich MC, Braziel RM, McGreevey L, Haley AD, Giese N, Druker BJ, Deininger MW. Effects of MLN518, a dual FLT3 and KIT inhibitor, on normal and malignant hematopoiesis. Blood 2004;104(9):2912–2918.

315. Kelly LM, Yu JC, Boulton CL, Apatira M, Li J, Sullivan CM, Williams I, Amaral SM, Curley DP, Duclos N, Neuberg D, Scarborough RM, Pandey A, Hollenbach S, Abe K, Lokker NA, Gilliland DG, Giese NA. CT53518, a novel selective FLT3 antagonist for the treatment of acute myelogenous leukemia (AML). Cancer Cell 2002;1(5):421–432.

316. DeAngelo DJ, Stone RM, Heaney ML, Nimer SD, Paquette RL, Klisovic RB, Caligiuri MA, Cooper MR, Lecerf JM, Karol MD, Sheng S, Holford N, Curtin PT, Druker BJ, Heinrich MC. Phase 1 clinical results with tandutinib (MLN518), a novel FLT3 antagonist, in patients with acute myelogenous leukemia or high-risk myelodysplastic syndrome: safety, pharmacokinetics, and pharmacodynamics. Blood 2006;108(12):3674–3681.

317. DeAngelo DJ, Amrein PC, Kovacsovics TJ, Klisovic RB, Powell BL, Cooper M, Webb IJ, Stone RM. Phase 1/2 study of tandutinib (MLN518) plus standard induction chemotherapy in newly diagnosed acute myelogenous leukemia (AML). ASH Annual Meeting Abstracts 2006;108(11):Abstr 158.

318. Shankar DB, Li J, Tapang P, Owen McCall J, Pease LJ, Dai Y, Wei RQ, Albert DH, Bouska JJ, Osterling DJ, Guo J, Marcotte PA, Johnson EF, Soni N, Hartandi K, Michaelides MR, Davidsen SK, Priceman SJ, Chang JC, Rhodes K, Shah N, Moore TB, Sakamoto KM, Glaser KB. ABT-869, a multitargeted receptor tyrosine kinase inhibitor: inhibition of FLT3 phosphorylation and signaling in acute myeloid leukemia. Blood 2007;109(8):3400–3408.

319. Zhou J, Pan M, Xie Z, Loh SL, Bi C, Tai YC, Lilly M, Lim YP, Han JH, Glaser KB, Albert DH, Davidsen SK, Chen CS. Synergistic antileukemic effects between ABT-869 and chemotherapy involve downregulation of cell cycle-regulated genes and c-Mos-mediated MAPK pathway. Leukemia 2008;22(1):138–146.

320. Heinrich MC, Rubin BP, Longley BJ, Fletcher JA. Biology and genetic aspects of gastrointestinal stromal tumors: KIT activation and cytogenetic alterations. Hum Pathol 2002;33(5):484–495.

321. Hirota S, Isozaki K, Moriyama Y, Hashimoto K, Nishida T, Ishiguro S, Kawano K, Hanada M, Kurata A, Takeda M, Muhammad Tunio G, Matsuzawa Y, Kanakura Y, Shinomura Y, Kitamura Y. Gain-of-function mutations of c-kit in human gastrointestinal stromal tumors. Science 1998;279(5350):577–580.

322. Corless CL, Fletcher JA, Heinrich MC. Biology of gastrointestinal stromal tumors. J Clin Oncol 2004;22(18):3813–3825.

323. Heinrich MC, Corless CL, Demetri GD, Blanke CD, von Mehren M, Joensuu H, McGreevey LS, Chen CJ, Van den Abbeele AD, Druker BJ, Kiese B, Eisenberg B, Roberts PJ, Singer S, Fletcher CD, Silberman S, Dimitrijevic S, Fletcher JA. Kinase mutations and imatinib response in patients with metastatic gastrointestinal stromal tumor. J Clin Oncol 2003;21(23):4342–4349.

324. Tian Q, Frierson HF Jr, Krystal GW, Moskaluk CA. Activating c-kit gene mutations in human germ cell tumors. Am J Pathol 1999;154(6):1643–1647.

325. Corless CL, McGreevey L, Haley A, Town A, Heinrich MC. KIT mutations are common in incidental gastrointestinal stromal tumors one centimeter or less in size. Am J Pathol 2002;160(5):1567–1572.

326. Heinrich MC, Griffith DJ, Druker BJ, Wait CL, Ott KA, Zigler AJ. Inhibition of c-kit receptor tyrosine kinase activity by STI 571, a selective tyrosine kinase inhibitor. Blood 2000;96(3):925–932.

327. Tuveson DA, Willis NA, Jacks T, Griffin JD, Singer S, Fletcher CD, Fletcher JA, Demetri GD. STI571 inactivation of the gastrointestinal stromal tumor c-KIT oncoprotein: biological and clinical implications. Oncogene 2001;20(36):5054–5058.

328. Joensuu H, Roberts PJ, Sarlomo-Rikala M, Andersson LC, Tervahartiala P, Tuveson D, Silberman S, Capdeville R, Dimitrijevic S, Druker B, Demetri GD. Effect of the tyrosine kinase inhibitor STI571 in a patient with a metastatic gastrointestinal stromal tumor. N Engl J Med 2001;344(14):1052–1056.

329. Demetri GD, von Mehren M, Blanke CD, Van den Abbeele AD, Eisenberg B, Roberts PJ, Heinrich MC, Tuveson DA, Singer S, Janicek M, Fletcher JA, Silverman SG, Silberman SL, Capdeville R, Kiese B, Peng B, Dimitrijevic S, Druker BJ, Corless C, Fletcher CD, Joensuu H. Efficacy and safety of imatinib mesylate in advanced gastrointestinal stromal tumors. N Engl J Med 2002;347(7):472–480.

330. van Oosterom AT, Judson I, Verweij J, Stroobants S, Donato di Paola E, Dimitrijevic S, Martens M, Webb A, Sciot R, Van Glabbeke M, Silberman S, Nielsen OS. Safety and efficacy of imatinib (STI571) in metastatic gastrointestinal stromal tumours: a phase I study. Lancet 2001;358(9291):1421–1423.

331. Verweij J, Casali PG, Zalcberg J, LeCesne A, Reichardt P, Blay JY, Issels R, van Oosterom A, Hogendoorn PC, Van Glabbeke M, Bertulli R, Judson I. Progression-free survival in gastrointestinal stromal tumours with high-dose imatinib: randomised trial. Lancet 2004;364(9440):1127–1134.

332. Blanke CD, Demetri GD, von Mehren M, Heinrich MC, Eisenberg B, Fletcher JA, Corless CL, Fletcher CD, Roberts PJ, Heinz D, Wehre E, Nikolova Z, Joensuu H. Long-term results from a randomized phase II trial of standard- versus higher-dose imatinib mesylate for patients with unresectable or metastatic gastrointestinal stromal tumors expressing KIT. J Clin Oncol 2008;26(4):620–625.

333. Hornick JL, Fletcher CD. The role of KIT in the management of patients with gastrointestinal stromal tumors. Hum Pathol 2007;38(5):679–687.

334. Ma Y, Zeng S, Metcalfe DD, Akin C, Dimitrijevic S, Butterfield JH, McMahon G, Longley BJ. The c-KIT mutation causing human mastocytosis is resistant to STI571 and other KIT kinase inhibitors; kinases with enzymatic site mutations show different inhibitor sensitivity profiles than wild-type kinases and those with regulatory-type mutations. Blood 2002;99(5):1741–1744.

335. Corless CL, Schroeder A, Griffith D, Town A, McGreevey L, Harrell P, Shiraga S, Bainbridge T, Morich J, Heinrich MC. PDGFRA mutations in gastrointestinal stromal tumors: frequency, spectrum and in vitro sensitivity to imatinib. J Clin Oncol 2005;23(23):5357–5364.

336. Beghini A, Ripamonti CB, Cairoli R, Cazzaniga G, Colapietro P, Elice F, Nadali G, Grillo G, Haas OA, Biondi A, Morra E, Larizza L. KIT activating mutations: incidence in adult and pediatric acute myeloid leukemia, and identification of an internal tandem duplication. Haematologica 2004;89(8):920–925.

337. Debiec-Rychter M, Cools J, Dumez H, Sciot R, Stul M, Mentens N, Vranckx H, Wasag B, Prenen H, Roesel J, Hagemeijer A, Van Oosterom A, Marynen P. Mechanisms of resistance to imatinib mesylate in gastrointestinal stromal tumors and activity of the PKC412 inhibitor against imatinib-resistant mutants. Gastroenterology 2005;128(2):270–279.

338. Antonescu CR, Besmer P, Guo T, Arkun K, Hom G, Koryotowski B, Leversha MA, Jeffrey PD, Desantis D, Singer S, Brennan MF, Maki RG, DeMatteo RP. Acquired resistance to imatinib in gastrointestinal stromal tumor occurs through secondary gene mutation. Clin Cancer Res 2005;11(11):4182–4190.

339. Heinrich MC, Corless CL, Blanke CD, Demetri GD, Joensuu H, Roberts PJ, Eisenberg BL, von Mehren M, Fletcher CD, Sandau K, McDougall K, Ou WB, Chen CJ, Fletcher JA.

Molecular correlates of imatinib resistance in gastrointestinal stromal tumors. J Clin Oncol 2006;24(29):4764–4774.

340. Wardelmann E, Merkelbach-Bruse S, Pauls K, Thomas N, Schildhaus HU, Heinicke T, Speidel N, Pietsch T, Buettner R, Pink D, Reichardt P, Hohenberger P. Polyclonal evolution of multiple secondary KIT mutations in gastrointestinal stromal tumors under treatment with imatinib mesylate. Clin Cancer Res 2006;12(6):1743–1749.

341. Heinrich M, Corless C, Liegl B, Fletcher CD, Raut C, Donsky R, Bertagnolli M, Harlow A, Demetri G, Fletcher J. Mechanisms of sunitinib malate (SU) resistance in gastrointestinal stromal tumors (GISTs). J Clin Oncol (Meeting Abstracts) 2007;25(18 Suppl):Abstr 10006.

342. Blackstein M, Huang X, Demetri G, Casali P, Garrett C, Schoffski P, Shah M, Verweij J, Baum C, DePrimo S. Evaluation of soluble KIT (sKIT) as a potential surrogate marker for TTP in sunitinib malate (SU)-treated patients (pts) with advanced GIST. J Clin Oncol (Meeting Abstracts) 2007;25(18 Suppl):Abstr 10007.

343. Blackstein M, Huang X, Demetri G, Casali P, Garrett C, Schoffski P, Shah M, Verweij J, Baum C, DePrimo S. Evaluation of soluble KIT (sKIT) as a potential surrogate marker for TTP in patients with advanced GIST receiving sunitinib. ASCO Gastrointestinal Cancer Symposium 2008. Abstr 19.

344. Schittenhelm MM, Shiraga S, Schroeder A, Corbin AS, Griffith D, Lee FY, Bokemeyer C, Deininger MW, Druker BJ, Heinrich MC. Dasatinib (BMS-354825), a dual SRC/ABL kinase inhibitor, inhibits the kinase activity of wild-type, juxtamembrane, and activation loop mutant KIT isoforms associated with human malignancies. Cancer Res 2006;66(1):473–481.

345. Evans TRJ, Morgan JA, van den Abbeele AD, McPherson IRJ, George S, Crawford D, Mastrullo JM, Cheng S, Fletcher JA, Demetri GD. Phase I dose-escalation study of the SRC and multi-kinase inhibitor BMS-354825 in patients (pts) with GIST and other solid tumors. J Clin Oncol (Meeting Abstracts) 2005;23(16 Suppl):Abstr 3034.

346. Morgan JAD, Wang D, MacPherson IRJ, LoRusso P, van den Abbeele AD, Brunton VG, Luo R, Voi M, Evans TRJ. A phase I study of dasatinib, a Src and multi-kinase inhibitor, in patients (pts) with GIST and other solid tumors. 18th EORTC-NCI-AACR Symposium on Molecular Targets and Cancer Therapeutics. Prague, Czech Republic; 2006. Abstr 383.

347. Guo T, Agaram NP, Wong GC, Hom G, D'Adamo D, Maki RG, Schwartz GK, Veach D, Clarkson BD, Singer S, DeMatteo RP, Besmer P, Antonescu CR. Sorafenib inhibits the imatinib-resistant KITT670I gatekeeper mutation in gastrointestinal stromal tumor. Clin Cancer Res 2007;13(16):4874–4881.

348. Guida T, Anaganti S, Provitera L, Gedrich R, Sullivan E, Wilhelm SM, Santoro M, Carlomagno F. Sorafenib inhibits imatinib-resistant KIT and platelet-derived growth factor receptor beta gatekeeper mutants. Clin Cancer Res 2007;13(11):3363–3369.

349. Wiebe L, Kasza KE, Maki RG, D'Adamo DR, Chow WA, Wade JL, Agamah E, Stadler WM, Vokes EE, Kindler HL. Activity of sorafenib (SOR) in patients (pts) with imatinib (IM) and sunitinib (SU)-resistant (RES) gastrointestinal stromal tumors (GIST): a phase II trial of the University of Chicago Phase II Consortium. J Clin Oncol (Meeting Abstracts) 2008;26(15 Suppl):Abstr 10502.

350. Von Mehren M, Reichardt P, Casali PG, Blay J, Debiec-Rychter M, Dumez H, Cheung W, Feifel B, Veronese M, Demetri G. A phase I study of nilotinib alone and in combination with imatinib (IM) in patients (pts) with imatinib-resistant gastrointestinal stromal tumors (GIST)—study update. J Clin Oncol (Meeting Abstracts) 2007;25(18 Suppl):Abstr 10023.

351. Yamada Y, Sawaki A, Nishida T, Komatsu Y, Kanda T, Doi T, Koseki M, Baba H, Asami Y, Ohtsu T. Phase II study of motesanib diphosphate (AMG 706) in Japanese patients (pts) with advanced gastrointestinal stromal tumors (GISTs) who developed progressive disease or relapsed while on imatinib mesylate. ASCO Gastrointestinal Symposium 2008.Abstr 107.

352. Bui BN, Blay J, Duffaud F, Hermine O, Le Cesne A. Preliminary efficacy and safety results of masitinib administered front line in patients with advanced GIST. A phase II study. J Clin Oncol (Meeting Abstracts) 2007;25(18 Suppl):Abstr 10025.

353. Schoffski P, de Jonge M, Dumez H, Brega NM, Abbattista A, Courtney R, Verweij J. Phase I safety and pharmacokinetic (PK) study of SU014813 (S) in combination with docetaxel (D) in patients (pts) with solid tumors (STs). J Clin Oncol (Meeting Abstracts) 2008;26(15 Suppl):Abstr 3554.

354. Heuer T. XL820 inhibits mutated forms of KIT associated with drug resistance. AACR-NCI-EORTC Conference on Molecular Targets and Cancer Therapeutics; 2007 October 22; San Francisco, CA. Abstr B237.

355. Stein M, Yazji S, Rodon J, Miles D, O'Rourke P, Papadopoulos K, Mita AC. A phase I dose-escalation study of the safety, pharmacokinetics and pharmacodynamics of XL820 administered orally daily (QD) or twice daily (BID) to patients (pts) with solid malignancies. AACR-NCI-EORTC International Conference on Molecular Targets and Cancer Therapeutics; 2007; San Francisco, CA. Abstr B69.

356. Matsui J, Yamamoto Y, Funahashi Y, Tsuruoka A, Watanabe T, Wakabayashi T, Uenaka T, Asada M. E7080, a novel inhibitor that targets multiple kinases, has potent antitumor activities against stem cell factor producing human small cell lung cancer H146, based on angiogenesis inhibition. Int J Cancer 2008;122(3):664–671.

357. Glen H, Boss D, Morrison R, Roelvink M, Wanders J, Mazur A, Gupta A, Das A, Evans T, Schellens J. A phase I study of E7080 in patients (pts) with advanced malignancies. J Clin Oncol (Meeting Abstracts) 2008;26(15 Suppl):Abstr 3526.

358. Joly A, Gerritsen ME. EXEL-2880, A Small-Molecule, Orally Available Tyrosine Kinase Inhibitor that Targets VEGFR and the HGF Receptor, C-MET. Potent Anti-Angiogenic and Anti-Tumor Effects in vitro and in vivo. Miami Nature Winter Biotech Symposium; 2006; Miami, FL.

359. Ross R, Srinivasan R, Vaishampayan U, Bukowski R, Rosenberg J, Eisenberg P, Logan T, Srinivas S, Stein M, Mueller T, Keer H. A Phase 2 study of the dual MET/VEGFR2 inhibitor XL880 in patients (pts) with papillary renal carcinoma (PRC). AACR-NCI-EORTC Conference on Molecular Targets and Cancer Therapeutics; 2007 October 22; San Francisco, CA. Abstr B249.

360. Jeay S, Munshi N, Hill J, Moussa M, Ashwell M, Leggett D, Li C. ARQ 197, a highly selective small molecular inhibitor of c-Met, with selective antitumor properties in a broad spectrum of human cancer cells. AACR Annual Meeting; 2007 April 14–18; Los Angeles, CA. Abstr 2369.

361. Li Y, Zhou W, Chen D, Li W, Jiang Z, Chen TT, Li C. Anti-metastatic activity of ARQ 197, a highly selective oral small molecule inhibitor of c-Met, in experimental metastatic models of colon cancer. AACR Annual Meeting; 2007 April 14–18; Los Angeles, CA. Abstr 2191.

362. Joly A. Simultaneous blockade of VEGF and HGF receptors results in potent anti-angiogenic and anti-tumor effects. 18th EORTC-NCI-AACR Symposium on Molecular Targets and Cancer Therapeutics; 2006; Prague, Czech Republic. Abstr 104.

363. Joly A. Simultaneous blockade of HGF and VEGF receptors results in potent anti-angiogenic and anti-tumor effects. 18th EORTC-NCI-AACR Symposium on Molecular Targets and Cancer Therapeutics; 2006; Prague, Czech Republic. Abstr 104.

364. Perera T, Lavrijssen T, Janssens B, Geerts T, King P, Mevellec L, Cummings M, Lu T, Johnson D, Page M. JNJ-38877605: a selective Met kinase inhibitor inducing regression of Met-driven tumor models. AACR Meeting Abstracts 2008;1: 4837.

365. Beaulieu N, Beaulieu C, Dupont I, Nguyen H, Chute I, Gravel S, Durand J, Robert M-F, Lefebvre S, Lu A, Dubay M, Rahil J, Isakovic L, Claridge S, Saavedra O, Raeppel S, Mannion M, Bernstein N, Zhan L, Gaudett F, Zhou N, Raeppel F, Granger M-C, Deziel R, Vaisburg A, Wang J, Besterman J, Macleod AR, Maroun CR. Preclinical development of MGCD265, a potent orally active c-met/VEGFR multi-target kinase inhibitor. 99th AACR Annual Meeting; 2008 April 12–16; San Diego, CA. Abstr 4838.

366. Zou HY, Li Q, Lee JH, Arango ME, McDonnell SR, Yamazaki S, Koudriakova TB, Alton G, Cui JJ, Kung PP, Nambu MD, Los G, Bender SL, Mroczkowski B, Christensen JG. An orally available small-molecule inhibitor of c-Met, PF-2341066, exhibits cytoreductive antitumor efficacy through antiproliferative and antiangiogenic mechanisms. Cancer Res 2007;67(9):4408–4417.

367. Christensen JG, Zou HY, Arango ME, Li Q, Lee JH, McDonnell SR, Yamazaki S, Alton GR, Mroczkowski B, Los G. Cytoreductive antitumor activity of PF-2341066, a novel inhibitor of anaplastic lymphoma kinase and c-Met, in experimental models of anaplastic large-cell lymphoma. Mol Cancer Ther 2007;6(12Pt 1):3314–3322.

368. Vitale G, Caraglia M, Ciccarelli A, Lupoli G, Abbruzzese A, Tagliaferri P, Lupoli G. Current approaches and perspectives in the therapy of medullary thyroid carcinoma. Cancer 2001;91(9):1797–1808.

369. Quayle FJ, Moley JF. Medullary thyroid carcinoma: including MEN 2A and MEN 2B syndromes. J Surg Oncol 2005;89(3):122–129.

370. Carlomagno F, Anaganti S, Guida T, Salvatore G, Troncone G, Wilhelm SM, Santoro M. BAY 43–9006 inhibition of oncogenic RET mutants. J Natl Cancer Inst 2006;98(5):326–334.

371. Brose MS, Nellore A, Paziana K, Ransone K, Redlinger M, Flaherty KT, Mandel SJ, Troxel AB, Loevner LA, Gupta-Abramson V. A phase II study of sorafenib in metastatic thyroid carcinoma. J Clin Oncol (Meeting Abstracts) 2008;26(15 Suppl):Abstr 6026.

372. Ravaud A, de la Fouchardiere C, Asselineau J, Klewin M, Nicoli-Sire P, Bournaud C, Delord J, Weryha G, Catargi B. Sunitinib in patients with refractory advanced thyroid cancer: the THYSU phase II trial. J Clin Oncol (Meeting Abstracts) 2008;26(15 Suppl):Abstr 6058.

373. Salgia R, Sherman S, Hong DS, Ng CS, Frye J, Janisch L, Ratain MJ, Kurzrock R. A phase I study of XL184, a RET, VEGFR2 and MET kinase inhibitor, in patients (pts) with advanced malignancies, including pts with medullary thyroid cancer (MTC). J Clin Oncol (Meeting Abstracts) 2008;26(15 Suppl):Abstr 3522.

374. Kurzrock R, Sherman S, Hong D, Ng C, Frye J, Janisch L, Ratain M, Salgia R. A phase 1 study of XL184, a MET, VEGFR2, and RET kinase inhibitor, administered orally to patients (pts) with advanced malignancies, including a subgroup of patients with medullary thyroid cancer (MTC). 20th AACR-NCI-EORTC symposium on Molecular Targets and Cancer Therapeutics 2008 October 21–24; Geneva, Switzerland. Abstr 379.

375. Carlomagno F, Vitagliano D, Guida T, Ciardiello F, Tortora G, Vecchio G, Ryan AJ, Fontanini G, Fusco A, Santoro M. ZD6474, an orally available inhibitor of KDR tyrosine kinase activity, efficiently blocks oncogenic RET kinases. Cancer Res 2002;62(24):7284–7290.

376. Carlomagno F, Guida T, Anaganti S, Vecchio G, Fusco A, Ryan AJ, Billaud M, Santoro M. Disease associated mutations at valine 804 in the RET receptor tyrosine kinase confer resistance to selective kinase inhibitors. Oncogene 2004;23(36):6056–6063.

377. Wells S, Gosnell J, Gagel R, Moley J, Pfister D, Sosa J, Skinner M, Krebs A, Hou J, Schlumberger M. Vandetanib in metastatic hereditary thyroid cancer: follow-up results of an open-label phase II trial. J Clin Oncol (Meeting Abstracts) 2007;25(18 Suppl):Abstr 6018.

378. Haddad RI, Krebs AD, Vasselli J, Paz-Ares LG, Robinson B. A phase II open-label study of vandetanib in patients with locally advanced or metastatic hereditary medullary thyroid cancer. J Clin Oncol (Meeting Abstracts) 2008;26(15 Suppl):Abstr 6024.

379. Sherman SI, Schlumberger MJ, Droz J, Hoffmann M, Wirth L, Bastholt L, Martins RG, Licitra L, Shi Y, Stepan DE. Initial results from a phase II trial of motesanib diphosphate (AMG 706) in patients with differentiated thyroid cancer (DTC). J Clin Oncol (Meeting Abstracts) 2007;25(18 Suppl):Abstr 6017.

380. Roberts WG, Ung E, Whalen P, Cooper B, Hulford C, Autry C, Richter D, Emerson E, Lin J, Kath J, Coleman K, Yao L, Martinez-Alsina L, Lorenzen M, Berliner M, Luzzio M, Patel N, Schmitt E, LaGreca S, Jani J, Wessel M, Marr E, Griffor M, Vajdos F. Antitumor activity and pharmacology of a selective focal adhesion kinase inhibitor, PF-562,271. Cancer Res 2008;68(6):1935–1944.

381. Bagi CM, Roberts GW, Andresen CJ. Dual focal adhesion kinase/Pyk2 inhibitor has positive effects on bone tumors: implications for bone metastases. Cancer 2008;112(10):2313–2321.

382. Siu LL, Burris HA, III, Mileshkin LR, Camidge DR, Eckhardt SG, Lamb A, Chen EX, Jones SF, Xu H, Fingert H. A phase I clinical, pharmacokinetic (PK) and pharmacodynamic (PD) evaluation of PF-00562271 targeting focal adhesion kinase (FAK) in patients (pts) with advanced solid tumors. J Clin Oncol (Meeting Abstracts) 2008;26(15 Suppl):Abstr 3534.

383. Massague J. TGFbeta in Cancer. Cell 2008;134(2):215–230.

384. Yingling JM, Shou J, Xia X, Chen Y, Yan L, Evans W, Paul D, Banks C, Foreman R, Goode R, Law K, Peng S-B, Uhlik M, Starling J. A small molecule inhibitor of TGF {beta} RI kinase potentiates VEGF dependent angiogenesis in vitro. Proc Am Assoc Cancer Res 2006;47:Abstr 250.

385. Calvo-Aller E, Baselga J, Glatt S, Cleverly A, Lahn M, Arteaga CL, Rothenberg ML, Carducci MA. First human dose escalation study in patients with metastatic malignancies to determine safety and pharmacokinetics of LY2157299, a small molecule inhibitor of the transforming growth factor-beta receptor I kinase. J Clin Oncol (Meeting Abstracts) 2008;26(15 Suppl):Abstr 14554.

CHAPTER 9

ANGIOKINASE INHIBITORS

9.1 INTRODUCTION

Antiangiogenic therapy was a concept first proposed by the late Judah Folkman in the early 1970s as a method to restrict tumor growth. The idea stemmed from Folkman's observations that suggested that tumor growth was angiogenesis dependent (1). While initially received with considerable skepticism, Folkman's hypothesis gradually gained support, due in no large part to his unending dedication, promotion, and research to support the clinical applications of angiogenesis inhibition. Now over thirty years later, a vast literature of both basic and clinical data support the concept that both tumor growth and tumor metastasis depend on the recruitment of new blood vessels. Tumor cells are thought to generate their own "angiogenic switch," promoting angiogenesis by oncogene-driven tumor expression of proangiogenic proteins such as VEGFA, FGF2, IL8, PDGF, and others. The hypoxic conditions associated with tumors also result in the activation of the transcription factor HIF1α, which in turn promotes upregulation of many proangiogenic factors. Moreover, the angiogenic switch results in the downregulation of endogenous inhibitors of angiogenesis such as thrombospondin. Well over 100 different angiogenesis-inhibiting drugs, antibodies, and biologics are now in various stages of clinical trials. Several of these have successfully progressed through clinical trials and are marketed for various cancer indications. Bevacizumab (Avastin®) was the first FDA approved therapy designed to inhibit angiogenesis. The original reagent, a monoclonal antibody that specifically binds to VEGFA (all splice variants), was produced in 1993 by Napoleone Ferrara and his colleagues at Genentech (2). After 7 years of clinical trials, the antibody was approved by the FDA for the first line treatment of patients with metastatic colorectal cancer in combination with intravenous 5-FU (2004). Other approvals followed, namely, second line treatment in combination with intravenous 5-FU of patients with metastatic colorectal cancer (2006), first line treatment in combination with carboplatin and paclitaxel in patients with unresectable, locally advanced, recurrent or metastatic nonsquamous, non small cell lung cancer (2006), and metastatic breast cancer in combination with paclitaxel chemotherapy (2008). More recently (May 2009), bevacizumab was also approved as therapy for patients with previously treated glioblastoma. The most common adverse events associated with bevacizumab across all trials were asthenia,

Targeting Protein Kinases for Cancer Therapy, by David J. Matthews and Mary E. Gerritsen
Copyright © 2010 John Wiley & Sons, Inc.

abdominal pain, headache, hypertension, diarrhea, nausea, vomiting, anorexia, stomatitis, constipation, upper respiratory infection, epistaxis, dypsnea, exfoliative dermatits, and proteinurea. There are currently more than 300 ongoing clinical trials involving bevacizumab in at least 20 different tumor types.

An emerging concept in antiangiogenic therapy is that antiangiogenic agents transiently "normalize" the abnormal structure and function of the tumor vasculature (for a more comprehensive review, see (3)). The vasculature of tumors is structurally and functionally abnormal, with leaky, tortuous, dilated, saccular, and haphazardly patterned blood vessels (recently reviewed in (4)). Pericytes are often loosely attached or absent, and the basement membrane is abnormal in appearance: unusually thickened in some instances and entirely absent in others. These abnormalities, in addition to the elevated hydrostatic pressure observed in large tumors, result in functional impairments in tumor blood flow and, as a consequence, impaired drug delivery to solid tumors. Hypoxia also plays a role in tumor drug resistance; for example, hypoxic tumor cells are more resistant to both radiation and cytotoxic drugs and have a higher metastatic potential. Hypoxia and low pH also impair the function of cytotoxic immune cells. Observations from both animal models as well as clinical studies now support the concept that downregulation of aberrant VEGF signaling (either by inhibiting the RTKs or by sequestering VEGF) selectively prunes the immature and leaky blood vessels, "normalizing" both their structure (less leaky, less dilated, and less tortuous) and function (decreased interstitial fluid pressure, increased tumor oxygenation, and improved drug delivery to the tumor cells). It has also become apparent that the "pruning" effects of anti-VEGF therapies are not restricted to the abnormal vasculature of tumors. In mice, for example, in 11 of the 17 healthy organs examined, sustained inhibition of VEGF signaling significantly (but reversibly) reduced the number of normal capillaries (5–7).

The observed preclinical effects of antiangiogenic agents are now being recapitulated in the clinic. A recent clinical study evaluated relative vessel size and permeability, tumor contrast enhancement and edema-associated parameters using a series of MRI protocols in a Phase II clinical trial of the angiokinase inhibitor cediranib in glioblastoma patients who had failed conventional therapy. These data demonstrated that cediranib induced vascular normalization in recurrent glioblastomas within 24 hours, and this effect lasted at least 28 days. A direct consequence of vascular normalization was alleviation of vasogenic edema. A striking observation was that tumor vessels returned to the abnormal state following drug "holidays" and "renormalized" after resumption of drug therapy (8). Thus antiangiogenic agents may create a favorable window of opportunity for chemotherapy and/or radiotherapy to work more effectively.

In contrast to cytotoxic tumor therapy, inhibition of angiogenesis generally does not lead to tumor regression but does promote long-term stable disease. Thus in many tumor types (with the possible exception of renal cell carcinoma), monotherapy results in only modest effects on patient survival. However, when used in combination with other therapeutic modalities, antiangiogenic drugs are beginning to show appreciable impacts on patient survival. Current challenges for these combination treatments are how to dose and schedule the antiangiogenic and cytotoxic drug combinations, and what the best combinations will be (Chapter 11). When angiogenesis inhibitors were first entering clinical studies, the expectation was that this class of anticancer agents might be essentially nontoxic. In one of his early reviews on the subject, Folkman predicted that "a specific inhibitor of angiogenesis is not likely to cause bone marrow suppression, gastrointestinal symptoms, or hair loss." He did have the wisdom to predict, however, that "this is not to say that such a drug has no other actions and no side effects" (9). Today, a recognizable pattern of side effects has emerged (at least with the VEGF-targeted therapies), the most prominent of which is hypertension. VEGF preferentially dilates small arterioles and venules and also induces the phosphorylation of eNOS, resulting in an increased production of endothelial nitric oxide; thus the common feature of hypertension relates to a direct, pharmacodynamic effect of drugs targeting VEGF or VEGF receptor signaling. In otherwise healthy patients, VEGF inhibition-induced hypertension is manageable with antihypertensive drugs. Rarefaction, which may also contribute to hypertension, also occurs in certain organs such as the thyroid gland and organs with fenestrated endothelium. In the case of the drug axitinib, retrospective analysis showed that the occurrence of diastolic blood pressure of ≥ 90 mm Hg was associated with longer overall survival across multiple tumor types, although statistical significance was only attained in cases of metastatic renal cell carcinoma (10). Many of the angiokinase inhibitors also induce proteinuria, cardiovascular events, and bleeding complications. An increased risk for transient ischemic attacks, stroke, angina pectoris, and myocardial infarctions also may be associated with drugs targeting the VEGF pathway. Fatal pulmonary bleedings have been observed in patients with centrally located squamous cell lung cancer, and it has been hypothesized that tumor cavitation, possibly as a result of antitumor activity, may underlie these events. Treatment with some angiokinase inhibitors has been associated with an increased rate of gastrointestinal perforations and/or the induction of various degrees of abdominal discomfort or pain. Another common side effect is hoarseness: precisely how VEGF antagonism results in this complication is largely unknown, although hypothyroidism has been postulated as one common cause. Increased fatigue is a common complaint in patients treated with angiogenesis inhibitors; again one possible cause of this is hypothyroidism. Hypothyroidism was found to occur in up to 50% of patients treated with sunitinib. Other common side effects include elevations in transaminase, neurological complications such as seizures, dizziness and ataxia, and hand–foot syndrome (recently reviewed in (11)).

Plasma angiogenic proteins have also been investigated in multiple trials. Plasma levels of VEGFA and PlGF are significantly increased in rectal cancer patients receiving bevacizumab, in glioblastoma patients treated with cediranib, in renal cell carcinoma patients treated with GSK-1363089/XL880, and in several trials with vatalanib and sunitinib (for a review, see (12)). Decreases in soluble VEGFR1 (sVEGFR1) have been observed in many of the aforementioned trials. In patients with recurrent glioblastoma, patients on cediranib who progressed on therapy had increased SDF1α and FGF2 (8). Circulating endothelial cells (CECs) (identified phenotypically as CD31[bright] CD34[+] CD45[−] ToPro3[−] mononuclear cells by flow cytometry) are emerging as a possible biomarker for antiangiogenic therapy. For example, in rectal cancer patients treated with bevacizumab, decreases in tumor vascular density were associated with a decrease in the number of viable CECs (13, 14). In glioblastoma patients, viable CEC levels were significantly higher in patients who experienced disease progression during cediranib therapy, compared to those without progression at day 112 (8).

To date at least two indications have shown significant clinical benefit with antiangiogenic monotherapy, namely, renal cell carcinoma (RCC) and hepatocellular carcinoma (HCC). It should be noted, however, that the drugs that have activity in this setting (sunitinib and sorafenib) have multiple targets and may have direct effects on tumor epithelial cells as well as on the tumor vasculature. The efficacy of antiangiogenic agents in other cancer types thus far seems to depend on the mix of RTKs targeted by a specific drug, combination with other cytotoxics, and the appropriate dosing schedule. The success of combination therapy is exemplified by the anti-VEGF antibody bevacizumab, which was approved as first and second line treatment in metastatic colorectal cancer with infusion-based 5-FU combination regimens, and in first line treatment of patients with locally advanced, metastatic or recurrent NSCLC in combination with platinum-based therapy. Nonetheless, randomized Phase III trials of bevacizumab with standard chemotherapy did not improve overall survival as second line treatment in chemorefractory metastatic breast cancer, nor as first line treatment in metastatic cancer.

The resistance of tumor cells that were initially responsive to a drug often arises through mutation or selection of surviving cancer cells. Similarly, resistance to antiangiogenic drugs may occur through either intrinsic or extrinsic mechanisms. Intrinsic resistance may occur as a consequence of tumor cells utilizing existing blood vessels in highly vascularized organs such as the lungs, or colonization of tumors by bone marrow-derived cells (e.g., $CD11b^+$ Gr^+ myeloid suppressor cells). Acquired resistance may arise from the redundant nature of proangiogenic factors. For example, following treatment with anti-VEGFR antibody, there is an upregulation of FGF2. Similarly, RTK inhibitors such as sunitinib can induce high levels of circulating PlGF and VEGF. G-CSF and SDF-1, which may recruit circulating endothelial cell progenitors as well as other proangiogenic accessory cells, are also upregulated (at least in mice) following sunitinib treatment. Some recent studies also suggest that certain angiokinase inhibitors may actually increase tumor invasiveness. In the following section, we review those "angiokinase inhibitors" that have progressed into later stage clinical trials (Phase II and above), to approval, and in some cases, those for which there is compelling Phase I data suggesting clinical benefit. Additional drugs for which early clinical studies have been reported are listed in Table 9.1. Some of the compounds depicted in Table 9.1 also have potent EGFR inhibitory activity and are discussed in more detail in Chapter 8.

9.2 ANGIOKINASE INHIBITORS

Sunitinib   Sunitinib (SU11248, Sutent®) is a pyrrole substituted 2-indolinone derivative (Figure 9.1) and an orally active inhibitor of VEGFR2, PDGFRβ, KIT, and FLT3. Reported in vitro (biochemical) IC_{50} values for VEGFR1, VEGFR2,

TABLE 9.1 Angiokinase Inhibitors in Development

Drug	Company	Targets	Structure[a]	Latest stage of development
Sunitinib (SU11248; Sutent®)	Pfizer	FLT3, KIT, PDGFR	Figure 9.1	Marketed
Sorafenib (BAY43-9006; Nexavar®)	Bayer	RAF, VEGFR2,3, FLT3, KIT, RET, PDGFR	Figure 9.1	Marketed
Vandetanib (ZD6474; Zactima®)	Astra Zeneca	EGFR, RET, VEGFR2	Figure 9.1	Phase III
Pazopanib (GW786034B)	GSK	VEGFR1,2,3, PDGFR, FGFR, CSF1R	Figure 9.1	Phase III
Motesanib diphosphate (AMG706)	Amgen/Takeda	KIT, PDGFR, VEGFR1,2,3, RET	Figure 9.1	Phase III[b]
Cediranib (AZD2171; Recentin®)	AstraZeneca	VEGFR1,2,3, KIT, PDGFR, FGFR, SRC, CSF1R	Figure 9.1	Phase III
Axitinib (AG-013736)	Pfizer	VEGFR1,2,3, KIT, PDGFRβ, CSF1R, ABL	Figure 9.1	Phase III
Brivanib alaninate (BMS-540215)	BMS	VEGFR2, FGFR1,2,3	Figure 9.1	Phase III
Vatalanib (PTK-ZK; PTK787)	Novartis	VEGFR1,2	Figure 9.1	Phase III
BMS-907351/XL184	Bristol Myers-Squibb/Exelixis	MET, RET, VEGFR, FLT3, KIT, TIE2	ND	Phase III
XL820	Exelixis	KIT, PDGFR, VEGFR2	ND	Phase II
XL647[c]	Exelixis	VEGFR1,2, EGFR	ND	Phase II
Masitinib (AB-1010)	AB Science	KIT, PDGFR	Figure 9.1	Phase II
TSU-68 (SU6668)	Pfizer	VEGFR2, PDGFRβ, Aurora-A,B, TBK1, KIT	Figure 9.2	Phase II
Telatinib (BAY57-9352)	Bayer	PDGFR, VEGFR2,3	Figure 9.2	Phase II
BIBF-1120 (Vargatef®)	Boehringer Ingelheim	VEGFR1,2,3, FGFR1,2,3, PDGFRα,β,SRC	Figure 9.2	Phase II
SU14813	Pfizer	VEGFR1,2, PDGFRβ, KIT, FLT3, CSF1R	Figure 9.2	Phase II
ABT-869	Abbot	VEGFR1,2,3, FLT3, PDGFRβ, CSF1R, KIT, TIE2	Figure 9.2	Phase II
AV-951	Aveo/Kirin	VEGFR1,2,3, PDGFR, KIT	Figure 9.2	Phase II
GW1363089 (XL880)	GSK/Exelixis	VEGFR1,2, MET	ND	Phase II

(continued)

TABLE 9.1 *(Continued)*

Drug	Company	Targets	Structure[a]	Latest stage of development
CP-547632 (OSI-632)	OSI/Pfizer	VEGFR2, FGFR	Figure 9.2	Phase II
AEE788[c]	Novartis	EGFR, HER2, VEGFR2	Figure 8.3	Phase I/II
CHIR-265/RAF-265[d]	Chiron	BRAF, CRAF,VEGFR2,3, FLT3, KIT, PDGFR	Figure 10.3	Phase I
BMS-690514[c]	BMS	EGFR, HER2, VEGFR2	Figure 8.3	Phase I
ZK-304709	Bayer-Schering	CDK1,2, and 4, VEGFR2	ND	Phase I
KRN-633	Kirin	FLT3, KIT, PDGFR, VEGFR1,2,3	Figure 9.3	Phase I
JNJ-26483327	Johnson and Johnson	EGFR, ERBB2, ERBB3, ERBB4, SRC, VEGFR3	Figure 9.3	Phase I
E-7080	Esai	KIT, VEGFR2	Figure 9.3	Phase I
Dovitinib (CHIR258/TKI258)	Chiron	FGFR, FLT3, KIT, PDGFR, VEGFR	Figure 9.3	Phase I
CEP-7055	Cephalon	VEGFR	Figure 9.3	Phase I
R-1530	Roche	VEGFR, FGFR, PDGFR	Figure 9.3	Phase I
CEP-11981	Cephalon	TEK, VEGFR	ND	Phase I
BAY73–4506	Bayer	RAF, VEGFR	ND	Phase I
CP-868596	Pfizer	PDGFR	Figure 9.3	Phase I
OSI-930	OSI	VEGFR, KIT	Figure 9.3	Phase I

[a]ND, not disclosed

[b]Phase III trial halted due to toxicity

[c]Discussed in EGFR targeted drugs

[d]Discussed in RAF targeted drugs.

532

VEGFR3, PDGFRα, PDGFRβ, CSF1R, FLT3, KIT, and RET are 15, 38, 30, 69, 55, 35, 21, >10, and 224 nM, respectively. The compound is a relatively weak inhibitor of FGFR1 (675 nM), SRC (1 μM), ABL (610 nM), and CDK1 (2.6 μM) (15). In cell-based assays, the compound inhibits VEGFR2 and PDGFRβ with IC_{50} values around 10 nM, and inhibits KIT receptor phosphorylation and cellular proliferation with IC_{50} values of 10–100 and 7 nM, respectively (16). In cultured TT cells (a medullary thyroid carcinoma cell line with an activating C634W RET mutation), sunitinib inhibited RET autophosphorylation with an IC_{50} of 100 nM (17). In vivo, when administered orally at 40 mg/kg, sunitinib inhibits VEGFR2 and PDGFRβ phosphorylation in xenografts for up to 12 hours, after which the inhibitory activity is not maintained. However, despite the lack of continuous inhibition of receptor phosphorylation, daily dosing effectively decreased mean tumor vascular density and inhibited tumor growth. In vivo, plasma levels of 125–250 nM sunitinib were required to inhibit the phosphorylation of VEGFR2 and PDGFRβ. Based on the initial animal efficacy studies, it was suggested that targeted therapeutic plasma levels of sunitinib should be above 125 nM (50 ng/mL) for 12 hours on a once-daily oral regimen in human clinical trials (15).

In humans, sunitinib is metabolized to an active N-desethyl metabolite, SU-012662, which demonstrates comparable biologic activity and potency (18). This metabolite is the result of Cyp3A4 metabolism in the liver, and clinical studies to evaluate this concluded that potent Cyp3A4 inducers (e.g., rifampin) or inhibitors (e.g., ketoconazole) should be avoided in patients receiving sunitinib.

A number of Phase I trials were performed, demonstrating that the absorption of the compound was slow ($T_{max} = 8$ h) and there was no effect of food on absorption. The half-life of the metabolite SU-012662 was 60–105 hours. Various dosing schedules were examined including a 2 week on/1 week off cycle, a 2 week on/2 week off cycle, and a 4 week on/2 week off cycle, as well as both daily dosing and every-other-day dosing. Dose-limiting toxicities of fatigue, asthenia, and thrombocytopenia were observed at 75 mg, regardless of dosing schedule, and the recommended Phase II dose of 50 mg was selected. The onset of fatigue generally occurred after 2 weeks of treatment and resolved during a 2 week rest period, supporting the utility of a discontinuous dosing schedule. Exposure to sunitinib correlated with an increase in diastolic blood pressure, an observation consistent with the effects of other agents (e.g., bevacizumab) that inhibit the VEGF pathway. Variations in PK parameters were observed with female sex, age, weight, race, Eastern Cooperative Oncology Group (ECOG) score, tumor type, and formulation. Of these, the most marked effects were observed in Asians, who demonstrate a 26% higher SU-012662 clearance relative to Caucasian patients. However, these differences were not considered large enough to require dose adjustment (19).

To assess biologic activity of sunitinib in the Phase I studies, a number of clinical observations and correlative assessments were performed. Hair depigmentation, a characteristic sign of inhibiting KIT, was frequently observed in sunitinib-treated patients and correlates with the cycles of drug treatment (20). Symptoms of VEGFR inhibition included mild hypertension and the development of painless distal subungual splinter hemorrhages after 2–4 weeks on therapy (21).

(Similar nonthrombotic/embolic splinter hemorrhages were also reported with sorafenib, another angiokinase inhibitor described later (21)). In a Phase I/II trial of GIST patients, monocytes, circulating endothelial cells, VEGF, and sVEGFR2 were modulated by sunitinib treatment. VEGF increased and sVEGFR2 decreased during treatment and rebounded toward baseline off treatment (22). The pattern and magnitude of changes in these two markers were similar between patients with clinical benefit and progressive disease, suggesting that VEGF and sVEGFR2 may be useful pharmacodynamic markers but may not predict clinical benefit in this indication. Patients with clinical benefit had significantly greater increases in circulating endothelial cells and small decreases in monocyte levels during cycle 1 of treatment, suggesting that these might be useful markers of sunitinib efficacy (22). In a Phase II study of RCC patients, plasma levels of VEGF, sVEGFR2, PlGF, and sVEGFR3 were monitored. Sunitinib treatment was associated with increases in VEGF and PlGF and decreases in sVEGFR2 and sVEGFR3 (23).

In a Phase I trial with sunitinib given orally daily for a 4 week on, 2 week off schedule in patients with advanced solid malignancies, early signs of efficacy were noted, with six objective responses (four partial responses and two stable diseases with intratumoral necrosis) in three cases of RCC, one neuroendocrine tumor, one stromal tumor, and one primary adenocarcinoma patient at doses of ≥ 50 mg/day. At higher doses (75 mg/day), tumor responses were often associated with reduced intratumoral vascularization and central tumor necrosis. Based on this and other evidence of antitumor activity, Phase II trials were initiated in patients with RCC, neuroendocrine tumors, and imatinib-resistant GIST. In two single-arm Phase II trials, sunitinib at 50 mg/d on a 4 week on, 2 week off schedule demonstrated a high response rate and prolonged time to tumor progression in patients with cytokine-refractory RCC. Sunitinib induced a response rate of 39–40% in both trials, with a median time to progression of 8.7 months and median survival of 16.4 months. There were also many patients in the trials (23–27%) who experienced stable disease for more than 3 months (24–26). Sunitinib was compared with IFNα in a Phase III trial: 750 patients with previously untreated, metastatic renal cell cacinoma were enrolled in a multicenter randomized Phase III trial to receive either repeated 6-week cycles of sunitinib (50 mg qd, 4 weeks on, 2 weeks off) or IFNα (9 MU subcutaneously 3 × week). The mean progression-free survival was significantly longer in the sunitinib group (11 months) compared with IFNα group (5 months); sunitinib was also associated with a higher objective response rate than was interferon α (31% vs. 6%, $p < 0.001$). The patients in the sunitinib group also reported a significantly better quality of life than did patients in the IFNα group (27). Sunitinib was given FDA approval for advanced RCC in January 2006.

Promising antitumor activity of sunitinib in other advanced malignances has also been noted in Phase I and II trials, including breast cancer, neuroendocrine tumors, colorectal cancer, sarcoma, thyroid cancer, melanoma, and NSCLC. Additional Phase II studies in RCC and GIST are ongoing to determine if continuous dosing (at doses less than 50 mg/d) of sunitinib is tolerated and produces a comparable clinical benefit. There are many actively recruiting clinical trials with sunitinib, including Phase III trials in breast, pancreatic, and colorectal cancers, as well as combination studies with other approved drugs such as paclitaxel, docitaxel, capecitabine, erlotinib, and FOLFIRI (www.clinicaltrials.gov).

Sorafenib   Sorafenib (BAY43–9006, Nexavar®) is a multikinase inhibitor of the biaryl urea class developed by Bayer and Onyx (Figure 9.1). In biochemical assays, sorafenib has been reported to inhibit CRAF, BRAF, BRAF V600E, VEGFR1, VEGFR2, VEGFR3 (mouse), PDGFRβ (mouse), FLT3, KIT, and p38 with IC_{50} values of 6, 22, 38, 26, 90, 20, 57, 33, 68, and 38 nM, respectively (28, 29). The compound also moderately inhibits FGFR1 (IC_{50} 580 nM), but has little to no inhibitory activity on ERK1, MEK1, EGFR, HER2, IGFR1, MET, PKB, PKA, CDK1/cyclin B, PKCα, PKCγ, or PIM1 (28). In cell-based assays the compound inhibited the MAPK pathway in colon, pancreatic, and breast tumor cell lines expressing mutant KRAS or wild-type or mutant BRAF. In contrast, NSCLC lines expressing mutant KRAS were insensitive to the compound. Sorafenib demonstrated antitumor activity in colon, breast, and non small cell lung xenograft models (28). In several xenograft models (e.g., A549, NCI-H460, Colo205), sorafenib inhibited growth but was not associated with a detectable reduction in phosphorylation of ERK, suggesting that the compound can inhibit growth of some tumor types by mechanisms independent of MAPK pathway inhibition, possibly through antivascular effects (28, 30). Other studies clearly demonstrated antiangiogenic activity of sorafenib (31–33), with reductions in microvessel area and microvessel density as well as disruption of the tumor vasculature.

Sorafenib inhibited imatinib-resistant KIT and PDGFRβ with mutations in the gatekeeper residue (KIT T670I; PDGFRβ T681I) but was less active on kinases with mutations in the activation loop (KIT D816V; PDGFRβ D850V)(34). Sorafenib also inhibits RET kinase function and oncogenic activity (35). The compound arrested the growth of NIH3T3 cells and RAT1 fibroblasts transformed by oncogenic RET, and also inhibited the growth of thyroid carcinoma cells that harbor spontaneously oncogenic RET alleles. In tumor xenograft studies with TT cells, sorafenib dosed at 60 mg/kg/day demonstrated significant tumor regression (35). Sorafenib also inhibits RET gatekeeper mutants (V904M/L) (36), and the evaluation of sorafenib in thyroid carcinoma is discussed further in Chapter 8. Sorafenib has been shown to downregulate the antiapoptotic protein MCL1 (myeloid cell leukemia sequence 1) and it is thought that this mechanism is responsible for the ability of the compound to induce apoptosis in various tumor cell lines (37, 38).

In Phase I studies to explore various dosing regimens, sorafenib was generally well tolerated and the recommended dose selected for future trials was 400 mg bid continuously (39–43). Higher doses were associated with dose-limiting toxicities including diarrhea, fatigue, and skin rash. In Phase I trials, 11 patients with metastatic RCC were evaluated for tumor response by the RECIST criteria. In one patient, early signs of antitumor activity were detected; the patient had a confirmed partial response that was sustained for 104 days with 600 mg bid sorafenib. Two additional RCC patients experienced stable disease of equal to or greater than 2-years duration. Combination trials with standard chemotherapies including oxaliplatin, 5-FU and leucovorin, paclitaxel/carboplatin, gemcitabine, doxorubicin,

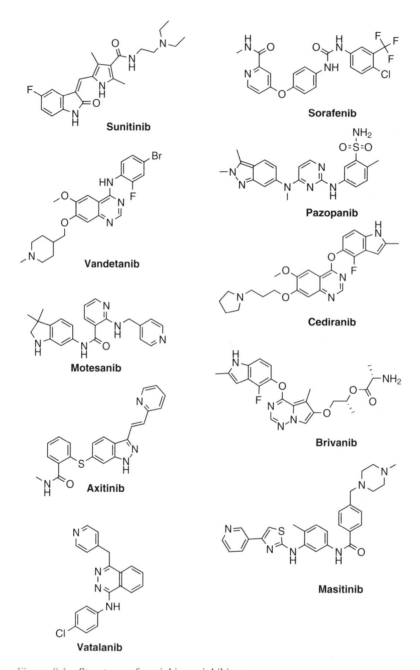

Figure 9.1 Structures of angiokinase inhibitors.

taxotere, CPT-11, and dacarbazine were also performed and the addition of sorafenib did not result in significant increases in toxicity over the chemotherapeutic agent alone (44–52).

Based on promising preliminary activity in RCC patients across the various Phase I trials, sorafenib monotherapy was evaluated in RCC by enriching for RCC patients in a randomized discontinuation Phase II trial. Out of 502 patients with multiple tumor types, a total of 202 RCC patients were evaluated. Sorafenib treatment significantly prolonged the median progression-free survival fourfold over placebo treatment (24 weeks vs. 6 weeks, $p = 0.0087$)(53).

A Phase III Treatment Approaches in Renal Cancer Global Evaluation Trial (TARGET) involved 903 patients with advanced RCC. In this randomized, controlled trial, sorafenib was associated with a twofold increase in median progression-free survival compared to placebo treatment (24 vs. 12 weeks, $p < 0.000001$) that was independent of gender, age, prior therapy, and a number of other variables. Patients receiving sorafenib had a 39% improvement in overall survival, although this did not reach the prespecified threshold for statistical significance. There was a low rate of partial response, although many of the treated patients did experience some degree of tumor shrinkage. The most common adverse events were dermatological (rash and hand–foot skin reaction), gastrointestinal (diarrhea), and fatigue. Mild hypertension was more prevalent in the sorafenib-treated patients. The results from the Phase II and III trial established oral sorafenib (400 mg bid) as a safe and effective treatment for metastatic RCC and formed the basis for FDA approval in December 2005 for the treatment of advanced RCC.

In one of the Phase I trials for sorafenib, a confirmed partial response was observed in a metastatic HCC patient (39). This response, and literature support for a role of VEGF and RAF/MEK/ERK signaling in HCC, prompted a Phase II study to further evaluate the efficacy, toxicity, and pharmacokinetics of sorafenib in advanced HCC. In a multicenter, international, uncontrolled Phase II trial in advanced HCC patients, single-agent sorafenib demonstrated modest efficacy. Of 137 patients treated, 3 patients achieved a partial response, 8 a minor response, and 46 had stable disease for at least 16 weeks (54). This promising data led to an international, Phase III, placebo-controlled Sorafenib HCC Assessment Randomized Protocol (SHARP) trial, which demonstrated that sorafenib significantly extended overall survival (OS) in patients with HCC versus placebo by 44% (HR = 0.69; p-value = 0.0006). This large randomized trial evaluated 602 liver cancer patients who had had no prior systemic therapy. Median OS was 10.7 months in the sorafenib-treated patients compared to 7.9 months in the placebo group (55). On November 16, 2007, the FDA approved sorafenib for the treatment of patients with unresectable HCC.

Evaluation of sorafenib in other indications thus far has been less successful. A Phase II trial of sorafenib as monotherapy in metastatic melanoma indicated the compound was minimally active, with few short-term responses in both mutant and wild-type BRAF metastatic melanoma (56). A clinical trial evaluating the benefit of combining sorafenib with carboplatin/paclitaxel chemotherapy for lung cancer was stopped early based on results from an interim analysis. In a subset of patients with squamous cell histology, the addition of sorafenib appeared to have a detrimental effect: patients with squamous cell taking all three drugs had a median overall survival of 8.9 months, compared with 13.6 months for patients taking just the two chemotherapy drugs. In the remainder of the patients with non squamous cell carcinoma, the median overall survival was 11.5 months in patients treated with the three drugs and 10.3 months in those treated with the two drugs. There was no increase in adverse bleeding events, in contrast to a previous study in which bevacizumab was added to chemotherapy in the same patient population (57).

There are many actively recruiting clinical trials with sorafenib. These include additional Phase I combination therapy trials, as well as Phase II and III trials of sorafenib as monotherapy or in combination with various chemotherapeutic regimens in many different cancers including melanoma, hepatocellular, pancreatic, biliary, renal, breast, glioblastoma, prostate, lymphoma, multiple myeloma, AML, myelodysplastic syndromes, NSCLC, SCLC, anaplastic thyroid, medullary thyroid, GIST, CLL, uveal melanoma, colorectal, head and neck, and neuroendocrine.

Vandetanib Vandetanib (ZD6474, Zactima®; Figure 9.1) is an orally administered heteroaromatic-substituted anilinoquinazoline in development by AstraZeneca. It was originally identified in a screen for VEGFR inhibitors. Vandetanib is an ATP-competitive inhibitor of VEGFR and inhibits the following kinases with submicromolar IC_{50} values (reported IC_{50} in parentheses): VEGFR2 (40 nM), RET (100 nM), VEGFR3 (110 nM), and EGFR (500 nM). It also has weak activity on VEGFR1 (1.6 μM), PDGFRβ (1.1 μM), FGFR1 (3.6 μM), and TIE2 (2.5 μM); IC_{50} values for MEK, CDK2, KIT, ERBB2, FAK, PDK1, AKT, and IGFR1 are all greater than 10 μM (58, 59). Vandetanib inhibits VEGF-stimulated human umbilical vein endothelial cell (HUVEc) proliferation with an IC_{50} of 60 nM and inhibits A549 and Calu-6 proliferation with IC_{50} values of 2.7 and 13.5 μM, respectively (58). Chronic once-daily oral administration of vandetanib produced a dose-dependent inhibition of tumor xenografts associated with inhibition of tumor angiogenesis (as assessed by CD31 staining); when administered to mice with established PC-3 tumors, vandetanib induced tumor regression, with the most dramatic effects produced in the largest tumors (58). In preclinical models, gemcitabine plus vandetanib interacted synergistically to inhibit pancreatic tumor cell proliferation (60, 61). Combination studies with radiation therapy also indicated additive to synergistic interactions with vandetanib (61–66).

As discussed in Chapter 8, vandetanib is a fairly potent inhibitor of RET, an RTK that was originally identified in 1985 as an oncogene activated by DNA rearrangement (67). Recently, somatic rearrangements in RET were identified in a cell line (EHMES-10) derived from a malignant pleural mesothelioma. EHMES-10 cells also overexpress VEGF. Vandetanib induced apoptosis of these cells in vitro and inhibited tumor growth in EHMES-10 xenografts (at least partly through suppression of angiogenesis)(68).

In two Phase I clinical trials, vandetanib was evaluated in patients with advanced solid tumors refractory to standard therapy (69, 70). One study recruited a Western population of 88 patients with a variety of solid tumors, although most were colorectal. A second study recruited 18 patients in Japan, most of whom had either non small cell lung cancer or colorectal cancer. At doses less than 300 mg/day the compound was well tolerated with generally mild and tolerable adverse events. Dose-limiting toxicity was observed at the 500 mg/d dose in the Western patients and 400 mg/d in the Japanese trial. The most common adverse events were rash and diarrhea, which were dose dependent, as well as proteinuria, hypertension, and asymptomatic QTc prolongation. In the first trial of Western patients, no objective responses were noted, although more than 40% of the patients had stable disease of at least 8 weeks duration. In the Japanese population, four of the patients with NSCLC dosed at 200–300 mg/day exhibited an objective response by RECIST criteria. The compound had a long terminal half-life (median values of 96 h in the Japan study and 130 h in the Western study), and biologically relevant plasma concentrations were achieved after a single dose ranging from 50 to 300 mg/day. Although vandetanib has a lower biochemical and cell-based potency than some of the other angiokinase inhibitors (Table 9.1), the promising PK properties of this compound encouraged further development.

A number of Phase II clinical trials were initiated to evaluate vandetanib at 100–300 mg/day dosing. Single-agent vandetanib was evaluated in a randomized Phase II trial involving 168 patients with locally advanced or metastatic NSCLC refractory to first or second line platinum-based therapies. In this trial, patients received either vandetanib (300 mg/d) or gefitinib (250 mg/d). Patients were dosed until evidence of disease progression or limiting toxicity was noted. Progression-free survival (PFS) was the primary endpoint. A statistically significantly improvement in PFS was observed in the vandetanib versus gefinitib arms (11 vs. 8.1 weeks, $p = 0.025$). Those patients progressing on either treatment had the option to cross over to the other treatment arm. Again, more of the patients switching from gefitinib to vandetanib (43% vs. 24%) experienced stable disease of 8 weeks or more. There was not a statistically significant difference in overall survival in the vandetanib arm (6.1 months) versus the gefitinib arm (7.4 months)(71).

The combination of vandetanib plus docetaxel was evaluated in a randomized, placebo-controlled Phase II study in NSCLC. The run in phase investigated the safety of vandetanib with docetaxel, with vandetanib 100 mg/d plus docetaxel 75 mg/m^2 every 3 weeks. In the absence of dose-limiting toxicity at week 4, the subsequent cohort received vandetanib 300 mg/day plus docetaxel. In the second stage of the trial, patients were randomized to one of three treatment groups: placebo/docetaxel, low-dose (100 mg/d) vandetanib plus docetaxel, and high-dose vandetanib (300 mg/d) plus docetaxel. Adverse events were not significantly increased with the addition of vandetanib. Overall mean time to disease progression was 18.7 and 17.0 weeks in the vandetanib 100-mg and 300-mg cohorts, versus 12 weeks in the placebo/docetaxel arm (72, 73); there were no statistically significant differences in mean overall survival between the three groups.

Vandetanib was also evaluated in a randomized, double-blind Phase II study, alone and in combination with carboplatin/paclitaxel (CP) as first line treatment for patients with locally advanced or metastatic (IIIB-IV) NSCLC. In this Phase II trial, 181 patients with advanced NSCLC were randomized to first line treatment with vandetanib, CP, or vandetanib + CP. Progression-free survival (PFS) was prolonged for vandetanib + CP versus CP. The objective response rates were 32%, 25%, and 7% for vandetanib + CP, vandetanib, and CP groups, respectively. Overall survival was not significantly different between groups. Exploratory subgroup analyses of vandetanib + CP versus CP suggested advantages for the 56 female patients. Biomarker analyses indicated that significant increases in plasma VEGF and decreases in sVEGFR2 occurred with treatment in the vandetanib arm, while IL12, IL1RA, MMP9, and MCP1 changed in the CP and vandetanib + CP arms (74, 75).

Based on the promising results seen in Phase II trials of vandetanib in NSCLC, Phase III trials were initiated. ZODIAC is a randomized, double-blind, international, multicenter Phase III study to assess the efficacy of vandetanib 100 mg once daily plus the standard docetaxel chemotherapy versus docetaxel alone in patients with locally advanced or metastatic NSCLC after failure of first line anticancer therapy. This study, enrolling a total of 1301 patients, showed a benefit in progression-free survival (PFS, the primary endpoint) and overall response rate with the vandetanib + docetaxel combination, but it showed no statistical increase in overall survival compared to docetaxel alone. The ZEAL trial is a Phase III parallel group, randomized, double-blind study evaluating vandetanib 100 mg once daily plus pemetrexed 500 mg/m^2 (every 3 weeks) compared with placebo plus pemetrexed as second line treatment in patients with locally advanced or metastatic NSCLC who have failed first line anticancer therapy. This study enrolled 534 patients, with the primary endpoint of PFS. Secondary endpoints were ORR and OS. In this trial, the vandetanib combination did not meet the primary endpoint, although there was benefit in ORR. The ZEST trial compared vandetanib (300 mg) to erlotinib (Tarceva$^®$) in a head-to-head study. A total of 1240 patients were enrolled, with PFS as the secondary endpoint. The study did not meet the primary objective of demonstrating a statistically significant benefit of vantetanib compared to erlotinib. In a preplanned non-inferiority analysis, however, vandetanib and erlotinib showed equivalent efficacy.

The use of vandetanib has also been explored in several other indications. In a Phase II study of vandetanib (300 mg/d) versus placebo in small cell lung cancer patients after complete or partial response to induction chemotherapy with or without radiation therapy, vandetanib failed to demonstrate efficacy as maintenance therapy (76). A multicenter Phase II trial of vandetanib monotherapy in 46 patients with previously treated metastatic breast cancer indicated that the compound was generally well tolerated but had limited activity in this patient population. There were no objective responses although one patient in the 300-mg cohort had stable disease ≥24 weeks (77). A Phase II trial of vandetanib dosed at 100 mg/day in patients with relapsed multiple myeloma also indicated that the therapy was well tolerated; however, there were no objective responses (as assessed by reduction in M protein) in this patient population (78).

Phase II data on vandetanib in patients with locally advanced or metastatic hereditary thyroid cancer (MTC) were recently disclosed. MTC is caused by activating germline mutations in the RET proto-oncogene, which is one of the molecular targets of vandetanib. The authors concluded that vandetanib at 100 mg has clinical activity in patients with metastatic hereditary MTC; confirmed partial responses were observed in 16% of patients, and stable disease of at least 24 weeks duration was observed in a further 52%. This study also monitored the biochemical response to therapy using the markers calcitonin (CTN) and carcinoembryonic antigen (CEA). Serum levels of CTN and CEA showed a sustained $\geq 50\%$ decrease from baseline in 16% and 5% of patients, respectively (79). An international, randomized placebo-controlled Phase III trial (ZETA) of 300-mg vandetanib in patients with locally advanced or metastatic MTC (hereditary or sporadic) is ongoing but not recruiting participants.

Phase I and II trials with vandetinib as monotherapy and also with various chemotherapy regimens are ongoing in gliomas, neuroblastoma, brain tumors, hereditary medullary thyroid carcinoma, ovarian, fallopian tube, and primary peritoneal cavity cancers, renal cancers, mesothelioma, breast cancer, prostate cancer, colorectal cancer, and esophageal cancer.

Pazopanib Pazopanib (GW786034B; Figure 9.1) is an orally available 2H-indazolylpyrimidine under development by GSK that inhibits VEGFR1, VEGFR2, and VEGFR3 with IC_{50} values of 10, 30, and 47 nM, respectively. The reported K_I for human VEGFR2 is 24 nM in biochemical assays. The compound also inhibits the activity of VEGFR2 from other species (dog, mouse, rat) with similar potencies to the human enzyme. Additionally, pazopanib has significant activity toward PDGFRα, PDGFRβ, and KIT, with IC_{50} values of 71, 84, and 74 nM, respectively, and modest activity on FGFR1 (140 nM), FGFR3 (130 nM), CSF1R (146 nM), LCK (411 nM), and ITK (430 nM). Five other kinases had IC_{50} values within tenfold of the VEGFR2 activity, namely, Aurora-A, CRAF, MLK1, PTK5, and TAO3. For 23 other serine/threonine and tyrosine kinases evaluated, pazopanib had IC_{50} values greater than 800 nM (80). In cell-based assays, pazopanib inhibited VEGF-induced VEGFR2 phosphorylation with an IC_{50} of 8 nM, as well as potently inhibiting KIT and PDGFRβ in other cell-based assays. Pazopanib inhibits VEGF-induced endothelial proliferation with an IC_{50} of 21.3 nM, much less than the IC_{50} observed for FGF-induced proliferation (720 nM). The compound had no antiproliferative activity on a wide variety of tumor cells ($IC_{50} > 10$ μM), but significant inhibition of VEGF-induced angiogenesis was observed in in vivo angiogenesis (mouse corneal pocket and matrigel plug) assays with 100 mg/kg pazopanib twice a day. Oral dosing of pazopanib showed a dose-dependent growth inhibition of a number of different tumor xenografts (Caki-2, BT474, NCI-HC322, HT29, A375P, and PC3), although melanoma (A375P), prostate carcinoma (PC-3), and breast carcinoma (BT474) showed a more modest inhibition compared to the other xenograft models. Detailed PK/PD studies indicated that steady state plasma concentrations of around 40 μM were required for the maximal PD effect (inhibition of VEGF-induced VEGFR2 phosphorylation in mouse lungs) (80).

These preclinical findings were used to select doses for a Phase I dose escalation study. The target steady state concentration of ≥ 40 μM was achieved in the majority of patients receiving ≥ 800 mg qd or 300 mg bid. A total of 56 patients with relapsed or refractory solid tumors were enrolled. The mean $t_{1/2}$ of the compound was approximately 35 h. Over a 22-day dosing period, there was a 1.5-to 3-fold accumulation of the drug at steady state. Pazopanib was relatively well tolerated, with the most common adverse events being nausea, hypertension, diarrhea, fatigue, anorexia, vomiting, and hair depigmentation. The largest change in blood pressure was observed at 800 mg and correlated with a plasma concentration at 24 h of greater than 20 μg/mL. Preliminary evidence of clinical benefit was also observed in all five RCC patients enrolled (one confirmed partial response and four stable disease/minor responses). Durable stable disease was also noted in several other solid tumors, with stable disease in one patient with Hurthle cell tumor, one GIST patient, and one chondrosarcoma patient for 92, 32, and >56 weeks, respectively. Based on pharmacokinetics, exposure, and trough concentrations, the recommended Phase II dosage was 800 mg/day, administered orally.

Pazopanib was shown to inhibit VEGF-stimulated signaling pathways in multiple myeloma (MM) cells as well as endothelial cells, and the combination of these two activities as thought to be responsible for the ability of this compound to promote MM cell apoptosis in vivo (81). Based on these observations, a multicenter Phase I/II trial with pazopanib alone in patients with relapsed or refractory MM was initiated.

A Phase II randomized discontinuation trial evaluated 800 mg qd pazopanib in patients with advanced or metastatic RCC, and efficacy data were reported on 255 patients. The response rate (CR + PR) was 34.5%. In the 55 patients with stable disease who were randomly assigned to pazopanib versus placebo, progression-free survival was 11.9 months in the pazopanib group versus 6.2 months in the placebo group (82). An ongoing Phase III trial, VEG105192 (a randomized, placebo controlled, multicenter international Phase III study), is evaluating pazopanib in patients with locally advanced and/or metastatic RCC who have either not been treated previously, failed prior therapy, or showed intolerance to cytokines. The primary endpoint is progression-free survival. This trial has apparently reached the efficacy cutoff, and analysis is ongoing. Another Phase III study is being conducted to compare the efficacy and safety of pazopanib in combination with lapatinib with that of lapatinib alone in subjects with inflammatory breast cancer whose tumors overexpress the ERBB2 protein. There are a number of actively recruiting clinical trials with pazopanib in a variety of cancers, both alone and in combination with lapatinib, and/or other chemotherapies.

Motesanib Diphosphate   Motesanib diphosphate, also known as AMG706, is a small molecule, orally active 2-amino nicotinamide derivative in development by Amgen (Figure 9.1). In February 2008, Amgen announced the establishment of a partnership with Takeda supporting the worldwide development and commercialization of motesanib diphosphate. The compound is a potent inhibitor of VEGFR1 ($IC_{50} = 2$ nM), VEGFR2 (3 nM), VEGFR3 (6 nM), and KIT (8 nM) and also inhibits PDGFR (84 nM) and RET (59 nM). The compound does not significantly inhibit 47 other kinases tested, including EGFR, SRC, and p38. In cell-based assays, motesanib diphosphate inhibited VEGF-induced HUVEc proliferation with an IC_{50} of 10 nM; in contrast, FGF2-induced HUVEc proliferation was not potently inhibited ($IC_{50} > 3$ μM). PDGF-induced proliferation and

SCF-induced KIT phosphorylation were also inhibited in cell-based assays, with IC_{50} values of 207 nM and 37 nM, respectively. In vivo, motesanib diphosphate inhibited VEGF-induced vascular permeability, VEGF-induced angiogenesis in the rat corneal pocket assay, and growth of A431 tumor xenografts. The mechanism of tumor xenograft inhibition was attributed to the antivascular activity of motesanib diphosphate since the compound did not inhibit A431 cell proliferation, and in vivo, tumor regression correlated with rapid loss of tumor vasculature. After 7 days of treatment with 75 mg bid of motesanib diphosphate, tumor vascular density (assessed by the endothelial marker, CD31) was dramatically reduced, with only a small rim of blood vessels visible on the periphery of the tumors. Extensive tumor cell necrosis was also observed. Additionally, at early time points (e.g., 48 h after compound administration), a significant increase in endothelial cell apoptosis was observed. These observations suggest that the primary mechanism of motesanib diphosphate is targeting of the tumor vasculature (83).

A Phase I dose finding study evaluated the safety, pharmacokinetics, and pharmacodynamics of motesanib diphosphate in 71 patients with refractory advanced solid tumors. The compound was administered at escalating doses of 50 to 175 mg qd or 25 mg bid for the first 21 days of a 28-day cycle. The 125-mg dose was also administered continuously, and the MTD was established as 125 mg qd continuously. Adverse events included fatigue, diarrhea, nausea, and hypertension. Plasma concentrations were dose proportional, without accumulation following multiple doses. In this Phase I trial, 5 patients had a partial response, and 35 had stable disease of at least 50 days duration. Measurement of serum biomarkers indicated that changes in tumor size correlated with increases in PlGF (placental growth factor) and decreases in sVEGFR2 (84).

Motesanib diphosphate was evaluated in a multicenter, open-label, single-arm study in patients with differentiated thyroid cancer (DTC) and MTC. Patients received 125 mg motesanib daily until disease progression or unacceptable toxicity. Initial results focused on the 93 patients with advanced, ^{131}I resistant DTC who had been enrolled in the trial. After a median follow-up of 52 days, motesanib diphosphate showed some clinical activity: a low rate of objective response (12%) and 24% of patients with durable (≥ 24 weeks) stable disease (85).

A Phase III study in advanced NSCLC evaluating the compound versus placebo in combination with chemotherapy was initiated, but in November 2008 the trial was halted on the advice of an independent data monitoring committee (IDMC), upon reports of higher than usual death rates among patients. The IDMC recommended resumption of enrollment in early 2009, pending modification of the study design.

Cediranib   Cediranib (AZD2171, Recentin®) is an orally bioavailable quinazoline derivative in development by AstraZeneca (Figure 9.1). This compound is a very potent inhibitor of VEGFR2 ($IC_{50} < 1$ nM) and also inhibits VEGFR1 (5 nM), VEGFR3 (≤ 3 nM), KIT (2 nM), PDGFRβ (5 nM), PDGFRα (36 nM), and FGFR1 (26 nM). Cediranib is also a modest inhibitor of SRC (130 nM), ABL (250 nM), and CSF1R (110 nM). It is much less active on EGFR, ERBB2, CDK2, CDK4, Aurora-A, Aurora-B, or MEK ($IC_{50} > 1$ μM). Cediranib inhibits

VEGF-stimulated HUVEc proliferation with an IC_{50} value of >1 nM, and comparisons with other VEGFR RTK inhibitors indicated that cediranib is a more potent inhibitor of VEGF–induced proliferation than PTK787, SU11248, and CP-547632. In HUVEc, cediranib showed selectivity of 275-fold for inhibition of VEGF-induced proliferation versus FGF2-induced proliferation, and selectivity of 125-fold versus inhibition of EGF-stimulated proliferation. In contrast cediranib inhibited tumor cell proliferation only at high concentrations (>3 μM). Cediranib inhibited endothelial sprouting in in vitro angiogenesis assays with IC_{50} values <1 nM, and inhibited VEGF-induced vessel formation in Matrigel plugs in vivo at concentrations as low as 1.5 mg/kg/day. When administered orally at a dose of 1.5 mg/kg qd, cediranib inhibited the growth of a number of different tumor xenografts. Immunohistochemical analysis of tumors indicated that cediranib administration reduced tumor vessel number and this occurred quite rapidly (86). In an orthotopic murine RCC model, cediranib dosed orally at 6.3 mg/kg qd demonstrated significant inhibition of primary tumor growth, reduced microvessel density, and also decreased lung metastases (87). Preclinical studies also indicated that cediranib improved the radiation response (88) and also showed synergistic to additive efficacy when combined with other chemotherapeutic regimens such as paclitaxel, irinotecan, and gefitinib (89–91).

Based on these promising preclinical data, cediranib was selected as a clinical candidate. Phase I dose escalation studies demonstrated that the compound was generally well tolerated, and several of these studies showed signs of clinical benefit. The most common dose-limiting toxicities were hypertension, fatigue, joint pain, dypsnea, increased ALT, and anorexia. A dose of 45 mg qd was selected as the recommended Phase II dose (92), although this dose was not tolerable in patients with advanced HCC (93) or in the majority of those with RCC (94). Additionally, in men with hormone-refractory prostate cancer, 20 mg/day was identified as the MTD (95). These observations as well as experience with other combination drugs indicated that dose modifications of cedarinib in combination studies might be required. In a Phase I study of cedarinib in combination with carboplatin and paclitaxel in patients with advanced NSCLC, a dose of 30 mg was found to be tolerable. This study showed encouraging antitumor activity, with all but one of the 20 patients in the trial showing signs of some tumor shrinkage (96). Phase I combination studies with various chemotherapies were also initiated, and signs of clinical efficacy were seen in some indications (97, 98).

Results from a number of Phase II studies now indicate that cediranib may have significant clinical activity in a number of tumor types. In recurrent ovarian cancer, several confirmed partial responses and prolonged stable disease were observed in patients treated with 30 mg/day cediranib (99, 100). Phase II data from a trial in patients with previously untreated metastatic renal cell cancer showed that cediranib had an encouraging disease control rate with 12/32 partial responses and 15/32 patients with stable disease (101). In a Phase II trial of docetaxel-resistant, castrate-resistant prostate cancer, cediranib monotherapy also appeared to show potential (102). Results from the NCI sponsored study at the Massachusetts General Hospital Cancer Center showed that 8 of the 31 patients (27.5%) treated with cedarinib with recurrent glioblastoma were alive and progression free at 6 months (historic controls are about 15%). This trial included patients with glioblastoma whose cancer had progressed following prior therapy with radiation, chemotherapy, and surgery. The median survival was 221 days, and progression-free survival average was 117 days. Over half of the patients had a reduction in swelling, and the compound also had a steroid-sparing effect in many of the patients enrolled (103). Cediranib had modest anticancer activity as monotherapy in recurrent small cell lung cancer (<20% response rate, the predefined target), although consideration to evaluate the compound as part of combination regimens may be underway (104). Across the trials the most common toxicities were fatigue, hypertension, diarrhea, and voice alteration. Multiple clinical trials with cediranib are actively recruiting, including Phase III trials in combination with standard chemotherapies in colorectal cancers, ovarian cancers, and glioblastoma.

Axitinib   Pfizer is developing axitinib (AG-013736; Figure 9.1), an orally available small molecule inhibitor with single-digit nanomolar IC_{50} values for VEGFR1, VEGFR2, VEGF3, KIT, and PDGFRβ. Axitinib is also a fairly potent inhibitor of CSF1R and ABL (105, 106). At subnanomolar concentrations, axitinib inhibits VEGF-stimulated endothelial proliferation and survival. The compound also demonstrated dose-dependent inhibition of tumor growth using a number of different xenograft models. The inhibition of tumor growth was associated with a significant decrease in microvessel density and tumor necrosis (107).

In Phase I clinical trials of axitinib, the compound was found to have dose-limiting toxicities of hypertension, hemoptysis, and stomatitis, and a recommended dose of 5 mg bid was selected (108). Administration of the compound in the fed state resulted in reduced exposure, and it was recommended that it be given in the fasted state. PK profiles in Caucasian and Japanese populations were similar, but exposure was reduced when coadministered with inducers of Cyp3A4. In vitro studies with human liver microsomes indicated that axitinib was metabolized by conversion to glucuronide metabolites, as well as oxidation by the Cyp3A4 and Cyp1A2 isozymes. The latter two CYP isoforms are known to be inducible and likely to exhibit variability in patients. Sustained tumor response was seen in renal cell cancer as well as in one patient with adenoid cystic cancer, and antitumor activity was also seen in lung cancer patients. Two patients with adenocarcinoma of the lung (NSCLC) developed fatal hemoptysis, and one was likely due to the drug: axitinib treatment may have led to the rapid breakdown of a blood vessel with tumor infiltration. Tumor necrosis with hemoptysis in centrally located lung lesions was also seen with bevacizumab (Avastin; anti-VEGF antibody) and may be a common complication of antiangiogenic treatment in this subset of patients.

A Phase II study of axitinib in patients with cytokine-refractory metastatic renal cell cancer demonstrated promising clinical activity in this indication. Of 52 patients enrolled, 2 complete and 21 partial responses were noted, for an objective response rate of 44.2%. The median response duration was 23 months. Treatment-related adverse events included diarrhea, hypertension, fatigue, nausea, and hoarseness but were generally manageable and controlled by dose modification and supportive care (109). Axitinib administration to patients with sorafenib-

or sunitinib-refractory metastatic renal cell cancer also appears to have antitumor activity (110).

Phase II data from a trial of axitinib in thyroid cancer patients also indicated clinical benefit in this patient population (111, 112). Thirty percent of patients had partial responses, and 42% had stable disease lasting more than 16 weeks. The most common adverse events were fatigue, stomatitis/mucositis, and hypertension. Responses were observed across every histological type. Drug administration was associated with a decrease in soluble VEGFR levels in the plasma, although this did not correlate with response. Axitinib also demonstrated promising activity in pancreatic cancer. In a Phase II, randomized, open-label, active control, parallel assignment trial of axitinib in combination with gemcitabine, data indicated that there was a reduced risk of death in the axitinib + gemcitabine treated patients, and this effect was even greater in a subgroup of patients with better performance status at trial entry (113). Axitinib has also demonstrated single-agent activity in Phase II trials in advanced non small cell lung cancer (114) and metastatic melanoma (115). However, axitinib had minimal biologic or clinical activity in elderly patients with AML or myelodysplastic syndrome (116).

A Phase III randomized study was initiated comparing gemcitabine plus axitinib versus gemcitabine alone for advanced pancreatic cancer: however, in January 2009 this study was halted after an independent monitoring board found no evidence for increased survival with axitinib. Single-agent Phase III trials in refractory metastatic renal cell cancer, and Phase II trials in doxorubicin-refractory or intolerant thyroid cancer are ongoing, as well as combination studies with other therapeutic regimens in metastatic colorectal cancer, and advanced lung cancer.

Vatalanib Vatalanib (PTK-ZK/PTK787/ZK222584; Figure 9.1) is a small molecule, orally active molecule that is being developed by Novartis for the potential treatment of MDS and AML. The compound is an inhibitor of VEGFR1, 2, and 3 (IC_{50} values of 77, 33, and 660 nM, respectively), as well as inhibiting KIT (730 nM), PDGFRβ (580 nM), and CSF1R (1.4 μM). In cell-based assays, vatalanib inhibits VEGF-induced VEGFR2 phosphorylation with IC_{50} values of 17 nM (endothelial cells) and 34 nM (CHO cells transfected with VEGFR2). The compound inhibited HUVEc proliferation, migration, and survival with IC_{50} values of 7.1, 58, and <10 nM, respectively, but did not inhibit the proliferation of A431 or DU 145 cells even at concentrations of up to 1 μM (117). Vatalanib inhibits tumor growth in several xenograft models, including A431 epidermoid carcinoma, Ls174T colon carcinoma, HT29 colon carcinoma, and PC-3 prostate carcinoma. The effect of the drug in these models is presumed not to be due to a direct effect on the tumor cells, but rather through the inhibition of angiogenesis, as indicated by reduction in microvessel density. Vatalanib does have direct inhibitory effects on multiple myeloma cells that express VEGFR1, inhibiting proliferation and cell migration.

Vatalanib was evaluated in a number of Phase I/II trials. As monotherapy, common adverse events were nausea, vomiting, fatigue, lethargy, hypertension, headache, dizziness, and diarrhea. Pharmacokinetic studies have shown that vatalanib is rapidly absorbed and has a half-life of 56 h. Absorbtion is influenced by food, and a high fat meal can increase the time to maximal absorption.

However, the differences in vatalanib exposure with food did not correlate with significant changes in the safety profile, suggesting that this effect may not be clinically relevant. Tumor reduction was not generally observed; monotherapy resulted primarily in stable disease and minor responses in CRC, GM, and RCC. Rapid changes in tumor blood flow were observed, as well as increases in serum VEGFA. Phase III trials in colorectal cancer were initiated in January 2003. Vatalanib was administered at an oral dose of 1250 mg qd, in combination with oxaliplatin in the FOLFOX4 regimen. CONFIRM 1 (Colorectal Oral Novel Therapy for the Inhibition of Angiogenesis and Retarding of Metastases in First Line) enrolled 1168 patients with previously untreated metastatic colorectal cancer. The outcomes evaluated were progression-free and overall survival benefit of daily vatalanib in combination with FOLFOX4 versus FOLFOX4 with placebo. The addition of vatalanib did not result in differences in the response rate (42% for FOLFOX4 plus vatalanib versus 45% for FOLFOX4 plus placebo). There was also no increase in progression-free survival, although there was a trend toward an improvement in the vatalanib arm ($p = 0.12$). A planned subset analysis suggested that in patients with elevated lactate dehydrogenase (LDH) a significant benefit in progression-free survival was observed ($p = 0.012$). The side effect profile was consistent with those for other antiangiogenic therapies, with adverse events including hypertension and thromboembolic events (118). CONFIRM 2 (Colorectal Oral Novel Therapy for the Inhibition of Angiogenesis and Retarding of Metastases in Second Line) enrolled 855 patients with metastatic colorectal cancer who had progressed after treatment with irinotecan. Vatalanib had no significant overall survival benefit, although in a subpopulation of patients with elevated baseline LDH levels, there was again a significant improvement in overall survival (119).

A number of clinical trials are ongoing or have recently been completed. Phase I/II trials include evaluation of vatalanib in various combination studies with standard of care chemotherapy in a number of indications including relapsed malignant glioma, NSCLC, pleural mesothelioma, AML, prostate cancer, metastatic breast cancer, and pancreatic cancer. Evaluation of vatalanib as monotherapy is also continuing in melanoma, age-related macular degeneration, multiple myeloma, VHL-related hemangioblastoma, mesothelioma, diffuse large cell lymphoma, imatinib-resistant GIST, and metastatic neuroendocrine tumors.

Brivanib Alaninate Bristol-Myers Squibb is developing brivanib alaninate (BMS-582664; Figure 9.1), an orally active prodrug of BMS-540215, which is a dual inhibitor of VEGFR2 and FGFR1, 2, and 3. The compound inhibits VEGFR2 with an IC_{50} of 26 nM, and FGFR1, 2, and 3 with IC_{50} values of 150, 125, and 68 nM, respectively. In vivo, the compound inhibits the growth of human lung carcinoma and colorectal cancer xenografts, through mechanisms involving inhibition of tumor vessel growth and direct inhibitory effects on cancer cell proliferation (120, 121).

In Phase I studies, the compound was well tolerated, with the adverse events being hypertension, fatigue, dizziness, and elevated liver enzymes. Partial responses were seen in two patients (administered with doses >600 mg) and six patients had stable disease for more than 6 months. A Phase II trial for HCC was initiated in

November 2006. This nonrandomized, open-label, active control trial evaluated oral daily administration of 800 mg of brivanib alaninate in patients with unresectable, locally advanced, or metastatic disease. The trial will enroll 185 patients and is expected to complete in May 2010.

A Phase III randomized study of cetuximab with or without brivanib alaninate in patients with metastatic colorectal carcinoma previously treated with combination chemotherapy is also ongoing. Patients (375 in each group) are randomized to receive either brivanib and cetuximab or cetuximab alone, with the primary endpoint being overall survival. A Phase I study found that brivanib in combination with full-dose cetuximab was well tolerated and did not enhance cetuximab-associated adverse events (122). The best antitumor activity observed in evaluable patients with colorectal cancer as measured by anatomical tumor evaluation and progression-free survival was in the subset of patients who had not received either EGFR or VEGFR inhibitors as prior therapy. The majority of patients who had durable stable disease or partial response anatomically had partial metabolic responses on FDG-PET at days 15 and 56. This study monitored collagen IV and sVEGFR2 as pharmacodynamic markers, and noted that changes in serum levels of these two biomarkers were dose related (123).

TSU-68   TSU-68 (SU6668; Figure 9.2) is a small molecule inhibitor licensed from Sugen (Pfizer) by Taiho Pharmaceutical Company (Japan). The compound inhibits VEGFR2, PDGFRβ, and FGFR1, with reported IC_{50} values of 3.9, 0.2, and 3.8 μM, respectively (124). In cell-based assays, TSU-68 inhibited VEGF-induced VEGFR2 phosphorylation in endothelial cells and PDGF-induced PDGFRβ phosphorylation in NIH-3T3 cells overexpressing PDGFRβ. TSU-88 also inhibited acidic FGF-induced phosphorylation of the FGFR1 substrate, FRS-2 at somewhat higher concentrations (>10 μM). TSU-68 inhibited VEGF-driven mitogenesis of HUVEcs in a dose-dependent manner, with a mean IC_{50} of 340 nM (125, 126). More recent proteomic studies revealed that TSU-68 also inhibited Aurora-B ($IC_{50} = 0.047$ μM), Aurora-A ($IC_{50} = 0.850$ μM), and TANK-binding kinase 1 (TBK1) ($IC_{50} = 1.4$ μM) (127), and another study demonstrated that TSU-68 also had inhibitory activity against KIT ($IC_{50} \approx 0.01$ μM) (124). The compound has been shown to inhibit the growth and induce regression of some xenograft models, effects mediated by suppression of tumor angiogenesis (125, 126) followed by apoptosis of tumor cells. TSU-88 also inhibited peritoneal dissemination of ovarian cancer, liver metastases of human colon cancer xenografts, and pulmonary metastases of breast cancer xenografts (128–130). Pharmacokinetic analysis of plasma samples showed that inhibition of VEGFR2 phosphorylation required sustained plasma concentrations ≥ 1 μg/mL.

Phase I clinical trials with TSU-68 indicated that the compound was tolerable with once-daily dosing, but when dosed twice daily yielded DLT consisting of fatigue, dyspnea, chest pain, and pericardial effusions. The compound had a short plasma half-life, and plasma concentrations exceeding those required to inhibit tyrosine kinase activity in preclinical models were seen on the first day but not following prolonged administration. Phase I studies of the agent administered intravenously were prematurely terminated due to chemical instability of the formulation. In

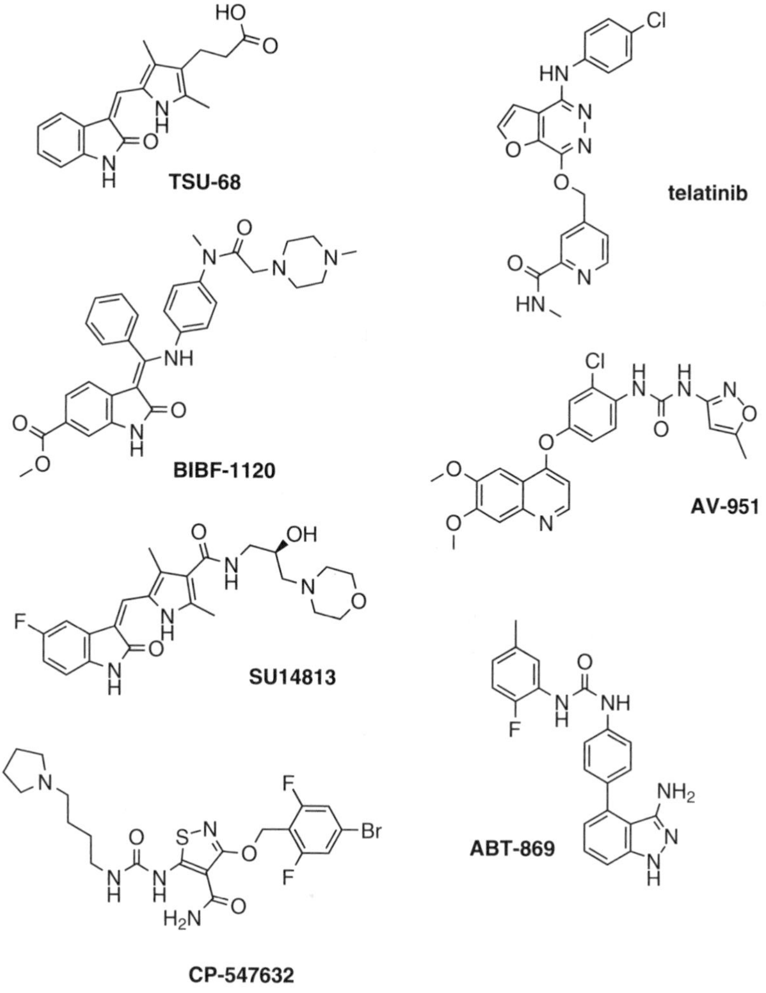

Figure 9.2 Structures of angiokinase inhibitors.

another Phase I trial, oral bioavailability was improved when administered under fed conditions and this increased exposure was associated with a lower tolerability with TSU-68 doses of 200 and 400 mg/m^2 given two or three times daily. In this second trial, reduced exposure was also seen at later time points, consistent with saturable absorption and metabolic induction (131). No objective responses were seen, although clinical benefit (disease stability, increased necrosis of liver metastases) was seen in some patients. The Taiho company website currently lists TSU-68 as being in Phase II clinical trials in breast cancer in Japan and Korea and hepatocellular cancer in Japan.

Telatinib   Telatinib (BAY57-9352; Figure 9.2) is a small molecule, orally active inhibitor in development by Bayer Yakuhin. Telatinib inhibits human VEGFR2, human VEGFR3, mouse PDGFR, and human KIT tyrosine kinase activity with IC_{50} values of 6, 4, 15, and 1 nM, respectively. This agent exhibits IC_{50} values of >10,000 nM for the inhibition of RAF, EGFR, ERBB2, FGFR1, p38α, FLT3, LCK, and BCR-ABL. In cell-based assays, telatinib inhibited VEGF-dependent receptor autophophorylation in mouse fibroblasts overexpressing human VEGFR2 ($IC_{50} = 19$ nM) and inhibited the proliferation of human endothelial cells with an IC_{50} value of 26 nM. The compound had no inhibitory activity on MDA-MB-231 breast carcinoma, LS174T colorectal carcinoma, HCT-116 colorectal carcinoma, or PC-3 prostate carcinoma cells. In mice, the compound exhibited good pharmaceutical properties and was shown to delay tumor growth and inhibit tumor angiogenesis.

In a Phase I, nonrandomized, continuous dose study of telatinib, patients with colorectal cancer were treated with 200, 1200, or 1500 mg telatinib bid for 108 days. Common treatment-related adverse events included diarrhea, hypertension, infection without neutropenia, fatigue, tumor pain, hepatic pain, increased bilirubin, and dyspnea. Stable disease was seen in many of the patients, although as monotherapy, no partial responses were observed. In this and another trial, increases in VEGF and decreases in sVEGFR2 were observed that reached plateaus at approximately 900 mg bid continuously administered, and a recommended Phase II dose of 900 mg bid was proposed. In patients with advanced solid tumors, telatinib (600 and 900 mg bid po) administered in combination with 75 mg/m² IV docetaxel produced a partial response in three patients and stable disease in six patients. In another Phase I trial, telatinib was evaluated in combination with irinotecan and capecitabine. Coadministration of the drugs did not alter exposure to the drugs. Partial response was reported as the best overall tumor response in 5/17 patients, suggesting possible activity of this combination, although it may also be associated with cardiac toxicity (132).

BIBF-1120   Boehringer Ingelheim is developing an oral capsule formulation of the indolinone derivative BIBF-1120 (Vargatef®; Figure 9.2). The compound is an inhibitor of VEGFR1, VEGFR2, VEGFR3, FGFR1, FGFR2, FGFR3, PDGFRα, and PDGFRβ with reported IC_{50} values of 34, 21, 13, 69, 37, 106, 59, and 65 nM, respectively. The compound also inhibits some of the SRC family kinases, for example, SRC, LCK, and LYN, with IC_{50} values of 156, 16, and 195 nM. The compound has IC_{50} values >1000 nM on IGF1R and the insulin receptor, and IC_{50} values >50,000 nM for EGFR, ERBB2, CDK1, and CDK2, and no activity when assayed at 10 μM on over 20 additional serine/threonine and tyrosine kinases. In cell-based assays, BIBF-1120 inhibited VEGF-stimulated HUVEc proliferation ($EC_{50} = 9$ nM), PDGF-stimulated bovine retinal pericyte proliferation ($EC_{50} = 76$ nM), and PDGF-stimulated human aortic smooth muscle cell proliferation ($EC_{50} = 55$ nM). However, the compound had little direct antiproliferative activity on tumor cells (FaDU, Calu-6, HeLa). BIBF-1120 inhibited VEGF-stimulated VEGFR2 phosphorylation in transiently transfected 3T3 cells with an IC_{50} of about 100 nM, and this inhibition was sustained for at least 32 hours following a 1-hour exposure to the drug. Similarly, the compound inhibited FGF2- and PDGF-stimulated signaling (MAPK pathway activation) in smooth muscle cells and pericytes. BIBF-1120 also demonstrated good antitumor activity in mouse xenograft models, with potent and long-lasting growth suppression and tumor regression associated with a reduction in tumor vessel density (both endothelial cells and pericytes). In vivo tumor regression was achieved even with intermittent dose schedules. When combined with suboptimal doses of docetaxel, BIBF-1120 results in improved antitumor efficacy compared to single-agent treatments (133, 134).

Phase I clinical trials began in 2004. In a dose escalation trial designed to determine safety, tolerability, and MTD, the dose of BIBF-1120 was escalated up to 450 mg qd and 300 mg bid (28 days on, 7 days off) (135, 136). Predominant drug-related adverse events were gastrointestinal in nature with mild to moderate intensity. Elevation of liver enzymes constituted the DLT. One patient showed a complete response at 200 mg qd, and for 2 patients, a partial response was observed at >200 mg bid. DCE-MRI measurements indicated that blood flow and permeability in metastasis were reduced by >40% in 24/42 evaluable patients. The exposure (AUC) to BIBF-1120 showed moderate to high variability and increased with dose. The maximal plasma concentrations were attained about 3 hours after drug ingestion. The agent was extensively distributed out of the blood, showing a high clearance, with a mean terminal half-life of 15 h. Other Phase I trials indicated that the compound was well tolerated and showed promising clinical activity. In a Phase II trial in patients with advanced, relapsed NSCLC, patients with good ECOG status experienced longer overall survival, longer progression-free survival, and a higher stable disease rate compared with the overall study population (137). Several combination trials of BIBF-1120 with BIBF-2992 (a EGFR inhibitor) are ongoing. A trial in idiopathic pulmonary fibrosis has also been initiated, and a Phase III clinical trial in non small cell lung cancer was opened in late 2008.

SU14813 Pfizer is developing SU14813 (Figure 9.2) as a small molecule, orally available agent for the treatment of cancer. The compound was originally identified at Sugen (later acquired by Pfizer) as part of a program targeting multiple split kinase domain receptor tyrosine kinases. SU14813 inhibits VEGFR1, VEGFR2, PDGFRβ, KIT, FLT3, and CSF1R with IC_{50} values ranging from 0.002 to 0.05 μM (138). The compound is a weak inhibitor of FGFR1, SRC, and MET (IC_{50} values of 3.5, 2.5, and 9 μM, respectively) and has minimal activity on EGFR ($IC_{50} > 20$ μM). In cell-based assays, SU14813 inhibited VEGF-dependent phosphorylation of VEGFR2 (transfected NIH-3T3 cells), PDGFRβ (transfected NIH-3T3 cells), KIT (Mo7e cells), and FLT3-ITD (MV-4-11 cells) as well as CSF1R (transfected NIH-3T3 cells) with IC_{50} values ranging from 6 to 50 nM. Consistent with these potent cell-based mechanistic data, the compound inhibited PDGF-dependent proliferation of NIH-3T3 cells overexpressing PDGFRβ, FLT3 ligand dependent proliferation of OC1-AML5 cells expressing wild-type FLT3, and autonomous proliferation of MV-4-11 cells (expressing constitutively active FLT3-ITD) with IC_{50} values ranging from 20 to 79 nM. SU14813 inhibited VEGF-stimulated but not FGF2-stimulated endothelial survival. In xenograft models using human and rat tumor cells, SU14813 exhibited dose-dependent antitumor activity, and tumor regression in two models 786-O (a PDGFR, VEGFR expressing cell line) and MV-4-11 (activated FLT3 dependent). Tumor growth inhibition was enhanced by combination with docetaxel. Overall, SU14813 is similar to sunitinib, with some differences in plasma kinetics (shorter half-life) and a lack of major detectable circulating metabolites. In mice, twice-daily doses of SU14183 were required to achieve plasma concentrations above the target concentration of 100–200 ng/mL, in contrast to a once-daily dose of sunitinib.

In Phase I studies, 77 patients with advanced solid malignancies were treated. The rate of grade 3 and 4 adverse events increased at doses above 100 mg, with hypertension and fatigue as the most common events, as well as diarrhea and thrombocytopenia. The maximal tolerated dose was determined to be 100 mg dosed continuously. SU14813 decreased plasma sVEGFR2 and sVEGFR3 in a dose-dependent manner, but levels rebounded when patients were off treatment. Plasma VEGF also tended to decrease and hair depigmentation was observed, consistent with the inhibition of KIT. One patient with RCC had a complete response, and 11 patients had a partial response (2 RCC, 2 thymoma, 2 NSCLC, 1 CRC, 4 other), and 14 patients had stable disease (median 178 d). These encouraging data suggested that SU14813 had durable responses across several tumor types (139).

A Phase I safety and pharmacokinetic study of SU14813 in combination with docetaxel was also recently disclosed. The conclusions were that the combination of SU14813 50 mg/day with docetaxel 75 mg/m^2 every 3 weeks was tolerable and active in patients with advanced solid tumors. The investigators reported an unexpected rate of long-term disease stabilization and partial responses, particularly in treatment-refractory malignant melanoma, GIST, and CUP (cancer of unknown primary origin)(140). Pfizer lists SU14813 as being in Phase II (September 2008) although there are no U.S. trials currently listed as ongoing or actively recruiting (www.clinicaltrials.gov, January 2009).

ABT-869   ABT-869 (Figure 9.2) is a small molecule inhibitor of VEGF and PDGF family receptor tyrosine kinases under joint development by Abbott and Genentech. The compound is a potent inhibitor of VEGFR1, VEGFR2, VEGFR3, FLT3, PDGFRβ, CSF1R (CSF1R), KIT, and TIE2 with biochemical IC$_{50}$ values of 3, 4, 190, 4, 66, 3, 14, and 179 nM, respectively. IC$_{50}$ values greater than 1 μM were observed for nonrelated RTKs and serine/threonine kinases. In cell-based mechanistic assays, the compound inhibited VEGFR2, PDGFRβ, KIT, and CSF1R with IC$_{50}$ values ranging from 2 to 30 nM. VEGF-stimulated VEGFR2 phosphorylation in human endothelial cells was inhibited with an IC$_{50}$ value of 0.2 nM. In MV-4-11 cells and Kasumi-1 cells, which have constitutively activated FLT3-ITD and KIT, respectively, ABT-869 inhibited cell proliferation with IC$_{50}$ values of 11 and 1 nM. In contrast, the compound only weakly inhibited the proliferation of tumor cells not driven by VEGF or PDGF RTKs (e.g., HT20 and MDA-MB-435 cells). ABT-869 inhibited angiogenesis and edema in vivo and exhibited efficacy against a number of xenograft models with ED$_{50}$ values of 3–10 mg/kg po (141). In a mouse xenograft model using the AML cell line MV-4-11 (FLT3-ITD), ABT-869 dosed at 3–10 mg/kg/day resulted in tumor regression.

A Phase I study was performed to determine maximum tolerated dose and toxicity profile and to assess pharmacokinetics and tumor response. ABT-869 had a $t_{1/2}$ of approximately 17 hours, and dose-limiting toxicities of fatigue, proteinuria, and hypertension were observed at doses as low as 0.3 mg/kg. Promising clinical activity was observed, with several partial responses and a number of patients with stable disease. A recommended dose of 0.25 mg/day was determined. ABT-869 induced dose-dependent changes in serum biomarkers (decrease in sVEGFR1, increase in PlGF and VEGF) consistent with antiangiogenic activity (142). However, serum biomarkers had limited value in predicting safety. Phase II clinical trials in RCC previously treated with sunitinib, HCC, non small cell lung cancer, metastatic breast cancer, and colorectal cancer are ongoing, and a Phase I trial involving patients with refractory or relapsed AML and myelodysplastic syndrome is planned. Combination studies with Tarcéva in solid tumors are also planned.

AV-951   Aveo is developing AV-951 (Figure 9.2) under license from Kirin Brewery. This is a quinoline urea based compound that inhibits VEGFR1, VEGFR2, VEGFR3, PDGFR, and KIT tyrosine kinases with IC_{50} values of 0.21, 0.16, 0.24, 1.63, and 1.72 nM, respectively (143). The compound also shows potent and selective inhibitory activity against VEGF-stimulated phosphorylation of VEGFRs, and downstream MAPK activation, but not FGF2- or EGF-induced MAPK activation. VEGF, but not FGF2, driven endothelial proliferation was inhibited by the compound. In contrast, the compound did not inhibit the in vitro growth of cancer cells up to 1 μM. Dosed orally in athymic mice and rats, AV-951 showed significant antitumor activity against human tumor xenografts derived from breast, colon, liver, lung, ovarian, pancreas, prostate, brain, and renal cancer cells. These effects were associated with a reduction in tumor vessel density and vascular permeability. In a Phase I dose escalation study, the compound was given orally on a 4 week on, 2 week off schedule (143). The maximal tolerated dose was determined to be 1.5 mg/day. Promising clinical activity was observed in renal, colon, and lung cancers. In a follow-up study, the compound was administered daily at 1, 1.5, and 2 mg/day. At 2 mg, DLTs consisting of grade 3 proteinuria, grade 3 ataxia, and grade 4 intracranial hemorrhage were seen. The primary toxicity observed at all dose levels was hypertension, which was dose dependent and managed with standard antihypertensive agents. Among nine patients with RCC, there were two confirmed partial responses at 2 mg and 1.5 mg (lasting 128 weeks and 42 weeks, respectively), and seven patients at doses of 1–2 mg with stable disease lasting >12 weeks. In addition, clinical benefit was observed in patients with colon and lung cancers.

A randomized, double-blind, placebo-controlled, randomized discontinuation Phase II trial in approximately 200 patients with RCC naive to VEGF targeted therapy has been initiated at more than 30 sites in Europe and India. In this trial, all patients receive 16 weeks of AV-951, after which time patients are evaluated for response, stable disease, or progressive disease. Those patients who experience a partial or complete response remain on therapy; those patients who experience stable disease are randomized to receive 12 weeks of AV-951 or placebo in a double-blind fashion. A Phase Ib trial in combination with temsirolimus, an approved mTOR inhibitor, in patients with metastatic RCC was initiated in November 2007.

A Phase Ib combination study with FOLFOX6 in patients with advanced colorectal cancer and other gastrointestinal cancers began in August 2008.

CP-547632 CP-547632 (OSI-632; Figure 9.2) is a novel isothiazole originally identified by OSI in collaboration with Pfizer. The compound is an orally active, potent inhibitor of VEGFR2 and FGFR (IC$_{50}$ values of 11 and 9 nM, respectively). The compound also inhibited TIE2 (IC$_{50}$ = 48 nM). The compound is ATP

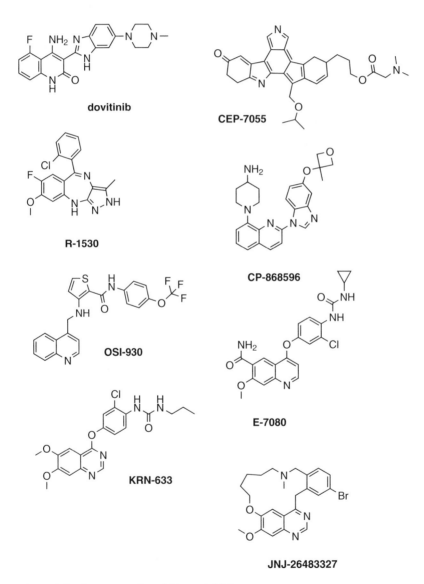

Figure 9.3 Structures of angiokinase inhibitors.

competitive, and 250–1000-fold less potent for PDGFRβ, IR, and EGFR. CP-547632 inhibits VEGF- and FGF2-stimulated thymidine incorporation into human endothelial cells with IC_{50} values of 14 and 53 nM, respectively. CP-547632 inhibited VEGF-stimulated VEGFR2 phosphorylation in porcine aortic endothelial cells transiently expressing hVEGFR2 with an IC_{50} of 6 nM. The in vivo effects of the compound were assessed to evaluate pharmacodynamic/pharmacokinetic relationships. The ability of the compound to inhibit the phosphorylation of VEGFR2 in vivo correlated with the blood plasma concentration of the compound, and a single oral dose of 50 mg/kg yielded plasma concentrations of ≈500 ng/mL for 12 hours (144). Phase I data reported for CP-547632 indicated that the compound had minimal side effects and no DLTs when administered as a single agent in patients with solid tumors (145). Combination treatment with paclitaxel/carboplatin and CP-547632 in advanced NSCLC patients led to a response rate of 20%, and 50% of the patients had stable disease (including three patients with unconfirmed partial responses). The compound has a half-life of about 30 hours and, at doses equal to or greater than 150 mg qd, achieved plasma concentrations within the range associated with angiogenesis in clinical models (146).

In a Phase II combination trial with paclitaxel/carboplatin in patients with advanced lung cancer, the combination was well tolerated at doses up to 200 mg CP-547632 qd. At 250 mg, dose-limiting toxicities of CP-547632 consisting of diarrhea and rash were observed. CP-547632 did not increase the ORR to chemotherapy alone in patients with advanced non small cell lung cancer (147). In May 2007, Pfizer returned full commercial rights for CP-547632 to OSI. Since CP-547632 has a different selectivity profile than OSI-930 (Figure 9.3), a VEGFR/KIT inhibitor currently in Phase I studies, OSI is evaluating the data and potential positioning of OSI-632 in their portfolio prior to making any decision on its potential future development.

REFERENCES

1. Folkman J. Tumor angiogenesis: therapeutic implications. N Engl J Med 1971;285(21):1182–1186.
2. Kim KJ, Li B, Winer J, Armanini M, Gillett N, Phillips HS, Ferrara N. Inhibition of vascular endothelial growth factor-induced angiogenesis suppresses tumour growth in vivo. Nature 1993;362(6423):841–844.
3. Jain RK. Normalization of tumor vasculature: an emerging concept in antiangiogenic therapy. Science 2005;307(5706):58–62.
4. Baluk P, Hashizume H, McDonald DM. Cellular abnormalities of blood vessels as targets in cancer. Curr Opin Genet Dev 2005;15(1):102–111.
5. Baffert F, Le T, Sennino B, Thurston G, Kuo CJ, Hu-Lowe D, McDonald DM. Cellular changes in normal blood capillaries undergoing regression after inhibition of VEGF signaling. Am J Physiol Heart Circ Physiol 2006;290(2):H547–559.
6. Kamba T, McDonald DM. Mechanisms of adverse effects of anti-VEGF therapy for cancer. Br J Cancer 2007;96(12):1788–1795.
7. Kamba T, Tam BY, Hashizume H, Haskell A, Sennino B, Mancuso MR, Norberg SM, O'Brien SM, Davis RB, Gowen LC, Anderson KD, Thurston G, Joho S, Springer ML, Kuo CJ, McDonald DM. VEGF-dependent plasticity of fenestrated capillaries in the normal adult microvasculature. Am J Physiol Heart Circ Physiol 2006;290(2):H560–576.

8. Batchelor TT, Sorensen AG, di Tomaso E, Zhang WT, Duda DG, Cohen KS, Kozak KR, Cahill DP, Chen PJ, Zhu M, Ancukiewicz M, Mrugala MM, Plotkin S, Drappatz J, Louis DN, Ivy P, Scadden DT, Benner T, Loeffler JS, Wen PY, Jain RK. AZD2171, a pan-VEGF receptor tyrosine kinase inhibitor, normalizes tumor vasculature and alleviates edema in glioblastoma patients. Cancer Cell 2007;11(1):83–95.

9. Folkman J. Seminars in Medicine of the Beth Israel Hospital, Boston. Clinical applications of research on angiogenesis. N Engl J Med 1995;333(26):1757–1763.

10. Rini BI, Schiller JH, Fruehauf JP, Cohen EE, Tarazi JC, Rosbrook B, Ricart AD, Olszanski AJ, Kim S, Spano J. Association of diastolic blood pressure (dBP) >= 90 mmHg with overall survival (OS) in patients treated with axitinib (AG- 013736). J Clin Oncol (Meeting Abstracts) 2008;26(15 Suppl):Abstr 3543.

11. Eskens FA, Verweij J. The clinical toxicity profile of vascular endothelial growth factor (VEGF) and vascular endothelial growth factor receptor (VEGFR) targeting angiogenesis inhibitors; a review. Eur J Cancer 2006;42(18):3127–3139.

12. Duda DG, Batchelor TT, Willett CG, Jain RK. VEGF-targeted cancer therapy strategies: current progress, hurdles and future prospects. Trends Mol Med 2007;13(6):223–230.

13. Willett CG, Boucher Y, Duda DG, di Tomaso E, Munn LL, Tong RT, Kozin SV, Petit L, Jain RK, Chung DC, Sahani DV, Kalva SP, Cohen KS, Scadden DT, Fischman AJ, Clark JW, Ryan DP, Zhu AX, Blaszkowsky LS, Shellito PC, Mino-Kenudson M, Lauwers GY. Surrogate markers for antiangiogenic therapy and dose-limiting toxicities for bevacizumab with radiation and chemotherapy: continued experience of a phase I trial in rectal cancer patients. J Clin Oncol 2005;23(31):8136–8139.

14. Willett CG, Boucher Y, di Tomaso E, Duda DG, Munn LL, Tong RT, Chung DC, Sahani DV, Kalva SP, Kozin SV, Mino M, Cohen KS, Scadden DT, Hartford AC, Fischman AJ, Clark JW, Ryan DP, Zhu AX, Blaszkowsky LS, Chen HX, Shellito PC, Lauwers GY, Jain RK. Direct evidence that the VEGF-specific antibody bevacizumab has antivascular effects in human rectal cancer. Nat Med 2004;10(2):145–147.

15. Mendel DB, Laird AD, Xin X, Louie SG, Christensen JG, Li G, Schreck RE, Abrams TJ, Ngai TJ, Lee LB, Murray LJ, Carver J, Chan E, Moss KG, Haznedar JO, Sukbuntherng J, Blake RA, Sun L, Tang C, Miller T, Shirazian S, McMahon G, Cherrington JM. In vivo antitumor activity of SU11248, a novel tyrosine kinase inhibitor targeting vascular endothelial growth factor and platelet-derived growth factor receptors: determination of a pharmacokinetic/pharmacodynamic relationship. Clin Cancer Res 2003;9(1):327–337.

16. Abrams TJ, Lee LB, Murray LJ, Pryer NK, Cherrington JM. SU11248 inhibits KIT and platelet-derived growth factor receptor beta in preclinical models of human small cell lung cancer. Mol Cancer Ther 2003;2(5):471–478.

17. Pfizer. Investigator's Brochure SU011248 New York, NY: Pfizer Global Research and Development; 2004.

18. Baratte S, Sarati S, Frigerio E, James CA, Ye C, Zhang Q. Quantitation of SU11248, an oral multi-target tyrosine kinase inhibitor, and its metabolite in monkey tissues by liquid chromatograph with tandem mass spectrometry following semi-automated liquid–liquid extraction. J Chromatogr A 2004;1024(1–2):87–94.

19. Houk B, Garrett M, Bello C. Population pharmacokinetics of SU011248 and its primary metabolite SU12662 in oncology patients and healthy volunteers. AACR Meeting Abstracts 2005 (Molecular Targets and Cancer Therapeutics, Philadelphia, PA).

20. Moss KG, Toner GC, Cherrington JM, Mendel DB, Laird AD. Hair depigmentation is a biological readout for pharmacological inhibition of KIT in mice and humans. J Pharmacol Exp Ther 2003;307(2):476–480.

21. Robert C, Faivre S, Raymond E, Armand JP, Escudier B. Subungual splinter hemorrhages: a clinical window to inhibition of vascular endothelial growth factor receptors? Ann Intern Med 2005;143(4):313–314.

22. Norden-Zfoni A, Desai J, Manola J, Beaudry P, Force J, Maki R, Folkman J, Bello C, Baum C, DePrimo SE, Shalinsky DR, Demetri GD, Heymach JV. Blood-based biomarkers of SU11248 activity and clinical outcome in patients with metastatic imatinib-resistant gastrointestinal stromal tumor. Clin Cancer Res 2007;13(9):2643–2650.

23. Deprimo SE, Bello CL, Smeraglia J, Baum CM, Spinella D, Rini BI, Michaelson MD, Motzer RJ. Circulating protein biomarkers of pharmacodynamic activity of sunitinib in patients with metastatic renal cell carcinoma: modulation of VEGF and VEGF-related proteins. J Transl Med 2007;5:32.

24. Motzer RJ, Michaelson MD, Redman BG, Hudes GR, Wilding G, Figlin RA, Ginsberg MS, Kim ST, Baum CM, DePrimo SE, Li JZ, Bello CL, Theuer CP, George DJ, Rini BI. Activity of SU11248, a multitargeted inhibitor of vascular endothelial growth factor receptor and platelet-derived growth factor receptor, in patients with metastatic renal cell carcinoma. J Clin Oncol 2006;24(1):16–24.

25. Motzer RJ, Michaelson MD, Rosenberg J, Bukowski RM, Curti BD, George DJ, Hudes GR, Redman BG, Margolin KA, Wilding G. Sunitinib efficacy against advanced renal cell carcinoma. J Urol 2007;178(5):1883–1887.

26. Motzer RJ, Rini BI, Bukowski RM, Curti BD, George DJ, Hudes GR, Redman BG, Margolin KA, Merchan JR, Wilding G, Ginsberg MS, Bacik J, Kim ST, Baum CM, Michaelson MD. Sunitinib in patients with metastatic renal cell carcinoma. JAMA 2006;295(21):2516–2524.

27. Motzer RJ, Hutson TE, Tomczak P, Michaelson MD, Bukowski RM, Rixe O, Oudard S, Negrier S, Szczylik C, Kim ST, Chen I, Bycott PW, Baum CM, Figlin RA. Sunitinib versus interferon alfa in metastatic renal-cell carcinoma. N Engl J Med 2007;356(2):115–124.

28. Wilhelm SM, Carter C, Tang L, Wilkie D, McNabola A, Rong H, Chen C, Zhang X, Vincent P, McHugh M, Cao Y, Shujath J, Gawlak S, Eveleigh D, Rowley B, Liu L, Adnane L, Lynch M, Auclair D, Taylor I, Gedrich R, Voznesensky A, Riedl B, Post LE, Bollag G, Trail PA. BAY 43–9006 exhibits broad spectrum oral antitumor activity and targets the RAF/MEK/ERK pathway and receptor tyrosine kinases involved in tumor progression and angiogenesis. Cancer Res 2004;64(19):7099–7109.

29. Wilhelm S, Carter C, Lynch M, Lowinger T, Dumas J, Smith RA, Schwartz B, Simantov R, Kelley S. Discovery and development of sorafenib: a multikinase inhibitor for treating cancer. Nat Rev Drug Discov 2006;5(10):835–844.

30. Sharma A, Trivedi NR, Zimmerman MA, Tuveson DA, Smith CD, Robertson GP. Mutant V599EB-Raf regulates growth and vascular development of malignant melanoma tumors. Cancer Res 2005;65(6):2412–2421.

31. Liu L, Cao Y, Chen C, Zhang X, McNabola A, Wilkie D, Wilhelm S, Lynch M, Carter C. Sorafenib blocks the RAF/MEK/ERK pathway, inhibits tumor angiogenesis, and induces tumor cell apoptosis in hepatocellular carcinoma model PLC/PRF/5. Cancer Res 2006;66(24):11851–11858.

32. Chang YS, Adnane J, Trail PA, Levy J, Henderson A, Xue D, Bortolon E, Ichetovkin M, Chen C, McNabola A, Wilkie D, Carter CA, Taylor IC, Lynch M, Wilhelm S. Sorafenib (BAY 43–9006) inhibits tumor growth and vascularization and induces tumor apoptosis and hypoxia in RCC xenograft models. Cancer Chemother Pharmacol 2007;59(5):561–574.

33. Adnane L, Trail PA, Taylor I, Wilhelm SM. Sorafenib (BAY 43–9006, Nexavar®), a dual-action inhibitor that targets RAF/MEK/ERK pathway in tumor cells and tyrosine kinases VEGFR/PDGFR in tumor vasculature. Methods Enzymol 2005;407:597–612.

34. Guida T, Anaganti S, Provitera L, Gedrich R, Sullivan E, Wilhelm SM, Santoro M, Carlomagno F. Sorafenib inhibits imatinib-resistant KIT and platelet-derived growth factor receptor beta gatekeeper mutants. Clin Cancer Res 2007;13(11):3363–3369.

35. Carlomagno F, Anaganti S, Guida T, Salvatore G, Troncone G, Wilhelm SM, Santoro M. BAY 43–9006 inhibition of oncogenic RET mutants. J Natl Cancer Inst 2006;98(5):326–334.

36. Caraglia M, Tassone P, Marra M, Budillon A, Venuta S, Tagliaferri P. Targeting Raf-kinase: molecular rationales and translational issues. Ann Oncol 2006;17(Suppl 7):vii124–127.

37. Yu C, Bruzek LM, Meng XW, Gores GJ, Carter CA, Kaufmann SH, Adjei AA. The role of Mcl-1 downregulation in the proapoptotic activity of the multikinase inhibitor BAY 43–9006. Oncogene 2005;24(46):6861–6869.

38. Rahmani M, Davis EM, Bauer C, Dent P, Grant S. Apoptosis induced by the kinase inhibitor BAY 43–9006 in human leukemia cells involves down-regulation of Mcl-1 through inhibition of translation. J Biol Chem 2005;280(42):35217–35227.

39. Strumberg D, Richly H, Hilger RA, Schleucher N, Korfee S, Tewes M, Faghih M, Brendel E, Voliotis D, Haase CG, Schwartz B, Awada A, Voigtmann R, Scheulen ME, Seeber S. Phase I clinical and pharmacokinetic study of the novel Raf kinase and vascular endothelial growth factor

receptor inhibitor BAY 43-9006 in patients with advanced refractory solid tumors. J Clin Oncol 2005;23(5):965–972.

40. Clark JW, Eder JP, Ryan D, Lathia C, Lenz HJ. Safety and pharmacokinetics of the dual action Raf kinase and vascular endothelial growth factor receptor inhibitor, BAY 43-9006, in patients with advanced, refractory solid tumors. Clin Cancer Res 2005;11(15):5472–5480.

41. Awada A, Hendlisz A, Gil T, Bartholomeus S, Mano M, de Valeriola D, Strumberg D, Brendel E, Haase CG, Schwartz B, Piccart M. Phase I safety and pharmacokinetics of BAY 43-9006 administered for 21 days on/7 days off in patients with advanced, refractory solid tumours. Br J Cancer 2005;92(10):1855–1861.

42. Moore M, Hirte HW, Siu L, Oza A, Hotte SJ, Petrenciuc O, Cihon F, Lathia C, Schwartz B. Phase I study to determine the safety and pharmacokinetics of the novel Raf kinase and VEGFR inhibitor BAY 43-9006, administered for 28 days on/7 days off in patients with advanced, refractory solid tumors. Ann Oncol 2005;16(10):1688–1694.

43. Strumberg D, Awada A, Hirte H, Clark JW, Seeber S, Piccart P, Hofstra E, Voliotis D, Christensen O, Brueckner A, Schwartz B. Pooled safety analysis of BAY 43-9006 (sorafenib) monotherapy in patients with advanced solid tumours: Is rash associated with treatment outcome? Eur J Cancer 2006;42(4):548–556.

44. Kupsch P, Henning BF, Passarge K, Richly H, Wiesemann K, Hilger RA, Scheulen ME, Christensen O, Brendel E, Schwartz B, Hofstra E, Voigtmann R, Seeber S, Strumberg D. Results of a phase I trial of sorafenib (BAY 43-9006) in combination with oxaliplatin in patients with refractory solid tumors, including colorectal cancer. Clin Colorectal Cancer 2005;5(3):188–196.

45. Figer A, Moscovici M, Bulocinic S, Radu P, Atsmon J, Shmuely E, Laba O, Gadish D, Brendel E, Schwartz B. Phase I trial of BAY 43-9006 in combination with 5-fluorouracil (5-FU) and leucovorin (LCV) in patients with advanced refractory solid tumors. Ann Oncol 2004;15:iii87.

46. Flaherty K, Brose M, Schuchter L, Tuveson D, Sosman J, Schiller J, Lee R, Schwartz B, O'Dwyer P. Sorafenib combined with carboplatin and paclitaxel for metastatic melanoma: PFS and response versus B-Raf status. Proc 4th Intl Symp Targeted Anticancer Ther, Amsterdam, The Netherlands, 2006:O.1111.

47. Siu LL, Awada A, Takimoto CH, Piccart M, Schwartz B, Giannaris T, Lathia C, Petrenciuc O, Moore MJ. Phase I trial of sorafenib and gemcitabine in advanced solid tumors with an expanded cohort in advanced pancreatic cancer. Clin Cancer Res 2006;12(1):144–151.

48. Richly H, Kupsch P, Passage K, Grubert M, Hilger RA, Voigtmann R, Schwartz B, Brendel E, Christensen O, Haase CG, Strumberg D. Results of a phase I trial of BAY 43-9006 in combination with doxorubicin in patients with primary hepatic cancer. Int J Clin Pharmacol Ther 2004;42(11):650–651.

49. Richly H, Henning BF, Kupsch P, Passarge K, Grubert M, Hilger RA, Christensen O, Brendel E, Schwartz B, Ludwig M, Flashar C, Voigtmann R, Scheulen ME, Seeber S, Strumberg D. Results of a phase I trial of sorafenib (BAY 43-9006) in combination with doxorubicin in patients with refractory solid tumors. Ann Oncol 2006;17(5):866–873.

50. Awada A, Hendlisz A, Gil T, Schwartz B, Bartholomeus B, Brendel E, de Valeriola D, Haase C, Delaunoit T, Piccart M. A phase I study of Bay 43-9006, a novel Raf kinase and VEGFR inhibitor, in combination with taxotere in patients with advanced solid tumors. Eur J Cancer Suppl 2004;2(8):Abstr 381.

51. Steinbild S, Baas F, Gmehling D, Brendel E, Christensen O, Schwartz B, Mross K. Phase I study of BAY 43-9006 (sorafenib), a Raf kinase and VEGFR inhibitor, combined with irinotecan (CPT-11) in advanced solid tumors. J Clin Oncol (Meeting Abstracts) 2005;23(16 Suppl):Abstr 3115.

52. Eisen T, Ahmad T, Gore ME, Marais R, Gibbens I, James MG, Schwartz B, Bergamini L. Phase I trial of BAY 43-9006 (sorafenib) combined with dacarbazine (DTIC) in metastatic melanoma patients. J Clin Oncol (Meeting Abstracts) 2005;23(16 Suppl):Abstr 7508.

53. Ratain MJ, Eisen T, Stadler WM, Flaherty KT, Kaye SB, Rosner GL, Gore M, Desai AA, Patnaik A, Xiong HQ, Rowinsky E, Abbruzzese JL, Xia C, Simantov R, Schwartz B, O'Dwyer PJ. Phase II placebo-controlled randomized discontinuation trial of sorafenib in patients with metastatic renal cell carcinoma. J Clin Oncol 2006;24(16):2505–2512.

54. Abou-Alfa GK, Schwartz L, Ricci S, Amadori D, Santoro A, Figer A, De Greve J, Douillard JY, Lathia C, Schwartz B, Taylor I, Moscovici M, Saltz LB. Phase II study of sorafenib in patients with advanced hepatocellular carcinoma. J Clin Oncol 2006;24(26):4293–4300.

55. Llovet J, Ricci S, Mazzaferro V, Hilgard P, Raoul J, Zeuzem S, Poulin-Costello M, Moscovici M, Voliotis D, Bruix J, for the SISG. Randomized phase III trial of sorafenib versus placebo in patients with advanced hepatocellular carcinoma (HCC). J Clin Oncol (Meeting Abstracts) 2007;25(18 Suppl):Abstr LBA1.

56. Min CJ, Liebes LF, Escalon J, Hamilton A, Yee H, Buckley MT, Wright JJ, Osman I, Polsky D, Pavlick AC. Phase II trial of sorafenib (S [BAY 43-9006]) in metastatic melanoma (MM) including detection of BRAF with mutant specific-PCR (MS-PCR) and altered proliferation pathways—final outcome analysis. J Clin Oncol (Meeting Abstracts) 2008;26(15 Suppl):Abstr 9072.

57. Herbst RS, Sandler AB. Non-small cell lung cancer and antiangiogenic therapy: what can be expected of bevacizumab? Oncologist 2004;9(Suppl 1):19–26.

58. Wedge SR, Ogilvie DJ, Dukes M, Kendrew J, Chester R, Jackson JA, Boffey SJ, Valentine PJ, Curwen JO, Musgrove HL, Graham GA, Hughes GD, Thomas AP, Stokes ES, Curry B, Richmond GH, Wadsworth PF, Bigley AL, Hennequin LF. ZD6474 inhibits vascular endothelial growth factor signaling, angiogenesis, and tumor growth following oral administration. Cancer Res 2002;62(16):4645–4655.

59. Carlomagno F, Vitagliano D, Guida T, Ciardiello F, Tortora G, Vecchio G, Ryan AJ, Fontanini G, Fusco A, Santoro M. ZD6474, an orally available inhibitor of KDR tyrosine kinase activity, efficiently blocks oncogenic RET kinases. Cancer Res 2002;62(24):7284–7290.

60. Conrad C, Ischenko I, Kohl G, Wiegand U, Guba M, Yezhelyev M, Ryan AJ, Barge A, Geissler EK, Wedge SR, Jauch KW, Bruns CJ. Antiangiogenic and antitumor activity of a novel vascular endothelial growth factor receptor-2 tyrosine kinase inhibitor ZD6474 in a metastatic human pancreatic tumor model. Anticancer Drugs 2007;18(5):569–579.

61. Bianco C, Giovannetti E, Ciardiello F, Mey V, Nannizzi S, Tortora G, Troiani T, Pasqualetti F, Eckhardt G, de Liguoro M, Ricciardi S, Del Tacca M, Raben D, Cionini L, Danesi R. Synergistic antitumor activity of ZD6474, an inhibitor of vascular endothelial growth factor receptor and epidermal growth factor receptor signaling, with gemcitabine and ionizing radiation against pancreatic cancer. Clin Cancer Res 2006;12(23):7099–7107.

62. Williams KJ, Telfer BA, Brave S, Kendrew J, Whittaker L, Stratford IJ, Wedge SR. ZD6474, a potent inhibitor of vascular endothelial growth factor signaling, combined with radiotherapy: schedule-dependent enhancement of antitumor activity. Clin Cancer Res 2004;10(24):8587–8593.

63. Shibuya K, Komaki R, Shintani T, Itasaka S, Ryan A, Jurgensmeier JM, Milas L, Ang K, Herbst RS, O'Reilly MS. Targeted therapy against VEGFR and EGFR with ZD6474 enhances the therapeutic efficacy of irradiation in an orthotopic model of human non-small-cell lung cancer. Int J Radiat Oncol Biol Phys 2007;69(5):1534–1543.

64. Gustafson DL, Frederick B, Merz AL, Raben D. Dose scheduling of the dual VEGFR and EGFR tyrosine kinase inhibitor vandetanib (ZD6474, Zactima) in combination with radiotherapy in EGFR-positive and EGFR-null human head and neck tumor xenografts. Cancer Chemother Pharmacol 2008;61(2):179–188.

65. Damiano V, Melisi D, Bianco C, Raben D, Caputo R, Fontanini G, Bianco R, Ryan A, Bianco AR, De Placido S, Ciardiello F, Tortora G. Cooperative antitumor effect of multitargeted kinase inhibitor ZD6474 and ionizing radiation in glioblastoma. Clin Cancer Res 2005;11(15):5639–5644.

66. Brazelle WD, Shi W, Siemann DW. VEGF-associated tyrosine kinase inhibition increases the tumor response to single and fractionated dose radiotherapy. Int J Radiat Oncol Biol Phys 2006;65(3):836–841.

67. Takahashi M, Ritz J, Cooper GM. Activation of a novel human transforming gene, ret, by DNA rearrangement. Cell 1985;42(2):581–588.

68. Ogino H, Yano S, Kakiuchi S, Yamada T, Ikuta K, Nakataki E, Goto H, Hanibuchi M, Nishioka Y, Ryan A, Sone S. Novel dual targeting strategy with vandetanib induces tumor cell apoptosis and inhibits angiogenesis in malignant pleural mesothelioma cells expressing RET oncogenic rearrangement. Cancer Lett 2008;265(1):55–66.

69. Holden SN, Eckhardt SG, Basser R, de Boer R, Rischin D, Green M, Rosenthal MA, Wheeler C, Barge A, Hurwitz HI. Clinical evaluation of ZD6474, an orally active inhibitor of VEGF and EGF receptor signaling, in patients with solid, malignant tumors. Ann Oncol 2005;16(8):1391–1397.

70. Mainami H, Eibi H, Thara Y, Sasaki N, Yamamoto Y, Yamada T, Tamura T, Saijo N. A phase I trial of an oral VEGF receptor tyrosine kinase inhibitor ZD6474, in Japanese patients with solid tumors. Proc Am Soc Clin Oncol 2003;24:Abstr 7062.

71. Natale RB, Bodkin D, Govindan R, Sleckman B, Rizvi N, Capo A, Germonpre P, Stockman P, Kennedy S, Ranson M. ZD6474 versus gefitinib in patients with advanced NSCLC: final results from a two-part, double-blind, randomized phase II trial. J Clin Oncol (Meeting Abstracts) 2006;24(18 Suppl):Abstr 7000.

72. Heymach JV, Johnson BE, Prager D, Csada E, Roubec J, Pesek M, Spasova I, Belani CP, Bodrogi I, Gadgeel S, Kennedy SJ, Hou J, Herbst RS. Randomized, placebo-controlled phase II study of vandetanib plus docetaxel in previously treated non small-cell lung cancer. J Clin Oncol 2007;25(27):4270–4277.

73. Heymach JV, Johnson BE, Prager D, Csada E, Roubec J, Pesek M, Spasova I, Hou J, Kennedy S, Herbst RS. A phase II trial of ZD6474 plus docetaxel in patients with previously treated NSCLC: follow-up results. J Clin Oncol (Meeting Abstracts) 2006;24(18 Suppl):Abstr 7016.

74. Hanrahan EO, Lin HY, Du DZ, Yan S, Kim ES, Lee JJ, Ryan AJ, Tran HT, Johnson BE, Heymach JV. Correlative analyses of plasma cytokine/angiogenic factor (C/AF) profile, gender and outcome in a randomized, three-arm, phase II trial of first-line vandetanib (VAN) and/or carboplatin plus paclitaxel (CP) for advanced non-small cell lung cancer (NSCLC). J Clin Oncol (Meeting Abstracts) 2007;25(18 Suppl):Abstr 7593.

75. Heymach J, Paz-Ares L, De Braud F, Sebastian M, Stewart DJ, Eberhardt W, Herbst RS, Krebs A, Langmuir P, Johnson BE. Randomized phase II study of vandetanib (VAN) alone or in combination with carboplatin and paclitaxel (CP) as first-line treatment for advanced non-small cell lung cancer (NSCLC). J Clin Oncol (Meeting Abstracts) 2007;25(18 Suppl):Abstr 7544.

76. Arnold AM, Seymour L, Smylie M, Ding K, Ung Y, Findlay B, Lee CW, Djurfeldt M, Whitehead M, Ellis P, Goss G, Chan A, Meharchand J, Alam Y, Gregg R, Butts C, Langmuir P, Shepherd F. Phase II study of vandetanib or placebo in small-cell lung cancer patients after complete or partial response to induction chemotherapy with or without radiation therapy: National Cancer Institute of Canada Clinical Trials Group Study BR.20. J Clin Oncol 2007;25(27):4278–4284.

77. Miller KD, Trigo JM, Wheeler C, Barge A, Rowbottom J, Sledge G, Baselga J. A multicenter phase II trial of ZD6474, a vascular endothelial growth factor receptor-2 and epidermal growth factor receptor tyrosine kinase inhibitor, in patients with previously treated metastatic breast cancer. Clin Cancer Res 2005;11(9):3369–3376.

78. Kovacs MJ, Reece DE, Marcellus D, Meyer RM, Matthews S, Dong R-P, Eisenhauer E. A phase II study of ZD6474, a vascular endothelial growth factor receptor (VEGFR) and epidermal growth factor receptor (EGFR) tyrosine kinase inhibitor (TKI) in patients with relapsed multiple myeloma (MM). ASH Annual Meeting Abstracts 2004;104(11):Abstr 3464.

79. Haddad RI, Krebs AD, Vasselli J, Paz-Ares LG, Robinson B. A phase II open-label study of vandetanib in patients with locally advanced or metastatic hereditary medullary thyroid cancer. J Clin Oncol (Meeting Abstracts) 2008; 26(15 Suppl):Abstr 6024.

80. Kumar R, Knick VB, Rudolph SK, Johnson JH, Crosby RM, Crouthamel MC, Hopper TM, Miller CG, Harrington LE, Onori JA, Mullin RJ, Gilmer TM, Truesdale AT, Epperly AH, Boloor A, Stafford JA, Luttrell DK, Cheung M. Pharmacokinetic–pharmacodynamic correlation from mouse to human with pazopanib, a multikinase angiogenesis inhibitor with potent antitumor and antiangiogenic activity. Mol Cancer Ther 2007;6(7):2012–2021.

81. Podar K, Tonon G, Sattler M, Tai YT, Legouill S, Yasui H, Ishitsuka K, Kumar S, Kumar R, Pandite LN, Hideshima T, Chauhan D, Anderson KC. The small-molecule VEGF receptor inhibitor pazopanib (GW786034B) targets both tumor and endothelial cells in multiple myeloma. Proc Natl Acad Sci U S A 2006;103(51):19478–19483.

82. Hutson TE, Davis ID, Machiels JH, de Souza PL, Baker K, Bordogna W, Westlund R, Crofts T, Pandite L, Figlin RA. Biomarker analysis and final efficacy and safety results of a phase II renal cell carcinoma trial with pazopanib (GW786034), a multi-kinase angiogenesis inhibitor. J Clin Oncol (Meeting Abstracts) 2008;26(15 Suppl):Abstr 5046.

83. Polverino A, Coxon A, Starnes C, Diaz Z, DeMelfi T, Wang L, Bready J, Estrada J, Cattley R, Kaufman S, Chen D, Gan Y, Kumar G, Meyer J, Neervannan S, Alva G, Talvenheimo J, Montestruque S, Tasker A, Patel V, Radinsky R, Kendall R. AMG 706, an oral, multikinase inhibitor that selectively targets vascular endothelial growth factor, platelet-derived growth factor, and kit receptors, potently inhibits angiogenesis and induces regression in tumor xenografts. Cancer Res 2006;66(17):8715–8721.

84. Rosen LS, Kurzrock R, Mulay M, Van Vugt A, Purdom M, Ng C, Silverman J, Koutsoukos A, Sun YN, Bass MB, Xu RY, Polverino A, Wiezorek JS, Chang DD, Benjamin R, Herbst RS. Safety, pharmacokinetics, and efficacy of AMG 706, an oral multikinase inhibitor, in patients with advanced solid tumors. J Clin Oncol 2007;25(17):2369–2376.

85. Sherman SI, Schlumberger MJ, Droz J, Hoffmann M, Wirth L, Bastholt L, Martins RG, Licitra L, Shi Y, Stepan DE. Initial results from a phase II trial of motesanib diphosphate (AMG 706) in patients with differentiated thyroid cancer (DTC). J Clin Oncol (Meeting Abstracts) 2007;25(18 Suppl):Abstr 6017.

86. Wedge SR, Kendrew J, Hennequin LF, Valentine PJ, Barry ST, Brave SR, Smith NR, James NH, Dukes M, Curwen JO, Chester R, Jackson JA, Boffey SJ, Kilburn LL, Barnett S, Richmond GH, Wadsworth PF, Walker M, Bigley AL, Taylor ST, Cooper L, Beck S, Jurgensmeier JM, Ogilvie DJ. AZD2171: a highly potent, orally bioavailable, vascular endothelial growth factor receptor-2 tyrosine kinase inhibitor for the treatment of cancer. Cancer Res 2005;65(10):4389–4400.

87. Drevs J, Esser N, Wedge S, Ogilvie D, Marme D. Effect of AZD2171, a highly potent VEGF receptor tyrosine kinase inhibitor, on primary tumor growth, metastasis and vessel density in murine renal cell carcinoma. Proc Am Assoc Cancer Res 2004;45:Abstr 4554.

88. Cao C, Albert JM, Geng L, Ivy PS, Sandler A, Johnson DH, Lu B. Vascular endothelial growth factor tyrosine kinase inhibitor AZD2171 and fractionated radiotherapy in mouse models of lung cancer. Cancer Res 2006;66(23): 11409–11415.

89. Denduluri N, Tan AR, Walshe J, Berman A, Yang SX, Chow CK, Swain SM. A pilot study to evaluate the vascular endothelial growth factor receptor tyrosine kinase inhibitor AZD2171 and chemotherapy in locally advanced and inflammatory breast cancer. Clin Breast Cancer 2005;6(5):460–463.

90. Furutani K, Komaki R, Imagumbai T, Onn A, Jacoby J, Massarelli E, Korshunova M, Ryan A, Jurgensmeier J, Herbst R, O'Reilly M. Targeted therapy against VEGFR-1,-2 and -3 by AZD2171 blocks tumor growth and angiogenesis, and enhances paclitaxel efficacy in an orthotopic lung cancer model. AACR Meeting Abstracts 2007 (98th Annual Meeting, Los Angeles, CA): 2121.

91. Dragoi AM, Fu X, Ivanov S, Zhang P, Sheng L, Wu D, Li GC, Chu WM. DNA-PKcs, but not TLR9, is required for activation of Akt by CpG-DNA. EMBO J 2005;24(4):779–789.

92. Drevs J, Siegert P, Medinger M, Mross K, Strecker R, Zirrgiebel U, Harder J, Blum H, Robertson J, Jurgensmeier JM, Puchalski TA, Young H, Saunders O, Unger C. Phase I clinical study of AZD2171, an oral vascular endothelial growth factor signaling inhibitor, in patients with advanced solid tumors. J Clin Oncol 2007;25(21):3045–3054.

93. Alberts S, Morlan B, Kim G, Pitot H, Quevedo F, Dakhil S, Gross H, Merchan J, Roberts L. NCCTG phase II trial (N044J) of AZD2171 for patients with hepatocellular carcinoma (HCC)–interim review of toxicity. Proceedings of the 2007 Gastrointestinal Cancers Symposium, Orlando, FL, January 19–21 2007:Abstract 186.

94. Sridhar SS, Hotte SJ, Mackenzie MJ, Kollmannsberger C, Haider MA, Pond GR, Chen EX, Srinivasan R, Ivy SP, Moore MJ. Phase II study of the angiogenesis inhibitor AZD2171 in first line, progressive, unresectable, advanced metastatic renal cell carcinoma (RCC): a trial of the PMH Phase II Consortium. J Clin Oncol (Meeting Abstracts) 2007;25(18 Suppl):Abstr 5093.

95. Ryan CJ, Stadler WM, Roth B, Hutcheon D, Conry S, Puchalski T, Morris C, Small EJ. Phase I dose escalation and pharmacokinetic study of AZD2171, an inhibitor of the vascular endothelial growth factor receptor tyrosine kinase, in patients with hormone refractory prostate cancer (HRPC). Invest New Drugs 2007;25(5):445–451.

96. Laurie SA, Gauthier I, Arnold A, Shepherd FA, Ellis PM, Chen E, Goss G, Powers J, Walsh W, Tu D, Robertson J, Puchalski TA, Seymour L. Phase I and pharmacokinetic study of daily oral AZD2171, an inhibitor of vascular endothelial growth factor tyrosine kinases, in combination with carboplatin and paclitaxel in patients with advanced non-small-cell

lung cancer: the National Cancer Institute of Canada clinical trials group. J Clin Oncol 2008;26(11):1871–1878.

97. Goss GD, Laurie S, Shepherd F, Leighl N, Chen E, Gauthier I, Reaume N, Feld R, Powers J, Seymour L. IND.175: phase I study of daily oral AZD2171, a vascular endothelial growth factor receptor inhibitor (VEGFRI), in combination with gemcitabine and cisplatin (G/C) in patients with advanced non-small cell lung cancer (ANSCLC): a study of the NCIC Clinical Trials Group. J Clin Oncol (Meeting Abstracts) 2007;25(18 Suppl):Abstr 7649.

98. Shields AF, Heath E, DeLuca P, Pilat M, Wozniak A, Gadgeel S, Puchalski T, Xu J, Liu Q, LoRusso P. AZD2171 in combination with various anticancer regimens: follow-up results of a phase I multi-cohort study. J Clin Oncol (Meeting Abstracts) 2007;25(18 Suppl):Abstr 3544.

99. Hirte HW, Vidal L, Fleming GF, Sugimoto AK, Morgan RJ, Biagi JJ, Wang L, McGill S, Ivy SP, Oza AM. A phase II study of cediranib (AZD2171) in recurrent or persistent ovarian, peritoneal or fallopian tube cancer: final results of a PMH, Chicago and California consortia trial. J Clin Oncol (Meeting Abstracts) 2008;26(15 Suppl):Abstr 5521.

100. Matulonis UA, Berlin ST, Krasner CN, Tyburski K, Lee J, Roche M, Ivy SP, Lenahan C, King M, Penson RT. Cediranib (AZD2171) is an active agent in recurrent epithelial ovarian cancer. J Clin Oncol (Meeting Abstracts) 2008;26(15 Suppl):Abstr 5501.

101. Sridhar SS, Mackenzie MJ, Hotte SJ, Mukherjee SD, Kollmannsberger C, Haider MA, Chen EX, Wang L, Srinivasan R, Ivy SP, Moore MJ. Activity of cediranib (AZD2171) in patients (pts) with previously untreated metastatic renal cell cancer (RCC). A phase II trial of the PMH Consortium. J Clin Oncol (Meeting Abstracts) 2008;26(15 Suppl):Abstr 5047.

102. Karakunnel JJ, Gulley JL, Arlen PM, Mulquin M, Wright JJ, Turkbey IB, Choyke P, Ahlers CM, Figg WD, Dahut WL. Phase II trial of cediranib (AZD2171) in docetaxel-resistant, castrate-resistant prostate cancer (CRPC). J Clin Oncol (Meeting Abstracts) 2008;26(15 Suppl):Abstr 5136.

103. Batchelor T, Sorensen G, Di Tomaso E, Duda D, Zhang W, Ancukiewicz M, Lahdenranta J, Louis DN, Plotkin S, Ivy P, Loeffler JS, Wen PY, Jain RK. A multidisciplinary phase II study of AZD2171 (cediranib), an oral pan-VEGF receptor tyrosine kinase inhibitor, in patients with recurrent glioblastoma. In: Proceedings of the 99th Annual Meeting of the American Society for Cancer Research, April 12–16, San Diego, CA, 2008:Abstr LB-247.

104. Ramalingam SS, Mack PC, Vokes EE, Longmate J, Govindan R, Koczywas M, Ivy SP, Belani CP, Gandara DR. Cediranib (AZD2171) for the treatment of recurrent small cell lung cancer (SCLC): A California Consortium phase II study (NCI # 7097). J Clin Oncol (Meeting Abstracts) 2008;26(15 Suppl):Abstr 8078.

105. Hu-Lowe D, Hallin M, Feeley R, Zhou H, Rewolinski D, Wickman G, Chen E, Kim YG, Riney S, Reed J, Heller D, Simmons B, Kania R, McTigue M, Neisman M, Gregory S, Shalinsky D, Bender S. Characterization of potency and activity of the VEGF/PDGF receptor tyrosine kinase inhibitor AG013736. Proceedings of the American Association of Cancer Research 2002;43:Abstr 5356.

106. Guo J, Marcotte PA, McCall JO, Dai Y, Pease LJ, Michaelides MR, Davidsen SK, Glaser KB. Inhibition of phosphorylation of the colony-stimulating factor-1 receptor (c-Fms) tyrosine kinase in transfected cells by ABT-869 and other tyrosine kinase inhibitors. Mol Cancer Ther 2006;5(4):1007–1013.

107. Wickman G, Hallin M, Amundson K, Acena A, Grazzini M, Dillon R, Herrmann M, Vekich S, Bender S, Shalinksy D, Hu-Lowe D. Further characterization of the potent VEGF/PDGF receptor tyrosine kinase inhibitor AG-013736 in preclinical tumor models for its antiangiogenesis and antitumor activity. Proceedings of the American Association of Cancer Research 2003;44:Abstr 3780.

108. Rugo HS, Herbst RS, Liu G, Park JW, Kies MS, Steinfeldt HM, Pithavala YK, Reich SD, Freddo JL, Wilding G. Phase I trial of the oral antiangiogenesis agent AG-013736 in patients with advanced solid tumors: pharmacokinetic and clinical results. J Clin Oncol 2005;23(24):5474–5483.

109. Rixe O, Bukowski RM, Michaelson MD, Wilding G, Hudes GR, Bolte O, Motzer RJ, Bycott P, Liau KF, Freddo J, Trask PC, Kim S, Rini BI. Axitinib treatment in patients with cytokine-refractory metastatic renal-cell cancer: a phase II study. Lancet Oncol 2007;8(11):975–984.

110. Dutcher JP, Wilding G, Hudes GR, Stadler WM, Kim S, Tarazi JC, Rosbrook B, Rini BI. Sequential axitinib (AG-013736) therapy of patients (pts) with metastatic clear cell renal cell cancer (RCC) refractory to sunitinib and sorafenib, cytokines and sorafenib, or sorafenib alone. J Clin Oncol (Meeting Abstracts) 2008;26(15 Suppl):Abstr 5127.

111. Kim S, Rosen LS, Cohen EE, Cohen RB, Forastiere A, Silva AM, Liau KF, Archer RL, Bycott P, Vokes EE. A phase II study of axitinib (AG-013736), a potent inhibitor of VEGFRs, in patients with advanced thyroid cancer. J Clin Oncol (Meeting Abstracts) 2006;24(18 Suppl):Abstr 5529.

112. Cohen EE, Vokes EE, Rosen LS, Kies MS, Forastiere AA, Worden FP, Kane MA, Liau KF, Shalinsky DR, Cohen RB. A phase II study of axitinib (AG-013736 [AG]) in patients (pts) with advanced thyroid cancers. J Clin Oncol (Meeting Abstracts) 2007;25(18 Suppl):Abstr 6008.

113. Spano J, Chodkiewicz C, Maurel J, Wong RP, Wasan HS, Pithavala YK, Bycott PW, Liau K, Kim S, Rixe O. A randomized phase II study of axitinib (AG-013736) and gemcitabine versus gemcitabine in advanced pancreatic cancer, preceded by a phase I component. J Clin Oncol (Meeting Abstracts) 2007;25(18 Suppl):Abstr 4551.

114. Schiller JH, Larson T, Ou SI, Limentani SA, Sandler AB, Vokes EE, Kim S, Liau KF, Bycott PW, Olszanski AJ. Efficacy and safety of axitinib (AG-013736; AG) in patients (pts) with advanced non-small cell lung cancer (NSCLC): a phase II trial. J Clin Oncol (Meeting Abstracts) 2007;25(18 Suppl):Abstr 7507.

115. Fruehauf JP, Lutzky J, McDermott DF, Brown CK, Pithavala YK, Bycott PW, Shalinsky D, Liau KF, Niethammer A, Rixe O. Axitinib (AG-013736) in patients with metastatic melanoma: a phase II study. J Clin Oncol (Meeting Abstracts) 2008;26(15 Suppl):Abstr 9006.

116. Giles FJ, Bellamy WT, Estrov Z, O'Brien SM, Verstovsek S, Ravandi F, Beran M, Bycott P, Pithavala Y, Steinfeldt H, Reich SD, List AF, Yee KW. The anti-angiogenesis agent, AG-013736, has minimal activity in elderly patients with poor prognosis acute myeloid leukemia (AML) or myelodysplastic syndrome (MDS). Leuk Res 2006;30(7):801–811.

117. Wood JM, Bold G, Buchdunger E, Cozens R, Ferrari S, Frei J, Hofmann F, Mestan J, Mett H, O'Reilly T, Persohn E, Rosel J, Schnell C, Stover D, Theuer A, Towbin H, Wenger F, Woods-Cook K, Menrad A, Siemeister G, Schirner M, Thierauch KH, Schneider MR, Drevs J, Martiny-Baron G, Totzke F. PTK787/ZK 222584, a novel and potent inhibitor of vascular endothelial growth factor receptor tyrosine kinases, impairs vascular endothelial growth factor-induced responses and tumor growth after oral administration. Cancer Res 2000;60(8):2178–2189.

118. Hecht JR, Trarbach T, Jaeger E, Hainsworth J, Wolff R, Lloyd K, Bodoky G, Borner M, Laurent D, Jacques C. A randomized, double-blind, placebo-controlled, phase III study in patients (pts) with metastatic adenocarcinoma of the colon or rectum receiving first-line chemotherapy with oxaliplatin/5-fluorouracil/leucovorin and PTK787/ZK 222584 or placebo (CONFIRM-1). J Clin Oncol (Meeting Abstracts) 2005;23(16 Suppl):Abstr LBA3.

119. Kohne C, Bajetta E, Lin E, Valle JW, Van Cutsem E, Hecht JR, Moore M, Germond CJ, Meinhardt G, Jacques C. Final results of CONFIRM 2: a multinational, randomized, double-blind, phase III study in 2nd line patients (pts) with metastatic colorectal cancer (mCRC) receiving FOLFOX4 and PTK787/ZK 222584 (PTK/ZK) or placebo. J Clin Oncol (Meeting Abstracts) 2007;25(18 Suppl):Abstr 4033.

120. Bhide RS, Cai ZW, Zhang YZ, Qian L, Wei D, Barbosa S, Lombardo LJ, Borzilleri RM, Zheng X, Wu LI, Barrish JC, Kim SH, Leavitt K, Mathur A, Leith L, Chao S, Wautlet B, Mortillo S, Jeyaseelan R Sr, Kukral D, Hunt JT, Kamath A, Fura A, Vyas V, Marathe P, D'Arienzo C, Derbin G, Fargnoli J. Discovery and preclinical studies of (R)-1-(4-(4-fluoro-2-methyl-1H-indol-5-yloxy)-5-methylpyrrolo[2,1-f][1,2,4]triazin-6-yloxy)propan-2-ol (BMS-540215), an in vivo active potent VEGFR-2 inhibitor. J Med Chem 2006;49(7):2143–2146.

121. Cai ZW, Zhang Y, Borzilleri RM, Qian L, Barbosa S, Wei D, Zheng X, Wu L, Fan J, Shi Z, Wautlet BS, Mortillo S, Jeyaseelan R Sr, Kukral DW, Kamath A, Marathe P, D'Arienzo C, Derbin G, Barrish JC, Robl JA, Hunt JT, Lombardo LJ, Fargnoli J, Bhide RS. Discovery of brivanib alaninate ((S)-((R)-1-(4-(4-fluoro-2-methyl-1H-indol-5-yloxy)-5-methylpyrrolo[2,1-f] [1,2,4]triazin-6-yloxy)propan-2-yl)2-aminopropanoate), a novel prodrug of dual vascular endothelial growth factor receptor-2 and fibroblast growth factor receptor-1 kinase inhibitor (BMS-540215). J Med Chem 2008;51(6):1976–1980.

122. Garrett CR, Siu LL, Giaccone G, El-Khoueiry A, Marshall J, LoRusso P, Velasquez L, Kollia G, He P, Feltquate D. A phase I study of BMS-582664 (brivanib alaninate), an oral dual inhibitor of VEGFR and FGFR tyrosine kinases, in combination with full-dose cetuximab in patients (pts) with advanced gastrointestinal malignancies (AGM) who failed prior therapy. ASCO Meeting Abstracts 2007;25(18 Suppl):Abstr 14018.

123. Garrett CR, Siu LL, El-Khoueiry AB, Buter J, Rocha-Lima CM, Marshall JL, Kollia G, Velasquez L, Syed S, Feltquate D. A phase I study of brivanib alaninate (BMS-582664), an oral dual inhibitor of VEGFR and FGFR tyrosine kinases, in combination with full dose cetuximab (BC) in patients (pts) with advanced gastrointestinal malignancies (AGM) who failed prior therapy. ASCO Meeting Abstracts 2008;26(15 Suppl):Abstr 4111.

124. Krystal GW, Honsawek S, Kiewlich D, Liang C, Vasile S, Sun L, McMahon G, Lipson KE. Indolinone tyrosine kinase inhibitors block Kit activation and growth of small cell lung cancer cells. Cancer Res 2001;61(9):3660–3668.

125. Laird AD, Christensen JG, Li G, Carver J, Smith K, Xin X, Moss KG, Louie SG, Mendel DB, Cherrington JM. SU6668 inhibits Flk-1/KDR and PDGFR beta in vivo, resulting in rapid apoptosis of tumor vasculature and tumor regression in mice. FASEB J 2002;16(7):681–690.

126. Laird AD, Vajkoczy P, Shawver LK, Thurnher A, Liang C, Mohammadi M, Schlessinger J, Ullrich A, Hubbard SR, Blake RA, Fong TA, Strawn LM, Sun L, Tang C, Hawtin R, Tang F, Shenoy N, Hirth KP, McMahon G, Cherrington. SU6668 is a potent antiangiogenic and antitumor agent that induces regression of established tumors. Cancer Res 2000;60(15):4152–4160.

127. Godl K, Gruss OJ, Eickhoff J, Wissing J, Blencke S, Weber M, Degen H, Brehmer D, Orfi L, Horvath Z, Keri G, Muller S, Cotten M, Ullrich A, Daub H. Proteomic characterization of the angiogenesis inhibitor SU6668 reveals multiple impacts on cellular kinase signaling. Cancer Res 2005;65(15):6919–6926.

128. Huang X, Wong MK, Yi H, Watkins S, Laird AD, Wolf SF, Gorelik E. Combined therapy of local and metastatic 4T1 breast tumor in mice using SU6668, an inhibitor of angiogenic receptor tyrosine kinases, and the immunostimulator B7.2-IgG fusion protein. Cancer Res 2002;62(20):5727–5735.

129. Machida S, Saga Y, Takei Y, Mizuno I, Takayama T, Kohno T, Konno R, Ohwada M, Suzuki M. Inhibition of peritoneal dissemination of ovarian cancer by tyrosine kinase receptor inhibitor SU6668 (TSU-68). Int J Cancer 2005;114(2):224–229.

130. Yorozuya K, Kubota T, Watanabe M, Hasegawa H, Ozawa S, Kitajima M, Chikahisa LM, Yamada Y. TSU-68 (SU6668) inhibits local tumor growth and liver metastasis of human colon cancer xenografts via anti-angiogenesis. Oncol Rep 2005;14(3):677–682.

131. Kitamura R, Asanoma H, Nagayama S, Otagiri M. Identification of human liver cytochrome P450 isoforms involved in autoinduced metabolism of the antiangiogenic agent (Z)-5-[(1,2-dihydro-2-oxo-3H-indol-3-ylidene)methyl]-2,4-dimethyl-1H-pyrrole-3-propanoic acid (TSU-68). Drug Metab Dispos 2008;36(6):1003–1009.

132. Witteveen P, Langenberg M, Verheul HM, Roodhart J, Roelvink M, van der Sar J, Brendel E, Laferriere N, Schellens JH, Voest EE. Phase I evaluation of telatinib, a VEGF receptor tyrosine kinase inhibitor, in combination with irinotecan and capecitabine in patients with advanced solid tumors. J Clin Oncol (Meeting Abstracts) 2008;26(15 Suppl):Abstr 2530.

133. Hilberg F, Roth GJ, Krssak M, Kautschitsch S, Sommergruber W, Tontsch-Grunt U, Garin-Chesa P, Bader G, Zoephel A, Quant J, Heckel A, Rettig WJ. BIBF 1120: triple angiokinase inhibitor with sustained receptor blockade and good antitumor efficacy. Cancer Res 2008;68(12):4774–4782.

134. Hilberg F, Tontsch-Grunt U, Colbatzky F, Heckel A, Lotz R, van Meel J, Roth G. BIBF1120 a novel, small molecule triple angiokinase inhibitor: profiling as a clinical candidate for cancer therapy. Eur J Cancer Suppl 2004;2:32– (Abstr 158).

135. Lee CP, Attard G, Poupard L, Nathan PD, de Bono JS, Temple GMR, Stefanic MF, Padhani AR, Judson IR, Rustin GJ. A phase I study of BIBF 1120, an orally active triple angiokinase inhibitor (VEGFR, PDGFR, FGFR) in patients with advanced solid malignancies. J Clin Oncol (Meeting Abstracts) 2005;23(16 Suppl):Abstr 3054.

136. Mross KB, Gmehling D, Frost A, Baas F, Strecker R, Hennig J, Stopfer P, Stefanic M, Stehle G, de Rossi L. A clinical phase I, pharmacokinetic (PK), and pharmacodynamic study of twice daily BIBF 1120 in advanced cancer patients. J Clin Oncol (Meeting Abstracts) 2005;23(16 Suppl):Abstr 3031.

137. von Pawel J, Kaiser R, Eschbach C, Love J, Staab A, Freiwald M, Bruno R, Stopfer P, Gatzemeier U, Reck M. Efficacy, safety and pharmacokinetic (PK) results of a phase II study with the triple angiokinase inhibitor BIBF 1120 in patients suffering from advanced non-small cell lung cancer (NSCLC). J Thorac Oncol 2008;3(4) Suppl 1: S9–S98, April 2008 (Abstr 1630).

138. Patyna S, Laird AD, Mendel DB, O'Farrell A M, Liang C, Guan H, Vojkovsky T, Vasile S, Wang X, Chen J, Grazzini M, Yang CY, Haznedar JO, Sukbuntherng J, Zhong WZ, Cherrington JM, Hu-Lowe D. SU14813: a novel multiple receptor tyrosine kinase inhibitor with potent antiangiogenic and antitumor activity. Mol Cancer Ther 2006;5(7):1774–1782.

139. Fiedler WM, Giaccone G, Lasch P, Van der Horst I, Brega NM, Raber S, Shalinsky D, Ljubmir V, Bokemeyer C, Boven E, Pfizer AST. Phase I trial of SU014813 in patients (pts) with advanced solid malignancies. J Clin Oncol (Meeting Abstracts) 2007;25(18 Suppl):Abstr 3521.

140. Schoffski P, de Jonge M, Dumez H, Brega NM, Abbattista A, Courtney R, Verweij J. Phase I safety and pharmacokinetic (PK) study of SU014813 (S) in combination with docetaxel (D) in patients (pts) with solid tumors (STs). J Clin Oncol (Meeting Abstracts) 2008;26(15 Suppl):Abstr 3554.

141. Albert DH, Tapang P, Magoc TJ, Pease LJ, Reuter DR, Wei RQ, Li J, Guo J, Bousquet PF, Ghoreishi-Haack NS, Wang B, Bukofzer GT, Wang YC, Stavropoulos JA, Hartandi K, Niquette AL, Soni N, Johnson EF, McCall JO, Bouska JJ, Luo Y, Donawho CK, Dai Y, Marcotte PA, Glaser KB, Michaelides MR, Davidsen SK. Preclinical activity of ABT-869, a multitargeted receptor tyrosine kinase inhibitor. Mol Cancer Ther 2006;5(4):995–1006.

142. Soo RA, McKeegan E, Chen CS, Thng CH, Koh TS, Laird D, Zhang K, Wong CI, Gupta N, Goh BC. The effect of varying doses of ABT-869 on biomarkers of angiogenesis and their correlation with pharmacodynamic outcome. J Clin Oncol (Meeting Abstracts) 2008;26(15 Suppl):Abstr 14535.

143. Eskens F, De Jong M, Esteves B, Cotreau M, Bhargava P, Ryan JJ, Van Doorn L, Isoe T, Hayashi K, Ekman, L, Burger H, Verweij J. Updated results from a phase I study of AV-951 (KRN951), a potent and selective VEGFR-1,2, and 3 tyrosine kinase inhibitor, in patients with advanced solid tumors. AACR Annual Meeting, April 12–16, 2008 San Diego, CA, Abstr LB-201.

144. Beebe JS, Jani JP, Knauth E, Goodwin P, Higdon C, Rossi AM, Emerson E, Finkelstein M, Floyd E, Harriman S, Atherton J, Hillerman S, Soderstrom C, Kou K, Gant T, Noe MC, Foster B, Rastinejad F, Marx MA, Schaeffer T, Whalen PM, Roberts WG. Pharmacological characterization of CP-547,632, a novel vascular endothelial growth factor receptor-2 tyrosine kinase inhibitor for cancer therapy. Cancer Res 2003;63(21):7301–7309.

145. Tolcher A, O'Leary J, DeBono J, Caulkins J, Moplus K, Sutula K, Ferrante K, Gualberto A, Noe D, Huberman M, Rowinsky E, Healey D. A phase I and biologic correlative study of an oral vascular endothelial growth factor receptor-2 (VEGFR-2) tyrosine kinase inhibitor, CP-547,632, in patients (pts) with advanced solid tumors. Proc Am Soc Clin Oncol 2002;21:Abstr 334.

146. Cohen RB, Simon G, Langer CJ, Schol JR, McHale J, Eisenberg P, Hainsworth JD, Liau KF, Healey D. Phase I trial of oral CP-547,632 (VEGFR2) in combination with paclitaxel (P) and carboplatin (C) in advanced non-small cell lung cancer (NSCLC). J Clin Oncol (Meeting Abstracts) 2004;22(14 Suppl):Abstr 3014.

147. Cohen RB, Langer CJ, Simon GR, Eisenberg PD, Hainsworth JD, Madajewicz S, Cosgriff TM, Pierce K, Xu H, Liau K, Healey D. A phase I/randomized phase II, non-comparative, multicenter, open label trial of CP-547,632 in combination with paclitaxel and carboplatin or paclitaxel and carboplatin alone as first-line treatment for advanced non-small cell lung cancer (NSCLC). Cancer Chemother Pharmacol 2007;60(1):81–89.

CHAPTER 10

INTRACELLULAR SIGNALING KINASE INHIBITORS

INITIAL DRUG discovery efforts targeting protein kinases were directed toward inhibiting tyrosine kinase receptors or, in some cases, the nonreceptor tyrosine kinases that act as proximal effectors for various cell surface receptors. However, there is substantial rationale for targeting many intracellular kinases in downstream intracellular pathways. Many of these kinases represent convergent signaling nodes downstream of multiple cell surface receptors, so inhibiting at this level in the pathway may be more effective than blocking a single receptor and may also help to block growth of tumors with activating mutations in intracellular signaling pathways. These same intracellular pathways have been widely implicated in resistance to chemotherapy, so inhibitors may have additional utility in combination with various genotoxic agents. This is particularly the case for inhibitors of cell cycle checkpoint kinases, which specifically target a known survival mechanism for tumor cells treated with DNA-damaging agents. Furthermore, aberrant regulation of cell cycle progression and mitosis is prevalent in almost all tumor cells, and various cell cycle and mitotic kinase inhibitors may be able to directly target this hallmark of cancer. In this chapter, we survey the many inhibitors of intracellular signal transduction pathways and cell cycle kinases that are currently being evaluated in the clinic.

10.1 mTOR INHIBITORS

Most of the mTOR inhibitors (Table 10.1) currently in clinical trials are derivatives of the macrolide antibiotic rapamycin (sirolimus), which was first isolated from *Streptomyces hygroscopicus* bacteria collected in Rapa Nui (Easter Island) in the 1970s (1–3). Members of this class of drugs are sometimes referred to as "rapalogs," and all are highly specific inhibitors of the mTORC1, or mTOR:Raptor complex (Chapter 5). Their mechanism of action is somewhat distinct from that of most of the kinase inhibitors discussed here, in that they primarily bind to

---

TABLE 10.1 mTOR Inhibitors

Drug	Company	Target(s)	Structure[a]	Latest stage of development
Rapamune/sirolimus/ rapamycin	Wyeth	mTORC1	Figure 10.1	Marketed (transplant rejection)
Torisel/temsirolimus/ CCI-779	Wyeth	mTORC1	Figure 10.1	Marketed
Everolimus/RAD001	Novartis	mTORC1	Figure 10.1	Phase III
Deforolimus/AP23573/ MK-8669	Ariad/Merck	mTORC1	Figure 10.1	Phase III
ABI-009 (Nab-rapamycin)	Abraxis	mTORC1	NA	Phase I
OSI-027	OSI Pharmaceuticals	mTORC1/ mTORC2	ND	Phase I
AZD8055	Astra-Zeneca	mTORC1/ mTORC2	ND	Phase I

[a] NA, not applicable; ND, not disclosed.

mTOR in complex with the immunophilin FKBP12 (4). X-ray crystallography shows that rapamycin bridges two hydrophobic regions on FKBP12 and the FRB (FKBP12:rapamycin binding) domain of mTOR, although the proteins do not appear to associate extensively with each other (5). This interaction does not directly inhibit the catalytic activity of mTOR but promotes dissociation of Raptor and thereby inhibits the association of mTOR with specific mTOR:Raptor substrates such as p70S6 kinase and 4E-BP1 (6, 7). These effects are manifest at nanomolar concentrations in cells: however, at higher concentrations rapamycin and its analogs may also elicit effects independent of FKBP12 (although still dependent on the mTOR FRB domain). Rapamycin and CCI-779 were recently shown to directly inhibit mTOR with an IC_{50} value of 1.7 μM and inhibited cellular proliferation independent of FKBP12 (8).

Although rapamycin was first shown to have anticancer activity in the early 1980s (9), it has been developed principally as an immunosuppressive agent and was approved by the FDA in 1999 for use in preventing kidney transplant rejection (10). Rapamycin has been widely used in preclinical studies and has been shown to inhibit the growth of many cancer cell lines grown in vitro and in vivo. The majority of studies indicate that rapamycin treatment elicits a cytostatic rather than cytotoxic effect: however, tumor cell apoptosis has been observed in some cell lines and objective responses have been observed clinically following treatment with rapalogs (11). Preclinical studies have also demonstrated robust modulation of specific phosphoproteins following treatment of cells in vitro and in vivo with mTOR inhibitors. In particular, rapamycin inhibits phosphorylation of the mTOR substrates 4E-BP1 and p70S6K, downregulating translation of mRNAs involved in tumor progression (such as MYC and cyclin D1) and inducing G1 cell cycle arrest.

The antitumor activity of rapamycin may also be partly due to inhibition of tumor angiogenesis, particularly in response to hypoxia, and mTOR inhibition may have profound effects in both tumor epithelial cells and tumor vascular endothelial cells. Multiple angiogenic growth factors converge on the intracellular PI3K/mTOR signaling pathways, and mTOR can promote the translation of the hypoxia-inducible transcription factor HIF1α—which in turn enhances the expression of many of the same vascular growth factors. This may be particularly relevant in the case of tumors bearing loss of function mutations in the von Hippel–Lindau (VHL) protein, which serves to block proteaseome-mediated destruction of HIF1α and thereby causes constitutive expression of proangiogenic growth factors. Such mutations are particularly prevalent in renal cell carcinoma and may underlie the promising clinical activity seen with mTOR inhibitors in this disease (see later discussion).

One potential impediment to obtaining optimal clinical responses with mTOR inhibitors is the presence of a negative feedback mechanism within the pathway, whereby inhibition of p70S6 kinase leads to upregulation of IGF1R-dependent signaling (via the insulin receptor substrate IRS-1) leading to activation of PI3K and its downstream effectors, including AKT, and mTOR itself (Chapter 5) (12–15). Although this may often lead to increased cellular survival and proliferation via upregulation of AKT and other PI3K-dependent kinases, the overall phenotypic effect may differ widely between different cell lines and tumor types. It has been suggested that, in some cell lines, chronic treatment with rapamycin leads to eventual downregulation of AKT signaling via a mechanism involving depletion of the mTOR:Rictor (TORC2) complex (16). Furthermore, recent evidence suggests that although rapamycin produces durable inhibition of S6 phosphorylation, its effect on 4E-BP1 is more transient and enables reinitiation of protein translation (17). These potential drawbacks of rapamycin-like compounds have prompted a search for ATP-competitive mTOR inhibitors that would be expected to inhibit both the mTOR:Raptor and mTOR:Rictor complexes. Two such inhibitors have recently advanced to clinical testing: OSI-027 (OSI Pharmaceuticals) and AZD8055 (AstraZeneca), although no further details are currently available. In addition, there are several inhibitors in Phase I trials that inhibit both PI3K and mTOR. An alternative strategy to circumvent the negative feedback mechanism may be to combine rapamycin analogs with inhibitors of IGF1R signaling.

10.1.1   Clinical Pharmacodynamics and Tolerability of mTOR Inhibitors

The modulation of mTOR pathway-related molecular markers seen in preclinical models has prompted investigation of these readouts for monitoring clinical activity of mTOR inhibitors (18–21). Key readouts downstream of mTOR include p70S6K, S6 ribosomal protein, and 4E-BP1, which have variously been evaluated with each of the rapalogs currently in clinical trials. In addition, effects on AKT phosphorylation, cyclin D1, and other proteins have also been measured. One important goal of these studies has been to determine whether surrogate tissues (most commonly skin and peripheral blood mononuclear cells) can be used as markers of drug activity in tumors, and whether there is any correlation with clinical benefit. A recent study of everolimus in patients with advanced tumors evaluated the pharmacodynamic effects of various dosing regimens (5/10 mg daily, or 20/50/70 mg weekly) on a broad range of biomarkers in tumor and skin tissue (20). Inhibition of mTOR signaling was observed at all dose levels and schedules in this study, with particularly pronounced effects on phosphorylation of S6 and eIF4G (and, to a lesser extent, 4E-BP1) in both skin and tumors after 22 days/3 weeks of dosing. In the weekly dosing regimens, peIF4G inhibition was only complete and sustained at the higher dose levels. Also of note, AKT phosphorylation was upregulated (although inconsistently between samples), consistent with earlier preclinical and clinical studies and with the IGF1R-mediated feedback loop within the PI3K/mTOR/S6K pathway (Chapter 5). Other pharmacodynamic studies with everolimus have highlighted p70S6K activity in PBMCs as a surrogate tissue.

A further important technique for evaluating effects on mTOR inhibitors in vivo is [^{18}F] deoxyglucose (FDG) positron emission tomography (PET) imaging. Since mTOR is a central integrator of cellular nutrient uptake and growth factor signaling, tumors with elevated mTOR function may have particular avidity for glucose (and the radiolabeled analog FDG). In particular, many glycolytic enzymes are regulated by the HIF1α transcription factor, which is activated via mTOR in response to hypoxic conditions. Preclinical studies suggest that mTOR inhibitors can downregulate uptake of FDG into tumors, leading to a decrease in FDG signal (22–24). FDG-PET responses have also been observed clinically. For example, sarcomas exhibit high levels of metabolic activity, and FDG tumor uptake was assessed in a study of the rapalog deforolimus in sarcoma patients (25). Scans were performed on day 1 and day 5, with dosing on a schedule of once-daily for 5 days (qd × 5) every 2 weeks. Nine out of 23 patients with elevated baseline FDG uptake showed a partial metabolic response (i.e., a reduction in tumor FDG-PET signal following treatment) and 5 of these patients reported symptomatic improvement. However, although some observations of FDG-PET response have been accompanied by decreases in tumor size, a metabolic response per se is not necessarily indicative of antitumor activity. Current evidence suggests that FDG-PET may be a useful noninvasive pharmacodynamic tool for demonstrating target inhibition, but it remains to be seen whether it has value in predicting response to therapy.

In general, mTOR inhibitor therapy has been well tolerated, whether administered orally or intravenously, or on a daily or weekly schedule. Although there may be a few specific differences between the different rapalogs, these toxicities are mostly consistent with those associated with administration of rapamycin (sirolimus) in transplant rejection. Common toxicities associated with administration of rapalogs include reversible mucositis/stomatitis, rash, fatigue, and hyperlipidemia; hematological adverse events include thrombocytopenia, neutropenia, and anemia (18, 19, 26–28).

Sirolimus (Rapamycin; Rapamune®) Sirolimus (rapamycin; Figure 10.1) is by far the most broadly used mTOR inhibitor in preclinical studies and there are myriad literature reports describing its activity in various cancer models, both in

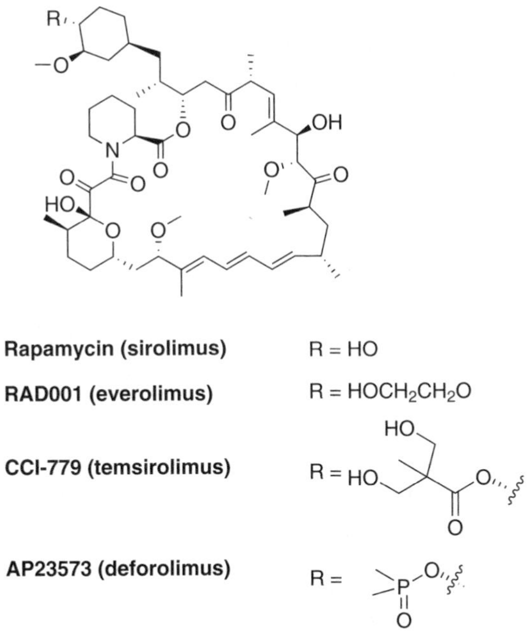

Rapamycin (sirolimus)   R = HO

RAD001 (everolimus)   R = HOCH₂CH₂O

CCI-779 (temsirolimus)   R =

AP23573 (deforolimus)   R =

Figure 10.1   Structures of mTOR inhibitors.

vitro and in vivo. Although oral Rapamune is only approved for prophylactic treatment of renal transplant rejection, sirolimus is also used in drug-eluting stents for angioplasty procedures. In addition, several off-label studies have explored its utility in the treatment of cancer. As an immunosuppressive agent, sirolimus is administered as a 2–8-mg oral daily dose, although a higher initial loading dose can be given. Steady state pharmacokinetics using a 2-mg dose demonstrate a C_{max} of ~15 ng/mL, C_{min} of ~7 ng/mL, and AUC of ~200 ng·h/mL, with a plasma half-life of 2–4 hours. In a Phase I dose-finding study of sirolimus in patients with solid tumors, two patients were shown to have a FDG-PET response to the drug and disease stabilization at daily doses of 6 and 9 mg (29). A second Phase I study evaluated weekly dosing of 10–60 mg and demonstrated that active drug levels similar to those obtained with a clinically relevant dose of temsirolimus (a sirolimus prodrug; see later discussion) could be achieved. The percentage change in plasma triglycerides after 4 weeks of dosing varied in a dose-dependent manner, suggesting that doubling of plasma triglycerides may be a useful guide to achieving a therapeutically relevant dose level. Two patients in this study (pancreatic and small cell lung cancer) experienced tumor regression (30). A pharmacodynamic analysis of sirolimus was also conducted in the neoadjuvant setting in patients with recurrent glioblastoma (31). In this Phase I study, 15 patients with confirmed PTEN-negative tumors were treated for 1 week prior to surgery, then after surgery until disease progression. Patients received 2-, 5-, or 10-mg daily doses of sirolimus, and tumor samples from historical samples and following 1-week treatment with sirolimus were analyzed for a variety of molecular markers. Overall, 2 patients showed a radiographic response. In all three dose groups, phosphorylation of S6 ribosomal protein was decreased following treatment; moreover, the extent of decrease correlated with inhibition of tumor cell proliferation as assessed by Ki67 staining. A subset of tumors showed induction of PRAS40 phosphorylation, suggesting that these tumors were upregulating AKT activity via the p70S6K-IRS1 feedback mechanism. Moreover, pPRAS40 induction was associated with shorter time-to-progression.

Temsirolimus (CCI-779; Torisel®)   Temsirolimus is a relatively soluble prodrug that is converted to rapamycin by hydrolysis of the ester (R group; Figure 10.1). Preclinical data have demonstrated activity in multiple tumor models, including breast, neuroectodermal, and glioma xenografts (32, 33), with some data suggesting that PTEN-deficient tumors (which have constitutive activation of PI3K and downstream signaling) may be more sensitive than isogenic tumors with functional PTEN (34). The drug has been evaluated in two Phase I studies using different schedules of intravenous administration: qd × 5 every 2 weeks (27) and once weekly (28). In the qd × 5 every 2 weeks schedule, 15 mg/m^2/ day was determined to be the maximum tolerated dose in heavily pretreated patients (although minimally pretreated patients tolerated doses of up to 24 mg/m^2). At 15 mg/m^2/ day, exposure of the active metabolite sirolimus was characterized by a C_{max} (on day 5) of 58 ng/mL and a long half-life (∼40 h). Temsirolimus was generally well tolerated, with mild to moderate asthenia, mucositis, nausea, and rash being the most common adverse events; grade 3 and 4 events included hyperglycemia (8%) and hypophosphatemia (11%). Six patients across all dose levels showed either a partial response or prolonged stable disease. For the once-weekly regimen, dose-limiting toxicities were observed at 220 mg/m^2. Toxicities were broadly consistent with those in the qd × 5 study, although mucositis and rash were more pronounced with weekly dosing. The high dose group (220 mg/m^2) was also notable for producing symptoms of bipolar disorder. Consistent with the higher dose of temsirolimus, exposure of sirolimus was higher for the weekly dose than for qd × 5, with C_{max} of 798 ng/mL and a half-life of 60.5 hours. Temsirolimus has been evaluated clinically in a wide variety of solid tumors and lymphomas, with the most promising results as a single agent in renal cell carcinoma, endometrial carcinoma, and mantle cell lymphoma. Although objective responses have also been seen with single-agent temsirolimus in other diseases, most of the more recent studies have been conducted in combination with other targeted and chemotherapy agents.

As discussed in Chapter 5 and above, the biology of renal cell carcinoma (RCC) presents a particularly promising opportunity for therapeutic intervention using mTOR inhibitors. A randomized, double-blind Phase II study of temsirolimus in advanced RCC evaluated three dose levels (25 mg, 75 mg, and 250 mg IV weekly) in 111 patients, with encouraging results. In agreement with Phase I studies, temsirolimus was quite well tolerated, with mild rash, mucositis, asthenia, and nausea being most frequently reported; grade 3 or 4 events included hyperglycemia (17%) and hypophosphatemia (13%). Seventy-one percent of patients across all dose groups achieved clinical benefit, including one with a complete response and seven with partial response (35). Of particular interest, a retrospective analysis suggested that patients in intermediate/high risk strata had improved survival relative to historical (interferon α (IFN)) treatment, whereas lower risk patients showed no such advantage. On the basis of these data, together with results from a Phase I/II study of everolimus in combination with IFN (36), a randomized Phase III study (the ARCC trial) was initiated in previously untreated metastatic RCC patients with at least three factors predictive of short survival (37). Three treatment regimens were evaluated: temsirolimus (25 mg IV weekly), IFN, and a combination of the two drugs. A total of 626 patients were enrolled, and temsirolimus demonstrated both improved progression-free and overall survival compared to IFN; the combination treatment showed improved progression-free survival but no change in overall survival compared to IFN alone. Temsirolimus was generally well tolerated in comparison to IFN and these data supported the approval of the drug (marketed as Torisel®) in 2007 for treatment of advanced RCC patients with poor prognosis.

Endometrial carcinoma is another disease with strong rationale for targeting the PI3K/mTOR axis; not only is there a high incidence of mutations in both PI3K and PTEN, but these mutations are frequently found to coexist in the same tumor cells (38). A 25-mg IV weekly dose of temsirolimus was evaluated in a small Phase II study in metastatic endometrial carcinoma, with encouraging results: among 28 evaluable patients, 7 partial responses were seen and 16 achieved stable disease. Of note, objective responses were seen in both PTEN-positive and PTEN-negative patients. Overall progression-free survival was 8 months (39).

Mantle cell lymphoma (MCL) is characterized by a chromosomal translocation driving overexpression of cyclin D1, the mRNA of which is under translational control of mTOR signaling. In a Phase II study of 35 patients with relapsed MCL, temsirolimus was dosed at 250 mg IV weekly. Substantial antitumor activity was observed, with 1 complete response, 12 partial responses, and a median duration of response in the responders of 6.9 months (40). More recently, a lower dose (25 mg IV weekly) was found to produce a similar response rate in this patient population (1 CR and 10 PRs out of 27 evaluable patients), but with lower myelosuppression than in the high dose study (41). A Phase III study was initiated in MCL in April 2005; enrollment has completed, but no data are yet available.

A Phase II study of temsirolimus was also conducted in 65 glioblastoma patients. In this study, 250-mg doses of temsirolimus were administered by weekly infusion. Dosing was complicated by the fact that concurrent administration of anticonvulsants substantially reduced the exposure of temsirolimus: however, drug levels consistent with activity in preclinical models were still achieved. Radiographic response was observed in 36% of patients and correlated with increased time to progression (5.4 months in responders compared to 1.9 months in nonresponders). Notably, responders also had high levels of phosphorylated p70S6K in baseline tumor samples, and development of hyperlipidemia also appeared to correlate with response (42). Given the high incidence of EGFR activation in glioblastoma (Chapter 3), there is strong rationale for combining EGFR inhibitors with mTOR inhibitors in this disease. A Phase I study combining erlotinib and temsirolimus in patients with malignant glioma was reported in 2007. The erlotinib dose was fixed at 150 mg daily, and temsirolimus was initially given as a 50-mg weekly infusion. However, despite excluding patients who required anticonvulsant therapy, the combination was poorly tolerated and no clear signs of clinical benefit were observed (43).

In breast cancer patients, temsirolimus was evaluated using a weekly infusion of 75 mg or 250 mg (44). Ten partial responses were seen among 109 patients and an additional five patients had disease stabilization for 24 weeks or more; efficacy was similar for the two dose levels. Adverse events were mostly the expected mucositis, rash, and nausea but were more pronounced in the higher dose group. In addition, 10% of patients in the high dose group (but none in the low dose group) experienced depression, mirroring the experience in the Phase I weekly dosing study (28). Temsirolimus has also been evaluated in advanced breast cancer patients in combination with the aromatase inhibitor letrozole. Both letrozole and mTOR inhibitors block expression of cyclin D1 at the transcriptional and translational levels, respectively; moreover, estrogen receptor and growth factor signaling pathways exhibit significant crosstalk, contributing to endocrine resistance (45, 46). A Phase II study in postmenopausal women with advanced breast cancer suggested that progression-free survival was higher in patients treated with intermittent oral temsirolimus (75 mg qd × 5 every 2 weeks) than for patients treated with letrozole alone (13.2 vs. 11.6 months) (47). However, a Phase III study combining letroloze with temsirolimus for first-line use in postmenopausal women with hormone-receptor positive metastatic breast cancer (HORIZON) was stopped early when interim data monitoring indicated that the combination treatment was unlikely to provide significant additional benefit compared to letrozole alone.

Other indications explored as single-agent therapy include melanoma and small cell lung cancer (48, 49). In both cases, some evidence for clinical activity was observed but response rates were only modest—3% in melanoma and 1.2% in small cell lung cancer. As of July 3, 2008, the NIH clinical trials database (www.clinicaltrials.gov) lists 73 studies with temsirolimus, most involving combination therapy. Agents combined with temsirolimus include angiogenesis inhibitors (bevacizumab, sunitinib, sorafenib, AV-951), EGF receptor inhibitors (erlotinib, pelitinib), chemotherapy (gemcitabine, carboplatin/paclitaxel, topotecan), and others such as imatinib, the proteasome inhibitor bortezomib, and the anti-IGF1R antibody IMC-A12.

Everolimus (RAD001)   Everolimus is approved in Europe and the United States as a drug for prevention of transplant rejection, but it has also seen significant development for the treatment of cancer. As in the case of temsirolimus and rapamycin, preclinical studies have shown significant antitumor activity in xenograft models. For example, both intermittent (twice-weekly) and daily dosing regimens were shown to be effective in a syngeneic rat pancreatic tumor model. Administration of everolimus produced inhibition of phosphorylation of the downstream mTOR substrates S6 and 4E-BP1, with inhibition of p70S6K sustained to at least 72 hours following a single dose (50). Preclinical data have also supported the combination of everolimus with various chemotherapy and targeted therapy agents.

For example, everolimus and the EGFR/VEGFR inhibitor AEE788 show greater antitumor activity in glioma models compared to either agent alone (51), and coadministration of everolimus and trastuzumab may be able to inhibit tumor growth in cancer cells with resistance to trastuzumab due to loss of PTEN function (52). Everolimus is orally available and has been evaluated in Phase I studies using both daily and weekly schedules (18, 20). Based on these studies, recommended doses are 5 mg or 10 mg/day, and 20 mg or 50 mg/week. The drug was generally well tolerated and a MTD was not established: observed toxicities were commensurate with those reported for other mTOR inhibitors and included stomatitis, neutropenia, hyperglycemia, and fatigue.

Like temsirolimus, everolimus has also been evaluated as a single agent in renal cell carcinoma and endometrial carcinoma. In the latter indication, everolimus was administered orally at 10 mg/day, in contrast to the weekly IV dose of temsirolimus. Forty-three percent of patients experienced clinical benefit, although no objective responses were recorded (53). In renal cell carcinoma, everolimus showed encouraging clinical activity in two Phase II studies, both of which used a 10-mg daily dosing schedule. In the first of these, everolimus was administered to patients with metastatic clear cell RCC (54). Out of 25 evaluable patients, 9 (33%) achieved a partial response with 70% showing some degree of tumor shrinkage. Toxicities were generally mild and included mucositis, skin rash, hyperglycemia, and hypophosphatemia. In a second study, 41 patients with metastatic RCC were enrolled and 12 partial responses were observed out of 37 evaluable for response (55). Nineteen patients had stable disease for at least 3 months, and tolerability was similar to that reported in the earlier RCC study. Based on these encouraging data, the RECORD-1 (Renal Cell cancer treatment with Oral RAD001 given Daily) Phase III trial was initated. This study enrolled RCC patients who had previously progressed following treatment with sunitinib and/or sorafenib. A total of 410 patients were assigned to receive either everolimus or placebo in combination with best supportive care. The trial was halted in February 2008 due to superior activity in the everolimus arm, and results subsequently presented showed that everolimus treatment produced a median progression-free survival of 4 months, compared to 1.9 months with placebo (56, 57). Moreover, all subgroups appeared to benefit from treatment, irrespective of prior therapy, risk factors, age, sex, or geographical region. Safety was broadly similar to that seen in earlier Phase II studies.

As of June 19, 2008, the NIH clinical trials database (www.clinicaltrials.gov) lists 165 studies involving everolimus. Although many of these studies are for transplant rejection, over 100 of them are for various oncology indications, including evaluation of everolimus as a single agent and in combination with a wide range of chemotherapy and other kinase inhibitors. One of the more advanced indications is treatment of neuroendocrine tumors. Most of these tumors can be classified by one of two subtypes: carcinoid or pancreatic islet tumors, both of which often secrete biogenic amines and/or peptide hormones resulting in a range of gastrointestinal and other symptoms. The somatostatin mimetic octreotide is frequently used for treatment of symptoms associated with this disease, and mTOR inhibitors have been evaluated both as single agents and in combination with octreotide in both pancreatic and carcinoid tumors. A Phase II study of weekly intravenous temsirolimus yielded a low response rate: 2 out of 37 patients (58). Somewhat higher activity was observed for daily oral dosing of everolimus (5 or 10 mg/day) in combination with depot octreotide. In a single-arm Phase II study of 60 patients (30 with carcinoid, 30 with pancreatic islet tumors), 17% had a partial response and 75% stable disease (of which a third had >15% reduction in tumor size), with a median progression-free survival of 59 weeks (59). These encouraging results are being further explored in the RADIANT-2 and RADIANT-3 Phase III studies, comparing depot octreotide + placebo with depot octreotide + everolimus in advanced carcinoid and advanced pancreatic islet tumors, respectively.

Early results from studies evaluating everolimus in non small cell lung cancer highlight the potential value of combination therapy. In two Phase II studies in patients with advanced non small cell lung carcinoma, oral everolimus was administered as a 10-mg single-agent daily dose (60), or as a 5-mg daily dose in combination with 250 mg/day gefitinib (61). Both studies employed a Simon two-stage design. The single-agent study showed that everolimus was well tolerated but produced only a low response rate: 5.3% in patients failing two or fewer chemotherapy regimens, and even lower (2.3%) in a similar population who had also progressed on EGFR inhibitor therapy. Based on these data, the trial did not advance to the second stage. The combination study enrolled two cohorts, one with no prior chemotherapy and one with prior cisplatin/carboplatin and docetaxel. In contrast to the single-agent study, objective responses were seen in 20% of chemotherapy naive and 15% of previously treated patients, prompting expansion of each arm of the study.

There have been many studies evaluating everolimus in breast cancer. A Phase II study in patients with metastatic breast cancer showed evidence of single-agent activity, with a potential benefit for daily dosing (10 mg/day; 3/18 objective responses) compared to weekly dosing (70 mg/week; 0/16 objective responses) (62). However, larger studies are needed to confirm these findings. There have also been multiple studies of everolimus in combination with other agents in breast cancer. In particular, there is strong rationale for the utility of mTOR inhibitors in patients with resistance to the anti-HER2 antibody trastuzumab, since trastuzumab resistance is frequently mediated by loss of PTEN and activation of PI3K/AKT signaling (63, 64). Two recent Phase Ib studies in heavily pretreated HER2+ patients with trastuzumab resistance showed encouraging activity. In the first of these studies, everolimus was evaluated in combination with vinorelbine and trastuzumab. Everolimus was administered at 5 mg/day, 20 mg/week, or 30 mg/week. Out of 22 patients treated, 1 complete response and 2 partial responses were noted, with no progression for at least 20 weeks at the time of reporting: moreover, 11 patients had stable disease of >4 months and most remained on study at the time of the report (65). Similarly striking data were presented in a similar population of patients treated with paclitaxel, trastuzumab, and 5 mg/day or 30 mg/week everolimus. Of 22 patients evaluated, 6 partial responses and 6 disease stabilizations were observed (66). In both of these studies, neutropenia was the most common dose-limiting toxicity.

As discussed earlier for temsirolimus, preclinical data also support the use of mTOR inhibitors in combination with letrozole for treatment of hormone receptor-positive breast cancer (67). Everolimus has shown evidence of clinical activity in combination with letrozole in a Phase I study of 18 metastatic breast cancer patients, with one durable complete response, one near-partial response, and prolonged stable disease (>12 months) in four additional patients (68). The experience with temsirolimus suggests that larger studies are warranted to confirm the utility of this approach: it is currently unclear whether the daily dosing employed in the everolimus study is more effective than the intermittent schedule used in the temsirolimus studies. Finally, a randomized neoadjuvant study comparing letrozole and everolimus to letrozole alone in hormone receptor-positive breast cancer showed a higher clinical response rate for the combination group (68% vs. 59%), and a significantly greater reduction in tumor cell proliferation as assessed by Ki67 immunohistochemistry (69). However, grade 3/4 adverse events were also higher in the combination arm, primarily hyperglycemia, stomatitis, interstitial lung disease/pneumonitis, and infections.

Deforolimus (renamed as ridaforolimus; AP23573, MK-8669) Deforolimus (Figure 10.1) is a solubilized, non-prodrug analog of rapamycin. Phase I studies were initially performed using daily intravenous administration for 5 days every 2 weeks (19). Doses from 3 to 28 mg/day were evaluated, and the MTD was 18.75 mg/day; mouth sores and dermatologic events were the most common toxicities observed. There were some encouraging signs of activity, with 18 of 27 evaluable patients experiencing some degree of tumor shrinkage and 4 confirmed partial responses. More recently, a Phase I study comparing seven oral dosing regimens was reported (70). Dose-limiting toxicity of mouth sores was consistent between these regimens and other safety signals were broadly consistent with those seen following intravenous administration. A comparison of toxicities and pharmacokinetics led to selection of 40 mg given qd × 5 in 28-day cycles as the optimal schedule.

Several patients in the Phase I trial of deforolimus had a diagnosis of sarcoma and all achieved some degree of clinical benefit (19), prompting a Phase II study of deforolimus (12.5 mg IV qd × 5 every 2 weeks) in 212 patients with advanced sarcoma (71). Four independent cohorts were enrolled: bone sarcoma, leiomyosarcoma, liposarcoma, and other types. Clinical benefit rates (partial response or stable disease) ranged from 23% to 33% across groups, with no clear difference in clinical benefit between subgroups. Five confirmed partial responses were observed and toxicities were relatively mild and consistent with previous studies (primarily mouth sores, fatigue, and rash). Based on the activity seen in this study, a Phase III placebo-controlled trial (SUCCEED) has been initiated using oral administration of deforolimus (www.clinicaltrials.gov, identifier NCT00538239). Like temsirolimus and everolimus, deforolimus has also shown activity in endometrial cancer. A Phase II study in advanced/recurrent endometrial carcinoma employed a dosing schedule of 12.5 mg deforolimus IV for five consecutive days every other week in 28-day cycles. Nine of 27 evaluable patients had clinical benefit, including 2 partial responses (72). There are also indications of activity in various leukemias and lymphomas (73), and an additional Phase I/II study is exploring the safety and tolerability of deforolimus in pediatric patients.

Other mTOR Inhibitors ABI-009 (Abraxis) is an albumin-encapsulated form of rapamycin, designed to enhance drug delivery and therapeutic index. In preclinical studies in rats, AB-009 was well tolerated at up to 90 mg/kg/dose on a q4d × 3 schedule (74). Phase I studies are in progress in patients with advanced solid tumors. Two additional small molecule mTOR inhibitors (OSI-027 and AZD8055) have also recently advanced to clinical testing, although no further details are currently available.

10.2 PI3K INHIBITORS

PI3K has attracted significant attention in recent years as a target for anticancer drugs, and several inhibitors of this lipid kinase (Table 10.2) have recently entered clinical trials (75). These drugs can broadly be divided into two groups: those that are specific for class I PI3K enzymes and those that also inhibit mTOR and other PI3K/PIKK family kinases.

BEZ235 BEZ235 (Novartis; Figure 10.2) is a dual inhibitor of PI3K and mTOR, with in vitro IC_{50} values of 4, 76, 5, and 7 nM toward $PI3K\alpha$, β, γ, δ, respectively, and an IC_{50} for mTOR inhibition of 6.75 or 31 nM, depending on the assay format used (76). The compound shows no crossreactivity with a diverse panel of 18 protein kinases and does not elicit cellular effects downstream of ATM or DNAPK. In vitro cellular assays show inhibition of pathway readouts downstream of PI3K and mTOR, resulting in antiproliferative activity and G1 cell cycle arrest. Antitumor activity was demonstrated as a single agent in various tumor xenograft models,

TABLE 10.2   PI3K Inhibitors

Drug	Company	Target(s)	Structure[a]	Latest stage of development
BEZ235	Novartis	PI3K, mTOR	Figure 10.2	Phase I
BGT226	Novartis	PI3K, mTOR	ND	Phase I
BKM120	Novartis	PI3K	ND	Phase I
XL765	Exelixis	PI3K, mTOR, DNAPK	ND	Phase I
XL147	Exelixis	PI3K	ND	Phase I
SF1126	Semafore	PI3K, mTOR, DNAPK	Figure 10.2	Phase I
GDC-0941	Piramed/Genentech	PI3K, mTOR	Figure 10.2	Phase I
PX-866	Oncothyreon	PI3K, mTOR, DNAPK	Figure 10.2	Phase I
GSK615	GlaxoSmithKline	PI3K, mTOR	ND	Phase I
CAL-101	Calistoga	PI3Kδ	ND	Phase I

[a]ND, not disclosed.

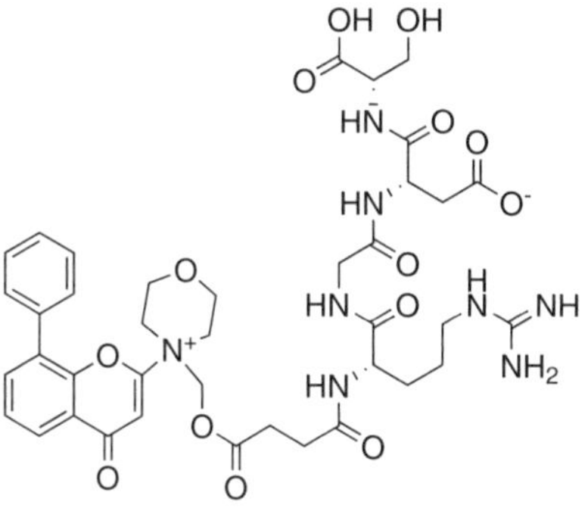

SF-1126

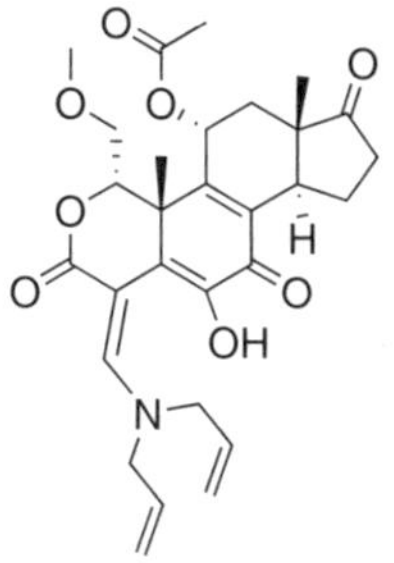

PX-866

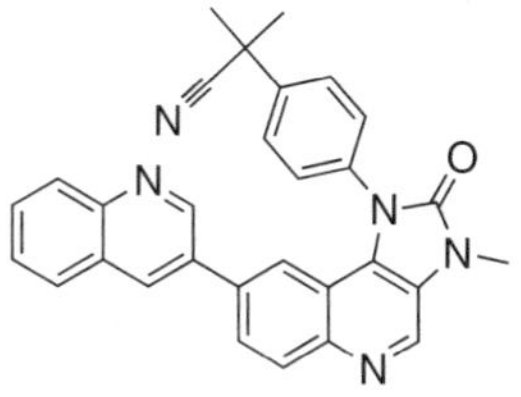

BEZ-235

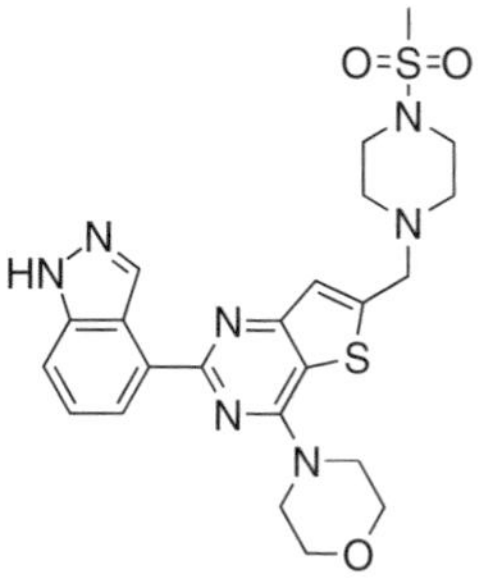

GDC-0941

Figure 10.2   Structures of PI3K inhibitors.

and in combination with temozolomide in U87MG xenografts (76, 77). One of the early concerns with development of PI3K pathway inhibitors was the potential for deleterious effects on glucose homeostasis, based on the fact that PI3K is a critical downstream regulator of insulin receptor signaling. An investigation of insulin pathway gene expression following BEZ235 administration in rats showed significant changes in multiple pathway-related genes after 2 weeks of treatment, but little or no change after 13 weeks. Both glucose and insulin levels were found to increase on the first day after dosing with 20 mg/kg BEZ235: however, after 13 weeks of treatment at this dose level glucose showed no change from vehicle and insulin may even have decreased (78). Collectively, these data suggest an adaptation mechanism that may mitigate the effects of PI3K inhibition on insulin signaling following chronic inhibition of PI3K inhibitors. Phase I studies of BEZ235 are in progress. Two additional PI3K inhibitors from Novartis, BGT226 (PI3K/mTOR) and BKM120 (PI3K), have also entered clinical trials but no further details are currently available.

SF1126   SF1126 (Semafore Pharmaceuticals) is a prodrug comprising the benzopyranone derivative LY294002 conjugated to an integrin-binding (RGDS) peptide (Figure 10.2). LY294002, widely referred to as the "Lilly compound," was identified by researchers at Eli Lilly in the mid-1990s (79) and has been extensively used in preclinical studies. LY294002 is a pan-PI3K inhibitor with IC_{50} values of 720, 306, 1600, and 1330 nM for PI3K α, β, γ, and δ, respectively (80), and also inhibits PIKK-related kinases (81). However, clinical development of LY294002 was precluded by poor pharmacological properties. The RGDS peptide of SF1126 is spontaneously cleaved from the active LY294002 moiety in plasma following subcutaneous, intravenous, or intramuscular dosing: however, tumor xenograft studies suggest that the RGDS peptide confers additional tumor growth inhibition compared to an analogous drug conjugate that does not target cell surface integrins. Tumor growth inhibition was demonstrated in multiple xenograft models including U87MG glioblastoma, PC-3 prostate carcinoma, MDA-MB-468 breast carcinoma, and LN229/LN229viii glioma (80). Two Phase I studies, in solid tumors and in multiple myeloma, were initiated in 2007.

XL765   XL765 (Exelixis) is an orally available inhibitor of PI3K that also inhibits the PIKK-related kinase mTOR. IC_{50} values were reported as 39, 113, 43, and 9 nM for PI3Kα, β, γ, and δ, respectively, with $\sim$150-nM activity toward mTOR and DNAPK and high selectivity versus a panel of >120 other kinases (82). XL765 was shown to suppress phosphorylation of PI3K and mTOR pathway markers (pAKT, pPRAS40, pp70S6K, and pS6) for up to 24 h following a single oral dose in an MCF-7 tumor xenograft model, correlating with decreased tumor cell proliferation and increased apoptosis. Tumor growth inhibition was demonstrated in MCF7 and A549 xenograft models, using various dosing schedules ranging from twice daily to twice weekly. Early results from a Phase I study indicated a preliminary maximum tolerated dose of 60 mg bid, with transaminitis as the main dose-limiting toxicity (83). A dose-dependent increase in plasma insulin was observed following XL765 administration but minimal treatment-related effects on glucose were evident, consistent with the lack of effect on glucose following chronic administration of BEZ235 (see earlier discussion). Pharmacodynamic analyses were conducted in hair, skin, PBMCs, and tumor tissue, all of which showed downregulation of PI3K pathway signaling. For example, phosphorylation of the AKT substrate PRAS40 in PBMCs was inhibited with $IC_{50} = 109$ ng/mL (plasma concentration of XL765). In hair samples, multiple pathway readouts were progressively inhibited throughout the dosing cycle and a correlation of pS6 phosphorylation with XL765 exposure was noted (84). Analysis of chondrosarcoma tumor biopsies taken at screening and after 28 days of dosing with XL765 showed downregulation of AKT, PRAS40, S6, and 4EBP1 phosphorylation (85). No objective responses were reported, but five patients achieved disease stabilization for 3 or more months (85).

XL147   XL147 (Exelixis) is an orally bioavailable inhibitor of the class I PI3K enzymes, with IC_{50} values of 39, 383, 36, and 23 nM for PI3Kα, β, γ and δ, respectively (86). XL147 is highly selective against other PIKK family enzymes and a panel of >130 human protein kinases. XL147 was shown to inhibit growth of multiple human tumor xenograft models, both as a single agent (86) and in combination with various chemotherapy and targeted therapeutic agents including paclitaxel, carboplatin, rapamycin, and erlotinib (87). Early clinical data indicated that oral doses of 30 mg and 60 mg (given daily for 21 days out of 28) were well tolerated and produced high plasma exposures (up to 15000 ng/mL after 21 days of dosing), with a terminal half-life between 2.5 and 8 days (86). Updated results from this study have been reported, indicating that dose escalation had proceeded to a MAD of 900 mg, with plasma concentrations on day 21 exceeding 100,000 ng/mL. Following one cycle of treatment, decreased phosphorylation of AKT, S6, and PRAS40 was found in tumor biopsies, and exposure-dependent PI3K pathway inhibition was also noted in hair and skin samples. In hair samples, for example, phosphorylation of multiple pathway proteins (AKT, PRAS40, S6, and 4EBP) was increasingly inhibited throughout the dosing cycle, with plasma IC_{50} values ranging from 27 to 42 μg/mL (84). Glucose levels were only minimally perturbed, although there was a trend toward increasing insulin levels at higher doses. Eight patients had prolonged stable disease, five of whom were on study for over 200 days (88).

GDC-0941 GDC-0941 (Genentech; Figure 10.2) is an orally available analog of PI-103, which is a dual PI3K/mTOR inhibitor developed by Piramed (now part of Roche) that has been used in multiple preclinical studies. However, GDC-0941 is a relatively specific inhibitor of class I PI3K enzymes, with IC_{50} values of 3, 33, 75, and 3 nM for PI3Kα, β, γ, and δ, respectively, and a K_I value of 580 nM for mTOR (89). In cellular assays in vitro, GDC-0941 induces time- and dose-dependent G1 cell cycle arrest in PC-3 cells. Dose-dependent apoptosis was reported in a subset of cell lines, particularly those with activating PI3K mutations. Antitumor activity was noted in several human tumor xenograft models, including single-agent activity in MDA-MB-361, PC-3, and NCI-H2122 tumors, and strong activity in combination with docetaxel in a MAXF401 breast cancer model. Two Phase I dose escalation clinical trials are in progress in the United States and the United Kingdom. As of September 2008, 27 patients had been enrolled in these studies and treated with doses ranging from 15 to 60 mg qd, or 30 mg bid. The $t_{1/2}$ ranged from 8 to 29 hours, and exposure was found to increase in a dose-proportional manner. Dose-dependent inhibition of AKT phosphorlyation in platelet-rich plasma was noted (90).

PX-866 PX-866 (Oncothyreon) is a semisynthetic analog of wortmannin, an irreversible PI3K inhibitor that binds to a lysine residue at the kinase active site (91–93). Wortmannin is active in tumor xenograft models but lacks the necessary stability and toxicological profile for successful clinical development. PX-866 (Figure 10.2) was identified as the most promising in a series of semisynthetic wortmannin analogs, based on in vitro and in vivo measurements of PI3K activity, pharmacokinetics, and toxicity. In Vitro, PX-866 inhibits recombinant PI3Kα, β, γ, and δ with IC_{50} values of 5.5, >300, 9, and 2.7 nM, respectively, and shows enhanced stability compared to wortmannin (94, 95). Inhibition of PI3K pathway signaling was demonstrated in HT29 cells, both in vitro and in xenograft tumors in nude mice, and antitumor activity was also noted in several xenograft models including HT29, OVCAR-3, and A549 (95). Both acute and long-term administration of PX-866 produced hyperglycemia in rodents, although this was reversible when dosing was halted (94). The hyperglycemia was associated with impaired glucose tolerance, which could be alleviated by administration of pioglitazone but not metformin. A Phase I clinical trial was initiated in 2008.

10.3 RAF KINASE INHIBITORS

Sorafenib   Sorafenib (Figure 10.3, Table 10.3; Onyx/Bayer) was the first drug with RAF-inhibitory properties to enter clinical trials: however, the fact that it shows antitumor activity in the absence of modulation of ERK phosphorylation suggests that many, if not most, of its effects are mediated by mechanisms other than RAF inhibition. In particular, sorafenib is a potent inhibitor of VEGF receptors, and further discussion of the preclinical and clinical profile of this drug can be found in Chapter 9. With the exception of sorafenib, all other clinical RAF inhibitors are at early stages of clinical evaluation.

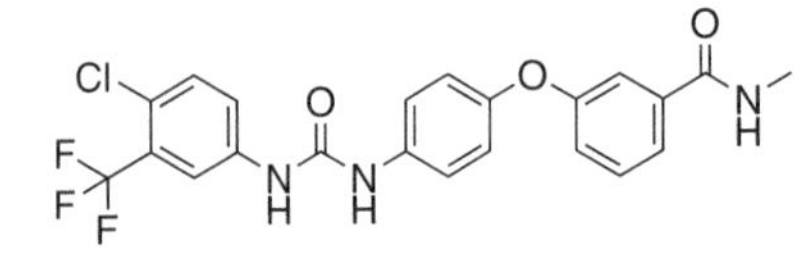

Sorafenib (BAY-43-9006)

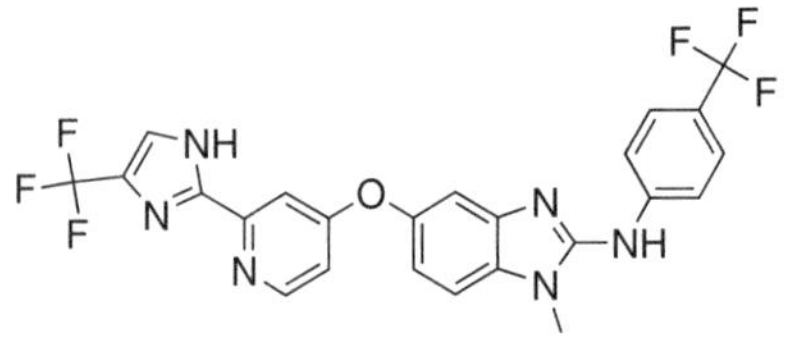

RAF-265

Figure 10.3   Structures of RAF inhibitors.

TABLE 10.3   RAF Kinase Inhibitors

Drug	Company	Target(s)	Structure[a]	Latest stage of development
Sorafenib (BAY43-9006; Nexavar®)	Onyx/Bayer	RAF, VEGFR2,VEGFR3, FLT3, KIT, RET, PDGFRβ	Figure 10.3	Approved
RAF265	Novartis	RAF, VEGFR2, PDGFRβ, KIT	Figure 10.3	Phase I
XL281	Exelixis/ Bristol-Myers Squibb	RAF	ND	Phase I
PLX4032/R-7204	Plexxikon/Roche	RAF	ND	Phase I

[a]ND, not disclosed.

XL281   XL281 (Exelixis/Bristol-Myers Squibb) is an orally available, highly specific inhibitor of the active forms of BRAF and CRAF, with IC_{50} values of 4.5 and 2.6 nM, respectively; the BRAF V600E mutant is inhibited with an IC_{50} of 6 nM (96). Inhibition of ERK and MEK phosphorylation was reported in HCT116 (KRAS mutant) and A375 (BRAF mutant) xenograft tumors, with ED_{50} values of 60–90 mg/kg. Tumor growth inhibition was demonstrated in HCT116, A375, and A431 xenograft models using various daily and intermittent dosing schedules. A Phase I dose escalation study of XL281 is in progress in patients with advanced solid tumors. Data have been reported for 30 patients with various malignancies including thyroid cancer, colorectal cancer, and melanoma. Doses administered ranged from 10 to 225 mg qd, given in 28-day cycles. The MAD was 225 mg, while 150 mg was declared the MTD; dose-limiting toxicities at 225 mg were fatigue, nausea, vomiting, and diarrhea. The 150-mg dose produced a C_{max} of 2620 ng/mL and the median half-life across all dose groups was 7.9 hours. Decreased ERK phosphorylation was reported in hair and skin samples from a patient treated at the 150-mg dose, and tumor biopsies from a patient with a sweat gland tumor showed reduced ERK and MEK phosphorylation together with reduced proliferation and increased apoptosis. A partial response was achieved in a patient with ocular melanoma, and 12 patients had stable disease for greater than 3 months (97).

PLX4032   PLX4032 (Plexxikon/Roche) is also a specific RAF inhibitor, with IC_{50} values against wild-type and V600E mutant BRAF of 100 nM and 31 nM, respectively (98, 99). Cellular inhibition of MEK phosphorylation, ERK phosphorylation, and antiproliferative activity were found to be selective for cells bearing the V600E mutation (e.g., Colo205, HT29), in contrast to cells with wild-type RAF (e.g., LoVo, HCT116). Correspondingly, antitumor activity was observed in HT29 but not in HCT116 xenograft models. Phase I clinical evaluation of PLX4032 is in progress: the study is recruiting patients with solid tumors and also includes a planned pharmacodynamic component in patients with malignant melanoma harboring a confirmed BRAF V600E mutation.

RAF265   Compared to the above inhibitors, RAF265 (Figure 10.3; Novartis) has a profile closer to that of sorafenib, in that it inhibits VEGFR2, KIT, and PDGFRβ in addition to RAF. Reported IC_{50} values are 70 nM for BRAF, 5 nM for CRAF, 70 nM for VEGFR2, and 20 nM for KIT. In addition, the BRAF V600E mutant is inhibited with an IC_{50} of 19 nM (100). Cellular activity against both wild-type and mutant RAF kinase is reported to be greater than that of sorafenib, with cells expressing the BRAF V600E mutant being particularly sensitive. Regression of xenograft tumors was observed in two melanoma models bearing the BRAF V600E mutation (A375 and MEXF-276), using various intermittent dosing schedules (dosing every 2 or 3 days); inhibition of KRAS mutant HCT116 tumors was also reported. In addition, RAF265 has effects on tumor microvessel density, likely due to its inhibition of VEGFR2 and/or PDGFRβ (100). RAF265 is currently in a Phase I clinical study in patients with locally advanced or metastatic melanoma.

10.4 MEK INHIBITORS

CI-1040 CI-1040 (PD184352; Figure 10.4) was discovered and developed by researchers at Pfizer as a highly specific, non-ATP-competitive inhibitor of MEK kinase (Table 10.4) and was the first such MEK inhibitor to enter clinical studies. CI-1040 binds to a pocket adjacent to the MEK ATP binding site (for more details of this binding mode, see Chapter 7). In preclinical studies, MEK1 was inhibited by CI-1040 in vitro with $IC_{50} = 17$ nM, and no appreciable activity was detected against other kinases. This activity produced potent intracellular inhibition of ERK phosphorylation in multiple cell lines and antiproliferative activity characterized by prominent G1 arrest. In vivo, a single dose of 150 mg/kg inhibited ERK phosphorylation in colon26 tumors for at least 6 hours following administration, and twice-daily dosing (up to 200 mg/kg) produced strong tumor growth inhibition

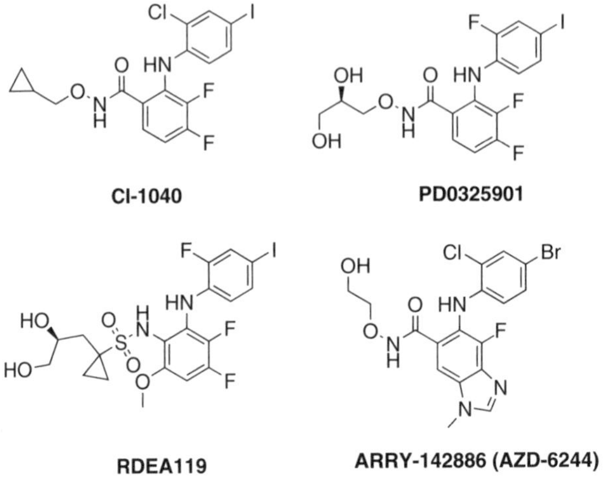

CI-1040   PD0325901

RDEA119   ARRY-142886 (AZD-6244)

Figure 10.4 Structures of MEK inhibitors.

TABLE 10.4 MEK Kinase Inhibitors

Drug	Company	Target	Structure[a]	Latest stage of development
CI-1040	Pfizer	MEK1	Figure 10.4	Phase II (discontinued)
PD0325901	Pfizer	MEK1	Figure 10.4	Phase II
AZD-6244 (ARRY-142886)	Array/AstraZeneca	MEK1/2	Figure 10.4	Phase II
GDC-0973 (XL518)	Exelixis/Genentech	MEK1	ND	Phase I
AZD-8330 (ARRY-704)	Array/AstraZeneca	MEK1	ND	Phase I
RDEA119	Ardea Biosciences	MEK1/2	Figure 10.4	Phase I

[a] ND, not disclosed.

(101). In early clinical studies the drug was quite well tolerated, with mild diarrhea, rash, fatigue, nausea, and vomiting being the main side effects: grade 3 asthenia was the dose-limiting toxicity. Several encouraging signs of clinical activity were seen, including a patient with pancreatic cancer who achieved a partial response for 355 days. However, metabolic stability was found to be a liability: CI-1040 undergoes extensive oxidative metabolism to form 14 metabolites (102). In particular, the O-alkyl hydroxamate moiety of CI-1040 is extensively hydrolyzed in vivo to form an inactive acidic metabolite, which reaches concentrations approximately 30-fold greater than those of CI-1040 itself (Figure 10.4). Due to this extensive metabolism, a high dose of 800 mg bid was selected for Phase II evaluation in patients with advanced non small cell lung, breast, colon, and pancreatic cancer. However, this study showed highly variable exposure to CI-1040 and inconsistent modulation of ERK phosphorylation in tumor biopsies. Perhaps as a result of the pharmacokinetic and metabolic liabilities, CI-1040 failed to demonstrate any objective responses and only 12% of patients showed disease stabilization: consequently, development was discontinued (103).

PD0325901 PD0325901 (Figure 10.4) was discovered by Pfizer as a second generation MEK inhibitor and improves on several of the liabilities of CI-1040. As well as demonstrating increased potency (in vitro $IC_{50} \approx 1$ nM) (104), PD0325901 has increased metabolic stability and better pharmacokinetic properties (although the O-alkyl hydroxamate moiety is still somewhat labile). In preclinical studies, PD0325901 demonstrates modulation of ERK phosphorylation and excellent antitumor activity at daily oral doses of 5 and 25 mg/kg, particularly in xenograft models harboring the BRAF V600E mutation (105). Preclinical pharmacokinetic/pharmacodynamic modeling showed that inhibition of ERK phosphorylation following treatment with PD0325901 declined rapidly as plasma levels of the drug declined and suggested that twice-daily dosing in humans might be preferable to daily dosing (106). Clinically, PD0325901 was dosed twice daily in Phase I studies, and some striking changes in ERK phosphorylation were observed in patient tumor samples (107, 108). However, modulation of ERK phosphorylation was not well correlated with dose level. Pharmacokinetics were also found to be significantly altered when dosed under fasting conditions compared to administration with food (107, 108). Clinically, dose-limiting toxicities of PD0325901 were reported as acneiform rash (observed at all dose levels), and additional toxicities included diarrhea, fatigue, nausea, and vomiting. Notably, a significant fraction of patients also reported visual disturbances and other symptoms suggestive of CNS involvement. Several patients, dosed using various schedules, were later reported to have experienced retinal vein occlusion (109). A pilot Phase II study in patients with advanced non small cell lung cancer was undertaken. The initial treatment schedule of 15 mg bid for 3 weeks on/1 week off was poorly tolerated, so additional breaks (no dosing on weekends) were introduced. No objective responses were seen but several patients had disease stabilization, although a significant incidence of visual disturbance was also noted in this study (110). Currently, the future development status of PD0325901 is unclear.

AZD-6244 AZD-6244/ARRY-142886 is being developed by Array Pharmaceuticals in collaboration with AstraZeneca. Its mechanism of action is similar to that of CI-1040 and PD0325901 in that it is a noncompetitive inhibitor: however, it is based on a benzimidazole core scaffold (Figure 10.4). AZD-6244 inhibits MEK1 with $IC_{50} = 14$ nM and, like CI-1040 and PD0325901, is noncompetitive with respect to ATP (111). Inhibition of cellular ERK phosphorylation was found to occur with similar potency to the in vitro IC_{50} for MEK1 inhibition. Inhibition of cellular proliferation in vitro seemed to be specific for cells with mutated BRAF, KRAS, or NRAS: however, in vivo tumor growth inhibition was demonstrated in both the HT29 model (BRAF V600E) and in BxPC3 tumors (which have no mutations in RAS or RAF), suggesting that some of the antitumor activity may be due to modulation of angiogenesis or other tumor:stromal interactions. Additional preclinical activity has been seen in various xenograft models, including lung cancer, colon cancer, pancreatic cancer and melanoma (112–115), thyroid cancer (116), and hepatocellular carcinoma (117), both as a single agent and in combination with other therapies.

Most of the clinical studies with AZD-6244 have been conducted using an orally administered suspension of the free base in an aqueous solution of sulfobutylether β-cyclodextrin. However, a recent Phase I trial evaluated a solid oral dose based on the hydrogen sulfate salt and found that the safety profile was similar to that of the suspension formulation, but exposure was more than twofold higher when comparing each formulation at the maximum tolerated dose (100 mg bid for the suspension, 75 mg bid for the solid) (118). The initial Phase I study established an MTD of 200 mg bid, and a dose of 100 mg bid was selected for future studies (119). The most prominent (and dose-limiting) toxicity was rash, occurring in 74% of patients treated; diarrhea, nausea, and fatigue were also evident. As with PD0325901, several patients experienced blurred vision, although there were no signs of overt neurotoxicity. ERK phosphorylation (induced ex vivo by phorbol ester treatment) was found to decrease in peripheral blood mononuclear cells from treated patients whereas skin biopsies were found to be difficult to interpret due to variability in baseline levels. Decreased ERK phosphorylation was also observed following treatment in 12 out of 19 tumor specimens examined, with some of the decreases approaching 100%; 9 out of 20 tumor samples also showed decreases in nuclear Ki67 antigen. The best response in this study was stable disease, observed for >5 months in 16% of patients. Although KRAS, NRAS, and BRAF mutational status was examined, the number of patients was too small to draw concrete conclusions.

Phase II studies of AZD-6244 were conducted in advanced melanoma, colorectal cancer, and non small cell lung cancer, diseases in which RAS/RAF/MEK/ERK pathway activation is strongly implicated (Chapter 5). In a randomized, open-label study in patients with advanced melanoma, 200 patients were enrolled and assigned to receive either AZD-6244 (100 mg/day) or temozolomide (200 mg/m^2 for 5 days, every 28 days). Clinical responses to AZD-6244 were observed (6 confirmed and 5 unconfirmed partial responses). However, the primary endpoint (progression-free survival) showed no difference between the two arms, nor in a planned subgroup analysis of patients with BRAF or NRAS mutations (120). Similarly, no difference in progression-free survival was seen in a randomized, open-label Phase II comparing AZD-6244 with capecitabine in colorectal cancer (121). For the 69 patients enrolled, the best response in the AZD-6244 arm was stable disease (29% of patients). Finally, AZD-6244 was compared with pemetrexed as second/third-line therapy for patients with advanced non small cell lung cancer. Forty patients received AZD-6244 and 44 received pemetrexed; there were 2 partial responses in each arm, and again no difference in primary endpoint.

GDC-0973/XL518   XL518 (Genentech/Exelixis) is a noncompetitive inhibitor of MEK1 ($IC_{50} \approx 1$ nM); activity against MEK2 is significantly lower ($IC_{50} \approx 200$ nM) (122). Consistent with other MEK inhibitors, XL518 potently inhibits ERK phosphorylation and proliferation in tumor cells, resulting in G1 arrest. Preclinical pharmacodynamic studies demonstrated durable inhibition of ERK phosphorylation in tumor tissue but not in brain tissue, and dose-dependent tumor growth inhibition and regression at oral doses of 0.3–10 mg/kg qd (122). Phase I studies were initiated in 2007, and preliminary results indicate that the drug is well tolerated at suspension doses of 0.05, 0.10, and 0.20 mg/kg and at a 10-mg fixed solid (capsule) dose (123). Genentech, Inc. has exercised its option to further develop and commercialize Exelixis's compound XL518.

RDEA119   RDEA119 (Figure 10.4; Ardea Biosciences) is another non-ATP-competitive MEK inhibitor that binds adjacent to the ATP binding site. In vitro IC_{50} values for MEK1 and MEK2 inhibition were reported as 19 and 47 nM, respectively. Preclinical data indicate potent inhibition of MEK phosphorylation, tumor cell growth, and G1 arrest, with tumor growth inhibition and regression in xenograft models at doses of 25–100 mg/kg administered daily. Like XL518, RDEA119 appears to have relatively low exposure and MEK inhibition in brain tissue compared to tumor tissue (124). The half-life of RDEA119 in mice is relatively short and in preclinical xenograft studies twice-daily dosing was found to be more effective than once-daily dosing. However, early pharmacokinetic results from a Phase I study in humans showed that half-life ranged from 16 to 26 hours (125). Phase I studies are ongoing. A second clinical candidate from Ardea, RDEA436, entered Phase I studies in 2008 (126).

10.5   CDK INHIBITORS

Alvocidib   Alvocidib (flavopiridol; Sanofi-Aventis, Figure 10.5), a synthetic flavone derivative originally isolated from the bark of the Indian tree *Dysoxylum binectariferum*, is a potent inhibitor of cyclin-dependent kinases (Table 10.5) in development by Sanofi-Aventis and the National Cancer Institute. Flavopiridol inhibits CDK1, CDK2, CDK4, CDK6, and CDK7 (in vitro IC_{50} values of approximately 30, 100, 20, 60, 100, and 10 nM, respectively), which function in regulating progression through the cell division cycle (Chapter 6). In addition, flavopiridol is a potent inhibitor of CDK9 (in vitro IC_{50} value of approximately

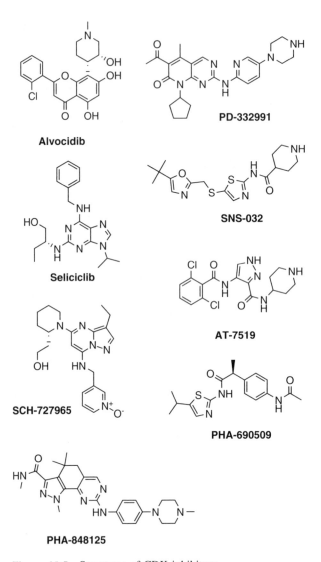

Figure 10.5 Structures of CDK inhibitors.

10 nM), which plays a critical role in the regulation of mRNA transcription via phosphorylation of RNAP polymerase II (127). In vitro studies have demonstrated that flavopiridol exerts cell cycle arrest and apoptosis-mediated cell death effects on diverse tumor cell types derived from solid and hematopoietic malignancies. Median to maximal induction levels of cell cycle arrest and cell apoptosis occur below 500 nM flavopiridol in most cell types (128). Sensitization to flavopiridol-induced cell death can be achieved by recruitment of cells into S phase prior to drug treatments (by either cell population synchronization or chemotherapy-induced S-phase delay). Cells treated with flavopiridol have

TABLE 10.5   CDK Inhibitors

Drug	Company	Target(s)	Structure[a]	Latest stage of development
Alvocidib	Sanofi-Aventis	CDK1, CDK2, CDK4, CDK6, CDK7	Figure 10.5	Phase III
Seliciclib	Cyclacel	CDK1, CDK2, CDK7, CDK9	Figure 10.5	Phase II
PD-332991	Pfizer/Onyx	CDK4, CDK6	Figure 10.5	Phase II
KRX-0601 (UCN-01)	Keryx	CHK1, PKC, PDK1, RSK1/RSK2, PRK2, PHK, CAMKKβ, AMPK, MARK3, PIM3, MST2, CDK1, CDK2, CDK4	Figure 10.6	Phase II
P-276-00	NPIL	CDK1, CDK2, CDK4, CDK9	ND	Phase II
SNS-032 (BMS-387032)	Sunesis	CDK2, CDK7, CDK9	Figure 10.5	Phase I
SCH-727965	Schering-Plough	CDK1, CDK2, CDK5, CDK9	Figure 10.5	Phase I
R-547	Hoffmann–La Roche	CDK1, CDK2, CDK3, CDK4, CDK5, CDK6, CDK7, CDK9	ND	Phase I
AT7519	Astex	CDK1, CDK2	Figure 10.5	Phase I
PHA-690509	Pfizer/Pharmacia	CDK2	Figure 10.5	Phase I
PHA-848125	Pfizer/Nerviano	CDK1, CDK2, CDK4, TRKA	Figure 10.5	Phase I
PHA-793887	Pfizer/Nerviano	Unknown	ND	Phase I
ZK-304709	Bayer Schering	CDK1, CDK2, PDGFRβ, VEGFR	ND	Phase I

[a] ND, not disclosed.

decreased expression of short-lived proteins as a consequence of CDK9 inhibition and blockade of RNA polymerase II mediated mRNA transcription—an activity that affects important cell growth and survival proteins. The antiapoptotic proteins MCL1 and XIAP, of the BCL2 family of survival proteins, are among the proteins whose expression decreases following exposure of cells to flavopiridol at concentrations that induce apoptosis (129, 130). Flavopiridol-induced mRNA and protein expression changes are aligned with cell death phenotypic responses, and the CDK9 inhibitory activity of flavopiridol recently has been recognized as an activity that contributes significantly to the antitumor growth properties of the drug. In vivo preclinical studies show xenograft tumor growth inhibition by flavopiridol in solid and hematopoietic tumor models as both a single agent and in combination with γ-radiation or chemotherapy. Models demonstrating single-agent activity include HNSCC (HN12), prostate cancer (PRXK1337 and PRXF1369), leukemia (HL-60), and rhabdoid (G401) tumors (131–134). Combination therapy activity has been observed preclinically in lung, colon, gastric, and glioma tumors.

Numerous Phase I clinical studies with flavopiridol have been completed, investigating drug safety, pharmacokinetics, and activity with different dosing and administration schedules as a mono- and combination therapy agent (135, 136). Initial trials utilized a continuous 72-hour intravenous administration; on the basis of preclinical data, prolonged maintenance of nanomolar level plasma drug concentrations were optimal for balancing drug activity and tolerability. However, due to disappointing activity in these trials, 1-hour infusion schedules were adopted to attain micromolar level plasma drug concentrations. Different 1-hour infusion administration schedules have been utilized with variable toxicities and tumor growth inhibition data. Stable disease and some partial response outcomes in both solid (lung, prostate, pancreas, renal, stomach, and esophagus) and hematopoietic (chronic lymphocytic leukemia) tumors provide evidence of drug activity (135, 137, 138). With 1-hour bolus administration schedules the dose-limiting toxicity is grade 3/4 neutropenia. Nonhematological toxicities that occur include nausea, vomiting, diarrhea, and fatigue (139–141).

Phase II studies with flavopiridol have demonstrated clinical activity in select studies, most significantly to date in CLL. However, management of drug-related toxicities in addition to ineffective clinical response data across a number of trials may limit the therapeutic opportunities for this drug. The most promising clinical activity to date has been observed in relapsed chronic lymphocytic leukemia patients, when flavopiridol was administered as a single agent by a 30-minute intravenous bolus followed by 4-hour continuous infusion (142, 143). With 62 patients enrolled and treated in this study, 26 patients have responded with a partial response and 4 complete responses have been observed. Dose-limiting toxicities in the form of acute tumor lysis syndrome and cytokine release syndrome have been managed by a decreased dosing frequency, prophylactic steroid administration, and establishing maximum white blood cell counts for patient eligibility. Flavopiridol has also shown clinical activity in MCL (1-hour daily infusion for 3 days every 21 days) and in AML (1-hour daily infusion for 3 days followed by ara-C day 6 and mitoxantrone day 9). A number of Phase II trials with flavopiridol have failed to demonstrate clinical activity and have been associated with significant toxicities. Single-agent studies of this type include metastatic renal cancer, metastatic androgen-independent prostate cancer, stage IV non small cell lung cancer, advanced gastric carcinoma, endometrial carcinoma, and soft tissue sarcoma (144–149). Combination therapy trials without flavopiridol activity include gemcitibine-refractory pancreatic cancer (docetaxol), paclitaxel-refractory esophageal cancer (paclitaxel), soft tissue sarcoma (doxorubicin), and advanced hepatocellular carcinoma (irinotecan). Most of the single-agent trials in which flavopiridol failed to demonstrate activity used a 72-hour continuous intravenous administration schedule, which has been demonstrated to be ineffective, although the endometrial cancer and soft tissue sarcoma trials utilized a 1-hour bolus infusion regimen. In trials where flavopiridol was administered as a 1-hour bolus, or a bolus followed by a 4-hour infusion, evidence of clinical activity has been observed. It remains to be determined how the confluence of antitumor activity and toxicity (mainly neutropenia and tumor lysis syndrome) will shape the utility of flavopiridol.

Seliciclib   Seliciclib (Cyclacel; Figure 10.5) inhibits CDK1, CDK2, CDK7, and CDK9 kinases with moderate potencies and is under current development by Cyclacel Pharmacueticals in Phase II non small cell lung cancer and nasopharyngeal cancer trials. In Vitro biochemical IC_{50} values for seliciclib against CDK2, CDK7, CDK9, and CDK1 are 0.1, 0.5, 0.8, and 2.7 μM, respectively (150). Seliciclib is administered orally, and in a solid tumor Phase I study dose-limiting toxicities (hypokalemia, rash, and fatigue) were observed at a dose level of 800 mg bid, given for 7 days in a 21-day cycle (151). Neutropenia and gastrointestinal toxicites are mild with Seliciclib. A Phase II non small cell lung cancer trail combining seliciclib with gemcitibine and cisplatin ended without evidence that Seliciclib contributed to the antitumor activity of the drug combination, although the combination was tolerated. A single-agent, randomized Phase II study with Seliciclib in non small cell lung cancer (APPRAISE) is ongoing, with dosing at 1200 mg bid for 3 days out of every 14 days, and a Phase I combination study of Seliciclib with erlotinib in non small cell lung cancer was initiated in 2008.

PD-332991   PD-332991 (Pfizer/Onyx; Figure 10.5) is a selective CDK4 and CDK6 inhibitor discovered by Onyx Pharmaceuticals and under current development by Pfizer. PD-332991 is a potent inhibitor of CDK4 (IC_{50} = 11 nM) and CDK6 (IC_{50} = 16 nM), by in vitro kinase assay, and inhibits xenograft tumor growth in Colo205 and MDA-MB-435 tumor xenograft models (152). Sustained suppression of Rb phosphorylation in tumor tissue is associated with the in vivo xenograft tumor growth efficacy of PD-332991, providing pharmacodynamic evidence of drug activity. A Phase I study of PD-332991 in patients with solid tumors was reported in 2007, in which the maximum tolerated dose and recommended Phase II dose was 125 mg qd × 21 days every 28 days by oral administration. The principal dose-limiting toxicity associated with PD-332991 is myelosuppression (153). A Phase I/II trial in patients with multiple myeloma was reported to be in progress in December 2007.

UCN-01 (KRX-0601)   KRX-0601, formerly UCN-01 (Figure 10.6; Kyowa Hakko/Keryx), is a staurosporine analog that inhibits a broad spectrum of kinases, including cyclin-dependent kinases CDK1, CDK2, and CDK4. Additional kinases inhibited by KRX-0601 include protein kinase C and CHK1 (see Section 10.6). Phase I and Phase II development is proceeding under the direction and sponsorship of the NCI. KRX-0601, administered intravenously by 72-hour continuous infusion every 4 weeks, has dose-limiting toxicities that include hyperglycemia, metabolic acidosis, pulmonary dysfunction, cardiac ischemia, atrial fibrillation, nausea, vomiting, and hypotension. Phase I trials have included single-agent (154) and combination studies with chemotherapies such as cisplatin (155). Current Phase I trials underway include combination treatment of solid tumors in combination with irinotecan or carboplatin, as well as CLL in combination with fludarabine. Phase II trials are also underway in melanoma, T-cell lymphoma, and (in combination with topotecan) small cell lung cancer. KRX-0601 inhibits a broad spectrum of kinases and the activity most relevant to the clinical activity is not clear at this time.

P-276-00   P-276-00, a flavone that inhibits cyclin-dependent kinases, is in Phase I and Phase II clinical development in patients with multiple myeloma by Nicholas Piramal India Limited. P-276-00 targets CDK9 with the greatest potency (20 nM), although it displays activity against CDK4 (63 nM), CDK1 (79 nM), and CDK2 (224 nM) with nanomolar IC_{50} values (156).

SNS-032   SNS-032 (Figure 10.5; Sunesis), formerly BMS-387032, is a CDK2, CDK7, and CDK9 inhibitor currently in Phase I development by Sunesis in patients with multiple myeloma (MM) and chronic lymphocytic leukemia (CLL). A Phase I trial in patients with advanced solid tumors concluded in 2007 with a report that the MTD is lower than the level of drug likely required to show single-agent activity, and nonclinical studies are being conducted to evaluate possible combination therapies (Sunesis Pharmaceuticals press release, March 9, 2007). SNS-032 is administered intravenously; initial clinical studies used a 1-hour infusion once per week for 3 weeks. Transient neutropenia is the primary dose-limiting toxicity associated with SNS-032. Gastrointestinal toxicity (nausea, vomiting, diarrhea, and anorexia) and transient liver aminase elevations are moderate (157). In a Phase I trial in patients with MM and CLL, SNS-032 is being administered with a loading dose followed by a 6-hour infusion weekly for 3 consecutive weeks every 28 days, a schedule that aims to sustain plasma drug concentrations for 6 hours at a level that inhibits 90% of in vitro cell growth (158).

SCH-727965   SCH-727965 (Figure 10.5; Schering-Plough) is a potent inhibitor of multiple CDKs that function in cell cycle and transcriptional regulation, with in vitro IC_{50} values of less than 10 nM for CDK1 (4 nM), CDK2 (1 nM), CDK5 (1 nM), and CDK9 (4 nM). SCH-727965 is currently in Phase I clinical development (159). In a dose escalation study, administration by 2-hour IV infusion on day 1 of a 21-day cycle led to a maximum tolerated dose of 58 mg/m^2, with the dose-limiting toxicity being neutropenia complicated by fever or infection. Elimination was rapid, with a terminal half-life of 1.5–3 hours.

AT7519   AT7519 (Figure 10.5; Astex) inhibits multiple CDKs affecting both cell cycle and transcription regulation and is in Phase I clinical development by Astex Pharmaceuticals. In Vitro biochemical IC_{50} values against these CDKs are reported to be less than 200 nM: CDK1 (190 nM), CDK2 (44 nM), CDK4 (67 nM), CDK5 (18 nM), and CDK9 (<10 nM). GSK3β also is inhibited by AT7519, with a biochemical IC_{50} value of 98 nM. In Phase I studies AT7519 is being administered intravenously by a 1-hour infusion on days one, two, three, four, and five of a 3-week cycle (160).

R-547   R-547 (Hoffmann–La Roche) potently inhibits many cell cycle and tran-scription regulatory cyclin-dependent kinases (IC_{50} values in parentheses): CDK1 (0.2 nM), CDK2 (0.4 nM), CDK3 (0.8 nM), CDK4 (1 nM), CDK5 (0.1 nM), CDK6 (4 nM), CDK7 (171 nM), and CDK9 (13 nM) (161, 162). A Phase I clinical study included investigation of 90-minute and 180-minute intravenous infusions, day 1 and day 8 every 21 days, with the conclusion that the 3-hour infusion schedule mitigates the most significant infusion-related toxicities and is the selected schedule for additional R-547 clinical investigation (162).

PHA-848125   PHA-848125 (Figure 10.5; Pfizer/Nerviano) is reported to inhibit CDK2 (32 nM), CDK1 (400 nM), CDK4 (160 nM), CDK5 (260 nM), and TrkA (50 nM) (163). Phase I oral administration using a 7-day on followed by 7-day off schedule identified a MTD of 200 mg/day with neurological dose-limiting toxicities (tremors and ataxia). The neurological effects are dose dependent (frequency and severity) and reversible upon drug discontinuation. The recommended Phase II dose is 150 mg/day, 7 days on followed by 7 days off. Alternate dose schedules that allow an increase in the administered dose are under investigation, for example, 4 days on followed by 3 days off for 3 weeks in a 4-week cycle.

10.6   CELL CYCLE CHECKPOINT KINASE INHIBITORS

Several checkpoint kinase inhibitors (Table 10.6) are currently in early stages of clinical evaluation (164, 165). The first of these—UCN-01—was initially identified as a PKC inhibitor and is relatively nonspecific. However, several more recent compounds have been introduced with the goal of abrogating cell cycle checkpoints that are induced following administration of chemotherapy, resulting in enhanced tumor cell death. The development of these agents presents several challenges over and above those of other kinase inhibitors in that they are only expected to show broad activity in combination with other agents. This presents regulatory challenges, as well as issues such as defining the optimal schedule for administration of the checkpoint inhibitor relative to the chemotherapy agent(s). Preliminary results from Phase I studies are beginning to emerge, although it will be difficult to assess whether this strategy provides true therapeutic benefit before randomized clinical trials are conducted comparing chemotherapy with and without administration of a checkpoint kinase inhibitor.

UCN-01   UCN-01 (KRX-0601; Kyowa Hakko/Keryx, Figure 10.6) has widely been used as a CHK1 kinase inhibitor in both in vitro and in vivo preclinical studies and has been evaluated as such in clinical trials. Many studies have shown abrogation of cell cycle checkpoints when UCN-01 is administered in combination with radiation (166–169) or various chemotherapy agents including SN38 (the active metabolite of irinotecan) (170), cisplatin (171, 172), temozolomide (173), mitomycin C (174), and gemcitabine (175). However, UCN-01 exhibits broad and potent crossreactivity with other kinases (including cyclin-dependent kinases; see Section 10.5) and a significant fraction of the compound's anticancer activity may

TABLE 10.6 Checkpoint Kinase Inhibitors

Drug	Company	Target(s)	Structure[a]	Latest stage of of development (combination)
UCN-01 (KRX-0601)	Keryx, Kyowa-Hakko	CHK1, PKC, PDK1, RSK1/RSK2, PRK2, PHK, CAMKK B, AMPK, MARK3, PIM3, MST2, CDK1, CDK2, CDK4	Figure 10.6	Phase I (cisplatin, irinotecan, 5-FU); II (topotecan)
XL844	Exelixis	CHK1, CHK2, VEGFR2, VEGFR3	ND	Phase I (gemcitabine)
PF-00477736	Pfizer	CHK1 > CHK2	Figure 10.6	Phase I (gemcitabine)
AZD7762	AstraZeneca	CHK1, CHK2	Figure 10.6	Phase I (gemcitabine, irinotecan)
CBP501	Takeda/CanBas	Substrate mimetic	Peptide	Phase I (cisplatin)
LY2603618	Icos/Lilly	No information available	ND	Phase I (pemetrexed)

[a] ND, not disclosed.

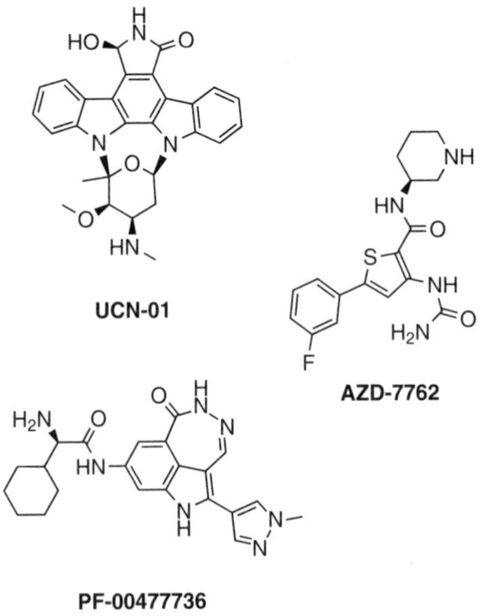

Figure 10.6 Structures of checkpoint kinase inhibitors.

be due to this crossreactivity. UCN-01 was initially identified as an inhibitor of PKC (176) and inhibits CHK1with in vitro $IC_{50} = 11$ nM (168). In addition to PKC and CHK1, UCN-01 has potent inhibitory activity toward RSK1/RSK2, PRK2, CaMKKβ, PHK, AMPK, MARK3, PIM3, MST2, and PDK1 (177).

Pharmacologically, UCN-01 is characterized by very high binding to human α1-acid glycoprotein and a very long elimination half-life in humans (200–400 h) (178). This may somewhat limit its clinical utility if the goal is to transiently inhibit cell cycle checkpoints following administration of chemotherapy. Nevertheless, UCN-01 has been evaluated in several clinical studies. Phase I dose-finding studies were performed using various dosing regimens including a 72-hour continuous infusion (154) and infusions of 1–3 hours (179). In a study of UCN-01 in combination with cisplatin, patients received cisplatin on day 1 and a continuous infusion of UCN-01 on days 2, 3, and 4 of a 28-day cycle. A constellation of diverse and severe dose-limiting toxicities (dysphagia, hypoxia, atrial fibrillation, renal failure, hyponatremia, and fatal infection) precluded escalation to an efficacious dose of cisplatin when combined with UCN-01 (180). A similar dosing schedule was used in a separate Phase I pharmacodynamic study of UCN-01 in combination with cisplatin (155). Serial tumor biopsies showed a marked reduction of cells in S/G2 phase following combination treatment, consistent with abrogation of cell cycle checkpoints. It is likely that future studies will use a more clinically acceptable 3-hour infusion schedule for UCN-01.

The combination of UCN-01 with 5-fluorouracil (5-FU) has also been investigated in humans (181). The mechanism of synergy with 5-FU may be somewhat different from the other chemotherapy agents discussed above, since UCN-01 suppresses expression of thymidylate synthase, one of the targets of 5-FU (182). 5-FU was given as a once-weekly 24-hour infusion per 4-week cycle, with UCN-01 (45 mg/m^2/ day) as a 72-hour infusion immediately following the first 5-FU dose in cycle 1 and a 36-hour infusion in subsequent cycles. 5-FU was dose-escalated from 250 to 2600 mg/m^2; no objective responses were seen but 8 patients had stable disease, 7 of whom had previously progressed on 5-FU therapy. UCN-01 was also studied in combination in a Phase I/II trial with topotecan in advanced recurrent ovarian cancer (183). Patients received topotecan (1 mg/m^2 over 30 min) on days 1–5 of a 3-week cycle, and UCN-01 on day 1 only (70 mg/m^2 over 3 hours in cycle 1, reduced to 35 mg/m^2 on subsequent cycles). Out of 29 patients treated, 3 had a partial response and 15 showed stable disease. Median time to progression was 3.3 months, with a median overall survival of 9.7 months. P53 status, H2AX phosphorylation, and Ki67 were assessed by serial biopsy in 7 patients, but no clear correlation was found with response or survival. These data are consistent with the expected activity of topotecan in this disease setting, suggesting little or no added benefit of UCN-01.

XL844   XL844 (Exelixis) is the only orally administered checkpoint kinase inhibitor currently undergoing clinical evaluation. The molecule is a potent inhibitor of CHK1 ($K_I = 2.2$ nM) and CHK2 ($K_I = 0.07$ nM) and also inhibits several other kinases including VEGFR3, VEGFR2, PDGFRβ, and FLT3 ($IC_{50} = 6$, 12, 25, and 28 nM, respectively) (184, 185). XL844 abrogates the S and/or G2 checkpoint induced by a variety of chemotherapy agents, including gemcitabine (184), daunorubicin (186), gamma radiation, cisplatin, and irinotecan/SN38 (185). This checkpoint inhibition results in potentiation of chemotherapy in clonogenic assays in vitro and/or enhanced tumor growth inhibition in xenograft models. In particular, XL844 shows no single-agent activity in a Panc-1 pancreatic carcinoma xenograft model but increases the gemcitabine-mediated tumor growth inhibition from 70% to >100% at well-tolerated doses (184). A Phase I dose escalation study was initiated with XL844 dosed orally in combination with intravenous gemcitabine, and preliminary results have been presented (187). Twenty-seven patients with various advanced solid tumors were treated for 2 weeks with XL844 alone (dosed on days 1 and 2), then for 3 weeks in combination with 800 mg/m^2 gemcitabine (with gemcitabine dosed first on day 1, followed by two doses of XL844 at 8 h and 24 h after gemcitabine). One patient experienced a serious adverse event of grade 4 thrombocytopenia in cohort 1 (0.8 mg/kg), and two patients dosed at 3.5 mg/kg had doses delayed due to neutropenia. One additional patient treated at 3.5 mg/kg died during the study treatment period. Other adverse events included nausea, fatigue, and vomiting. The mean half-life of XL844 was 2–4.5 hours, and there was no apparent pharmacokinetic interaction with gemcitabine. One patient (endometrial carcinoma) had a confirmed partial response, and 10 additional patients had stable disease for greater than 3 months. In December 2008, Exelixis reported that further development of XL844 would be suspended.

PF-00477736 PF-00477736 (Figure 10.6; Pfizer) is a somewhat selective CHK1 inhibitor, with ~100-fold greater in vitro potency toward CHK1 compared to CHK2 (K_I values 0.49 and 47 nM, respectively). This molecule is also a nanomolar inhibitor of several other kinases including VEGFR2, FMS, YES, Aurora-A, FGFR3, and FLT3 (IC$_{50}$ values 8, 10, 14, 23, 23, and 25 nM, respectively). In vitro, PF-00477736 was shown to potentiate the activity of multiple genotoxic agents in cell survival assays, including gemcitabine, SN38, carboplatin, doxorubicin, and mitomycin C. In vivo, PF-00477736 produced increased tumor growth inhibition in combination with gemcitabine or irinotecan (188). Intriguingly, PF-00477736 also shows in vivo (but not in vitro) potentiation of the mitotic spindle poison docetaxel (189). The role of CHK1 in the mitotic spindle checkpoint is less well characterized than its role in the S and G2/M checkpoints, and at least one paper suggests that CHK1 is required for efficient cell killing by taxol (190). Nevertheless, the data reported for PF-00477736 suggest that CHK1 inhibitors may have utility in combination with antimicrotubule agents as well as DNA-damaging agents. PF-00477736 is currently in a Phase I clinical trial in combination with gemcitabine.

AZD7762 AZD7762 (Figure 10.6; AstraZeneca) is a potent inhibitor of CHK1 and CHK2, with IC$_{50}$ values of 5 nM and <10 nM, respectively (191). It is selective against a broad panel of kinases but shows crossreactivity with SRC family kinases (< tenfold selective compared to CHK1/CHK2). AZD7762 is highly potent in cellular assays (IC$_{50}$ ≈ 10 nM), leading to cell cycle checkpoint inhibition following treatment of cells with gemcitabine or irinotecan. This checkpoint inhibition is manifest as a potentiation of cell killing in vitro, and of tumor growth inhibition in H460 and SW620 xenograft models. Two Phase I studies of AZD7762 are in progress, in combination with gemcitabine and irinotecan, respectively.

CBP501   CBP501 is a dodecapeptide designed to mimic the CDC25C substrate of checkpoint kinases. It is reported to inhibit CHK1 and CHK2 with IC$_{50}$ values of 3.4 and 6.5 μM, respectively, with additional activity against MAPKAPK2 (0.9 μM) and C-TAK1 (1.3 μM) (192). In vitro and in vivo studies showed that G2 checkpoint induced by bleomycin or cisplatin was inhibited by treatment of cells with CBP501, resulting in enhanced cell killing in clonogenic assays and tumor growth inhibition in xenograft models. A Phase I study of CBP501 in combination with cisplatin was recently reported (193). Thirty patients were treated with CBP501 alone, and 33 patients with the combination of CBP501 and cisplatin. CBP501 was administered as a 1-hour infusion on days 1, 8, and 15 of a 4-week schedule; in the combination study, cisplatin was given as a 1-hour infusion starting 1 hour after the CBP501 infusion. Adverse events were principally allergic reaction to the CBP501 infusion, which was dose limiting in the combination arm of the study at doses of 25 mg/m^2 CBP501 and 75 mg/m^2 cisplatin. C_{max} and AUC for CBP501 were dose proportional over the range evaluated. In the combination arm, one partial response (endometrial carcinoma) and five cases of disease stabilization were noted, two of which were in platinum-resistant ovarian cancer patients. An additional study is in progress evaluating CBP501 in combination with cisplatin/pemetrexed in mesothelioma.

10.7   MITOTIC KINASE INHIBITORS

10.7.1   PLK Inhibitors

BI 2536   BI 2536 (Figure 10.7; Boehringer Ingelheim) is a very potent and highly selective inhibitor of PLK family kinases (Table 10.7). In Vitro, it is somewhat specific for PLK1 compared to PLK2 and PLK3 (IC$_{50}$ values 0.83, 3.5, and 9.0 nM, respectively) and has little activity against a panel of 63 other protein kinases (194). Treatment of tumor cells with BI 2536 produces a constellation of mitotic defects, including delayed prophase, monopolar mitotic spindle formation, and prometaphase arrest, culminating in mitotic catastrophe (195). In preclinical tumor xenograft models, BI 2536 was dosed by weekly or twice-weekly intravenous injection and produced substantial tumor growth inhibition in several models (194). Tumor growth inhibition was found to correlate with increased mitotic fraction (as assessed by mitotic index and phosphohistone H3 (pHisH3) staining and induction of apoptosis.

In Phase I clinical studies, BI 2536 was administered as an IV infusion using several alternative dosing schedules. A Phase I study in patients with advanced solid tumors evaluated two different schedules, dosing either on day 1 or on days

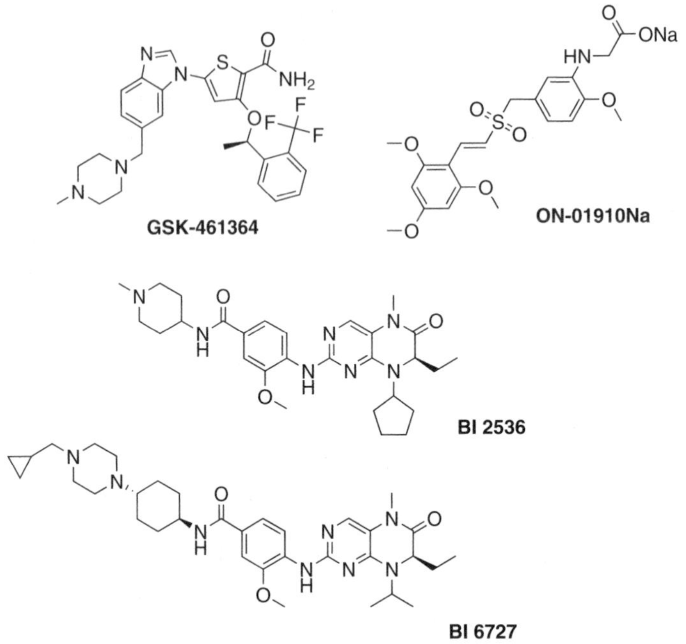

GSK-461364

ON-01910Na

BI 2536

BI 6727

Figure 10.7 Structures of PLK inhibitors.

TABLE 10.7 PLK (Polo-like Kinase) Inhibitors

Drug	Company	Target(s)	Structure	Latest stage of development
BI 2536	Boehringer Ingelheim	PLK1, PLK2, PLK3	Figure 10.7	Phase II
BI 6727	Boehringer Ingelheim	PLK1	Figure 10.7	Phase I
ON01910.Na	Onconova	PLK1, PDGFR, ABL, VEGFR1	Figure 10.7	Phase I
GSK-461364	GlaxoSmithKline	PLK1	Figure 10.7	Phase I

1–3 of a 3-week cycle (196). Neutropenia was the principal dose-limiting toxicity, with additional adverse events of alopecia, nausea, anorexia, vomiting, fatigue, and mucositis. The maximum tolerated single dose was 200 mg, whereas dose-limiting toxicities were observed at 70 mg using the intensified dosing schedule. In a separate study, dosing on days 1 and 8 of a 3-week cycle, the maximum tolerated dose was 100 mg, again limited by neutropenia (197). A Phase I dose escalation study of BI 2536 has also been conducted in combination with pemetrexed (198).

In a randomized Phase II study, two dose schedules of BI 2536 were evaluated in patients with advanced non small cell lung cancer (199). The drug was administered as a 60-minute IV infusion, either at 200 mg on day 1 or at 50 (amended to 60) mg on days 1–3 of a 21-day cycle. For the 95 patients treated, fatigue, nausea, and neutropenia were the main toxicities. Median progression-free survival was 7 and 8.2 weeks for the single and triple infusion groups, respectively, with no statistically significant difference: however, almost 50% of patients had stable disease 16 weeks after the start of therapy and median overall survival was 28.7 weeks. In addition, four patients achieved a partial response; however, two deaths on study (sepsis and pulmonary hemorrhage) were deemed to be potentially related to treatment. A second PLK inhibitor from Boehringer Ingelheim, BI 6727, is also in early stage clinical trials. BI 6727 was administered as a 1-hour intravenous infusion once every 3 weeks at dose levels of 12–450 mg. The compound has a very long half-life in humans (110 h). Dose-limiting toxicities were mainly hematological and occurred at dose levels of 350–450 mg; the recommended Phase II dose is 300 mg. An encouraging rate of disease stabilization and two partial responses were seen in the Phase I study (200).

ON01910.Na   ON01910.Na (Figure 10.7; Onconova) is distinct from many other kinase inhibitors discussed here in that it is substrate competitive rather than ATP competitive, with an IC_{50} of ~ 10 nM for PLK1 (201). Some crossreactivity was observed with PDGFR, ABL, and VEGFR1 (IC_{50} 18–42 nM) and somewhat less potently with CDK1, PLK2, SRC, and FYN (IC_{50} 155–260 nM). Notably, PLK3 was not inhibited. In tumor cells, ON01910.Na treatment produced multipolar spindles and misaligned chromosomes, leading to apoptosis with IC_{50} values ranging from 50 to 100 nM. In contrast, normal human epithelial cells, endothelial cells, and fibroblasts were highly resistant to drug-induced apoptosis. Activity was demonstrated in several mouse xenograft tumor models both as a single agent and in combination with oxaliplatin, doxorubicin, or gemcitabine. In an ongoing Phase I study, the drug was administered as a weekly 24-hour infusion and was well tolerated at doses from 250 to 2750 mg/m^2 (202).

GSK-461364   GSK-461364 (Figure 10.7; GlaxoSmithKline) is a potent inhibitor of PLK1 ($K_I = 2.2$ nM) and is >100-fold selective with respect to PLK2, PLK3, and 48 other kinases tested (203). Treatment of 120 cell lines with GSK-461364 led to growth inhibition with an IC_{50} of <100 nM in over 90% of cases, with a net cytostatic response in about 40% and net cell death in 45% of cell lines tested. As expected for a PLK1 inhibitor, G2/M arrest and mitotic perturbation were observed (204). Mitotic arrest was also observed in vivo, and tumor growth delay and/or regression was observed in a Colo205 xenograft model following intraperitoneal dosing at 50 mg/kg q2d or q4d (205). Phase I studies with intravenous administration of GSK-461364 were initiated in 2007.

10.7.2 Aurora Kinase Inhibitors

VX680 (MK-0457/tozasertib)   VX680 (Figure 10.8; Vertex/Merck) was the first Aurora kinase inhibitor (Table 10.8) to enter clinical studies. Preclinical data showed it to be a potent inhibitor of all Aurora kinases, with IC_{50} values of 0.6,

18, and 4.6 nM for Aurora-A, -B, and -C, respectively (206). The compound was found to be quite selective against a panel of 55 other kinases, with only FLT3 showing significant crossreactivity ($K_1 = 30$ nM); more recently, activity against JAK2 kinase has been reported (207). Tumor cells treated with VX680 in vitro showed inhibition of phosphohistone H3 (pHisH3) phosphorylation, retarded mitotic progression, and an increased fraction with $\geq$ 4N DNA content. Inhibition of proliferation and induction of apoptosis were demonstrated both in vitro and in tumor xenograft models in vivo (using twice-daily intraperitoneal dosing). Additional interest in the clinical application of VX680 was generated by the discovery that it also inhibits both the wild-type and (imatinib-resistant) T315I mutant forms of BCR-ABL, with IC_{50} values of 10 and 30 nM, respectively (208, 209). VX680 was found to have particularly potent activity against various leukemia cell lines and displayed in vitro evidence of synergy with chemotherapy agents and other BCR-ABL inhibitors in leukemia cells (210). The FLT3 activity of VX680 lends further support to its potential application in hematological malignancies, as activating FLT3 mutations are frequently found in AML (Chapter 3).

In a Phase I study of VX680, patients with advanced solid tumors received a 5-day continuous infusion of drug every 28 days (211). Dose-limiting toxicity of neutropenia was observed at 12 mg/m^2/h, establishing 10 mg/m^2/h as the maximum tolerated dose. There were no objective responses, although two patients had stable disease for six cycles of treatment. Myelosuppression was also seen in a Phase I study in hematological malignancies: in this case VX680 was administered as a 5-day infusion every 2–3 weeks at doses up to 28 mg/m^2/h. Several encouraging signs of clinical activity were observed, including objective responses in 11 of 14 evaluable CML patients who all had the BCR-ABL T315I resistance mutation (207, 212, 213), and pharmacodynamic studies in samples from CML and AML patients showed evidence for increased apoptosis in leukemia cells (214). In addition, activity was seen in patients with JAK2-transformed myeloproliferative disease (215, 216). A pivotal study of VX680 was initiated in January 2007 in patients with T315I mutant CML and Ph+ ALL; however, this trial was suspended in November 2007 following evidence of QTc prolongation.

PHA-739358 Like VX680, PHA-739358 (Figure 10.8; Nerviano/Pfizer) is another pan-Aurora inhibitor that also shows crossreactivity with both wild-type and mutant BCR-ABL (217, 218). In vitro IC_{50} values were reported as 13, 79, and 61 nM for Aurora-A, -B, and -C, respectively, and binding affinities for wild-type and T315I ABL were determined as 14 and 5 nM, respectively (217, 219). Several other kinases are also targets of PHA-739358, including FGFR1, RET, and TRKA (IC_{50} values 47, 31, and 31 nM, respectively). Cellular inhibition of these kinases was confirmed and, as in the case of VX680, in vitro treatment with PHA-739358 produced an increase in $\geq$ 4N DNA content and inhibition of tumor cell proliferation. Intravenous administration using a twice-daily schedule produced strong antitumor activity in mouse xenograft models, correlating with inhibition of pHisH3 phosphorylation and accumulation of p53 and p21 (217). In a Phase I study, PHA-739358 was administered as a 24-hour infusion every

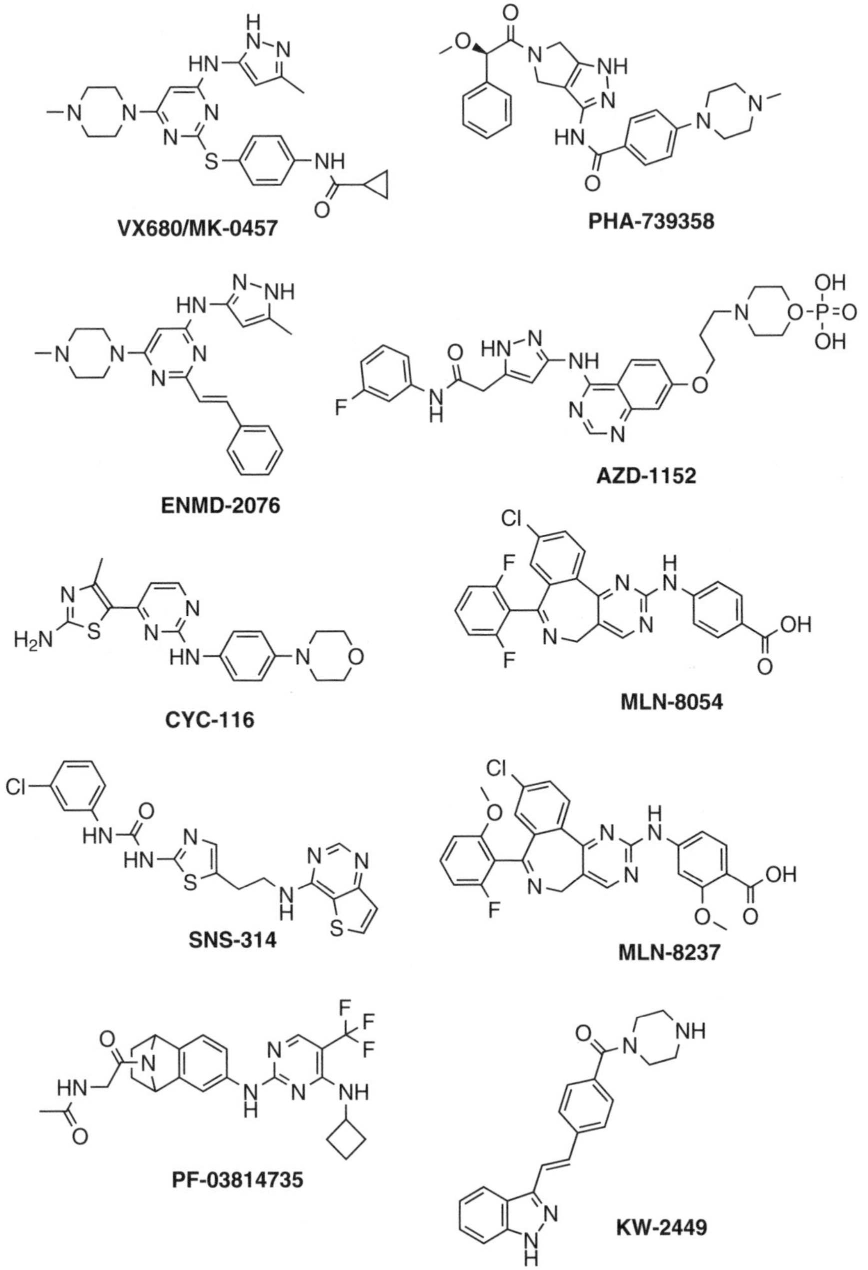

Figure 10.8 Structures of Aurora inhibitors.

TABLE 10.8   Aurora Kinase Inhibitors

Drug	Company	Target(s)	Structure[a]	Latest stage of development
Tozasertib (VX680/MK-0457)	Vertex/Merck	Aurora-A, Aurora-B, Aurora-C, FLT3, JAK2, ABL	Figure 10.8	Phase II (discontinued)
PHA-739358	Pfizer	Aurora-A, Aurora-B, Aurora-C, FGFR1, RET, TRKA	Figure 10.8	Phase II
AZD-1152	AstraZeneca	Aurora-B	Figure 10.8	Phase I/II
AT9283	Astex	Aurora-A, Aurora-B, TYK2, JAK2, JAK3, RSK2, RET, MER, YES, GSK3β	Figure 8.5	Phase I/II
MLN8054	Millennium	Aurora-A	Figure 10.8	Phase I
MLN8237	Millennium	Aurora-A	Figure 10.8	Phase I
PF-03814735	Pfizer	Aurora-A, Aurora-B	Figure 10.8	Phase I
CYC-116	Cyclacel	Aurora-A, Aurora-B, Aurora-C, VEGFR2, FLT3	Figure 10.8	Phase I
KW-2449	Kyowa-Hakko	Aurora-A, FLT3, FGFR1, ABL	Figure 10.8	Phase I
ENMD-2076	Entremed	Aurora-A	Figure 10.8	Phase I
R-763	Rigel/Serono	Aurora-A, Aurora-B	ND	Phase I
SNS-314	Sunesis	Aurora-A, Aurora-B, Aurora-C	Figure 10.8	Phase I

[a] ND, not disclosed.

14 days (220). Since neutropenia appears to be a common dose-limiting toxicity for Aurora inhibitors, the drug was evaluated with and without concurrent G-CSF therapy. In both cases the dose-limiting toxicity was neutropenia: however, the maximum tolerated dose was higher with G-CSF administration (750 mg/m^2) than without (500 mg/m^2). Nine out of 42 patients experienced disease stabilization for >3 months, with one patient (small cell lung carcinoma, treated with G-CSF) showing a partial response lasting 23 weeks. Skin biopsies (collected predose and at 30 minutes before the end of infusion) showed decreased histone H3 phosphorylation in most patients.

AZD-1152   AZD-1152 (Figure 10.8; AstraZeneca) is a prodrug that is rapidly converted in vivo to the active drug (termed AZD-1152-HQPA) (221). It was developed to specifically inhibit Aurora-B, for which it is highly selective: in vitro IC_{50} values are 0.37 nM and 1368 nM for Aurora-B and -A kinases, respectively (222). The phenotypic effects of AZD-1152 on cells mirror those of the pan-Aurora kinase inhibitors: inhibition of pHisH3 is accompanied by polyploidy, loss of cell viability, and induction of apoptosis (223).

   Continuous infusion of AZD-1152 in mice bearing xenograft tumors produced tumor growth inhibition and, in some cases, regression. Also, myelosuppression was observed in hematopoietic tissue (consistent with the effects of Aurora inhibition on cycling cells); however, this effect was reversible on cessation of dosing (223). Activity was also demonstrated in leukemia cells in vitro and in vivo: furthermore, the antitumor activities of several genotoxic agents were potentiated by coadministration of AZD-1152 (222). Multiple Phase I studies have been initiated to evaluate different intravenous dosing schedules in patients with advanced solid tumors and leukemias.

MLN8054   MLN8054 (Figure 10.8; Millennium/Takeda) is a specific inhibitor of Aurora-A ($IC_{50} = 4$ nM), with relatively weak Aurora-B activity ($IC_{50} = 172$ nM). This selectivity was recapitulated in cellular assays, with inhibition of Aurora-A autophosphorylation ($IC_{50} = 44$ nM) being significantly more potent than inhibition of the Aurora-B substrate pHisH3 ($IC_{50} = 5700$ nM) (224). In vitro treatment of tumor cells with MLN8054 led to accumulation of cells in G2/M with abnormal mitotic spindles, and subsequent defects in chromosomal segregation may underlie the antitumor activity of this drug (224, 225). Treatment with higher doses of drug led to cells with >4N DNA content, possibly reflecting the influence of Aurora-B. MLN8054 is orally available, and once-daily or twice-daily oral dosing produced robust antitumor activity: moreover, immunohistochemical analysis of tumors showed that this activity was consistent with inhibition of Aurora-A rather than Aurora-B (224). Although neutropenia was observed following 21-day dosing in nude mice, neutrophil counts recovered when treatment was stopped. In a Phase I dose escalation study, MLN8054 was administered orally once daily for 7 consecutive days out of a 21-day cycle. A dose-limiting toxicity of reversible somnolence was observed at doses of 20 and 40 mg, resulting from crossreactivity with the benzodiazepine receptor. This prompted evaluation of divided doses on a four-times-a-day schedule, which yielded a maximum tolerated dose of 45 mg/day. However, there was no evidence of target modulation in skin biopsies and no myelosuppression, suggesting that this dose and schedule is insufficient to achieve pharmacodynamic activity in humans. Studies are continuing with an extended dosing period (14 days) and coadminstration of the stimulant methylphenidate. A second Aurora-A inhibitor from Millennium, MLN8237, is also currently in Phase I.

AT9283   AT9283 (Figure 8.5; Astex) is a multitargeted kinase inhibitor with potent activity ($IC_{50} < 10$ nM) against Aurora-A, Aurora-B, TYK2, JAK2, RSK2, RET, MER, YES, and GSK3β. This inhibitor is discussed further under JAK2 inhibitors (Chapter 8).

PF-03814735 PF-03814735 (Figure 10.8; Pfizer) is an orally available inhibitor of Aurora-A and Aurora-B, with IC_{50} values of 0.8 and 5 nM, respectively. In a Phase I study in patients with advanced solid tumors, PF-03814735 was administered for 5 or 10 consecutive days in 3-week treatment cycles. In the 5-day schedule, the maximum tolerated dose was 80 mg/day; dose-limiting toxicity was febrile neutropenia. No objective responses were observed, but two patients were treated for at least four cycles (226).

KW-2449 KW-2449 (Figure 10.8; Kyowa Hakko) is an orally available multikinase inhibitor with activity against FLT3, FGFR1, and ABL kinases in addition to Aurora-A; Aurora-B and Aurora-C activity has not been reported. A Phase I dose escalation study is being conducted in patients with acute leukemia, treatment-resistant/intolerant CML, and myelodysplastic syndrome (227).

CYC-116 CYC-116 (Figure 10.8; Cyclacel) is a pan-Aurora aminopyrimidine-based inhibitor (IC_{50} values 44, 19, and 65 nM for Aurora-A, -B, and -C, respectively) with additional activity against VEGFR2 ($IC_{50} = 69$ nM) and FLT3 ($IC_{50} = 88$ nM). Cellular assays show inhibition of Aurora-A and Aurora-B phosphorylation and abnormal mitotic spindle formation (228). In Vivo, CYC-116 promotes polyploidy in tumor cells and also inhibits tumor angiogenesis (229). Phase I studies are currently in progress.

10.8 PROTEIN KINASE C INHIBITORS

Enzastaurin Enzastaurin (Figure 10.9; Eli Lilly) is a bisindolylmaleimide derivative that was originally developed as an inhibitor of PKCβ (Table 10.9). It inhibits PKCβ with $IC_{50} = 6$ nM and is also active against PKCα, PKCγ, and PKCε (IC_{50} values 39, 83, and 110 nM, respectively), as well as PKCδ and PKCθ (230). Antiproliferative activity was observed in PC-3, HCT116, and U87MG cell-based assays, with induction of apoptosis in HCT116 and U87MG cells. This activity was associated with inhibition of GSK3β and ribosomal S6 protein phosphorylation. Mice bearing HCT116 xenograft tumors were dosed orally with enzastaurin at 75 mg twice daily, suppressing GSK3β phosphorylation and reducing tumor growth (230). Enzastaurin was also found to inhibit growth of tumor cell lines with differential sensitivities to EGFR inhibitors and produced synergistic growth inhibition when combined with gefitinib in cellular assays and tumor xenografts (231). Further preclinical activity has been observed in multiple myeloma cells (232, 233) and in combination with radiation in pancreatic carcinoma cells (234).

In a Phase I dose escalation study, the drug was dosed orally and was well tolerated at up to 700 mg/day. Several incidences of asymptomatic QTc prolongation were reported as dose-limiting toxicities: otherwise, only grade 1/2 toxicities were noted. A maximum tolerated dose was not defined, although 525 mg was proposed as the recommended Phase II dose based on saturation of exposure. There were no objective responses (235). Phase II studies with enzastaurin have been pursued in a number of indications including B-cell lymphoma, glioma, and NSCLC.

Enzastaurin   Figure 10.9   Structure of PKC inhibitor.

TABLE 10.9   PKC inhibitors

Drug	Company	Target(s)	Structure	Latest stage of development
Enzastaurin (LY317615)	Eli Lilly	PKCα, PKCβ, PKCγ, PKCε, PKCδ, PKCθ	Figure 10.8	Phase III

Given the rationale for involvement of PKC in diffuse large B-cell lymphoma, a Phase II study was initiated in this disease. Fifty-five patients who had relapsed on previous therapy received 500 mg enzastaurin daily for 28-day cycles. Responses were encouraging: 12 patients remained progression-free after two cycles, of whom 8 were progression-free after four cycles. Four patients had long-term responses of 20+ to 50+ cycles, 3 of whom had a complete response. A Phase III trial is in progress, combining standard CHOP/rituxan induction chemotherapy with enzastaurin consolidation therapy in patients with newly diagnosed, high-risk DLBCL. Another trial evaluated enzastaurin in relapsed or refractory mantle cell lymphoma. Sixty patients received 500 mg daily, and although no objective responses were seen, 22 patients were progression-free after three cycles and 6 were progression-free for 6 months or more (236).

Encouraging preliminary data were presented in a trial of enzastaurin for recurrent high grade glioma: of 87 evaluable patients, 20 had an objective radiographic response and 6 had stable disease. Tolerability was good, with two incidences of thrombocytopenia (grade 3 and 4) being the main toxicities (237). However, these data were not recapitulated in a subsequent Phase III trial in glioblastoma, and further development in this indication was suspended.

REFERENCES

1. Baker H, Sidorowicz A, Sehgal SN, Vezina C. Rapamycin (AY-22,989), a new antifungal antibiotic. III. in vitro and in vivo evaluation. J Antibiot (Tokyo) 1978;31(6):539–545.
2. Sehgal SN, Baker H, Vezina C. Rapamycin (AY-22,989), a new antifungal antibiotic. II. Fermentation, isolation and characterization. J Antibiot (Tokyo) 1975;28(10):727–732.

3. Vezina C, Kudelski A, Sehgal SN. Rapamycin (AY-22,989), a new antifungal antibiotic. I. Taxonomy of the producing streptomycete and isolation of the active principle. J Antibiot (Tokyo) 1975;28(10):721–726.

4. Brown EJ, Albers MW, Shin TB, Ichikawa K, Keith CT, Lane WS, Schreiber SL. A mammalian protein targeted by G1-arresting rapamycin-receptor complex. Nature 1994;369(6483):756–758.

5. Choi J, Chen J, Schreiber SL, Clardy J. Structure of the FKBP12-rapamycin complex interacting with the binding domain of human FRAP. Science 1996;273(5272):239–242.

6. Lawrence JC, Lin TA, McMahon LP, Choi KM. Modulation of the protein kinase activity of mTOR. Curr Top Microbiol Immunol 2004;279:199–213.

7. Oshiro N, Yoshino K, Hidayat S, Tokunaga C, Hara K, Eguchi S, Avruch J, Yonezawa K. Dissociation of raptor from mTOR is a mechanism of rapamycin-induced inhibition of mTOR function. Genes Cells 2004;9(4):359–366.

8. Shor B, Zhang WG, Toral-Barza L, Lucas J, Abraham RT, Gibbons JJ, Yu K. A new pharmacologic action of CCI-779 involves FKBP12-independent inhibition of mTOR kinase activity and profound repression of global protein synthesis. Cancer Res 2008;68(8):2934–2943.

9. Sehgal SN. Sirolimus: its discovery, biological properties, and mechanism of action. Transplant Proc 2003;35(3 Suppl): 7S–14S.

10. Miller JL. Sirolimus approved with renal transplant indication. Am J Health Syst Pharm 1999;56(21):2177–2178.

11. Dancey JE. Therapeutic targets: MTOR and related pathways. Cancer Biol Ther 2006; 5(9):1065–1073.

12. Harrington LS, Findlay GM, Gray A, Tolkacheva T, Wigfield S, Rebholz H, Barnett J, Leslie NR, Cheng S, Shepherd PR, Gout I, Downes CP, Lamb RF. The TSC1-2 tumor suppressor controls insulin-PI3K signaling via regulation of IRS proteins. J Cell Biol 2004;166(2):213–223.

13. O'Reilly KE, Rojo F, She QB, Solit D, Mills GB, Smith D, Lane H, Hofmann F, Hicklin DJ, Ludwig DL, Baselga J, Rosen N. mTOR inhibition induces upstream receptor tyrosine kinase signaling and activates Akt. Cancer Res 2006;66(3):1500–1508.

14. Wan X, Harkavy B, Shen N, Grohar P, Helman LJ. Rapamycin induces feedback activation of Akt signaling through an IGF-1R-dependent mechanism. Oncogene 2007;26(13):1932–1940.

15. Carracedo A, Ma L, Teruya-Feldstein J, Rojo F, Salmena L, Alimonti A, Egia A, Sasaki AT, Thomas G, Kozma SC, Papa A, Nardella C, Cantley LC, Baselga J, Pandolfi PP. Inhibition of mTORC1 leads to MAPK pathway activation through a PI3K-dependent feedback loop in human cancer. J Clin Invest 2008;118(9):3065–3074.

16. Sarbassov DD, Ali SM, Sengupta S, Sheen JH, Hsu PP, Bagley AF, Markhard AL, Sabatini DM. Prolonged rapamycin treatment inhibits mTORC2 assembly and Akt/PKB. Mol Cell 2006;22(2):159–168.

17. Choo AY, Yoon SO, Kim SG, Roux PP, Blenis J. Rapamycin differentially inhibits S6Ks and 4E-BP1 to mediate cell-type-specific repression of mRNA translation. Proc Natl Acad Sci U S A 2008;105(45):17414–17419.

18. O'Donnell A, Faivre S, Burris HA 3rd, Rea D, Papadimitrakopoulou V, Shand N, Lane HA, Hazell K, Zoellner U, Kovarik JM, Brock C, Jones S, Raymond E, Judson I. Phase I pharmacokinetic and pharmacodynamic study of the oral mammalian target of rapamycin inhibitor everolimus in patients with advanced solid tumors. J Clin Oncol 2008;26(10):1588–1595.

19. Mita MM, Mita AC, Chu QS, Rowinsky EK, Fetterly GJ, Goldston M, Patnaik A, Mathews L, Ricart AD, Mays T, Knowles H, Rivera VM, Kreisberg J, Bedrosian CL, Tolcher AW. Phase I trial of the novel mammalian target of rapamycin inhibitor deforolimus (AP23573; MK-8669) administered intravenously daily for 5 days every 2 weeks to patients with advanced malignancies. J Clin Oncol 2008;26(3):361–367.

20. Tabernero J, Rojo F, Calvo E, Burris H, Judson I, Hazell K, Martinelli E, Ramon y Cajal S, Jones S, Vidal L, Shand N, Macarulla T, Ramos FJ, Dimitrijevic S, Zoellner U, Tang P, Stumm M, Lane HA, Lebwohl D, Baselga J. Dose- and schedule-dependent inhibition of the mammalian target of rapamycin pathway with everolimus: a phase I tumor pharmacodynamic study in patients with advanced solid tumors. J Clin Oncol 2008;26(10):1603–1610.

21. Tanaka C, O'Reilly T, Kovarik JM, Shand N, Hazell K, Judson I, Raymond E, Zumstein-Mecker S, Stephan C, Boulay A, Hattenberger M, Thomas G, Lane HA. Identifying optimal biologic doses

of everolimus (RAD001) in patients with cancer based on the modeling of preclinical and clinical pharmacokinetic and pharmacodynamic data. J Clin Oncol 2008;26(10):1596–1602.

22. Majumder PK, Sellers WR. Akt-regulated pathways in prostate cancer. Oncogene 2005;24(50):7465–7474.

23. Wei LH, Su H, Hildebrandt IJ, Phelps ME, Czernin J, Weber WA. Changes in tumor metabolism as readout for mammalian target of rapamycin kinase inhibition by rapamycin in glioblastoma. Clin Cancer Res 2008;14(11):3416–3426.

24. Thomas GV, Tran C, Mellinghoff IK, Welsbie DS, Chan E, Fueger B, Czernin J, Sawyers CL. Hypoxia-inducible factor determines sensitivity to inhibitors of mTOR in kidney cancer. Nat Med 2006;12(1):122–127.

25. Sankhala KK, Chawla SP, Iagaru A, Dellamaggiora R, Chua V, Daly S, Bedrosian CL, Edwards GK, Cohen S, Demetri GD, for the APSSG. Early response evaluation of therapy with AP23573 (an mTOR inhibitor) in sarcoma using [^{18}F]2-fluoro-2-deoxy-D-glucose (FDG) positron emission tomography (PET) scan. J Clin Oncol (Meeting Abstracts) 2005;23(16 Suppl):Abstr 9028.

26. Tabernero J, Rojo F, Burris H, Casado E, Macarulla T, Jones S, Dimitrijevic S, Hazell K, Shand N, Baselga J. A phase I study with tumor molecular pharmacodynamic (MPD) evaluation of dose and schedule of the oral mTOR-inhibitor everolimus (RAD001) in patients (pts) with advanced solid tumors. J Clin Oncol (Meeting Abstracts) 2005;23(16 Suppl): Abstr 3007.

27. Hidalgo M, Buckner JC, Erlichman C, Pollack MS, Boni JP, Dukart G, Marshall B, Speicher L, Moore L, Rowinsky EK. A phase I and pharmacokinetic study of temsirolimus (CCI-779) administered intravenously daily for 5 days every 2 weeks to patients with advanced cancer. Clin Cancer Res 2006;12(19):5755–5763.

28. Raymond E, Alexandre J, Faivre S, Vera K, Materman E, Boni J, Leister C, Korth-Bradley J, Hanauske A, Armand JP. Safety and pharmacokinetics of escalated doses of weekly intravenous infusion of CCI-779, a novel mTOR inhibitor, in patients with cancer. J Clin Oncol 2004;22(12):2336–2347.

29. Jimeno A, Kulesza P, Cusatis G, Howard A, Khan Y, Messersmith W, Laheru D, Garrett-Mayer E, Baker SD, Hidalgo M. Pharmacodynamic-guided, modified continuous reassessment method (mCRM)-based, dose finding study of rapamycin in adult patients with solid tumors. J Clin Oncol (Meeting Abstracts) 2006;24(18 Suppl):Abstr 3020.

30. Ratain MJ, Napoli KL, Moshier KK, Jiang X, Fleming GF, Gajewski TF, Jacobsen E, Cohen EE. A phase 1b study of oral rapamycin (sirolimus) in patients with advanced malignancies. J Clin Oncol (Meeting Abstracts) 2007;25(18 Suppl):Abstr 3510.

31. Cloughesy TF, Yoshimoto K, Nghiemphu P, Brown K, Dang J, Zhu S, Hsueh T, Chen Y, Wang W, Youngkin D, Liau L, Martin N, Becker D, Bergsneider M, Lai A, Green R, Oglesby T, Koleto M, Trent J, Horvath S, Mischel PS, Mellinghoff IK, Sawyers CL. Antitumor activity of rapamycin in a phase I trial for patients with recurrent PTEN-deficient glioblastoma. PLoS Med 2008;5(1):e8.

32. Geoerger B, Kerr K, Tang CB, Fung KM, Powell B, Sutton LN, Phillips PC, Janss AJ. Antitumor activity of the rapamycin analog CCI-779 in human primitive neuroectodermal tumor/medulloblastoma models as single agent and in combination chemotherapy. Cancer Res 2001;61(4):1527–1532.

33. Yu K, Toral-Barza L, Discafani C, Zhang WG, Skotnicki J, Frost P, Gibbons JJ. mTOR, a novel target in breast cancer: the effect of CCI-779, an mTOR inhibitor, in preclinical models of breast cancer. Endocr Relat Cancer 2001;8(3):249–258.

34. Neshat MS, Mellinghoff IK, Tran C, Stiles B, Thomas G, Petersen R, Frost P, Gibbons JJ, Wu H, Sawyers CL. Enhanced sensitivity of PTEN-deficient tumors to inhibition of FRAP/mTOR. Proc Natl Acad Sci U S A 2001;98(18):10314–10319.

35. Atkins MB, Hidalgo M, Stadler WM, Logan TF, Dutcher JP, Hudes GR, Park Y, Liou SH, Marshall B, Boni JP, Dukart G, Sherman ML. Randomized phase II study of multiple dose levels of CCI-779, a novel mammalian target of rapamycin kinase inhibitor, in patients with advanced refractory renal cell carcinoma. J Clin Oncol 2004;22(5):909–918.

36. Motzer RJ, Hudes GR, Curti BD, McDermott DF, Escudier BJ, Negrier S, Duclos B, Moore L, O'Toole T, Boni JP, Dutcher JP. Phase I/II trial of temsirolimus combined with interferon alfa for advanced renal cell carcinoma. J Clin Oncol 2007;25(25):3958–3964.

37. Hudes G, Carducci M, Tomczak P, Dutcher J, Figlin R, Kapoor A, Staroslawska E, Sosman J, McDermott D, Bodrogi I, Kovacevic Z, Lesovoy V, Schmidt-Wolf IG, Barbarash O, Gokmen E, O'Toole T, Lustgarten S, Moore L, Motzer RJ. Temsirolimus, interferon alfa, or both for advanced renal-cell carcinoma. N Engl J Med 2007;356(22):2271–2281.

38. Oda K, Stokoe D, Taketani Y, McCormick F. High frequency of coexistent mutations of PIK3CA and PTEN genes in endometrial carcinoma. Cancer Res 2005;65(23):10669–10673.

39. Oza AM, Elit L, Biagi J, Chapman W, Tsao M, Hedley D, Hansen C, Dancey J, Eisenhauer E. Molecular correlates associated with a phase II study of temsirolimus (CCI-779) in patients with metastatic or recurrent endometrial cancer–NCIC IND 160. J Clin Oncol (Meeting Abstracts) 2006;24(18 Suppl):Abstr 3003.

40. Witzig TE, Geyer SM, Ghobrial I, Inwards DJ, Fonseca R, Kurtin P, Ansell SM, Luyun R, Flynn PJ, Morton RF, Dakhil SR, Gross H, Kaufmann SH. Phase II trial of single-agent temsirolimus (CCI-779) for relapsed mantle cell lymphoma. J Clin Oncol 2005;23(23):5347–5356.

41. Ansell SM, Inwards DJ, Rowland KM Jr, Flynn PJ, Morton RF, Moore DF Jr, Kaufmann SH, Ghobrial I, Kurtin PJ, Maurer M, Allmer C, Witzig TE. Low-dose, single-agent temsirolimus for relapsed mantle cell lymphoma: a phase 2 trial in the North Central Cancer Treatment Group. Cancer 2008;113(3):508–514.

42. Galanis E, Buckner JC, Maurer MJ, Kreisberg JI, Ballman K, Boni J, Peralba JM, Jenkins RB, Dakhil SR, Morton RF, Jaeckle KA, Scheithauer BW, Dancey J, Hidalgo M, Walsh DJ. Phase II trial of temsirolimus (CCI-779) in recurrent glioblastoma multiforme: a North Central Cancer Treatment Group Study. J Clin Oncol 2005;23(23):5294–5304.

43. Robins HI, Wen PY, Chang SM, Kuhn J, Lamborn K, Cloughesy T, Glibert MR, Yung WK, Dancey J, Prados MD. Phase I study of erlotinib and CCI-779 (temsirolimus) for patients with recurrent malignant gliomas (MG) (NABTC 04-02). J Clin Oncol (Meeting Abstracts) 2007;25(18 Suppl):Abstr 2057.

44. Chan S, Scheulen ME, Johnston S, Mross K, Cardoso F, Dittrich C, Eiermann W, Hess D, Morant R, Semiglazov V, Borner M, Salzberg M, Ostapenko V, Illiger HJ, Behringer D, Bardy-Bouxin N, Boni J, Kong S, Cincotta M, Moore L. Phase II study of temsirolimus (CCI-779), a novel inhibitor of mTOR, in heavily pretreated patients with locally advanced or metastatic breast cancer. J Clin Oncol 2005;23(23):5314–5322.

45. Schiff R, Massarweh SA, Shou J, Bharwani L, Mohsin SK, Osborne CK. Cross-talk between estrogen receptor and growth factor pathways as a molecular target for overcoming endocrine resistance. Clin Cancer Res 2004;10(1Pt 2): 331S–336S.

46. Yue W, Wang JP, Conaway MR, Li Y, Santen RJ. Adaptive hypersensitivity following long-term estrogen deprivation: involvement of multiple signal pathways. J Steroid Biochem Mol Biol 2003;86(3–5):265–274.

47. Carpenter JT, Roche H, Campone M, Colomer R, Jagiello-Gruszfeld A, Moore L, D'Amore M, Kong S, Boni J, Baselga J. Randomized 3-arm, phase 2 study of temsirolimus (CCI-779) in combination with letrozole in postmenopausal women with locally advanced or metastatic breast cancer. J Clin Oncol (Meeting Abstracts) 2005;23(16 Suppl):Abstr 564.

48. Margolin K, Longmate J, Baratta T, Synold T, Christensen S, Weber J, Gajewski T, Quirt I, Doroshow JH. CCI-779 in metastatic melanoma: a phase II trial of the California Cancer Consortium. Cancer 2005;104(5):1045–1048.

49. Pandya KJ, Dahlberg S, Hidalgo M, Cohen RB, Lee MW, Schiller JH, Johnson DH. A randomized, phase II trial of two dose levels of temsirolimus (CCI-779) in patients with extensive-stage small-cell lung cancer who have responding or stable disease after induction chemotherapy: a trial of the Eastern Cooperative Oncology Group (E1500). J Thorac Oncol 2007;2(11):1036–1041.

50. Boulay A, Zumstein-Mecker S, Stephan C, Beuvink I, Zilbermann F, Haller R, Tobler S, Heusser C, O'Reilly T, Stolz B, Marti A, Thomas G, Lane HA. Antitumor efficacy of intermittent treatment schedules with the rapamycin derivative RAD001 correlates with prolonged inactivation of ribosomal protein S6 kinase 1 in peripheral blood mononuclear cells. Cancer Res 2004;64(1):252–261.

51. Goudar RK, Shi Q, Hjelmeland MD, Keir ST, McLendon RE, Wikstrand CJ, Reese ED, Conrad CA, Traxler P, Lane HA, Reardon DA, Cavenee WK, Wang XF, Bigner DD, Friedman HS, Rich JN. Combination therapy of inhibitors of epidermal growth factor receptor/vascular endothelial

growth factor receptor 2 (AEE788) and the mammalian target of rapamycin (RAD001) offers improved glioblastoma tumor growth inhibition. Mol Cancer Ther 2005;4(1):101–112.

52. Lu CH, Wyszomierski SL, Tseng LM, Sun MH, Lan KH, Neal CL, Mills GB, Hortobagyi GN, Esteva FJ, Yu D. Preclinical testing of clinically applicable strategies for overcoming trastuzumab resistance caused by PTEN deficiency. Clin Cancer Res 2007;13(19):5883–5888.

53. Slomovitz BM, Lu KH, Johnston T, Munsell M, Ramondetta LM, Broaddus RR, Coleman RL, Walker C, Gershenson DM, Burke TW, Wolf J. A phase II study of oral mammalian target of rapamycin (mTOR) inhibitor, RAD001 (everolimus), in patients with recurrent endometrial carcinoma (EC). J Clin Oncol (Meeting Abstracts) 2008;26(15 Suppl):Abstr 5502.

54. Amato RJ, Misellati A, Khan M, Chiang S. A phase II trial of RAD001 in patients (pts) with metastatic renal cell carcinoma (MRCC). ASCO Meeting Abstracts 2006;24(18 Suppl): 4530.

55. Jac J, Giessinger S, Khan M, Willis J, Chiang S, Amato R. A phase II trial of RAD001 in patients (pts) with metastatic renal cell carcinoma (MRCC). ASCO Meeting Abstracts 2007;25(18 Suppl): 5107.

56. Motzer RJ, Escudier B, Oudard S, Hutson TE, Porta C, Bracarda S, Grunwald V, Thompson JA, Figlin RA, Hollaender N, Urbanowitz G, Berg WJ, Kay A, Lebwohl D, Ravaud A. Efficacy of everolimus in advanced renal cell carcinoma: a double-blind, randomised, placebo-controlled phase III trial. Lancet 2008;372(9637):449–456.

57. Motzer RJ, Escudier B, Oudard S, Porta C, Hutson TE, Bracarda S, Hollaender N, Urbanowitz G, Kay A, Ravaud A. RAD001 vs placebo in patients with metastatic renal cell carcinoma (RCC) after progression on VEGFR-TKI therapy: results from a randomized, double-blind, multicenter phase-III study. J Clin Oncol (Meeting Abstracts) 2008;26(15 Suppl):Abstr LBA5026.

58. Duran I, Kortmansky J, Singh D, Hirte H, Kocha W, Goss G, Le L, Oza A, Nicklee T, Ho J, Birle D, Pond GR, Arboine D, Dancey J, Aviel-Ronen S, Tsao MS, Hedley D, Siu LL. A phase II clinical and pharmacodynamic study of temsirolimus in advanced neuroendocrine carcinomas. Br J Cancer 2006;95(9):1148–1154.

59. Yao JC, Phan A, Chang DZ, Wolff RA, Jacobs C, Mares JE, Gupta S, Meric-Bernstam F, Rashid A. Phase II study of RAD001 (everolimus) and depot octreotide (sandostatin LAR) in advanced low grade neuroendocrine carcinoma (LGNET). J Clin Oncol (Meeting Abstracts) 2007;25(18 Suppl):Abstr 4503.

60. Papadimitrakopoulou V, Soria JC, Douillard JY, Giaccone G, Wolf J, Crino L, Cappuzzo F, Sharma S, Gross SH, Shepherd FA. A phase II study of RAD001 (R) (everolimus) monotherapy in patients (pts) with advanced non-small cell lung cancer (NSCLC) failing prior platinum-based chemotherapy (C) or prior C and EGFR inhibitors (EGFR-I). ASCO Meeting Abstracts 2007;25(18 Suppl): 7589.

61. Kris MG, Riely GJ, Azzoli CG, Heelan RT, Krug LM, Pao W, Milton DT, Moore E, Rizvi NA, Miller VA. Combined inhibition of mTOR and EGFR with everolimus (RAD001) and gefitinib in patients with non-small cell lung cancer who have smoked cigarettes: a phase II trial. ASCO Meeting Abstracts 2007;25(18 Suppl): 7575.

62. Ellard S, Gelmon KA, Chia S, Clemons M, Kennecke H, Norris B, McIntosh L, Seymour L. A randomized phase II study of two different schedules of RAD001C in patients with recurrent/metastatic breast cancer. J Clin Oncol (Meeting Abstracts) 2007;25(18 Suppl):Abstr 3513.

63. Nagata Y, Lan KH, Zhou X, Tan M, Esteva FJ, Sahin AA, Klos KS, Li P, Monia BP, Nguyen NT, Hortobagyi GN, Hung MC, Yu D. PTEN activation contributes to tumor inhibition by trastuzumab, and loss of PTEN predicts trastuzumab resistance in patients. Cancer Cell 2004;6(2):117–127.

64. Berns K, Horlings HM, Hennessy BT, Madiredjo M, Hijmans EM, Beelen K, Linn SC, Gonzalez-Angulo AM, Stemke-Hale K, Hauptmann M, Beijersbergen RL, Mills GB, van de Vijver MJ, Bernards R. A functional genetic approach identifies the PI3K pathway as a major determinant of trastuzumab resistance in breast cancer. Cancer Cell 2007;12(4):395–402.

65. Jerusalem GH, Dieras V, Cardoso F, Bergh J, Fasolo A, Rorive A, Manlius C, Pylvaenaeinen I, Sahmoud T, Gianni L. Multicenter phase I clinical trial of daily and weekly RAD001 in combination with vinorelbine and trastuzumab in patients with HER2-overexpressing metastatic breast cancer with prior resistance to trastuzumab. J Clin Oncol (Meeting Abstracts) 2008;26(15 Suppl):Abstr 1057.

66. Andre F, Campone M, Hurvitz SA, Vittori L, Pylvaenaeinen I, Sahmoud T, O'Regan RM. Multicenter phase I clinical trial of daily and weekly RAD001 in combination with weekly paclitaxel and trastuzumab in patients with HER2-overexpressing metastatic breast cancer with prior resistance to trastuzumab. J Clin Oncol (Meeting Abstracts) 2008;26(15 Suppl):Abstr 1003.

67. Boulay A, Rudloff J, Ye J, Zumstein-Mecker S, O'Reilly T, Evans DB, Chen S, Lane HA. Dual inhibition of mTOR and estrogen receptor signaling in vitro induces cell death in models of breast cancer. Clin Cancer Res 2005;11(14):5319–5328.

68. Awada A, Cardoso F, Fontaine C, Dirix L, De Greve J, Sotiriou C, Steinseifer J, Wouters C, Tanaka C, Zoellner U, Tang P, Piccart M. The oral mTOR inhibitor RAD001 (everolimus) in combination with letrozole in patients with advanced breast cancer: results of a phase I study with pharmacokinetics. Eur J Cancer 2008;44(1):84–91.

69. Baselga J, van Dam PA, Greil R, Gardner H, Bandaru R, Molloy B, Steinseifer J, Phillips P, Dixon JM, Rugo HS. Improved clinical and cell cycle response with an mTOR inhibitor, daily oral RAD001 (everolimus) plus letrozole versus placebo plus letrozole in a randomized phase II neoadjuvant trial in ER+ breast cancer. J Clin Oncol (Meeting Abstracts) 2008;26(15 Suppl):Abstr 530.

70. Mita MM, Britten CD, Poplin E, Tap WD, Carmona A, Yonemoto L, Wages DS, Bedrosian CL, Rubin EH, Tolcher AW. Deforolimus trial 106—a phase I trial evaluating 7 regimens of oral deforolimus (AP23573, MK-8669). J Clin Oncol (Meeting Abstracts) 2008;26(15 Suppl):Abstr 3509.

71. Chawla SP, Tolcher AW, Staddon AP, Schuetze SM, D'Amato GZ, Blay JY, Sankhala KK, Daly ST, Rivera VM, Demetri GD. Updated results of a phase II trial of AP23573, a novel mTOR inhibitor, in patients (pts) with advanced soft tissue or bone sarcomas. ASCO Meeting Abstracts 2006;24(18 Suppl): 9505.

72. Colombo N, McMeekin S, Schwartz P, Kostka J, Sessa C, Gehrig P, Holloway R, Braly P, Matei D, Einstein M. A phase II trial of the mTOR inhibitor AP23573 as a single agent in advanced endometrial cancer. J Clin Oncol (Meeting Abstracts) 2007;25(18 Suppl):Abstr 5516.

73. Rizzieri DA, Feldman E, Moore JO, Roboz GJ, DiPersio JF, Gabrail N, Stock W, Rivera VM, Albitar M, Bedrosian CL, Giles F. A phase 2 clinical trial of AP23573, an mTOR inhibitor, in patients with relapsed or refractory hematologic malignancies. ASH Annual Meeting Abstracts 2005;106(11):2980.

74. Trieu V, De T, Desai N. Toxicology and safety pharmacology of nanoparticle albumin-bound (nab) rapamycin (ABI-009). AACR Meeting Abstracts 2008;2008(1 Annual Meeting): 5732.

75. Maira SM, Voliva C, Garcia-Echeverria C. Class IA phosphatidylinositol 3-kinase: from their biologic implication in human cancers to drug discovery. Expert Opin Ther Targets 2008;12(2):223–238.

76. Maira SM, Stauffer F, Brueggen J, Furet P, Schnell C, Fritsch C, Brachmann S, Chene P, De Pover A, Schoemaker K, Fabbro D, Gabriel D, Simonen M, Murphy L, Finan P, Sellers W, Garcia-Echeverria C. Identification and characterization of NVP-BEZ235, a new orally available dual phosphatidylinositol 3-kinase/mammalian target of rapamycin inhibitor with potent in vivo antitumor activity. Mol Cancer Ther 2008;7(7):1851–1863.

77. Serra V, Markman B, Scaltriti M, Eichhorn PJ, Valero V, Guzman M, Botero ML, Llonch E, Atzori F, Di Cosimo S, Maira M, Garcia-Echeverria C, Parra JL, Arribas J, Baselga J. NVP-BEZ235, a dual PI3K/mTOR inhibitor, prevents PI3K signaling and inhibits the growth of cancer cells with activating PI3K mutations. Cancer Res 2008;68(19):8022–8030.

78. Marrer E, Maira S-M, Garcia-Echeverria C, Schnell C. Integrative approaches to investigate the molecular basis of the in vivo activity of NVP-BEZ235, a dual pan-PI3K/mTOR inhibitor. AACR Meeting Abstracts 2008 (99th AACR Annual Meeting—Apr 12–16, San Diego, CA): 215.

79. Vlahos CJ, Matter WF, Hui KY, Brown RF. A specific inhibitor of phosphatidylinositol 3-kinase, 2-(4-morpholinyl)-8-phenyl-4H-1-benzopyran-4-one (LY294002). J Biol Chem 1994;269(7):5241–5248.

80. Garlich JR, De P, Dey N, Su JD, Peng X, Miller A, Murali R, Lu Y, Mills GB, Kundra V, Shu HK, Peng Q, Durden DL. A vascular targeted pan phosphoinositide 3-kinase inhibitor prodrug, SF1126, with antitumor and antiangiogenic activity. Cancer Res 2008;68(1):206–215.

81. Izzard RA, Jackson SP, Smith GC. Competitive and noncompetitive inhibition of the DNA-dependent protein kinase. Cancer Res 1999;59(11):2581–2586.

82. Laird AD. XL765 targets tumor growth, survival, and angiogenesis in preclinical models by dual inhibition of PI3K and mTOR. AACR Meeting Abstracts 2007 (Molecular Targets and Cancer Therapeutics, Oct 22–26, San Francisco, CA): B250.

83. Papadopoulos KP, Markman B, Tabernero J, Patnaik A, Heath EI, DeCillis A, Laird D, Aggarwal SK, Nguyen L, LoRusso PM. A phase I dose-escalation study of the safety, pharmacokinetics (PK), and pharmacodynamics (PD) of a novel PI3K inhibitor, XL765, administered orally to patients (pts) with advanced solid tumors. J Clin Oncol (Meeting Abstracts) 2008;26(15 Suppl):Abstr 3510.

84. Laird AD, Sillman A, Sun B, Mengistab A, Wu B, Chu F, Lee M, Cancilla B, Martini J-F, Nguyen L, Aggarwal SK, Bentzien F. Evaluation of peripheral blood cells and hair as surrogate tissues for clinical trial pharmacodynamic assessment of XL147 and XL765, inhibitors of the PI3K signaling pathway. 20th EORTC-NCI-AACR Symposium on Molecular Targets and Cancer Therapeutics; 2008 Oct 21–24; Geneva, Switzerland.

85. Markman B, LoRusso PM, Patnaik A, Elisabeth Heath E, Laird AD, van Leeuwen B, Papadopoulos KP, Baselga J. A phase 1 dose-escalation study of the safety, pharmacokinetics and pharmaco-dynamics of XL765, a novel inhibitor of PI3K and mTOR, administered orally to patients with solid tumors. 20th EORTC-NCI-AACR Symposium on Molecular Targets and Cancer Therapeutics 2008 Oct 21–24; Geneva, Switzerland.

86. Shapiro G, Edelman G, Calvo E, Aggarwal S, Laird A. Targeting aberrant PI3K pathway signaling with XL147, a potent, selective and orally bioavailable PI3K inhibitor. AACR Meeting Abstracts 2007 (Molecular Targets and Cancer Therapeutics, Oct 22–26, San Francisco, CA): C205.

87. Foster P. Potentiating the antitumor effects of chemotherapy with the selective PI3K inhibitor XL147. AACR Meeting Abstracts 2007 (Molecular Targets and Cancer Therapeutics, Oct 22–26, San Francisco, CA): C199.

88. Calvo E, Edelman G, Baselga J, Kwak E, Scheffold C, Nguyen L, Shapiro GI. A phase 1 dose-escalation study of the safety, pharmacokinetics and pharmacodynamics of XL147, a novel PI3K inhibitor administered orally to patients with advanced solid tumors. 20th EORTC-NCI-AACR Symposium on Molecular Targets and Cancer Therapeutics 2008 Oct 21–24; Geneva, Swizerland.

89. Friedman L. GDC-0941, a potent, selective, orally bioavailable inhibitor of class I PI3K. American Association for Cancer Research Annual Meeting; 2008; San Diego, CA. Abstr LB-110.

90. Lorusso P, Sarker D, Von Hoff D, Tibes R, Derynck MK, Ware JA, Yan Y, Demetri G, De Bono J, Wagner AJ. Pre-clinical evaluation of efficacy and PK/PD biomarkers of GDC-0941, a potent class1 PI3K inhibitor. 20th EORTC-NCI-AACR Symposium on Molecular Targets and Cancer Therapeutics; 21–24 Oct 2008; Geneva, Swizerland.

91. Powis G, Bonjouklian R, Berggren MM, Gallegos A, Abraham R, Ashendel C, Zalkow L, Matter WF, Dodge J, Grindey G, et al. Wortmannin, a potent and selective inhibitor of phosphatidylinositol-3-kinase. Cancer Res 1994;54(9):2419–2423.

92. Walker EH, Pacold ME, Perisic O, Stephens L, Hawkins PT, Wymann MP, Williams RL. Structural determinants of phosphoinositide 3-kinase inhibition by wortmannin, LY294002, quercetin, myricetin, and staurosporine. Mol Cell 2000;6(4):909–919.

93. Wymann MP, Bulgarelli-Leva G, Zvelebil MJ, Pirola L, Vanhaesebroeck B, Waterfield MD, Panayotou G. Wortmannin inactivates phosphoinositide 3-kinase by covalent modification of Lys-802, a residue involved in the phosphate transfer reaction. Mol Cell Biol 1996;16(4):1722–1733.

94. Ihle NT, Paine-Murrieta G, Berggren MI, Baker A, Tate WR, Wipf P, Abraham RT, Kirkpatrick DL, Powis G. The phosphatidylinositol-3-kinase inhibitor PX-866 overcomes resistance to the epidermal growth factor receptor inhibitor gefitinib in A-549 human non-small cell lung cancer xenografts. Mol Cancer Ther 2005;4(9):1349–1357.

95. Ihle NT, Williams R, Chow S, Chew W, Berggren MI, Paine-Murrieta G, Minion DJ, Halter RJ, Wipf P, Abraham R, Kirkpatrick L, Powis G. Molecular pharmacology and antitumor activity of PX-866, a novel inhibitor of phosphoinositide-3-kinase signaling. Mol Cancer Ther 2004;3(7):763–772.

96. Malek S. Selective inhibition of Raf results in down regulation of the Ras/Raf/MEK/ERK pathway and inhibition of tumor growth in vivo. 18th EORTC-NCI-AACR Symposium on Molecular Targets and Cancer Therapeutics; 2006 Nov 7–10; Prague, Czech Republic.

97. Schwartz GK, Salim Yazji S, Mendelson DS, Dickson MA, Johnston SH, Wang EW, Shannon P, Pace L, Gordon MS. A phase 1 study of XL281, a potent and selective inhibitor of RAF kinases, administered orally to patients (pts) with advanced solid tumors 20th EORTC-NCI-AACR Symposium on Molecular Targets and Cancer Therapeutics; 2008 Oct 21–24; Geneva, Swizerland.

98. Tsai J, Zhang J, Bremer R, Artis R, Hirth P, Bollag G. Development of a novel inhibitor of oncogenic b-raf. Proc Am Assoc Cancer Res; 2006 Apr 1. Abstr 2412.

99. Lee JT, Kong J, Smalley KS, Tsai J, Cho H, Bollag G, Herlyn M. Antitumor activity of PLX4032, a novel B-Raf V600E Inhibitor. 18th EORTC-NCI-AACR Symposium on Molecular Targets and Cancer Therapeutics; 2006 Nov 7–10; Prague, Czech Republic.

100. Stuart D, Aardalen K, Venetsanakos E, Nagel T, Wallroth M, Batt D, Ramurthy S, Poon D, Faure M, Lorenzana E, Salangsang F, Dove J, Garrett E, Aikawa M, Kaplan A, Amiri P, Renhowe P. RAF265 is a potent Raf kinase inhibitor with selective anti-proliferative activity in vitro and in vivo. AACR Meeting Abstracts 2008;2008(99th AACR Annual Meeting, Apr 12–16, San Diego, CA):4876.

101. Sebolt-Leopold JS, Dudley DT, Herrera R, Van Becelaere K, Wiland A, Gowan RC, Tecle H, Barrett SD, Bridges A, Przybranowski S, Leopold WR, Saltiel AR. Blockade of the MAP kinase pathway suppresses growth of colon tumors in vivo. Nat Med 1999;5(7):810–816.

102. Lorusso PM, Adjei AA, Varterasian M, Gadgeel S, Reid J, Mitchell DY, Hanson L, DeLuca P, Bruzek L, Piens J, Asbury P, Van Becelaere K, Herrera R, Sebolt-Leopold J, Meyer MB. Phase I and pharmacodynamic study of the oral MEK inhibitor CI-1040 in patients with advanced malignancies. J Clin Oncol 2005;23(23):5281–5293.

103. Rinehart J, Adjei AA, Lorusso PM, Waterhouse D, Hecht JR, Natale RB, Hamid O, Varterasian M, Asbury P, Kaldjian EP, Gulyas S, Mitchell DY, Herrera R, Sebolt-Leopold JS, Meyer MB. Multicenter phase II study of the oral MEK inhibitor, CI-1040, in patients with advanced non-small-cell lung, breast, colon, and pancreatic cancer. J Clin Oncol 2004;22(22):4456–4462.

104. Sebolt-Leopold JS, Herrera R. Targeting the mitogen-activated protein kinase cascade to treat cancer. Nat Rev Cancer 2004;4(12):937–947.

105. Solit DB, Garraway LA, Pratilas CA, Sawai A, Getz G, Basso A, Ye Q, Lobo JM, She Y, Osman I, Golub TR, Sebolt-Leopold J, Sellers WR, Rosen N. BRAF mutation predicts sensitivity to MEK inhibition. Nature 2006;439(7074):358–362.

106. Koup JR, Liu J, Loi C-M, Howard C, Van Becelaere K, Przybranowski S, Walton J, Sebolt-Leopold J, Merriman R. PK/PD modeling of biomarker (p-ERK) response and tumor growth to PD 0325901 in a human tumor xenograft mouse model. Proc Amer Assoc Cancer Res; 2004. Abstr 5409.

107. Lorusso P, Krishnamurthi S, Rinehart JR, Nabell L, Croghan G, Varterasian M, Sadis SS, Menon SS, Leopold J, Meyer MB. A phase 1–2 clinical study of a second generation oral MEK inhibitor, PD 0325901 in patients with advanced cancer. J Clin Oncol (Meeting Abstracts) 2005;23(16 Suppl):Abstr 3011.

108. Menon SS, Whitfield LR, Sadis S, Meyer MB, Leopold J, Lorusso PM, Krishnamurthi S, Rinehart JR, Nabell L, Croghan G. Pharmacokinetics (PK) and pharmacodynamics (PD) of PD 0325901, a second generation MEK inhibitor after multiple oral doses of PD 0325901 to advanced cancer patients. J Clin Oncol (Meeting Abstracts) 2005;23(16 Suppl):Abstr 3066.

109. LoRusso P, Krishnamurthi S, Rinehart J, Nabell L, Croghan G, Chapman P, Selaru P, Kim S, Ricart A, Wilner K. Clinical aspects of a phase I study of PD-0325901, a selective oral MEK inhibitor, in patients with advanced cancer. AACR Meeting Abstracts 2007;2007(3 Molecular Targets Meeting): B113.

110. Haura E, Larson T, Stella P, Bazhenova L, Miller V, Cohen R, Eisenberg P, Selaru P, Wilner K, Ricart A, Gadgeel S. A pilot phase II study of PD-0325901, an oral MEK inhibitor, in previously treated patients with advanced non-small cell lung cancer. AACR Meeting Abstracts 2007;2007(3 Molecular Targets Meeting): B110.

111. Yeh TC, Marsh V, Bernat BA, Ballard J, Colwell H, Evans RJ, Parry J, Smith D, Brandhuber BJ, Gross S, Marlow A, Hurley B, Lyssikatos J, Lee PA, Winkler JD, Koch K, Wallace E. Biological

characterization of ARRY-142886 (AZD6244), a potent, highly selective mitogen-activated protein kinase kinase 1/2 inhibitor. Clin Cancer Res 2007;13(5):1576–1583.

112. Davies BR, Logie A, McKay JS, Martin P, Steele S, Jenkins R, Cockerill M, Cartlidge S, Smith PD. AZD6244 (ARRY-142886), a potent inhibitor of mitogen-activated protein kinase/extracellular signal-regulated kinase kinase 1/2 kinases: mechanism of action in vivo, pharmacokinetic/pharmacodynamic relationship, and potential for combination in preclinical models. Mol Cancer Ther 2007;6(8):2209–2219.

113. Haass NK, Sproesser K, Nguyen TK, Contractor R, Medina CA, Nathanson KL, Herlyn M, Smalley KS. The mitogen-activated protein/extracellular signal-regulated kinase kinase inhibitor AZD6244 (ARRY-142886) induces growth arrest in melanoma cells and tumor regression when combined with docetaxel. Clin Cancer Res 2008;14(1):230–239.

114. Lee P, Wallace E, Yeh T, Poch G, Litwiler K, Pheneger T, Lyssikatos J, Winkler J. ARRY-142886, a potent and selective MEK inhibitor: III) Efficacy in murine xenograft models correlates with decreased ERK phosphorylation. Proc Am Assoc Cancer Res 2004;45:Abstr 3890.

115. Wallace E, Yeh T, Lyssikatos J, Winkler J, Lee P, Marlow A, Hurley B, Marsh V, Bernat B, Evans R, Colwell H, Ballard J, Morales T, Smith D, Brandhuber B, Gross S, Poch G, Litwiler K, Hingorani G, Otten J, Sullivan F, Blake J, Pheneger T, Goyette M, Koch K. Preclinical development of ARRY-142886, a potent and selective MEK inhibitor. Proc Am Assoc Cancer Res 2004;45:Abstr 3891.

116. Ball DW, Jin N, Rosen DM, Dackiw A, Sidransky D, Xing M, Nelkin BD. Selective growth inhibition in BRAF mutant thyroid cancer by the mitogen-activated protein kinase kinase 1/2 inhibitor AZD6244. J Clin Endocrinol Metab 2007;92(12):4712–4718.

117. Huynh H, Chow PK, Soo KC. AZD6244 and doxorubicin induce growth suppression and apoptosis in mouse models of hepatocellular carcinoma. Mol Cancer Ther 2007;6(9):2468–2476.

118. Agarwal R, Banerji U, Camidge DR, Brown KH, Cantarini MV, Morris C, Desar IM, van Herpen CM. The first-in-human study of the solid oral dosage form of AZD6244 (ARRY-142886): a phase I trial in patients (pts) with advanced cancer. J Clin Oncol (Meeting Abstracts) 2008;26(15 Suppl):Abstr 3535.

119. Adjei AA, Cohen RB, Franklin W, Morris C, Wilson D, Molina JR, Hanson LJ, Gore L, Chow L, Leong S, Maloney L, Gordon G, Simmons H, Marlow A, Litwiler K, Brown S, Poch G, Kane K, Haney J, Eckhardt SG. Phase I pharmacokinetic and pharmacodynamic study of the oral, small-molecule mitogen-activated protein kinase kinase 1/2 inhibitor AZD6244 (ARRY-142886) in patients with advanced cancers. J Clin Oncol 2008;26(13):2139–2146.

120. Dummer R, Robert C, Chapman PB, Sosman JA, Middleton M, Bastholt L, Kemsley K, Cantarini MV, Morris C, Kirkwood JM. AZD6244 (ARRY-142886) vs temozolomide (TMZ) in patients (pts) with advanced melanoma: an open-label, randomized, multicenter, phase II study. J Clin Oncol (Meeting Abstracts) 2008;26(15 Suppl):Abstr 9033.

121. Lang I, Adenis A, Boer K, Escudero P, Kim T, Valladares M, Sanders N, Pover G, Douillard J. AZD6244 (ARRY-142886) versus capecitabine (CAP) in patients (pts) with metastatic colorectal cancer (mCRC) who have failed prior chemotherapy. J Clin Oncol (Meeting Abstracts) 2008;26(15 Suppl):Abstr 4114.

122. Johnston S. XL518, a potent selective orally bioavailable MEK1 inhibitor, downregulates the RAS/RAF/MEK/ERK pathway in vivo, resulting in tumor growth inhibition and regression in preclinical models. AACR Meeting Abstracts 2007;2007(Molecular Targets and Cancer Therapeutics, San Francisco, CA): C209.

123. Rosen LS, Galatin P, Fehling JM, Laux I, Dinolfo M, Frye J, Laird D, Sikic BI. A phase 1 dose-escalation study of XL518, a potent MEK inhibitor administered orally daily to subjects with solid tumors. J Clin Oncol 2008;26(15 Suppl):Abstr 14585.

124. Weingarten P, Hamatake R, Gunawan S, Yeh L-T, Kim H, Tieu K, Larson G, Lai C, Iverson C, Vo T, Yan S, Vernier J-M. RDEA119: a potent and highly selective MEK inhibitor for the treatment of cancer. AACR Meeting Abstracts 2007;2007(Molecular Targets and Cancer Therapeutics):Abstr B120.

125. Hamatake R, Iverson C, Yeh L-T, Dadson C, Tieu K, Vernier J-M, Quart B. RDEA119, a potent and highly specific MEK inhibitor is efficacious in mouse tumor xenograft studies. AACR Meeting Abstracts 2008(99th AACR Annual Meeting, San Diego, CA):Abstr 4878.

126. Hamatake R, Iverson C, Larson G, Lai C, Weingarten P, Vo T, Yan S, Yeh L-T, Dadson C, Tieu K, Vernier J-M, Quart B. RDEA436, a novel MEK inhibitor with favorable pharmacokinetic properties. AACR Meeting Abstracts 2008 (99th AACR Annual Meeting, San Diego, CA):Abstr 4895.

127. Sedlacek HH. Mechanisms of action of flavopiridol. Crit Rev Oncol Hematol 2001; 38(2):139–170.

128. Shapiro GI, Koestner DA, Matranga CB, Rollins BJ. Flavopiridol induces cell cycle arrest and p53-independent apoptosis in non-small cell lung cancer cell lines. Clin Cancer Res 1999;5(10):2925–2938.

129. Ma Y, Cress WD, Haura EB. Flavopiridol-induced apoptosis is mediated through up-regulation of E2F1 and repression of Mcl-1. Mol Cancer Ther 2003;2(1):73–81.

130. Rosato RR, Almenara JA, Kolla SS, Maggio SC, Coe S, Gimenez MS, Dent P, Grant S. Mechanism and functional role of XIAP and Mcl-1 down-regulation in flavopiridol/vorinostat antileukemic interactions. Mol Cancer Ther 2007;6(2):692–702.

131. Arguello F, Alexander M, Sterry JA, Tudor G, Smith EM, Kalavar NT, Greene JF Jr, Koss W, Morgan CD, Stinson SF, Siford TJ, Alvord WG, Klabansky RL, Sausville EA. Flavopiridol induces apoptosis of normal lymphoid cells, causes immunosuppression, and has potent antitumor activity in vivo against human leukemia and lymphoma xenografts. Blood 1998;91(7):2482–2490.

132. Drees M, Dengler WA, Roth T, Labonte H, Mayo J, Malspeis L, Grever M, Sausville EA, Fiebig HH. Flavopiridol (L86-8275): selective antitumor activity in vitro and activity in vivo for prostate carcinoma cells. Clin Cancer Res 1997;3(2):273–279.

133. Patel V, Senderowicz AM, Pinto D Jr, Igishi T, Raffeld M, Quintanilla-Martinez L, Ensley JF, Sausville EA, Gutkind JS. Flavopiridol, a novel cyclin-dependent kinase inhibitor, suppresses the growth of head and neck squamous cell carcinomas by inducing apoptosis. J Clin Invest 1998;102(9):1674–1681.

134. Smith ME, Cimica V, Chinni S, Challagulla K, Mani S, Kalpana GV. Rhabdoid tumor growth is inhibited by flavopiridol. Clin Cancer Res 2008;14(2):523–532.

135. Byrd JC, Peterson BL, Gabrilove J, Odenike OM, Grever MR, Rai K, Larson RA. Treatment of relapsed chronic lymphocytic leukemia by 72-hour continuous infusion or 1-hour bolus infusion of flavopiridol: results from Cancer and Leukemia Group B study 19805. Clin Cancer Res 2005;11(11):4176–4181.

136. Shapiro GI. Preclinical and clinical development of the cyclin-dependent kinase inhibitor flavopiridol. Clin Cancer Res 2004;10(12Pt 2): 4270s–4275s.

137. Schwartz GK, O'Reilly E, Ilson D, Saltz L, Sharma S, Tong W, Maslak P, Stoltz M, Eden L, Perkins P, Endres S, Barazzoul J, Spriggs D, Kelsen D. Phase I study of the cyclin-dependent kinase inhibitor flavopiridol in combination with paclitaxel in patients with advanced solid tumors. J Clin Oncol 2002;20(8):2157–2170.

138. Senderowicz AM, Headlee D, Stinson SF, Lush RM, Kalil N, Villalba L, Hill K, Steinberg SM, Figg WD, Tompkins A, Arbuck SG, Sausville EA. Phase I trial of continuous infusion flavopiridol, a novel cyclin-dependent kinase inhibitor, in patients with refractory neoplasms. J Clin Oncol 1998;16(9):2986–2999.

139. Fornier MN, Rathkopf D, Shah M, Patil S, O'Reilly E, Tse AN, Hudis C, Lefkowitz R, Kelsen DP, Schwartz GK. Phase I dose-finding study of weekly docetaxel followed by flavopiridol for patients with advanced solid tumors. Clin Cancer Res 2007;13(19):5841–5846.

140. Tan AR, Headlee D, Messmann R, Sausville EA, Arbuck SG, Murgo AJ, Melillo G, Zhai S, Figg WD, Swain SM, Senderowicz AM. Phase I clinical and pharmacokinetic study of flavopiridol administered as a daily 1-hour infusion in patients with advanced neoplasms. J Clin Oncol 2002;20(19):4074–4082.

141. Whitlock JA, Krailo M, Reid JM, Ruben SL, Ames MM, Owen W, Reaman G. Phase I clinical and pharmacokinetic study of flavopiridol in children with refractory solid tumors: a Children's Oncology Group Study. J Clin Oncol 2005;23(36):9179–9186.

142. Byrd JC, Lin TS, Dalton JT, Wu D, Phelps MA, Fischer B, Moran M, Blum KA, Rovin B, Brooker-McEldowney M, Broering S, Schaaf LJ, Johnson AJ, Lucas DM, Heerema NA, Lozanski G, Young DC, Suarez JR, Colevas AD, Grever MR. Flavopiridol administered using a pharmacologically

derived schedule is associated with marked clinical efficacy in refractory, genetically high-risk chronic lymphocytic leukemia. Blood 2007;109(2):399–404.

143. Christian BA, Grever MR, Byrd JC, Lin TS. Flavopiridol in the treatment of chronic lymphocytic leukemia. Curr Opin Oncol 2007;19(6):573–578.

144. Grendys EC Jr, Blessing JA, Burger R, Hoffman J. A phase II evaluation of flavopiridol as second-line chemotherapy of endometrial carcinoma: a Gynecologic Oncology Group study. Gynecol Oncol 2005;98(2):249–253.

145. Liu G, Gandara DR, Lara PN Jr, Raghavan D, Doroshow JH, Twardowski P, Kantoff P, Oh W, Kim K, Wilding G. A phase II trial of flavopiridol (NSC #649890) in patients with previously untreated metastatic androgen-independent prostate cancer. Clin Cancer Res 2004;10(3):924–928.

146. Morris DG, Bramwell VH, Turcotte R, Figueredo AT, Blackstein ME, Verma S, Matthews S, Eisenhauer EA. A phase II study of flavopiridol in patients with previously untreated advanced soft tissue sarcoma. Sarcoma 2006;2006:64374.

147. Schwartz GK, Ilson D, Saltz L, O'Reilly E, Tong W, Maslak P, Werner J, Perkins P, Stoltz M, Kelsen D. Phase II study of the cyclin-dependent kinase inhibitor flavopiridol administered to patients with advanced gastric carcinoma. J Clin Oncol 2001;19(7):1985–1992.

148. Shapiro GI, Supko JG, Patterson A, Lynch C, Lucca J, Zacarola PF, Muzikansky A, Wright JJ, Lynch TJ Jr, Rollins BJ. A phase II trial of the cyclin-dependent kinase inhibitor flavopiridol in patients with previously untreated stage IV non-small cell lung cancer. Clin Cancer Res 2001;7(6):1590–1599.

149. Stadler WM, Vogelzang NJ, Amato R, Sosman J, Taber D, Liebowitz D, Vokes EE. Flavopiridol, a novel cyclin-dependent kinase inhibitor, in metastatic renal cancer: a University of Chicago Phase II Consortium study. J Clin Oncol 2000;18(2):371–375.

150. MacCallum DE, Melville J, Frame S, Watt K, Anderson S, Gianella-Borradori A, Lane DP, Green Sr. Seliciclib (CYC202, R-Roscovitine) induces cell death in multiple myeloma cells by inhibition of RNA polymerase II-dependent transcription and down-regulation of Mcl-1. Cancer Res 2005;65(12):5399–5407.

151. Benson C, White J, De Bono J, O'Donnell A, Raynaud F, Cruickshank C, McGrath H, Walton M, Workman P, Kaye S, Cassidy J, Gianella-Borradori A, Judson I, Twelves C. A phase I trial of the selective oral cyclin-dependent kinase inhibitor seliciclib (CYC202; R-Roscovitine), administered twice daily for 7 days every 21 days. Br J Cancer 2007;96(1):29–37.

152. Fry DW, Harvey PJ, Keller PR, Elliott WL, Meade M, Trachet E, Albassam M, Zheng X, Leopold WR, Pryer NK, Toogood PL. Specific inhibition of cyclin-dependent kinase 4/6 by PD 0332991 and associated antitumor activity in human tumor xenografts. Mol Cancer Ther 2004;3(11):1427–1438.

153. O'Dwyer PJ, LoRusso P, DeMichele A, Gupta V, Barbi A, Dials H, Chen I, Courtney R, Wilner K, Schwartz GK. A phase I dose escalation trial of a daily oral CDK 4/6 inhibitor PD-0332991. J Clin Oncol (Meeting Abstracts) 2007;25(18 Suppl):Abstr 3550.

154. Sausville EA, Arbuck SG, Messmann R, Headlee D, Bauer KS, Lush RM, Murgo A, Figg WD, Lahusen T, Jaken S, Jing X, Roberge M, Fuse E, Kuwabara T, Senderowicz AM. Phase I trial of 72-hour continuous infusion UCN-01 in patients with refractory neoplasms. J Clin Oncol 2001;19(8):2319–2333.

155. Perez RP, Lewis LD, Beelen AP, Olszanski AJ, Johnston N, Rhodes CH, Beaulieu B, Ernstoff MS, Eastman A. Modulation of cell cycle progression in human tumors: a pharmacokinetic and tumor molecular pharmacodynamic study of cisplatin plus the Chk1 inhibitor UCN-01 (NSC 638850). Clin Cancer Res 2006;12(23):7079–7085.

156. Joshi KS, Rathos MJ, Joshi RD, Sivakumar M, Mascarenhas M, Kamble S, Lal B, Sharma S. in vitro antitumor properties of a novel cyclin-dependent kinase inhibitor, P276-00. Mol Cancer Ther 2007;6(3):918–925.

157. Jones S, Burris HA, Kies M, Willcutt N, Degen P, Bai S, Mauro D, Decillis A, Youssoufian H, Papadimitrakopoulou V. A phase I study to determine the safety and pharmacokinetics (PK) of BMS-387032 given intravenously every three weeks in patients with metastatic refractory solid tumors. Proc Am Soc Clin Oncol 2003;22:Abstr 798.

158. Goldberg Z, Wierda W, Chen R, Plunkett W, Coutre S, Badros A, Popplewell L, Fox J, Hoch U. A phase 1 trial of SNS-032, a potent and specific CDK 2, 7 and 9 inhibitor, in chronic lymphocytic

leukemia and multiple myeloma. 13th Congress of the European Hematology Association; 2008 Jun 12–15; Copenhagen, Denmark. Abstr 0792.

159. Shapiro GI, Bannerji R, Small K, Black S, Statkevich P, Abutarif M, Moseley J, Yao S, Takimoto CH, Mita MM. A phase I dose-escalation study of the safety, pharmacokinetics (PK) and pharmacodynamics (PD) of the novel cyclin-dependent kinase inhibitor SCH 727965 administered every 3 weeks in subjects with advanced malignancies. J Clin Oncol (Meeting Abstracts) 2008;26(15 Suppl):Abstr 3532.

160. Mahadevan D, Plummer R, Squires MS, Rensvold D, Dragovich T, Adams J, Lock V, Smith D, Von Hoff DD, Calvert H. A dose escalation, pharmacokinetic, and pharmacodynamic study of AT7519, a cyclin-dependent kinase inhibitor in patients with refractory solid tumors. J Clin Oncol (Meeting Abstracts) 2008;26(15 Suppl):Abstr 3533.

161. DePinto W, Chu XJ, Yin X, Smith M, Packman K, Goelzer P, Lovey A, Chen Y, Qian H, Hamid R, Xiang Q, Tovar C, Blain R, Nevins T, Higgins B, Luistro L, Kolinsky K, Felix B, Hussain S, Heimbrook D. in vitro and in vivo activity of R547: a potent and selective cyclin-dependent kinase inhibitor currently in phase I clinical trials. Mol Cancer Ther 2006;5(11):2644–2658.

162. Diab S, Eckhardt S, Tan A, Frenette G, Gore L, Depinto W, Grippo J, DeMario M, Mikulski S, Papadimitrakopoulou S. A phase I study of R547, a novel, selective inhibitor of cell cycle and transcriptional cyclin dependent kinases (CDKs). J Clin Oncol (Meeting Abstracts) 2007;25(18 Suppl):Abstr 3528.

163. Tibes R, Jimeno A, Von Hoff DD, Walker R, Pacciarini MA, Scaburri A, Fiorentini F, Borad MJ, Jameson GS, Hidalgo M. Phase I dose escalation study of the oral multi-CDK inhibitor PHA-848125. J Clin Oncol (Meeting Abstracts) 2008;26(15 Suppl):Abstr 3531.

164. Ashwell S, Zabludoff S. DNA damage detection and repair pathways—recent advances with inhibitors of checkpoint kinases in cancer therapy. Clin Cancer Res 2008;14(13):4032–4037.

165. Janetka JW, Ashwell S, Zabludoff S, Lyne P. Inhibitors of checkpoint kinases: from discovery to the clinic. Curr Opin Drug Discov Dev 2007;10(4):473–486.

166. Xiao HH, Makeyev Y, Butler J, Vikram B, Franklin WA. 7-Hydroxystaurosporine (UCN-01) preferentially sensitizes cells with a disrupted TP53 to gamma radiation in lung cancer cell lines. Radiat Res 2002;158(1):84–93.

167. Hu B, Zhou XY, Wang X, Zeng ZC, Iliakis G, Wang Y. The radioresistance to killing of A1-5 cells derives from activation of the Chk1 pathway. J Biol Chem 2001;276(21):17693–17698.

168. Busby EC, Leistritz DF, Abraham RT, Karnitz LM, Sarkaria JN. The radiosensitizing agent 7-hydroxystaurosporine (UCN-01) inhibits the DNA damage checkpoint kinase hChk1. Cancer Res 2000;60(8):2108–2112.

169. Wang Q, Fan S, Eastman A, Worland PJ, Sausville EA, O'Connor PM. UCN-01: a potent abrogator of G2 checkpoint function in cancer cells with disrupted p53. J Natl Cancer Inst 1996;88(14):956–965.

170. Tse AN, Schwartz GK. Potentiation of cytotoxicity of topoisomerase I poison by concurrent and sequential treatment with the checkpoint inhibitor UCN-01 involves disparate mechanisms resulting in either p53-independent clonogenic suppression or p53-dependent mitotic catastrophe. Cancer Res 2004;64(18):6635–6644.

171. Bunch RT, Eastman A. Enhancement of cisplatin-induced cytotoxicity by 7-hydroxystaurosporine (UCN-01), a new G2-checkpoint inhibitor. Clin Cancer Res 1996;2(5):791–797.

172. Mack PC, Gandara DR, Lau AH, Lara PN Jr, Edelman MJ, Gumerlock PH. Cell cycle-dependent potentiation of cisplatin by UCN-01 in non-small-cell lung carcinoma. Cancer Chemother Pharmacol 2003;51(4):337–348.

173. Hirose Y, Berger MS, Pieper RO. Abrogation of the Chk1-mediated G(2) checkpoint pathway potentiates temozolomide-induced toxicity in a p53-independent manner in human glioblastoma cells. Cancer Res 2001; 61(15):5843–5849.

174. Sugiyama K, Shimizu M, Akiyama T, Tamaoki T, Yamaguchi K, Takahashi R, Eastman A, Akinaga S. UCN-01 selectively enhances mitomycin C cytotoxicity in p53 defective cells which is mediated through S and/or G(2) checkpoint abrogation. Int J Cancer 2000; 85(5):703–709.

175. Shi Z, Azuma A, Sampath D, Li YX, Huang P, Plunkett W. S-phase arrest by nucleoside analogues and abrogation of survival without cell cycle progression by 7-hydroxystaurosporine. Cancer Res 2001;61(3):1065–1072.

176. Tamaoki T, Nakano H. Potent and specific inhibitors of protein kinase C of microbial origin. Biotechnology (NY) 1990;8(8):732–735.

177. Bain J, Plater L, Elliott M, Shpiro N, Hastie CJ, McLauchlan H, Klevernic I, Arthur JS, Alessi DR, Cohen P. The selectivity of protein kinase inhibitors: a further update. Biochem J 2007;408(3):297–315.

178. Fuse E, Kuwabara T, Sparreboom A, Sausville EA, Figg WD. Review of UCN-01 development: a lesson in the importance of clinical pharmacology. J Clin Pharmacol 2005;45(4):394–403.

179. Dees EC, Baker SD, O'Reilly S, Rudek MA, Davidson SB, Aylesworth C, Elza-Brown K, Carducci MA, Donehower RC. A phase I and pharmacokinetic study of short infusions of UCN-01 in patients with refractory solid tumors. Clin Cancer Res 2005;11(2Pt 1):664–671.

180. Lara PN Jr, Mack PC, Synold T, Frankel P, Longmate J, Gumerlock PH, Doroshow JH, Gandara DR. The cyclin-dependent kinase inhibitor UCN-01 plus cisplatin in advanced solid tumors: a California cancer consortium phase I pharmacokinetic and molecular correlative trial. Clin Cancer Res 2005;11(12):4444–4450.

181. Kortmansky J, Shah MA, Kaubisch A, Weyerbacher A, Yi S, Tong W, Sowers R, Gonen M, O'Reilly E, Kemeny N, Ilson DI, Saltz LB, Maki RG, Kelsen DP, Schwartz GK. Phase I trial of the cyclin-dependent kinase inhibitor and protein kinase C inhibitor 7-hydroxystaurosporine in combination with fluorouracil in patients with advanced solid tumors. J Clin Oncol 2005;23(9):1875–1884.

182. Hsueh CT, Kelsen D, Schwartz GK. UCN-01 suppresses thymidylate synthase gene expression and enhances 5-fluorouracil-induced apoptosis in a sequence-dependent manner. Clin Cancer Res 1998;4(9):2201–2206.

183. Welch S, Hirte HW, Carey MS, Hotte SJ, Tsao MS, Brown S, Pond GR, Dancey JE, Oza AM. UCN-01 in combination with topotecan in patients with advanced recurrent ovarian cancer: a study of the Princess Margaret Hospital Phase II consortium. Gynecol Oncol 2007;106(2):305–310.

184. Matthews DJ, Yakes FM, Chen J, Tadano M, Bornheim L, Clary DO, Tai A, Wagner JM, Miller N, Kim YD, Robertson S, Murray L, Karnitz LM. Pharmacological abrogation of S-phase checkpoint enhances the anti-tumor activity of gemcitabine in vivo. Cell Cycle 2007;6(1):104–110.

185. Matthews D. In vitro and in vivo potentiation of cytotoxic therapy by XL844, an orally bioavailable inhibitor of Chk1 and Chk2. AACR Meeting Abstracts 2007;2007(Molecular Targets and Cancer Therapeutics, San Francisco, CA):Abstr B228.

186. Matthews DJ. Dissecting the roles of CHK1 and CHK2 in mitotic catastrophe using chemical genetics. 18th EORTC-NCI-AACR Symposium on Molecular Targets and Cancer Therapeutics; 2006; Prague, Czech Republic. Abstr 344.

187. Tse AN, Salim Yazji S, Naing A, Matthews DJ, Schwartz GK, Lawhorn K, Kurzrock R. Phase I study of XL844, a novel Chk1 and Chk2 kinase inhibitor, in combination with gemcitabine in patients with advanced malignancies 20th EORTC-NCI-AACR Symposium on Molecular Targets and Cancer Therapeutics; 2008; Geneva, Swizerland.

188. Blasina A, Hallin J, Chen E, Arango ME, Kraynov E, Register J, Grant S, Ninkovic S, Chen P, Nichols T, O'Connor P, Anderes K. Breaching the DNA damage checkpoint via PF-00477736, a novel small-molecule inhibitor of checkpoint kinase 1. Mol Cancer Ther 2008;7(8):2394–2404.

189. Hallin M, Zhang C, Yan Z, Arango M, Chen E, Kraynov E, Anderes K. PF-00477736 an inhibitor of Chk1 enhances the antitumor activity of docetaxel indicating a role for Chk1 in the mitotic spindle checkpoint. AACR Meeting Abstracts 2007(98th AACR Annual Meeting, Los Angeles, CA):Abstr 4373.

190. Zachos G, Black EJ, Walker M, Scott MT, Vagnarelli P, Earnshaw WC, Gillespie DA. Chk1 is required for spindle checkpoint function. Dev Cell 2007;12(2):247–260.

191. Zabludoff SD, Deng C, Grondine MR, Sheehy AM, Ashwell S, Caleb BL, Green S, Haye HR, Horn CL, Janetka JW, Liu D, Mouchet E, Ready S, Rosenthal JL, Queva C, Schwartz GK, Taylor KJ, Tse AN, Walker GE, White AM. AZD7762, a novel checkpoint kinase inhibitor, drives checkpoint abrogation and potentiates DNA-targeted therapies. Mol Cancer Ther 2008;7(9):2955–2966.

192. Sha SK, Sato T, Kobayashi H, Ishigaki M, Yamamoto S, Sato H, Takada A, Nakajyo S, Mochizuki Y, Friedman JM, Cheng FC, Okura T, Kimura R, Kufe DW, Vonhoff DD, Kawabe T. Cell cycle phenotype-based optimization of G2-abrogating peptides yields CBP501 with a unique mechanism of action at the G2 checkpoint. Mol Cancer Ther 2007;6(1):147–153.

193. Wong BY, Shapiro GI, Gordon MS, Borad MJ, Eder JP, Tibes R, Mendelson DS, Wasserman E, Kawabe T, Sharma S. Phase I studies of CBP501, a novel G2 checkpoint abrogator, alone and combined with cisplatin (CDDP) in advanced solid tumor patients (pts). J Clin Oncol (Meeting Abstracts) 2008;26(15 Suppl):Abstr 2528.

194. Steegmaier M, Hoffmann M, Baum A, Lenart P, Petronczki M, Krssak M, Gurtler U, Garin-Chesa P, Lieb S, Quant J, Grauert M, Adolf GR, Kraut N, Peters JM, Rettig WJ. BI 2536, a potent and selective inhibitor of polo-like kinase 1, inhibits tumor growth in vivo. Curr Biol 2007;17(4):316–322.

195. Lenart P, Petronczki M, Steegmaier M, Di Fiore B, Lipp JJ, Hoffmann M, Rettig WJ, Kraut N, Peters JM. The small-molecule inhibitor BI 2536 reveals novel insights into mitotic roles of polo-like kinase 1. Curr Biol 2007;17(4):304–315.

196. Munzert G, Steinbild S, Frost A, Hedborn S, Rentschler J, Kaiser R, Trommeshauser D, Hoffmann M, Steegmaier M, Mross K. A phase I study of two administration schedules of the Polo-like kinase 1 inhibitor BI 2536 in patients with advanced solid tumors. ASCO Meeting Abstracts 2006;24(18 Suppl):Abstr 3069.

197. Hofheinz R, Hochhaus A, Al-Batran S, Nanci A, Reichardt V, Trommeshauser D, Hoffmann M, Steegmaier M, Munzert G, Jager E. A phase I repeated dose escalation study of the Polo-like kinase 1 inhibitor BI 2536 in patients with advanced solid tumours. ASCO Meeting Abstracts 2006;24(18 Suppl):Abstr 2038.

198. Ellis PM, Chu QS, Leighl NB, Laurie SA, Trommeshauser D, Hanft G, Munzert G, Gyorffy S. A phase I dose escalation trial of BI 2536, a novel Plk1 inhibitor, with standard dose pemetrexed in previously treated advanced or metastatic non-small cell lung cancer (NSCLC). J Clin Oncol (Meeting Abstracts) 2008;26(15 Suppl):Abstr 8115.

199. Von Pawel J, Reck M, Digel W, Kortsik C, Thomas M, Frickhofen N, Schuler M, Gaschler-Markefski B, Hanft G, Sebastian M. Randomized phase II trial of two dosing schedules of BI 2536, a novel Plk-1 inhibitor, in patients with relapsed advanced or metastatic non-small-cell lung cancer (NSCLC). J Clin Oncol (Meeting Abstracts) 2008;26(15 Suppl):Abstr 8030.

200. Schoffski P, Awada A, Dumez H, Gil T, et al. A phase I single dose escalation study of the novel Polo-like kinase 1 inhibitor BI 6727 in patients with advanced solid tumours. 20th EORTC-NCI-AACR Symposium on Molecular Targets and Cancer Therapeutics; 2008 Oct 21–24; Geneva, Swizerland.

201. Gumireddy K, Reddy MV, Cosenza SC, Boominathan R, Baker SJ, Papathi N, Jiang J, Holland J, Reddy EP. ON01910, a non-ATP-competitive small molecule inhibitor of Plk1, is a potent anticancer agent. Cancer Cell 2005;7(3):275–286.

202. Vainshtein JM, Ghalib MH, Kumar M, Chaudhary I, Maniar M, Taft DR, Cosenza S, Reddy EP, Goel S, Mani S. Phase I study of ON 01910.Na, a novel polo-like kinase 1 pathway modulator, administered as a weekly 24-hour continuous infusion in patients with advanced cancer. J Clin Oncol (Meeting Abstracts) 2008;26(15 Suppl):Abstr 2515.

203. Erskine S, Madden L, Hassler D, Smith G, Copeland R, Gontarek R. Biochemical characterization of GSK461364: a novel, potent, and selective inhibitor of Polo-like kinase-1 (Plk1). AACR Meeting Abstracts 2007(98th AACR Annual Meeting, Los Angeles, CA): 3257.

204. Laquerre S, Sung C-M, Gilmartin A, Courtney M, Ho M, Salovich J, Cheung M, Kuntz K, Huang P, Jackson J. A potent and selective Polo-like kinase 1 (Plk1) inhibitor (GSK461364) induces cell cycle arrest and growth inhibition of cancer cell. AACR Meeting Abstracts 2007(98th AACR Annual Meeting, Los Angeles, CA):Abstr 5389.

205. Sutton D, Diamond M, Faucette L, Giardiniere M, Zhang S, Gilmartin A, Salovich J, Cheung M, Kuntz K, Laquerre S, Huang P, Jackson J. Efficacy of GSK461364, a selective Plk1 inhibitor, in human tumor xenograft models. AACR Meeting Abstracts 2007(98th AACR Annual Meeting, Los Angeles, CA):Abstr 5388.

206. Harrington EA, Bebbington D, Moore J, Rasmussen RK, Ajose-Adeogun AO, Nakayama T, Graham JA, Demur C, Hercend T, Diu-Hercend A, Su M, Golec JM, Miller KM. VX-680, a potent and selective small-molecule inhibitor of the Aurora kinases, suppresses tumor growth in vivo. Nat Med 2004;10(3):262–267.

207. Giles FJ, Cortes J, Jones D, Bergstrom D, Kantarjian H, Freedman SJ. MK-0457, a novel kinase inhibitor, is active in patients with chronic myeloid leukemia or acute lymphocytic leukemia with the T315I BCR-ABL mutation. Blood 2007;109(2):500–502.

208. Carter TA, Wodicka LM, Shah NP, Velasco AM, Fabian MA, Treiber DK, Milanov ZV, Atteridge CE, Biggs WH 3rd, Edeen PT, Floyd M, Ford JM, Grotzfeld RM, Herrgard S, Insko DE, Mehta SA, Patel HK, Pao W, Sawyers CL, Varmus H, Zarrinkar PP, Lockhart DJ. Inhibition of drug-resistant mutants of ABL, KIT, and EGF receptor kinases. Proc Natl Acad Sci U S A 2005;102(31):11011–11016.

209. Cheetham GM, Charlton PA, Golec JM, Pollard Jr. Structural basis for potent inhibition of the Aurora kinases and a T315I multi-drug resistant mutant form of Abl kinase by VX-680. Cancer Lett 2007;251(2):323–329.

210. Hoover RR, Harding MW. Synergistic activity of the Aurora kinase inhibitor MK-0457 (VX-680) with idarubicin, Ara-C, and inhibitors of BCR-ABL. ASH Annual Meeting Abstracts 2006;108(11):Abstr 1384.

211. Rubin EH, Shapiro GI, Stein MN, Watson P, Bergstrom D, Xiao A, Clark JB, Freedman SJ, Eder JP. A phase I clinical and pharmacokinetic (PK) trial of the Aurora kinase (AK) inhibitor MK-0457 in cancer patients. J Clin Oncol (Meeting Abstracts) 2006;24(18 Suppl):Abstr 3009.

212. Bergstrom DA, Clark JB, Xiao A, Griffiths M, Falcon S, Pollard J, Freedman SJ, Giles F. MK-0457, a novel multikinase inhibitor, inhibits BCR-ABL activity in patients with chronic myeloid leukemia (CML) and acute lymphocytic leukemia (ALL) with the T315I BCR-ABL mutation. ASH Annual Meeting Abstracts 2006;108(11):Abstr 637.

213. Giles F, Cortes J, Bergstrom DA, Xiao A, Bristow P, Jones D, Verstovsek S, Thomas D, Kantarjian H, Freedman SJ. MK-0457, a novel Aurora kinase and BCR-ABL inhibitor, is active against BCR-ABL T315I mutant chronic myelogenous leukemia (CML). ASH Annual Meeting Abstracts 2006;108(11):Abstr 163.

214. Tibes R, Giles F, McQueen T, Bergstrom DA, Freedman SJ, Andreeff M. Translational in vivo and in vitro studies in patients (pts) with acute myeloid leukemia (AML), chronic myeloid leukemia (CML) and myeloproliferative disease (MPD) treated with MK-0457 (MK), a novel Aurora kinase, Flt3, JAK2, and Bcr-Abl inhibitor. ASH Annual Meeting Abstracts 2006;108(11):Abstr 1362.

215. Giles F, Bergstrom DA, Garcia-Manero G, Kornblau S, Andreeff M, Kantarjian H, Jones D, Freedman SJ, Verstovsek S. MK-0457 is a novel Aurora kinase and Janus kinase 2 (JAK2) inhibitor with activity in transformed JAK2-positive myeloproliferative disease (MPD). ASH Annual Meeting Abstracts 2006;108(11):Abstr 4893.

216. Giles F, Freedman SJ, Xiao A, Borthakur G, Garcia-Manero G, Wierda W, Kornblau SM, O'Brien S, Bergstrom DA, Rizzieri DA. MK-0457, a novel multikinase inhibitor, has activity in refractory AML, including transformed JAK2 positive myeloproliferative disease (MPD), and in Philadelphia-positive ALL. ASH Annual Meeting Abstracts 2006;108(11):Abstr 1967.

217. Carpinelli P, Ceruti R, Giorgini ML, Cappella P, Gianellini L, Croci V, Degrassi A, Texido G, Rocchetti M, Vianello P, Rusconi L, Storici P, Zugnoni P, Arrigoni C, Soncini C, Alli C, Patton V, Marsiglio A, Ballinari D, Pesenti E, Fancelli D, Moll J. PHA-739358, a potent inhibitor of Aurora kinases with a selective target inhibition profile relevant to cancer. Mol Cancer Ther 2007;6(12Pt 1):3158–3168.

218. Fancelli D, Moll J, Varasi M, Bravo R, Artico R, Berta D, Bindi S, Cameron A, Candiani I, Cappella P, Carpinelli P, Croci W, Forte B, Giorgini ML, Klapwijk J, Marsiglio A, Pesenti E, Rocchetti M, Roletto F, Severino D, Soncini C, Storici P, Tonani R, Zugnoni P, Vianello P. 1,4,5,6-Tetrahydropyrrolo[3,4-c]pyrazoles: identification of a potent Aurora kinase inhibitor with a favorable antitumor kinase inhibition profile. J Med Chem 2006;49(24):7247–7251.

219. Modugno M, Casale E, Soncini C, Rosettani P, Colombo R, Lupi R, Rusconi L, Fancelli D, Carpinelli P, Cameron AD, Isacchi A, Moll J. Crystal structure of the T315I Abl mutant in complex with the Aurora kinases inhibitor PHA-739358. Cancer Res 2007;67(17):7987–7990.

220. Cohen RB, Jones SF, von Mehren M, Cheng J, Spiegel DM, Laffranchi B, Mariani M, Spinelli R, Magazzu D, Burris HA III. Phase I study of the pan Aurora kinases (AKs) inhibitor PHA-739358 administered as a 24h infusion without/with G-CSF in a 14-day cycle in patients with advanced solid tumors. J Clin Oncol (Meeting Abstracts) 2008;26(15 Suppl):Abstr 2520.

221. Mortlock AA, Foote KM, Heron NM, Jung FH, Pasquet G, Lohmann JJ, Warin N, Renaud F, De Savi C, Roberts NJ, Johnson T, Dousson CB, Hill GB, Perkins D, Hatter G, Wilkinson RW, Wedge SR, Heaton SP, Odedra R, Keen NJ, Crafter C, Brown E, Thompson K, Brightwell S, Khatri L, Brady MC, Kearney S, McKillop D, Rhead S, Parry T, Green S. Discovery, synthesis, and in vivo activity of a new class of pyrazoloquinazolines as selective inhibitors of Aurora B kinase. J Med Chem 2007;50(9):2213–2224.

222. Yang J, Ikezoe T, Nishioka C, Tasaka T, Taniguchi A, Kuwayama Y, Komatsu N, Bandobashi K, Togitani K, Koeffler HP, Taguchi H, Yokoyama A. AZD1152, a novel and selective Aurora B kinase inhibitor, induces growth arrest, apoptosis, and sensitization for tubulin depolymerizing agent or topoisomerase II inhibitor in human acute leukemia cells in vitro and in vivo. Blood 2007;110(6):2034–2040.

223. Wilkinson RW, Odedra R, Heaton SP, Wedge SR, Keen NJ, Crafter C, Foster JR, Brady MC, Bigley A, Brown E, Byth KF, Barrass NC, Mundt KE, Foote KM, Heron NM, Jung FH, Mortlock AA, Boyle FT, Green S. AZD1152, a selective inhibitor of Aurora B kinase, inhibits human tumor xenograft growth by inducing apoptosis. Clin Cancer Res 2007;13(12):3682–3688.

224. Manfredi MG, Ecsedy JA, Meetze KA, Balani SK, Burenkova O, Chen W, Galvin KM, Hoar KM, Huck JJ, LeRoy PJ, Ray ET, Sells TB, Stringer B, Stroud SG, Vos TJ, Weatherhead GS, Wysong DR, Zhang M, Bolen JB, Claiborne CF. Antitumor activity of MLN8054, an orally active small-molecule inhibitor of Aurora A kinase. Proc Natl Acad Sci U S A 2007;104(10):4106–4111.

225. Hoar K, Chakravarty A, Rabino C, Wysong D, Bowman D, Roy N, Ecsedy JA. MLN8054, a small-molecule inhibitor of Aurora A, causes spindle pole and chromosome congression defects leading to aneuploidy. Mol Cell Biol 2007;27(12):4513–4525.

226. Jones SF, Burris HA III, Dumez H, Infante JR, Fowst C, Gerletti P, Xu H, Jakubczak J, Mellaerts N, Schoffski P. Phase I accelerated dose-escalation, pharmacokinetic (PK) and pharmacodynamic study of PF-03814735, an oral Aurora kinase inhibitor, in patients with advanced solid tumors: preliminary results. J Clin Oncol (Meeting Abstracts) 2008;26(15 Suppl):Abstr 2517.

227. Cortes J, Roboz GJ, Kantarjian H, Feldman E, Karp J, Pollack A, Sandy K, Rao N, Akinaga S, Levis M. A phase I dose escalation study of KW-2449, an oral multi-kinase inhibitor against FLT3, Abl, FGFR1 and Aurora in patients with relapsed/refractory AML, treatment resistant/intolerant CML, ALL and MDS. ASH Annual Meeting Abstracts 2007;110(11):Abstr 909.

228. Griffiths G, Scaerou F, Midgley C, McClue S, Tosh C, Jackson W, MacCallum D, Wang S, Fischer P, Glover D, Zheleva D. Anti-tumor activity of CYC116, a novel small molecule inhibitor of Aurora kinases and VEGFR2. AACR Meeting Abstracts 2008;2008(99th AACR Annual Meeting, San Diego, CA):Abstr 5644.

229. Hajduch M, Vydra D, Dzubak P, Dziechciarkova M, Stuart I, Zheleva D. in vivo mode of action of CYC116, a novel small molecule inhibitor of Aurora kinases and VEGFR2. AACR Meeting Abstracts 2008;2008(99th AACR Annual Meeting, San Diego, CA):Abstr 5645.

230. Graff JR, McNulty AM, Hanna KR, Konicek BW, Lynch RL, Bailey SN, Banks C, Capen A, Goode R, Lewis JE, Sams L, Huss KL, Campbell RM, Iversen PW, Neubauer BL, Brown TJ, Musib L, Geeganage S, Thornton D. The protein kinase C beta-selective inhibitor, enzastaurin (LY317615.HCl), suppresses signaling through the AKT pathway, induces apoptosis, and suppresses growth of human colon cancer and glioblastoma xenografts. Cancer Res 2005;65(16):7462–7469.

231. Gelardi T, Caputo R, Damiano V, Daniele G, Pepe S, Ciardiello F, Lahn M, Bianco R, Tortora G. Enzastaurin inhibits tumours sensitive and resistant to anti-EGFR drugs. Br J Cancer 2008;99(3):473–480.

232. Rizvi MA, Ghias K, Davies KM, Ma C, Weinberg F, Munshi HG, Krett NL, Rosen ST. Enzastaurin (LY317615), a protein kinase C beta inhibitor, inhibits the AKT pathway and induces apoptosis in multiple myeloma cell lines. Mol Cancer Ther 2006;5(7):1783–1789.

233. Podar K, Raab MS, Zhang J, McMillin D, Breitkreutz I, Tai YT, Lin BK, Munshi N, Hideshima T, Chauhan D, Anderson KC. Targeting PKC in multiple myeloma: in vitro and in vivo effects of the novel, orally available small-molecule inhibitor enzastaurin (LY317615.HCl). Blood 2007;109(4):1669–1677.

234. Spalding AC, Watson R, Davis ME, Kim AC, Lawrence TS, Ben-Josef E. Inhibition of protein kinase Cbeta by enzastaurin enhances radiation cytotoxicity in pancreatic cancer. Clin Cancer Res 2007;13(22Pt 1):6827–6833.

235. Carducci MA, Musib L, Kies MS, Pili R, Truong M, Brahmer JR, Cole P, Sullivan R, Riddle J, Schmidt J, Enas N, Sinha V, Thornton DE, Herbst RS. Phase I dose escalation and pharmacokinetic study of enzastaurin, an oral protein kinase C beta inhibitor, in patients with advanced cancer. J Clin Oncol 2006;24(25):4092–4099.

236. Morschhausser F, Wolf M, Seymour J, Tilly H, Pfreundschuh M, Kluin-Nelemans H, Raemaekers J, van't Veer MB, Milpied N, Cartron G, Pezzutto A, Spencer A, Darstein C, Thornton D, Dreyling M, Reyes F. Phase II study of enzastaurin in the treatment of relapsed/refractory mantle cell lymphoma. ASH Annual Meeting Abstracts 2006;108(11):Abstr 2450.

237. Fine HA, Kim L, Royce C, Draper D, Haggarty I, Ellinzano H, Albert P, Kinney P, Musib L, Thornton D. Results from phase II trial of enzastaurin (LY317615) in patients with recurrent high grade gliomas. J Clin Oncol (Meeting Abstracts) 2005;23(16 Suppl):Abstr 1504.

CHAPTER 11

CURRENT CHALLENGES AND FUTURE DIRECTIONS

I N EARLIER chapters, we described many of the diverse oncology drug discovery targets residing within the human protein kinase family. Some of these have been successfully targeted by small molecule and/or antibody-based therapeutics: others are in the early stages of clinical proof-of-concept studies, whereas a further (and potentially larger) subset of targets remains to be explored. Although there have been some notable successes, it has become obvious that no kinase inhibitor is a "magic bullet." There remain liabilities with even the most successful drugs, and as we move forward one of our challenges is to optimize the use of currently available inhibitors as well as to explore new therapeutic avenues. In this final chapter, we review some of the impediments to therapeutic efficacy of kinase inhibitors, most notably the diverse mechanisms that can prevent *ab initio* antitumor response or lead to acquired drug resistance. One of the key issues in optimizing the use of inhibitors is the development of combination therapies: we discuss some of the challenges and benefits associated with this approach and review some of the successes and failures of kinase inhibitor combination treatments in the clinic. We conclude by surveying two areas that will undoubtedly be of paramount importance as the field advances: systems biology and translational medicine. Although seemingly disparate disciplines (the first emerging from the synthesis of mathematics and engineering with cell biology, the second lying at the interface of preclinical pharmacology and clinical oncology), these two areas are inextricably related and offer the promise of greater understanding and therapeutic benefit in targeting protein kinases for cancer therapy.

11.1 KINASE INHIBITOR DRUG RESISTANCE

As kinase inhibitors continue to advance through clinical trials and become more widely used, the issue of resistance to these agents is receiving increasing attention.

Drug resistance is not, of course, unique to kinase inhibitors (nor to molecularly targeted therapeutics in general) and can arise as a consequence of such classical mechanisms as metabolic inactivation, reduced bioavailability, modulation of cellular pumps or active transporters, and defects in immune system function. However, resistance to targeted therapy may also result from additional mechanisms, such as selection of cells bearing mutations in the target gene that render them insensitive to the drug. As we shall see, in some cases this mutational resistance may not only be specific to a given kinase inhibitor but may depend on the specific binding mode of the inhibitor to its target. Additional resistance mechanisms with particular relevance to targeted therapies include activation or upregulation of alternative pathways that bypass the targeted one, or upregulation and/or constitutive activation of signaling molecules downstream from the target, thus negating the effects of target inhibition.

We may define two major forms of drug resistance: intrinsic (primary) resistance, which prevents the drug from eliciting an initial response, and acquired (secondary) resistance, whereby a tumor may initially respond to the drug but eventually becomes refractory to therapy. In the case of intrinsic resistance, there are some indications that we may be able to define sensitivity and resistance factors in advance and thereby tailor therapies to patients who are most likely to benefit. These factors may include specific genetic lesions and molecular biomarkers but, in some cases, may also correlate with clinical characteristics such as disease histology, patient ethnicity, and sex. The case of acquired resistance presents an added layer of complexity, since tumors may adopt one (or several) of many diverse mechanisms in order to escape the effects of a given kinase inhibitor. Figure 11.1 summarizes some of the basic mechanisms believed to account for drug resistance at the level of the tumor cells themselves. In the first scheme (corresponding to intrinsic resistance), all of the cells in the tumor possess some characteristic(s) that render them insensitive to the drug and therapy has no effect on tumor growth. Such characteristics may include lack of dependence on the targeted pathway and activation of downstream or alternative pathways in tumor cells but may also involve the tumor microenvironment and interactions with neighboring cells. In the second scheme, a subpopulation of tumor cells expresses high levels of the *MDR1* gene, which encodes a pump that actively exports the drug out of the cell and prevents it from hitting the target at the required concentrations. (The reverse scenario may be envisaged, whereby an active transport protein plays a key role in delivering drug into the cell; in this case, downregulation of the transporter may promote drug resistance.) This may represent a mechanism of intrinsic resistance but may also promote acquired resistance if exposure to the drug modulates the expression of the transporter proteins. In the third scheme, the tumor contains a subpopulation of tumor cells—tumor stem cells—that are resistant to the action of the drug. Upon drug treatment most of the tumor cells are killed, leaving behind the stem cells. Over time, the stem cells remain viable and can repopulate the tumor with tumor cells at various degrees of differentiation. In the final scheme, a subpopulation of cells expresses a mutation in the target (or alternatively has an activated downstream or parallel pathway) that renders the cells resistant to drug

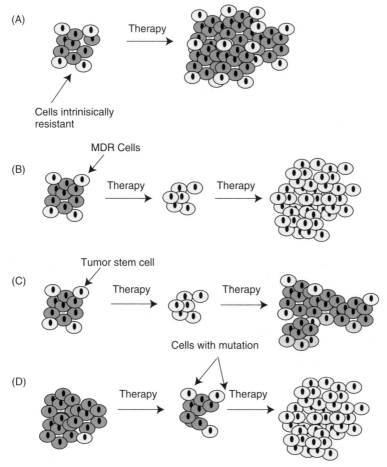

Figure 11.1 Mechanisms of drug resistance. (A) Intrinsic resistance: cells do not respond to therapy. (B) Outgrowth of cells expressing high levels of xenobiotic transporter proteins. (C) Therapy results in selection of a population of cells ("cancer stem cells") that can expand, differentiate, and repopulate the tumor. (D) Mutational resistance can occur either by selecting for a preexisting population of cells with a drug resistance mutation, or by promotion of drug resistance mutations in genetically unstable tumor cells in response to therapy.

treatment. These cells may be present in the original tumor, but at very low frequency. Alternatively, the mutation may arise in genetically unstable tumor cells at some time during the course of therapy. Drug treatment selects for those cells bearing the mutation/activation such that the therapy leads to a population of tumor cells exhibiting drug resistance.

We discuss both classical and target-dependent mechanisms of drug resistance with particular emphasis on two molecular targets, BCR-ABL and EGFR, together with the BCR-ABL inhibitor imatinib and the EGFR inhibitors gefitinib and erlotinib. Imatinib has impressive effects in chronic myelogenous leukemia

(CML) patients (Chapter 8) and has revolutionized the treatment of this disease. However, resistance is now a well-recognized problem, particularly so in the more advanced phases of the disease. Imatinib resistance can be classified as BCR-ABL dependent or independent. Intrinsic (also called primary) resistance is defined by the NCCN (National Comprehensive Cancer Network) guidelines as failure to achieve any level of cytogenetic response (CyR) at 6 months, major CyR at 12 months, or complete CyR at 18 months. The rate of intrinsic resistance to imatinib is estimated at 16% of patients with newly diagnosed chronic phase CML. After 24 months about 24% fail to achieve a complete CyR (1). The incidence of acquired (secondary) resistance is in the range of 17% and is greater in patients with more advanced stages of CML (2). First generation inhibitors of EGFR such as erlotinib have also demonstrated clinical benefit in several diseases, in particular, non small cell lung cancer (NSCLC). However, the success of these agents has been somewhat less dramatic than that of imatinib in CML. The initial rate of objective response to EGFR inhibitors in unselected NSCLC patients is only ~10%: in other words, there is a high degree of intrinsic resistance. Although some of the initial responses are dramatic (including some complete responses), patients inevitably become refractory to therapy. For example, in the pivotal clinical study of erlotinib in locally advanced or metastatic NSCLC after failure of at least one prior chemotherapy regimen, the median duration of response was 34.3 weeks (3). Thus there is a compelling need to understand the molecular factors and clinical characteristics that give rise to primary resistance, and the mechanisms whereby tumors become refractory to therapy over time.

11.1.1 Efflux Pumps and Drug Transporters

The *MDR1* gene belongs to the ABC superfamily and encodes PGP (P-glycoprotein, ABCB1), one of a family of multidrug resistance (MDR) proteins that are known to pump a wide range of structurally diverse drugs out of cells (4). As well as being expressed on tumor cells, PGP is found on the apical surface of intestinal epithelial cells and in many other organs, where it is important for protecting tissues from the potentially harmful effects of xenobiotics. Imatinib is a substrate of PGP and may also be a substrate for the transport protein ABCG2, (BCRP) although this has been debated (5–8). Overexpression of *MDR1* in the AR230 CML cell line results in resistance to imatinib, which can be reversed by PGP inhibitors (9). Dulucq and co-workers (10) analyzed the three most relevant SNPs of *MDR1* in 90 CML patients treated with imatinib. The results suggested that patients homozygous for the allele 1236T were more likely to achieve a major molecular response (85%) versus 47.7% for the other genotypes. One of the haplotypes (1236C-2677C-3435C) was statistically linked to less frequent major molecular responses. The authors concluded that *MDR1* polymorphisms could contribute to heterogeneity in imatinib plasma levels and in molecular responses to therapy. ABCB1 is also expressed in most GISTs, although expression has not been correlated with initial responses of these tumors to imatinib (11).

The EGFR inhibitor gefitinib is not a substrate of PGP but inhibits its activity, along with that of ABCG2 (12, 13). Consequently, although PGP overexpression does not confer resistance to gefitinib, coadministration of gefinitib with other drugs that are PGP substrates may affect their uptake and activity in tumor cells. This may be of benefit in increasing the intracellular concentrations of, for example, coadministered chemotherapy drugs in tumor cells. However, given the role of PGP in mediating intestinal uptake, care is warranted in order to ensure that this effect does not produce dangerously high levels of coadministered drugs due to inhibition of PGP-mediated efflux (14). Similar effects on PGP and ABCG2 may be mediated by the EGFR inhibitor erlotinib (15), although there is a report that erlotinib may in fact be a substrate for PGP (16).

In contrast to the drug efflux promoted by PGP and other MDR proteins, the active transport protein OCT-1 (organic cation transport protein 1) has been reported to promote the cellular uptake of imatinib in CML cells, thus playing an important role in delivering the drug to tumor cells (17). Conversely, the structurally related inhibitor nilotinib showed no such dependence on OCT-1 (18). The cellular activity of imatinib in patient samples (as assessed by inhibition of phosphorylation of the ABL substrate CRKL) was shown to correlate with imatinib uptake and retention; an inhibitor of OCT-1 reduced imatinib uptake, suggesting that intrinsic resistance to imatinib may be at least in part due to OCT-1 activity (18). Further characterization showed that 85% of patients with high OCT-1 achieved major molecular response (MMR) by 24 months, versus 45% with low levels of OCT-1 activity (19).

11.1.2 Other DMPK Factors

In addition to MDR transporters, a number of other factors relating to the absorption, distribution, metabolism, and excretion (ADME) properties of molecules may contribute to drug resistance. A thorough review of these issues is outside the scope of this book: however, we briefly consider here two representative examples.

Sequestration of drug molecules by specific plasma proteins can have a substantial effect on drug disposition, and differing expression levels or allelic variants of these plasma proteins contribute to the variable on-target activity observed for many drugs in vivo. The plasma protein $\alpha 1$–acid glycoprotein (AGP) has been shown to bind to imatinib at physiological concentrations of the drug, and coadministration of drugs that compete for binding to AGP improves the therapeutic efficacy of imaitnib in mouse models (20). This finding has been mirrored in patient samples, where AGP levels were found to correlate with plasma levels and addition of AGP during ex vivo treatment of CML blasts with imatinib dramatically reduced the cellular levels of the drug (21, 22). Furthermore, imatinib has been reported to bind with different affinity to different genetic variants of AGP, potentially adding more variability to in vivo pharmacokinetic/pharmacodynamic correlations (23).

Polymorphisms in the cytochrome P450 (CYP450) oxidative metabolism enzymes is also a major source of interpatient variability in drug exposure, and characterization of CYP450 pharmacogenomics for various drugs has received increasing attention in recent years (24). CYP450 3A4 has been implicated in the metabolism of imatinib, and induction or inhibition of this enzyme leads to decreased or increased levels of imatinib, respectively (25). However, since polymorphisms in CYP450 3A4 are not common, it is not clear that this will have a significant impact on clinical resistance.

11.1.3 Target Mutation

By far, the most common mechanism of resistance to imatinib appears to be the emergence of point mutations in the ABL kinase domain. Disease progression beyond the chronic phase of CML has long been associated with the acquisition of chromosomal abnormalities not observed in the initial Ph chromosome-positive population, changes that are thought to be due to the genomic instability that characterizes the Ph-positive clone. Many studies have now documented the emergence of CML tumor cells with amino acid substitutions that render the resulting kinase insensitive to imatinib inhibition. The original observation of such mutations occurred at about the same time as the elucidation of the co-crystal structure of ABL bound to imatinib (26), which demonstrated that an inactive conformation of the kinase domain was critical for imatinib binding (Chapter 7). Resistance mutations may broadly be divided into three classes. One class of mutations affects residues that are in close contact with the imatinib binding site, directly interfering with drug binding. This class includes the commonly observed substitution of the "gatekeeper" residue, T315, which forms a hydrogen bond with imatinib within the ATP binding pocket (27). Replacement of the threonine with isoleucine eliminates the oxygen atom needed to form the hydrogen bond and induces a steric clash with imatinib (Figure 11.2). The second class of mutations involves residues that are important determinants of the activation state of the kinase. Since imatinib preferentially binds to the inactive (DFG-out) form of the kinase, mutations that destabilize the inactive form or stabilize the active form will tend to diminish imatinib binding. The remaining mutations are less well characterized and most likely have other indirect effects on the imatinib binding site and/or the kinase

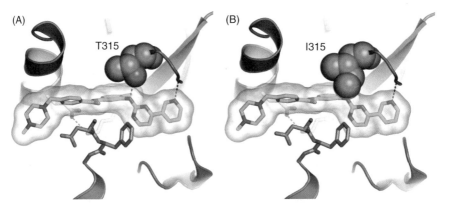

Figure 11.2   Inhibition of imatinib binding by the T315I mutant form of ABL kinase. (A) Imatinib binds to the ABL active site and makes a hydrogen bond with the side chain of T315. (B) Substitution of isoleucine at residue 315 impinges on the imatinib binding site, causing loss of affinity. Figure based on PDB accession code 2HYY.

domain conformation. Some of these mutations may also modulate interactions of the kinase with other cellular components, thereby upregulating cellular function in a manner independent from intrinsic enzymatic activity.

At present, more than 50 different mutations have been reported, although the majority of them occur at seven sites: G250, Y253, E255, T315, M351, F359, and H396 (See Appendix XVI). Many of the more common mutations destabilize the inactive, closed conformation of ABL required for imatinib binding, raising the possibility that one might overcome these resistance mutations with an inhibitor that binds to the active, open conformation of ABL. Dasatinib (originally developed as a SRC kinase inhibitor) met most of these requirements, although it can still be overcome by the T315I gatekeeper mutation. Several small molecule inhibitors that have activity against T315I ABL are currently in early clinical trials (Chapter 8).

How these drug-resistant mutations arise is not entirely clear and may differ depending on the nature and stage of the disease. In the case of CML, it is likely that they may be present in a proliferating stem cell early in the course of disease (prior to drug treatment), but may offer little survival advantage until exposure to imatinib. Imatinib treatment results in selective pressure for clones that are resistant to the drug. Several observations fit with this model, including (i) the finding that the time from initiation of imatinib treatment to the detection of a mutation is often quite short; (ii) two of the more frequent mutations (M351T and H396P) actually exhibit reduced enzymatic function compared with wild-type ABL, and T315I may also have reduced transforming activity (28); and (iii) mutations in ABL have been found prior to imatinib treatment (29–34).

The gatekeeper residue in EGFR is also a threonine residue (T790), and emergence of mutations at this position is an important determinant of acquired resistance to EGFR inhibitor therapy. About 50% of NSCLC patients who progress following treatment with erlotinib or gefitinib are found to have tumors harboring a T790M mutation, and an allele encoding this mutant has also been identified as a rare susceptibility factor for inherited lung cancer (35). Cells expressing the T790M form of EGFR have a proliferative advantage over cells expressing similar levels of wild-type receptor, and hence the mechanism of T790M resistance may be distinct from that of the T315I mutation in BCR-ABL (36). Although this mutation was initially thought to sterically hinder drug binding, its effect is more likely to be due to increasing the affinity of the kinase for ATP, thus not only promoting EGFR signaling but making it more difficult for ATP-competitive drugs to compete for binding (37). A different resistance mutation, D761Y in exon 19, has also been found in a patient with acquired resistance to gefitinib (38). In the case of EGFR in lung cancer, the prominent T790M drug resistance mutation has been detected in treatment-naive patients and thus may be selected for during drug treatment as described earlier for imatinib.

Early clinical data on mutational resistance to kinase inhibitors has clearly indicated some key "hot spots" that may have particular significance for the emergence of resistance, perhaps most notably the gatekeeper residue. This raises the possibility that drug designers may be able to proactively address the potential for drug resistance, perhaps by specifically screening or counterscreening for inhibitors that block key mutants as well as the wild-type enzyme. It would be even more desirable to have an in vitro method for predicting the susceptibility of these drugs to target-driven resistance. Such a method has in fact already been applied successfully to a number of clinically relevant inhibitors, including imatinib and dasatinib, and the results have recapitulated the observations from treatment of patients. The basic experimental design for these experiments is shown in Figure 11.3. The target protein is cloned into a suitable expression vector (typically a retroviral transfer construct) and passaged in a mutagenic *E. coli* strain (or subjected to chemical mutagenesis), generating a library of expression vectors encoding mutant proteins. This library is introduced into a cellular background that is dependent on the introduced target protein kinase for survival: hence the only clones that grow are those that successfully express functional kinases. Cells are then treated with a dose of drug that inhibits the wild-type receptor, such that cells expressing the wild-type kinase cannot survive. Following a suitable selection period, the only surviving cells will be those that express a functional mutant kinase domain that is resistant to the drug. DNA sequencing can then be used to identify the mutations, and the mutant proteins can be recloned and expressed for further characterization. Although the discovery of a mutation in such an experiment does not guarantee

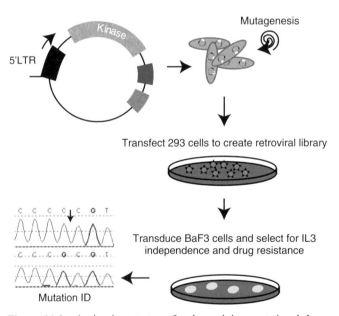

Figure 11.3 An in vitro strategy for determining mutational drug resistance. The kinase gene is subjected to random mutagenesis, either by exposure to a chemical mutagen or by passaging in an error-prone strain of *E. coli*. The resulting plasmids are used to create a retroviral mutant kinase expression library, which in turn is used to transducer a cytokine-dependent mammalian cell line. Upon cytokine withdrawal these cells are dependent on the expressed kinase for survival. When cells are treated with drug, only clones expressing functional, drug-resistant kinases will survive.

that it will be of clinical relevance, this approach nevertheless provides a framework for predicting and understanding various functional classes of mutation and the degree of susceptibility of a given drug to mutational resistance.

Pioneering studies using this approach were conducted by Azam et al. (39), using a library of BCR-ABL mutant proteins expressed in BaF3 cells. Treatment of the cellular library with imatinib resulted in isolation of over 60 mutations in the kinase domain alone, including each of the major classes of mutation that had hitherto been found in patient samples. Mutations were found throughout the kinase domain and were associated with disruption at the drug/ATP binding site, modulation of the activation state, and altering contacts with the regulatory SH2 and SH3 domains of the protein. Additional mutations were also identified outside the kinase domain, and collectively these data supported the emerging view that, in addition to mutations that directly interfere with drug binding, mutations affecting the activation state of the kinase could also impact the ability of imatinib to block enzyme activity. A similar study was conducted with the second generation BCR-ABL inhibitor dasatinib (40). In contrast to imatinib, only ten mutations were found at six distinct amino acids, most prominently at residues T315 (mutation to I, A) and F317 (mutation to V, L, I, S). Moreover, the changes in IC_{50} values for mutant BCR-ABL dependent cell growth (relative to wild-type BCR-ABL) were modest, with the exception of mutations at T315. These data are consistent with the much narrower mutational resistance profile of dasatinib that has emerged with clinical use. More recently, the irreversible EGFR inhibitor CL-387,785 and the EGFR/ERBB2 inhibitors lapatinib and XL647 have been subjected to similar analyses (41, 42). In the case of CL-387,785, a randomly mutagenized EGFR library was constructed in the background of the L585R activating mutation and the T790M resistance mutation. Twenty-nine distinct amino acid substitutions were found in 14 residues with the most prevalent being E931G, followed by L658P, L655H, and H773L. These mutations caused a shift in cellular IC_{50} for CL-387,785 ranging from 5.4- to 18.6-fold relative to the parental cells, but interestingly a different irreversible ERBB inhibitor was relatively unaffected. The E931 mutation is thought to interfere with the asymmetrical EGFR:EGFR dimer interface that has been shown to be important in receptor activation ((43); see also Chapter 2). A separate study of lapatinib and XL647 was designed to search for potential resistance mutations in ERBB2 rather than EGFR (42). Mutations were generated in the background of an activating (V659E) mutation in ERBB2. Seventeen lapatinib resistance mutations were recovered, the most common of which was T798M, which is structurally equivalent to the T790M mutation in EGFR. Other substitutions conferring significant lapatinib resistance included L755S and T733I, two mutations that had previously been detected in human gastric tumors. In contrast, the only mutation isolated in screens with XL647 was L785F, which was associated with a modest degree of drug resistance.

11.1.4 Target Overexpression and Activation

Amplification of BCR-ABL or increased expression of BCR-ABL mRNA leads to an increased level of protein, and this has been shown to restore oncogenic signaling in the presence of imatinib. Sometimes this kind of resistance can be overcome by increasing the imatinib dose, although in this case dose-limiting toxicity/intolerance of imatinib may be problematic. Although BCR-ABL amplification has been reported in CML, it appears to be a relatively infrequent cause of imatinib resistance (27, 44–47).

In general, target overexpression is an unreliable predictor of drug resistance. For example, in the case of EGFR receptor abundance does not correlate with resistance to EGFR inhibitors; in fact, EGFR overexpression may in some cases indicate sensitivity to such inhibitors, since tumor cells with amplified and/or overexpressed EGFR may be more dependent on EGFR signaling than those with more normal levels of receptor expression (Chapter 8). However, in other cases hyperactivation of receptors may represent an important resistance mechanism. In addition to mutational activation (discussed previously) and overexpression, this may also be mediated by various other mechanisms. For example, ADAM family metalloproteinases are responsible for cleavage of multiple EGFR ligands and may promote constitutive receptor signaling in the face of small molecule inhibition. In this case, the combination of EGFR inhibitors with ADAM inhibitors in tumor cells may have a synergistic effect in blocking tumor cell growth (48). Another potential resistance mechanism may involve changes in receptor trafficking following inhibitor treatment, as has been demonstrated in an in vitro selection experiment using the EGFR inhibitor gefitinib (49). Gefitinib-resistant clones were found to have no additional EGFR pathway mutations and EGFR expression was unaffected: however, receptor internalization was increased. Interestingly, these gefitinib-resistance cells retained sensitivity to several irreversible EGFR inhibitors. The authors speculate that the resistance mechanism may depend on dissociation of EGFR:gefitinib complexes in intracellular vesicles, while the irreversible inhibitors remain bound to the receptor under these conditions.

11.1.5 Downstream Pathway Activation

Another BCR-ABL independent mechanism of imatinib resistance is the constitutive activation of downstream signaling molecules, rendering the tumor cells insensitive to BCR-ABL inhibition. The upregulation/activation of SRC family kinases (SFKs) is thought to play a role in resistance to imatinib and related compounds. For example, imatinib-resistant CML cell lines that did not have BCR-ABL resistance mutations overexpressed LYN and HCK; moreover, the combination of SFK and BCR-ABL inhibition has been reported to induce a greater degree of apoptosis compared to BCR-ABL inhibition alone (50–53).

The PI3K/PTEN pathway plays a key role in mitogenic, growth, and survival signaling downstream of RTKs, and failure to downregulate PI3K pathway signaling despite robust inhibition of EGFR phosphorylation is a key characteristic of EGFR inhibitor resistance (54–56). In such cases, a mutation in the intracellular signaling network often overrides the signal emanating from cell surface receptors. Possible mechanisms of resistance include activating mutations in PI3K and loss of PTEN function (by deletion, mutation, or promoter methylation), which are prevalent in many tumor types (Chapter 5). KRAS mutation is also an important determinant of resistance to EGFR inhibitors. In NSCLC, activating EGFR and KRAS mutations appear to be largely mutually exclusive, although it is consequently not clear if resistance is primarily due to the lack of a sensitizing mutation or receptor-independent pathway activation via mutant KRAS (57).

11.1.6   Redundant Receptors/Pathways

The antitumor activity of a specific kinase inhibitor may be circumvented if cells possess redundant mechanisms for activating the same pathway, or if parallel pathways can functionally substitute for the inhibited one. This may apply particularly to RTKs, where related family members may perform overlapping functions and inhibiting one receptor may not be sufficient to downregulate signaling through downstream intracellular pathways. For example, the ability of ERBB family receptors to form heterodimeric complexes (Chapter 3) may be an important determinant of resistance to EGFR inhibitors. Expression of a mutationally activated form of the ERBB2 receptor was found to phosphorylate EGF receptors and confer substantial resistance to the EGFR inhibitors erlotinib and gefitinib (58), and activation of the kinase-dead ERBB3 may play a particularly important role in maintaining receptor signaling in cancer cells, particularly via the PI3K pathway (59). In addition to other ERBB family members, several other RTKs as well as nonkinase receptors have been implicated in mediating resistance to ERBB inhibitors. For example, two studies found that the *MET* gene was amplified in about 20% of tumor samples from patients with acquired resistance to EGFR inhibitors (60, 61). Amplification of *MET* was found to be more prevalent in tumors with acquired resistance compared with tumors from untreated patients, some of which also harbored the T790M acquired resistance mutation (61). Interestingly, the activation of PI3K in cells with amplified *MET* was found to be mediated by ERBB3 (60). Crosstalk between EGFR and MET has also been demonstrated recently in breast cancer cells, which represent a tumor type that shows little response (and therefore has intrinsic resistance) to EGFR inhibitors (62). In the presence of the EGFR inhibitor gefitinib, MET was found to be highly phosphorylated and to mediate the phosphorylation of EGFR and cellular proliferation through the activity of SRC kinase. The insulin-like growth factor receptor 1 (IGF1R) has also been implicated in resistance to EGFR inhibitors (63, 64). In preclinical models, combining IGF1R inhibition with small molecule inhibitors of EGFR results in enhanced antitumor activity, as inhibition of either receptor alone promotes activation of the other (65).

The occurrence of receptor "switching"—altering dependence from one growth factor receptor family to another—is associated with the invasive properties of tumors. Several years ago, it was noted that sensitivity to EGFR inhibitors (and potentially inhibitors of other RTKs such as IGF1R) is intimately related to the phenomenon of epithelial–mesenchymal transition (EMT), a form of transcriptional reprogramming whereby epithelial tumor cells lose their epithelial character and express features more consistent with cells of mesenchymal origin (66). This is a major event in the progression of tumors, endowing malignant cells with highly invasive and metastatic properties so that they can migrate from the primary tumor to distal metastatic niches where they may implant, revert to an epithelial phenotype, and resume neoplastic growth. Thomson and colleagues (67) showed that sensitivity to the EGFR inhibitor erlotinib correlated with the degree of epithelial character. Cells expressing the epithelial marker E-cadherin were markedly more sensitive to erlotinib compared with cells expressing mesenchymal markers such as vimentin and/or fibronectin, both in vitro and in xenograft models. A similar result was derived by Yauch and co-workers (68), who used gene microarray analysis to show that erlotinib-sensitive cells expressed an epithelial-like gene signature whereas resistant cells expressed mesenchymal characteristics. In this same report, a retrospective analysis of a small subset of patients enrolled in the TRIBUTE clinical study (comparing erlotinib plus chemotherapy to chemotherapy alone) showed that, although time to progression was not statistically significant between the two arms of the study overall, patients whose tumors expressed E-cadherin had substantially longer time to progression in the erlotinib + chemotherapy arm compared to chemotherapy alone. Paradoxically, persistent signaling through EGFR, IGF1R, MET, and other kinases can promote EMT, so the same pathways that confer sensitivity to small molecule inhibitors may also allow tumors to escape from their effects. Although cells that have undergone EMT are no longer dependent on EGFR, they may express receptors that are characteristic of mesodermal cells such as PDGFRα/β. Hence effective antitumor strategies may need to address both of these mechanisms in order to block both epithelial-directed and mesenchymal-directed pathways.

Receptor switching may also apply to RTKs involved in angiogenesis. In studies using a mouse T47D breast cancer xenograft model with inducible VEGF expression, VEGF activity was found to be essential for establishing tumor growth, but other angiogenic factors including FGF were implicated in supporting growth of established tumors (69). In an angiogenic model of pancreatic islet cell carcinogenesis, blockade of both VEGFR signaling in endothelial cells and PDGFR signaling in pericytes was shown to be more effective than either therapy alone, both in preventing tumor formation and in regressing established tumors (70). Furthermore, the same model was used to demonstrate that blockade of VEGFR signaling may be circumvented by induction of alternative proangiogenic factors in tumors, particularly FGF (71). This observation may have clinical relevance: in a clinical trial of the VEGFR inhibitor cediranib in glioblastoma patients, patients who relapsed following cediranib treatment were found to have elevated plasma levels of FGF2 (72). In order to dissect the relative importance of various receptor tyrosine kinases to the activity of the "angiokinase" inhibitor sunitinib, Potapova et al. (73) compared the efficacy of sunitinib with that of a selective VEGFR inhibitor (SU10944) and imatinib, which inhibits PDGFR. In most tumor models studied, the activity of sunitinib was similar to the combined effect of SU10944 and imatinib and was much greater than that of either SU10944 or imatinib alone. Resistance to VEGF inhibitors may also be mediated by non-RTK pathways. In particular, VEGF induces the Notch ligand DLL4 and the Notch signaling pathway works in parallel with RTK-directed angiogenic signaling to promote vascular maturation. Inhibition of Notch signaling actually leads to an increase in angiogenic sprouting, but due to the malformation of these new vessels, vascular function is compromised. In preclinical models, inhibition of the Notch pathway leads to tumor growth inhibition in tumors that are insensitive to anti-VEGF therapy (74, 75). Hence there is reason to believe that multifactorial blockade of angiogenic factors and/or their receptors will be necessary to produce robust and durable antitumor activity, highlighting the advantage of targeting multiple receptors simultaneously, either with a multitargeted small molecule or by combining separate, specific inhibitors.

There is increasing evidence that RTKs which at first appear to be functionally distinct may in fact work together to activate intracellular signaling pathways and confer resistance to therapies that target a single receptor. Evaluation of RTK phosphorylation status in glioma cells revealed that the vast majority of cell lines and primary tumor samples had three or more activated receptors, including EGFR, ERBB3, PDGFRα, and MET (76). Furthermore, only modest effects were seen with single (and relatively specific) small molecule inhibitors, whereas combination treatments led to more profound inhibition of downstream signaling kinases (such as AKT and p70S6K) and a concomitant decrease in cell survival. As discussed previously, the MET receptor may play a particularly prominent role in resistance to RTK inhibitors, in addition to its role in promoting survival invasion and metastasis. Finally, crosstalk between RTK and non-RTK pathways has also been implicated in therapeutic resistance. Chronic treatment of BT474 breast carcinoma cells with the EGFR/ERBB2 inhibitor lapatinib resulted in upregulation of estrogen receptor (ER) and progesterone receptor (PR) expression and a switch in cellular survival mechanism from ERBB receptors to codependence on ERBB2 and ER (77). Together, these data provide a rationale for the relatively low clinical responses to some single-agent RTK inhibitors and point to the need for combinatorial therapies to both prevent and treat drug resistance.

11.2 COMBINATION THERAPY WITH KINASE INHIBITORS

The genesis and progression of several tumor types can be attributed to aberrant activation of a single molecular target, and in these cases inhibition of that target may be sufficient to produce significant antitumor activity. The most prominent example of this is the use of imatinib in CML, where the disease is overwhelmingly driven by constitutive activity of the BCR-ABL fusion protein. Other kinases implicated as drivers of specific diseases include KIT (gastrointestinal stromal tumors), PDGFRα (hypereosinophilic syndrome), ALK (anaplastic large cell lymphoma), and JAK2 kinase (various myeloproliferative diseases such as polycythemia vera, essential thrombocythemia, and myelofibrosis). However, these examples are the exception rather than the rule, and in most tumor types it is likely that inhibiting a single kinase (or even a constellation of kinases using a multitargeted inhibitor) will not be universally efficacious in treating cancer. The reasons for this stem from the inherent plasticity of tumor cells, which can adapt to different environmental stresses (including chemotherapy and targeted therapies) to remodel intracellular pathways and find a way to survive. Indeed, due to their varied histories and microenvironments, different tumor masses in the same patient may be driven by different signaling pathways even if they arose from the same primary lesion, and there may even be substantial variability within different regions of a single solid tumor.

The concept of combining cancer drugs to improve antitumor activity is not new. Pioneering studies in the 1960s showed that when different chemotherapy agents were administered to leukemia patients, the combination regimen was well tolerated and outcomes were improved compared to single-agent therapies (78). The general guiding principle behind this strategy is that tumors cells that escape from a single cytotoxic treatment may be less likely to simultaneously escape from two cytotoxic treatments with different mechanisms of action. Alternatively, two agents with similar mechanisms of action may be more effective in combination if they have different large-organ toxicities that allow the combined effective drug dose to be escalated above the maximum tolerated dose for any one agent. The advent of kinase inhibitors that specifically target various receptors and intracellular pathways opens up new vistas for combination therapies, offering the possibility of specifically targeting mechanisms that are implicated in both intrinsic and acquired resistance to both chemotherapy and to other targeted agents. In this case, the rationale for combination is driven more by underlying biochemical mechanisms than by toxicological considerations. Our understanding of the myriad intracellular pathways acting in tumor cells has made tremendous strides and allows us to make some predictions about which combinations may be effective—but this knowledge is still incomplete, and so ideally we would like to test all feasible combinations in the hope of uncovering both predicted and unexpected synergies between agents. However, it is abundantly clear that there are not enough cancer patients in the world to test all combinations in the clinic, even if this were practically, financially, and ethically feasible. It is therefore necessary to make some judicious choices about which combinations to pursue, using both theoretical considerations and data from both in vitro and in vivo preclinical studies. Key factors to consider are the following.

- Which agent (or multidrug chemotherapy regimen) should be selected for combination with a given kinase inhibitor? This choice may be partly driven by preclinical data and partly by clinical considerations. The widespread availability of laboratory automation has made it possible to test combinations of many different agents at varying doses in cell-based assays, in a cost-efficient and timely manner. Various data analysis methods have been applied to such data in order to discriminate additive effects from those that are truly synergistic (79, 80). However, in vitro data may not be recapitulated in vivo and, conversely, some compelling synergistic activities may only be observable in the context of the complex microenvironments of tumors. Hence, although in vitro studies may provide some means of prioritizing combinations, in vivo data are particularly useful and may additionally convey useful information regarding any toxicities that may arise. Indeed, one of the key criteria for selecting a combination is that any synergy should be selective for tumor cells and not exacerbate systemic toxicities toward normal cells. It should also be noted that some drug combinations, while supported by preclinical data, may be impractical from a clinical point of view if the established drug/regimen is not approved or widely used in a given indication. Developing clinical strategies to evaluate combinations of investigational agents presents a further challenge from both a regulatory and intellectual property standpoint.

- Which disease(s) and patient population(s) should be studied? Again, although preclinical data may be of some use, clinical and regulatory considerations are important. In some cases, the initial clinical trial design may be driven by the currently approved indication(s) for the combination agent in question. For example, combination studies with the nucleoside analog gemcitabine may suggest utility in pancreatic cancer where gemcitabine is approved for single-agent therapy. (In this example, although gemcitabine is also approved in other diseases such as ovarian, breast, and non small cell lung cancer, these indications are in combination with other chemotherapy agents, which adds a further layer of complication to trial design and interpretation of results.)

- What dose and schedule of each drug should be employed? To date, most clinical trial designs for kinase inhibitors in oncology have adopted a "more is better" approach, aiming to find the dose and schedule that allows for the maximum (often continuous) exposure to the drug that is compatible with an acceptable tolerability profile. However, for some drugs this may not be the optimal strategy, particularly when incorporated into a combination regimen involving one or more additional agents. The dose level, dose schedule (e.g., continuous vs. intermittent), and relative timing of administration for each component of the combination therapy are important factors that may need to be optimized.

11.2.1 Angiogenesis Inhibitors and Chemotherapy

Although targeting angiogenesis was initially viewed as a strategy for "starving" a tumor, the prevailing view is that an equal or greater effect may be derived from the normalization of tumor vasculature, which may increase the efficiency of chemotherapy delivery. A similar argument applies to combining angiogenesis inhibitors with radiation, in which case the increased tumor oxygenation leads to increased levels of reactive oxygen species and increased tumor tissue damage. Jain (81) has proposed that, following administration of angiogenesis inhibitors, a "window of opportunity" exists during the vascular normalization process. At low doses and early times, there is little effect on tumor vessels and hence little augmentation of chemotherapeutic efficacy. Conversely, at higher doses and times there may be excessive cytotoxicity to normal tissues and/or pruning of the tumor vasculature, thus rendering chemo/radiotherapy either intolerable or ineffective. The time frame for optimal chemotherapy/radiation dosing may be as short as a few days, and so the relative timing and dose intensity of angiogenesis inhibitors and chemo/radiotherapy is of paramount importance. Nevertheless, the anti-VEGF antibody bevacizumab produces prolonged suppression of VEGF signaling and has demonstrated significantly improved patient outcomes in a variety of settings. Bevacizumab is approved in combination with 5-FU-based chemotherapy regimens in first or second line treatment of metastatic colorectal cancer, in combination with carboplatin and paclitaxel for treatment of metastatic NSCLC, and in combination with paclitaxel for treatment of chemotherapy-naive patients with HER2-negative metastatic breast cancer (82–84). As reviewed in Chapter 9, there are now multiple examples of small molecule angiokinase inhibitors showing encouraging activity in combination with chemotherapy in clinical studies. To cite one example, sorafenib has shown promising activity in combination with multiple chemotherapeutic agents (85). In a double-blind study in chemotherapy-naive patients with advanced melanoma, the combination of sorafenib with dacarbazine (DTIC) produced a 50% improvement in progression-free survival for the combination compared with dacarbazine alone, as well as improvements in response rate and duration of response (86). The combination was tolerable, although higher incidences of thrombocytopenia and neutropenia were observed for the combination compared to dacarbazine alone. However, similar improvements were not observed for sorafenib in combination with paclitaxel/carboplatin as second line treatment of melanoma in a randomized Phase III trial (87). Additional promising activity has been observed in combination with gemcitabine in ovarian cancer (88).

11.2.2 Survival Pathway Inhibitors and Chemotherapy/Targeted Therapy

The activation of prosurvival signals has been implicated in resistance to both chemotherapy and targeted agents. For example, many preclinical studies have implicated the PI3K pathway (in particular, AKT signaling) as a major mediator of chemotherapy resistance, supporting the use of PI3K pathway inhibitors in combination with chemotherapy. Although clinical experience with targeted therapies is less well established than for chemotherapy, there are clear indications that PI3K/AKT signaling plays a role in limiting the efficacy of these agents as well: for example, failure to downregulate PI3K signaling is clinically correlated with lack of response to anti-ERBB2 therapy. The combination of RTK inhibitors with chemotherapy has been explored as one means of attenuating PI3K-dependent survival signaling, and direct PI3K pathway inhibitors have also recently begun clinical evaluation. The optimal dosing regimen to use in such combination regimens is open to debate, since there is evidence that the commonly used single-agent dosing schedule RTK inhibitors may not be optimal in combination therapy. For example, Solit and co-workers (89) evaluated the combination of the EGFR inhibitor gefitinib with paclitaxel in a mouse xenograft model and found that pulsatile, high-dose administration of gefitinib prior to paclitaxel was significantly more effective than a lower, continuous dose. This is consistent with the "oncogenic shock" hypothesis, suggesting that there is a window during which the proapoptotic effects of RTK inhibition outweigh the prosurvival signals that can also be mediated by receptor inhibition (90).

There are now multiple clinical examples where targeted agents have been combined with other targeted agents or with chemotherapy. The results of these studies have been mixed: despite several examples of improved survival when kinase inhibitors have been added to standard therapies, other studies have shown no such improvement. Multiple studies with the EGFR inhibitors erlotinib and gefitinib in NSCLC showed no improvement in survival compared to chemotherapy alone (91–94). These disappointing results may be due to the fact that the patient populations addressed in these studies were not selected for responsiveness to EGFR inhibitors (Chapter 8). Alternatively, as noted earlier, these data may reflect the fact that combination doses and regimens have not been widely explored. Very recently, Riely and co-workers (95) have addressed this issue and reported encouraging data using an alternative dosing schedule of erlotinib in combination with carboplatin and paclitaxel in stage IIIB/IV NSCLC. This study focused on current or former smokers—a population that generally does not respond as well to EGFR inhibitors as nonsmokers. Patients received either 150 mg erlotinib (the standard daily dose) for 2 days before chemotherapy, or a much higher dose of 1500 mg erlotinib for 2 days prior to or after chemotherapy. Response rates were greater for patients receiving the higher doses, and those receiving erlotinib prior to chemotherapy had the highest response rate overall and longer survival compared to those receiving erlotinib after chemotherapy.

Earlier stage studies have addressed the combination of EGFR inhibitors with VEGFR inhibitors. There is substantial preclinical rationale for this strategy (reviewed in (96)). EGFR signaling drives multiple intracellular signaling pathways, including expression of VEGF, and so EGFR signaling may both directly promote tumor cell proliferation and indirectly support tumor growth through recruitment of tumor vasculature; conversely, VEGF signaling may represent one escape mechanism for tumors that initially respond to anti-EGFR therapy (see Section 11.1.6). In the clinic, bevacizumab has been evaluated in combination with erlotinib in patients with stage IIIB/IV NSCLC (97). Forty patients were enrolled, and bevacizumab was dosed every 3 weeks, whereas erlotinib was given daily. This regimen was quite well tolerated and there were 8 partial responses and a further 26 patients with stable disease. A comparison of bevacizumab–erlotinib with bevacizumab–chemotherapy in NSCLC patients who had progressed following prior chemotherapy confirmed the benefit of adding bevacizumab to chemotherapy alone, but also suggested that similar benefit could be derived with bevacizumab–erlotinib but with a more favorable toxicity profile (98). Encouraging data for the combination of bevacizumab and erlotinib have also been obtained in metastatic clear cell renal carcinoma (99).

11.2.3 DNA Damage Checkpoint Inhibitors and Chemotherapy

Checkpoint kinases have been implicated as a major resistance mechanism that limits the efficacy of chemotherapy and radiotherapy (see Chapters 6 and 10), and this has spurred the development of several checkpoint kinase inhibitors that are in early stage clinical trials. There is some reason to believe that these inhibitors may be efficacious as single agents, as rapidly dividing tumor cells with substantial genomic derangement and instability may be more dependent on checkpoint kinases for productive cell cycle progression compared to normal cells. However, the primary utility of these drugs is anticipated to be in combination with other therapeutic modalities, specifically those that induce DNA damage and invoke a checkpoint response. As in the case of angiogenesis inhibitors, timing and dose intensity are critical: in order to potentiate the effect of cytotoxic agents, checkpoint kinase inhibitors must be administered so as to suppress the cell cycle arrest induced by chemotherapy. Preclinical studies can be of some guidance, but optimal clinical schedules will ultimately depend on careful consideration of human pharmacokinetics and pharmacodynamics of both the chemotherapy agent and checkpoint inhibitor, which may differ substantially from animal (rodent) models.

11.2.4 RTK Switching: Targeting Receptor Redundancy

As discussed in Section 11.1.6, activation of alternative receptor tyrosine kinase signaling is implicated in resistance to RTK inhibitors, so coadministration of multiple RTK inhibitors might be expected to have greater efficacy than a single inhibitor. In practice, this strategy is somewhat complicated by the increased toxicity that might be expected to arise from administration of multiple agents: it is clearly self-defeating if the dose of one or both agents has to be lowered to below efficacious levels in order for the combination to be tolerated. It is also not clear whether continuous administration of both agents is necessarily the best strategy, or if pretreatment with one drug may lead to sensitization to the second. There are several examples of this approach in preclinical models. The *MET* gene was found to be amplified in tumor samples from lung cancer patients with acquired resistance to EGFR inhibitors, some of which also bore the T790M resistance mutation (61). This feature is also present in the NCI-H820 cell line, and growth of this cell line was inhibited by the MET/VEGFR inhibitor XL880 (GSK1363089), but not by reversible or irreversible EGFR inhibitors (61). IGF1R has also been proposed as a mediator of resistance to EGFR inhibitors. A gefitinib-resistant derivative of the A431 squamous cell carcinoma cell line was found to have reduced IGFBP3 and IGFBP4 expression, hyperphosphorylated IGF1R, and constitutive signaling to PI3K, rendering it insensitive to EGFR inhibitors (100). Sensitivity to gefitinib was found to be restored by addition of either recombinant IGFBP3, a small molecule IGF1R inhibitor (AEW541), or a neutralizing anti-IGF1R antibody. Most notably, when the parental A431 cells were grown as tumor xenografts, treatment with either gefitinib or the anti-IGF1R antibody MK-0646 produced tumor growth inhibition, but tumors regrew when treatment was withdrawn. In contrast, coadministration of both EGFR and IGF1R inhibitors produced prolonged suppression of tumor growth for at least 30 days after treatment was stopped (100). In a separate study, the combination of small molecule IGF1R and EGFR inhibitors (PQIP and erlotinib, respectively) was shown to synergistically inhibit growth and promote apoptosis in multiple tumor epithelial cells; cells that had undergone EMT, however, were less responsive, consistent with the downregulation of epithelial receptors discussed previously (65). The insulin receptor may be an important alternative means of resistance in some cellular contexts (101).

11.3   SYSTEMS BIOLOGY AND TRANSLATIONAL MEDICINE

Small molecule and antibody-directed drug discovery efforts over the past 10–20 years have produced an ever-increasing toolkit of kinase inhibitors, which are now available for basic research and, increasingly, clinical studies. Although we have made great progress in understanding the role of specific kinases in cellular homeostasis as well as tumor growth and progression, understanding the relationships between all of these potential molecular targets presents a formidable challenge. The field of systems biology—broadly defined as the study of the emergent properties of multiple interacting proteins and pathways—is gaining increasing attention as we try to decipher these relationships (102). The complexity of the myriad protein:protein interactions within the cell and their associated feedback inhibition/activation activities means that there are almost certainly emergent properties of the system as a whole that are difficult or impossible to discern from examination of a single protein (or even a single pathway). We have already encountered several such mechanisms. Notable examples include the myriad connections between the PI3K and RAS/MAPK pathways (Chapter 5), including feedback inhibition of PI3K signaling through activation of mTORC1 and p70S6 kinase, activation of AKT by the mTORC2 complex, inhibition of RAF by AKT, and the convergence of PDK1 and ERK signaling through p90RSK (Figure 5.1). Several fundamental questions can be addressed using systems-based approaches to tumor cell biology.

- How are various kinases and their associated signaling networks connected to each other—logistically, spatially, and temporally? The most direct means of probing these questions is by examining protein abundance and, in particular, protein phosphorylation in tumor cells. Although analysis of multiple readouts in multiple samples on a timescale of minutes to hours is not feasible in the clinic, such experiments are tractable using cell culture and may be able to offer important insights into the kinetics of signal pathway flux under basal conditions and in response to, for example, mitogen stimulation.

- How does perturbation of specific nodes within these networks (e.g., inhibition by a drug) change the flux through these pathways? Inhibition of one kinase/pathway may lead to inhibition or activation of other pathways (including the pathway that has been inhibited!) and this modulation may occur in a time-dependent manner. Moreover, tumor cells may behave differently from normal cells. The flexibility of cellular signaling networks is necessary for a single genome to be able to encode all of the operations necessary for metazoan development and homeostasis. Cellular signaling is remarkably robust in the face of perturbation, and this robustness is important in preventing unabated growth and tumor formation. However, once neoplastic growth has taken hold, the same robustness and flexibility may become liabilities in tumor cells, allowing them to proliferate despite genomic derangement and facilitating "intracellular rewiring," allowing the cells to access alternative signaling pathways and contributing to acquired therapeutic resistance. This underlies many of the paradoxes to which we have alluded in earlier chapters, whereby a protein that is associated with tumor prevention may also under the right circumstances behave as a tumor growth enhancer.

• What factors confer sensitivity to a given inhibitor, and what biomarkers indicate that (i) target inhibition has been achieved and (ii) this target inhibition produces a therapeutic response? As well as providing insight into the wiring (and rewiring) of phosphorylation cascades in tumor cells, these questions lead us to the field of translational medicine (Section 11.3.3), which has received increasing attention in recent years. The goals of this cross-disciplinary enterprise are to use data from preclinical studies to guide the design and interpretation of clinical studies, and conversely to obtain data from genetic profiling, biomarker analysis, and other methodologies in clinical studies that can help to formulate and validate hypotheses regarding therapeutic intervention. Some of the central questions to address are how to predict which patients will benefit most from a given therapy, how to measure the on-target activity of the therapy, and what, if any, biomarkers correlate with antitumor activity. It is important to note that biomarkers correlating with target inhibition and those that correlate with antitumor activity may be quite distinct from each other, and that the same degree of target inhibition in two tumors may produce significantly different outcomes depending on the associated genetic and microenvironmental contexts.

11.3.1 Classification of Tumors and Prediction of Response: Expression Profiling

The emergence of "gene chip" analysis in recent years has had a significant impact on how we think about classification of tumor types and has the potential to assist in both prognosis and selection of therapy (103). This technology involves the selective hybridization of nucleic acids from tumor cell samples to a microarray of DNA probes, and variations of the technique enable the estimation of the relative abundance of various mRNA transcripts, changes in gene copy number, and mapping of single nucleotide polymorphisms. Breast cancer has been one of the most thoroughly examined tumor types using these methods and will be considered here as an example. Historically, tumors have been classified according to multiple pathophysiological factors, including tumor histology, grade, size, and lymph node involvement. More recently, additional molecular metrics have been employed including estrogen/progesterone receptor (ER/PR) expression, and gene amplification and/or immunohistochemical analysis of ERBB2/HER2. Indeed, the approval of the anti-ERBB2 antibody trastuzumab was restricted to patients whose tumors showed high expression of the ERBB2 receptor as determined by immunohistochemistry and/or fluorescence in situ hybridization (FISH) analysis.

Genome-wide expression analysis has allowed clinical outcomes to be correlated with tumor expression profiles and enabled tumor types to be categorized on a molecular basis rather than by pathology and tumor grade. In a series of landmark studies, hierarchical clustering analysis was applied to gene expression data from multiple sets of surgical breast tumor specimens (104–107). These analyses showed that tumors could be classified into several distinct subtypes: luminal/ER-positive (further classified as type A and B), ERBB2-positive, basal-like, and normal breast-like (Figure 11.4). Notably, these subtypes (which were derived from a purely empirical approach) included ER-positive and ERBB2-positive tumors, which had previously been identified by more traditional biochemical and cellular analysis of tumor biology. This classification was consistent across independent data sets and, moreover, could be correlated with tumor recurrence and patient survival (106, 107). Additional gene expression signatures have been derived and shown to have prognostic value in breast cancer (108–112), and at least two commercially available diagnostic tools (Oncotype DX and Mammaprint) are now available to predict the risk of recurrence in breast cancer patients. Stratification of patients by outcome may be improved by combining gene expression profiling with copy number analysis, which also reveals potential therapeutic targets that are deregulated by high-level amplification in specific tumor subtypes (113).

The ability of gene expression signatures to classify tumors among different subtypes suggests that a similar approach may be able to indicate which therapy to choose for a given tumor. Although such investigations are still in early stages and have not been thoroughly validated, there are some indications that expression signatures may be able to predict response to chemotherapy (111, 114–116). From the point of view of targeted therapeutics, there are some intriguing data regarding the importance of different pathways in tumors. Bild and co-workers (117) constructed cell lines with mutational activation of various pathways (including RAS, SRC, and β-catenin) in human mammary epithelial cells and derived associated oncogene signatures from gene chip expression analysis of these cells. The expression signatures were applied to lung, ovarian, and breast tumor samples and enabled various patterns of concerted pathway deregulation to be associated with survival (e.g., tumors with predicted elevation of both SRC and β-catenin pathways were associated with particularly poor prognosis in breast and ovarian tumors). Moreover, the in vitro response of breast cancer cell lines to targeted therapies showed close correlation with the predicted probability of target deregulation. For example, cell lines exhibiting a strong SRC activity signature were more sensitive to the SRC inhibitor SU6656 than cell lines exhibiting signatures from other pathways. Gene expression signatures for PTEN loss and AKT activation in breast tumors have also been reported (118, 119). Similar methods have been used to develop gene expression signatures for predicting sensitivity and resistance to various chemotherapy agents (120). In several cases, resistance was correlated with deregulation of specific kinase signaling pathways: PI3K was implicated in resistance to docetaxel and SRC pathway was associated with topotecan resistance. In both cases, cell lines with a high probability of pathway activation were more likely to respond to a PI3K or SRC kinase inhibitor than cell lines without pathway deregulation, suggesting additional utility of expression profiling in selecting second line or combination therapies for drug-resistant tumors.

Two recent studies of signaling pathway deregulation in clinical breast cancer samples specifically compared expression profiles between younger (<45 years) and older (>65 years) women, and between good and poor prognosis groups within these populations (121, 122). Overall, younger women were found to be more likely to have lower expression of ER and PR, but higher expression of EGFR

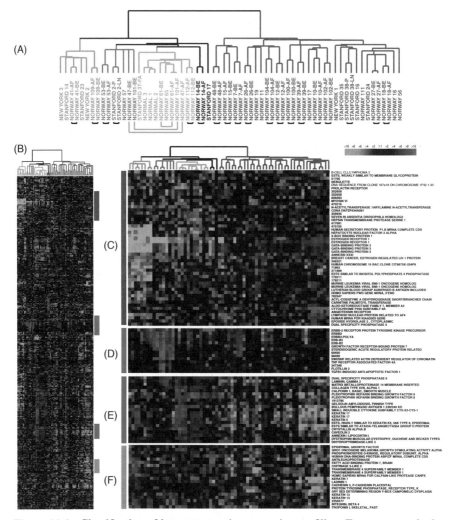

Figure 11.4 Classification of breast tumors by expression profiling. Twenty-two paired tumor samples (in most cases, obtained from the same patient before and after doxorubicin chemotherapy) were subjected to gene expression analysis. A subset of 496 genes were selected that showed significantly greater variability between different tumors than between paired samples of the same tumor. Clustering analysis based on this subset was applied to 65 tumor samples (including the paired samples) and the resulting dendrogram is shown in (A) paired samples are indicated by bars underneath the dendrogram. Coloring of the branches is as follows: basal-like, orange; ERBB2-positive, magenta; normal breast-like, green; luminal epithelial/estrogen receptor-positive, blue. Part (B) shows a scaled-down representation of the entire gene expression clustering diagram. Parts (C–F) show the gene clusters for various subtypes, with colors corresponding to those in panel (A): (C) luminal epithelial/estrogen receptor-positive; (D) ERBB2-positive; (E) basal epithelial cell-related; (F) second basal epithelial-like cluster. Reprinted by permission from Macmillan Publishers Ltd, reference (104), copyright © 2000.

and ERBB2 compared to older women. Multiple oncogenic pathways were also found to be more prevalent in the younger population, supporting the contention that breast cancer in young women is, from a molecular pathway perspective, a distinct disease compared to breast cancer in older women (122). In younger women, high expression of PI3K pathway components (along with MYC and β-catenin) confers poor prognosis, although, curiously, in a background of PI3K, MYC, and β-catenin deregulation, SRC and E2F deregulation appear to correlate with better prognosis. In contrast, poor prognosis in older patients correlates with SRC and E2F deregulation but PI3K, MYC, and β-catenin appear less important (in fact, PI3K upregulation is essentially absent in the cluster with the poorest prognosis). Moreover, in older patients high RAS and low E2F actually correlate with better prognosis (121). Collectively, these data suggest that PI3K pathway therapy may be more effective in younger women, whereas SRC inhibition might be more useful in older patients. Much additional validation needs to be done, but the studies discussed above suggest that molecular classification of tumors by expression analysis may be useful in assigning specific targeted therapy to patients on an individual basis—thus advancing toward the much-discussed goal of "personalized medicine."

11.3.2 Phosphoprotein Analysis, Kinomics, and Systems-Based Approaches

Preclinical investigations into the role of kinases in cancer and the development of inhibitors are critically dependent on methods for measuring cellular substrate phosphorylation. Historically, these techniques have focused on interrogation of a single kinase or determination of the kinase(s) responsible for phosphorylating a given substrate. These methods remain vitally important and are among the primary tools for dissecting molecular pathways and characterizing the effects of drug molecules. Several emerging methods are directed at more global surveys of cellular phosphorylation. This is a challenging undertaking: it is estimated that at least one-third of all intracellular proteins are post-translationally modified by phosphorylation (123). However, the potential rewards are also significant, as these studies can provide insight into pathway modulation and feedback mechanisms at the level of kinase targets and substrates, often in a time-dependent manner. In keeping with the recent proliferation of "-omics" nomenclatures, the global application of such techniques is often termed kinomics, a branch of the more general proteomics (124). As the volume of protein phosphorylation data continues to increase, methods for cataloging and using this information are increasingly important. For example, Scansite (scansite.mit.edu) is a program that uses an empirically derived substrate motif for a given kinase in conjunction with online protein databases to predict potential cellular substrates (125, 126). Several databases of phosphorylation sites have been created in recent years, including phosida (www.phosida.com) and phosphosite (www.phosphosite.org).

The classical techniques used for detecting and investigating intracellular protein phosphorylation include various immunological detection methods such as Western blotting, in situ immunofluorescent/immunohistochemical analysis, and microtiter plate-based assays (ELISA). A large number of antibodies are now commercially available, including both monoclonal and polyclonal reagents with selectivities ranging from highly specific to highly degenerate. In general, phosphotyrosine residues are more immunogenic than phosphoserine and phosphothreonine, and the generation of highly selective reagents for detecting the substrates of serine/threonine kinases has therefore been more challenging than for tyrosine kinases. Radiolabeling (usually involving the transfer of radiolabeled γ-phosphate from ATP) is another classical method that has been used to great effect in conjunction with peptide mapping techniques to discover substrates for a given kinase (127). Consensus substrate sequences can also be determined using peptide library arrays, phage display technology, and chemical genetic approaches (128).

Mass spectrometry (MS) has played an important role in identifying specific kinase substrates (129). One of the principal technical challenges in these studies has been obtaining phosphorylated peptides in sufficient quantity to enable quantitative detection by MS. Several enrichment methods have been employed. In the case of tyrosine kinases, immunocapture techniques have been effective. Other methods that are also applicable to serine/threonine phosphorylated substrates include strong cation exchange (SCX) and immobilized metal affinity chromatography (IMAC), which can selectively enrich cell lysates for phosphorylated proteins. Global application of MS techniques can lead to the identification (and in some cases quantitation) of thousands of protein phosphorylation substrates. For example, Salomon et al. (130) employed a large scale phosphotyrosine mapping strategy whereby cell lysates taken from different treatments/time points were immunoprecipitated with antiphosphotyrosine antibodies and subjected to tryptic digestion. Tryptic digests were further enriched by chemical modification and chromatography before being subjected to HPLC/MS analysis. The results provided a global temporal analysis of the cellular tyrosine phosphorylation events following activation of T-cell receptor signaling in Jurkat cells and also highlighted many changes in CML cells following treatment with the ABL inhibitor imatinib (130). Using the SCX enrichment method, Beausoleil et al. (131) investigated phosphorylation of serine/threonine residues in nuclear extracts from HeLa cells. Over 2000 sites were identified in almost 1000 proteins. A further advance was made by Mann and colleagues, who pioneered the temporal analysis of tyrosine kinase signaling networks using the SILAC (stable isotope-labeled amino acids in cell culture) method (132, 133). Cells were cultured in the presence of distinct isotopically labeled amino acid mixtures, resulting in a unique mass "fingerprint" for corresponding proteins within each cell population. Cell populations were subjected to different treatments (e.g., plus or minus EGF), then the lysates were extracted, enriched for phosphotyrosine-containing proteins, and subjected to tryptic digest analysis. The isotopic labeling allowed the relative abundance of a given phosphoprotein to be determined and compared before and after treatment. In a refinement of this method, a more complex isotopic labeling protocol enabled multiple timepoints to be assessed, thereby providing a temporal picture of the tyrosine phosphorylation dynamics following EGF stimulation (134). This approach was further extended to include substrates of serine/threonine kinases, resulting in the detection of 6600 phosphorylation sites on 2244 distinct proteins in HeLa cells. Following EGF stimulation, distinct profiles of phosphorylation dynamics were found to exist for various classes of protein, including RTKs and their immediate downstream effectors, intracellular signaling cascades, terminal effectors, and negative regulators of EGF signaling (135).

More recently, the same philosophy that guided development of DNA microarrays has been applied to protein analysis. Reverse phase protein arrays (RPPAs) have emerged as a means of measuring multiple phosphoprotein responses to cellular stimulation and kinase inhibition (136, 137). In these arrays, analytes (e.g., cell lysates following stimulation or drug treatment) are immobilized at various dilutions and probed with a solution phase antibody. Detection can be highly sensitive (as little as attogram amounts of purified protein). The ability to quantify many samples in parallel makes RPPAs potentially useful for both mechanistic studies (such as measuring a time course of cellular pathway flux in response to different activators or inhibitors) and characterization of multiple clinical samples. A recent investigation of the effects of MEK inhibitors in breast cancer cells nicely illustrates the power of combining expression profiling with proteomic analysis to correlate the effects of pathway inhibition with molecular signatures of tumor cells (138). Using two structurally distinct small molecule inhibitors and existing mRNA expression profiles, a subset of basal cell tumors were found to be particularly sensitive to MEK inhibition, whereas luminal subtypes were generally more resistant. Expression of genes involved in ERK/MAPK signaling was associated with sensitivity, whereas genes involved in the PI3K pathway were associated with resistance. (Incidentally, only a fraction of the genes associated with sensitivity were found to be common to both inhibitors, underlining the importance of using multiple compounds to probe a given pathway where possible.) The results of gene expression studies were recapitulated by proteomic analyses using both traditional Western blotting as well as reverse phase protein array technology: sensitivity was associated with expression of basal cell markers and resistance with luminal cell markers. Of particular note, inhibition of MEK was found to promote a time-dependent upregulation of EGFR phosphorylation and subsequent downstream signaling through PI3K and AKT. Combining MEK and PI3K inhibitors produced profound G1 arrest through inhibition of cyclin D, although cells with wild-type p53 responded by triggering apoptosis. Collectively, these data point the way toward selecting subpopulations of breast cancer patients who might benefit most from MEK inhibitor therapy, as well as supporting the combination of MEK inhibitors with EGFR or PI3K pathway inhibitors (138).

11.3.3 Translational Medicine

Translational medicine is the broad term given to preclinical and clinical studies that guide the development of clinical strategies for drug treatment. This endeavor, bridging the worlds of basic research, drug discovery, and clinical science, is an increasingly important aspect of drug discovery and development. Kinase inhibitors in oncology have received particular attention as academic researchers, drug companies, and clinicians alike strive to determine the best ways to use these emerging drugs. Translational medicine means different things to different people, but in the context of oncology it includes generation of preclinical pharmacodynamic and efficacy data with therapeutic agents (in both cell culture and in vivo models), correlation of genomic and proteomic tumor cell profiles with drug activity, and measurement of pharmacodynamics in response to preclinical and clinical drug treatment, using readouts in both tumor tissue and surrogate compartments. As well as using preclinical experiments to suggest clinical strategies (such as optimal dosing regimens and pharmacodynamic metrics of compound activity), both preclinical and clinical data may be directed toward identifying specific diseases and patient populations that might derive the most benefit from a given therapeutic agent. There are currently only a few cases where a priori assessments of molecular markers have been used to select patients for therapy, most notably the use of trastuzumab in ERBB2-positive patients as mentioned previously. It is increasingly clear, however, that selecting patients solely on the basis of primary tumor origin (even with additional histological stratification) does not, in general, indicate which molecular pathways are the most appropriate for therapeutic intervention in a given individual. Although the promise of personalized medicine has received much attention in both the scientific and popular press, the prevailing paradigm in many (if not most) clinical studies is still to test new drugs in broad, unselected populations, in the hope of uncovering perhaps unexpected signals of activity. As translational medicine continues to gather momentum, perhaps this situation will change as more examples of the predictive power of preclinical models, expression profiles, and proteomic signatures are clinically validated. Going forward, one of the key challenges for translational research will be to use preclinical data in planning clinical studies but to then capture as much data from clinical samples as possible in order to gain more insight into mechanisms of intrinsic and acquired resistance to therapies, returning to the laboratory to test hypotheses that are driven by data from real patients.

Biomarkers   "Biomarker," like "translational medicine," has myriad definitions and as such has the potential to cause confusion. In the most general sense, a biomarker is an indicator of a biological state. This may refer to the genetic or phenotypic characterization of a tumor (e.g., a gene expression profile, the presence or absence of a given mutation as determined by DNA sequencing, or proliferation index as measured by the Ki67 antigen (139)). In this case, the biomarker may have prognostic significance or may indicate susceptibility to a given therapeutic agent. Another definition of biomarker is some indicator that changes upon drug treatment, such as protein phosphorylation in a tumor or surrogate tissue, increase or decrease of a serum protein, or the presence or absence of an imaging signal (e.g., fluorodeoxyglucose positron emission tomography (FDG-PET (140)). This definition may even extend to clinical signs, such as the transient hair depigmentation observed on inhibition of KIT (141, 142) and hypertension following treatment with angiokinase inhibitors (143). It should be noted that there is substantial overlap between the above definitions: for example, Ki67 is broadly used as a measurement of drug treatment and FDG-PET has utility in determining the basal metabolic state of a tumor. Next, we discuss the application of various biomarkers to angiogenesis and PI3K/mTOR pathway inhibitors. We will use *pharmacodynamic marker* to refer to an indicator of in vivo target modulation by a drug; it is important that this should be distinguished from a *surrogate endpoint marker*, which refers to an indicator of clinical response or lack of response (144).

Clinical experience with the angiokinase inhibitor sunitinib provides some excellent examples of the utility of biomarker studies as both pharmacodynamic and surrogate endpoint markers (reviewed in (145)). Plasma levels of several proangiogenic growth factors (e.g., VEGFA, PlGF, SCF) and their receptors are modulated in response to antiangiogenic therapy and can provide evidence of in vivo target inhibition. Following 4 weeks of sunitinib therapy in a Phase II study in advanced renal cell carcinoma, plasma levels of VEGF and PlGF were elevated in 40–50% of patients. Conversely, levels of the soluble ectodomain of VEGFR2 (sVEGFR2) were found to decrease in all patients tested, and sVEGFR3 was also decreased in most cases (146). Following a 2-week period off drug, these levels returned to near baseline, providing strong evidence that these changes reflect the pharmacodynamics of sunitinib activity (Figure 11.5). Moreover, changes in VEGF, sVEGFR2, and sVEGFR3 were more pronounced in patients showing an objective response compared to patients with stable or progressive disease. Similar trends in plasma protein levels were seen in studies of sunitinib in metastatic breast cancer (147), gastrointestinal stromal tumors (148), and neuroendocrine tumors (149), and for some plasma proteins there were indications that baseline plasma levels as well as changes in response to treatment were associated with survival. Although this suggests that these assessments may be useful surrogate endpoint markers, the correlation is not perfect and it is likely that multiple independent biomarker measurements will have to be integrated in order to generate a robust prognostic signal. In a nice example of the "lab bench to the bedside and back" philosophy underpinning translational research, analogous plasma protein assays were conducted in *nontumor-bearing* mice following treatment with sunitinib. The observed changes in plasma proteins were similar to those seen in cancer patients, suggesting that the clinically observed changes are not necessarily reflective of tumor biology. Circulating endothelial cells have also shown promise as markers of antiangiogenic drug activity and, like plasma growth factors, may also have prognostic significance (150). Various imaging techniques are also seeing increasing use for monitoring tumor glucose uptake (FDG-PET) and tumor vascularization (DCE-MRI; dynamic contrast-enhanced magnetic resonance imaging). These methods are noninvasive and provide compelling evidence of target inhibition and insight into tumor function in response to therapy. However, they remain costly and there is to date no clear evidence that FDG-PET or DCE-MRI responses are correlated with objective decreases in tumor size or survival. Further examples of plasma protein modulation and other biomarkers for additional angiokinase inhibitors are discussed in Chapter 9.

The PI3K/mTOR signaling pathways have received significant attention in recent years, and inhibitors of various targets within these pathways have the potential for both single-agent therapy and sensitization to other therapeutic modalities (Chapters 5 and 10). Many phosphoprotein readouts within this pathway have been used as pharmacodynamic markers in preclinical models and are increasingly being used in clinical studies. These include phosphorylation of AKT and its substrates (such as PRAS40), phosphorylation of the mTOR substrate p70S6K and its substrate S6 ribosomal protein, and phosphorylation of IRS1, a substrate of p70S6K that is involved in feedback inhibition of PI3K/mTOR signaling (151). As discussed in Chapter 5, this feedback loop may have significant implications for the efficacy of mTORC1 inhibitors, since downstream inhibition of p70S6K may actually promote AKT signaling and subsequent growth, proliferation, and

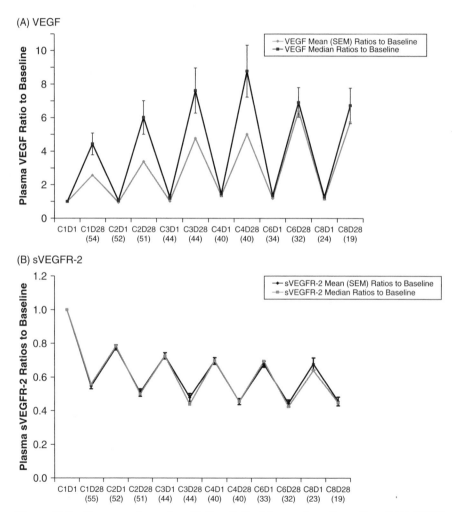

Figure 11.5 Plasma markers of sunitinib activity. Mean and median ratios of (A) VEGF, (B) sVEGFR2, and (C) PlGF are shown relative to baseline (predose) levels. Error bars indicate the standard error in the mean (SEM). Letters and numbers below each data point indicate cycle/day of sample (e.g., C1D1 = cycle 1, day 1), and the numbers in parentheses indicate the number of samples assessed. Reprinted from (146), under the terms of the Creative Commons Attribution License (http://creativecommons.org/licenses/by/2.0/).

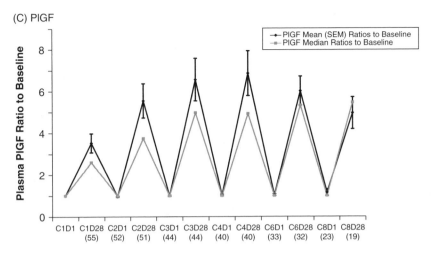

Figure 11.5 (*Continued*)

survival signaling (152). Indeed, AKT activation has been reported in patients treated with everolimus (153), suggesting that caution is warranted in using these inhibitors even though preclinical studies with rapamycin and related molecules have shown impressive antitumor activity. The effects of intervention at different points in the PI3K/AKT/mTOR pathway have been modeled using mathematical models adapted from the field of control engineering theory (102). Although these models are substantial simplifications that exclude many important cellular effects, they can provide insight into the strengths and liabilities of targeting one pathway node versus another and the value of simultaneously inhibiting multiple targets within the pathway. In the presence of active signaling through IGF1R and PI3K, inhibition of mTOR alone leads to hyperactivation of IRS1 and exacerbates a "one-way on-switch," whereby constitutive signaling occurs even if upstream receptor signaling is withdrawn (102).

Potential mechanisms to circumvent both the feedback activation of AKT by mTOR inhibitors include combination therapies either with inhibitors of IGF1R (which drives signaling to PI3K via IRS1) or with direct inhibitors of the PI3K pathway. The translation of pharmacodynamic markers from preclinical to clinical studies has recently been demonstrated in a Phase I study of the dual PI3K/mTOR inhibitor XL765. In preclinical studies, treatment of tumor-bearing nude mice produced strong and durable inhibition of phosphoprotein readouts along the PI3K and mTOR signaling pathways (154). In a Phase I clinical study of XL765, phosphorylation of various PI3K and mTOR pathway proteins was assessed in patient samples (155, 156). Modulation of pathway protein phosphorylation was observed in tumor tissue as well as surrogate compartments (hair, skin, and peripheral blood). For example, analysis of tumor biopsies from a chondrosarcoma patient taken at screening and after 28 days of dosing with XL765 showed downregulation of AKT, PRAS40, S6, and 4EBP1 phosphorylation. In PBMC samples taken from multiple patients, phosphorylation of the AKT substrate PRAS40 was inhibited with $IC_{50} = 109$ ng/mL (plasma concentration of XL765). Assessment of target inhibition in easily accessible surrogate tissues such as blood, hair, and skin may be particularly useful in that they are usually amenable to much more frequent sampling compared to tumor tissue. In this study, for example, hair samples were taken from some patients on several days throughout the dosing cycle, and immuno-histochemical analysis showed that multiple pathway readouts were increasingly inhibited as the dosing cycle proceeded (157). Additional evidence for pathway modulation was provided by measurement of plasma insulin. A comparison across all dose levels in the Phase I study indicated a dose-dependent increase in plasma insulin levels although plasma glucose was minimally impacted, even in patients where elevated insulin levels were observed (155). Together, these data provide an example of what has been called a "pharmacological audit trail," allowing correlations of drug exposure with target modulation, phenotypic effects, and, ultimately, clinical outcome (158).

11.4   CONCLUSIONS

The last few years have been exciting ones for the development of kinase inhibitors in cancer therapy. Since the introduction of imatinib for treatment of CML in 2001, an avalanche of small molecule kinase inhibitors has descended into the oncology clinic, offering the promise of novel, targeted therapies that specifically block signaling pathways supporting tumor growth. Large randomized clinical trials have demonstrated that kinase inhibitors have improved the survival and quality of life for cancer patients, and multiple inhibitors are now approved by the FDA and regulatory agencies across the world. As outlined earlier, however, substantial challenges remain. The very specificity of kinase inhibitors for selected cellular targets means that they are likely to be most beneficial (or in some cases only beneficial) in tumors that depend on those targets for survival. As discussed previously, a classically defined disease setting such as breast cancer—even a histologically defined subset of breast cancer—may in fact represent a constellation of different diseases with different molecular underpinnings. There are some encouraging signs that techniques such as gene expression profiling, copy number analysis, proteomics, and plasma protein biomarker analysis may have prognostic value, but these data need to be converted into cost-effective, tractable solutions with validation data from prospective clinical studies. Drug resistance is also emerging as a major challenge, and the coming years will undoubtedly see the clinical translation of strategies to overcome this, either through the advancement of inhibitors designed to overcome such liabilities or with combination therapies and alternate dosing regimens.

Addressing the above challenges inevitably involves translation of preclinical data to the clinical setting, and it is worth reminding ourselves of the strengths and liabilities of current drug discovery technology. Although cell-based and animal model studies have been instrumental in supporting the advancement of drugs into the clinic, there are many case examples where exciting preclinical data has not been recapitulated in humans. There are many potential reasons for this disconnect.

Tumor xenograft models are derived from a relatively clonal cell population, and while the inherent instability of many cancer cell lines will result in some heterogeneity, real human tumors are likely to be much more genetically diverse and able to respond to therapy by "rewiring" molecular pathways. Also, tumor:stromal interactions will be substantially different in a mouse xenograft model compared to a real human tumor, which might lead to overestimation or underestimation of antitumor activity for a given drug. Engineered mouse models with defined genetic lesions that give rise to targeted tumor growth may be more realistic, but to date these systems have typically been slower, more challenging, and more costly to use as tools for drug discovery compared to human tumor xenograft models. There are also compound-specific issues such as drug metabolism and disposition and different toxicity profiles. Collectively, these data remind us that although preclinical models are useful for guiding clinical studies, they cannot recapitulate all the features of the human disease. As a corollary to the above, one wonders how many promising human therapeutics have never reached the clinic because of failure to show promising results in a mouse xenograft model: while it is common for a promising preclinical compound to show disappointing results in the clinic, the reverse situation is almost never encountered because compounds with disappointing xenograft tumor growth inhibition data are unlikely to be advanced, even if there is strong rationale for inhibition of their cognate target(s).

Notwithstanding the challenges outlined above, the prospects for the successful treatment of cancers that hitherto have had only dismal prognoses are increasingly bright. Modern techniques of rapid drug discovery and optimization, coupled with an ever improving understanding of the molecular basis of cancer, continue to generate innovative approaches to cancer therapy. Targeted kinase inhibitors are already making incremental improvements in patient survival across a broad range of tumor types, and the growing armamentarium of targeted pathway inhibitors, combined with pharmacogenomic and proteomic tumor profiling, offers the promise of individually tailored cancer treatments. These advances will continue to translate into increasing survival rates, offering hope and improved outcomes for patients and their families.

REFERENCES

1. O'Brien SG, Guilhot F, Larson RA, Gathmann I, Baccarani M, Cervantes F, Cornelissen JJ, Fischer T, Hochhaus A, Hughes T, Lechner K, Nielsen JL, Rousselot P, Reiffers J, Saglio G, Shepherd J, Simonsson B, Gratwohl A, Goldman JM, Kantarjian H, Taylor K, Verhoef G, Bolton AE, Capdeville R, Druker BJ. Imatinib compared with interferon and low-dose cytarabine for newly diagnosed chronic-phase chronic myeloid leukemia. N Engl J Med 2003;348(11):994–1004.
2. Druker BJ, Guilhot F, O'Brien SG, Gathmann I, Kantarjian H, Gattermann N, Deininger MW, Silver RT, Goldman JM, Stone RM, Cervantes F, Hochhaus A, Powell BL, Gabrilove JL, Rousselot P, Reiffers J, Cornelissen JJ, Hughes T, Agis H, Fischer T, Verhoef G, Shepherd J, Saglio G, Gratwohl A, Nielsen JL, Radich JP, Simonsson B, Taylor K, Baccarani M, So C, Letvak L, Larson RA. Five-year follow-up of patients receiving imatinib for chronic myeloid leukemia. N Engl J Med 2006;355(23):2408–2417.

3. Shepherd FA, Rodrigues Pereira J, Ciuleanu T, Tan EH, Hirsh V, Thongprasert S, Campos D, Maoleekoonpiroj S, Smylie M, Martins R, van Kooten M, Dediu M, Findlay B, Tu D, Johnston D, Bezjak A, Clark G, Santabarbara P, Seymour L. Erlotinib in previously treated non-small-cell lung cancer. N Engl J Med 2005;353(2):123–132.

4. Nooter K, Stoter G. Molecular mechanisms of multidrug resistance in cancer chemotherapy. Pathol Res Pract 1996;192(7):768–780.

5. Shukla S, Sauna ZE, Ambudkar SV. Evidence for the interaction of imatinib at the transport-substrate site(s) of the multidrug-resistance-linked ABC drug transporters ABCB1 (P-glycoprotein) and ABCG2. Leukemia 2008;22(2):445–447.

6. Brendel C, Scharenberg C, Dohse M, Robey RW, Bates SE, Shukla S, Ambudkar SV, Wang Y, Wennemuth G, Burchert A, Boudriot U, Neubauer A. Imatinib mesylate and nilotinib (AMN107) exhibit high-affinity interaction with ABCG2 on primitive hematopoietic stem cells. Leukemia 2007;21(6):1267–1275.

7. Burger H, van Tol H, Boersma AW, Brok M, Wiemer EA, Stoter G, Nooter K. Imatinib mesylate (STI571) is a substrate for the breast cancer resistance protein (BCRP)/ABCG2 drug pump. Blood 2004;104(9):2940–2942.

8. Houghton PJ, Germain GS, Harwood FC, Schuetz JD, Stewart CF, Buchdunger E, Traxler P. Imatinib mesylate is a potent inhibitor of the ABCG2 (BCRP) transporter and reverses resistance to topotecan and SN-38 in vitro. Cancer Res 2004;64(7):2333–2337.

9. Mahon FX, Belloc F, Lagarde V, Chollet C, Moreau-Gaudry F, Reiffers J, Goldman JM, Melo JV. MDR1 gene overexpression confers resistance to imatinib mesylate in leukemia cell line models. Blood 2003;101(6):2368–2373.

10. Dulucq S, Bouchet S, Turcq B, Lippert E, Etienne G, Reiffers J, Molimard M, Krajinovic M, Mahon FX. Multidrug resistance gene (MDR1) polymorphisms are associated with major molecular responses to standard-dose imatinib in chronic myeloid leukemia. Blood 2008;112(5):2024–2027.

11. Theou N, Gil S, Devocelle A, Julie C, Lavergne-Slove A, Beauchet A, Callard P, Farinotti R, Le Cesne A, Lemoine A, Faivre-Bonhomme L, Emile JF. Multidrug resistance proteins in gastrointestinal stromal tumors: site-dependent expression and initial response to imatinib. Clin Cancer Res 2005;11(21):7593–7598.

12. Leggas M, Panetta JC, Zhuang Y, Schuetz JD, Johnston B, Bai F, Sorrentino B, Zhou S, Houghton PJ, Stewart CF. Gefitinib modulates the function of multiple ATP-binding cassette transporters in vivo. Cancer Res 2006;66(9):4802–4807.

13. Kitazaki T, Oka M, Nakamura Y, Tsurutani J, Doi S, Yasunaga M, Takemura M, Yabuuchi H, Soda H, Kohno S. Gefitinib, an EGFR tyrosine kinase inhibitor, directly inhibits the function of P-glycoprotein in multidrug resistant cancer cells. Lung Cancer 2005;49(3):337–343.

14. Yang CH, Huang CJ, Yang CS, Chu YC, Cheng AL, Whang-Peng J, Yang PC. Gefitinib reverses chemotherapy resistance in gefitinib-insensitive multidrug resistant cancer cells expressing ATP-binding cassette family protein. Cancer Res 2005;65(15):6943–6949.

15. Shi Z, Peng XX, Kim IW, Shukla S, Si QS, Robey RW, Bates SE, Shen T, Ashby CR Jr, Fu LW, Ambudkar SV, Chen ZS. Erlotinib (Tarceva, OSI-774) antagonizes ATP-binding cassette subfamily B member 1 and ATP-binding cassette subfamily G member 2-mediated drug resistance. Cancer Res 2007;67(22):11012–11020.

16. Marchetti S, de Vries NA, Buckle T, Bolijn MJ, van Eijndhoven MA, Beijnen JH, Mazzanti R, van Tellingen O, Schellens JH. Effect of the ATP-binding cassette drug transporters ABCB1, ABCG2, and ABCC2 on erlotinib hydrochloride (Tarceva) disposition in in vitro and in vivo pharmacokinetic studies employing $BCRP^{-/-}/Mdr1a/1b^{-/-}$ (triple-knockout) and wild-type mice. Mol Cancer Ther 2008;7(8):2280–2287.

17. Thomas J, Wang L, Clark RE, Pirmohamed M. Active transport of imatinib into and out of cells: implications for drug resistance. Blood 2004;104(12):3739–3745.

18. White DL, Saunders VA, Dang P, Engler J, Zannettino AC, Cambareri AC, Quinn SR, Manley PW, Hughes TP. OCT-1-mediated influx is a key determinant of the intracellular uptake of imatinib but not nilotinib (AMN107): reduced OCT-1 activity is the cause of low in vitro sensitivity to imatinib. Blood 2006;108(2):697–704.

19. White DL, Saunders VA, Dang P, Engler J, Venables A, Zrim S, Zannettino A, Lynch K, Manley PW, Hughes T. Most CML patients who have a suboptimal response to imatinib have low OCT-1 activity: higher doses of imatinib may overcome the negative impact of low OCT-1 activity. Blood 2007;110(12):4064–4072.

20. Gambacorti-Passerini C, Barni R, le Coutre P, Zucchetti M, Cabrita G, Cleris L, Rossi F, Gianazza E, Brueggen J, Cozens R, Pioltelli P, Pogliani E, Corneo G, Formelli F, D'Incalci M. Role of alpha 1 acid glycoprotein in the in vivo resistance of human BCR-ABL(+) leukemic cells to the abl inhibitor STI571. J Natl Cancer Inst 2000;92(20):1641–1650.

21. Gambacorti-Passerini C, Zucchetti M, Russo D, Frapolli R, Verga M, Bungaro S, Tornaghi L, Rossi F, Pioltelli P, Pogliani E, Alberti D, Corneo G, D'Incalci M. Alpha 1 acid glycoprotein binds to imatinib (STI571) and substantially alters its pharmacokinetics in chronic myeloid leukemia patients. Clin Cancer Res 2003;9(2):625–632.

22. Larghero J, Leguay T, Mourah S, Madelaine-Chambrin I, Taksin AL, Raffoux E, Bastie JN, Degos L, Berthaud P, Marolleau JP, Calvo F, Chomienne C, Mahon FX, Rousselot P. Relationship between elevated levels of the alpha 1 acid glycoprotein in chronic myelogenous leukemia in blast crisis and pharmacological resistance to imatinib (Gleevec) in vitro and in vivo. Biochem Pharmacol 2003;66(10):1907–1913.

23. Fitos I, Visy J, Zsila F, Mady G, Simonyi M. Selective binding of imatinib to the genetic variants of human alpha 1-acid glycoprotein. Biochim Biophys Acta 2006;1760(11):1704–1712.

24. van Schaik RH. CYP450 pharmacogenetics for personalizing cancer therapy. Drug Resist Updat 2008;11(3):77–98.

25. Cohen MH, Williams G, Johnson JR, Duan J, Gobburu J, Rahman A, Benson K, Leighton J, Kim SK, Wood R, Rothmann M, Chen G, U KM, Staten AM, Pazdur R. Approval summary for imatinib mesylate capsules in the treatment of chronic myelogenous leukemia. Clin Cancer Res 2002;8(5):935–942.

26. Schindler T, Bornmann W, Pellicena P, Miller WT, Clarkson B, Kuriyan J. Structural mechanism for STI-571 inhibition of abelson tyrosine kinase. Science 2000;289(5486):1938–1942.

27. Gorre ME, Mohammed M, Ellwood K, Hsu N, Paquette R, Rao PN, Sawyers CL. Clinical resistance to STI-571 cancer therapy caused by BCR-ABL gene mutation or amplification. Science 2001;293(5531):876–880.

28. Griswold IJ, MacPartlin M, Bumm T, Goss VL, O'Hare T, Lee KA, Corbin AS, Stoffregen EP, Smith C, Johnson K, Moseson EM, Wood LJ, Polakiewicz RD, Druker BJ, Deininger MW. Kinase domain mutants of Bcr-Abl exhibit altered transformation potency, kinase activity, and substrate utilization, irrespective of sensitivity to imatinib. Mol Cell Biol 2006;26(16):6082–6093.

29. Wei Y, Hardling M, Olsson B, Hezaveh R, Ricksten A, Stockelberg D, Wadenvik H. Not all imatinib resistance in CML are BCR-ABL kinase domain mutations. Ann Hematol 2006;85(12):841–847.

30. Willis SG, Lange T, Demehri S, Otto S, Crossman L, Niederwieser D, Stoffregen EP, McWeeney S, Kovacs I, Park B, Druker BJ, Deininger MW. High-sensitivity detection of BCR-ABL kinase domain mutations in imatinib-naive patients: correlation with clonal cytogenetic evolution but not response to therapy. Blood 2005;106(6):2128–2137.

31. Sorel N, Bonnet ML, Guillier M, Guilhot F, Brizard A, Turhan AG. Evidence of ABL-kinase domain mutations in highly purified primitive stem cell populations of patients with chronic myelogenous leukemia. Biochem Biophys Res Commun 2004;323(3):728–730.

32. Roche-Lestienne C, Preudhomme C. Mutations in the ABL kinase domain pre-exist the onset of imatinib treatment. Semin Hematol 2003;40(2 Suppl 2):80–82.

33. Hofmann WK, Komor M, Wassmann B, Jones LC, Gschaidmeier H, Hoelzer D, Koeffler HP, Ottmann OG. Presence of the BCR-ABL mutation Glu255Lys prior to STI571 (imatinib) treatment in patients with Ph+ acute lymphoblastic leukemia. Blood 2003;102(2):659–661.

34. Kang HY, Hwang JY, Kim SH, Goh HG, Kim M, Kim DW. Comparison of allele specific oligonucleotide–polymerase chain reaction and direct sequencing for high throughput screening of ABL kinase domain mutations in chronic myeloid leukemia resistant to imatinib. Haematologica 2006;91(5):659–662.

35. Bell DW, Gore I, Okimoto RA, Godin-Heymann N, Sordella R, Mulloy R, Sharma SV, Brannigan BW, Mohapatra G, Settleman J, Haber DA. Inherited susceptibility to lung cancer may be associated with the T790M drug resistance mutation in EGFR. Nat Genet 2005;37(12):1315–1316.

36. Pao W, Miller VA, Politi KA, Riely GJ, Somwar R, Zakowski MF, Kris MG, Varmus H. Acquired resistance of lung adenocarcinomas to gefitinib or erlotinib is associated with a second mutation in the EGFR kinase domain. PLoS Med 2005;2(3): e73.

37. Yun CH, Mengwasser KE, Toms AV, Woo MS, Greulich H, Wong KK, Meyerson M, Eck MJ. The T790M mutation in EGFR kinase causes drug resistance by increasing the affinity for ATP. Proc Natl Acad Sci U S A 2008;105(6):2070–2075.

38. Balak MN, Gong Y, Riely GJ, Somwar R, Li AR, Zakowski MF, Chiang A, Yang G, Ouerfelli O, Kris MG, Ladanyi M, Miller VA, Pao W. Novel D761Y and common secondary T790M mutations in epidermal growth factor receptor-mutant lung adenocarcinomas with acquired resistance to kinase inhibitors. Clin Cancer Res 2006;12(21):6494–6501.

39. Azam M, Latek RR, Daley GQ. Mechanisms of autoinhibition and STI-571/imatinib resistance revealed by mutagenesis of BCR-ABL. Cell 2003;112(6):831–843.

40. Burgess MR, Skaggs BJ, Shah NP, Lee FY, Sawyers CL. Comparative analysis of two clinically active BCR-ABL kinase inhibitors reveals the role of conformation-specific binding in resistance. Proc Natl Acad Sci U S A 2005;102(9):3395–3400.

41. Yu Z, Boggon TJ, Kobayashi S, Jin C, Ma PC, Dowlati A, Kern JA, Tenen DG, Halmos B. Resistance to an irreversible epidermal growth factor receptor (EGFR) inhibitor in EGFR-mutant lung cancer reveals novel treatment strategies. Cancer Res 2007;67(21):10417–10427.

42. Trowe T, Boukouvala S, Calkins K, Cutler RE Jr, Fong R, Funke R, Gendreau SB, Kim YD, Miller N, Woolfrey JR, Vysotskaia V, Yang JP, Gerritsen ME, Matthews DJ, Lamb P, Heuer TS. EXEL-7647 inhibits mutant forms of ErbB2 associated with lapatinib resistance and neoplastic transformation. Clin Cancer Res 2008;14(8):2465–2475.

43. Zhang X, Gureasko J, Shen K, Cole PA, Kuriyan J. An allosteric mechanism for activation of the kinase domain of epidermal growth factor receptor. Cell 2006;125(6):1137–1149.

44. Phan CL, Megat Baharuddin PJ, Chin LP, Zakaria Z, Yegappan S, Sathar J, Tan SM, Purushothaman V, Chang KM. Amplification of BCR-ABL and t(3;21) in a patient with blast crisis of chronic myelogenous leukemia. Cancer Genet Cytogenet 2008;180(1):60–64.

45. Campbell LJ, Patsouris C, Rayeroux KC, Somana K, Januszewicz EH, Szer J. BCR/ABL amplification in chronic myelocytic leukemia blast crisis following imatinib mesylate administration. Cancer Genet Cytogenet 2002;139(1):30–33.

46. Morel F, Bris MJ, Herry A, Calvez GL, Marion V, Abgrall JF, Berthou C, Braekeleer MD. Double minutes containing amplified bcr-abl fusion gene in a case of chronic myeloid leukemia treated by imatinib. Eur J Haematol 2003;70(4):235–239.

47. Hochhaus A, Kreil S, Corbin AS, La Rosee P, Muller MC, Lahaye T, Hanfstein B, Schoch C, Cross NC, Berger U, Gschaidmeier H, Druker BJ, Hehlmann R. Molecular and chromosomal mechanisms of resistance to imatinib (STI571) therapy. Leukemia 2002;16(11):2190–2196.

48. Witters L, Scherle P, Friedman S, Fridman J, Caulder E, Newton R, Lipton A. Synergistic inhibition with a dual epidermal growth factor receptor/HER-2/neu tyrosine kinase inhibitor and a disintegrin and metalloprotease inhibitor. Cancer Res 2008;68(17):7083–7089.

49. Kwak EL, Sordella R, Bell DW, Godin-Heymann N, Okimoto RA, Brannigan BW, Harris PL, Driscoll DR, Fidias P, Lynch TJ, Rabindran SK, McGinnis JP, Wissner A, Sharma SV, Isselbacher KJ, Settleman J, Haber DA. Irreversible inhibitors of the EGF receptor may circumvent acquired resistance to gefitinib. Proc Natl Acad Sci U S A 2005;102(21):7665–7670.

50. Dai Y, Rahmani M, Corey SJ, Dent P, Grant S. A Bcr/Abl-independent, Lyn-dependent form of imatinib mesylate (STI-571) resistance is associated with altered expression of Bcl-2. J Biol Chem 2004;279(33):34227–34239.

51. Donato NJ, Wu JY, Stapley J, Gallick G, Lin H, Arlinghaus R, Talpaz M. BCR-ABL independence and LYN kinase overexpression in chronic myelogenous leukemia cells selected for resistance to STI571. Blood 2003;101(2):690–698.

52. Donato NJ, Wu JY, Stapley J, Lin H, Arlinghaus R, Aggarwal BB, Shishodia S, Albitar M, Hayes K, Kantarjian H, Talpaz M. Imatinib mesylate resistance through BCR-ABL independence in chronic myelogenous leukemia. Cancer Res 2004;64(2):672–677.

53. Okabe S, Tauchi T, Ohyashiki K. Characteristics of dasatinib- and imatinib-resistant chronic myelogenous leukemia cells. Clin Cancer Res 2008;14(19):6181–6186.

54. Engelman JA, Janne PA, Mermel C, Pearlberg J, Mukohara T, Fleet C, Cichowski K, Johnson BE, Cantley LC. ErbB-3 mediates phosphoinositide 3-kinase activity in gefitinib-sensitive non-small cell lung cancer cell lines. Proc Natl Acad Sci U S A 2005;102(10):3788–3793.

55. Janmaat ML, Kruyt FA, Rodriguez JA, Giaccone G. Response to epidermal growth factor receptor inhibitors in non-small cell lung cancer cells: limited antiproliferative effects and absence of apoptosis associated with persistent activity of extracellular signal-regulated kinase or Akt kinase pathways. Clin Cancer Res 2003;9(6):2316–2326.

56. Sordella R, Bell DW, Haber DA, Settleman J. Gefitinib-sensitizing EGFR mutations in lung cancer activate anti-apoptotic pathways. Science 2004;305(5687):1163–1167.

57. Kosaka T, Yatabe Y, Endoh H, Kuwano H, Takahashi T, Mitsudomi T. Mutations of the epidermal growth factor receptor gene in lung cancer: biological and clinical implications. Cancer Res 2004;64(24):8919–8923.

58. Wang SE, Narasanna A, Perez-Torres M, Xiang B, Wu FY, Yang S, Carpenter G, Gazdar AF, Muthuswamy SK, Arteaga CL. HER2 kinase domain mutation results in constitutive phosphorylation and activation of HER2 and EGFR and resistance to EGFR tyrosine kinase inhibitors. Cancer Cell 2006;10(1):25–38.

59. Sergina NV, Rausch M, Wang D, Blair J, Hann B, Shokat KM, Moasser MM. Escape from HER-family tyrosine kinase inhibitor therapy by the kinase-inactive HER3. Nature 2007;445(7126):437–441.

60. Engelman JA, Zejnullahu K, Mitsudomi T, Song Y, Hyland C, Park JO, Lindeman N, Gale CM, Zhao X, Christensen J, Kosaka T, Holmes AJ, Rogers AM, Cappuzzo F, Mok T, Lee C, Johnson BE, Cantley LC, Janne PA. MET amplification leads to gefitinib resistance in lung cancer by activating ERBB3 signaling. Science 2007;316(5827):1039–1043.

61. Bean J, Brennan C, Shih JY, Riely G, Viale A, Wang L, Chitale D, Motoi N, Szoke J, Broderick S, Balak M, Chang WC, Yu CJ, Gazdar A, Pass H, Rusch V, Gerald W, Huang SF, Yang PC, Miller V, Ladanyi M, Yang CH, Pao W. MET amplification occurs with or without T790M mutations in EGFR mutant lung tumors with acquired resistance to gefitinib or erlotinib. Proc Natl Acad Sci U S A 2007;104(52):20932–20937.

62. Tao Y, Pinzi V, Bourhis J, Deutsch E. Mechanisms of disease: signaling of the insulin-like growth factor 1 receptor pathway—therapeutic perspectives in cancer. Nat Clin Pract Oncol 2007;4(10):591–602.

63. Jones HE, Goddard L, Gee JM, Hiscox S, Rubini M, Barrow D, Knowlden JM, Williams S, Wakeling AE, Nicholson RI. Insulin-like growth factor-I receptor signalling and acquired resistance to gefitinib (ZD1839; Iressa) in human breast and prostate cancer cells. Endocr Relat Cancer 2004;11(4):793–814.

64. Chakravarti A, Loeffler JS, Dyson NJ. Insulin-like growth factor receptor I mediates resistance to anti-epidermal growth factor receptor therapy in primary human glioblastoma cells through continued activation of phosphoinositide 3-kinase signaling. Cancer Res 2002;62(1):200–207.

65. Buck E, Eyzaguirre A, Rosenfeld-Franklin M, Thomson S, Mulvihill M, Barr S, Brown E, O'Connor M, Yao Y, Pachter J, Miglarese M, Epstein D, Iwata KK, Haley JD, Gibson NW, Ji QS. Feedback mechanisms promote cooperativity for small molecule inhibitors of epidermal and insulin-like growth factor receptors. Cancer Res 2008;68(20):8322–8332.

66. Thiery JP. Epithelial-mesenchymal transitions in tumour progression. Nat Rev Cancer 2002;2(6):442–454.

67. Thomson S, Buck E, Petti F, Griffin G, Brown E, Ramnarine N, Iwata KK, Gibson N, Haley JD. Epithelial to mesenchymal transition is a determinant of sensitivity of non-small-cell lung carcinoma cell lines and xenografts to epidermal growth factor receptor inhibition. Cancer Res 2005;65(20):9455–9462.

68. Yauch RL, Januario T, Eberhard DA, Cavet G, Zhu W, Fu L, Pham TQ, Soriano R, Stinson J, Seshagiri S, Modrusan Z, Lin CY, O'Neill V, Amler LC. Epithelial versus mesenchymal phenotype determines in vitro sensitivity and predicts clinical activity of erlotinib in lung cancer patients. Clin Cancer Res 2005;11(24Pt 1):8686–8698.

69. Yoshiji H, Harris SR, Thorgeirsson UP. Vascular endothelial growth factor is essential for initial but not continued in vivo growth of human breast carcinoma cells. Cancer Res 1997;57(18):3924–3928.

70. Bergers G, Song S, Meyer-Morse N, Bergsland E, Hanahan D. Benefits of targeting both pericytes and endothelial cells in the tumor vasculature with kinase inhibitors. J Clin Invest 2003;111(9):1287–1295.

71. Casanovas O, Hicklin DJ, Bergers G, Hanahan D. Drug resistance by evasion of antiangiogenic targeting of VEGF signaling in late-stage pancreatic islet tumors. Cancer Cell 2005;8(4):299–309.

72. Batchelor TT, Sorensen AG, di Tomaso E, Zhang WT, Duda DG, Cohen KS, Kozak KR, Cahill DP, Chen PJ, Zhu M, Ancukiewicz M, Mrugala MM, Plotkin S, Drappatz J, Louis DN, Ivy P, Scadden DT, Benner T, Loeffler JS, Wen PY, Jain RK. AZD2171, a pan-VEGF receptor tyrosine kinase inhibitor, normalizes tumor vasculature and alleviates edema in glioblastoma patients. Cancer Cell 2007;11(1):83–95.

73. Potapova O, Laird AD, Nannini MA, Barone A, Li G, Moss KG, Cherrington JM, Mendel DB. Contribution of individual targets to the antitumor efficacy of the multitargeted receptor tyrosine kinase inhibitor SU11248. Mol Cancer Ther 2006;5(5):1280–1289.

74. Noguera-Troise I, Daly C, Papadopoulos NJ, Coetzee S, Boland P, Gale NW, Lin HC, Yancopoulos GD, Thurston G. Blockade of Dll4 inhibits tumour growth by promoting non-productive angiogenesis. Nature 2006;444(7122):1032–1037.

75. Ridgway J, Zhang G, Wu Y, Stawicki S, Liang WC, Chanthery Y, Kowalski J, Watts RJ, Callahan C, Kasman I, Singh M, Chien M, Tan C, Hongo JA, de Sauvage F, Plowman G, Yan M. Inhibition of Dll4 signalling inhibits tumour growth by deregulating angiogenesis. Nature 2006;444(7122):1083–1087.

76. Stommel JM, Kimmelman AC, Ying H, Nabioullin R, Ponugoti AH, Wiedemeyer R, Stegh AH, Bradner JE, Ligon KL, Brennan C, Chin L, Depinho RA. Coactivation of receptor tyrosine kinases affects the response of tumor cells to targeted therapies. Science 2007;318(5848):287–290.

77. Xia W, Bacus S, Hegde P, Husain I, Strum J, Liu L, Paulazzo G, Lyass L, Trusk P, Hill J, Harris J, Spector NL. A model of acquired autoresistance to a potent ErbB2 tyrosine kinase inhibitor and a therapeutic strategy to prevent its onset in breast cancer. Proc Natl Acad Sci U S A 2006;103(20):7795–7800.

78. Frei E 3rd, Karon M, Levin RH, Freireich EJ, Taylor RJ, Hananian J, Selawry O, Holland JF, Hoogstraten B, Wolman IJ, Abir E, Sawitsky A, Lee S, Mills SD, Burgert EO Jr, Spurr CL, Patterson RB, Ebaugh FG, James GW 3rd, Moon JH. The effectiveness of combinations of antileukemic agents in inducing and maintaining remission in children with acute leukemia. Blood 1965;26(5):642–656.

79. Chou TC. Theoretical basis, experimental design, and computerized simulation of synergism and antagonism in drug combination studies. Pharmacol Rev 2006;58(3):621–681.

80. Greco WR, Bravo G, Parsons JC. The search for synergy: a critical review from a response surface perspective. Pharmacol Rev 1995;47(2):331–385.

81. Jain RK. Normalization of tumor vasculature: an emerging concept in antiangiogenic therapy. Science 2005;307(5706):58–62.

82. Hurwitz H, Fehrenbacher L, Novotny W, Cartwright T, Hainsworth J, Heim W, Berlin J, Baron A, Griffing S, Holmgren E, Ferrara N, Fyfe G, Rogers B, Ross R, Kabbinavar F. Bevacizumab plus irinotecan, fluorouracil, and leucovorin for metastatic colorectal cancer. N Engl J Med 2004;350(23):2335–2342.

83. Miller K, Wang M, Gralow J, Dickler M, Cobleigh M, Perez EA, Shenkier T, Cella D, Davidson NE. Paclitaxel plus bevacizumab versus paclitaxel alone for metastatic breast cancer. N Engl J Med 2007;357(26):2666–2676.

84. Sandler A, Gray R, Perry MC, Brahmer J, Schiller JH, Dowlati A, Lilenbaum R, Johnson DH. Paclitaxel-carboplatin alone or with bevacizumab for non-small-cell lung cancer. N Engl J Med 2006;355(24):2542–2550.

85. Dal Lago L, D'Hondt V, Awada A. Selected combination therapy with sorafenib: a review of clinical data and perspectives in advanced solid tumors. Oncologist 2008;13(8):845–858.

86. McDermott DF, Sosman JA, Gonzalez R, Hodi FS, Linette GP, Richards J, Jakub JW, Beeram M, Tarantolo S, Agarwala S, Frenette G, Puzanov I, Cranmer L, Lewis K, Kirkwood J, White JM,

Xia C, Patel K, Hersh E. Double-blind randomized phase II study of the combination of sorafenib and dacarbazine in patients with advanced melanoma: a report from the 11715 Study Group. J Clin Oncol 2008;26(13):2178–2185.

87. Agarwala SS, Keilholz U, Hogg D, Robert C, Hersey P, Eggermont A, Grabbe S, Gonzalez R, Patel K, Hauschild A. Randomized phase III study of paclitaxel plus carboplatin with or without sorafenib as second-line treatment in patients with advanced melanoma. J Clin Oncol (Meeting Abstracts) 2007;25(18 Suppl):Abstr 8510.

88. Welch S, Hirte H, Elit L, Schilder RJ, Pond G, Kovacs J, Wright J, Oza AM. CA-125 response as a marker of clinical benefit in patients with recurrent ovarian cancer treated with gemcitabine and sorafenib—a trial of the PMH Phase II Consortium. J Clin Oncol (Meeting Abstracts) 2007;25(18 Suppl):Abstr 5519.

89. Solit DB, She Y, Lobo J, Kris MG, Scher HI, Rosen N, Sirotnak FM. Pulsatile administration of the epidermal growth factor receptor inhibitor gefitinib is significantly more effective than continuous dosing for sensitizing tumors to paclitaxel. Clin Cancer Res 2005;11(5):1983–1989.

90. Sharma SV, Fischbach MA, Haber DA, Settleman J. "Oncogenic shock": explaining oncogene addiction through differential signal attenuation. Clin Cancer Res 2006;12(14Pt 2): 4392s–4395s.

91. Giaccone G, Herbst RS, Manegold C, Scagliotti G, Rosell R, Miller V, Natale RB, Schiller JH, Von Pawel J, Pluzanska A, Gatzemeier U, Grous J, Ochs JS, Averbuch SD, Wolf MK, Rennie P, Fandi A, Johnson DH. Gefitinib in combination with gemcitabine and cisplatin in advanced non-small-cell lung cancer: a phase III trial—INTACT 1. J Clin Oncol 2004;22(5):777–784.

92. Herbst RS, Giaccone G, Schiller JH, Natale RB, Miller V, Manegold C, Scagliotti G, Rosell R, Oliff I, Reeves JA, Wolf MK, Krebs AD, Averbuch SD, Ochs JS, Grous J, Fandi A, Johnson DH. Gefitinib in combination with paclitaxel and carboplatin in advanced non-small-cell lung cancer: a phase III trial—INTACT 2. J Clin Oncol 2004;22(5):785–794.

93. Gatzemeier U, Pluzanska A, Szczesna A, Kaukel E, Roubec J, De Rosa F, Milanowski J, Karnicka-Mlodkowski H, Pesek M, Serwatowski P, Ramlau R, Janaskova T, Vansteenkiste J, Strausz J, Manikhas GM, Von Pawel J. Phase III study of erlotinib in combination with cisplatin and gemcitabine in advanced non-small-cell lung cancer: the Tarceva Lung Cancer Investigation Trial. J Clin Oncol 2007;25(12):1545–1552.

94. Herbst RS, Prager D, Hermann R, Fehrenbacher L, Johnson BE, Sandler A, Kris MG, Tran HT, Klein P, Li X, Ramies D, Johnson DH, Miller VA. TRIBUTE: a phase III trial of erlotinib hydrochloride (OSI-774) combined with carboplatin and paclitaxel chemotherapy in advanced non-small-cell lung cancer. J Clin Oncol 2005;23(25):5892–5899.

95. Riely GJ, Rizvi NA, Kris MG, Milton DT, Solit DB, Rosen N, Senturk E, Azzoli CG, Brahmer JR, Sirotnak FM, Seshan VE, Fogle M, Ginsberg M, Miller VA, Rudin CM. Randomized phase II study of pulse erlotinib before or after carboplatin and paclitaxel in current or former smokers with advanced non-small-cell lung cancer. J Clin Oncol 2009;27(2):264–270.

96. Tabernero J. The role of VEGF and EGFR inhibition: implications for combining anti-VEGF and anti-EGFR agents. Mol Cancer Res 2007;5(3):203–220.

97. Herbst RS, Johnson DH, Mininberg E, Carbone DP, Henderson T, Kim ES, Blumenschein G Jr, Lee JJ, Liu DD, Truong MT, Hong WK, Tran H, Tsao A, Xie D, Ramies DA, Mass R, Seshagiri S, Eberhard DA, Kelley SK, Sandler A. Phase I/II trial evaluating the anti-vascular endothelial growth factor monoclonal antibody bevacizumab in combination with the HER-1/epidermal growth factor receptor tyrosine kinase inhibitor erlotinib for patients with recurrent non-small-cell lung cancer. J Clin Oncol 2005;23(11):2544–2555.

98. Herbst RS, O'Neill VJ, Fehrenbacher L, Belani CP, Bonomi PD, Hart L, Melnyk O, Ramies D, Lin M, Sandler A. Phase II study of efficacy and safety of bevacizumab in combination with chemotherapy or erlotinib compared with chemotherapy alone for treatment of recurrent or refractory non small-cell lung cancer. J Clin Oncol 2007;25(30):4743–4750.

99. Hainsworth JD, Sosman JA, Spigel DR, Edwards DL, Baughman C, Greco A. Treatment of metastatic renal cell carcinoma with a combination of bevacizumab and erlotinib. J Clin Oncol 2005;23(31):7889–7896.

100. Guix M, Faber AC, Wang SE, Olivares MG, Song Y, Qu S, Rinehart C, Seidel B, Yee D, Arteaga CL, Engelman JA. Acquired resistance to EGFR tyrosine kinase inhibitors in cancer cells is mediated by loss of IGF-binding proteins. J Clin Invest 2008;118(7):2609–2619.

101. Jones HE, Gee JM, Barrow D, Tonge D, Holloway B, Nicholson RI. Inhibition of insulin receptor isoform-A signalling restores sensitivity to gefitinib in previously de novo resistant colon cancer cells. Br J Cancer 2006;95(2):172–180.

102. Araujo RP, Liotta LA, Petricoin EF. Proteins, drug targets and the mechanisms they control: the simple truth about complex networks. Nat Rev Drug Discov 2007;6(11):871–880.

103. Chung CH, Bernard PS, Perou CM. Molecular portraits and the family tree of cancer. Nat Genet 2002;32 Suppl: 533–540.

104. Perou CM, Sorlie T, Eisen MB, van de Rijn M, Jeffrey SS, Rees CA, Pollack JR, Ross DT, Johnsen H, Akslen LA, Fluge O, Pergamenschikov A, Williams C, Zhu SX, Lonning PE, Borresen-Dale AL, Brown PO, Botstein D. Molecular portraits of human breast tumours. Nature 2000;406(6797):747–752.

105. Perou CM, Jeffrey SS, van de Rijn M, Rees CA, Eisen MB, Ross DT, Pergamenschikov A, Williams CF, Zhu SX, Lee JC, Lashkari D, Shalon D, Brown PO, Botstein D. Distinctive gene expression patterns in human mammary epithelial cells and breast cancers. Proc Natl Acad Sci U S A 1999;96(16):9212–9217.

106. Sorlie T, Perou CM, Tibshirani R, Aas T, Geisler S, Johnsen H, Hastie T, Eisen MB, van de Rijn M, Jeffrey SS, Thorsen T, Quist H, Matese JC, Brown PO, Botstein D, Eystein Lonning P, Borresen-Dale AL. Gene expression patterns of breast carcinomas distinguish tumor subclasses with clinical implications. Proc Natl Acad Sci U S A 2001;98(19):10869–10874.

107. Sorlie T, Tibshirani R, Parker J, Hastie T, Marron JS, Nobel A, Deng S, Johnsen H, Pesich R, Geisler S, Demeter J, Perou CM, Lonning PE, Brown PO, Borresen-Dale AL, Botstein D. Repeated observation of breast tumor subtypes in independent gene expression data sets. Proc Natl Acad Sci U S A 2003;100(14):8418–8423.

108. Wang Y, Klijn JG, Zhang Y, Sieuwerts AM, Look MP, Yang F, Talantov D, Timmermans M, Meijer-van Gelder ME, Yu J, Jatkoe T, Berns EM, Atkins D, Foekens JA. Gene-expression profiles to predict distant metastasis of lymph-node-negative primary breast cancer. Lancet 2005;365(9460):671–679.

109. van de Vijver MJ, He YD, van't Veer LJ, Dai H, Hart AA, Voskuil DW, Schreiber GJ, Peterse JL, Roberts C, Marton MJ, Parrish M, Atsma D, Witteveen A, Glas A, Delahaye L, van der Velde T, Bartelink H, Rodenhuis S, Rutgers ET, Friend SH, Bernards R. A gene-expression signature as a predictor of survival in breast cancer. N Engl J Med 2002;347(25):1999–2009.

110. Paik S, Shak S, Tang G, Kim C, Baker J, Cronin M, Baehner FL, Walker MG, Watson D, Park T, Hiller W, Fisher ER, Wickerham DL, Bryant J, Wolmark N. A multigene assay to predict recurrence of tamoxifen-treated, node-negative breast cancer. N Engl J Med 2004;351(27):2817–2826.

111. Paik S, Tang G, Shak S, Kim C, Baker J, Kim W, Cronin M, Baehner FL, Watson D, Bryant J, Costantino JP, Geyer CE Jr, Wickerham DL, Wolmark N. Gene expression and benefit of chemotherapy in women with node-negative, estrogen receptor-positive breast cancer. J Clin Oncol 2006;24(23):3726–3734.

112. Buyse M, Loi S, van't Veer L, Viale G, Delorenzi M, Glas AM, d'Assignies MS, Bergh J, Lidereau R, Ellis P, Harris A, Bogaerts J, Therasse P, Floore A, Amakrane M, Piette F, Rutgers E, Sotiriou C, Cardoso F, Piccart MJ. Validation and clinical utility of a 70-gene prognostic signature for women with node-negative breast cancer. J Natl Cancer Inst 2006;98(17):1183–1192.

113. Chin K, DeVries S, Fridlyand J, Spellman PT, Roydasgupta R, Kuo WL, Lapuk A, Neve RM, Qian Z, Ryder T, Chen F, Feiler H, Tokuyasu T, Kingsley C, Dairkee S, Meng Z, Chew K, Pinkel D, Jain A, Ljung BM, Esserman L, Albertson DG, Waldman FM, Gray JW. Genomic and transcriptional aberrations linked to breast cancer pathophysiologies. Cancer Cell 2006;10(6):529–541.

114. Chang JC, Wooten EC, Tsimelzon A, Hilsenbeck SG, Gutierrez MC, Elledge R, Mohsin S, Osborne CK, Chamness GC, Allred DC, O'Connell P. Gene expression profiling for the prediction of therapeutic response to docetaxel in patients with breast cancer. Lancet 2003;362(9381):362–369.

115. Dressman HK, Hans C, Bild A, Olson JA, Rosen E, Marcom PK, Liotcheva VB, Jones EL, Vujaskovic Z, Marks J, Dewhirst MW, West M, Nevins JR, Blackwell K. Gene expression profiles of multiple breast cancer phenotypes and response to neoadjuvant chemotherapy. Clin Cancer Res 2006;12(3Pt 1):819–826.

116. Folgueira MA, Carraro DM, Brentani H, Patrao DF, Barbosa EM, Netto MM, Caldeira JR, Katayama ML, Soares FA, Oliveira CT, Reis LF, Kaiano JH, Camargo LP, Vencio RZ, Snitcovsky

IM, Makdissi FB, e Silva PJ, Goes JC, Brentani MM. Gene expression profile associated with response to doxorubicin-based therapy in breast cancer. Clin Cancer Res 2005;11(20):7434–7443.

117. Bild AH, Yao G, Chang JT, Wang Q, Potti A, Chasse D, Joshi MB, Harpole D, Lancaster JM, Berchuck A, Olson JA Jr, Marks JR, Dressman HK, West M, Nevins JR. Oncogenic pathway signatures in human cancers as a guide to targeted therapies. Nature 2006;439(7074):353–357.

118. Saal LH, Johansson P, Holm K, Gruvberger-Saal SK, She QB, Maurer M, Koujak S, Ferrando AA, Malmstrom P, Memeo L, Isola J, Bendahl PO, Rosen N, Hibshoosh H, Ringner M, Borg A, Parsons R. Poor prognosis in carcinoma is associated with a gene expression signature of aberrant PTEN tumor suppressor pathway activity. Proc Natl Acad Sci U S A 2007;104(18):7564–7569.

119. Creighton CJ. A gene transcription signature of the Akt/mTOR pathway in clinical breast tumors. Oncogene 2007;26(32):4648–4655.

120. Potti A, Dressman HK, Bild A, Riedel RF, Chan G, Sayer R, Cragun J, Cottrill H, Kelley MJ, Petersen R, Harpole D, Marks J, Berchuck A, Ginsburg GS, Febbo P, Lancaster J, Nevins JR. Genomic signatures to guide the use of chemotherapeutics. Nat Med 2006;12(11):1294–1300.

121. Anders CK, Acharya CR, Hsu DS, Broadwater G, Garman K, Foekens JA, Zhang Y, Wang Y, Marcom K, Marks JR, Mukherjee S, Nevins JR, Blackwell KL, Potti A. Age-specific differences in oncogenic pathway deregulation seen in human breast tumors. PLoS ONE 2008;3(1): e1373.

122. Anders CK, Hsu DS, Broadwater G, Acharya CR, Foekens JA, Zhang Y, Wang Y, Marcom PK, Marks JR, Febbo PG, Nevins JR, Potti A, Blackwell KL. Young age at diagnosis correlates with worse prognosis and defines a subset of breast cancers with shared patterns of gene expression. J Clin Oncol 2008;26(20):3324–3330.

123. Cohen P. The role of protein phosphorylation in human health and disease. The Sir Hans Krebs Medal Lecture. Eur J Biochem 2001;268(19):5001–5010.

124. Johnson SA, Hunter T. Kinomics: methods for deciphering the kinome. Nat Methods 2005;2(1):17–25.

125. Obenauer JC, Cantley LC, Yaffe MB. Scansite 2.0: proteome-wide prediction of cell signaling interactions using short sequence motifs. Nucleic Acids Res 2003;31(13):3635–3641.

126. Yaffe MB, Leparc GG, Lai J, Obata T, Volinia S, Cantley LC. A motif-based profile scanning approach for genome-wide prediction of signaling pathways. Nat Biotechnol 2001;19(4):348–353.

127. Cohen P, Knebel A. KESTREL: a powerful method for identifying the physiological substrates of protein kinases. Biochem J 2006;393(Pt 1):1–6.

128. Manning BD, Cantley LC. Hitting the target: emerging technologies in the search for kinase substrates. Sci STKE 2002;2002(162): PE49.

129. Mann M, Ong SE, Gronborg M, Steen H, Jensen ON, Pandey A. Analysis of protein phosphorylation using mass spectrometry: deciphering the phosphoproteome. Trends Biotechnol 2002;20(6):261–268.

130. Salomon AR, Ficarro SB, Brill LM, Brinker A, Phung QT, Ericson C, Sauer K, Brock A, Horn DM, Schultz PG, Peters EC. Profiling of tyrosine phosphorylation pathways in human cells using mass spectrometry. Proc Natl Acad Sci U S A 2003;100(2):443–448.

131. Beausoleil SA, Jedrychowski M, Schwartz D, Elias JE, Villen J, Li J, Cohn MA, Cantley LC, Gygi SP. Large-scale characterization of HeLa cell nuclear phosphoproteins. Proc Natl Acad Sci U S A 2004;101(33):12130–12135.

132. Ong SE, Blagoev B, Kratchmarova I, Kristensen DB, Steen H, Pandey A, Mann M. Stable isotope labeling by amino acids in cell culture, SILAC, as a simple and accurate approach to expression proteomics. Mol Cell Proteomics 2002;1(5):376–386.

133. Blagoev B, Kratchmarova I, Ong SE, Nielsen M, Foster LJ, Mann M. A proteomics strategy to elucidate functional protein–protein interactions applied to EGF signaling. Nat Biotechnol 2003;21(3):315–318.

134. Blagoev B, Ong SE, Kratchmarova I, Mann M. Temporal analysis of phosphotyrosine-dependent signaling networks by quantitative proteomics. Nat Biotechnol 2004;22(9):1139–1145.

135. Olsen JV, Blagoev B, Gnad F, Macek B, Kumar C, Mortensen P, Mann M. Global, in vivo, and site-specific phosphorylation dynamics in signaling networks. Cell 2006;127(3):635–648.

136. Nishizuka S, Charboneau L, Young L, Major S, Reinhold WC, Waltham M, Kouros-Mehr H, Bussey KJ, Lee JK, Espina V, Munson PJ, Petricoin E 3rd, Liotta LA, Weinstein JN. Proteomic

profiling of the NCI-60 cancer cell lines using new high-density reverse-phase lysate microarrays. Proc Natl Acad Sci U S A 2003;100(24):14229–14234.

137. Sheehan KM, Calvert VS, Kay EW, Lu Y, Fishman D, Espina V, Aquino J, Speer R, Araujo R, Mills GB, Liotta LA, Petricoin EF 3rd, Wulfkuhle JD. Use of reverse phase protein microarrays and reference standard development for molecular network analysis of metastatic ovarian carcinoma. Mol Cell Proteomics 2005;4(4):346–355.

138. Mirzoeva OK, Das D, Heiser LM, Bhattacharya S, Siwak D, Gendelman R, Bayani N, Wang NJ, Neve RM, Guan Y, Hu Z, Knight Z, Feiler HS, Gascard P, Parvin B, Spellman PT, Shokat KM, Wyrobek AJ, Bissell MJ, McCormick F, Kuo WL, Mills GB, Gray JW, Korn WM. Basal subtype and MAPK/ERK kinase (MEK)-phosphoinositide 3-kinase feedback signaling determine susceptibility of breast cancer cells to MEK inhibition. Cancer Res 2009;69(2):565–572.

139. Gerdes J, Schwab U, Lemke H, Stein H. Production of a mouse monoclonal antibody reactive with a human nuclear antigen associated with cell proliferation. Int J Cancer 1983;31(1):13–20.

140. Stahl A, Wieder H, Piert M, Wester HJ, Senekowitsch-Schmidtke R, Schwaiger M. Positron emission tomography as a tool for translational research in oncology. Mol Imaging Biol 2004;6(4):214–224.

141. Moss KG, Toner GC, Cherrington JM, Mendel DB, Laird AD. Hair depigmentation is a biological readout for pharmacological inhibition of KIT in mice and humans. J Pharmacol Exp Ther 2003;307(2):476–480.

142. Routhouska S, Gilliam AC, Mirmirani P. Hair depigmentation during chemotherapy with a class III/V receptor tyrosine kinase inhibitor. Arch Dermatol 2006;142(11):1477–1479.

143. Rixe O, Billemont B, Izzedine H. Hypertension as a predictive factor of sunitinib activity. Ann Oncol 2007;18(6):1117.

144. Fleming TR, DeMets DL. Surrogate end points in clinical trials: are we being misled? Ann Intern Med 1996;125(7):605–613.

145. DePrimo SE, Bello C. Surrogate biomarkers in evaluating response to anti-angiogenic agents: focus on sunitinib. Ann Oncol 2007;18 (Suppl 10): x11–19.

146. Deprimo SE, Bello CL, Smeraglia J, Baum CM, Spinella D, Rini BI, Michaelson MD, Motzer RJ. Circulating protein biomarkers of pharmacodynamic activity of sunitinib in patients with metastatic renal cell carcinoma: modulation of VEGF and VEGF-related proteins. J Transl Med 2007;5: 32.

147. Deprimo SE, Friece C, Huang X, Smeraglia J, Sherman L, Collier M, Baum C, Elias AD, Burstein HJ, Miller KD. Effect of treatment with sunitinib malate, a multitargeted tyrosine kinase inhibitor, on circulating plasma levels of VEGF, soluble VEGF receptors 2 and 3, and soluble KIT in patients with metastatic breast cancer. J Clin Oncol (Meeting Abstracts) 2006;24(18 Suppl):Abstr 578.

148. Norden-Zfoni A, Desai J, Manola J, Beaudry P, Force J, Maki R, Folkman J, Bello C, Baum C, DePrimo SE, Shalinsky DR, Demetri GD, Heymach JV. Blood-based biomarkers of SU11248 activity and clinical outcome in patients with metastatic imatinib-resistant gastrointestinal stromal tumor. Clin Cancer Res 2007;13(9):2643–2650.

149. Bello C, Deprimo SE, Friece C, Smeraglia J, Sherman L, Tye L, Baum C, Meropol NJ, Lenz H, Kulke MH. Analysis of circulating biomarkers of sunitinib malate in patients with unresectable neuroendocrine tumors (NET): VEGF, IL-8, and soluble VEGF receptors 2 and 3. J Clin Oncol (Meeting Abstracts) 2006;24(18 Suppl):Abstr 4045.

150. Bertolini F, Shaked Y, Mancuso P, Kerbel RS. The multifaceted circulating endothelial cell in cancer: towards marker and target identification. Nat Rev Cancer 2006;6(11):835–845.

151. Harrington LS, Findlay GM, Gray A, Tolkacheva T, Wigfield S, Rebholz H, Barnett J, Leslie NR, Cheng S, Shepherd PR, Gout I, Downes CP, Lamb RF. The TSC1-2 tumor suppressor controls insulin-PI3K signaling via regulation of IRS proteins. J Cell Biol 2004;166(2):213–223.

152. Sun SY, Rosenberg LM, Wang X, Zhou Z, Yue P, Fu H, Khuri FR. Activation of Akt and eIF4E survival pathways by rapamycin-mediated mammalian target of rapamycin inhibition. Cancer Res 2005;65(16):7052–7058.

153. O'Reilly KE, Rojo F, She QB, Solit D, Mills GB, Smith D, Lane H, Hofmann F, Hicklin DJ, Ludwig DL, Baselga J, Rosen N. mTOR inhibition induces upstream receptor tyrosine kinase signaling and activates Akt. Cancer Res 2006;66(3):1500–1508.

154. Laird AD. XL765 targets tumor growth, survival, and angiogenesis in preclinical models by dual inhibition of PI3K and mTOR. AACR Meeting Abstracts 2007(Molecular Targets and Cancer Therapeutics, Oct 22–26, San Francisco, CA): B250.

155. Papadopoulos KP, Markman B, Tabernero J, Patnaik A, Heath EI, DeCillis A, Laird D, Aggarwal SK, Nguyen L, LoRusso PM. A phase I dose-escalation study of the safety, pharmacokinetics (PK), and pharmacodynamics (PD) of a novel PI3K inhibitor, XL765, administered orally to patients (pts) with advanced solid tumors. J Clin Oncol (Meeting Abstracts) 2008;26(15 Suppl):Abstr 3510.

156. Markman B, LoRusso PM, Patnaik A, Elisabeth Heath E, Laird AD, van Leeuwen B, Papadopoulos KP, Baselga J. A phase 1 dose-escalation study of the safety, pharmacokinetics and pharmacodynamics of XL765, a novel inhibitor of PI3K and mTOR, administered orally to patients with solid tumors. 20th EORTC-NCI-AACR Symposium on Molecular Targets and Cancer Therapeutics; 2008 Oct 21–24; Geneva, Switzerland.

157. Laird AD, Sillman A, Sun B, Mengistab A, Wu B, Chu F, Lee M, Cancilla B, Martini J-F, Nguyen L, Aggarwal SK, Bentzien F. Evaluation of peripheral blood cells and hair as surrogate tissues for clinical trial pharmacodynamic assessment of XL147 and XL765, inhibitors of the PI3K signaling pathway. 20th EORTC-NCI-AACR Symposium on Molecular Targets and Cancer Therapeutics; 2008 Oct 21–24; Geneva, Switzerland.

158. Workman P. How much gets there and what does it do?: The need for better pharmacokinetic and pharmacodynamic endpoints in contemporary drug discovery and development. Curr Pharm Des 2003;9(11):891–902.

LIST OF ABBREVIATIONS

Term or Abbreviation	Definition
(p70) S6K	(p70) S6 kinase
(p90) RSK	(p90) ribosomal S6 kinase
4E-BP	eIF4E binding protein
5-FU	5-fluorouracil
5-UTR	5′ untranslated region
9-1-1 complex	Rad9-Hus1-Rad1
AACR	American Association for Cancer Research
AAK1	AP2 associated kinase 1
AATK	apoptosis-associated tyrosine kinase
ABL1	v-abl Abelson murine leukemia viral oncogene homolog 1
ABL2	v-abl Abelson murine leukemia viral oncogene homolog 2 (arg, Abelson-related gene)
ACVR1/1B/1C/2A/2B	activin A receptor, type I/IB/IC/IIA/IIB
ACVRL1	activin A receptor type II-like 1
ADAM	a disintegrin and metalloproteinase
ADCK1/2/4/5	aarF domain containing kinase 1/2/4/5
ADN	adenosine
ADRBK1/2	adrenergic, beta, receptor kinase 1/2
Ag	antigen
Ajuba	a LIM domain protein that functions as a histone-deactylase dependent corepressor
AKT	AKR mouse thymoma kinase
AKT1/2/3	v-akt murine thymoma viral oncogene homolog 1/2/3
AL	acute leukemia
ALBL	acute lymphoblastic B-cell leukemia
ALCL	anaplastic large cell lymphoma
ALK	anaplastic lymphoma kinase (Ki-1)
ALL	acute lymphocytic leukemia

Targeting Protein Kinases for Cancer Therapy, by David J. Matthews and Mary E. Gerritsen
Copyright © 2010 John Wiley & Sons, Inc.

ALP1	amphiphysin
ALPK1/2/3	alpha-kinase 1/2/3
ALS2CR2	amyotrophic lateral sclerosis 2 (juvenile) chromosome region, candidate 2
ALTL	acute lymphoblastic T-cell leukemia
AMHR2	anti-Mullerian hormone receptor, type II
AMKL	acute megakaryocytic leukemia
AML	acute myeloid leukemia
AMLAMDS	acute myeloid leukemia associated with MDS
AMLTR	acute myeloid leukemia therapy related
AMP	adenosine monophosphate
ANG	angiopoietin
ANKK1	ankyrin repeat and kinase domain containing 1
AP-1	activator protein 1
APAF-1	apoptotic protease activating factor 1
APC	anaphase promoting complex (mitosis), or adenomatous polyposis coli (tumor suppressor)
APC/C	anaphase promoting complex/cyclosome
APL	acute promyelocytic leukemia
AR	amphiregulin
ARAF	v-raf murine sarcoma 3611 viral oncogene homolog
ARF	ADP ribosylation factor
ARG	Abelson-related gene
ARTN	artemin
ASCO	American Society for Clinical Oncology
ASF	anti-silencing factor, also known as SF2/ASF, a splicing protein
ASH	American Society for Hematology
ASK	activator of S-phase kinase
AT	ataxia telangiectasia
ATCLL	adult T-cell lymphoma-leukemia
ATM	ataxia telangiectasia mutated (includes complementation groups A, C, and D)
ATP	adenosine triphosphate
ATR	ataxia telangiectasia and Rad3-related kinase
ATRIP	ATR interacting protein
AUC	area under the curve
AURKA	Aurora kinase A/B/C
AXL	a receptor tyrosine kinase
BAK	bcl-2 antagonist killer 1

BAX	bcl-2 associated X protein
BCC	basal cell carcinoma
BCKDK	branched chain ketoacid dehydrogenase kinase
BCL	B-cell lymphoma unspecified
BCL2	B-cell lymphoma gene 2
BCLXL	bcl-2-like 1
BCR	breakpoint cluster region
BH3	bcl-2 homology 3
bHLH	basic helix–loop–helix transcription factor
bid	bis in die; twice-daily dosing
BIM	bcl-2-like 4
BIP	GRP78, a molecular chaperone
BL	Burkitt lymphoma
BLK	B lymphoid tyrosine kinase
BMP	bone morphogenetic protein
BMP2K	BMP2 inducible kinase
BMPR1A/1B/2	bone morphogenetic protein receptor, type IA/IB/II (serine/threonine kinase)
BMX	BMX nonreceptor tyrosine kinase
borealin	a member of the chromosomal passenger complex of Aurora-B
BPCML	blast phase chronic myeloid leukemia
BPPCV	blast phase polycythemia vera
BPET	blast phase erythroleukemia
BRAF	v-raf murine sarcoma viral oncogene homolog B1
BRCA1	breast cancer 1, early onset
BRD2/3/4	bromodomain containing 2/3/4
BRDT	bromodomain, testis-specific
BRK	PTK6, protein tyrosine kinase 5
BRSK1	BR serine/threonine kinase 1/2
BTC	betacellulin
BTK	Bruton agammaglobulinemia tyrosine kinase
BUB1	BUB1 budding uninhibited by benzimidazoles 1 homolog
BUB1B/BUBR1	BUB1 budding uninhibited by benzimidazoles 1 homolog β
C/EBP	CCAAT/enhancer binding protein
C9orf96	chromosome 9 open reading frame 96
CABC1	chaperone, ABC1 activity of bc1 complex homolog (*S. pombe*)

CABLES	connecting CDK5 with c-ABL
CAKβ	cell adhesion kinase β; PYK2, CADTK, RAFTK
C-ALCL	CD30+ anaplastic large cell lyphoma
C-TAK1	see MARK3
CAMK1/1D/1G	calcium/calmodulin-dependent protein kinase I/ID/IG
CAMK2A/B/D/G	calcium/calmodulin-dependent protein kinase (CaM kinase) II α/β/δ/γ
CAMK4	calcium/calmodulin-dependent protein kinase IV
CAMKK1	calcium/calmodulin-dependent protein kinase kinase 1, alpha
CAMKK2	calcium/calmodulin-dependent protein kinase kinase 2, beta
CAMKV	CaM kinase-like vesicle-associated
cAMP	cyclic AMP
CARS-ALK	cysteinyl-tRNA synthase–ALK fusion protein
CASK	calcium/calmodulin-dependent serine protein kinase (MAGUK family)
CBL	Cas-Br-M ectopic retroviral transforming sequence
CBLB	Cas-Br-M ectopic retroviral transforming sequence B
CBP	cyclic amp response element binding protein
CCR	chemokine receptor
CCRK	cell cycle related kinase
CCVw	clathrin coated vesicles
CDC	cell division and control
CDC2	cell division cycle 2, G1 to S and G2 to M
CDC2L1	cell division cycle 2-like 2 (PITSLRE proteins)
CDC2L5	cell division cycle 2-like 5 (cholinesterase-related cell division controller)
CDC2L6	cell division cycle 2-like 6 (CDK8-like)
CDC42BPA/B/G	CDC42 binding protein kinase α/β/γ (DMPK-like)
CDC7	cell division cycle 7 homolog
CDCH	cyclin-dependent protein kinase H
CDH1	E-cadherin
CDK1–10	cyclin-dependent kinase 1–10
CDKL1/2/3/4/5	cyclin-dependent kinase-like 1/2/3/4/5 (CDC2-related kinase)
CDKN2	cyclin-dependent kinase inhibitor 2A
cDNA	complementary DNA copy of mRNA
CEA	carcinoembryonic antigen
CEC	circulating endothelial cell

CELHS	chronic eosinophilic leukemia-hypereosinophilic syndrome
CENP-A/E	centromere protein A/E
CEP	circulating endothelial progenitor cell
CFC	cardio-facio-cutaneous syndrome, a developmental disorder
CGH	comparative genomic hybridization
CHED	cholinesterase-related cell division controller
CHEK1	CHK1 checkpoint homolog (*S. pombe*)
CHEK2	CHK2 checkpoint homolog (*S. pombe*)
CHK1	checkpoint kinase 1
CHK2	checkpoint kinase 2
CHUK	conserved helix–loop–helix ubiquitous kinase
CIP4	thyroid hormone receptor interactor 8
CIT	citron (rho-interacting, serine/threonine kinase 21)
CKII	casein kinase II
CLK1/2/3/4	CDC-like kinase 1/2/3/4
CLLSLL	chronic lymphocytic leukemia–small lymphocytic lymphoma
CMGC	CDK/MAPK/GSK/CDK-like kinase group
CML	chronic myeloid leukemia
CMML	chronic myelomonocytic leukemia
CNK	connector-enhancer of KSR, a scaffolding protein
CNL	chronic neutrophilic leukemia
CNS	central nervous system
COL1A1	collagen type 1, alpha 1
CP	carboplatin/paclitaxel
CR	complete response; may also refer to a cysteine-rich region
CRAF	v-raf1 murine leukemia viral oncogene homolog 1
CRC	colorectal cancer
CREB	cAMP response element binding protein
CREM-τ	cAMP responsive element modulator
CRIC	conserved region in CNK
CRK/CRKII	v-crk sarcoma virus CT10 oncogene homolog adaptor protein
CRKL	CRK-like
CRKRS	Cdc2-related kinase, arginine/serine-rich; CDK12+B1005
CRM1	exportin 1

CSF1	colony stimulating factor
CSF1R	colony stimulating factor 1 receptor, formerly McDonough feline sarcoma viral (v-fms) oncogene homolog
CSK	c-terminal src kinase
CSNK1A1	casein kinase 1, α1
CSNK1A1L	casein kinase 1, α1-like
CSNK1D/E	casein kinase 1, δ/ε
CSNK1G1/2/3	casein kinase 1, γ1/2/3
CSNK2A1	casein kinase 2, α1 polypeptide
CSNK2A2	casein kinase 2, α′ polypeptide
CT (CAT)	computed tomography (computed axial tomography)
CTD	C terminal domain
CUP	cancer of unknown primary
CYP	cytochrome P450
DAG	diacylglycerol
DALK	*Drosophila I ALK*
DAP5	EIF4G2 eukaryotic transcription iniation factor 4, gamma 2
DAPK1/2/3	death-associated protein kinase 1
DC	dendritic cell
DCLK1/2/3	double cortin and CaM kinase-like 1/2/3
DDR1/2	discoidin domain receptor family 1/2
DFS	disease-free survival
DFSB	dermatofibrosarcoma protuberans
Diablo	direct IAP binding protein with low P_i
disabled	PTB domain containing adaptor protein from *Drosophila*
DISC	death-inducing signaling complex
DLBCL	diffuse large B-cell lymphoma
DLT	dose-limiting toxicity
DMPK	dystrophia myotonica-protein kinase
DN	dominant negative
DNA	deoxyribonucleic acid
DNAPK	DNA-dependent protein kinase
DOK	docking protein
DOK-R	docking protein 2 or docking protein R
DOUBLETIME	*Drosophila* clock gene, a kinase that regulates the subcellular localization of the gene *period*
DP-1	dimerization partner 1 transcription factor

DPK1	DNA-dependent serine/threonine protein kinase
DS-ALL	Down syndrome ALL
DS-BCP-ALL	Down syndrome B-cell precursor ALL
DSBs	double strand breaks
DYRK1A/1B/2/3/4	dual-specificity tyrosine-(Y)-phosphorylation regulated kinase 1A/1B/2/3/4
E2F	transcription factor activating adenovirus E2 gene
EBV	Epstein–Barr virus
ECD	extracellular domain
ECM	extracellular matrix
EDG3	endothelial differentiation gene-3, S1P13
EEF2K	eukaryotic elongation factor-2 kinase
EGF	epidermal growth factor
EGFR	epidermal growth factor receptor (ERBB1)
EIF2AK1/2/3/4	eukaryotic translation initiation factor 2-alpha kinase 1/2/3/4
eIF4E	eukaryotic translation initiation factor 4E
ELMO	engulfment and cell motility
Emi-1	early mitotic inhibitor-1
EML4-ALK	echinoderm microtubule-associated protein-like 4–ALK fusion protein
EMT	epithelial–mesenchymal transition
Enigma	PDZ and LIM domain 7, PDLIM7
EORTC	European Organization for Research and Treatment of Cancer
EPH	ephrin
EPHA1/2/3/4/5/6/7/8/10	EPH receptor 1/2/3/4/5/6/7/8/10
EPHB1/2/3/4/6	EPH receptor B1/2/3/4/6
EPHR	ephrin receptor
EPO(R)	erythropoietin (receptor)
EPR	epiregulin
EPS8	EGFR pathway substrate 8
ER	endoplasmic reticulum; estrogen receptor
ERBB1/2/3/4	v-erb-b2 erythroblastic leukemia viral oncogene homolog 1/2/3/4, neuro/glioblastoma-derived oncogene homolog (avian)
ERG	ets-related gene
ERK	extracellular signal-related kinase
ERN1/2	endoplasmic reticulum to nucleus signaling 1/2
ES	embyronic stem cell

ET	essential thrombocythemia
ETS	v-ets erthyroblastosis virus E26 homolog
ETV6-PDGFRA	ETS-related gene 6–ALK fusion protein
Ewings	Ewing's sarcoma–peripheral primitive neuroectodermal tumor
EWS	Ewing's sarcoma breakpoint region 1
EWS-FLI1	EWS-FLI1 fusion protein
FACS	fluorescence-activated cell sorting
FAK	focal adhesion kinase
FASTK	Fas-activated serine/threonine kinase
FAT	focal adhesion targeting domain
FATC	a FRAP, ATP, TRRAP C-terminal domain, thought to play a role in redox-dependent structural and cellular stability
FBX07	F-box only protein 7
FDA	U.S. Food and Drug Administration
FER	fer (fps/fes related) tyrosine kinase (phosphoprotein NCP94)
FERM	4.1, ezrin, radixin, moesin domain
FES	feline sarcoma oncogene
FGF(R)	fibroblast growth factor (receptor)
FGFR1/2/3/4	fibroblast growth factor receptor 1/2/3/4
FGR	Gardner–Rasheed feline sarcoma viral (v-fgr) oncogene homolog
FHA	forkhead associated
FIPIL1-PDGFRA	FIP1-like1-PDGFRA fusion protein
FISH	fluorescence in situ hybridization
FKPB12	FK506 binding protein of 12 kDa
FL	follicular lymphoma (B1892); FLT3 ligand
FLG	filaggrin
FLJ23356	hypothetical protein FLJ23356
FLJ25006	hypothetical protein FLJ25006
FLT	fms-like tyrosine kinase
FLT1	fms-related tyrosine kinase 1 (vascular endothelial growth factor/vascular permeability factor receptor); VEGFR1
FLT3	fms-related tyrosine kinase 3
FLT4	fms-related tyrosine kinase 4; VEGFR3
FMS	proto-oncogene that codes for the MCSF (CSF1) receptor

FOLFIRI	folinic acid, fluorouracil, and irinotecan (chemotherapy)
FOLFOX4	folinic acid, oxaliplatin, and fluorouracil (chemotherapy)
FOXO3a	forkead homeobox type O 3a
FRAP1	FK506 binding protein 12–rapamycin associated protein 1
FRB	FKPB12 binding domain
FRK	fyn-related kinase
FRS2	fibroblast receptor substrate 2
FT&UO	fibrous tissue and uncertain origin
FTL2	FGFR1
FYN	FYN oncogene related to SRC, FGR, YES
G1	gap 1 phase (of cell cycle)
G2	gap 2 phase (of cell cycle)
GAB	grb2 associated binding protein
GAK	cyclin G–associated kinase
GAP	GTPase activating protein
GBM	glioblastoma multiforme
GDNF	glial cell-derived neurotrophic growth factor
GEF	guanine nucleotide exchange factor
GF	growth factor
GFRs	growth factor receptors
GH	growth hormone
GI	gastrointestinal
GIST	gastrointestinal stromal tumor
GLUT4	SLC2A4, glucose transporter
GM-CSF	granulocyte macrophage colony stimulating factor
GPCR	G protein-coupled receptor
GPI	glycosylphosphatidylinositol
GRB2	growth factor bound 2
GRK1/4/5/6/7	G protein-coupled receptor kinase 1/4/5/6/7
GSF3	granulocyte colony stimulating factor 3
GSG2	germ cell associated 2 (haspin)
GSK3α	glycogen synthase kinase 3 alpha
GSK3β	glycogen synthase kinase 3 beta
GTPase	guanosine triphosphate hydrolase
GUCY2C	guanylate cyclase 2C (heat stable enterotoxin receptor)
GUCY2D	guanylate cyclase 2D, membrane (retina-specific)

GUCY2F	guanylate cyclase 2F, retinal
H&E	hematoxylin and eosin
H&L	hematopoietic and lymphoid tissue
HAT	histone acetyltransferase
HB-EGF	heparin binding–EGF
HBX	hepatitis BV X protein; homeobox
HCC	hepatocellular carcinoma
HCK	hematopoietic cell kinase
HCL	hairy cell leukemia
HEAT	Huntington elongation factor 1A protein
HEK	human embryonic kidney
Hem. Neo.	hematopoietic neoplasm
HER1/2/3/4	human epidermal growth factor receptor 1/2/3/4; same as ERBB1/2/3/4
HES	hairy enhancer of split
HEXIM1	hexamethylene-induced protein
HGF	hepatocyte growth factor, also called scatter factor
Hh	hedgehog
HIC-5	TGFβ 1-induced transcript 1
HIF	hypoxia-inducible factor
HIPK1/2/3/4	homeodomain interacting protein kinase 1
HL	Hodgkin's lymphoma
HMG1	high mobility group 1
HNSCC	head and neck squamous cell carcinoma
HPRC+A24	hereditary papillary renal carcinoma
HSC	hematopoietic stem cell
HSP70	heat shock 70-kDa protein
HSP73	heat shock protein 8, 70-kDa protein
HSP90	heat shock 90-kDa protein
HSPA8	HSP73 gene
HSPB8	heat shock 22-kDa protein 8
HSPG	heparan sulfate proteoglycan
HTLV	human T-cell lymphotrophic virus
HTS	high throughput screening
HU	hydroxyurea
HUNK	hormonally upregulated Neu-associated kinase
Hus1	protein, part of a DNA damage responsive complex, checkpoint homolog of *S. pombe*
IAP	inhibitor of apoptosis

IC_{50}	concentration required to obtain 50% inhibition
ICC	interstitial cells of Cajal
ICK	intestinal cell (MAK-like) kinase
IFN	interferon
IGF1	insulin-like growth factor 1
IGF1R	insulin-like growth factor 1 receptor
IGFBP	IGF binding protein
IK3-1	interactor-1 with CDK3
IKBKB/E	inhibitor of κ light polypeptide gene enhancer in B-cells, kinase β/ε
IKK	IκB kinase
ILK	integrin-linked kinase
IMT	inflammatory myofibroblastic tumor
INCENP	inner centromer protein
INSR	insulin receptor
INSRR	insulin receptor-related receptor
ip	intraperitoneal (route of drug administration)
IP3	inositol (1,4,5)-triphosphate
IR	insulin receptor
IRAK1/2/3/4	interleukin-1 receptor-associated kinase 1/2/3/4
IRES	internal ribosome entry site
IRK	insulin receptor kinase
IRS	insulin receptor signaling protein
ITD	internal tandem duplication/repeat
ITK	IL2-inducible T-cell kinase
IV	intravenous (route of drug administration)
JAK	Janus kinase
JAK1/2/3	Janus kinase 1/2/3
Jeb	Jelly Belly, a *Drosophila* protein that is a ligand for DALK
JIP	MAPK8(JNK) interacting protein
JM	juxtamembrane
JMML	juvenile myelomonocytic leukemia
JNK	MAPK8; Janus kinase
KALRN	kalirin, RhoGEF kinase
kb	kilobase
kDa	kilodalton
KD	kinase domain
KDR	kinase insert domain receptor (a type III receptor tyrosine kinase); VEGFR2

KGF	keratinocyte growth factor (FGFR7)
KGFR	keratinocyte growth factor receptor (FGFR2IIIb)
KIAA0999	KIAA0999 protein
KIAA1804	mixed lineage kinase 4
KID	kinase insert domain
KIF5B-PDGFRA	kinesin family member 5 B–PDGFRA fusion protein
KIT	v-kit Hardy–Zuckerman 4 feline sarcoma viral oncogene homolog
KL	kit ligand
KSR1/2	kinase suppressor of ras 1/2
KU	an autoantigen consisting of 70- and 80-kDa polypeptides; regulatory component of DNA-PK
L domain	leucine-rich region
LAR	leuokcyte common antigen-related tyrosine phosphatase
LATS1	LATS, large tumor suppressor, homolog 1/2 (*Drosophila*)
LBD	ligand binding domain
LCK	lymphocyte-specific protein tyrosine kinase
LIM	Lin-1, Isl-1, Mec3 zinc finger domain
LIMK1/2	LIM domain kinase 1/2
LKB	STK11; a serine/threonine kinase; mutations of which cause Peutz–Jeghers syndrome
LMB	leptomycin
LMP	low molecular weight proteins
LMTK2/3	lemur tyrosine kinase 2
LOC646643	similar to protein kinase Bsk146
LOC91461	hypothetical protein BC007901
LOK	STK10, serine/threonine kinase 10
LRRK1/2	leucine-rich repeat kinase 1/2
LTK	leukocyte tyrosine kinase
Lymph. Neo.	lymphoid neoplasm
LYN	v-yes-1 Yamaguchi sarcoma viral related oncogene homolog
M	molar; mitosis
MA	mastocytoma
MAD	maximum administered dose
MAD1/2	a basic helix–loop–helix leucine zipper protein; mitotic arrest deficient-like protein 1/2
MAK	male germ cell-associated kinase
MAPK	mitogen-activated protein kinase

MAP2K	mitogen-activated protein kinase kinase
MAP3K	mitogen-activated protein kinase kinase kinase
MAP4K	mitogen-activated protein kinase kinase kinase kinase
MAPKAPK	mitogen-activated protein kinase-activated protein kinase
MARCKS	myristolyated alanine-rich protein kinase C substrate
MARK1/2/3/4	MAP/microtubule affinity-regulating kinase 1/2/3/4
MAST1/2/3/4	microtubule associated serine/threonine kinase 1/2/3/4
MASTL	microtubule-associated serine/threonine kinase-like
MAT1	ménage-a-trois protein; methionine adensyl transferase 1 alpha
MATK	megakaryocyte-associated tyrosine kinase
MBD	methylated DNA-binding domain
MCAK	kinesin family member 2C
MCH	mast cell hyperplasia
MCL1	mantle cell lymphoma 1; myeloid cell leukemia sequence 1
MCM2/3	minichromosome maintenance complex component 2/3
MCN	mast cell neoplasm
M-CSF	macrophage colony stimulating factor
MDCK	Mandin–Darby canine kidney
MDM2	mouse double minute chromosome 2
MDMX	homolog of MDM2; a ring finger ubiquitin ligase
MDR	multidrug resistance
MDS	myelodysplastic syndrome
MDSTR	myelodysplastic syndrome therapy-related
MED	mediator
MEF	myocyte enhancer factor; mouse embryonic fibroblast
MEK	MAPK/ERK kinase
MELK	maternal embryonic leucine zipper kinase
MEN	multiple endocrine neoplasia
MEN-2A	multiple endocrine neoplasia-2A
Mena	mammalian enabled
MERLIN	a protein involved in neurofibromatosis, type 2
MERTK	c-mer proto-oncogene tyrosine kinase
MET	met proto-oncogene (hepatocyte growth factor receptor)
MF	myelofibrosis
MFSS	mycosis fungoides–Sézary syndrome
MGC16169	hypothetical protein MGC16169

MGC42105	hypothetical protein MGC42105
MGUS	monoclonal gammopathy of undetermined significance
MINK1	misshapen-like kinase 1 (zebrafish)
MKNK1/2	MAP kinase interacting serine/threonine kinase 1/2
MLH1	MutL homolog 1
MLK5	mixed lineage kinase 5
MLKL	mixed lineage kinase domain-like
MM	multiple myeloma
MMAC1	mutated in multiple cancers
MMM	myeloid metaplasia
MMP	matrix metalloproteinase
MMR	MSI/mismatch repair
MMTV	mouse mammary tumor virus
MNK1	MAPK interacting kinase
MOS	v-mos Moloney murine sarcoma viral oncogene homolog
MPD	myeloproliferative disease
MPL	receptor for erythropoietin
MPNST	malignant peripheral nerve sheath tumor
Mre11	meiotic recombination 11 homolog
MRK	male germ cell-associated kinase
MRN	Mre11-Rad50-Nbs1
mRNA	messenger RNA
MSH2	mutS homolog 2
mSIN1	microsatellite instability
MSK	mitogen and stress-activated kinase
MSP	macrophage stimulating protein
MST1R	macrophage stimulating 1 receptor (c-met-related tyrosine kinase)
MST2	serine/threonine kinase 3 (STK3)
MST4	serine/threonine protein kinase MST4
MTC	medullary thyroid carcinoma
MTD	maximum tolerated dose
mTOR	mammalian target of rapamycin
mTORC1	mammalian target of rapamycin complex 1
mTORC2	mammalian target of rapamycin complex 2
MUSK	muscle, skeletal, receptor tyrosine kinase
MYLK	myosin, light chain kinase
MYLK2	myosin light chain kinase 2, skeletal muscle
MYLK3	MLCK protein

MYLK4	hypothetical protein LOC340156
MYO3A/3B	myosin IIIA/IIIB
MYT1	myelin transcription factor 1
N-	N (amino) terminus
NBSI	nibrin (NLR2; pyrin family containing 2)
NCI	National Cancer Institute
NCK	novel cytoplasmic protein; an adaptor protein
NEK1-11	NIMA related kinase 1–11
NELF	negative elongation factor
NES	nuclear export signal
NF	neurofibromatosis
NF1/2	neurofibromin 1
NFκB	nuclear factor κB
NGF	nerve growth factor
NHEJ	nonhomologous end joining
NHL	non Hodgkin's lymphoma
NIMA	never-in-mitosis-A
NK	natural killer
NKTCL	NK T-cell lymphoma
NLK	nemo-like kinase
NLS	nuclear localization (import) sequence
NMR	nuclear magnetic resonance
NOD/SCID	non-obese diabetic/severe combined immunodeficient
NOXA	NADPH oxidase activator
NPM	nucleophosmin
NPM-ALK	nucleophosmin–ALK fusion protein
NPR1	natriuretic peptide receptor A/guanylate cyclase A (atrionatriuretic peptide receptor A)
NPR2	natriuretic peptide receptor B/guanylate cyclase B (atrionatriuretic peptide receptor B)
NRBP1/2	nuclear receptor binding protein 1/2
NRG	neuregulin
NRK	Nik-related kinase
NSCLC	non small cell lung carcinoma
NTD	N-terminal domain
NTRK1/2/3	neurotrophic tyrosine receptor, kinase, type 1/2/3
NUAK1/2	NUAK family, SNF1-like kinase, 1/2
OBSCN	obscurin, cytoskeletal calmodulin and titin-interacting RhoGEF

OPN	osteopontin
OXSR1	oxidative-stress responsive 1
p	short arm of a chromosome; a phosphorylated protein
p	probablility of an event
p120ctn	CTNND1, catenin-associated protein delta 1
p130CAS	BCAR, breast cancer anti-estrogen resistance 1
p190RHOGAP	RHOGTPase activating protein
p300/CBP	p300/CREB binding protein, a coactivator
PA	plasmacytoma; phosphatidic acid
PAI-1	plasminogen activator inhibitor-1
PAK1–7	p21/Cdc42/Rac1-activated kinase 1–7 (homolog of yeast STE20)
PAR6	partitioning defective 6
PASK	PAS domain containing serine/threonine kinase
PBK	PDZ binding kinase
PBS	phosphate buffered saline
pCAF	p300/CBP associated factor
PCM	plasma cell myeloma
PCTK1/2/3	PCTAIRE protein kinase 1
PCV	polycythemia vera
PD	pharmacodynamic; progressive disease
PD2	PAF1, RNA polymerase II associated factor
PDCDR	DECR2, 2,4-dienoyl CoA reductase 2, peroxisomal
PDGF(R)	platelet-derived growth factor (receptor)
PDGFRα	platelet-derived growth factor receptor, alpha polypeptide
PDGFRβ	platelet-derived growth factor receptor, beta polypeptide
PDIK1L	PDLIM1 interacting kinase 1-like
PDK1	3-phosphoinositide-dependent kinase 1; may also be used as the abbreviation for pyruvate dehydrogenase kinase, isozyme 1
PDK2	3-phosphoinositide-dependent kinase 2, generally accepted to be mTORC2; may also be used as the abbreviation for pyruvate dehydrogenase kinase, isozyme 2
PDPK1	3-phosphoinositide-dependent kinase 1
PEST	a protein degradation signal
PET	positron emission tomography
PFS	progression-free survival

PFTK1	PFTAIRE protein kinase 1
PFTK2	amyotrophic lateral sclerosis 2 (juvenile) chromosome region, candidate 7
PH	pleckstrin homology (PIP3 binding) domain
Ph+	Philadelphia chromosome positive
PHKG1	phosphorylase kinase, gamma 1 (muscle)
PHKG2	phosphorylase kinase, $\gamma 2$ (testis)
PHLPP	PH domain and leucine-rich repeat phosphatase
PHOX-BEMI	domains that mediate protein:protein interactions via the formation of homo- or heterodimers
PI	phosphatidylinositol
PI3K	phosphatidylinositol-3 kinase
PIF	prolactin inhibiting factor; $5'$ to $3'$ DNA helicase homolog
PIK3R4	phosphoinositide-3 kinase, regulatory subunit 4, p150
PIKE-A	phosphatidylinositol-3 kinase enhancer isoform A
PIKK	phosphatidylinositol-3 kinase-related kinase
PIM1/2/3	proviral integration of MMLV kinase 1/2/3
PINK1	PTEN-induced putative kinase 1
PIP$_2$	phosphatidylinositol(4,5)bisphosphate
PIP$_3$	phosphatidylinositol(3,4,5)trisphosphate
PK	pharmacokinetics
PKA/B/C	protein kinase A/B/C
PKMYT1	protein kinase, membrane associated tyrosine/threonine 1
PKN1	protein kinase N1/2/3
PL2F	promyelocytic leukemia zinc finger protein
PLC/D	phospholipase C/D
PlGF	placental growth factor
PLK1/2/3/4	polo-like kinase 1 (*Drosophila*)
PMA	phorbol-12-myristate-13-acetate
PMBL	primary mediastinal B-cell lymphoma
PMF	primary myelofibrosis
PML	promyelocytic leukemia
PMN	polymorphonuclear leukocytes
PNCK	pregnancy upregulated nonubiquitously expressed CaM kinase
po	oral (route of drug administration)
pol	polymerase
pol II	RNA polymerase II

POSH	plenty of SH3; a protein with a RING finger and four SH3 domains
PP1/2A	protein phosphatase 1/2A
PR	partial response
PRAGMIN	homolog of rat pragma of Rnd2
PRAS40	AKT1 substrate, proline rich
PRKAA1/2	protein kinase, AMP-activated, α1/2 catalytic subunit
PRKACA/B/G	protein kinase, cAMP-dependent, catalytic, α/β/γ
PRKCA/B/D/E/G/ H/I/Q/Z	protein kinase C α/β/δ/ε/γ/η/ι/θ/ζ
PRKD1/2/3	protein kinase D1/2/3
PRKDC	protein kinase, DNA-activated, catalytic polypeptide
PRKG1	protein kinase, cGMP-dependent, type 1
PRKG2	protein kinase, cGMP-dependent, type 2
PRKX	protein kinase, X-linked
PRKY	protein kinase, Y-linked
PRL	prolactin
Pro-B ALL	pro-B-cell acute lymphocytic leukemia
PROTOR	protein observed with Rictor-1
PRPF4B	PRP4 pre-mRNA processing factor 4 homolog B (yeast)
PS	phosphatidyl serine
PSA	prostate specific antigen
PSKH1/2	protein serine kinase H1/2
PSTAIRE	a consensus amino acid sequence proline serine threonine alanine isoleucine arginine glutamine
PTB	polypyrimidine tract binding protein
PTC	papillary thyroid carinoma
PTCL	peripheral T-cell lymphoma unspecified
P-TEFb	positive transcription factor elongation factor b
PTEN	phosphatase and tensin homolog deleted on chromosome 10
PTK2/2B/5/6/7	PTK2 protein tyrosine kinase 2/2 β/5/6/7
PTN	pleiotrophin
PTP (1b)	phosphotyrosine phosphatase (1b)
PUMA	Bcl binding component 3
PV	polycythemia vera
PXK	PX domain containing serine/threonine kinase
PYK2	protein tyrosine kinase 2
q	long arm of a chromosome

qd	quaque die; daily dosing
qPCR	quantitative polymerase chain reaction
QTc	corrected QT interval (electrocardiogram)
RabBP	rab binding protein kinase 2 beta
RAC1	ras-related C3 botulinum substrate 1
RACK	receptor for activated C kinase
Rad1/3/9/41/50	rad1 homolog (repair endonuclease)
RAF1	v-raf-1 murine leukemia viral oncogene homolog 1
RAGE	renal tumor antigen
RAL	ras-related antigen
RALGDS	ral GDP dissociation stimulator
RalGEF	ral guanine exchange factor
RAN	ras-related nuclear GTP binding protein
RANBP	ran binding protein
RanGTPase	Ran GTPase
Raptor	regulator-associated protein of mTOR
RAR	retinoic acid receptor
Rb	retinoblastoma protein
RBD	ras binding domain
RCC1	regulator of chromosome condensation 1
REDD1/2	DNA-damage-inducible transcript
RET	rearranged during transfection; ret proto-oncogene
Rheb	ras homolog enriched in brain
RHE-PDGFRA	rearranged in hypereosinophilia; fusion with PDGFRA
RHO	rhodopsin
Rictor	rapamycin-insensitive companion of mTOR
RIOK1	RIO kinase 1/2/3 (yeast)
RIPK1/2/3/4/5	receptor (TNFRSF)-interacting serine–threonine kinase 1/2/3/4/5
RNAi	RNA interference
RNAPII	RNA polymerase II
RNASEL	ribonuclease L (2′,5′-oligoisoadenylate synthetase-dependent)
RNPS1	RNA binding protein S1
ROCK1/2	Rho-associated, coiled-coil containing protein kinase 1/2
RON	recepteur d'origine Nantais
ROR1/2	receptor tyrosine kinase-like orphan receptor 1/2
ROS	reactive oxygen species

ROS1	v-ros UR2 sarcoma virus oncogene homolog 1 (avian)
RPA	replication protein A
RPS6KA1/2/3/4/5/6	ribosomal protein S6 kinase, 90 kDa, polypeptide 1
RPS6KB1	ribosomal protein S6 kinase, 70 kDa, polypeptide 1
RPS6KB2	ribosomal protein S6 kinase, 70 kDa, polypeptide 2
RPS6KC1	ribosomal protein S6 kinase, 52 kDa, polypeptide 1
RPS6KL1	ribosomal protein S6 kinase-like 1
RR	relative risk
RSK1/2/3/4	p90 ribosomal S6 kinase 1/2/3/4
RSV	Rous sarcoma virus
RT	reverse transcriptase
RTK	receptor tyrosine kinase
RYK	RYK receptor-like tyrosine kinase
S	DNA synthesis phase of cell cycle
S1P	sphingosine-1-phosphate
S6	protein 6 of the small ribosomal subunit
SADDAM	severe achondroplasia with developmental delay and acanthosis nigricans
SAM	sterile alpha motif and leucine zipper containing kinase AZK
SBK1	SH3 binding domain kinase 1
sc	subcutaneous
SC35	RRM containing SR protein; regulates alternative splicing
SCC	small cell carcinoma
SCCHN	squamous cell carcinoma of the head and neck
SCF	stem cell factor
SCK	SHC, SRC homology 2 domain containing
SCLC	small cell lung carcinoma
SCYL1	SCY1-like 1/2/3 (*S. cerevisiae*)
SDF-1	stroma-derived factor -1
SEA	S13 erythroblastosis oncogene homolog
SEC3IL1-ALK	exocyst complement component 1 (EXOC1)–ALK fusion protein
SEMA	structural domain of semaphorins characterized by a conserved set of cystein residues
semaphorins	a class of secreted and membrane proteins that act as axonal growth cone guidance molecules
SF	scatter factor; splicing factor + B24
SF1	steroidogenic factor 1
SGK1	serum/glucocorticoid regulated kinase 1/2/3

SGK269	KIAA2002 protein
SH1	src homology 1 domain (kinase domain)
SH2	src homology 2 domain
SH3	src homology 3 domain
SHB	src homology 2 domain containing adaptor protein
SHC	src homology 2 domain containing transforming protein 1
SHP	SH2 containing phosphatase
shRNA	small hairpin RNA
siRNA	small interfering RNA
SLK	STE20-like kinase (yeast)
SLUG	SNAI2; snail homolog 2
SM	systemic mastocytosis
SMAD	homolog of the *Drosophila* protein, mothers against decapentaplegic
SMG1	PI3 K-related kinase SMG-1
sn	small nuclear
SNAIL	SNAI1, snail homolog 1, a Zn finger protein
SNF1LK	SNF1-like kinase
SNF1LK2	SNF1-like kinase 2
SNP	single nucleotide polymorphism
SNRK	SNF-related kinase
SNT1	syntrophin, alpha 1 (SNTA1)
SOCS1	suppressor of cytokine signaling 1 + B650
SOS	son of sevenless
SPEG	similar to aortic preferentially expressed gene 1
SQCC	squamous cell carcinoma
SR	serine and arginine rich
SRC	v-src sarcoma (Schmidt–Ruppin A-2) viral oncogene homolog (avian)
SRM	SRC-related kinase lacking C-terminal regulatory tyrosine and N-terminal myristoylation sites
SRPK1	SFRS protein kinase 1/2/3
ss	single stranded (DNA or RNA)
STAT	signal transducer and activator of transcription
STK	serine/threonine kinase, homolog of yeast STE20
STLK5	STE20-related kinase 5
STLK6	STE20-related kinase 6
STRADA	protein kinase LYK5
STRN-PDGFRA	striatin–PDGFRA fusion protein

STYK1	serine/threonine/tyrosine kinase 1
SWI/SNF	switch/sucrose nonfermentable; nucleosome remodeling
SYK	spleen tyrosine kinase
t	referring to a chromosomal translocation
$t_{1/2}$	half-life
TACE	TNF converting enzyme
TAF1	TAF1 RNA polymerase II, TATA box binding protein (TBP)-associated factor, 250 kDa
TAF1L	TAF1-like RNA polymerase II, TATA box binding protein (TBP)-associated factor, 210 kDa
TAK1	MAP3K7
T-ALL	T-cell acute lymphocytic leukemia
TANK	TRAF family member associated NFκB activator
TAO3	thousand and one amino acid protein 3
TAOK1/2/3	thousand and one amino acid kinase 1/2/3
TAP	trasporter with antigen processing
TBK1	TANK-binding kinase 1
TEC	tec protein tyrosine kinase
TEK	TIE2
TEL-FGFR3	fusion of TEL (member of the ETS transcription factor family) with FGFR3
TESK1/2	testis-specific kinase 1/2
TEX14	testis expressed sequence 14
TF	transcription factor
TFIIH	transcription factor IIH
TGCTs	testicular germ cell tumors
TGFα/β	transforming growth factor α/β
TGF-βR	transforming growth factor β receptor
TGFβR1	transforming growth factor, beta receptor I (activin A receptor type II-like kinase, 53 kDa)
TGFβR2	transforming growth factor, beta receptor II (70/80 kDa)
TIAM	T-cell lymphoma invasion and metastasis
TIE1	tyrosine kinase with immunoglobulin-like and EGF-like domains 1
TIE2	tyrosine kinase with immunoglobulin-like and EGF-like domains 2
TK	tyrosine kinase
TKK	tokkaebi

TKL	avian homolog of LCK; a family of kinases including RAF, MLK, LIMK, RIPK, and TGFβR
TKS13	tyrsoine kinase substrate 13
TKS202	tyrsoine kinase substrate 202
TKS5	tyrsoine kinase substrate 5
TLK1/2	tousled-like kinase 1
TLS	translocated in liposarcoma
TLS-ERG	TLS-v-ets erythroblastosis virus E26 homology fusion protein
TM	transmembrane
TMP4	tropomyosin 4, partner of a fusion protein with ALK
TNF	tumor necrosis factor
TNIK	TRAF2 and NCK interacting kinase
TNK1/2	tyrosine kinase, nonreceptor, 1/2
TNNI3K	TNNI3 interacting kinase
TopBP1	topoisomerase binding protein 1
TP53RK	TP53 regulating kinase
TPO	thrombopoietin
TPR-MET	translocated promoter region−MET fusion protein
TPX2	targeting protein for XKLP2
TRAPP2	transport protein particle 2
TRIB1/2/3	tribbles homolog 1/2/3 (*Drosophila*)
TRIM24	tripartite motif-containing 24
TRIM28	tripartite motif-containing 28
TRIM33	tripartite motif-containing 33
TRIO	triple functional domain (PTPRF interacting)
TRPM6/7	transient receptor potential cation channel, subfamily M, member 6/7
TRRAP	transformation/transcription domain-associated protein
TSC1	tuberous sclerosis complex 1 (Hamartin)
TSC2	tuberous sclerosis complex 2 (Tuberin)
TSSK1B/2/3/4/6	testis-specific serine kinase 1B/2/3/4/6
TTBK1/2	tau tubulin kinase 1/2
TTK	TTK protein kinase
TTN	titin
TTP	time to progression
TUNEL	terminal deoxynucleotidyl transferase-mediated dUTP nick end labeling
TWIST	homolog of the *Drosophila* twist transcription factor
TXK	TXK tyrosine kinase
TYK2	tyrosine kinase 2

TYRO	protein tyrosine kinase
TYRO3	TYRO3 protein tyrosine kinase
UHMK1	U2AF homology motif (UHM) kinase 1
ULK1/2/3/4	unc-51-like kinase 1 (*C. elegans*)
VAV	a guanine nucleotide exchange factor
VEGF(R)	vascular endothelial growth factor (receptor)
VHL	von Hippel–Lindau factor
VPS34	vacuolar protein sorting 34, a phosphatidylinositol-3 kinase thought to play a role in protein sorting and autophagy
VPS35p	an endosomal component of the membrane-associated retromer complex
VRAP	VEGF receptor-associated protein
VRK1/23	vaccinia related kinase 1/2/3
WAF	cyclin-dependent kinase inhibitor also known as p21CIP/WAF
WASP	Wiscott–Aldrich syndrome (eczema thrombocytopenia)
WBC	white blood cell
WEE1	WEE1 homolog (*S. pombe*)
WEE2	hypothetical protein FLJ40852
WIP	WAS/WASL interacting protein family member 1 (WIPF1)
WNK1/2/3/4	WNK lysine-deficient protein kinase 1/2/3/4
WNT	wingless type MMTV integration site family member 1
WT	wild type
XIAP	X-chromosome-linked inhibitor of apoptosis
XPD	ERCC5 xeroderma pigmentosum
YES1	v-yes-1 Yamaguchi sarcoma viral oncogene homolog 1
YSK4	yeast Sps1/Ste20-related kinase 4 (*S. cerevisiae*)
ZAK	sterile alpha motif and leucine zipper containing kinase AZK
ZAP70	zeta-chain (TCR) associated protein kinase 70 kDa

INDEX

Targeting Protein Kinases for Cancer Therapy, by David J. Matthews and Mary E. Gerritsen
Copyright © 2010 John Wiley & Sons, Inc.